D1582939

BREASTFEEDING ANSWERS *Made Simple*

A Guide for Helping Mothers

BREASTFEEDING ANSWERS
Made Simple
A Guide for Helping Mothers

Nancy Mohrbacher, IBCLC, FILCA
co-author of *The Breastfeeding Answer Book* & *Breastfeeding Made Simple*

Breastfeeding Answers Made Simple

A Guide for Helping Mothers

Nancy Mohrbacher, IBCLC, FILCA

Hale Publishing, L.P.

1712 N. Forest St.

Amarillo, TX 79106-7017

806-376-9900

800-378-1317

www.iBreastfeeding.com

www.hale-publishing.com

Library of Congress Control Number: 2010926441

ISBN-13: 978-0-9845039-0-2

Table of Contents

Part III. Mother

Appendices

Dedication

This book is dedicated to my mother Patricia Black, whose death during this project broke my heart. I will always miss you.

Acknowledgements

My sincere thanks goes to all the mothers and babies who allowed me to journey with them down the path of breastfeeding. It was a true privilege to learn from you and to share your joys and sorrows.

I am also grateful to the many amazing individuals who played a vital role in the creation of this book. First and foremost, my eternal thanks goes to Kathleen Kendall-Tackett, my editor and greatest supporter. Without your encouragement, expertise in publishing, and timely help in shepherding this book through its phases, it might never have happened. You are a remarkable woman and I feel truly blessed to have you in my life as colleague, coauthor, and, most important, friend.

Thanks also to Tom Hale, who saw the value in this project from the start. Your willingness to provide the necessary resources—access to research and the time and energy of your publishing staff—helped me transform this book from a dream to a reality.

I also extend my sincere thanks to the rest of the Hale Publishing staff, Janet Rourke, Alicia Ingram, Christian Bressler, and Quetha Hale, who devoted countless hours to this book. I will always be grateful for your hard work.

My thanks also goes to Jennifer Carr and Dustin Epstein, who allowed me to scale back my role at Ameda Breastfeeding Products, which gave me the time I needed to research and write. I will always be grateful for your generous support.

No one can be an expert on everything, so I extend my gratitude to the world-class clinicians and researchers who generously took the time to review my chapters and provide invaluable feedback. They include Suzanne Colson, RN, RM, PhD, Nils Bergman, MB, ChB, MPH, DCH, MD, Catherine Watson Genna, BS, IBCLC, Diana West, IBCLC, Miriam Labbok, MD, MPH, FACPM, FABM, IBCLC, Karleen Gribble, BRurSC, PhD, Barbara Wilson-Clay, BS, IBCLC, FILCA, Diane Wiessinger, MS, IBCLC, Kathleen Kendall-Tackett, Phd, IBCLC, Gill Rapley, RM, RHV, MSc, Lawrence Gartner, MD, FAAP, Susan Burger, MHS, PhD, IBCLC, Laurie Nommsen-Rivers, PhD, RD, IBCLC, Kirsten Berggren, PhD, IBCLC, Marsha Walker, RN, IBCLC, Hilary Flower, BA, MA, Lisa Marasco, MA, IBCLC, FILCA, Cheryl Lovelady, PhD, RD, Carol Wagner, MD, Christina Smillie, MD, FAAP, IBCLC, FABM, and Kerstin Hedberg Nyqvist, RN, PhD, IBCLC.

I also extend my thanks to those who provided the images for this book. Special thanks to my beautiful and talented daughter-in-law Anna Mohrbacher, an in-demand artist who made the time to create line drawings especially for these pages. I am so grateful you squeezed me in! Thanks also to Christian Bressler, graphic artist for Hale Publishing, who created several original images for this book. Thanks, too, to Catherine Watson Genna, BS, IBCLC, a gifted lactation consultant and wonderful friend who generously allowed me to reprint 11 of her clinical photos, most from her amazing books, *Supporting Sucking Skills in Breastfeeding Infants* and *Selecting and Using Breastfeeding Tools.* Your help and support meant the world to me! Thanks also to Barbara Wilson-Clay, BS, IBCLC, FILCA and Kay Hoover, MEd, IBCLC, FILCA, who kindly gave me permission to reprint several photos from their fabulous book, *The Breastfeeding Atlas.*

And last but never least, I thank my family. Out of love for me, my son Carl suggested this project, for which I will always be grateful. He and his brothers Peter and Ben gave me welcome support through the two long years it took to finish this project. I am also grateful to my husband of 33 years, Michael, who was (mostly) patient and understanding above and beyond the call of duty.

Introduction

I had my initial encounter with breastfeeding help in June of 1980 when I attended my first La Leche League meeting. I was 5 months pregnant with my oldest child, and I arrived feeling curious about motherhood and wondering if I would be able to make breastfeeding work.

That was also the night I fell in love with breastfeeding. It happened as I watched a mother and her 3-week-old baby interact at the breast. In my mind's eye, I can still see her stroking, smiling, and talking to her newborn girl while they stared into each other's eyes. I was stunned by how alive that tiny baby was to her mother's overtures! Others had told me that newborns were incapable of real interaction, but that mother and baby proved them wrong. Although I didn't know it then, what I witnessed that night was the "right-brain connection" described in Chapter 1, and after that experience, I would never be the same. I don't remember a word that mother said to the group, but the impression she left on me was indelible. I knew immediately this was the kind of intimacy I wanted with my own baby. When I left that meeting, I was confident that with this group's help I would be able to breastfeed, and I felt even more excited about becoming a mother.

After that meeting and many more, I went on to breastfeed my three sons and threw my heart and soul into helping other mothers. In 1982, before breastfeeding was a career choice, I became a La Leche League leader. In 1984, I began reading lactation research and reporting on breastfeeding trends in the articles I wrote for La Leche League publications (in those days I wrote with pen on yellow pad and typed final drafts on a typewriter). In 1991, with my co-author Julie Stock, I finished the first edition of *The Breastfeeding Answer Book* (my first work on a computer) and joined a new profession as a board-certified lactation consultant. In 1993, I founded and ran what became a large Chicago-area private lactation practice that over the next 10 years helped thousands of families. Since 2003 as a lactation consultant for Ameda Breastfeeding Products, I have had the privilege of supporting those "in the trenches" helping mothers by organizing educational programs attended by more than 10,000 U.S. healthcare professionals and presented by some of the most innovative researchers and thinkers in breastfeeding.

In the years since my first La Leche League meeting, approaches to breastfeeding help have undergone radical shifts, which are described in detail in this book. When I began helping mothers in 1982, our mainstays were basic information, encouragement, and faith that breastfeeding worked. Most often that was enough. Over time, though, we acquired more skills and tools. With the benefit of research and after much trial and error, our technical understanding of breastfeeding increased, and our focus shifted to teaching mothers specific techniques, which we discovered could improve breastfeeding comfort and milk transfer. These techniques, which are described in Chapters 1, 3, and the "Techniques" appendix, often pulled breastfeeding couples back from the brink of premature weaning, and as more mothers breastfed, our new skills enabled us to help them overcome increasingly more complicated breastfeeding challenges. But the way we taught breastfeeding to the average mother became more complicated, too. In the years I taught breastfeeding classes for a Chicago-area OB-GYN practice, I spent a third of my class time describing positioning and latching (attachment) techniques in sitting and side-lying positions while the pregnant mothers practiced with dolls. During these years, breastfeeding initiation rates rose, but perhaps at least partly due to these teaching strategies, many mothers gave up early because they found breastfeeding "too difficult."

Now, however, we are coming full circle. Since the 2003 *Breastfeeding Answer Book* was published, exciting research (from Suzanne Colson in the U.K., Nils Bergman in South Africa, Kerstin Hedberg Nyqvist in Sweden, and many others) has provided profound insights into new ways we can both improve breastfeeding outcomes and simplify the way we help mothers. Strategies like laid-back breastfeeding and skin-to-skin contact offer the best of both worlds by making breastfeeding easier while enhancing the mother-baby relationship. We are also learning much more about breastfeeding norms, enabling us to better distinguish normal variations from problems and provide research-based answers to common questions. New insights into breastfeeding norms can be found in Chapter 1, "Basic Breastfeeding Dynamics," Chapter 2, "Breastfeeding Rhythms," Chapter 4, "Solid Foods," Chapter 5, "Weaning from the Breast," Chapter 6, "Weight Gain and Growth " (including the new WHO Growth Standards), Chapter 10, "Making Milk," Chapter 11, "Milk Expression and Storage," Chapter 12, "Sexuality, Fertility, and Contraception," Chapter 13, "Nutrition, Exercise, and Lifestyle Issues," and Chapter 14, "Pregnancy and Tandem Nursing." (For simplicity's sake, in these pages baby is referred to as "he" while mother is, of course, "she.")

Research since 2003 has increased our understanding of both simple and complex breastfeeding dynamics. The better we understand the forces that underlie breastfeeding (sometimes called its "natural laws"), the better we can help those with common and unusual challenges. See, for example, Chapter 1, "Basic Breastfeeding Dynamics," for illustrations of both laid-back and other feeding positions for mothers with twins, triplets, or more and Chapter 10, "Making Milk," for strategies for making abundant milk for even higher-order multiples. See Chapter 3, "Challenges at the Breast," for ways to make breastfeeding work for the baby with unusual oral anatomy. See Chapter 8, "Health Issues—Baby," for breastfeeding approaches to try when baby is ill or has chronic health issues. See Chapter 9, "The Preterm Baby," for the research and strategies that resulted in exclusive breastfeeding (not just human-milk feeding) among 85% of Swedish 36-week-old preterm babies. See Chapter 15, "Employment," for new approaches to help working mothers maintain milk production long-term. See Chapter 16, "Relactation, Induced Lactation, and Emergencies," for research-based insights into stimulating milk production in these unusual situations. See Chapters 17 and 18, "Nipple Pain and Other Issues" and "Breast Issues," for an overview of common and unusual causes of nipple pain and trauma and anatomical breast and nipple issues that can affect breastfeeding in mothers with inadequate glandular tissue (hypoplasia), a history of breast surgery (including breast lifts), flat and inverted nipples, and even gestational gigantomastia, a disabling condition of pregnancy that some believe is becoming more common. See Chapter 19, "Health Issues—Mother," for the research on stress-relieving effects of breastfeeding, the protection breastfeeding provides for many maternal illnesses, and strategies for managing breastfeeding when a mother has an acute or chronic illness or is physically challenged. Newly understood basic breastfeeding dynamics makes it possible for us to help simplify breastfeeding for average and not-so-average mothers.

My personal philosophy of breastfeeding help has always been "Do what works, and don't do what doesn't work." Yet as simple as this sounds, many mothers and clinicians continue the same strategies even after it is clear they're not working. When using this book, please remember this "do what works" philosophy. After a fair trial, if one of the many strategies in these pages isn't working, move on to the next. Differences in personal preferences, cultural beliefs, anatomy, and physiology make each mother-baby couple unique, so a "one-size-fits-all" or "cookbook" approach to breastfeeding help will not do justice to mothers and babies.

Another important point to keep in mind as we promote breastfeeding and offer our help is that what initially drew many of us to breastfeeding was not the wonders of human milk (which are considerable and also described in these pages), but the miraculous way breastfeeding deepens the bond between mother and baby. Breastfeeding's real power and draw lies in the profound intimacy I witnessed between that mother and her newborn at my first La Leche League meeting. Experiencing that—even second-hand—created a hunger in me for that intimacy with my own newborn. Experiencing it myself was my main motivation for helping other mothers feel that same amazing magic.

Let us keep our eye on that prize. Approaching breastfeeding help with intimacy and attachment as a focus enables us to better reinforce mothers' instincts and leave them feeling empowered rather than incompetent. My hope is that *Breastfeeding Answers Made Simple* will give you the tools you need to both help mothers breastfeed and enhance their bond with their babies. Many of the new insights in these pages take us back to our roots, but this time with a greater understanding of the underlying forces at work. We are entering an exciting time in breastfeeding. The best is definitely yet to come, both for us and for the mothers we help.

For Nancy's continuing commentary on breastfeeding research and trends, follow her blog at www.NancyMohrbacher.com.

Foreword

There was a time when the choice between bottle feeding with formula and breastfeeding was a lifestyle choice. The choice was seen as purely nutritional, and any artificial substance that resembled human milk and resulted in babies gaining weight was obviously good. After that, lists of "pros and cons" for each could be presented to mothers in an objective way. Anybody suggesting breastfeeding was better was labeled as biased, and ignored.

We now know that breastfeeding is a great deal more than just "food" or nutrition. From the moments after birth newborn behaviors have been studied, and these are entirely focused on the breast. The human newborn has amazing competencies. All undrugged and undisturbed healthy newborns will attach themselves to a breast. In my own research, I have suggested that this birth behavior has nothing to do with nutrition at all. Rather it is an innate neural program that the newborn must express in order for it to ensure all its basic biological needs.

From latest neuroscience we now know that it is the sensory stimulations provided by the maternal environment that are essential to keep this brain development program moving forward. Breastfeeding is perhaps the unique time when every single sensation is provided in an integrated manner, and these sensations might be seen as the brain's real "food"! This should then be seen in the longer-term perspective, which is that the brain's objective is to make the baby into a social being. Future social and emotional intelligence is built on this early relationship. Nancy summarizes this so perfectly in the very opening line of this book: "Breastfeeding is part of an intimate relationship."

Of course mother's milk as such has inestimable nutritional value. The behavior of breastfeeding I have suggested is 90% brain-wiring, and only 10% nutrition. I could say the same for mother's milk: the components in the milk are 10% for energy and growth (some of which uniquely brain growth), but 90% for protection. Babies fed artificial formula will obviously grow and gain weight, but they are short-changed on both the brain wiring, brain growth and the protection.

For a long time studies have shown human milk "might be better." But since formula was regarded as normal and healthy in itself, conclusions would at best allow that "human milk is better". In fact, depriving the baby of the sensations to the brain, and protection to the body, means "bottle and formula are worse," and worse means it does cause harm. Recent studies, and meta-analyses of many studies, are now clear on this matter: breastfeeding and breast milk have major impacts on development and health! Breastfeeding is no longer a simple lifestyle choice; it is a public health priority. Our culture is slowly waking up to this fact. The problem is that for some hundred years we have made breastfeeding difficult, and even unattractive! Our drugs and our hospital practices combine to confuse both babies and mothers, and derail the early start that would make it easy. This is the real world in which now live--and why this book is essentialfor anybody with the wellbeing of babies and mothers at heart.

It deals with all the breastfeeding complexities and practicalities of both our culture and our health systems. Quite apart from just the weight of this book in your hands (put it on the table), a quick look at the index will show you that the scope of problems covered are even more than you had imagined. Nevertheless, every piece of advice and instruction comes with balanced and evidence-based references, over and above much wisdom and practical experience in helping mothers and babies. With the unique layout you will find it to be accessible and user friendly.

Try it. Think of any breastfeeding problem (common or unusual), scan the content pages, or look up the index, and you will quickly find your answer. With this book you will be equipped to better manage any breastfeeding question that needs an answer!

Dr Nils Bergman

MB ChB, DCH, MPH, MD

Basic Breastfeeding Dynamics

Chapter

1

SUPPORTING VERSUS TEACHING

Breastfeeding is part of an intimate relationship, rather than a skill to be learned.

Both mother and baby bring an inborn hardwiring to breastfeeding that we have only begun to understand. Learning to breastfeed is not an intellectual process, like learning to drive a car (see the later section "The Mother's Role). Breastfeeding is part of a mother's intimate relationship with her baby.

In years past, many prenatal breastfeeding classes taught mothers specific breastfeeding positions, sometimes using dolls for practice. Thanks to new insights, we know now that there are basic problems with this approach.

Too much information can make breastfeeding more difficult.

Teaching a mother specific movements or positions can sometimes be helpful when there are breastfeeding difficulties. But teaching normal breastfeeding as if every mother has a problem can make early learning more difficult and create problems where none existed.

In a randomized trial of 160 first-time mothers in Australia, the mothers were assigned to one of two groups (Henderson, Dickinson, Evans, McDonald, & Paech, 2003). In the first 24 hours after birth, one group received one-on-one positioning and attachment training (the experimental group). The other group did not receive this training. Although the mothers who received the training reported less nipple pain on the 2nd day in the hospital, these mothers had a trend toward lower breastfeeding rates and less satisfaction with breastfeeding at 3 and 6 months. The researchers noted:

> ...[A] possible unintended consequence of the emphasis on instruction and assessment of positioning and attachment may have been to raise anxiety in first-time mothers....The physical and psychological events of childbirth may also influence the amount of information a new mother can process. Therefore this intervention may have contributed to a feeling that breastfeeding was too difficult for women in the experimental group (Henderson et al., 2003, p. 241).

A Brazilian study found that teaching mothers breastfeeding techniques after birth had no effect on breastfeeding exclusivity (de Oliveira et al., 2006). A U.K. study found that even when breastfeeding technique was taught after birth using a "hands off" approach, breastfeeding duration did not increase (Wallace et al., 2006).

• •

When supporting normal breastfeeding, suggest the mother focus on getting comfortable and give encouragement rather than instructions.

Instructions trigger thinking, which can take a mother's focus off her baby and may even cause her to question her instincts. Too much information at the wrong time leaves some mothers feeling overwhelmed. Finding a comfortable, private place where a mother can interact freely with her baby allows her to tap into the hardwiring described in this chapter and find her own best approach to breastfeeding. Encouraging each mother to find her own way can enhance both her self-confidence and the mother-baby relationship.

BABY'S INBORN FEEDING BEHAVIORS

Practice Changes as Understanding Grows

As our understanding of the newborn's role in breastfeeding has changed, so too has our approach to supporting mother and baby.

Until 2 decades ago, the human newborn was considered by most to be completely helpless. Then in 1987 as an experiment, Swedish researchers asked mothers not to interact with their babies immediately after birth. They discovered that if laid tummy down on the mother's abdomen, the newborn could make his own way to the mother's breast and breastfeed without help (Widstrom et al., 1987). In this study and others that followed, researchers replicated these same conditions and discovered that some of the reflexes that were once thought to be useless, such as the stepping reflex, were actually a part of a newborn's hardwiring, and under the right circumstances, made it possible for him to make his own way to the breast (Matthiesen, Ransjo-Arvidson, Nissen, & Uvnas-Moberg, 2001; Righard & Alade, 1990). These findings and others have changed the way we understand the newborn. We now know that, like every other mammal, when born healthy, our babies have inborn reflexes to help them feed.

Our understanding of these inborn feeding behaviors affects our response. For example, some of these reflexes were once wrongly thought to undermine breastfeeding. To prevent newborns from being "their own worst enemy" at the breast, many were swaddled to restrict hand and arm movements. Mothers were taught to move babies quickly onto the breast when they opened wide, rather than waiting until their baby was ready to take the breast. A better understanding of how a baby's feeding reflexes contribute to breastfeeding makes it possible for us to foster birthing practices and postpartum environments that encourage rather than sabotage these reflexes and find better ways to support mothers and babies as they learn to breastfeed.

• •

At first, these feeding behaviors were thought to be fragile and short-lived, but now we know they can be triggered for months and even years.

In a classic Swedish study, researchers noted two interventions that derailed babies' journey to the breast after birth (Righard & Alade, 1990):

- Separating babies from their mothers for 20 minutes for bath and measurements
- Giving mothers pethidine (Demerol), a pain medication, during labor

When one of these interventions occurred, about half of the babies were unable to make their way to the breast and feed well. When both of these interventions occurred, none of the babies went to the breast and fed well. Many assumed from this study that these reflexes faded within the first day of life and had little impact on later breastfeeding.

One of the first to describe these behaviors as long-lasting was U.S. pediatrician Christina Smillie (Smillie, 2008). When she began helping mothers with breastfeeding problems, she noticed that when babies were held upright with their torso in contact with their mother's chest, they all exhibited similar breast-seeking behaviors. This occurred with full-term and preterm babies, young babies and older babies.

Being new to breastfeeding, Smillie had few preconceived notions, and her fresh eyes led to new insights. Smillie observed that these feeding behaviors persisted long after the newborn period.

> Although I have seen babies as old as 10 months learn to feed for the first time in this manner, it is much easier in the first 3 months of life. Once infants reach 4 or 5 month of age, when developmentally they are more and more distractible, their curiosity and high activity can interfere with the behavioral state that allows them to follow through on their instincts for the breast (Smillie, 2008).

In Australia, these breast-seeking behaviors have been observed in adopted children 8 months to 12 years old (Gribble, 2005).

• •

When both mother and baby take an active role during breastfeeding, this simplifies the process and enhances their relationship. Positive experiences at the breast reinforce effective feeding, which can prevent problems. Encouraging rather than suppressing these feeding behaviors can also help overcome breastfeeding problems, such as breast refusal, which may arise from negative associations at the breast. See the chapter, "Challenges at the Breast."

When a mother supports her baby's breast-seeking behaviors, it reinforces positive breastfeeding dynamics and can help overcome problems.

What Inborn Feeding Behaviors Look Like

Twenty inborn reflexes have been identified that help babies get to the breast and feed.

Until recently, only a small number of feeding reflexes—rooting, sucking, and swallowing—had been formally identified. To learn more, British midwife Suzanne Colson videotaped 40 British and French mothers and babies during the first month after birth (S. D. Colson, Meek, & Hawdon, 2008). Twenty-four hours of videotaped breastfeeding footage from 93 separate breastfeeding episodes was analyzed to identify inborn feeding behaviors (or "primitive neonatal reflexes") and to better understand their contribution to breastfeeding.

These 20 inborn behaviors (Table 1.1) appeared to have two primary purposes: to find and take the breast and to transfer milk. One new insight the researchers discovered was a strong "foot to mouth connection," with the mother's stroking of the baby's feet triggering reflexive movements of the baby's toes and feet and active sucking at the breast. The baby's gestational age, age when videotaped, ethnicity, and state of alertness had no effect on the triggering of these reflexes.

Table 1.1 Primitive Neonatal Reflexes by Function

Reflex	Purpose
Hand to mouth	Finding/taking breast
Finger flex/extend	Finding/taking breast
Mouth gape	Finding/taking breast
Tongue dart, tick	Finding/taking breast
Arm cycle	Finding/taking breast
Leg cycle	Finding/taking breast
Foot/hand flex	Finding/taking breast
Head lift	Finding/taking breast
Head right	Finding/taking breast
Head bob/nod	Finding/taking breast
Root	Finding/taking breast
Placing	Finding/taking breast
Palmar grasp	Finding/taking breast, milk transfer
Plantar grasp	Finding/taking breast, milk transfer
Babinski toe fan	Finding/taking breast, milk transfer
Step (withdrawal)	Finding/taking breast, milk transfer
Crawl	Finding/taking breast, milk transfer
Suck	Milk transfer
Jaw jerk	Milk transfer
Swallow	Milk transfer

(Colson et al., 2008)

Feeding behaviors vary from baby to baby and from position to position.

The U.K. researchers described in the previous point found that not all babies used all these reflexes at all feedings (S. D. Colson et al., 2008). And the number of feeding behaviors observed varied with the mother's body position, with the semi-reclining—or "laid-back"—positions producing the most feeding behaviors. For more, see the later section, "Body Positions."

U.S. pediatrician Christina Smillie also described variations in how different babies go to the breast (Smillie, 2007, 2008). Some use their whole body to slowly crawl to the breast, other move quickly. Smillie calls these behaviors the "searching response" (Smillie, 2008).

These behaviors are seen in preterm babies as young as 29 weeks.

These inborn feeding behaviors are a part of an infant's survival skills. As such, they are present in all babies, not just those born healthy and full-term. Studies from Sweden confirm that preterm babies born as early as 29 weeks gestation can make their own way to the breast and suckle. (K. H. Nyqvist, 2008; K. H. Nyqvist, Ewald, & Sjoden, 1996; K. H. Nyqvist, Ewald, U., Sjoden, P., 1998; K. H. Nyqvist, Sjoden, & Ewald, 1999). For details see the chapter, "The Preterm Baby."

Several Swedish studies found that even when mothers are specifically instructed not to interact with their babies after birth, mothers' hormonal levels change with their babies' actions (Matthiesen et al., 2001; Righard & Alade, 1990; Widstrom et al., 1987). One Swedish study videotaped the movements 10 babies made between an unmedicated birth and the first breastfeeding to determine which behaviors all newborns have in common (Matthiesen et al., 2001). At the same time, they measured the mothers' blood oxytocin levels. Oxytocin has wide-ranging physical effects on mothers, including milk let-down and uterine contractions, and has a calming and relationship-enhancing effect.

The baby's feeding behaviors affect the mother's hormonal levels and prepare her body for breastfeeding.

After birth, all the study babies did the following in this order: opened their eyes, massaged the breast, put hand to mouth, rooted, put moistened hand to the breast which caused the mother's nipple to become erect, extended their tongue and licked the nipple, and finally breastfed. These actions increased the mothers' blood oxytocin levels and the researchers concluded:

Babies' behaviors at the breast increases their mothers' blood oxytocin levels.

> Newborns use their hands as well as their mouths to stimulate maternal oxytocin release after birth, which may have significance for uterine contraction, milk ejection, and mother-infant interaction (Matthiesen et al., 2001).

In all feeding positions, finding and taking the breast is triggered mainly by touch and usually happens in the same sequence:

The touch of the breast on the baby's chin and cheeks helps him locate the nipple, take the breast, and begin feeding.

- Baby finds the nipple by rooting (moving his head from side to side with an open mouth).
- The touch of his chin on the breast stimulates him to open his mouth wide (gape).
- He then drops his tongue and extends its tip over his lower lip as he takes the breast and begins to suckle (Genna, 2008).

After taking the breast, feeding is easier if the baby can tilt his head back slightly. Both adults and babies find swallowing easier with the head slightly tilted back because this opens the throat. Australian midwife and lactation consultant Rebecca Glover refers to this as the "instinctive feeding position" (Glover, 2008).

The DVD "Baby-Led Breastfeeding: The Mother-Baby Dance" illustrates some of the various ways individual babies use their cheeks and chin to make their way to the nipple (Smillie, 2007). Some babies drop slowly to the breast, with their cheek lightly touching it. Some lunge quickly, turning their head only when their cheek touches the nipple. Others crawl slowly, using their whole body. Some make their way by touching each cheek alternately to the breast as they make their way.

Helpful DVDs

- **Baby-led Breastfeeding: The Mother-Baby Dance**
- **Biological Nursing: Laid-back Breastfeeding**

The DVD, "Biological Nurturing: Laid-Back Breastfeeding" (S. Colson, 2008) demonstrates graphically how gravity can make the process of taking the breast easier or more difficult. See the later section "Body Positions."

The baby draws milk from the breast by dropping his tongue and creating a vacuum.

Early research suggested that babies use a of their tongue to compress the breast and press milk into their mouth (Woolridge, 1986). More recent research indicates that most milk flow occurs during times of peak vacuum when the baby drops his tongue (Geddes, Kent, Mitoulas, & Hartmann, 2008). Rather than the milk being compressed out of the breast, it appears to be drawn out by vacuum.

How deeply the nipple goes into the baby's mouth can affect mother's comfort and milk flow during breastfeeding, as well as how actively baby suckles.

If the baby takes the nipple shallowly into his mouth with the nipple pressed against the front of his hard palate, this can result in nipple pain or trauma and slow milk flow. If the milk flow is slow enough, the baby may not gain weight well, suckle inactively, or fall asleep quickly.

According to ultrasound studies of healthy, thriving babies during normal breastfeeding, the nipple extends on average to within about 5 mm of the junction of the baby's hard and soft palates (Geddes et al., 2008; Jacobs, Dickinson, Hart, Doherty, & Faulkner, 2007). Some have nicknamed this area in the baby's mouth (Figure 1.1) the "comfort zone" (Mohrbacher & Kendall-Tackett, 2005).

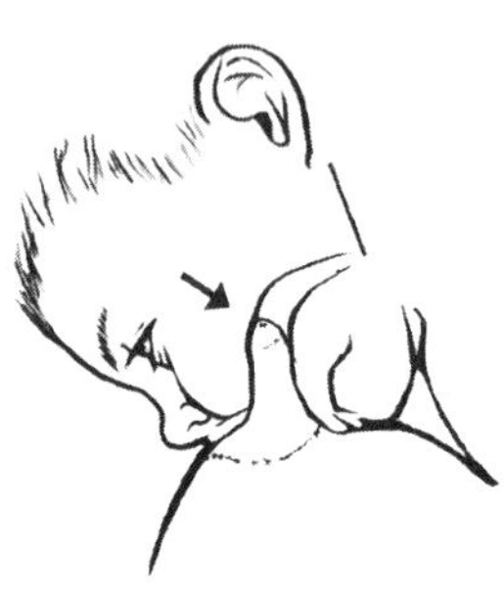

Figure 1.1. The comfort zone.
©2005 Peter Mohrbacher, used with permission

Triggers for Breast-Seeking Behaviors

A baby's breast-seeking behaviors are primarily triggered and maintained by the touch of the baby's chest, tummy, and legs against his mother's body.

The way mothers naturally hold their babies for cuddling triggers babies' breast-seeking behaviors. U.K. midwife and researcher Suzanne Colson suggests that a mother hold her baby "so that baby's face, neck, chest, tummy, and legs are closely flexed around a body contour, offering unrestricted access to the breast" (S. Colson, 2003).

U.S. pediatrician Christina Smillie suggests mothers hold their baby with his torso against her chest (Smillie, 2008). From there, the baby begins making his way to the breast. Smillie has observed that if a mother is upright and part of the baby's torso loses contact with her body, such as when the baby curls up or moves away, these behaviors stop. If this happens, the upright mother can bring the baby's torso in close contact with her body to restimulate these behaviors (Smillie, 2008).

Hunger and thirst may play a role in a baby seeking the breast and feeding.

A young baby's reflexes can be triggered even when he is not hungry, but if enough time goes by since the last breastfeeding, the biochemistry of hunger begins to play a role. When a baby's blood sugar drops, the first sign of hunger may be to put his hands to his mouth, perhaps chewing or sucking on his hand. If he cannot get to the breast, he will finally start to cry.

The baby can move to the breast more easily if his legs, feet, and soles can brush against the mother's thighs or another nearby object.

The stimulation of her baby's feet, either by the mother or by contact with something else in the environment, appears to help stimulate a baby's movement toward the breast. When the mother is in a semi-reclining, laid-back position and the top of her baby's feet brush against her body, this releases the stepping reflex, which can help a baby get to the breast. U.K. midwife and researcher Suzanne Colson noted that when semi-reclined mothers had their hands free, they often "spontaneously stroked their baby's feet triggering toe fanning and toe grasping," which appeared at the same time to release their baby's lip and tongue reflexes (S. D. Colson, Meek, & Hawdon, 2008a). This same behavior was not seen when mothers were sitting upright (possibly because the mothers didn't have a free hand in these positions). If a baby's body is tummy down with legs draped over the mother's side, pillows or other objects can also stimulate this response (S. Colson, 2007).

When a baby's cheek is touched, it causes him to turn his head in that direction, which can either help or hinder breastfeeding.

The rooting response is part of a baby's inborn feeding behaviors. This helps a baby locate the nipple and take it into his mouth. This can help a baby get to the breast. It can also be a barrier if a mother accidentally triggers this response by touching his cheek with her fingers, causing him to turn away from the breast.

Hearing, smell, and sight play a role in orienting the baby to the breast.

In their book, Your Amazing Newborn (2000), Marshall and Phyllis Klaus note that shortly after birth, a healthy full-term newborn will make eye contact, will turn toward his mother's voice, and can recognize his mother's smell.

Many studies have found that babies use smell to orient themselves to their mother and to the breast. One overview of the literature described several studies (Porter & Winberg, 1999). In one, breast pads were suspended over a baby's face, one clean and one with the smell of the mother's breast (Macfarlane, 1975). Babies consistently turned to the pad with their mother's smell. Another study found that even 2-week-old exclusively formula-fed babies turned first to smell a pad with an unfamiliar mother's milk on it over a pad with the more familiar smell of formula (Porter, Makin, Davis, & Christensen, 1991). In another study of 30 newborns and their mothers, one breast was washed with an odorless soap just before the newborn was placed between the mother's breasts after birth and allowed to choose which breast to go to (Varendi, Porter, & Winberg, 1994). Twenty-two babies (73%) preferred the unwashed breast. The authors noted that the infants' attraction to breast odors clearly influenced their behaviors and were "analogous to the role of 'nipple search pheromone' in guiding young rabbits and piglets to the nipple" (Porter & Winberg, 1999). In a more recent study in which the mother was not present, babies 36 to 72 hours old were placed tummy down in a warming bed. A breast pad was placed 17 cm away from the babies' nose (Varendi & Porter, 2001). Within 3 minutes, 18 of the 22 babies (85%) made their way to the breast pad with the mother's scent on it. Only 3 of the 22 babies (15%) made their way to the control pad. Being on their abdomen made it possible for these babies to get to the pads. In addition to helping a baby find the nipple, the smell of the mother's breast increases sucking during breastfeeding (Russell, 1976).

Pediatrician T. Berry Brazelton found that newborn babies will turn toward the sound of their mothers' voices, and even prefer her voice to others talking at the same time (Brazelton, 1995). Newborns have also been found to respond better to their mother's face than to other faces (Fifer & Moon, 1994).

Barriers to Breast-Seeking Behaviors

Some labor medications, separation of mother and baby, and swaddling may interfere with baby's breast-seeking behaviors.

For details, see the next chapter, "Breastfeeding Rhythms."

If a hungry newborn does not feel his mother's body against his torso, he may become confused and frustrated.

Even if a baby is close enough to see his mother, without the feel of her body against his torso, he can easily become disoriented (Smillie, 2008).

When the back of a baby's head is pushed, he will usually push back, which can undermine breastfeeding.

Pushing on the back of a baby's head is sometimes done in upright breastfeeding positions to move a baby toward the breast or to keep a baby on the breast. However, tilting the baby's head forward, chin to chest, makes swallowing more difficult (Glover, 2008) and pushing the baby's nose into the breast makes breathing more difficult, neither of which promotes effective breastfeeding. Most babies react negatively when their heads are pushed.

THE MOTHER'S ROLE

Encourage the mother to think of breastfeeding as something she and her baby work out in their own way.

Some mothers approach breastfeeding with worries about doing everything "right" or are nervous because they think of breastfeeding as their first critical test of motherhood. Although it may seem logical that giving mothers breastfeeding instructions would alleviate some of their worries, this can take a mother's focus off her baby and may even create problems.

Due to the popularity of upright and side-lying feeding positions, breastfeeding was once considered primarily the mother's job. When gravity pulls baby's body away from the mother, much more effort and dexterity are needed to achieve comfortable and effective breastfeeding, especially during the early learning period. However, research indicates that the use of a semi-reclining, or laid-back, position simplifies early breastfeeding (see the later section "Body Positions"). Researchers have concluded that when babies feed on their tummies, breastfeeding is much less of struggle, and suggest that human newborns are meant to be "tummy feeders," like puppies and hamsters.

Babies have reflexes that help them breastfeed

Rather than giving a mother breastfeeding instructions, it may be more helpful to let a mother know that her baby is born with reflexes to help him breastfeed, which can:

- Make breastfeeding less stressful for her.
- Build her confidence in breastfeeding.
- Enhance her relationship with her baby.
- Support a more positive breastfeeding dynamic, which makes it easier and more enjoyable for her and her baby (S. Colson, 2007; Smillie, 2008).

• •

Knowing [illegible] her baby's inborn feeding behaviors helps a mother better interpret and support them.

Some mothers mistakenly interpret their babies' inborn feeding behaviors as signs that breastfeeding isn't working. For example, in one study (S. D. Colson et al., 2008b), mothers made the following comments:

- My baby prefers sucking on his hand.
- He fights the breast.
- He does not like breastfeeding.

If a baby bats at the breast or struggles because he doesn't feel the touch he needs to orient himself, a mother may misunderstand, believing this means her baby doesn't want to breastfeed. She may even worry that her baby doesn't like her. The inborn feeding behaviors remain the same, but a mother's reactions to them will vary with her understanding.

Hardwiring and Learned Behavior

For mothers, breastfeeding may be partly learned and partly innate.

Mothers have biological triggers and innate responses, too. Without even thinking, a mother's body helps regulate her baby's body temperature (Chiu, Anderson, & Burkhammer, 2005; Kimura & Matsuoka, 2007). Each breast can even maintain a different temperature when a set of twins—each with a different thermal need—rests on each breast (Ludington-Hoe et al., 2006).

The hormone oxytocin, released during breastfeeding and skin-to-skin contact, makes most mothers feel like touching and stroking their babies. Some of these behaviors may have an innate component. U.S. pediatrician Christina Smillie noted strong similarities in the way the mothers in her practice touch and stroke their babies (Smillie, 2008).

Mothers are also hard-wired to breastfeed.

In one U.K. study (S. D. Colson et al., 2008), the researchers noted that many of the mothers who were videotaped during breastfeeding made the same movements to trigger their babies' inborn reflexes. For example, when the mothers were in a semi-reclining, laid-back position with their hands free, they often helped their baby get into the same type of vertical position used in neurological exams and used their fingers to stroke their baby's feet, triggering toe fanning and toe grasping, which released lip and tongue reflexes and helped the baby take the breast and feed. The researchers wrote that the mothers "appeared to trigger instinctively the right reflex at the right time" (S. D. Colson et al., 2008) and suggested that some aspects of breastfeeding may be innate for mothers as well.

But while babies' behaviors are reflex-driven, mothers can over-think breastfeeding. Unlike other mammals, a human mother can use her intellect to overrule her innate behaviors and emotions. In fact, engaging a mother's intellect can even alter her hormonal state, making it more difficult for her to know what her body is telling her (S. Colson, 2008). This is why is it so important for those supporting the mother after birth to engage her intellect as little as possible when breastfeeding is going well (also see next chapter).

Right-Brained Learning

When we think and act, we use both sides of our brain—left and right—which are joined by the corpus collosum and, therefore, work together. However, certain modes of thinking are more associated with one side of the brain than with the other. For example, the left brain is associated with planning ahead and the logical, sequential, rational, and analytical. The right brain, on the other hand, is associated with relationships, being in-the-moment, the intuitive, and the holistic. Newborns use their right brains because their left brains are not yet well developed. Some suggest that during early postpartum, a mother's right brain may become dominant to make it possible for her to connect better with her baby (Smillie, 2008).

After birth, helping strategies that are more right-brained in their approach are more consistent with a mother's enhanced right-brain function.

During the early weeks, many mothers report difficulty following instructions, remembering facts, and keeping track of time, all primarily governed by the left brain. Some researchers have referred to this phenomenon as a "cognitive deficiency" (Eidelman, Hoffmann, & Kaitz, 1993).

However, for the survival of the species, mothers must want to care for their newborns, and it is the right brain that governs a mother's emotions. This may explain in part why the right brain appears to take a more active role in the early weeks. Rather than referring to this as a "cognitive deficiency," it may be more accurate to say that new mothers have "enhanced right brain function."

Mothers and babies are more right-brained after birth.

For this reason, U.S. pediatrician Christina Smillie suggests that using a right-brained approach to supporting breastfeeding is more consistent with a new mother's physiology. In her quest for a better understanding of babies' inborn feeding behaviors, she found scientific backing for this in the neurobehavioral literature (Smillie, 2008), particularly in the work of U.S. neuropsychoanalyst Allan Schore.

Schore integrated research from several fields to describe an emotional right-brain connection (which he called "affective synchrony") between mother and baby, and described its importance to a baby's development (Schore, 2001). Schore noted that when mothers and babies interact—talk, look into each other's eyes, and touch—these behaviors create a direct right-brain to right-brain connection that makes it possible for a mother to help regulate her baby's state and his autonomic nervous system. At first, the resonance between a mother and baby's right brains helps a baby settle and stay calm. As he gets older and his attachment to his mother grows, this right-brain connection also helps him learn to regulate emotions.

With this information, Smillie began supporting and encouraging a right-brained connection in her practice. She noticed that the babies became more coordinated and proficient at feeding, and the mothers became more confident. She also noticed that this right-brain connection helped solve some of their breastfeeding problems, and she became more effective at helping mothers meet their breastfeeding goals.

A right-brain approach to supporting breastfeeding makes it easier for a mother to be responsive to her baby and to focus on their relationship.

To distinguish between left-brained and right-brained learning, think of left-brain as "head" knowledge and right-brain as "heart" or "body" knowledge. Some learning is best done with books and classes. Other learning is best done in other ways. Learning to ride a bicycle, for example, is best learned with the right brain by "feel."

In some ways, breastfeeding is similar. The "feel" that guides mothers as they learn to breastfeed comes from the physiological responses that draw mother and baby to one another. It's why they love to look at each other, touch each other, and interact. Much of this behavior is guided by the right brain, where emotion lies. Breastfeeding is a natural outcome of this right-brain interaction between mother and baby.

Along these lines, U.K. midwife and researcher Suzanne Colson developed an approach to breastfeeding that she calls "biological nurturing" (S. Colson, 2005, 2007). To start, she suggests that a mother lean back and get comfortable, with good arm and body support, and that she give her baby unrestricted access to the breast. The baby lies tummy down on the mother's body, so gravity keeps him in close contact and makes it easy for him to make his way to the breast. For more details, see the section "Body Positions."

U.S. pediatrician Christina Smillie (2008) also emphasizes to mothers that "there is no one right way to do this" and focuses instead on:

- Displaying confidence that breastfeeding will work.
- Encouraging the mother to talk to her baby.
- Reassuring the mother that her baby's actions are normal.

Her main message to each mother is that "her job is not to learn to breastfeed or to make her baby learn. Her job is to get comfortable and help her baby stay calm, relaxed, and comfortable (Smillie, 2008).

Susan Burger, a U.S. lactation consultant in New York City, offers insights into the value of mother's intuition and the downsides of prescriptive approaches and over-thinking:

> Most of what infants need is careful observation and empathy. I've seen how mothers' observational skills or just plain intuitive guesswork actually works quite well at times to develop creative adaptations. I spend more and more time watching and trying to understand what mothers and babies are actually doing before I ever touch or advise.
>
> Sitting on mats at a support group, mothers would complain how much more painful it was to feed at home. On the floor, they would slump back a bit and lean against pillows without analyzing about the 'proper' positions. The subtle adjustments that they made on the floor when they didn't have the 'proper' chair made a huge difference for some of them.
>
> Most of what happens in the Manhattan culture I deal with is too much trying to 'analyze' the 'proper' way to do things and then mothers feeling frustrated because they can't 'analyze' the way they used to, instead of letting go and observing the relationship with their babies unfold and how their babies respond to their actions (Burger, 2008).

If it is necessary to touch mother or baby, always ask permission first.

If a mother requests help or if touch is needed, asking first helps mothers feel respected and in control. A Swedish study examined 10 mothers' reactions to hands-on versus hands-off breastfeeding help (Weimers, Svensson, Dumas, Naver, & Wahlberg, 2006). The mothers reported that when hands-on breastfeeding help was given without first asking permission, it felt almost brutal, unpleasant, and like a violation of their integrity. When someone else squeezed their breast into their baby's mouth, they considered it a negative experience that they did not want repeated. The mothers considered hands-off approaches more positive and more effective at enhancing their feelings of competence.

GETTING MOTHER AND BABY IN SYNC

When mother and baby experience a right-brain connection, the whole becomes greater than the sum of their parts.

Baby's State, Readiness, and the Right-Brain Connection

A baby's state of alertness affects his ability to breastfeed.

One infant assessment guide, the Neonatal Behavior Assessment Scale (Brazelton, 1995), describes six infant states:

- Deep sleep
- Light sleep
- Drowsy
- Quiet alert
- Fussy
- Crying

Before breastfeeding, a fussy or crying baby will most likely first need to calm down. However, research confirms that babies can breastfeed in any of the other states, and there may even be advantages to putting babies to breast when they are drowsy or asleep. One study of 12 late preterm babies, 35 to 37 weeks gestation, found that when sleeping babies were kept in their mothers' arms and the mothers gave them cues to feed, these babies took the breast and fed well at some feedings without completely waking (S. Colson, DeRooy, L., Hawdon, J., 2003).

The DVD "Biological Nurturing: Laid-Back Breastfeeding" illustrates how inborn feeding reflexes continue to be triggered when babies are asleep (S. Colson, 2008). It recommends putting babies having breastfeeding problems (such as breast refusal) on their mothers' semi-reclined bodies while they're asleep. U.K. researcher Suzanne Colson has found that because sleep "blunts" feeding reflexes, this can make breastfeeding go more smoothly, even in upright positions. Babies can organize sucking and swallowing with breathing more easily when drowsy or asleep.

Whenever possible, suggest breastfeeding begin before baby starts crying.

One of the most common questions new parents ask is how to know when to feed their baby. Although many parenting books describe how a new parent learns over time to tell the difference between a "hungry cry" and a "tired cry," babies should ideally be fed before they are crying at all. In its policy statement on breastfeeding, the American Academy of Pediatrics describes crying as "a late indicator of hunger" and suggests breastfeeding before a baby gets to this point (Gartner et al., 2005). It recommends breastfeeding whenever babies show any of these early feeding cues:

- Increased alertness
- Physical activity
- Mouthing (including putting hand to mouth)
- Rooting (turning head side to side as cheeks are touched)

Especially in the early weeks, when mother and baby are getting comfortable with breastfeeding, it can be a real advantage to breastfeed whenever the baby will accept the breast, whether he's hungry or not. Because a newborn's feeding reflexes can be triggered at any time, encourage the mother to put her baby to breast whenever she wants to relieve breast fullness (to prevent engorgement) or if she just wants that closeness with her baby. The more babies breastfeed, the more quickly they become comfortable with it. Frequent feedings in the early weeks are also associated with positive health outcomes and a healthy milk production (see next chapter).

A right-brained connection between mother and baby can trigger a "charmed" state, which improves a baby's coordination.

U.S. pediatrician Christina Smillie (2008) discovered this dynamic in the neurobehavioral literature (Smillie, 2008). French neurologists had been looking for ways to simplify infant neurological exams and noticed that when babies were engaged through eye contact, talking, and touch, their coordination markedly improved, and they could do motor tasks far beyond their age expectations (Amiel-Tison, 1983). These researchers suggested that when babies appeared "charmed" by others, this "communicative state" was different from states previously identified. In this state, infants appeared to be "liberated" from many distracting reflexive behaviors, which made it possible for them to better control their actions. One remarkable photo from this study showed a 17-day-old "charmed" infant (with just a little head support provided by two of the researcher's fingers) sitting upright and reaching for a toy.

Similarly, U.S. neuropsychoanalyst Allan Schore described how when mothers and babies talk, look into each other's eyes, and touch, this interaction can create a direct right-brain to right-brain connection that allows a mother to help regulate her baby's state. He called the resonance between a mother and baby's right brains "affective synchrony," which he said allows the newborn's immature systems to be "co-regulated by the caregiver's more mature and differentiated nervous system" (Schore, 2001).

This information helped Smillie better understand the role of the mother-baby relationship to successful breastfeeding. By encouraging mothers to focus on their babies rather than learning specific breastfeeding techniques, the babies became more coordinated when they went to the breast and fed better (Smillie, 2008).

Body Positions

Teaching specific breastfeeding positions is a left-brain approach that has drawbacks.

When breastfeeding positions are named and taught, breastfeeding may seem unnecessarily complicated to mothers. Smillie notes that we don't teach bottle-feeding positions (e.g., "the highchair hold," "the carseat hold"). We trust that when mothers feed their babies by bottle, they will find their own comfortable feeding positions. She suggests the same should be true when supporting breastfeeding.

There are no right or wrong feeding positions.

Another drawback to standardized positions is that it causes some mothers to focus on the wrong things. When a mother worries about doing specific positions "right" or tries to duplicate a position learned in a book or a class, it makes her less responsive to her baby.

• •

If mothers want information about positioning, focus instead on the dynamics that work for or against breastfeeding.

There are no "right" or "wrong," "proper" or "improper" feeding positions. However, some aspects of body positions can work for or against breastfeeding. For example, gravity works with mothers and babies in semi-reclining, laid-back positions, whereas in upright or side-lying positions, mothers must work against gravity to keep their babies' bodies against theirs. Rather than teaching specific positions, it may be more helpful for mothers to know about these basic dynamics.

Mothers and babies come in different shapes and sizes, and there are hundreds of possible feeding positions. This is a much more helpful message than implying that mothers are limited to just a few positions or being too directive about how mothers should hold their babies. It boosts a new mother's confidence in her own abilities when she finds her best positions on her own and when she and her baby work this out without outside help. As some research has found, teaching positioning and attachment skills may inadvertently decrease breastfeeding satisfaction and duration over the long term (Henderson et al., 2003).

• •

Another helpful focus is on creating an environment conducive to breastfeeding.

Rather than teaching positioning and attachment skills during the early weeks of breastfeeding, suggest the mother create an environment that enhances her hormonal response to her baby, which is linked to increased duration of breastfeeding (Nissen et al., 1996). Some ways to do this include:

- Insuring the mother's privacy, warmth, and comfort.
- Respecting her choices and reinforcing what she does right.
- Enhancing her feeling of competence as she learns to care for her newborn by minimizing information/teaching unless absolutely necessary.

Instruction can disrupt a mother's ability to tap into and trust her natural responses, which may ultimately undermine breastfeeding.

• •

There is no need to vary positions at every feeding unless there is a special need.

In the past, some mothers were told to routinely vary their positions at each feeding. This idea became popular at a time when nipple pain and trauma were thought to be a normal part of breastfeeding and was based on the premise that using different positions would more evenly spread the pain and damage, making breastfeeding more tolerable.

With a better understanding of the causes of nipple trauma, this recommendation no longer makes sense, except in special situations, such as babies with tongue tie, unusual palates, or other anatomical differences that make breastfeeding painful.

Gravity Can Help or Hinder

In one U.K. study (S. D. Colson et al., 2008), researchers noted that when mothers sat upright, gravity pulled their baby's body away, and some of the babies' inborn reflexes worked against breastfeeding. Arm cycling, which babies use as a hunger cue, became 'breast boxing," which mothers interpreted as a sign their babies did not want to breastfeed. Startling occurred more often in upright positions, causing some babies to arch or fling themselves away.

Upright and side-lying breastfeeding positions are commonly taught, but laid-back positions can make the early learning period easier.

But when mothers assumed a semi-reclining "biological nurturing" position, these same reflexes more often worked for breastfeeding rather than against it. The researchers suggested that, like hamsters and puppies, the human newborn is meant to be a "tummy feeder" rather than a "back feeder" (needing pressure along his back to hold him against his mother's body). When the baby lies tummy down on the mother's semi-reclined body, the mother has one or both hands free and baby needs little or no support. There are no gaps between mother and baby, and baby's chin naturally comes in contact with mother's body. In this position, the babies were also more effective at taking milk for longer periods (S. Colson, personal communicator, January 22, 2009).

Babies' reflexes can work against breastfeeding.

Especially during the early weeks, a semi-reclined or laid-back position may be easier for mothers and babies than other positions. One way to think about this is to compare the semi-reclined position to training wheels on a bicycle, which, at first, help new riders keep their balance as they learn a new skill. As Colson and colleagues wrote:

> ...mothers' bodies provided a foundation, their arms the boundaries, their fingers stroking guidance, triggering and channeling the number and type of [inborn reflexes] needed to help the baby latch and feed (S. D. Colson et al., 2008a, p. 446)

Rather than the mother working against gravity to keep her baby's body pressed against hers, gravity does it for her. When the mechanics of breastfeeding are easier to manage, a "right-brain enhanced" mother can keep the focus on her baby, rather than on all the steps she needs to remember. For mothers giving birth in a hospital, an adjustable hospital bed makes this easy by allowing them to adjust their angle of recline to whatever works best for them and their babies.

• •

The positive effects of gravity on mothers' and babies' inborn feeding behaviors promote good breastfeeding dynamics almost automatically. Colson's research found:

Laid-back breastfeeding makes learning "latch-on techniques" unnecessary for most mothers.

> ...there was no need to line up nose to nipple and wait for mouth gape or to assess tongue position as suggested by those teaching [positioning and attachment] skills. Gravity pulled the baby's chin and tongue forward. Together the anti-gravity reflexes often triggered the degree of mouth opening needed to achieve pain-free, neonatal self-attachment

> even when the baby appeared to be in light sleep (S. D. Colson et al., 2008, p. 448).

• •

As babies grow and their mothers begin to breastfeed in public places, modified versions of laid-back positions or any other positions can be used.

In an article written for mothers, Colson explains that mothers can use these laid-back positions anywhere by simply shifting their hips forward in a chair (Figure 1.2):

> The movement is in the pelvis, not the shoulders. Some mothers prefer to sit slightly forward during latch and then lean back to maintain a comfortable nursing position. As soon as you lean back slightly, changing from ischial to sacral sitting, on a sofa at home or on a chair at the coffee shop, your baby has more space and can curl down around or obliquely across our body. Therefore, the degree to which you lean back during [semi-reclining] is up to you and often depends on your immediate environment (S. Colson, 2007, p. 46).

Colson notes that as babies grow, mothers naturally tailor their positions to the environment they're in, and that some mothers may prefer to use other positions, either early in breastfeeding or later on.

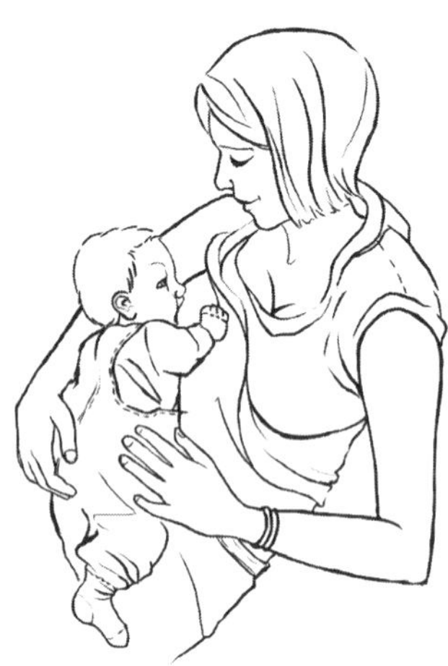

Figure 1.2. Laid-back position.
©2010 Anna Mohrbacher, used with permission

Use Comfort as a Guide

Mothers should choose their own feeding position based on comfort.

How is comfort defined? A comfortable position for a mother is one that is pain-free and easy to maintain for up to an hour, with no neck strain, relaxed shoulders, and good body support (S. Colson, 2005). Suggest the mother think about how she watches her favorite television show.

Although a laid-back position makes this easy to achieve, in any position, pillows and cushions can be used to provide enough support to allow a mother to relax. One of the ways Colson defines a comfortable "biological nurturing position" is one that allows mother and baby to fit together like the pieces of a puzzle. Encourage the mother to experiment until she finds a comfortable feeding position and to keep experimenting with positions as her baby grows.

Baby's comfort and coordination while breastfeeding may be affected by his position while in the womb.

For some time after birth, a baby's position in the womb may influence his comfort while he breastfeeds. Although many consider it important for baby's shoulders, torso, hips, and legs to be in a straight line during breastfeeding, if a baby was in a posterior position or had his arms or legs extended in the womb, he may not feel comfortable breastfeeding with his body in a straight line during the early weeks. This is another reason it is best not to be too specific about feeding positions and to encourage mother and baby to find their own.

The DVD, "Biological Nurturing: Laid-Back Breastfeeding" illustrates this with a baby who was born in a frank breech position (S. Colson, 2008). When the mother tried to breastfeed sitting upright, the baby kept one leg splayed straight up between him and his mother, making it impossible to pull him close enough to the mother's body. When she tried to move the baby's legs down, the baby held his legs straight and his body at an angle. When she laid her baby tummy down on her semi-reclined body with the bed supporting his legs, they finally relaxed and he was able to breastfeed comfortably.

Getting comfortable in upright and side-lying positions can be challenging.

Providing good body support in upright and side-lying positions can be tricky. A mother needs to insure that her baby's torso, hips, and legs stay in contact with her body (no gaps) and baby's shoulder and hips are well-supported. See Figures 1.3, 1.4, and 1.5 for examples of upright feeding positions that require mothers to apply pressure to their babies' backs and in some, support their baby's weight throughout the feeding.

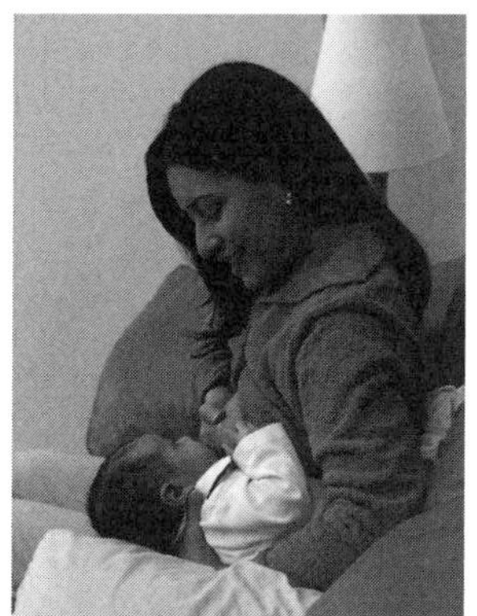

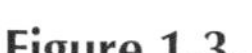

Figure 1.3.

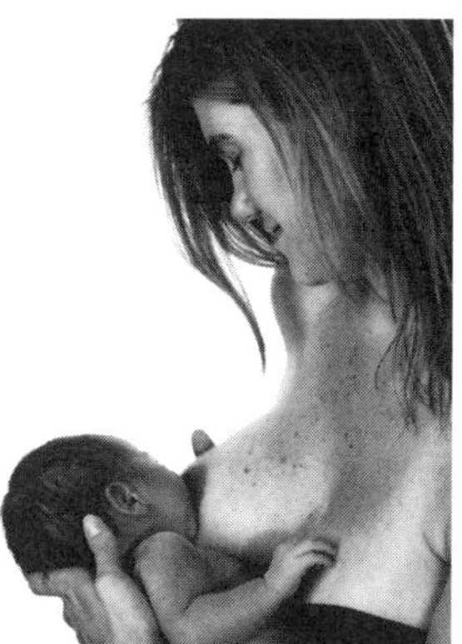

Figure 1.4.

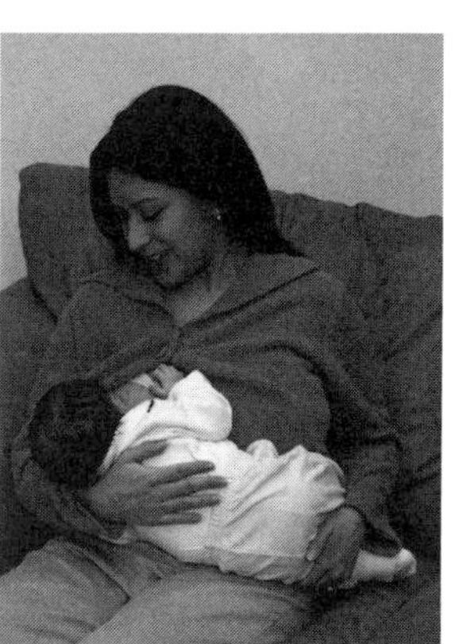

Figure 1.5.

Upright feeding positions.
©2010 Ameda, used with permission

When a baby's hips and torso are well supported, his head and neck coordination improves. "Lips follow hips" is an expression used by some physical and occupational therapists to describe how hip support affects a baby's ability to feed. A baby's head and neck control during breastfeeding depend in part on good support of his hips (Marmet, 2008).

To increase comfort in laid-back positions, two adjustments a mother can make are the baby's "lie" and her angle of recline.

In semi-reclining "biological nurturing" positions, the baby's body can lie in three general directions in relation to the mother's body (S. Colson, 2008; S. D. Colson et al., 2008a). Colson refers to these "lies" using the same terms that describe babies' positions in the womb: "longitudinal," "transverse," and "oblique." Because the breast is round and there are 360 degrees in a circle, it is possible for a baby to assume at least 270 different positions in relation to the mother's body.

If needed, another adjustment a mother can make to increase her and her baby's comfort during breastfeeding is to adjust how far she leans back. In some cases, either leaning back more or sitting up more may make breastfeeding easier.

Mothers who give birth by cesarean section can use laid-back positions that keep the baby away from their incision.

To avoid pain, these mothers can avoid using a "longitudinal lie" until their incision is healed. Colson wrote:

> Many mothers find that after a cesarean section, draping the baby over their shoulder or across their abdomen, so baby's torso and feet are supported by pillows on the bed and do not interfere with the wound, enables the baby to self-attach, and the mother to relax comfortably (S. Colson, 2007, p. 45).

As examples, see Figures 1.6, 1.7, and 1.8.

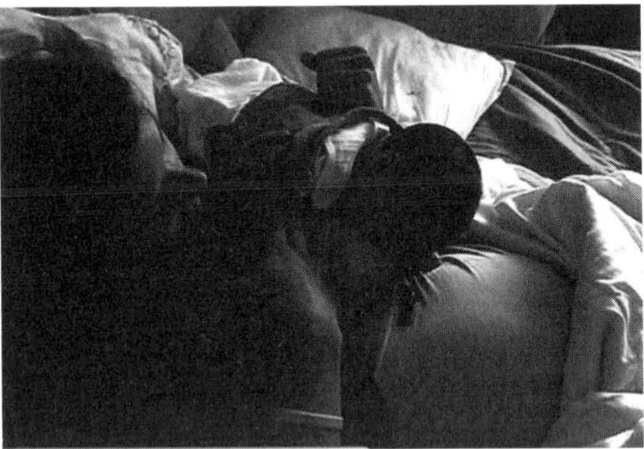

Figure 1.6. Laid back position that can be comfortably used after a cesarean section.
©Suzanne Colson, RN, RM, PhD, used with permission

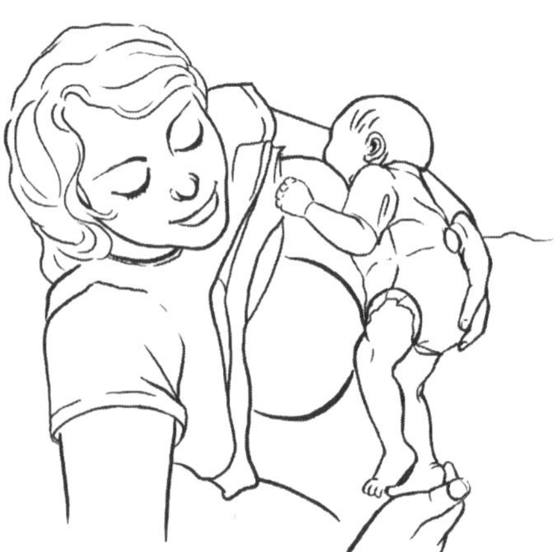

Figure 1.7.
©2010 Anna Mohrbacher, used with permission

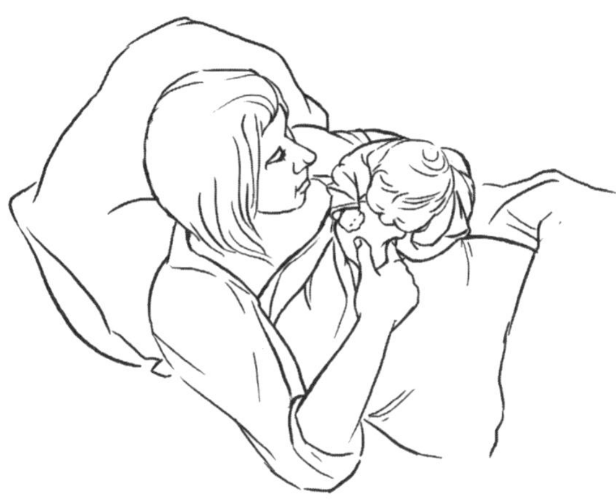

Figure 1.8.
©2010 Anna Mohrbacher, used with permission

Breastfeeding Two Babies

There are many positions in which mothers of multiples can breastfeed two babies at once.

Mothers of twins, triplets, or more often prefer to breastfeed two babies together at some feedings and separately at others. Breastfeeding two babies together can be a big time-saver, and it may be more effective at increasing a mother's prolactin levels, which can contribute to increased milk production, especially in the early weeks.

Figure 9 illustrates some of the many ways two babies can be positioned for breastfeeding. Encourage the mother to use the positions that feel most natural and comfortable for her and her babies.

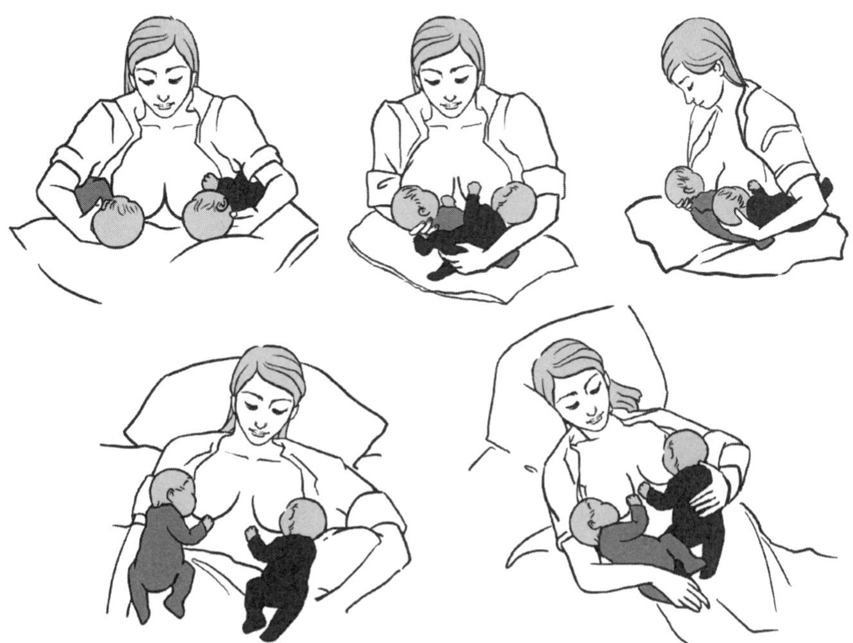

Figure 1.9. Different ways to position two babies at the breast.
©2010 Anna Mohrbacher, used with permission

Breast Support and Shaping

Some women support their breast during feedings; others do not. Some vary this from feeding to feeding.

Depending on the mother's body position and the relationship of the baby's body to the breast, a mother may or may not provide breast support during breastfeeding. This is best left to the mother's discretion. Colson wrote:

> The need to hold can change daily, even from feed to feed. Mothers are the best people to decide this and routine instruction about holding their breasts, still or otherwise, may inhibit their instinctual behaviors (S. Colson, 2005, p. 30).

If an upright mother supports her breast, suggest she keep it close to its natural height.

The closer the mother's breast is to its natural height, the less work it is for her to maintain it during feedings. If a mother with large breasts decides to provide support, suggest she focus on supporting just the part of her breast near the nipple and areola, as this is the area the baby needs to manage during breastfeeding. For more strategies for large-breasted women, see the chapter "Challenges at the Breast."

If a baby needs a little help in taking the breast, suggest the mother first try breast shaping.

Shaping the breast means gently squeezing the breast tissue to make it easier for the baby to take. This can sometimes help, but only if the breast is squeezed into an oval shaped to fit more easily into the baby's mouth (wider at the corners and narrower between upper and lower jaw). To do this, suggest the mother keep her thumb and fingers parallel to baby's lips as she gently squeezes (Figure 1.10). For the baby still having trouble taking the breast, see the chapter, "Challenges at the Breast."

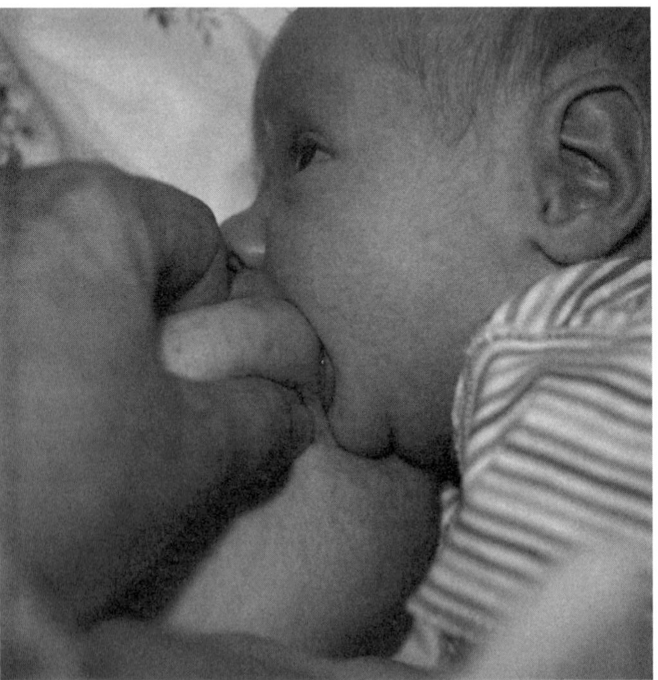

Figure 1.10. Breast sandwich.

B. Wilson-Clay and K. Hoover, The Breastfeeding Atlas, 4th ed. 2008

How Feedings End

For the baby who is thriving, suggest the mother breastfeed on one breast until her baby comes off on his own, and then offer the other breast.

Some babies are fast feeders and some are slow feeders. Although there may be "average" feeding lengths for babies of different ages, not all babies are average. If a baby is thriving, there is no advantage to timing feedings or switching breasts after a specific number of minutes. Encourage the mother to allow her baby to finish the first breast before offering the other breast. If the baby falls asleep while breastfeeding and comes off, she can offer the other breast when he awakens. For more details on feeding frequency and length, see the next chapter.

• •

If the mother wants to take the baby off the breast before he ends the feeding, suggest she first break the suction.

To avoid nipple pain or trauma, suggest the mother insert a clean finger quickly into the corner of baby's mouth, between his gums, so that he can't bear down on the breast as he comes off.

CHECKLIST

If the baby is not taking the breast well, first review the basics.

- Is gravity working for or against breastfeeding in the position mother is using?
- If semi-reclined, has the mother tried different angles of recline and different lies for her baby?
- Are the baby's feet in contact with either the mother's body or something else?
- Has the baby been given the chance to first lie on his mother's body in a position of his choosing and go to breast in his own time?
- Is the baby crying and needs to be calmed?
- Has the mother tried breastfeeding while her baby is asleep or drowsy?
- Would baby benefit from breast support or shaping?

If more strategies are needed, see the chapter "Challenges at the Breast."

RESOURCES FOR PARENTS

Websites

http://www.biologicalnurturing.com/pdfs/Poster%20for%20web%20site-locked.pdf. A simple, illustrated brochure for parents on "biological nurturning."

Videos

Colson, S. (2008). *Biological nurturing: Laid-back breastfeeding*. Available from www.biologicalnurturing.com.

Righard, L. (1995). *Delivery Self-Attachment*. Available from www.geddesproduction.com

Smillie, C. (2007). *Baby-led breastfeeding: The mother-baby dance*. Available from www.geddesproduction.com.

Books

Klaus, M.H., & Klaus, P. (1995). Your Amazing Newborn. Reading, MA: Perseus Books.

Mohrbacher, N., & Kendall-Tackett, K. (2005). *Breastfeeding made simple: Seven natural laws for nursing mothers*. Oakland, CA: New Harbinger Publications.

REFERENCES

Amiel-Tison, C., & Grenier, A. (1983). Expression of liberated motor activity (LMA) following manual immobilization of the head (J. Steichen, P. Steichen-Asch, & C.P. Braun, Trans.). In C. Amiel-Tison & A. Grenier (Eds.), *Neurologic evaluation of the newborn and the infant* (pp. 87-109). New York, NY: Masson Publishing.

Brazelton, T. B., & Nugent, J. K. (1995). Neonatal behavioral assessment scale. London, UK: MacKeith Press.

Burger, S. (2008). Right-brain enhancement. New York, New York: Lactnet.

Chiu, S. H., Anderson, G. C., & Burkhammer, M. D. (2005). Newborn temperature during skin-to-skin breastfeeding in couples having breastfeeding difficulties. *Birth, 32*(2), 115-121.

Colson, S. (2003). Cuddles, biological nurturing, exclusive breastfeeding and public health. *Journal of the Royal Society of Health, 123*(2), 76-77.

Colson, S. (2005). Maternal breastfeeding positions: have we got it right? (2). *The Practising Midwife, 8*(11), 29-32.

Colson, S. (2007). Biological nurturing (1). A non-prescriptive recipe for breastfeeding. *The Practising Midwife, 10*(9), 42, 44, 46-47.

Colson, S. (2008). *Biological nurturing: Laid-back breastfeeding*. Hythe, Kent, UK: The Nurturing Project.

Colson, S., DeRooy, L., Hawdon, J. (2003). Biological nurturing increases duration of breastfeeding for a vulnerable cohort. *MIDIRS Midwifery Digest, 13*(1), 92-97.

Colson, S. D., Meek, J. H., & Hawdon, J. M. (2008a). Optimal positions for the release of primitive neonatal reflexes stimulating breastfeeding. *Early Human Development, 84*(7), 441-449.

de Oliveira, L. D., Giugliani, E. R., do Espirito Santo, L. C., Franca, M. C., Weigert, E. M., Kohler, C. V., et al. (2006). Effect of intervention to improve breastfeeding technique on the frequency of exclusive breastfeeding and lactation-related problems. *Journal of Human Lactation, 22*(3), 315-321.

Eidelman, A. I., Hoffmann, N. W., & Kaitz, M. (1993). Cognitive deficits in women after childbirth. *Obstetrics and Gynecology, 81*(5 (Pt 1)), 764-767.

Fifer, W. P., & Moon, C. M. (1994). The role of mother's voice in the organization of brain function in the newborn. *Acta Paediatrica Supplement, 397*, 86-93.

Gartner, L. M., Morton, J., Lawrence, R. A., Naylor, A. J., O'Hare, D., Schanler, R. J., et al. (2005). Breastfeeding and the use of human milk. *Pediatrics, 115*(2), 496-506.

Geddes, D. T., Kent, J. C., Mitoulas, L. R., & Hartmann, P. E. (2008). Tongue movement and intra-oral vacuum in breastfeeding infants. *Early Human Development, 84*(7), 471-477.

Genna, C. W. (2008). Breastfeeding: normal sucking and swallowing. In C. W. Genna (Ed.), *Supporting sucking skills in breastfeeding infants* (pp. 1-41). Boston, MA: Jones and Bartlett.

Glover, R., Wiessinger, D. (2008). The infant-mother breastfeeding conversation: Helping when they lose the thread. In C. W. Genna (Ed.), *Supporting sucking skills in breastfeeding infants* (pp. 97-129). Boston, MA: Jones and Bartlett.

Gribble, K. D. (2005). Post-institutionalized adopted children who seek breastfeeding from their new mothers. *Journal of Prenatal and Perinatal Psychology and Health 19*(3), 217-234.

Henderson, J. J., Dickinson, J. E., Evans, S. F., McDonald, S. J., & Paech, M. J. (2003). Impact of intrapartum epidural analgesia on breast-feeding duration. *Australia and New Zealand Journal of Obstetrics and Gynaecology, 43*(5), 372-377.

Jacobs, L. A., Dickinson, J. E., Hart, P. D., Doherty, D. A., & Faulkner, S. J. (2007). Normal nipple position in term infants measured on breastfeeding ultrasound. *Journal of Human Lactation, 23*(1), 52-59.

Kimura, C., & Matsuoka, M. (2007). Changes in breast skin temperature during the course of breastfeeding. *Journal of Human Lactation, 23*(1), 60-69.

Ludington-Hoe, S. M., Lewis, T., Morgan, K., Cong, X., Anderson, L., & Reese, S. (2006). Breast and infant temperatures with twins during shared kangaroo care. *Journal of Obstetric, Gynecologic, and Neonatal Nursing, 35*(2), 223-231.

Macfarlane, A. (1975). Olfaction in the development of social preferences in the human neonate. In R. O. C. Porter, M. (Ed.), *Parent-infant interactions* (pp. 103-113). New York, New York: Elsevier.

Marmet, C., Shell, E. (2008). Therapeutic positioning for breastfeeding. In C. W. Genna (Ed.), *Supporting sucking skills in breastfeeding infants* (pp. 305-325). Boston, MA: Jones and Bartlett.

Matthiesen, A. S., Ransjo-Arvidson, A. B., Nissen, E., & Uvnas-Moberg, K. (2001). Postpartum maternal oxytocin release by newborns: effects of infant hand massage and sucking. *Birth, 28*(1), 13-19.

Mohrbacher, N., & Kendall-Tackett, K. (2005). *Breastfeeding made simple: Seven natural laws for nursing mothers.* Oakland, CA: New Harbinger Publications.

Nissen, E., Uvnas-Moberg, K., Svensson, K., Stock, S., Widstrom, A. M., & Winberg, J. (1996). Different patterns of oxytocin, prolactin but not cortisol release during breastfeeding in women delivered by caesarean section or by the vaginal route. *Early Human Development, 45*(1-2), 103-118.

Nyqvist, K. H. (2008). Early attainment of breastfeeding competence in very preterm infants. *Acta Paediatrica, 97*(6), 776-781.

Nyqvist, K. H., Ewald, U., & Sjoden, P. O. (1996). Supporting a preterm infant's behaviour during breastfeeding: a case report. *Journal of Human Lactation, 12*(3), 221-228.

Nyqvist, K. H., Ewald, U., Sjoden, P. (1998). Supporting a preterm infant's behaviour during breastfeeding: A case report. *Journal of Human Lactation, 12*(3), 221-228.

Nyqvist, K. H., Sjoden, P. O., & Ewald, U. (1999). The development of preterm infants' breastfeeding behavior. *Early Human Development, 55*(3), 247-264.

Porter, R. H., Makin, J. W., Davis, L. B., & Christensen, K. M. (1991). An assessment of the salient olfactory environment of formula-fed infants. *Physiology and Behavior, 50*(5), 907-911.

Porter, R. H., & Winberg, J. (1999). Unique salience of maternal breast odors for newborn infants. *Neuroscience and Biobehavioral Reviews, 23*(3), 439-449.

Righard, L., & Alade, M. O. (1990). Effect of delivery room routines on success of first breast-feed. *Lancet, 336*(8723), 1105-1107.

Russell, M. J. (1976). Human olfactory communication. Nature, 260(5551), 520-522.

Schore, A. N. (2001). The effects of a secure attachment relationship on right brain development, affect regulation, and infant mental health. *Infant Mental Health Journal, 22*, 7-66.

Smillie, C. (Writer) (2007). *Baby-led breastfeeding:* The Mother-Baby Dance: Geddes Productions.

Smillie, C. (2008). How infants learn to feed: A neurobehavioral model. In C. W. Genna (Ed.), *Supporting sucking skills in breastfeeding infants* (pp. 79-95). Boston, MA: Jones and Bartlett.

Varendi, H., & Porter, R. H. (2001). Breast odour as the only maternal stimulus elicits crawling towards the odour source. *Acta Paediatrica, 90*(4), 372-375.

Varendi, H., Porter, R. H., & Winberg, J. (1994). Does the newborn baby find the nipple by smell? *Lancet, 344(*8928), 989-990.

Wallace, L. M., Dunn, O. M., Alder, E. M., Inch, S., Hills, R. K., & Law, S. M. (2006). A randomised-controlled trial in England of a postnatal midwifery intervention on breast-feeding duration. *Midwifery, 22*(3), 262-273.

Weimers, L., Svensson, K., Dumas, L., Naver, L., & Wahlberg, V. (2006). Hands-on approach during breastfeeding support in a neonatal intensive care unit: a qualitative study of Swedish mothers' experiences. *International Breastfeeding Journal, 1*, 20.

Widstrom, A. M., Ransjo-Arvidson, A. B., Christensson, K., Matthiesen, A. S., Winberg, J., & Uvnas-Moberg, K. (1987). Gastric suction in healthy newborn infants. Effects on circulation and developing feeding behaviour. *Acta Paediatrica Scandinavica, 76*(4), 566-572.

Woolridge, M. W. (1986). The 'anatomy' of infant sucking. *Midwifery, 2*(4), 164-171.

Breastfeeding Rhythms

Chapter 2

Breastfeeding rhythms encompass many aspects of feeding: how often and long baby goes to breast, whether baby takes one breast or more, the day and night changes in feeding frequency, and how these variables change over time as baby matures. Both biology and culture affect breastfeeding rhythms.

"Breastfeeding rhythm" is the natural fluctuations in feeding patterns over time.

BIRTH PRACTICES AND BREASTFEEDING

Whether a birth is easy or difficult, ecstatic or traumatic, it is a life-changing event that profoundly influences the rhythms of early breastfeeding. Practices that prolong labor include keeping a laboring woman immobile and on her back, letting the woman labor alone, withholding food and drink, induction of labor by drugs, using forceps and/or vacuum extractor, and performing cesarean deliveries (Smith, 2008; Smith, 2010).

Practices that prolong labor or make birth more stressful can undermine early breastfeeding.

Research has found an association between stressful birth—either physically or psychologically—and delay in increased milk production (Beck & Watson, 2008; Chen, Nommsen-Rivers, Dewey, & Lonnerdal, 1998; Dewey, 2001; Dewey, Nommsen-Rivers, Heinig, & Cohen, 2003). This may be due to the elevated levels of cortisol in a mother's bloodstream after a long, stressful, or difficult birth (Grajeda & Perez-Escamilla, 2002). One U.S. study found that more than 1 hour spent pushing during stage II labor was associated with delayed milk increase (Dewey et al., 2003). An association also has been found between mild to moderate postpartum hemorrhage during birth and decreased milk production (Willis & Livingstone, 1995).

A stressful birth can undermine lactogenesis II.

If a mother considers her birth traumatic, her intention to breastfeed may also be affected. One internet study surveyed 52 women worldwide and found that experiencing birth trauma either gave mothers a stronger motivation to breastfeed (49) or influenced them to decide against it (3) (Beck & Watson, 2008). Those who were more motivated felt a determination to breastfeed to "make up" for the birth to themselves or their baby or to prove themselves as a mother. On the negative side, some of these mothers considered their breasts as "one more thing to be violated." They felt the need to take a time-out to heal mentally, perceived breastfeeding as another painful ordeal, experienced flashbacks from birth that intruded on breastfeeding, or felt a "disturbing detachment" from their baby. The researchers concluded that mothers traumatized by their birth would benefit from ongoing one-on-one support to establish breastfeeding.

Establishing a definitive cause-and-effect relationship between labor medications and breastfeeding problems is challenging, in part because most women are unlikely to agree to participate in research that randomly assigns them to a "medicated labor" or "non-medicated labor" group. While some studies have not found an association between labor analgesia and breastfeeding (Chang & Heaman, 2005; Radzyminski, 2003), some indicate that pain relievers or

Labor medications may affect baby's alertness, breast-seeking behaviors, and feeding effectiveness.

anesthesia during labor and delivery can contribute to breastfeeding problems by delaying the first breastfeeding, sedating babies, suppressing feeding behaviors, and decreasing baby's motor coordination.

In one large Australian study, researchers followed 1,260 mothers for 24 weeks (Torvaldsen, Roberts, Simpson, Thompson, & Ellwood, 2006). Women who had epidural anesthesia were twice as likely to stop breastfeeding within the first 24 weeks as those who used non-pharmacological pain-relieving techniques during labor. Another Australian study of 992 first-time mothers also found a significant association among the women who delivered vaginally between epidural anesthesia and shorter breastfeeding duration, even when comparing mothers who had intended to have an epidural but did not receive one (Henderson, Dickinson, Evans, McDonald, & Paech, 2003). A U.K. study found a dose-response relationship between the amount of the drug fentanyl used as part of epidural anesthesia and bottle-feeding at hospital discharge (Jordan, Emery, Bradshaw, Watkins, & Friswell, 2005). One U.S. double-blind, randomized study examined the effects of different doses of fentanyl as part of an epidural in 177 mothers who had previously breastfed and had requested an epidural (Beilin, Bodian et al. 2005). They were randomly assigned to one of three groups: no fentanyl, an intermediate dose, or a high dose. On their first day of life, babies' neurobehavioral scores were lowest in the high-dose group, and at 6 weeks, more of the mothers in the high-

Epidural anesthesia can shorten breastfeeding duration.

In a large retrospective cohort, a U.K. study of 48,366 women found a 6% to 8% reduction in breastfeeding at 48 hours among mothers given synthetic oxytocin (pitocin) to prevent hemorrhage after birth. This effect was strongest in women whose labor was induced or augmented or who received epidural or spinal anesthesia (Jordan et al., 2009).

Four Swedish studies found an association between the following labor medications and a suppression of babies' inborn feeding behaviors:

- Meperidine, also known as Demerol or pethidine (Nissen et al., 1997; Ransjo-Arvidson et al., 2001; Righard & Alade, 1990)
- Bupivacaine (Ransjo-Arvidson et al., 2001)
- Mepivacaine via pudendal block (Ransjo-Arvidson et al., 2001)
- Epidural anesthesia (Wiklund, Norman, Uvnas-Moberg, Ransjo-Arvidson, & Andolf, 2007)

A U.S. study also found an association between epidural anesthesia and diminished neonatal sucking (Riordan, Gross, Angeron, Krumwiede, & Melin, 2000).

One Swedish study found that several types of analgesics given in labor (even those given via pudendal block) were associated with more infant crying, fewer breast-seeking behaviors, and less suckling (Ransjo-Arvidson et al., 2001). Another Swedish study found that when a laboring woman received 100 mg of pethidine (Demerol) close to delivery, it was associated with delayed and depressed rooting and suckling (Nissen et al., 1997). A U.S. study found that during their entire first month of life babies whose mothers received epidurals were measurably less alert, less able to orient themselves, and had less organized movements than the babies whose mothers gave birth without pain medication (Sepkoski, Lester, Ostheimer, & Brazelton, 1992).

A classic Swedish study found reduced or absent feeding behaviors and ineffective first breastfeeding more common among babies whose mothers received pethidine during labor than among those who didn't (Righard & Alade, 1990). The same effect was found when the babies were taken away from their mothers for 20 minutes for a bath and measurements before their first breastfeeding. In babies whose mothers either received pethidine during labor or were separated before the first breastfeeding, about half did not go to the breast or breastfeed well. Nearly all babies (16 of 17) from unmedicated labors who were kept with their mothers made their way to the breast on their own and fed well. None of the babies (19 of 19) from the medicated labors who were separated for 20 minutes went to breast on their own and fed well.

Emotional support the mother receives during labor is associated with earlier breastfeeding.

A mother's desire to breastfeed and care for her baby may be enhanced by emotional support she is given during labor. One study of 209 first-time mothers in Nigeria found that the time to the first breastfeeding after birth was significantly shorter among the mothers who had a companion with them during labor (Morhason-Bello, Adedokun, & Ojengbede, 2009). Time to first breastfeeding is associated with longer duration of breastfeeding and greater infant survival (see next section).

A cesarean birth makes breastfeeding more physically challenging, so after a surgical delivery a mother will probably need help feeding comfortably.

A Swedish study found that on the 2nd day of life mothers who had caesarean deliveries had lower levels of oxytocin pulsatility and lower levels of blood prolactin than mothers who delivered vaginally (Nissen et al., 1996). Some studies have found an association between caesarean delivery and delayed lactation, but it is unclear whether this is a result of the physical stress of a surgical delivery or a delay in the first breastfeeding and fewer early feedings. One researcher wrote:

> Cesarean delivery may (Dewey, Nommsen-Rivers et al. 2003; Evans, Evans et al. 2003) or may not (Kulski, Smith, & Hartmann, 1981; Patel, Liebling, & Murphy, 2003) be associated with significant delay in milk 'coming in.' There is evidence from one small study (Sozmen, 1982) that women who delivered by caesarean and offered the breast sooner were able to feed colostrum sooner and their milk came in sooner than women who offered their infants the breast later (Rasmussen, 2007, p. 392).

Mothers can breastfeed after a cesarean birth but may require extra assistance.

In New Zealand, 153 mothers took part in semi-structured interviews about breastfeeding, and their responses indicated that a caesarean birth made breastfeeding a greater physical challenge, but that their commitment and persistence helped them to sustain breastfeeding over time (Manhire, Hagan, & Floyd, 2007). See p. 46- "Gravity Can Help or Hinder" for breastfeeding positions that can make early breastfeeding easier for mothers after a surgical delivery. U.K. research has found that positioning help can be key for these mothers (Cakmak & Kuguoglu, 2007).

ESTABLISHING BREASTFEEDING

The early postpartum period is a vulnerable time for breastfeeding and for the mother-baby relationship.

For most mammals, early postpartum is a sensitive period that has long-term effects on the mother-baby relationship. As one example, separation of mother and baby after birth causes many mammalian mothers to reject their newborns (D. Wiessinger, personal communication, December 6, 2008). To care for her baby, an animal mother must feel the sensations of birth and experience the touch, taste, and smell of her newborn. When any of these are missing, her attachment to her newborn can be disrupted. Human mothers can override these innate responses, but during this vulnerable time, postpartum practices should be tailored to support—rather than undermine—the natural forces at work. This sensitive period requires particular care.

The First 2 Hours

After birth, suggest the mother find a private, hormone-enhancing environment where she and her baby are kept together skin-to-skin.

Breastfeeding is a physical part of the intimate relationship between a mother and baby, so the ideal environment after birth is one that enhances their feelings of intimacy. Like birth, early breastfeeding works best when a mother can attend to her baby without distraction. French obstetrician Michel Odent described the strong link between the physiology of birth and breastfeeding, which supports the importance in the first hour after birth of keeping mother and baby together and protecting their privacy (Odent, 2008). U.K. midwife and researcher Suzanne Colson takes this one step further by suggesting that it is not just the first hour after birth that is critical, but the first weeks of life and that the primary role of the breastfeeding supporter is to promote a hormone-enhancing environment. The intimacy of the environment is key to enhancing the release of the mother's and baby's reciprocal behaviors, which are one way they get to know one another. Just as the third stage of labor is about seeing the baby for the first time and not just about delivering the placenta, breastfeeding provides a biological intimacy that helps mothers and babies establish their relationship (S. Colson, personal communication, January 22, 2009).

The primary role of the breastfeeding supporter is to promote the hormone-enhancing environment.

In one Australian study, researchers created a special private room designed to enhance comfort and relaxation (called a "Snoezelen room"), where mothers could take their babies to be alone or receive one-on-one help. The mothers reported that in this private setting, their anxiety decreased and they were better able to focus on their baby. One mother wrote:

> I wanted to experiment and explore it on my own because I'm not a complete idiot, sometimes you just need a chance to try it for yourself. You want some time out to yourself to see if you can do it yourself and I knew that in that space I was just going to have some time to find out for myself and not have any interruptions (Hauck, Summers, White, & Jones, 2008, p. 20)

As described in more detail in the next section, mother-baby skin-to-skin contact during the first hours after birth improves infant stability and provides the triggers for early breastfeeding. The American Academy of Pediatrics recommends: "Healthy infants should be placed and remain in direct skin-to-skin contact with their mothers immediately after delivery until the first feeding is accomplished" (Gartner et al., 2005, p. 498).

In some parts of the world, delaying the first breastfeeding longer than 2 hours increases the risk of illness and death. A study done in rural Ghana estimated that 16% of neonatal deaths could be prevented if all newborns were breastfed from the first day of life, and 22% could be prevented if all newborns started breastfeeding within the first hour after birth (Edmond et al., 2006).

Breastfeeding in the first hour or two after birth is associated with infant survival, longer breastfeeding duration, and more milk intake later.

Encouraging breastfeeding within the first hour after birth is one of the "Ten Steps" of the World Health Organization and UNICEF's Baby-Friendly Hospital Initiative. Research has found a positive association with hospital compliance with these Ten Steps and an increase in breastfeeding initiation and duration (Merten, Dratva, & Ackermann-Liebrich, 2005; Rosenberg, Stull, Adler, Kasehagen, & Crivelli-Kovach, 2008). One U.S. study surveyed more than 2,000 mothers to examine the effect of hospital practices on breastfeeding duration (Murray, Ricketts, & Dellaport, 2007). Breastfeeding within the first hour was one of the five hospital practices associated with longer breastfeeding duration. The other four were: baby received only mother's milk, rooming-in (no separation of mother and baby), no pacifier use, and receipt of a telephone number for breastfeeding help after discharge. However, only 18.7% of the U.S. mothers surveyed experienced all five of these practices at their hospital. A Japanese survey of 318 mothers also found a positive association between breastfeeding within the first 2 hours after birth and breastfeeding at 4 months (Nakao, Moji, Honda, & Oishi, 2008).

Breastfeeding the first 1 to 2 hours after birth increases the rate of infant survival.

A study done in Russia with a team of Swedish, Russian, and Canadian researchers examined the effects of postpartum practices on 176 mothers and their newborns (Bystrova, Widstrom et al., 2007). This study found a positive association between the timing of the first feeding and milk intake on Day 4. Newborns who breastfed for the first time within 2 hours of birth took on average 55% more milk on Day 4 (284 mL), as compared with the babies whose first feeding occurred more than 2 hours after birth (184 mL). The researchers noted that the babies who fed within the first 2 hours weighed more on average and were born closer to term than those babies who did not.

To better understand babies' instinctive behaviors after birth and the hormonal effects of early mother-baby interactions, Swedish researchers videotaped 10 mothers and babies after an unmedicated birth (Matthiesen, Ransjo-Arvidson, Nissen, & Uvnas-Moberg, 2001). At the same time, they measured the mothers' blood levels of oxytocin, the hormone responsible for milk ejection and uterine contraction that also enhances emotional closeness. The following are the behaviors all 10 babies had in common with the median time after birth they occurred:

A baby's early breast-seeking behaviors increase the mother's blood oxytocin levels, which may help prepare her body for breastfeeding.

- 6 min.—Opened their eyes
- 11 min.—Began massaging the breast
- 12 min.—Put hand to mouth
- 21 min.—Rooted at the breast
- 25 min.—Put their moistened hand to the breast; mothers' nipple became erect

- 27 min.—Stretched their tongue out and began licking the nipple
- 80 min—Began breastfeeding

The mother's oxytocin levels rose with these behaviors, and the researchers concluded that "newborns use their hands as well as their mouths to stimulate maternal oxytocin release after birth, which may have significance for uterine contraction, milk ejection, and mother-infant interaction" (Matthiesen et al., 2001, p. 13).

Separation of mother and baby after birth can inhibit baby's breast-seeking behaviors.

In a classic 1990 Swedish study described in detail in the previous section, some study babies were taken from their mothers for 20 minutes before their first breastfeeding for a bath and measurements. When they were reunited, half of the babies did not demonstrate these inborn feeding behaviors (Righard & Alade, 1990). In the mothers who also received the pain-reliever pethidine (Demerol) during labor, none of the babies exhibited breast-seeking behaviors.

The First Few Days

Togetherness, Separation, and Newborn Stability

The first hours after birth may be a sensitive period during which skin-to-skin contact is important to infant stability and early breastfeeding.

Many factors affect feeding rhythm on the first day of life. In addition to the birth, another major influencer is how much time baby spends on his mother's body, which is key to infant stability and is the stimulus for inborn feeding behaviors. During this time of rapid adjustment from womb to world, the newborn needs help staying warm. For the first time, he begins to breathe air and to feed intermittently, rather than receiving oxygen and food continuously through the umbilical cord. Research suggests that at this vulnerable time skin-to-skin contact smoothes baby's transition and that separation is a major stressor, which among other things contributes to breastfeeding problems.

Based on a review of 30 studies involving 1,925 mothers and babies, a Cochrane Review article concluded that babies in early skin-to-skin contact after birth interacted more with their mothers, stayed warmer, cried less, and were more likely to breastfeed and breastfeed longer (Moore, Anderson, & Bergman, 2007). The authors wrote: "this time may represent a psychophysiologically 'sensitive period' for programming future behavior" and skin-to-skin contact was also noted to have "no apparent short or long-term negative effects."

Early skin-to-skin contact is the most effective way to stabilize and maintain newborn temperature.

In Western countries, many assume that babies need to spend time in infant warmers before being given to their mothers, but research has found this strategy counterproductive. In a Swedish study of 50 healthy full-term babies, the researchers found that both the babies in the skin-to-skin contact group and the separated group had a rapid increase in temperature between 5 and 10 minutes after birth, but that the skin-to-skin contact group continued to have a slow, steady increase in temperature, whereas the temperatures of the separated group leveled off after 30 minutes (Christensson et al., 1992). They suggest the separated group used vasoconstriction to conserve heat, which requires energy and could be responsible for this difference in temperature.

One study of 176 mothers and babies done in Russia with a team of Swedish, Russian, and Canadian researchers compared outcomes in four groups of babies (Bystrova et al., 2003):

1. Kept in skin-to-skin contact for 30 to 120 minutes after birth
2. Held in arms wearing clothes
3. Separated from their mothers at birth and returned to their mothers after 2 hours
4. Taken to the hospital nursery at birth and only returned at set feeding times

In each group, some babies were swaddled and some wore clothes. The researchers reported that skin-to-skin contact reduced "the stress of being born" and found the babies kept skin-to-skin after birth had the highest body temperatures. The lowest temperatures were in the separated and swaddled babies, with their feet their coldest body part.

A U.S. study of 48 full-term newborns 24 to 48 hours old who were having breastfeeding problems found that even with feeding problems, skin-to-skin contact effectively prevented hypothermia (Chiu, Anderson, & Burkhammer, 2005).

Skin-to-skin contact helps stabilize infant temperature.

A preliminary U.S. study of two sets of preterm twins found that mothers' breasts appear to respond independently to their babies' temperature needs (Ludington-Hoe et al. 2006). These mothers placed one twin on each breast in skin-to-skin contact. Both sets of twins stayed warm and their body temperatures increased, but amazingly each breast responded differently to the babies' differing thermal needs. For example, if the twin on the right breast needed more warmth, that breast became warmer. At the same time, if the twin on the left breast was too warm, that breast became cooler.

Due to the large body of research that supports its efficacy, skin-to-skin contact is being recommended as an alternative to the use of an infant warmers for the treatment of mild hypothermia (Galligan 2006).

• •

When a newborn mammal is separated from his mother, he emits a distinctive distress cry and experiences predictable physiological changes. South African physician and researcher Nils Bergman decided to investigate these changes after he conducted a study of preterm babies in Zimbabwe that found an increase in survival rates in very low birthweight babies from 10% to 50% when they were kept in skin-to-skin contact with their mothers after birth (Bergman & Jurisoo, 1994). He found the explanation he was looking for in animal studies. Human newborns—like other mammals—have inborn physiological programming that is key to survival and growth (Bergman, 2008). Using biologists' terminology, he referred to the newborn's changing environments (womb, mother's body, family, the larger world) as "habitats," with the mother's body being baby's natural "habitat" after birth. The feel of the mother's body acts as a trigger for the behaviors and responses necessary for physiological regulation and optimal growth.

When separated from their mothers, newborn mammals—including human newborns—display predictable stress responses that can cause instability.

If a newborn is removed from his normal habitat—his mother's body—this triggers different responses. Bergman explains that in all mammal babies there are three basic physiological programs governed by the hindbrain that are key to survival: nutrition, reproduction, and defense. They regulate hormones, nerves, and muscles that affect the entire body. However, at any given time only one of these programs can run. If the defense program is running, the body shuts off the nutrition program and with it growth.

When a newborn is removed from his mother's body, he goes into defense mode, beginning with a distinctive cry known as the "separation distress call" (Christensson, Cabrera, Christensson, Uvnas-Moberg, & Winberg, 1995). Biologists refer to the set of behaviors during mother-baby separation as the "protest-despair response." If the baby's cries are unanswered, he goes into the despair mode, where to increase the odds of survival, his body uses less energy by decreasing his heart rate, breathing rate, and body temperature (Alberts, 1994). In this mode, his stress hormones increase as the baby physically prepares to fight for survival, shutting down gut function, digestion, and growth.

In contrast, when a newborn is held in skin-to-skin with his mother, the nutrition program is activated. Research found that skin-to-skin contact decreases blood levels of stress hormones by 74% (Modi & Glover, 1996; Mooncey, 1997). The amazing increase in preterm survival rates, Bergman explained, is the direct result of the baby remaining in the right habitat (touching his mother), which turns on the program that enhances baby's physiological regulation. In this program he has a lower level of stress hormones, his gut more easily processes food, and his heart rate and breathing are not elevated or slowed. These behaviors also lead to the successful beginning of breastfeeding because this mother-baby body contact elicits nurturing behaviors in the mother, enhances their bond, and triggers the baby's inborn feeding reflexes.

Early separation of mothers and babies increases infant instability in several ways.

The physiological changes described in the previous point that occur when a newborn is separated from his mother include:

- Lower infant body temperature (Bergman, Linley, & Fawcus, 2004; Bystrova, Matthiesen, Vorontsov et al., 2007; Bystrova et al., 2003)
- Lower blood glucose levels (Christensson et al., 1992)
- Agitated state, with more crying, higher levels of stress hormones, and less sleep (Christensson, Cabrera et al. 1995; Michelsson, Christensson, Rothganger, & Winberg, 1996; Ferber & Makhoul, 2004)
- More breastfeeding problems (Christensson et al., 1992)
- Decreased intake of mother's milk (Bystrova, Matthiesen, Widstrom et al., 2007)

One Swedish study of 29 full-term healthy newborns found that separated babies cried 10 times more than babies kept in skin-to-skin contact with their mothers (Michelsson et al., 1996). Another Swedish study of 50 full-term babies found that in the first 90 minutes after birth separated babies had lower skin temperatures, more rapid breathing and heart rate, and lower blood sugar levels than babies kept skin-to-skin with their mothers and that the differences in blood glucose levels were unrelated to feeding (Christensson et al., 1992). The researchers suggested that to conserve body heat the babies in the separated

Separation from their mothers is stressful for babies.

group used vasoconstriction, which could lower blood glucose levels. This means some of the conditions that put newborns at risk, such as hypothermia and hypoglycemia, may be caused or made worse by early separation.

In one Israeli study, after birth all of its 47 healthy babies were put on their mothers' chest for 10 to 15 minutes and then dried, weighed, and dressed (Ferber & Makhoul, 2004). The babies receiving skin-to-skin contact were returned to their mothers after 15 to 20 minutes and put in skin-to-skin contact for an hour. The other babies were taken to the nursery for an hour and did not receive skin-to-skin contact. Four hours later, the researchers noted significant differences between the groups. When compared to the babies separated in the nursery, the babies in the skin-to-skin group:

- Stayed in quiet sleep longer, indicating better brain stem control
- Were calmer and cried less, indicating better state control
- Had fewer purposeless movements, indicating more motor control
- Showed more flexed rather than extended muscles, indicating less distress

Although the skin-to-skin contact lasted only an hour, the difference between the two groups persisted for more than 4 hours.

• •

Skin-to-skin contact after birth can help overcome breastfeeding problems and is associated with longer duration of exclusive breastfeeding.

Two U.S. studies have found that skin-to-skin contact can help overcome early breastfeeding problems (Chiu, Anderson, & Burkhammer, 2008; Meyer & Anderson, 1999). In a one-group, prospective exploratory study of 48 healthy, ethnically diverse mothers, four sessions of skin-to-skin contact while breastfeeding during the first 2 days was found to be a successful intervention (Chiu et al., 2008). Despite having early breastfeeding problems, 81% of these mothers were still breastfeeding at a 1-month follow-up call. Time spent before breastfeeding in skin-to-skin contact has been found to act as a stress-reliever and to lower blood pressure in mothers (Jonas et al., 2008).

A Polish study of 1,250 children found that skin-to-skin contact longer than 20 to 30 minutes after birth was associated with a longer duration of exclusive breastfeeding (Mikiel-Kostyra, Mazur, & Boltruszko, 2002). In this study, skin-to-skin contact was one of several hospital practices supportive of breastfeeding, such as rooming-in with no separation longer than 1 hour. This study also found that skin-to-skin contact of less than 20 minutes had a more limited influence on duration of breastfeeding.

Early Breastfeeding

On their first day, newborns may want to breastfeed often or seem disinterested in feeding.

What happens in the first day of life will not "make or break" long-term milk production, but throughout a newborn's first week, the number of feedings in the first 24 hours can have a significant effect on health outcomes, such as weight loss and bilirubin levels.

Birth and postpartum practices can profoundly influence breastfeeding rhythms during the first 24 hours. In the introduction to her 2001 article on breastfeeding patterns during the first 60 hours, Australian researcher Stephanie Benson describes her granddaughter's breastfeeding pattern after an unmedicated home birth. It began with an early first feeding at which she breastfed for 2 to 3 minutes.

> An hour later she had a second breastfeed which lasted much longer and after about 60 minutes we decided to detach her. This was the beginning of a very long night. The baby roused and demanded a feed every 30-40 minutes and continued this whether we left her in bed with her mother, or wrapped her and put her in the cot or whether I took her and cuddled her! Early the next morning she shared a warm bath with her mum, where she again fed and then slipped into deep sleep that lasted 4½ hours. Then began a new pattern of feeding where she fed every 2 to 4 hours (Benson, 2001, p. 27).

In her work as a hospital midwife, Benson noted that after medicated labors and routine separation many babies were very difficult to awaken and did not feed well during the first days. Where labor medication and separation are routine, sleepy and disinterested babies may seem to be the norm, and babies with a strong desire to breastfeed may be viewed as problematic. Benson wrote that some members of her hospital staff considered the babies who wanted to breastfeed like her home-birthed granddaughter "overly demanding, particularly at night."

Defining "A Feeding"

Especially at first, the sensory experience of breastfeeding may be as important as the milk the newborn receives.

There are many ways to define a breastfeeding. At its essence, breastfeeding is an intimate act between mother and baby that enhances their relationship and provides the baby with food and other ingredients needed for normal growth and development. Many mothers depend as much on the calming, comforting aspects of breastfeeding as they do on the milk it provides.

The sensory stimulation at the breast is also important to mother and baby. Some researchers consider the smell and touch a baby experiences as important to stability and neurodevelopment as the milk he receives. The neurological effects of skin-to-skin contact and breastfeeding are the focus of South African public health physician and researcher Nils Bergman. According to Bergman, during a baby's journey to the breast, the mother's smell, taste, and touch activate nerve pathways that lead to a baby's amygdala, the seat of emotional memory in the brain, and stimulate the baby's limbic system, which helps regulate his autonomic nervous system, improving stability. Based on a large body of research, Bergman suggests that breastfeeding and uninterrupted skin-to-skin contact after birth are vital for optimal newborn brain wiring (Bergman, 2008).

Breastfeeding is an intimate act between mother and baby that enhances their relationship and provides the food babies need.

• •

A more "feeding-oriented" definition of a breastfeeding is when baby takes milk from one breast.

When focusing on the milk-feeding aspect of breastfeeding, any definition of a feeding will be based at least in part on the needs of the definer. One group of Swedish researchers, whose study's focus was time, defined a breastfeeding as at least 2 minutes spent at the breast, with at least 30 minutes in between (Aarts, Hornell, Kylberg, Hofvander, & Gebre-Medhin, 1999; Hornell, Aarts, Kylberg, Hofvander, & Gebre-Medhin, 1999).

An Australian research team used another definition better suited to its goals, defining a breastfeeding as whenever a baby takes milk from one breast (Kent et al., 2006). This group examined breastfeeding patterns among 71 exclusively breastfed 1- to 6-month-old babies and needed to distinguish whether babies took one breast or more and measured milk intake from left and right breast. In this study, if a baby went longer than 30 minutes before wanting to feed again, this was considered an "unpaired" feeding. If baby took both breasts within 30 minutes, this was considered a "paired" feeding. If after taking both breasts baby took the first breast again within 30 minutes, this was considered a "clustered" feeding. They defined a "meal" as an unpaired breastfeeding, two paired breastfeedings, or three clustered breastfeedings.

• •

Cultural beliefs affect what mothers consider "a feeding."

Breastfeeding rhythms vary among mothers and also vary considerably from place to place. As U.S. researcher Kathleen Kennedy noted, a "breastfeeding" means something very different to mothers in different cultures (Kennedy, 2010). A Western mother, for example, may consider a "breastfeeding" a lengthy, ritualized activity that involves changing the baby's diaper, making herself a drink, turning off her phone, settling into a certain chair, and then putting her baby to breast for an extended time. Many Western attitudes about feeding, such as the belief that babies should feed at set intervals every few hours, are based on bottle-feeding norms. In contrast, a mother in a developing country may keep her baby on her body, putting him to breast at the slightest cue for just a few minutes 15 to 20 times each day. These two babies may have about the same daily milk intake, but the immense cultural differences in their feeding rhythms affect early breastfeeding.

Health Outcomes and Early Breastfeeding

When a baby breastfeeds well, more feedings in the first 24 hours are associated with more milk intake and less weight loss days later.

The number of times a baby breastfeeds on the first day of life affects how quickly a mother's milk production increases. One Japanese study of 140 mothers and babies after vaginal births found that the babies who had breastfed 7 to 11 times on their first day consumed 86% more milk on Day 3 than the babies who breastfed fewer than seven times (Yamauchi & Yamanouchi, 1990). The babies who breastfed more on the first day also lost less weight initially and began regaining their birthweight more quickly. The difference in milk intake between these two groups continued to be significant through the 5th day of life.

• •

More feedings on the first day is also associated with fewer cases of exaggerated newborn jaundice on Day 6.

Exaggerated newborn jaundice can affect breastfeeding rhythm because elevated bilirubin levels can make a baby sleepy and less responsive. But frequent feedings on the first day can help prevent exaggerated newborn jaundice later. Research has found an association between number of feedings on the first day of life and bilirubin levels on Day 6. This is because colostrum—the first milk—acts as a laxative, so more breastfeeding stimulates the passage of more bilirubin-rich stools before the bilirubin can be reabsorbed by the baby's intestines. For more details, see the chapter "Hypoglycemia and Jaundice." The Japanese study described in the previous point found that frequency of breastfeeding during a baby's first 24 hours correlated significantly both with frequency of meconium passage and bilirubin levels on Day 6 (Yamauchi & Yamanouchi, 1990). The fewer times the babies breastfed during their first 24 hours, the more likely they were to have bilirubin levels higher than 14 mg/dL on Day 6:

- 28.1% who fed two or fewer times
- 24.5% who fed three to four times
- 15.2% who fed five to six times
- 11.8% who fed seven to eight times
- 0% of those who fed nine or more times

Feeding often is one part of the picture; feeding effectively is another part.

In the Japanese study described in the previous points, its babies clearly breastfed effectively, but in other studies, some babies did not. In one U.S. study of 73 mothers and babies, the researchers noted that the baby who had the most feedings per day (12) lost the most weight and was 30% below birthweight on Day 11 (Shrago, Reifsnider, & Insel, 2006, p. 200). They wrote that frequent breastfeeding "...particularly when associated with low bowel output strongly suggests the need for evaluation of baby's weight, the mother milk's supply, and the baby's ability to remove milk from the breasts" (Shrago, Reifsnider et al. 2006, p. 200). See the chapter, "Weight Gain and Growth" for ways to evaluate a baby's milk intake at the breast.

Rooming-In

Rooming-in is associated with greater breastfeeding frequency and better weight gain.

To encourage frequent breastfeeding, it only makes sense for mother and baby to stay together and spend as much time as possible with baby on mother's body, so baby's inborn feeding behaviors are triggered. Research has found a positive association between rooming-in, more frequent feedings, and better weight gain (Yamauchi & Yamanouchi, 1990; Bystrova, Matthiesen et al., 2007; Bystrova, Widstrom et al., 2007).

Caring for a baby in a hospital nursery is associated with less mother's milk consumed, more formula given, and greater weight loss.

A study done in Russia with a team of Swedish, Russian, and Canadian researchers of 176 mothers and babies found a negative association between nursery care and milk intake on Day 4 (Bystrova, Matthiesen, Widstrom et al., 2007). When compared with babies kept with their mothers, babies cared for in the hospital nursery:

Rooming-in is associated with more frequent feeding and greater weight gain.

- Ingested less mother's milk—on Day 4, an average of 37% less milk (162 mL vs. 255 mL) as compared with the babies who roomed-in with their mothers
- Lost more weight
- Received more formula

Overcoming Barriers to Early Breastfeeding

After a hospital birth, even when babies are sleepy, there are strategies that can promote frequent feedings.

About 2 hours after birth, newborns often go into a long sleep stretch, especially when mother and baby are separated. But to reach a goal of 8 to 12 feedings during the first day, it may first be necessary to let go of the assumption that newborns should breastfeed at regular intervals (such as every 2 hours). To encourage frequent feedings, take advantage of newborns' natural inclination to "cluster" their feedings together during some parts of the day. Suggest the mother keep her baby on her body in laid-back positions (see Chapter 1) and offer the breast several times whenever the baby is awake and alert.

Another effective strategy is not to assume that the baby has to be awake and alert to breastfeed, and bring the baby to the breast while drowsy or in a light asleep. One U.K. study found that when kept on their mothers' bodies in laid-back breastfeeding positions, late preterm babies could breastfeed very effectively during sleep (Colson, DeRooy, & Hawdon, 2003). Helping a sleeping baby to the breast can also be an effective strategy for babies having trouble breastfeeding, as their inborn feeding reflexes may be more muted during sleep, and they may take the breast more easily then (Colson, 2008).

• •

Because interruptions by others can be a barrier to breastfeeding, some birthing facilities have structured private times for mothers and babies.

One U.S. study found that in a university hospital during the 12 hours between 8 am and 8 pm on the first day of life, mothers and babies were interrupted by door openings and phone calls an average of 54 times (Morrison, Ludington-Hoe et al., 2006). Because of the nearly constant influx of visitors, phone calls, and hospital staff, the mothers reported that they felt rushed with breastfeeding and that they did not have enough quiet, uninterrupted time with their newborns. Half of the episodes of alone time were only 9 minutes long or less, with 1 minute being the most common length of time mothers and babies were alone together. The study mothers reported they were uncomfortable breastfeeding with visitors present and said they would have breastfed more if they'd had more privacy.

To encourage more early breastfeeding, some birthing facilities have instituted "nap times" or "sacred hours" during the day, when visitors and phone calls are not allowed and hospital staff is instructed to not interrupt mothers and babies.

• •

The attitude hospital staff conveys about night rooming-in can influence mothers' choices.

Step 7 of the World Health Organization and UNICEF's Baby-Friendly Hospital Initiative recommends that mothers and babies stay together day and night. In one Swedish study of 132 mothers, more of the mothers who chose to send their newborns to the hospital nursery at night thought the staff believed their babies should stay in the nursery (Svensson, Matthiesen, & Widstrom, 2005). Research has found that new mothers who are breastfeeding are more likely to go along with others' desires than mothers who are not breastfeeding (Uvnas-Moberg, Widstrom, Nissen, & Bjorvell, 1990). Of the mothers who chose to keep their babies with them at night, 93% felt positively about the experience, which was counter to how the hospital staff thought the mothers felt. Of those mothers who didn't keep their babies with them, 73% thought night rooming-in was a good idea. The researchers suggested that hospital staff may mistakenly believe that when babies are with mothers at night, they will cry as much as they would when kept in the hospital nursery. Research has found that mothers and babies actually get more sleep when together than when separated at night (Keefe 1988; Waldenstrom & Swenson 1991).

• •

Hospital sleeping arrangements that give mothers easy access to their babies result in more breastfeeding.

After vaginal births with no opiate analgesia, one U.K. study randomly assigned 64 mothers and babies to one of three different sleep locations during their first 2 days (Ball, Ward-Platt, Heslop, Leech, & Brown, 2006). When ready to sleep, the study mothers placed their newborns:

1. In a separate stand-alone crib/cot in their room.
2. In bed with them.

3. In a side-car bed closed on three sides and attached to the mother's bed for easy access.

The researchers videotaped the sleep episodes to evaluate the effects of the different sleep locations on infant safety, breastfeeding frequency, and mothers' sleep.

Previous studies of older babies found breastfeeding frequency was three times greater among mothers and babies sleeping together (McKenna, Mosko, & Richard, 1997), and these researchers also found that the babies placed in the mother's bed or in the side-car attempted to breastfeed and actually breastfed significantly more times than the mothers whose babies were in the stand-alone crib/cot. The median frequency per hour of attempted feeds was 1.3 in the mother's bed, 2.1 in the side-car, and 0.7 in the stand-alone crib, and frequency of actual feeds was 1.2 in the mother's bed, 1.3 in the side-car, and 0.5 in the stand-alone crib.

Regarding mothers' sleep, this study found no difference in sleep duration among the three groups, even when they shared a bed.

Regarding infant safety, "potential risk exposures" such as breathing risk, overheating, falling, entrapment, and overlaying were evaluated. None of the newborns in the study experienced any adverse events, but researchers identified more potential risks among those who slept in their mothers' beds than in the other two groups. However, each sleep setting had some potential risk exposures. Among the babies in the stand-alone crib/cot group, for example, the researchers found: "...all of whose observed bouts of airway covering occurred while sleeping in the stand-alone cots and were all related to swaddling" (Ball et al., 2006, p. 1008).

Side-car sleeping arrangements may provide the safest sleeping environment while also increasing feeding frequency.

The researchers concluded that the side-car crib appeared to be the best of the three sleep options, increasing breastfeeding frequency while providing a safe sleep setting.

• •

Formula supplements given without a medical reason are a barrier to frequent early breastfeeding.

One U.K. qualitative study found that hospital staff may supplement newborns due to a desire to protect new mothers from tiredness or distress (Cloherty, Alexander, & Holloway, 2004). However, the short-term "help" of giving newborns unnecessary supplements can lead to long-term breastfeeding problems in several ways. Supplements can replace or delay breastfeeding by leaving baby full and disinterested in breastfeeding for long periods, which can delay a mother's milk production. They can increase a baby's expectations of how much milk to expect, especially when more than 1 ounce is fed, leaving baby unsatisfied when he returns to the breast. If a feeding bottle is used, this may alter the way baby suckles at the breast (Righard, 1998). One U.S. study of 280 mothers and babies found that when the newborn received any fluids other than mother's milk during the first 48 hours of life, this could affect breastfeeding throughout the baby's first week (Dewey et al., 2003). In this study, babies supplemented with any other fluid were two to three times more likely to display sub-optimal breastfeeding behaviors on Days 3 and 7.

Swaddling/Bundling

Swaddling, also known as bundling, has been practiced historically in many parts of the world. Research has found that swaddled babies arouse less and sleep longer (Franco et al., 2005), which in the early hours and days after birth can mean less breastfeeding. Although there is much research on swaddling, in a review of the research, every randomized control trial compared swaddling with practices involving separation from mother, such as keeping babies in incubators or giving them a pacifier or massage (van Sleuwen, Engelberts et al. 2007). None of the studies compared swaddling to being held or carried by the mothers.

Babies who are swaddled sleep longer and arouse less, which can decrease early breastfeeding frequency.

• •

In a U.S. study of 21 newborns after a vaginal birth, researchers compared two groups (Moore & Anderson, 2007). One group was laid naked skin-to-skin tummy down on the mother's body immediately after birth, given a short examination, and returned to the mother for 2 hours. The other group was shown briefly to the mother after birth, examined, and swaddled with hands free and returned to the mother. The group placed skin-to-skin for most of their first 2 hours showed earlier feeding behaviors, more competent suckling during their first breastfeeding, and established effective breastfeeding earlier.

Swaddling after birth is associated with less competent early suckling and later establishment of breastfeeding.

• •

Research done in Russia with a team of Canadian, Russian, and Swedish researchers on 176 mothers and babies found that several newborn stressors had a more profound negative effect when newborns were also swaddled (Bystrova, Matthiesen, Widstrom et al., 2007; Bystrova, Widstrom et al., 2007; Bystrova et al., 2003).

Swaddling may compound the negative effects of other newborn stressors.

Separation during the first 2 hours after birth caused more measurable negative effects in the swaddled babies. Among the babies taken to the nursery for the first 2 hours after birth and then returned to their mothers for the rest of the hospital stay, the swaddled babies had a significantly greater weight loss on their 3rd, 4th, and 5th days.

Ongoing separation during the hospital stay. Among one group of newborns kept in the hospital nursery between feedings (the "nursery group"), some were swaddled and some were not. The swaddled newborns in the nursery group had the lowest foot temperature of any of the babies in any of the study groups. Newborns who were both separated and swaddled also consumed less mother's milk overall, these mothers produced less milk on Day 4, and they had a shorter duration of breastfeeding overall (Bystrova, Matthiesen, Widstrom et al., 2007).

Formula supplements and ongoing separation. The only babies in the study who received formula were some of those in the nursery group. The supplemented and unsupplemented babies in the nursery group consumed similar amounts of milk daily, but the supplemented newborns who were also swaddled lost significantly more weight on Days 3, 4, and 5 as compared with the newborns who were either not swaddled or not supplemented. The researchers suggested possible reasons for this greater weight loss:

Swaddling is associated with greater weight loss, shorter duration of breastfeeding and lower infant temperature.

- Swaddling may be physically stressful because activity is severely limited.

- Receiving less touch may compromise growth, as was found in one study of preterm babies (Ferber et al., 2002).
- Growth hormones in mother's milk are missing in formula and bottle-feeding releases less of the gastrointestinal hormone cholecystokinin (Marchini, Simoni, Bartolini, & Linden, 1993).

If there is a concern about the baby's temperature, an alternative to swaddling is putting blankets over mother and baby.

If the room is cool, warmed or unwarmed blankets over both mother and baby can help keep them both warm while stimulating inborn feeding behaviors (Galligan, 2006; Ludington-Hoe, Ferreira, Swinth, & Ceccardi, 2003; WHO, 2003).

Regular swaddling in the early months increases the risks of overheating, respiratory infection, hip dysplasia, and SIDS when babies sleep prone.

Parents often adopt practices at home that have been modeled in the hospital. Even if swaddling is not verbally promoted, if it is done after birth, parents may go home thinking they should continue this practice. When babies are swaddled routinely during the first few months of life, some negative health outcomes have been found.

Greater risk of respiratory illness. One study of 186 babies in Turkey and China found that babies who were routinely swaddled for their first 3 months were four times more likely to develop pneumonia and other respiratory infections compared with babies who were not swaddled (Yurdakok, Yavuz, & Taylor, 1990).

Greater risk of hip dysplasia. When babies are swaddled tightly and their legs cannot bend and flex, this creates a greater risk of hip dysplasia, sometimes called "developmental dysplasia" (Sahin, Akturk et al. 2004; van Sleuwen, Engelberts et al. 2007).

Greater risk of SIDS in prone sleeping position. One Australian case-control study that compared 22 babies who died of sudden infant death syndrome (SIDS) to 213 babies who did not found that swaddled babies laid face down to sleep (prone) were at 12 times greater risk for SIDS than babies laid face up, compared to a three times greater risk in babies laid face down who were not swaddled (Ponsonby, Dwyer, Gibbons, Cochrane, & Wang, 1993).

Greater risk of overheating. If also in warm surroundings, swaddled babies are at risk of overheating, which in rare cases has been fatal (van Gestel, L'Hoir, ten Berge, Jansen, & Plotz, 2002).

Feeding Amounts and Newborn Stomach Size

On their first day, newborns take on average about 7 mL of colostrum per breastfeeding, with this amount increasing each day.

Before birth, a baby never feels hunger. After birth, intermittent feeding is a new experience. To make this transition easier, mother's breasts provide small, gradually increasing amounts of milk. The amount of colostrum a newborn receives at the breast during the first day varies greatly from one mother and baby to another. An Australian study of nine babies found that milk intake on the first day ranged from 7 to 123 mL, with an average daily intake of 37 mL and average breastfeeding of 7 mL (Saint, Smith, & Hartmann, 1984). By the 2nd day, a Dutch study of 18 mothers and babies estimated the average milk intake per feeding was 14 mL, with a range of daily intake of 44 to 335 mL (Houston, Howie, & McNeilly, 1983). When breastfeeding is going normally, each day during the first week of life, the baby takes more milk as the mother's milk production increases. For more details, see p. 401- "Making Milk during the First Year and Beyond."

In parts of the world where bottle-feeding is the norm, some wrongly consider the small amount of colostrum available in the early days to be insufficient. But small feedings have advantages for the newborn.

For the newborn, small feedings have advantages over larger ones.

Newborns are born with excess fluids that need to be shed. After floating in amniotic fluid for 9 months, babies are born with more fluids in their tissues than they need, which is one reason most babies lose weight in the early days. In U.S. hospitals 25 years ago, it was standard practice for newborns to be given nothing by mouth for the first 24 hours, in part because healthcare providers assumed that overhydrated newborns didn't need to be fed. This extra tissue fluid at birth gives babies some "practice time" to learn to breastfeed well before their need for fluids is greater.

Newborns have small stomachs. Stomach size varies by birthweight, with larger babies having larger stomachs (Naveed, Manjunath, & Sreenivas, 1992; Scammon & Doyle, 1920), but even a large baby can only hold a relatively small amount of milk at first (Table 2.1).

Table 2.1. Newborn Stomach Capacity by Weight

Average Newborn Weight	Average Stomach Capacity mL (Scammon)	Average Stomach Capacity mL (Naveed)
1.5-2.0 kg (3.3-4.4 lbs.)	22	14
2.0-2.5 kg (4.4-5.5 lbs.)	30 (~1 oz.)	17
2.5-3.0 kg (5.5-6.6 lbs.)	30	20
3.0-3.5 kg (6.6-7.7 lbs.)	35	n/a
3.5-4.0 kg (7.7-8.8 lbs.)	35	n/a
4.0+ kg (8.8+ lbs.)	38	n/a

Adapted from (Naveed et al., 1992; Scammon, 1920)

Newborn stomachs don't stretch. In one U.S. study, researchers found that during the first day of life, the walls of a newborn's stomach stay firm and don't yet stretch as they will later (Zangen et al., 2001). By 3 days of age, as the baby takes more small, frequent feedings, his stomach begins to expand more easily to hold more milk.

Although new parents are sometimes encouraged to fill their babies as full as possible to help them stay satisfied or sleep longer, there are several problems with this approach.

Supplementing a newborn with too much milk has short- and long-term drawbacks.

Newborns are at greater risk of allergy sensitization from non-human milks. In the early weeks, giving non-human milks is not recommended unless there is a medical indication (Gartner et al., 2005), in part because a newborn's gut junctions are more open and permeable than they will be later. Introducing foreign proteins during this vulnerable time increases the risk of allergy sensitization (Host, Husby, & Osterballe, 1988). As a baby's gut matures, his gut junctions become tighter and this risk decreases. Giving non-human milks also changes a newborn's gut flora to more closely resemble that of an adult, which puts him at greater risk of infection (Mountzouris, McCartney, & Gibson, 2002).

Raising baby's milk-intake expectations. Even when expressed mother's milk is used as a supplement, only small amounts consistent with breastfeeding norms should be given. Giving a baby too much milk can leave him feeling dissatisfied later by the smaller amounts he receives at the breast, which can lead to breastfeeding problems.

Overfeeding during the first week is associated with obesity later in life. One U.S. study followed 653 formula-fed babies from birth to age 20 to 32 years and found that babies' weight gain in the first week of life was associated with adult overweight. The researchers suggested that birth to 8 days may be a "critical period" during which human physiology is programmed. They concluded that: "In formula fed infants, weight gain during the first week of life may be a critical determinant for the development of obesity several decades later" (Stettler et al., 2005, p. 1897). For more details, see p. 207- "Growth from Birth to 12 Months."

Hormonal Complexion

On the 2nd day, a mother's blood oxytocin levels are associated with breastfeeding duration.

U.K. midwife and researcher Suzanne Colson has coined the term "hormonal complexion" to describe the outward signs of a mother's blood oxytocin levels (Colson, 2005). She encouraged healthcare providers and breastfeeding supporters to observe these signs as one indicator of how well breastfeeding is going. A mother's hormonal levels are significant because high oxytocin pulsatility on the 2nd day has been associated with an increase in breastfeeding duration (Nissen et al., 1996). The hormone oxytocin is released during breastfeeding and plays a role in enhancing intimacy in the mother-baby relationship (Uvnas-Moberg, 2003). Signs of high oxytocin pulsatility include:

- Mother looking as if she's in "another world"
- Flushed face or glow
- Looking sleepy or relaxed
- Closed eyes with a smile or half-smile

Hormonal complexion is the outward signs of a mother's oxytocin levels.

According to Colson, when these signs are observed, care should be taken not to talk to the mother or engage her intellect, as this can alter her hormonal state. If needed, right-brained approaches to breastfeeding help, as described in the first chapter, will be least disruptive.

Feeding Patterns and Night Feedings

Most babies are born with their days and nights mixed up and feed more often at night.

Breastfeeding patterns in the first 60 hours of life were documented in an Australian study of 37 mothers and babies after an unmedicated vaginal birth (Benson, 2001). The researchers found that the newborns breastfed the fewest times from 3 a.m. to 9 a.m. Feeding frequency increased throughout the day with the most feedings occurring between 9 p.m. to 3 a.m.

Realistic expectations about feeding frequency at night are helpful during the early weeks. This is even more vital after a hospital birth when mothers and babies are discharged on the 2nd day. If new parents are unaware that frequent night feedings should be expected during this time and they didn't have night rooming-in in the hospital, they may mistakenly assume that their babies' desire to feed so often at night is a sign of a breastfeeding problem, which can lead to unnecessary supplementation.

An excellent one-page handout for parents is "Baby's Second Night," written by Jan Barger, RN, MA, IBCLC, which describes the breast as the "closest thing to home" the newborn knows in a scary new world and is available from: www.lactationeducationconsultants.com.

• •

Encourage parents to choose sleep options that minimize disruptions and make breastfeeding easier.

For details, see the last section "Night Feedings" at the end of this chapter.

• •

Babies' breastfeeding rhythm and diaper output may change as their mother's milk production increases.

With increasing milk production around the 3rd or 4th day, many mothers find that their baby's breastfeeding patterns change, with feedings becoming shorter and babies being satisfied for longer stretches. The color of their stools also may begin to change from black meconium to green transitional stools. Some babies may even have yellow stools at this stage (Shrago et al., 2006). For more details, see p. 214- "Other Signs of Milk Intake."

The First 40 Days

Feeding Intensity and Milk Production

During the first 40 days, suggest mothers can expect their babies to breastfeed intensively until full milk production is established.

Breastfeeding rhythms change over the weeks, months, and years as baby grows. As with early feeding rhythms, some changes are rooted in biology and some in culture. The first 40 days after birth is a time when a mother's body is primed and ready to make milk. Although hormones play a role in initiating milk production, the major driver is the rhythm and effectiveness of breast drainage, either by breastfeeding or expressing milk, also known as "autocrine control" (for more details, see the chapter, "Making Milk"). So when a baby is breastfeeding effectively, the baby's feeding rhythm is the main driver of the mother's rate of milk production. By the end of this first 40 days, a mother will produce just about as much milk as her baby will ever need. During this time, suggest the mother expect her baby to breastfeed at irregular intervals, "clustering" or bunching his feedings close together during some parts of the day.

The first 40 days after birth is when a mother's body is primed and ready to make milk.

The 1st week. With frequent breastfeeding, by the end of the first week, a mother's milk production has increased more than ten-fold—from an average of a little more than 1 ounce (37 mL) per day total on the first day to about 10 to 19 ounces (280 to 576 mL) per day by Day 7 (Ingram, Woolridge, Greenwood, & McGrath, 1999). During this same time, the baby's stomach expands and can comfortably hold about 1 to 2 ounces (30 to 59 mL) of milk at a feeding. With rapid growth, baby's stomach grows along with milk production.

The 2nd and 3rd weeks. With frequent feedings, the mother's milk supply continues to build. Now baby can hold about 2 to 3 ounces (59 to 89 mL) at a feeding and takes about 20 to 25 ounces (591 to 750 mL) of milk per day. At this stage, babies often increase the number and length of breastfeedings to increase a mother's milk production to meet his growing needs. These periods of longer, more frequent feedings are sometimes called "growth spurts."

The 4th and 5th weeks. Babies now take an average of about 3 to 4 ounces (89 to 118 mL) per feeding, and daily milk intake has increased to an average of about 25 to 35 ounces (750 to 1035 mL) per day (Kent et al., 2006). At 1 month, most mothers produce nearly as much milk per day as their breastfed baby will ever need. Because babies' growth and metabolic rate slow as they age, they continue to need about the same amount of milk from 1 month to 6 months of age. (For more details, see p. 203 -"Growth from Birth to 12 Months.")

But not every baby is average. One study of 71 1- to 6-month-old exclusively breastfed babies found a large range of daily milk intake among healthy, thriving babies, from 15.5 to 43 ounces, or 440 to 1220 g (Kent et al., 2006).

• •

Encourage the mother to arrange for extra help during this hectic time, so she can focus on her baby and on breastfeeding.

If a mother expects breastfeeding to be intense during the first 40 days, she can plan ahead to get help with meals, household chores, and any older children. Perhaps equally important, with a good understanding of normal breastfeeding patterns during this time, she will be less likely to assume something is wrong because her baby wants to breastfeed so often. Emphasize that after this "adjustment period," typically babies begin to take more milk in less time and number of feedings per day decrease, which will make breastfeeding easier to fit into her life.

Mother Care

The postpartum practices of some traditional societies that nurture new mothers have been found to help prevent the "baby blues" and postpartum depression.

Many cultures consider the first 40 days a time to care for new mothers. Many Hispanics refer to it as "la cuarentena." In years past in the U.S., it was called the "lying-in" period. In contrast, many Western mothers today are encouraged to "get back to normal" quickly, which can compromise both breastfeeding and new mothers' feelings of well-being.

After studying postpartum practices in many cultures, anthropologists Gwen Stern and Larry Kruckman noted in their 1983 cross-cultural review (Stern & Kruckman, 1983) that postpartum depression, including the "baby blues," were almost unheard of in some traditional societies. In contrast, in developed countries like the U.S., 50% to 85% of new mothers have the "baby blues," and 15% to 25% experience the more severe postpartum depression. These authors found that all the cultures with a low incidence of baby blues and postpartum depression had several practices in common to support new mothers.

Mothering the mother in the first 40 days can prevent postpartum mood disorders.

The postpartum period is seen as different and distinct. In almost all the societies studied, the postpartum period is considered a time distinct from normal life. During this time, experienced mothers help new mothers learn to care for their babies.

New mothers rest and are cared for in seclusion. During this time, new mothers are seen as especially vulnerable, so social seclusion is widely practiced. While they rest, they are expected to restrict their normal activities separate from others, which promotes frequent breastfeeding. This is a time to rest, regain strength, and learn baby care.

Mothers are relieved of household duties. In order for seclusion and mandated rest to be practical, mothers' normal workload must be taken on by someone else. In these cultures, someone else takes care of older children and household duties. Some women stay in their parents' homes during this time, where help is more available.

A woman's new status is publicly recognized. In these cultures, much personal attention is given to the mother, often described as "mothering the mother." In some places, the new status of the mother is recognized through social rituals, such as bathing, washing of hair, massage, binding of the abdomen, and other types of personal care.

In many Western cultures, new mothers receive greater concern and support before their baby is born. After birth, the focus on the mother vanishes. A new mother in the U.S. is usually discharged from a hospital 24 to 48 hours after a vaginal birth and 2 to 4 days after a cesarean birth. She may or may not have anyone to help her at home--chances are no one at the hospital has even asked. Her partner will probably return to work within the week, and she is left alone to feed herself, teach herself to breastfeed, and recover from birth. Those who gave her attention during pregnancy are no longer there, and the people who come to visit are often more interested in the baby. There is the unspoken understanding that she is not to "bother" her medical caregivers unless there is a medical reason.

Encourage mothers to adopt as many of these practices as they can during the first 40 days.

Caring for a newborn—especially a first baby—takes far more time and work than most mothers expect. The combination of hormonal shifts, physical discomfort, lack of sleep, body changes, and the intensity of being on call day and night are some of the reasons many Western women find breastfeeding overwhelming and the postpartum period stressful. If a mother lives in a country without help provided through the national healthcare system, encourage her to seek help from family and friends or to seek professional services available to postpartum women. Another valuable source of support is mother support groups—both live and online—which can alleviate the isolation many Western mothers feel after birth.

Mothers are often surprised--and dismayed-- by the intensity of the first few weeks postpartum.

FEEDING RHYTHMS AS BABY GROWS

Biology and Culture

Although many consider humans in a different category from other mammals, our biology profoundly influences us. When it comes to feeding rhythms, in general, the more mature the newborn mammal is at birth and the more protein and fat in its mother's milk, the less often that species' newborn is fed. Each of the more than 4,000 species of mammals falls into one of these general categories: mammals whose mothers are in intermittent contact with their newborns (cache, follow, and nest mammals) and mammals whose mothers and newborns are in continuous contact (Kirsten, Bergman, & Hann, 2001; Lozoff & Brittenham, 1979).

The natural feeding pattern of each type of mammal varies by its maturity at birth and the composition of its milk.

Cache mammals. These include the deer, the rabbit, and the seal. Seal mothers may leave their babies on shore for up to several days at a time as they hunt for fish in the sea. Land mammals in this category stash their newborns in a safe place (the "cache") and leave them for as many as 12 hours at a time. Their milk is very high in fat and protein to sustain the newborns for the long periods their mother is away.

Humans are carry mammals, which means they are to be carried constantly and fed around the clock.

Follow mammals. These include the giraffe and cow. Their newborns are mature enough at birth to follow their mothers around and feed. They feed more often than the cache mammals and their milk is lower in fat and protein.

Nest mammals. These include the dog and cat. These mothers leave their litter of newborns together (in a "nest") and return every few hours to feed. Their milk is correspondingly lower in fat and protein.

Carry mammals. Also referred to as continuous contact mammals, this group includes the apes and marsupials, like the kangaroo. These mammals are the most immature at birth, need to be held against their mother's body to stay warm, and are carried constantly. Their milk has the lowest levels of fat and protein, and as a result, they need to be fed often around the clock.

Human beings are in this last group. With our larger brains and smaller pelvises, we are born very early. At birth our brains are less mature than most other mammals, so our heads do not become too big to fit through our mothers' narrow pelvis. Most other mammals are born at about 80% of adult brain growth, but humans are born at less than 50%, with most brain growth occurring after birth. We also know that humans are carry mammals because human milk is among the lowest in fat and protein content of all mammalian milks. From the composition of our milk and our immaturity at birth, it is clear that from a biological standpoint human newborns are meant to be carried constantly and fed often around the clock.

• •

During most of history, frequent breastfeeding and constant carrying have been the human norm.

Breastfeeding and baby-care practices of hunter-gatherer societies provide a good idea of "natural human feeding rhythms" independent of cultural influences. These practices reflect how human babies were fed for more than 99% of human history. In an article comparing baby-care practices worldwide, U.S. pediatricians Betsy Lozoff and Gary Brittenham wrote: "If all human history were represented by an hour, the last 1/100th of a second would represent the 200 years of industrialization" (Lozoff & Brittenham, 1979, p. 479). Hunter-gatherer societies like the !Kung tribe in Botswana and Namibia and the people living in North Fore in the Highlands of New Guinea still live this ancient way. Among hunter-gatherers, similar breastfeeding patterns are reported, whether babies are born in Botswana, New Guinea, or to the Aboriginal tribes in Australia (Konner & Worthman, 1980; Hartmann, 2007). Babies born to hunter-gatherer cultures typically are carried on their mothers' bodies and breastfeed for a few minutes several times each hour for the first 2 years of life (Stuart-Macadam, 1995).

• •

Many breastfed babies do not conform to feeding and sleeping expectations of Western culture.

Western parenting recommendations are often based on bottle-feeding norms, with babies expected to stay full for hours after feedings and to sleep alone for long stretches at night (Ezzo & Bucknam, 2006; Ferber, 2006). While some breastfed babies can be convinced to follow these feeding and sleeping patterns, many do not easily conform to these expectations. In an Australian study of 71 exclusively breastfed 1- to 6-month-old babies, 11 feedings per day was average, with no differences in feeding frequency between 1 and 6 months (Kent et al., 2006; Thomas & Foreman, 2005). Number of daily feedings among these babies ranged from 6 to 18. In a U.S. study (Thomas & Foreman, 2005), nearly 30% of the babies 4 to 10 weeks old fed 13 or more times in 24 hours. For differences in sleep patterns among breastfed and formula-fed babies, see the later section "Night Feedings."

Rhythm Versus Schedule

Feeding schedules are recommended to breastfeeding mothers in some Western societies.

As described in the previous section, human babies are born expecting constant carrying and frequent feedings. Human babies' hardwiring hasn't changed since the stone age, so there is often a disconnect between modern expectations and babies' needs. Feeding schedules and "sleep training" are recent developments that are an outgrowth of bottle-feeding norms and are part of an approach to child-rearing sometimes referred to as "scientific mothering." This approach became popular in the early 20th century and was based on the beliefs of behaviorist psychologists, such as John Watson (Mohrbacher & Kendall-Tackett, 2005). Although many of these underlying beliefs have been proven wrong by science, when the natural feeding patterns of a breastfed baby are in conflict with cultural beliefs, this creates anxiety among new parents and can lead to breastfeeding problems and premature weaning.

Feeding schedules and sleep training are recent developments in human history and are an outgrowth of bottle-feeding norms.

Despite being disproved by science, some of scientific mothering's basic tenets have become a part of Western cultural beliefs and actively undermine breastfeeding. Ideas like "babies cry to manipulate adults" and "responding to a baby's cries encourages crying" are believed by many. However, the opposite has been proven true in studies around the world. In the U.S., longitudinal studies compared mothers who are responsive to their babies during infancy and mothers who were less responsive and found that babies who were responded to promptly cried less (Bates, Maslin, & Frankel, 1985; Crockenberg & McClusky, 1986). More recent research done in the U.K. and Denmark found the same (St James-Roberts et al., 2006).

Parenting beliefs can also be tested by observing cultures untouched by industrialization and scientific mothering, such as the !Kung, a hunter-gatherer tribe in which babies sleep with their mothers and are held most of the time. Their mothers often wear them in a carrier on their bodies, where the babies have near constant access to their mothers' breasts and breastfeed at will. !Kung babies rarely cry, and as toddlers, they have been found to be more independent than their U.S. counterparts (Konner, 1976).

• •

Feeding schedules are more compatible with bottle-feeding norms than breastfeeding.

Due to the bottle's faster, more consistent flow, babies fed by bottle tend to take more at a feeding and feed fewer times per day, which establishes an "overfeeding" pattern early in life, increasing the risk of childhood obesity (Taveras et al., 2004; Li, Fein, & Grummer-Strawn, 2008). In Western cultures where bottle-feeding has been common for several generations, new parents and their families may be more familiar with bottle-feeding norms and may attempt to apply those norms to breastfeeding. Bottle-feeding a baby "by the clock" works for more babies because a reluctant feeder can sometimes be "forced" to feed by pushing the firm bottle nipple into the back of baby's mouth, which triggers active sucking. But a baby cannot (and should not) be forced to breastfeed, so these same strategies will not work when a baby is breastfed.

Flexibility in feeding is important when breastfeeding because it allows a baby to adjust a mother's mother production as needed. If a mother's breast gave the same amount of milk day and night, and if all mothers produced milk at the exactly the same rate and had the same storage capacity, a prescribed feeding schedule could work. But that's not the reality (see next section), which is why flexibility in feeding is important.

A mother's breast storage capacity (see p. 399- "Breast Storage Capacity"), which varies considerably among mothers, has a major effect on how often her baby needs to feed to grow and gain weight, as well as to keep her rate of milk production steady. This individual variation can have a profound effect on a baby's feeding rhythm (see later section "Rhythm and Storage Capacity").

Daily Milk Ebb and Flow

Many breastfed babies feed more often in the evening and less often in the morning.

In Western cultures, breastfeeding mothers report that time of day influences feeding rhythm. When babies are fed less often than the human norm, a mother's milk production may have a natural ebb and flow over the course of the day.

Morning abundance. As newborns turn their days and night around to be more in tune with the rest of the family, they breastfeed less often at night (Kent et al., 2006), which means more milk accumulates in a mother's breasts by morning. Also, when researchers measure the hormonal levels of breastfeeding women, they find that prolactin, the hormone long thought to be related to milk production, is at its highest level in the middle of the night (Neville, 1999).

Evening low ebb. In the evening, many Western babies breastfeed more often to get the milk they need. Experienced breastfeeding mothers know that the baby who was happily full for hours between feedings in the morning is often the same baby who wants to feed every hour, every half hour, or even continuously during the evening. Called "the witching hour" in the U.S. and "hell hour" in Australia, this feeding frenzy often happens just about the time a mother's thoughts turn to getting dinner on the table. In some cases, these frequent feedings may continue all evening. One Israeli study that analyzed the milk expressed for 22 preterm babies (Lubetzky, Mimouni, Dollberg, Salomon, & Mandel, 2007) over 7 weeks found a consistent "circadian variation" in the fat content of the mothers' milk, with milk fat levels being higher during the evening (when the mothers' breasts were less full overall) as compared to the morning (when the breasts were fuller), which reflected this difference in milk volumes by time of day.

• •

No matter what the feeding intervals, overall babies get about the same the amount of fat.

Some mothers worry that if their baby breastfeeds often he won't get the fatty hindmilk he needs. However, U.S. and Australian researchers have found that as long as a baby is breastfeeding effectively, no matter what his feeding rhythm, he will receive about the same amount of fat over the course of a day (Casey, Neifert, Seacat, & Neville, 1986; Kent, 2007) . This is because the baby who breastfeeds more often gets foremilk higher in fat and hindmilk lower in fat than the baby who breastfeeds less often (Figure 2.1).

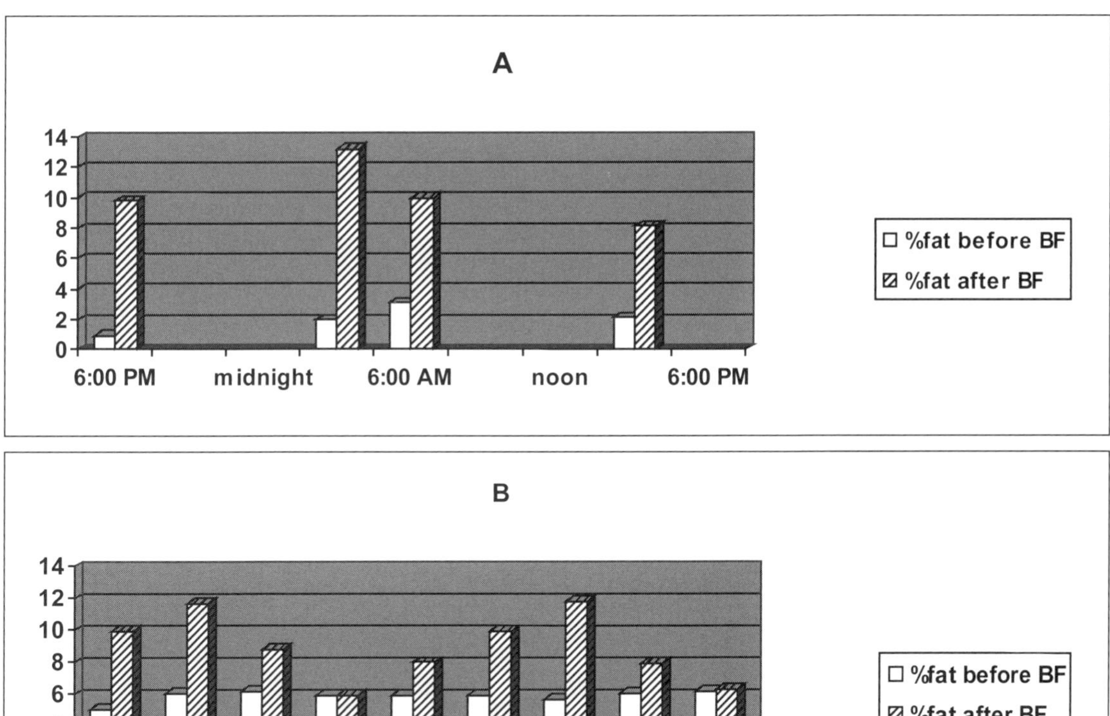

Figure 2.1. Percentage of fat in the milk before and after breastfeeding with longer (A) and shorter (B) feeding intervals (Kent, 2007).

Exclusively breastfed babies are usually happy to take milk from the breast no matter what the ebb and flow of daily milk production. What's most important to a baby's weight gain and growth is the total amount of milk received every 24 hours. On average, babies take about 25 ounces (750 mL) per day (Kent et al., 2006). As far as growth is concerned, it doesn't matter if a baby takes 1 ounce (30 mL) every hour or 3 ounces (89 mL) every 3 hours, as long as he receives enough milk overall. In fact, researchers have found that whether babies practice the frequent feedings of the hunter-gatherers or the longer intervals of Western societies, they take about the same amount of milk each day (Hartmann, 2007).

Whatever the feeding rhythm, overall daily milk intake is what's most important to a baby's growth.

Rhythm and Storage Capacity

A baby's breastfeeding rhythm will be determined in part by how much milk his stomach can hold and how much milk is available from the mother's breast. Baby's stomach size is determined in part by age, with a newborn's stomach capable of holding on average about 1 ounce (30 mL) of milk at birth and stomach size increasing with age (see Table 1 on p. 71 of this chapter).

Two physical dynamics that affect feeding rhythm are baby's stomach size and mother's breast storage capacity.

The other part of the equation is how much milk is available from the breast during feeding. Since humans are "carry" mammals and intended to feed often, large feedings and long intervals between feedings were not part of Nature's design for our babies. From the mother's side, human breasts were not designed with large milk storage areas, like the cistern in a cow's udder. So when breastfeeding proceeds naturally and babies feed often, there is no need for the breasts to store much milk.

Western cultural beliefs, however, influence many mothers and babies to test these boundaries. When mothers follow left-brained breastfeeding "rules" and encourage their babies to feed as infrequently as possible, this tests many mothers' milk-storage limits, which can lead to discomfort and mastitis. As more milk fills the breasts, internal pressure increases. When this pressure is combined with the accumulation of a whey protein or peptide in the milk referred to as feedback inhibitor of lactation (FIL), this slows the rate of milk production (Prentice, 1989). As described in detail in the "Making Milk" chapter, drained breasts make milk faster and full breasts make milk slower.

The term "breast storage capacity" refers to the maximum amount of milk available to the baby when the breast is at its fullest. Because this volume of milk varies—sometimes greatly—from mother to mother, this concept helps explain why feeding rhythms can vary so much from one mother-baby pair to another. One Australian study of 71 mothers and babies found a breast storage capacity range among its mothers of 74 to 382 g (2.6 to 12.9 oz.) per breast (Kent et al., 2006), while another Australian study (Daly, Owens, & Hartmann, 1993) found an even broader range among its mothers, from 81 to 606 mL (2.7 to 20.5 oz.).

Storage capacity dictates one breast or two, number of feedings per day, and whether babies continue to need night feedings.

Breast storage capacity is not related to breast size, which is usually determined by the amount of fatty tissue in the breasts. This means that smaller-breasted mothers could have a large storage capacity and large-breasted women could have a small storage capacity.

• •

Babies of Western mothers with large storage capacities may thrive on one breast per feeding and fewer feedings per day.

One breast or two. One breast per feeding may be plenty for a 3-month-old baby whose mother can comfortably hold 4 ounces (118 mL) of milk or more in each breast. Even if many hours pass before the baby takes that breast again, with a large storage capacity a mother can comfortably hold more milk, so her milk production may not slow as a result. In fact, spacing out larger feedings may help prevent the opposite problem—an overabundant milk supply. (For details, see the chapter, "Making Milk.")

Number of feedings per day may also be affected by storage capacity. Between 1 and 6 months of age, the Western baby typically takes on average about 3 to 4 ounces (76 to 118 mL) of milk per feeding (Kent et al., 2006), so to get enough milk over 24 hours he needs to breastfeed on average about eight times. But as his stomach grows and stretches, he can take more milk at a feeding. If a mother also has a large storage capacity, this may lead to the need for fewer feedings. Since the amount of milk a baby needs in a day stays about the same from months 1 to 6 (see next section), if he increases his milk intake at feedings, his number of feedings per day will drop. So if a mother has a large storage capacity, her baby may have previously needed to breastfeed eight times per day to get 25 ounces (750 mL) per day, but as he grows he may only need to feed six times per day to get the same amount of milk. One Australian study of 71 mothers and babies between 1 and 6 months found an inverse relationship been milk consumed at each feeding and the number of breastfeedings per day (Kent et al., 2006).

Mothers with small storage capacities can produce plenty of milk for their babies. Australian researchers found that all of the study babies whose mothers had a small storage capacity gained weight well (Kent et al., 2006). There were no issues with low milk supply or slow weight gain, but they had different feeding rhythms.

With a small storage capacity, in order to grow well and thrive, the baby may need both breasts per feeding and more feedings per day.

One difference in feeding rhythm is that more often these babies take both breasts at a breastfeeding and drain the breast more completely (Kent, 2007). On average, babies take one breast at some feedings and both breasts at some feedings (Kent et al., 2006), but mothers with a small storage capacity are not average.

Small storage capacity may also influence the number of feedings needed per day. Doing the math explains why. After 1 month of age, a baby needs on average 25 ounces (750 mL) of milk per day. If the most he can take at a breastfeeding is a little more than 2 ounces (74 mL) of milk per breast, he will need to breastfeed at least 12 times to get this daily volume. If he can take 3 ounces (89 mL) of milk per feeding, he will need at least eight feedings in a day. As one researcher wrote: "There is a significant tendency for babies of mothers with smaller storage capacities to feed more frequently than babies of mothers with larger storage capacities" (Kent, 2007, p. 568).

On average, babies take one breast at some feedings and both breasts at some feedings.

In general, it is best to let a mother and baby work out their own best feeding rhythm without too many "rules" imposed, as babies whose mothers have a very large storage capacity may do best on one breast per feeding, whereas babies whose mothers are on the other end of the storage capacity spectrum may do better when they take both breasts. In an Australian study of 71 exclusively 1- to 6-month-old babies in which 775 feedings were monitored, 53% of the feedings were "unpaired," meaning babies were happy with one breast for at least 1 hour, 44% of the feedings were "paired," meaning both breasts were taken within a 30-minute period, and 3% of the feedings were "clustered," meaning the baby took both breasts plus the first breast a second time during the "meal."

Milk Intake as Baby Grows

Despite rapid growth, the amount of milk a breastfed baby takes per day from 1 to 6 months of age remains remarkably stable.

At around 5 weeks of age, a breastfed baby reaches his peak daily milk intake of about 25 to 35 ounces (750 to 1035 mL) of milk per day, and this stays roughly the same until he begins solid foods at 6 months and his need for milk decreases. Because babies' growth and metabolic rate slows as they age, they continue to need about the same amount of milk from 1 month to 6 months of age. (For more details, see the chapter, "Weight Gain and Growth.")

There is a significant difference in the amount of milk a breastfeeding baby takes as compared with a baby fed formula.

On average, formula-fed babies consume much more milk per feeding and per day compared to breastfed babies: 15% more milk at 3 months, 23% more at 6 months, 20% more at 9 months, and 18% more at 12 months (Heinig, Nommsen, Peerson, Lonnerdal, & Dewey, 1993). Researchers noted that breastfed babies continued to gain less weight even after solid foods were started, and if availability of food was the reason, they could have consumed more solids to make up for the difference, but they didn't (Dewey, Heinig, Nommsen, & Lonnerdal, 1991). It is helpful for mothers to know about this difference in intake because sometimes they assume they need to pump as much milk for a feeding as their formula-feeding friends' babies take from the bottle.

The reasons for this difference are explained in detail on p. 206. It is due in part to the differences in the milk itself, as formula is missing hormones, such as leptin and adiponectin, which help babies regulate appetite and energy metabolism (Li et al. , 2008). Also, overfeeding that occurs with the fast flow of the bottle increases the risk of obesity later in life (Li et al., 2008; Taveras et al., 2004).

The Western advice to expect the number of feedings per day to decrease as babies grow is based on bottle-feeding norms.

The Western familiarity with bottle-feeding is most likely at the root of the common but erroneous advice given to breastfeeding mothers to eliminate feedings as their babies get older and heavier. Just as mothers of an earlier era were motivated to toilet train their babies within the first year to lighten their laundry loads, eliminating feedings by encouraging larger and fewer feedings from the bottle helps to eliminate some of the housekeeping work of bottle-feeding. But this is not good advice for breastfeeding mothers.

Mothers should not drop feedings as babies get older and heavier.

This approach also doesn't factor in differences in breast storage capacity. Doing the math explains why. As previously explained, a breastfed baby continues to need about the same amount of milk from 1 to 6 months, on average 25 ounces (750 mL) per day. If his mother has a small storage capacity and the most the baby can take at a feeding is 3 ounces (89 mL) and he needs a daily average of 25 ounces (750 mL), he will need at least eight feedings per day. What will happen if his mother attempts to drop some feedings as he grows? The baby's daily milk intake decreases because it is impossible for the baby to take more milk at each feeding to make up for the dropped feeding(s). And his mother's milk production would likely slow. In this case, with fewer feedings the baby's weight gain may slow or stop. Depending on the number of feedings dropped, he may even lose weight.

The Australian study of 71 exclusively breastfed 1- to 6-month-olds found that the average number of feedings—11 per day—did not vary by baby's age (Kent et al., 2006).

After 1 year, breastfeeding rhythm varies from child to child and from place to place.

By the time the breastfeeding baby is 15 months old and is eating many other foods, the baby will need less mother's milk, but may still breastfeed often for comfort and closeness. In Australia and the U.S., mothers' daily milk production at 15 months was measured at between 95 and 315 mL per day (Kent, Mitoulas, Cox, Owens, & Hartmann, 1999; Neville et al., 1991). However, in Zaire, where breastfeeding older babies is the norm, research found that at 30 months mothers produced on average of 300mL per day (Hennart, Delogne-Desnoeck, Vis, & Robyn, 1981). For more details on breastfeeding expectations for older babies, see the chapter "Weaning from the Breast."

PACIFIERS/DUMMIES

Pacifiers/dummies are not recommended during the first month of breastfeeding.

Because babies are given pacifiers to prolong the intervals between feedings, during the intense first 40 days of breastfeeding, this can alter feeding rhythm by decreasing the number of feedings per day (see later point), potentially decreasing a mother's milk production. Even health organizations that recommend pacifier use to prevent SIDS (see next section) recommend delaying its introduction until after the first month of breastfeeding, when milk production is established (AAP, 2005).

• •

In some places, mothers are cautioned not to let their baby "use the breast as a pacifier."

Where breastfeeding is not the cultural norm, pacifiers are sometimes recommended to keep the baby calm and achieve longer intervals between feedings. In the U.S., the pacifier is considered by many to be a baby's preferred source of comfort, and mothers are cautioned to limit their baby's time at the breast, so their baby doesn't "use the breast as a pacifier." Because the suckling at the breast is a newborn's natural source of comfort and pre-dates the pacifier, it is more accurate to say that babies "use the pacifier as the breast," rather than the reverse.

There are risks to pacifier use during normal breastfeeding.

Although there are some special situations when a pacifier can be a helpful tool, such as the preterm baby whose digestion is improved when sucking on a pacifier while fed by gavage tube (Field et al., 1982; Medoff-Cooper & Ray, 1995) or the baby with feeding problems who needs help learning to suckle effectively (Wilson-Clay & Hoover, 2008), there are also risks to pacifier use during normal breastfeeding, which the following points describe.

• •

Pacifier use is associated with a shorter duration of breastfeeding, earlier return of fertility, and several negative health outcomes.

Decrease in exclusive breastfeeding and earlier weaning. Many studies have found an association between pacifier use and shorter duration of breastfeeding (Ullah & Griffiths, 2003). One U.S. randomized clinical controlled trial of 700 breastfed newborns 36 to 42 weeks gestation found that introduction of pacifiers in the first 4 weeks of life caused a significant decrease in exclusive breastfeeding and shortened overall duration (Howard et al., 2003). A 2005 survey of child-care practices in 17 countries noted a dose-response effect on intensity of pacifier use and breastfeeding exclusivity, as well as an association between pacifier use and shorter duration of breastfeeding (Nelson, Yu, & Williams, 2005). A 2008 survey of maternity-care practices in about 2,000 U.S. hospitals also found a significant association between early pacifier use in the hospital and shortened breastfeeding duration (DiGirolamo, Grummer-Strawn, & Fein, 2008). A U.S. prospective cohort study of 265 mothers and babies found the mothers using pacifiers from birth were 1.5 times more likely to breastfeed for a shorter time than mothers who did not use pacifiers (Howard et al., 1999). Brazilian studies found a two to three times shorter breastfeeding duration among pacifier users, but in Brazil mothers use pacifiers to wean from the breast, so the higher rate may be due in part to this practice (Barros et al., 1995; Victora, Tomasi, Olinto, & Barros, 1993).

Researchers have questioned whether some mothers introduce a pacifier because they want to breastfeed less often or on a schedule, which can lead to reduced milk production and earlier weaning (Howard et al., 1999). Others questioned whether pacifiers are started because there is a breastfeeding problem, which might be the real cause of earlier weaning (Kramer et al., 2001; Victora, Behague, Barros, Olinto, & Weiderpass, 1997).

A New Zealand prospective cohort study of 349 mothers and babies noted a relationship between intensity of pacifier use and breastfeeding duration (Vogel, Hutchison, & Mitchell, 2001). Its researchers found that breastfeeding duration was shortened only when pacifiers were used daily, but not if the pacifier was used less often.

Fewer feedings per day. One possible mechanism for these negative effects on breastfeeding outcomes is that especially during the first month mothers who use pacifiers regularly on average breastfeed fewer times per day. One U.S. prospective cohort study found that at 2 weeks mothers using pacifiers breastfed on average eight times per day compared with nine times per day when the pacifier was not used and noted that fewer feedings can lead to breastfeeding problems later, such as insufficient milk production (Howard et al., 1999). An Australian prospective cohort study of 556 mothers and babies found that at 6 weeks mothers using pacifiers breastfed on average 6.9 times per day as compared with 7.4 feedings per day among those not using a pacifier (Binns & Scott, 2002). This study found that after controlling for breastfeeding problems and many other variables, pacifier use at 2 weeks was associated with reduced breastfeeding duration up to 6 months. A Swedish descriptive, longitudinal, prospective study of 506 mothers and babies found that at 2, 4, 6, 8, and 10 weeks, babies taking pacifiers breastfed fewer times per day than those who did not (Aarts et al., 1999).

Increased incidence of ear infection. Many studies have found an association between regular pacifier use and increased incidence of ear infection (Lubianca Neto, Hemb, & Silva, 2006; Ullah & Griffiths, 2003). One Finnish prospective randomized controlled trial of 484 children found a 29% reduction in ear infections in the group whose parents limited pacifier use to bedtime only, as compared to the other group who used pacifiers freely throughout the day (Niemela, Pihakari, Pokka, & Uhari, 2000). A U.S. prospective cohort study of 1375 babies also found a positive association between pacifier use and ear infection (Warren, Levy, Kirchner, Nowak, & Bergus, 2001). A Dutch prospective cohort study of 495 children from birth to 4 years (Rovers et al., 2008) found pacifier use to be a risk factor for recurring ear infections. Overall, there appears to be a 1.2 to 2-fold increased risk of ear infection associated with pacifier use (AAP, 2005). Some theories on the cause for this include increased saliva from suckling carries more organisms to the Eustachian tubes and non-nutritive sucking causes abnormal function of the Eustachian tubes, moving organisms from the mouth to the middle ear.

Increased incidence of candida/thrush. Pacifiers, like everything else that enters a baby's mouth, can carry candida, the fungus that causes thrush. An overgrowth of candida can occur when a pacifier is shared among children or can cause reinfection if a child uses a pacifier contaminated with candida after being treated for thrush. As part of a large survey, Finnish researchers analyzed the saliva of 166 healthy children and found a greater incidence of candida in those who used a pacifier (Ollila, Niemela, Uhari, & Larmas, 1997). A U.K. prospective cohort study of 95 healthy children found nearly twice as many cases of candida among those using pacifiers as compared with those who did not (Sio, Minwalla, George, & Booth, 1987). The researchers suggest that using a pacifier may prevent a child from effectively clearing sugar from his mouth.

Increased risk of mouth malformation and dental caries. A Spanish prospective cohort study of 1297 children found an association between pacifier use and a narrowed dental arch, which can lead to the need for orthodontia later (Aznar, Galan, Marin, & Dominguez, 2006). Other studies in other countries have found similar results (Warren, Levy, Nowak, & Tang, 2000; Zardetto, Rodrigues, & Stefani, 2002). A Finnish study also found an association between pacifier use and higher levels of the bacteria in the mouth that causes dental caries (Ollila et al., 1997).

Earlier return to fertility. The time spent using a pacifier decreases the amount of time spent suckling at the breast, influencing the hormonal balance that suppresses ovulation after birth. One U.K. prospective cohort study of 85 breastfeeding mothers found pacifier use associated with lower postpartum progesterone levels and an earlier return of menstruation (Ingram, Hunt, Woolridge, & Greenwood, 2004).

• •

Based on a meta-analysis of the research, the American Academy of Pediatrics' Task Force on Sudden Infant Death Syndrome recommended that to prevent SIDS all babies, whether breastfeeding or not, be given a pacifier when they go to sleep for naps and at bedtimes (Hauck, Omojokun, & Siadaty, 2005). However, they make one exception:

To prevent SIDS, one U.S. health organization recommends all breastfed babies older than 1 month be given a pacifier while going to sleep.

> For breastfed infants, delay pacifier introduction until 1 month of age to ensure that breastfeeding is firmly established (AAP, 2005, p. 1252).

When the Task Force analyzed the research, it found that as compared with the babies who did not use a pacifier, babies who went to sleep with a pacifier (even if it fell out as they slept) had 71% less risk of dying from SIDS during that sleep (Chapman, 2006). The Task Force suggested several possible mechanisms: sucking makes babies more arousable, pacifier use encourages a more forward position of the tongue preventing blockage of the baby's airway, and the effect pacifier use has in keeping baby on his back during sleep.

Pacifiers should not be used by breastfeeding infants at all until they are at least 1 month of age.

But could breastfeeding alone produce these same effects? After conducting their own research on SIDS in the Netherlands, Dutch researchers recommended pacifier use at sleep times only for bottle-fed babies (L'Hoir et al., 1999). As researcher and *Journal of Human Lactation* editor, M. Jane Heinig wrote in response:

> If sucking is associated with this arousal effect, it follows that the breastfed child who feeds during the night would be afforded the same protection. However, at this time, this mechanism has not been established, and fewer than half the studies included in the meta-analysis collected data on breastfeeding practices (Heinig & Banuelos, 2006, p. 8).

Breastfeeding is considered protective of SIDS, but with the limited information available in the studies used in this meta-analysis, it is currently impossible to evaluate whether these recommendations are valid only for bottle-fed babies or whether they also are appropriate for breastfed babies (Ip et al., 2007).

Despite known negative outcomes, many birthing facilities continue to give pacifiers to full-term, healthy newborns.

Despite the documented negative breastfeeding and health outcomes and the directive of Step 9 of the Baby Friendly Hospital Initiative: "Give no pacifiers or artificial nipples to breastfeeding infants," many birthing facilities continue to give newborns pacifiers in the days after birth. In a 2008 survey of maternity-care practices in U.S. hospitals, nearly 56% of the nearly 2000 hospitals that responded routinely gave their newborns pacifiers (DiGirolamo et al., 2008). In an earlier U.S. survey of 2093 Colorado mothers about hospital practices, 52% said their baby was given a pacifier during their hospital stay (Murray et al., 2007). Not only can this practice affect breastfeeding while mother and baby are in the hospital, but it models this practice, increasing the chances that the parents will continue to give the pacifier after hospital discharge.

NIGHT FEEDINGS

Sleep Patterns

To help newborns learn to take their longest sleep stretch at night, keep stimulation at night to a minimum.

Most babies are born with their days and nights mixed up, and many have one long 4- to 5-hour sleep stretch, which may happen at any time (Benson, 2001). There is no need to wake a baby during this longer sleep stretch unless he is feeding fewer than eight times in 24 hours or the parents want to try to encourage him to sleep longer at night.

To gradually help a baby shift his longest sleep period from day to night, suggest parents start by reducing stimulation at night:

- Keep lights low—for just enough light to see, leave on a closet light with door partly closed or use a nightlight
- Keep sound and movements to a minimum
- Change diapers only when necessary—when baby is soaked or has passed a stool

Over time this will help baby sleep more at night and be more alert during the day. In one U.S. study of 37 mothers and babies 4 to 10 weeks old, 78% of the babies took their longest sleep stretch at night (Thomas & Foreman, 2005).

To get her rest, encourage a mother to find a breastfeeding position in which she can sleep and to sleep when her baby sleeps.

When the mother learns to breastfeed in a side-lying or semi-reclining position, she can use her breastfeeding time to catch up on her rest. In one U.S. study of 20 breastfeeding mothers, mothers were less fatigued after breastfeeding in a side-lying position than after breastfeeding upright (Milligan, Flenniken, & Pugh, 1996). A semi-reclining position allows a mother to support her baby's weight with her body, which offers this same benefit (Colson, 2008).

Mothers are often encouraged to "sleep when the baby sleeps" in order to avoid fatigue, but one U.S. study found that many mothers were using this time to do other things, rather than catching up on their rest (Thomas & Foreman, 2005). Encourage any tired mother to take advantage of her baby's sleep time to get some extra sleep.

Fatigue is a fact of life for new parents no matter how a baby is fed. Some mothers think weaning will help them get more rest, but research has found that when mothers stop breastfeeding, their fatigue level does not change (Wambach, 1998). In fact, breastfeeding mothers appear to get more sleep.

Mothers, who exclusively breastfeed, sleep deeper and get more sleep than other mothers.

Exclusively breastfeeding mothers (and their partners) get more sleep. Some parents think that giving their babies formula at night will help them sleep longer. However, one U.S. study of 133 new mothers and fathers during the first 3 months found that mothers who exclusively breastfeed averaged 40 to 45 minutes more sleep at night than those who also gave their babies infant formula (Doan, Gardiner, Gay, & Lee, 2007). For more details, see the next point.

Breastfeeding mothers spend more time in deep sleep. An Australian study of 31 women, 12 who were breastfeeding, 12 age-matched women without infants, and seven bottle-feeding mothers, found that mothers who exclusively breastfeed had "a marked alteration in their sleep architecture," giving them longer periods of a type of deep sleep known as slow-wave sleep (SWS) than bottle-fed mothers with babies the same age (Blyton, Sullivan, & Edwards, 2002). The researchers concluded that "enhanced SWS may be another important factor to support breastfeeding in the postnatal period" (Blyton et al., 2002, p. 297).

Giving breastfed babies formula or solid foods does not appear to help them sleep longer, and may even have the opposite effect.

Giving formula results in less sleep. In the study mentioned in the previous point that found exclusively breastfeeding mothers averaged 40 to 45 minutes more sleep at night during the first 3 months, the authors wrote:

> ...formula feeding not only failed to improve parent sleep, but actually resulted in parents getting less sleep, even when fathers helped during the night with supplementation feedings (Doan et al., 2007, p. 204).

The researchers thought this was due to time spent preparing bottles and the disruption of sleep mothers experienced even when their partner fed the baby. They found that when mothers handled all night feedings they (and their partners) slept more than when night feedings were shared. Another U.S. study that compared 72 breastfeeding and non-breastfeeding families during the first month found that both the mothers and fathers in exclusively breastfeeding families got slightly more sleep overall than in families not breastfeeding, with mothers sleeping 384 minutes versus 364 minutes and fathers sleeping 407 minutes versus 386 minutes (Gay, Lee, & Lee, 2004).

Giving cow's milk alters a baby's sleep metabolism. A Brazilian study of 62 8-month-old babies found that babies' energy metabolism increased when they received cow's milk, the main ingredient of most infant formulas (Haisma et al., 2005).

Giving solids does not help babies "sleep through the night." This popular belief appears to have no basis in fact. Two studies found no difference in the sleep patterns of babies after solid foods, such as cereal, were started (Keane, 1988; Macknin, Medendorp, & Maier, 1989). About the same number of babies in these studies began sleeping more at night whether they received the solids or not. The researchers wrote: "Infants' ability to sleep through the night is a developmental and adaptive process that occurs regardless of the timing of introduction of cereal" (Macknin et al., 1989, p. 1068).

A mother's breast storage capacity can affect a baby's need to breastfeed at night.

As described in the previous section "Rhythm and Storage Capacity," this individual difference can affect how often a baby needs to breastfeed to thrive. It can also affect the longest interval between feedings and, therefore, a baby's need to breastfeed at night.

Mothers with a large storage capacity. This baby may take more milk per feeding and may take fewer feedings per day. He is more likely to "sleep through the night" at an earlier age than other babies. Yet even with longer stretches between feedings at night, this mother may not feel uncomfortably full by morning, since her breasts can hold more milk. So she may be able to maintain her milk production in spite of longer stretches between feedings.

Mothers with a small storage capacity. For this baby, night feedings may need to continue for many months. Because this baby has access to less milk per feeding, he may need night feedings to get enough milk overall. Because breast fullness causes milk production to slow, this mother may need to breastfeed at night to continue to make enough milk. In an Australian study of 71 mothers and babies, all the babies of the mothers with the smallest storage capacity breastfed during the night (Kent et al., 2006). If a mother with a small storage capacity tries to encourage her baby to sleep longer with "sleep training," this may undermine breastfeeding by slowing both milk production and the baby's weight gain.

Sleep patterns vary in babies fed by breast and bottle.

Western expectations of infant sleep are based on research conducted on non-breastfeeding babies put to sleep in a separate room (McKenna, Ball, & Gettler, 2007). Based on this research, many parents believe that at night their babies should sleep alone for long stretches by the time they are 3 to 4 months old. Research comparing breastfeeding and non-breastfeeding babies found that breastfed babies are more wakeful and sleep for shorter stretches than non-breastfeeding babies and that these differences in sleep patterns are apparent as early as 1 month (Ball, 2003; Quillin & Glenn, 2004). An Australian study found that at 2 to 3 months of age breastfed babies were significantly more easily aroused from active sleep than formula-fed babies (Horne, Parslow, Ferens, Watts, & Adamson, 2004).

Night wakings are more common in breastfed vs. bottle-fed infants.

In an Australian study of 71 mothers and exclusively breastfed babies, 64% of the 1- to 6-month-old babies breastfed between 10 p.m. and 4 a.m., and the number of night feedings did not vary by age (Kent et al., 2006). In other words, the 6-month-old babies were waking as often at night to breastfeed as the 1-month-old babies. The researchers noted that because the babies "…have a relatively small stomach capacity and/or a rapid gastric emptying time," they have a legitimate physical need to breastfeed at night (Kent et al., 2006, p. e393). A mother's storage capacity (see previous point) will also influence whether night feedings are needed to maintain milk production.

As described in the previous section "Biology and Culture," our babies are born expecting continuous contact and frequent feedings around the clock for their first years. There are also many reasons other than hunger that babies wake at night to breastfeed, even into the toddler years: teething, restlessness from rapid growth and development, individual differences in babies' normal sleep patterns, and loneliness.

One U.S. study of 32 breastfeeding mothers and babies followed into their 2nd year found that the breastfeeding babies and toddlers did not conform to the expected sleep patterns of non-breastfed babies and that these differences were even more pronounced among babies who slept with their parents (Elias, Nicolson, Bora, & Johnston, 1986). Rather than beginning to have long stretches of unbroken sleep after about 4 months of age, the breastfeeding babies continued to wake frequently, which was comparable to sleep patterns of breastfed babies in developing countries. The researchers concluded that as breastfeeding becomes more common in Western society, expectations of babies' sleep/wake patterns may need to be revised and wrote: "It seems ironic that, although night waking is so much less frequent in infants cared for in the Western style, it presents so much more of a problem for parents" (Elias et al., 1986, p. 327). After the first 8 weeks or so, night-feedings are considered by some in Western cultures to be an imposition on adults that should be discouraged, rather than a normal and natural part of infancy.

• •

With the adoption of the Western idea that babies "should" sleep undisturbed for long stretches, a whole industry has arisen to help parents solve infant "sleep problems." As part of this way of thinking, during the last 2 decades, the idea has become popular in the U.S. that it is better for babies to learn to fall asleep alone and soothe themselves back to sleep when they wake at night. If they don't, parents are told that their children may be at greater risk for "sleep problems," which supposedly afflict up to 45% of babies (Anders & Eiben, 1997). Anthropologist and researcher, James McKenna, acknowledges the double-bind parents are put in when they are told they should never let a baby fall asleep at the breast or in their arms, because:

The long-term effects of "sleep training" and "parent-directed feedings" are unknown.

> ...[This is] the very context within which the infants' falling asleep evolved and is practically impossible to prevent! Parents are taught that to establish lifelong 'healthy' sleep habits, their infants 'need' and 'should' be 'trained' to sleep alone. Yet, according to the 2000 National Sleep Foundation Survey in the United States, 62% of American adults whose parents probably followed these general Dr. Spock-inspired recommendations currently report difficulties falling and staying asleep... (McKenna & McDade, 2005, p. 140).

This idea has caused many parents to question whether they should breastfeed at night and comfort their children when they wake. Some proponents of "sleep training" (Ferber, 2006) and "parent-directed feeding" and sleeping schedules (Ezzo & Bucknam, 2006), advise parents to allow babies as young as 8 weeks old to "cry it out" until they fall asleep at naptimes and bedtime, which they say may take hours at first.

Although some babies can be "trained" to adopt sleep patterns appropriate for older children and adults, no research exists on the long-term physical and psychological effects of these practices, which is important before these practices are implemented, since their goals are radically different from natural human feeding and sleeping patterns (Lozoff & Brittenham, 1979; Nelson et al., 2001).

Where Should Babies Sleep?

If a mother is exhausted, explore with her sleep options that make breastfeeding easier and are less disruptive of her sleep.

When a baby's sleep patterns do not conform to cultural expectations, parents may become frustrated and upset. The mother may wonder what she is doing "wrong" to cause her baby's night-waking and be concerned that unless she does something to "correct" this, she may not be caring for her baby properly.

If an exhausted mother is worried that her baby's frequent waking is not "normal," acknowledge her frustrations and concerns. Assure her that night waking is normal in breastfed babies and discuss ways to make night feedings easier and allow her to get more sleep while meeting her baby's needs. For example, if the baby sleeps in a crib in another room, share with her the recommendations to keep the baby in her room at night (see next point), which will make it easier for her to hear her baby stir before he has fully awakened and begun to cry. Most mothers and babies fall back to sleep more quickly if they have not been fully awakened.

Many different sleeping arrangements can make night feedings easier:

- A bassinet or cradle next to the parents' bed
- Baby's crib attached to the parents' bed in a "side-car" arrangement
- A "co-sleeper" bed that attaches to the parents' bed (Ball et al., 2006)
- Baby put to sleep on a mattress on the floor away from the walls in the parents' room, so the mother can lie down and sleep while breastfeeding the baby and return to her own bed if she wishes after the baby goes back to sleep.
- Baby sleeps in the parents' bed, either for part of the night—after he awakens the first time—or for the whole night

Encourage the mother to do what works best for her family and share with her the safe and unsafe sleeping practices in Table 2.2, so she can find a workable solution that does not put her baby at risk.

To prevent SIDS, most health organizations recommend during their first 6 months that at night babies sleep on their backs in their parents' room.

These two recommendations have become generally accepted around the world as effective SIDS-prevention strategies, and parents everywhere are encouraged to follow them. As a result, during the last decade SIDS rates have dropped dramatically. For a review of the literature that supports both "back to sleep" and sleeping in the parents' room, see the American Academy of Pediatrics' Task Force on Sudden Infant Death Syndrome (SIDS) policy statement (AAP, 2005).

Bed-sharing is common in many cultures with low SIDS rates and is associated with more sleep and better breastfeeding outcomes.

Babies' needs are the same worldwide, but cultural beliefs on where babies should sleep vary. Western health organizations promote close but separate sleep surfaces for babies (AAP, 2005), but in a study by anthropologists of more than 100 societies, U.S. middle-class parents were the only ones who expected their babies to sleep alone (Latz, Wolf, & Lozoff, 1999).

In most cultures where breastfeeding is the norm, mothers and babies sleep next to each other at night so that the baby can breastfeed often with the least disruption of sleep. Parents in these cultures expect babies to wake frequently to feed at night until they have matured enough to outgrow this behavior, which may take years. A wakeful baby—even a wakeful older baby or toddler—is considered neither unusual nor a problem to be solved. As researchers studying infant sleep in Thailand wrote: "All infants normally arouse briefly on average 4 to 6 times throughout the night" (Anuntaseree et al., 2008, p. 565).

When mothers and babies sleep next to each other, mothers get more sleep.

A study conducted in Japan, where bedsharing is the norm, examined the sleep practices of 101 first-time parents to determine whether fathers slept better separate from mother and baby or if they slept better in bed with mother and baby and found that fathers slept better with mother and baby (Yamazaki, Lee et al. 2005). U.S. research indicates that mothers get more sleep when they share a bed with their baby then when they sleep alone (Quillin & Glenn, 2004).

Research conducted worldwide has found an association between bedsharing and more frequent, longer, and more exclusive breastfeeding (Baddock, Galland, Bolton, Williams, & Taylor, 2006; Ball et al., 2006; Blair & Ball, 2004; Buswell & Spatz, 2007; Horsley et al., 2007; McKenna et al., 2007; McKenna et al., 1997).

• •

In Western cultures, some recommend against bed-sharing without distinguishing between safe and unsafe sleeping practices and other risk factors.

Bedsharing is considered by some to be potentially dangerous. In 2005, the American Academy of Pediatrics' Task Force on Sudden Infant Death Syndrome released a policy statement recommending that new parents put their babies to sleep in a "separate but proximate sleeping environment," ideally a separate crib or bassinet in their room (AAP, 2005). In its backhanded acknowledgement of the proven safety of co-sleeping in Eastern cultures, this Task Force wrote that bedsharing: "*...as practiced in the United States and other Western countries* [emphasis added], is more hazardous than the infant sleeping on a separate sleep surface..." (AAP, 2005, p. 1252).

But when looking at bedsharing cross-culturally, these hazards are not apparent. Bedsharing is the cultural norm in the Far East, and countries with the greatest incidence of bedsharing (such as China, Vietnam, Cambodia, and Thailand) have the lowest incidence of SIDS. In Japan, as bedsharing becomes more common, SIDS rates are decreasing. Yet as Asian immigrants to the U.S. begin to adopt Western child-care practices, their previously low SIDS rates increase (Grether, Schulman et al., 1990; McKenna & McDade, 2005).

One reason Western SIDS researchers don't see the issue this way is their failure to control for unsafe sleep surfaces and other known risk factors for SIDS. As U.S. authors wrote:

> The problem with studies that do show an increase in SIDS related to bedsharing is that they do not uniformly control for unsafe bedsharing practices such as parental alcohol consumption, as in Tappin, Ecob, and Brooke (2005) who chose not to include alcohol as a factor; smoking (which often occurs with alcohol use) (Carpenter et al., 2004); unsafe sleeping surfaces, overcrowding, and many other factors (Morgan, Groer, & Smith, 2006, p. 686).

Yet even with U.S. health organizations recommending against bedsharing, research indicates that large numbers of U.S. parents still do it, and that as breastfeeding rates increase the numbers are growing. One U.S. study found that in 45% of the study's 8,453 families their babies had spent some time in an adult bed in the past 2 weeks and that this practice is increasing (Willinger, Ko, Hoffman, Kessler, & Corwin, 2003). A more recent U.S. study found 42% of its

2,300 families were bedsharing at 2 weeks, 34% at 3 months, and 27% at 12 months.

• •

Attempting to avoid bedsharing can inadvertently lead to dangerous sleeping practices.

When new parents are encouraged to exclusively breastfeed and also to avoid bedsharing, they may ask themselves the next logical question: "What is the alternative?" In an article written for U.S. pediatricians, Laura Wilwerding, MD, FAAP wrote that if a new mother is advised not to sleep with her baby:

> ...she may get out of bed at night and nurse or bottle-feed her baby in another location with no intention of sleeping. The result in the sleep-deprived mother is often inadvertently sleeping on a couch or recliner. This is far more dangerous to the infant than a firm adult mattress (Wilwerding, 2008, p. 3).

Mothers can easily become exhausted from spending their nights breastfeeding upright while trying to avoid falling asleep. Some mothers find themselves nodding off after several night feedings and nearly dropping their baby or falling asleep somewhere more dangerous than an adult bed. After experiences like these, many begin to see bedsharing as a safer alternative.

But putting parents in this quandary may also put breastfeeding at risk. As one British researcher explained, parents may view their choices as:

> (1) feeding the baby formula (or formula plus some 'heavy' indigestible substance, such as cereal or baby rice) so that he or she does not require frequent (or any) night feeding; (2) undertake an 'infant-training' program...to encourage them to lengthen their sleep bouts until they 'sleep through the night' (midnight to 5:00 AM); or (3) sleep next to the baby, allowing easy access to breasts, and eliminating the need for either mother or baby to wake fully for breastfeeds (Ball, 2003, pp. 185-186).

An alternative to issuing a blanket recommendation against bedsharing is to recommend parents adopt the Eastern bedsharing practices that make bedsharing safe (Table 2.2). The Academy of Breastfeeding Medicine, a physicians' organization, took a step in this direction by issuing safe sleeping guidelines for parents that can be applied to all sleep options. After reviewing the research, this organization concluded "There is currently not enough evidence to support routine recommendations against bedsharing" (ABM, 2008, p. 41).

Table 2.2. Safe and Unsafe Sleeping Practices

Safe sleeping practices:

- Put baby on his back to sleep
- Sleep on a firm, flat surface, such as a firm mattress on the floor away from walls or a "co-sleeper" baby bed or crib that attaches to an adult bed
- Tuck in any blankets around the mattress to avoid covering the baby's head
- Dress baby in a warm sleeper if the room is cold

Unsafe sleeping practices

- Exposing baby to smoke, either from a mother who smokes or environmental smoke from others
- Sleeping with baby on a sofa, couch, daybed, or waterbed or with pillows or loose bedding near baby
- Sleeping in a bed with an adjacent space that could trap baby
- Putting baby face down (prone) or on his side for sleeping
- Sharing a bed with other children or an adult who has consumed alcohol, sedatives, or other mind-altering drugs
- Leaving baby alone on an adult bed

Adapted from (ABM, 2008)

RESOURCES FOR PARENTS

Websites

www.breastfeedingmadesimple.com

DVDs

Righard, L. (1995). *Delivery self-attachment.* Available from www.geddesproduction.com.

Smillie, C. (2007). *Baby-led breastfeeding: The mother-baby dance.* Available from www.geddesproduction.com.

Books

Kendall-Tackett, K. (2005). *Hidden feelings of motherhood.* Amarillo, TX: Hale Publishing.

Klaus, M.H., & Klaus, P. (1995). *Your amazing newborn.* Reading, MA: Perseus Books.

Mohrbacher, N., & Kendall-Tackett, K. (2005). *Breastfeeding made simple: Seven natural laws for nursing mothers.* New Harbinger Publications: Oakland, CA.

REFERENCES

AAP. (2005). The changing concept of Sudden Infant Death Syndrome: Diagnostic coding shifts, controversies regarding the sleeping environment, and new variables to consider in reducing risk. *Pediatrics, 116*(5), 1245-1255.

Aarts, C., Hornell, A., Kylberg, E., Hofvander, Y., & Gebre-Medhin, M. (1999). Breastfeeding patterns in relation to thumb sucking and pacifier use. *Pediatrics, 104*(4), e50.

ABM. (2008). ABM clinical protocol #6: Guideline on co-sleeping and breastfeeding. Revision, March 2008. *Breastfeeding Medicine, 3*(1), 38-43.

Alberts, J. R. (1994). Learning as adaptation of the infant. *Acta Paediatrica Suppl, 397*, 77-85.

Anders, T. F., & Eiben, L. A. (1997). Pediatric sleep disorders: a review of the past 10 years. *Journal of the American Academy of Child and Adolescent Psychiatry, 36*(1), 9-20.

Anuntaseree, W., Mo-suwan, L., Vasiknanonte, P., Kuasirikul, S., Ma-a-lee, A., & Choprapawan, C. (2008). Night waking in Thai infants at 3 months of age: association between parental practices and infant sleep. *Sleep Medicine, 9*(5), 564-571.

Aznar, T., Galan, A. F., Marin, I., & Dominguez, A. (2006). Dental arch diameters and relationships to oral habits. *Angle Orthodontist, 76*(3), 441-445.

Baddock, S. A., Galland, B. C., Bolton, D. P., Williams, S. M., & Taylor, B. J. (2006). Differences in infant and parent behaviors during routine bed sharing compared with cot sleeping in the home setting. *Pediatrics, 117*(5), 1599-1607.

Ball, H. L. (2003). Breastfeeding, bed-sharing, and infant sleep. *Birth, 30*(3), 181-188.

Ball, H. L., Ward-Platt, M. P., Heslop, E., Leech, S. J., & Brown, K. A. (2006). Randomised trial of infant sleep location on the postnatal ward. *Archives of Disease in Childhood, 91*(12), 1005-1010.

Barros, F. C., Victora, C. G., Semer, T. C., Tonioli Filho, S., Tomasi, E., & Weiderpass, E. (1995). Use of pacifiers is associated with decreased breast-feeding duration. *Pediatrics, 95*(4), 497-499.

Bates, J. E., Maslin, C. A., & Frankel, K. A. (1985). Attachment security, mother-child interaction, and temperament as predictors of behavior-problem ratings at age three years. *Monographs of the Society for Research in Child Development, 50*(1-2), 167-193.

Beck, C. T., & Watson, S. (2008). Impact of birth trauma on breast-feeding: a tale of two pathways. *Nursing Research, 57*(4), 228-236.

Beilin, Y., Bodian, C.A., Weiser, J., Hossain, S., Arnold, I., Feierman, D.E., et al. (2005). Effect of labor epidural analgesia with and without fentanyl on infant breast-feeding: a prospective, randomized, double-blind study. *Anesthesiology, 103*(6), 1211-1217.

Benson, S. (2001). What is normal? A study of normal breastfeeding dyads during the first sixty hours of life. *Breastfeeding Review, 9*(1), 27-32.

Bergman, N. (2008). Breastfeeding and perinatal neuroscience. In C. W. Genna (Ed.), *Supporting sucking skills in breastfeeding infants* (pp. 43-56). Boston, MA: Jones and Bartlett.

Bergman, N. J., & Jurisoo, L. A. (1994). The 'kangaroo-method' for treating low birthweight babies in a developing country. *Tropical Doctor, 24*(2), 57-60.

Bergman, N. J., Linley, L. L., & Fawcus, S. R. (2004). Randomized controlled trial of skin-to-skin contact from birth versus conventional incubator for physiological stabilization in 1200- to 2199-gram newborns. *Acta Paediatrica, 93*(6), 779-785.

Binns, C. W., & Scott, J. A. (2002). Using pacifiers: what are breastfeeding mothers doing? *Breastfeeding Review, 10*(2), 21-25.

Blair, P. S., & Ball, H. L. (2004). The prevalence and characteristics associated with parent-infant bed-sharing in England. *Archives of Disease in Childhood, 89*(12), 1106-1110.

Blyton, D. M., Sullivan, C. E., & Edwards, N. (2002). Lactation is associated with an increase in slow-wave sleep in women. *Journal of Sleep Research, 11*(4), 297-303.

Buswell, S. D., & Spatz, D. L. (2007). Parent-infant co-sleeping and its relationship to breastfeeding. *Journal of Pediatric Health Care, 21*(1), 22-28.

Bystrova, K., Matthiesen, A. S., Vorontsov, I., Widstrom, A. M., Ransjo-Arvidson, A. B., & Uvnas-Moberg, K. (2007). Maternal axillar and breast temperature after giving birth: effects of delivery ward practices and relation to infant temperature. *Birth, 34*(4), 291-300.

Bystrova, K., Matthiesen, A. S., Widstrom, A. M., Ransjo-Arvidson, A. B., Welles-Nystrom, B., Vorontsov, I., et al. (2007). The effect of Russian Maternity Home routines on breastfeeding and neonatal weight loss with special reference to swaddling. *Early Human Development, 83*(1), 29-39.

Bystrova, K., Widstrom, A. M., Matthiesen, A. S., Ransjo-Arvidson, A. B., Welles-Nystrom, B., Vorontsov, I., et al. (2007). Early lactation performance in primiparous and multiparous women in relation to different maternity home practices. A randomised trial in St. Petersburg. *International Breastfeeding Journal, 2*, 9.

Bystrova, K., Widstrom, A. M., Matthiesen, A. S., Ransjo-Arvidson, A. B., Welles-Nystrom, B., Wassberg, C., et al. (2003). Skin-to-skin contact may reduce negative consequences of "the stress of being born": a study on temperature in newborn infants, subjected to different ward routines in St. Petersburg. *Acta Paediatrica, 92*(3), 320-326.

Cakmak, H., & Kuguoglu, S. (2007). Comparison of the breastfeeding patterns of mothers who delivered their babies per vagina and via cesarean section: an observational study using the LATCH breastfeeding charting system. *International Journal of Nursing Studies, 44*(7), 1128-1137.

Carpenter, R. G., Irgens, L. M., Blair, P. S., England, P. D., Fleming, P., Huber, J., et al. (2004). Sudden unexplained infant death in 20 regions in Europe: case control study. *Lancet, 363*(9404), 185-191.

Casey, C. E., Neifert, M. R., Seacat, J. M., & Neville, M. C. (1986). Nutrient intake by breast-fed infants during the first five days after birth. *American Journal of Diseases of Children, 140*(9), 933-936.

Chang, Z. M., & Heaman, M. I. (2005). Epidural analgesia during labor and delivery: effects on the initiation and continuation of effective breastfeeding. *Journal of Human Lactation, 21*(3), 305-314.

Chapman, D. J. (2006). Is pacifier use protective against Sudden Infant Death Syndrome. *Journal of Human Lactation, 22*(1), 129-130.

Chen, D. C., Nommsen-Rivers, L., Dewey, K. G., & Lonnerdal, B. (1998). Stress during labor and delivery and early lactation performance. *American Journal of Clinical Nutrition, 68*(2), 335-344.

Chiu, S. H., Anderson, G. C., & Burkhammer, M. D. (2005). Newborn temperature during skin-to-skin breastfeeding in couples having breastfeeding difficulties. *Birth, 32*(2), 115-121.

Chiu, S. H., Anderson, G. C., & Burkhammer, M. D. (2008). Skin-to-skin contact for culturally diverse women having breastfeeding difficulties during early postpartum. *Breastfeeding Medicine, 3*(4), 231-237.

Christensson, K., Cabrera, T., Christensson, E., Uvnas-Moberg, K., & Winberg, J. (1995). Separation distress call in the human neonate in the absence of maternal body contact. *Acta Paediatrica, 84*(5), 468-473.

Christensson, K., Siles, C., Moreno, L., Belaustequi, A., De La Fuente, P., Lagercrantz, H., et al. (1992). Temperature, metabolic adaptation and crying in healthy full-term newborns cared for skin-to-skin or in a cot. *Acta Paediatrica, 81*(6-7), 488-493.

Cloherty, M., Alexander, J., & Holloway, I. (2004). Supplementing breast-fed babies in the UK to protect their mothers from tiredness or distress. *Midwifery, 20*(2), 194-204.

Colson, S. (2005). Maternal breastfeeding positions: have we got it right? (2). *Practicing Midwife, 8*(11), 29-32.

Colson, S. (2008). *Biological Nurturing: laid-back breastfeeding*. Hythe, Kent, UK: The Nurturing Project.

Colson, S., DeRooy, L., & Hawdon, J. (2003). Biological Nurturing increases duration of breastfeeding for a vulnerable cohort. *MIDIRS Midwifery Digest, 13*(1), 92-97.

Crockenberg, S., McCluskey, K. (1986). Change in maternal behaivor during the baby's first year of life. *Child Development, 57*, 746-753.

Daly, S. E., Owens, R. A., & Hartmann, P. E. (1993). The short-term synthesis and infant-regulated removal of milk in lactating women. *Experimental Physiology, 78*(2), 209-220.

Dewey, K. G. (2001). Maternal and fetal stress are associated with impaired lactogenesis in humans. *Journal of Nutrition, 131*(11), 3012S-3015S.

Dewey, K. G., Heinig, M. J., Nommsen, L. A., & Lonnerdal, B. (1991). Adequacy of energy intake among breast-fed infants in the DARLING study: relationships to growth velocity, morbidity, and activity levels. Davis Area Research on Lactation, Infant Nutrition and Growth. *Journal of Pediatrics, 119*(4), 538-547.

Dewey, K. G., Nommsen-Rivers, L. A., Heinig, M. J., & Cohen, R. J. (2003). Risk factors for suboptimal infant breastfeeding behavior, delayed onset of lactation, and excess neonatal weight loss. *Pediatrics, 112*(3 Pt 1), 607-619.

DiGirolamo, A. M., Grummer-Strawn, L. M., & Fein, S. B. (2008). Effect of maternity-care practices on breastfeeding. *Pediatrics, 122 Suppl 2*, S43-49.

Doan, T., Gardiner, A., Gay, C. L., & Lee, K. A. (2007). Breast-feeding increases sleep duration of new parents. *Journal of Perinatal and Neonatal Nursing, 21*(3), 200-206.

Edmond, K. M., Zandoh, C., Quigley, M. A., Amenga-Etego, S., Owusu-Agyei, S., & Kirkwood, B. R. (2006). Delayed breastfeeding initiation increases risk of neonatal mortality. *Pediatrics, 117*(3), e380-386.

Elias, M. F., Nicolson, N. A., Bora, C., & Johnston, J. (1986). Sleep/wake patterns of breast-fed infants in the first 2 years of life. *Pediatrics, 77*(3), 322-329.

Evans, K. C., Evans, R. G., Royal, R., Esterman, A. J., & James, S. L. (2003). Effect of caesarean section on breast milk transfer to the normal term newborn over the first week of life. *Archives of Disease in Childhood. Fetal and Neonatal Edition, 88*(5), F380-382.

Ezzo, G., & Bucknam, R. (2006). *On becoming babywise.* Sisters, OR: Parent-Wise Solutions, Inc.

Ferber, R. (2006). *Solve your child's sleep problems.* London, England: Dorling Kindersley.

Ferber, S. G., Kuint, J., Weller, A., Feldman, R., Dollberg, S., Arbel, E., et al. (2002). Massage therapy by mothers and trained professionals enhances weight gain in preterm infants. *Early Human Development, 67*(1-2), 37-45.

Ferber, S. G., & Makhoul, I. R. (2004). The effect of skin-to-skin contact (kangaroo care) shortly after birth on the neurobehavioral responses of the term newborn: a randomized, controlled trial. Pediatrics, 113(4), 858-865.

Field, T., Ignatoff, E., Stringer, S., Brennan, J., Greenberg, R., Widmayer, S., et al. (1982). Nonnutritive sucking during tube feedings: effects on preterm neonates in an intensive care unit. *Pediatrics, 70*(3), 381-384.

Franco, P., Seret, N., Van Hees, J. N., Scaillet, S., Groswasser, J., & Kahn, A. (2005). Influence of swaddling on sleep and arousal characteristics of healthy infants. *Pediatrics, 115*(5), 1307-1311.

Galligan, M. (2006). Proposed guidelines for skin-to-skin treatment of neonatal hypothermia. MCN; *American Journal of Maternal Child Nursing, 31*(5), 298-304; quiz 305-296.

Gartner, L. M., Morton, J., Lawrence, R. A., Naylor, A. J., O'Hare, D., Schanler, R. J., et al. (2005). Breastfeeding and the use of human milk. *Pediatrics, 115*(2), 496-506.

Gay, C. L., Lee, K. A., & Lee, S. Y. (2004). Sleep patterns and fatigue in new mothers and fathers. *Biological Research for Nursing, 5*(4), 311-318.

Grajeda, R., & Perez-Escamilla, R. (2002). Stress during labor and delivery is associated with delayed onset of lactation among urban Guatemalan women. *Journal of Nutrition, 132*(10), 3055-3060.

Grether, J.K., Schulman, J., & Croen, L.A. (1990). Sudden infant death syndrome among Asians in California. *The Journal of Pediatrics, 116*(4), 525-528.

Haisma, H., Wells, J. C., Coward, W. A., Filho, D. D., Victora, C. G., Vonk, R. J., et al. (2005). Complementary feeding with cow's milk alters sleeping metabolic rate in breast-fed infants. *Journal of Nutrition, 135*(8), 1889-1895.

Hartmann, P. E. (2007). Mammary gland: Past, present, and future. In T. W. Hale & P. E. Hartmann (Eds.), *Hale & Hartmann's textbook of human lactation.* Amarillo, TX: Hale Publishing.

Hauck, F. R., Omojokun, O. O., & Siadaty, M. S. (2005). Do pacifiers reduce the risk of sudden infant death syndrome? A meta-analysis. *Pediatrics, 116*(5), e716-723.

Hauck, Y. L., Summers, L., White, E., & Jones, C. (2008). A qualitative study of Western Australian women's perceptions of using a Snoezelen room for breastfeeding during their postpartum hospital stay. *International Breastfeeding Journal, 3*, 20.

Heinig, M. J., & Banuelos, J. (2006). American Academy of Pediatrics task force on sudden infant death syndrome (SIDS) statement on SIDS reduction: friend or foe of breastfeeding? *Journal of Human Lactation, 22*(1), 7-10.

Heinig, M. J., Nommsen, L. A., Peerson, J. M., Lonnerdal, B., & Dewey, K. G. (1993). Energy and protein intakes of breast-fed and formula-fed infants during the first year of life and their association with growth velocity: the DARLING Study. *American Journal of Clinical Nutrition, 58*(2), 152-161.

Henderson, J. J., Dickinson, J. E., Evans, S. F., McDonald, S. J., & Paech, M. J. (2003). Impact of intrapartum epidural analgesia on breast-feeding duration. *Australian and New Zealand Journal of Obstetrics and Gynaecology, 43*(5), 372-377.

Hennart, P., Delogne-Desnoeck, J., Vis, H., & Robyn, C. (1981). Serum levels of prolactin and milk production in women during a lactation period of thirty months. *Clinical Endocrinology, 14*(4), 349-353.

Horne, R. S., Parslow, P. M., Ferens, D., Watts, A. M., & Adamson, T. M. (2004). Comparison of evoked arousability in breast and formula fed infants. *Archives of Disease in Childhood, 89*(1), 22-25.

Hornell, A., Aarts, C., Kylberg, E., Hofvander, Y., & Gebre-Medhin, M. (1999). Breastfeeding patterns in exclusively breastfed infants: a longitudinal prospective study in Uppsala, Sweden. *Acta Paediatrica, 88*(2), 203-211.

Horsley, T., Clifford, T., Barrowman, N., Bennett, S., Yazdi, F., Sampson, M., et al. (2007). Benefits and harms associated with the practice of bed sharing: a systematic review. *Archives of Pediatrics and Adolescent Medicine, 161*(3), 237-245.

Host, A., Husby, S., & Osterballe, O. (1988). A prospective study of cow's milk allergy in exclusively breast-fed infants. Incidence, pathogenetic role of early inadvertent exposure to cow's milk formula, and characterization of bovine milk protein in human milk. *Acta Paediatrica Scandinavica, 77*(5), 663-670.

Houston, M. J., Howie, P. W., & McNeilly, A. S. (1983). Factors affecting the duration of breast feeding: 1. Measurement of breast milk intake in the first week of life. *Early Human Development, 8*(1), 49-54.

Howard, C. R., Howard, F. M., Lanphear, B., deBlieck, E. A., Eberly, S., & Lawrence, R. A. (1999). The effects of early pacifier use on breastfeeding duration. *Pediatrics, 103*(3), E33.

Howard, C. R., Howard, F. M., Lanphear, B., Eberly, S., deBlieck, E. A., Oakes, D., et al. (2003). Randomized clinical trial of pacifier use and bottle-feeding or cupfeeding and their effect on breastfeeding. *Pediatrics, 111*(3), 511-518.

Ingram, J., Hunt, L., Woolridge, M., & Greenwood, R. (2004). The association of progesterone, infant formula use and pacifier use with the return of menstruation in breastfeeding women: a prospective cohort study. *European Journal of Obstetrics, Gynecology, and Reproductive Biology, 114*(2), 197-202.

Ingram, J. C., Woolridge, M. W., Greenwood, R. J., & McGrath, L. (1999). Maternal predictors of early breast milk output. *Acta Paediatrica, 88*(5), 493-499.

Ip, S., Chung, M., Raman, G., Chew, P., Magula, N., DeVine, D., et al. (2007). Breastfeeding and maternal and infant health outcomes in developed countries. *Evidence Report - Technology Assessment (Full Report)*(153), 1-186.

Jonas, W., Nissen, E., Ransjo-Arvidson, A. B., Wiklund, I., Henriksson, P., & Uvnas-Moberg, K. (2008). Short- and long-term decrease of blood pressure in women during breastfeeding. *Breastfeeding Medicine, 3*(2), 103-109.

Jordan, S., Emery, S., Bradshaw, C., Watkins, A., & Friswell, W. (2005). The impact of intrapartum analgesia on infant feeding. *British Journal of Obstetrics and Gynaecology, 112*(7), 927-934.

Jordan, S., Emery, S., Watkins, A., Evans, J. D., Storey, M., & Morgan, G. (2009). Associations of drugs routinely given in labour with breastfeeding at 48 hours: analysis of the Cardiff Births Survey. *British Journal of Obstetrics and Gynaecology, 116*(12), 1622-1629; discussion 1630-1622.

Keane, V., et al. (1988). Do solids help baby sleep through the night? *American Journal of Diseases of Children, 142*, 404-405.

Keefe, M. R. (1988). The impact of infant rooming-in on maternal sleep at night. *Journal of Obstetrics, Gynecologic, and Neonatal Nursing, 17*(2), 122-126.

Kennedy, K. I. (2010). Fertility, sexuality, and contraception during lactation. In J. Riordan & K. Wambach (Eds.), *Breastfeeding and human lactation* (4th ed., pp. 705-736). Boston, MA: Jones and Bartlett.

Kent, J. C. (2007). How breastfeeding works. *Journal of Midwifery & Women's Health, 52*(6), 564-570.

Kent, J. C., Mitoulas, L., Cox, D. B., Owens, R. A., & Hartmann, P. E. (1999). Breast volume and milk production during extended lactation in women. *Experimental Physiology, 84*(2), 435-447.

Kent, J. C., Mitoulas, L. R., Cregan, M. D., Ramsay, D. T., Doherty, D. A., & Hartmann, P. E. (2006). Volume and frequency of breastfeedings and fat content of breast milk throughout the day. *Pediatrics, 117*(3), e387-395.

Kirsten, G. F., Bergman, N. J., & Hann, F. M. (2001). Kangaroo mother care in the nursery. *Pediatric Clinics of North America, 48*(2), 443-452.

Konner, M. (1976). Maternal care, infant behavior and development among the !Kung. In R. B. Lee & I. DeVore (Eds.), *Kalahari hunter-gatherers: studies of the !Kung San and their neighbors*. Cambridge, MA: Harvard University Press.

Konner, M., & Worthman, C. (1980). Nursing frequency, gonadal function, and birth spacing among !Kung hunter-gatherers. *Science, 207*(4432), 788-791.

Kramer, M. S., Barr, R. G., Dagenais, S., Yang, H., Jones, P., Ciofani, L., et al. (2001). Pacifier use, early weaning, and cry/fuss behavior: a randomized controlled trial. *Jounral of the American Medical Association, 286*(3), 322-326.

Kulski, J. K., Smith, M., & Hartmann, P. E. (1981). Normal and caesarian section delivery and the initiation of lactation in women. *Australian Journal of Experimental Biology and Medical Science, 59*(4), 405-412.

L'Hoir, M. P., Engelberts, A. C., van Well, G. T., Damste, P. H., Idema, N. K., Westers, P., et al. (1999). Dummy use, thumb sucking, mouth breathing and cot death. *European Journal of Pediatrics, 158*(11), 896-901.

Latz, S., Wolf, A. W., & Lozoff, B. (1999). Cosleeping in context: sleep practices and problems in young children in Japan and the United States. *Archives of Pediatrics and Adolescent Medicine, 153*(4), 339-346.

Li, R., Fein, S. B., & Grummer-Strawn, L. M. (2008). Association of breastfeeding intensity and bottle-emptying behaviors at early infancy with infants' risk for excess weight at late infancy. *Pediatrics, 122 Suppl 2*, S77-84.

Lozoff, B., & Brittenham, G. (1979). Infant care: cache or carry. *Journal of Pediatrics, 95*(3), 478-483.

Lubetzky, R., Mimouni, F. B., Dollberg, S., Salomon, M., & Mandel, D. (2007). Consistent circadian variations in creamatocrit over the first 7 weeks of lactation: a longitudinal study. *Breastfeeding Medicine, 2*(1), 15-18.

Lubianca Neto, J. F., Hemb, L., & Silva, D. B. (2006). Systematic literature review of modifiable risk factors for recurrent acute otitis media in childhood. *Jornal de Pediatria, 82*(2), 87-96.

Ludington-Hoe, S. M., Ferreira, C., Swinth, J., & Ceccardi, J. J. (2003). Safe criteria and procedure for kangaroo care with intubated preterm infants. *Journal of Obstetric, Gynecologic, and Neonatal Nursing, 32*(5), 579-588.

Ludington-Hoe, S.M., Lewis, T., Morgan, K., Cong, X., Anderson, L., Reese, S. (2006). Breast and infant temperatures with twins during shared Kangaroo Care. *Journal of Obstetrics, Gynecologic, and Neonatal Nursing, 35*(2), 223-231.

Macknin, M. L., Medendorp, S. V., & Maier, M. C. (1989). Infant sleep and bedtime cereal. *American Journal of Diseases of Children, 143*(9), 1066-1068.

Manhire, K. M., Hagan, A. E., & Floyd, S. A. (2007). A descriptive account of New Zealand mothers' responses to open-ended questions on their breast feeding experiences. *Midwifery, 23*(4), 372-381.

Marchini, G., Simoni, M. R., Bartolini, F., & Linden, A. (1993). The relationship of plasma cholecystokinin levels to different feeding routines in newborn infants. *Early Human Development, 35*(1), 31-35.

Matthiesen, A. S., Ransjo-Arvidson, A. B., Nissen, E., & Uvnas-Moberg, K. (2001). Postpartum maternal oxytocin release by newborns: effects of infant hand massage and sucking. *Birth, 28*(1), 13-19.

McKenna, J. J., Ball, H. L., & Gettler, L. T. (2007). Mother-infant cosleeping, breastfeeding and sudden infant death syndrome: what biological anthropology has discovered about normal infant sleep and pediatric sleep medicine. *American Journal of Physical Anthropology, Suppl 45*, 133-161.

McKenna, J. J., & McDade, T. (2005). Why babies should never sleep alone: a review of the co-sleeping controversy in relation to SIDS, bedsharing and breast feeding. *Paediatric Respiratory Reviews, 6*(2), 134-152.

McKenna, J. J., Mosko, S. S., & Richard, C. A. (1997). Bedsharing promotes breastfeeding. *Pediatrics, 100*(2 Pt 1), 214-219.

Medoff-Cooper, B., & Ray, W. (1995). Neonatal sucking behaviors. *Image - the Journal of Nursing Scholarship, 27*(3), 195-200.

Merten, S., Dratva, J., & Ackermann-Liebrich, U. (2005). Do baby-friendly hospitals influence breastfeeding duration on a national level? *Pediatrics, 116*(5), e702-708.

Meyer, K., & Anderson, G. C. (1999). Using kangaroo care in a clinical setting with fullterm infants having breastfeeding difficulties. *MCN; American Journal of Maternal Child Nursing, 24*(4), 190-192.

Michelsson, K., Christensson, K., Rothganger, H., & Winberg, J. (1996). Crying in separated and non-separated newborns: sound spectrographic analysis. *Acta Paediatrica, 85*(4), 471-475.

Mikiel-Kostyra, K., Mazur, J., & Boltruszko, I. (2002). Effect of early skin-to-skin contact after delivery on duration of breastfeeding: a prospective cohort study. *Acta Paediatrica, 91*(12), 1301-1306.

Milligan, R. A., Flenniken, P. M., & Pugh, L. C. (1996). Positioning intervention to minimize fatigue in breastfeeding women. *Applied Nursing Research, 9*(2), 67-70.

Modi, N., & Glover, V. (1996). Non-pharmacological reduction of hypercortisolaemia in preterm infants. *Infant Behavior and Development, 21*, 86.

Mohrbacher, N., & Kendall-Tackett, K. (2005). *Breastfeeding made simple: seven natural laws for nursing mothers*. Oakland, CA: New Harbinger Publications.

Mooncey, S. (1997). The effect of mother-infant skin-to-skin contact on plasma cortisol and beta-endorphin concentrations in preterm newborns. *Infant Behavior and Development, 20*, 553.

Moore, E. R., & Anderson, G. C. (2007). Randomized controlled trial of very early mother-infant skin-to-skin contact and breastfeeding status. *Journal of Midwifery & Women's Health, 52*(2), 116-125.

Moore, E. R., Anderson, G. C., & Bergman, N. (2007). Early skin-to-skin contact for mothers and their healthy newborn infants. *Cochrane Database of Systematic Reviews*(3), CD003519.

Morgan, K. H., Groer, M. W., & Smith, L. J. (2006). The controversy about what constitutes safe and nurturant infant sleep environments. *Journal of Obstetric, Gynecologic, and Neonatal Nursing, 35*(6), 684-691.

Morhason-Bello, I. O., Adedokun, B. O., & Ojengbede, O. A. (2009). Social support during childbirth as a catalyst for early breastfeeding initiation for first-time Nigerian mothers. *International Breastfeeding Journal, 4*, 16.

Morrison, B., Ludington-Hoe, S., Anderson, G.C. (2006). Interruptions to breastfeeding dyads on postpartum day 1 in a university hospital. *Journal of Obstetrics, Gynecologic, and Neonatal Nursing, 35*(6), 709-716.

Mountzouris, K. C., McCartney, A. L., & Gibson, G. R. (2002). Intestinal microflora of human infants and current trends for its nutritional modulation. *British Journal of Nutrition, 87*(5), 405-420.

Murray, E. K., Ricketts, S., & Dellaport, J. (2007). Hospital practices that increase breastfeeding duration: results from a population-based study. *Birth, 34*(3), 202-211.

Nakao, Y., Moji, K., Honda, S., & Oishi, K. (2008). Initiation of breastfeeding within 120 minutes after birth is associated with breastfeeding at four months among Japanese women: A self-administered questionnaire survey. *International Breastfeeding Journal, 3*, 1.

Naveed, M., Manjunath, C. S., & Sreenivas, V. (1992). An autopsy study of relationship between perinatal stomach capacity and birthweight. *Indian Journal of Gastroenterology, 11*(4), 156-158.

Nelson, E. A., Taylor, B. J., Jenik, A., Vance, J., Walmsley, K., Pollard, K., et al. (2001). International Child Care Practices Study: infant sleeping environment. *Early Human Development, 62*(1), 43-55.

Nelson, E. A., Yu, L. M., & Williams, S. (2005). International Child Care Practices study: breastfeeding and pacifier use. *Journal of Human Lactation, 21*(3), 289-295.

Neville, M. C. (1999). Physiology of lactation. *Clinics in Perinatology, 26*(2), 251-279, v.

Neville, M. C., Allen, J. C., Archer, P. C., Casey, C. E., Seacat, J., Keller, R. P., et al. (1991). Studies in human lactation: milk volume and nutrient composition during weaning and lactogenesis. *American Journal of Clinical Nutrition, 54*(1), 81-92.

Niemela, M., Pihakari, O., Pokka, T., & Uhari, M. (2000). Pacifier as a risk factor for acute otitis media: A randomized, controlled trial of parental counseling. *Pediatrics, 106*(3), 483-488.

Nissen, E., Uvnas-Moberg, K., Svensson, K., Stock, S., Widstrom, A. M., & Winberg, J. (1996). Different patterns of oxytocin, prolactin but not cortisol release during breastfeeding in women delivered by caesarean section or by the vaginal route. *Early Human Development, 45*(1-2), 103-118.

Nissen, E., Widstrom, A. M., Lilja, G., Matthiesen, A. S., Uvnas-Moberg, K., Jacobsson, G., et al. (1997). Effects of routinely given pethidine during labour on infants' developing breastfeeding behaviour. Effects of dose-delivery time interval and various concentrations of pethidine/norpethidine in cord plasma. *Acta Paediatrica, 86*(2), 201-208.

Odent, M. (2008). *Birth and breastfeeding: rediscovering the needs of women during pregnancy and childbirth*. London, England: Rudolf Steiner Press.

Ollila, P., Niemela, M., Uhari, M., & Larmas, M. (1997). Risk factors for colonization of salivary lactobacilli and Candida in children. *Acta Odontologica Scandinavica, 55*(1), 9-13.

Patel, R. R., Liebling, R. E., & Murphy, D. J. (2003). Effect of operative delivery in the second stage of labor on breastfeeding success. *Birth, 30*(4), 255-260.

Ponsonby, A. L., Dwyer, T., Gibbons, L. E., Cochrane, J. A., & Wang, Y. G. (1993). Factors potentiating the risk of sudden infant death syndrome associated with the prone position. *New England Journal of Medicine, 329*(6), 377-382.

Prentice, A. (1989). Evidence for local feedback control of human milk secretion. . *Biochem Soc Trans, 17*, 489-492.

Quillin, S. I., & Glenn, L. L. (2004). Interaction between feeding method and co-sleeping on maternal-newborn sleep. *Journal of Obstetric, Gynecologic, and Neonatal Nursing, 33*(5), 580-588.

Radzyminski, S. (2003). The effect of ultra low dose epidural analgesia on newborn breastfeeding behaviors. *Journal of Obstetric, Gynecologic, and Neonatal Nursing, 32*(3), 322-31.

Ransjo-Arvidson, A. B., Matthiesen, A. S., Lilja, G., Nissen, E., Widstrom, A. M., & Uvnas-Moberg, K. (2001). Maternal analgesia during labor disturbs newborn behavior: effects on breastfeeding, temperature, and crying. *Birth, 28*(1), 5-12.

Rasmussen, K. M. (2007). Maternal obesity and the outcome of breastfeeding. In T. W. Hale & P. E. Hartmann (Eds.), *Hale & Hartmann's textbook of human lactation* (pp. 387-402). Amarillo, TX: Hale Publishing.

Righard, L. (1998). Are breastfeeding problems related to incorrect breastfeeding technique and the use of pacifiers and bottles? *Birth, 25*(1), 40-44.

Righard, L., & Alade, M. O. (1990). Effect of delivery room routines on success of first breast-feed. Lancet, 336(8723), 1105-1107.

Riordan, J., Gross, A., Angeron, J., Krumwiede, B., & Melin, J. (2000). The effect of labor pain relief medication on neonatal suckling and breastfeeding duration. *Journal of Human Lactation, 16*(1), 7-12.

Rosenberg, K. D., Stull, J. D., Adler, M. R., Kasehagen, L. J., & Crivelli-Kovach, A. (2008). Impact of hospital policies on breastfeeding outcomes. *Breastfeeding Medicine, 3*(2), 110-116.

Rovers, M. M., Numans, M. E., Langenbach, E., Grobbee, D. E., Verheij, T. J., & Schilder, A. G. (2008). Is pacifier use a risk factor for acute otitis media? A dynamic cohort study. *Family Practice, 25*(4), 233-236.

Sahin, F., Aktürk, A., Beyazova, U., Cakir, B., Boyunaga, O., Tezcan, S., et al. (2004). Screening for developmental dysplasia of the hip: results of a 7-year follow-up study. *Pediatrics International, 46*(2), 162-166.

Saint, L., Smith, M., & Hartmann, P. E. (1984). The yield and nutrient content of colostrum and milk of women from giving birth to 1 month post-partum. *British Journal of Nutrition, 52*(1), 87-95.

Scammon, R. E., Doyle, L.O. (1920). Observations on the capacity of the stomach in the first ten days of postnatal life. *American Journal of Diseases of Children, 20*, 516-538.

Sepkoski, C. M., Lester, B. M., Ostheimer, G. W., & Brazelton, T. B. (1992). The effects of maternal epidural anesthesia on neonatal behavior during the first month. *Developmental Medicine and Child Neurology, 34*(12), 1072-1080.

Shrago, L. C., Reifsnider, E., & Insel, K. (2006). The Neonatal Bowel Output Study: indicators of adequate breast milk intake in neonates. *Pediatric Nursing, 32*(3), 195-201.

Sio, J. O., Minwalla, F. K., George, R. H., & Booth, I. W. (1987). Oral candida: is dummy carriage the culprit? *Archives of Disease in Childhood, 62*(4), 406-408.

Smith, L. (2008). Why Johnny can't suck: Impact of birth practices on infant suck. In C. W. Genna (Ed.), *Supporting sucking skills in breastfeeding infants* (pp. 57-77). Boston, MA: Jones and Bartlett.

Smith, L. J. (2010). *Impact of birthing practices on breastfeeding* (2nd ed.). Boston, MA: Jones and Bartlett.

Sozmen, M. (1982). Effects of early suckling o cesarean-born babies on lactation. *Biology of the Neonate, 62*, 67-68.

St James-Roberts, I., Alvarez, M., Csipke, E., Abramsky, T., Goodwin, J., & Sorgenfrei, E. (2006). Infant Crying and Sleeping in London, Copenhagen and When Parents Adopt a "Proximal" Form of Care. *Pediatrics, 117*(6), e1146-1155.

Stern, G., & Kruckman, L. (1983). Multi-disciplinary perspectives on post-partum depression: an anthropological critique. *Social Science and Medicine, 17*(15), 1027-1041.

Stettler, N., Stallings, V. A., Troxel, A. B., Zhao, J., Schinnar, R., Nelson, S. E., et al. (2005). Weight gain in the first week of life and overweight in adulthood: a cohort study of European American subjects fed infant formula. *Circulation, 111*(15), 1897-1903.

Stuart-Macadam, P. (1995). Breastfeeding in prehistory. In P. Stuart-Macadam & K. A. Dettwyler (Eds.), *Breastfeeding: biocultural perspectives* (pp. 75-99). New York, NY: Aldine de Gruyter.

Svensson, K., Matthiesen, A. S., & Widstrom, A. M. (2005). Night rooming-in: who decides? An example of staff influence on mother's attitude. *Birth, 32*(2), 99-106.

Tappin, D., Ecob, R., & Brooke, H. (2005). Bedsharing, roomsharing, and sudden infant death syndrome in Scotland: a case-control study. *The Journal of Pediatrics, 147*(1), 32-37

Taveras, E. M., Scanlon, K. S., Birch, L., Rifas-Shiman, S. L., Rich-Edwards, J. W., & Gillman, M. W. (2004). Association of breastfeeding with maternal control of infant feeding at age 1 year. *Pediatrics, 114*(5), e577-583.

Thomas, K. A., & Foreman, S. W. (2005). Infant sleep and feeding pattern: effects on maternal sleep. *Journal of Midwifery & Women's Health, 50*(5), 399-404.

Torvaldsen, S., Roberts, C. L., Simpson, J. M., Thompson, J. F., & Ellwood, D. A. (2006). Intrapartum epidural analgesia and breastfeeding: a prospective cohort study. *International Breastfeeding Journal, 1*, 24.

Ullah, S., & Griffiths, P. (2003). Does the use of pacifiers shorten breastfeeding duration in infants? *British Journal of Community Nursing, 8*(10), 458-463.

Uvnas-Moberg, K. (2003). The oxytocin factor: tapping the hormone of calm, love, and healing. Cambridge, MA: Da Capo Press.

Uvnas-Moberg, K., Widstrom, A.-M., Nissen, E., & Bjorvell, H. (1990). Personality traits in women 4 days postpartum and their correlation with plasma levels of oxytocin and prolactin. *Journal of Psychosomatic Obstetrics and Gynaecology, 11*(4), 261-273.

van Gestel, J. P., L'Hoir, M. P., ten Berge, M., Jansen, N. J., & Plotz, F. B. (2002). Risks of ancient practices in modern times. *Pediatrics, 110*(6), e78.

van Sleuwen, B. E., Engelberts, A. C., Boere-Boonekamp, M.M., Kuis, W., Schulpen, T.W., & L'Hoir, M.P. (2007). Swaddling: a systemic review. *Pediatrics, 120*(4), e1097-1106.

Victora, C. G., Behague, D. P., Barros, F. C., Olinto, M. T., & Weiderpass, E. (1997). Pacifier use and short breastfeeding duration: cause, consequence, or coincidence? *Pediatrics, 99*(3), 445-453.

Victora, C. G., Tomasi, E., Olinto, M. T., & Barros, F. C. (1993). Use of pacifiers and breastfeeding duration. *Lancet, 341*(8842), 404-406.

Vogel, A. M., Hutchison, B. L., & Mitchell, E. A. (2001). The impact of pacifier use on breastfeeding: a prospective cohort study. *Journal of Paediatrics and Child Health, 37*(1), 58-63.

Waldenström, U., & Swenson, A. (1991). Rooming-in at night in the postpartum ward. *Midwifery, 7*(2), 82-89.

Wambach, K. A. (1998). Maternal fatigue in breastfeeding primiparae during the first nine weeks postpartum. *Journal of Human Lactation, 14*(3), 219-229.

Warren, J. J., Levy, S. M., Kirchner, H. L., Nowak, A. J., & Bergus, G. R. (2001). Pacifier use and the occurrence of otitis media in the first year of life. *Pediatric Dentistry, 23*(2), 103-107.

Warren, J. J., Levy, S. M., Nowak, A. J., & Tang, S. (2000). Non-nutritive sucking behaviors in preschool children: a longitudinal study. *Pediatric Dentistry, 22*(3), 187-191.

WHO. (2003). *Integrated management of pregnancy and childbirth: Pregnancy, childbirth, postpartum & newborn care.* Geneva, Switzerland: World Health Organization.

Wiklund, I., Norman, M., Uvnas-Moberg, K., Ransjo-Arvidson, A. B., & Andolf, E. (2007). Epidural analgesia: Breast-feeding success and related factors. *Midwifery*.

Willinger, M., Ko, C. W., Hoffman, H. J., Kessler, R. C., & Corwin, M. J. (2003). Trends in infant bed sharing in the United States, 1993-2000: the National Infant Sleep Position study. *Archives of Pediatrics and Adolescent Medicine, 157*(1), 43-49.

Willis, C. E., & Livingstone, V. (1995). Infant insufficient milk syndrome associated with maternal postpartum hemorrhage. *Journal of Human Lactation, 11*(2), 123-126.

Wilson-Clay, B., & Hoover, K. (2008). *The breastfeeding atlas* (4th ed.). Manchaca, TX: LactNews Press.

Wilwerding, L. (2008). Minimize bed-sharing risks for mom and baby. *American Academy of Pediatrics' Section on Breastfeeding Newsletter*(Summer), 3.

Yamauchi, Y., & Yamanouchi, I. (1990). Breast-feeding frequency during the first 24 hours after birth in full-term neonates. *Pediatrics, 86*(2), 171-175.

Yurdakok, K., Yavuz, T., & Taylor, C. E. (1990). Swaddling and acute respiratory infections. *American Journal of Public Health, 80*(7), 873-875.

Zangen, S., Di Lorenzo, C., Zangen, T., Mertz, H., Schwankovsky, L., & Hyman, P. E. (2001). Rapid maturation of gastric relaxation in newborn infants. *Pediatric Research, 50*(5), 629-632.

Zardetto, C. G., Rodrigues, C. R., & Stefani, F. M. (2002). Effects of different pacifiers on the primary dentition and oral myofunctional strutures of preschool children. *Pediatric Dentistry, 24*(6), 552-560.

Challenges at the Breast

Chapter 3

SAFEGUARDING BREASTFEEDING

A variety of difficulties can make breastfeeding challenging, such as when a baby takes the breast, but doesn't settle and feed contentedly or when he breastfeeds well at some feedings, but not at others. Among the most challenging is the baby who consistently refuses the breast. These and other feeding problems can usually be overcome, but to safeguard breastfeeding, first the baby must be fed, the mother's milk production must be protected, and some careful detective work must be done to find the cause.

Challenges at the breast include many different types of feeding problems.

When a mother can easily soothe and satisfy her baby, her self-confidence is enhanced. The opposite is also true. Struggles with breastfeeding undermine a mother's feelings of competence and self-worth, as well as her desire to continue breastfeeding. One Canadian study found that no matter what the baby's age the less control mothers felt they had over breastfeeding, the weaker their intentions to continue and the earlier they weaned (Rempel, 2004). In one U.S. study, a mother's overall satisfaction with breastfeeding was tied in part to her infant's satisfaction, with babies rated as "unsettled" at the breast lowering a mother's overall satisfaction score, which was associated with earlier weaning (Isabella & Isabella, 1994). Another U.S. study of 288 women reported that during the first 12 weeks after birth "Mothers who discontinued exclusive breastfeeding were more likely to have experienced problems with their infant latching on or sucking..." (Taveras et al., 2004, p. e283).

Difficult breastfeeding and breast refusal are stressful and demoralizing to a mother and can lead to premature weaning.

Feeding problems can increase mothers' stress levels and lead to premature weaning.

When there are feeding problems, a mother's feelings may run high. She may be frustrated and upset. She may be worried that her baby's behavior means he is rejecting her. She may worry about her ability to care for her baby. She may feel anxious about her baby's health. She may feel guilty, believing that her baby's behavior is somehow her fault or that she has not given her baby good care. She may feel like a failure.

Giving the mother an outlet to express her worries, fears, and doubts may make it easier for her to discuss and evaluate her situation. Assure her that her baby needs her now more than ever, that there are reasons for her baby's behavior, and that the problem can likely be overcome.

Feed the Baby

Gather some basic information to determine whether supplements may be needed.

Ask the mother her baby's age, weight, diaper output, and how many times each day breastfeeding goes well and at which feedings. One of the mother's first concerns is likely to be how to make sure her baby gets the milk he needs. This and her comfort should be the top priorities. The specifics will determine how this is done. For example, the needs of a 10-month-old baby on a nursing strike may be met with expressed milk in a cup along with solid foods, while his mother expresses milk to keep herself comfortable and works to get him back to the breast.

Because being stressed by hunger can weaken a baby and compromise his effectiveness at the breast, in some situations part of getting breastfeeding going smoothly may involve feeding the baby either expressed milk or a substitute. The strategy of withholding milk until the baby "gets hungry enough" will put some babies at risk for dehydration.

There are several ways to gauge whether the baby needs a supplement. The most reliable is the baby's weight gain. For healthy weight gain by age, see p. 205- Table 6.1 in "Weight Gain and Growth"] and see also p. 234 for "When and How to Supplement."

Food for the baby and mother's comfort should be the top priorities.

A less reliable gauge of milk intake—but one that can be helpful in combination with weight checks—is diaper output. In the first week of life, some aspects of diaper output can provide good clues about whether the baby is receiving the milk he needs. A transition to yellow stools by Day 6 or earlier was associated with acceptable levels of weight loss and earlier weight gain (Shrago, Reifsnider, & Insel, 2006). Day 4 breastfeeding *inadequacy* was predicted by less than three stools per day along with the mother's perception that her milk had not yet increased within 72 hours postpartum (Nommsen-Rivers, Heinig, Cohen, & Dewey, 2008). However, breastfeeding was actually going well with 41% of the mothers with these indicators.

Although diaper output is not as accurate as weight gain in determining whether a baby is getting enough milk, it can be used as a rough gauge between weight checks. During the first 6 weeks or so, daily stool output can be a helpful sign of whether milk intake is adequate. An average is at least four stools the diameter of a U.S. quarter (2.5 cm) or larger (Shrago et al., 2006). If the baby is having fewer stools but gaining weight well, this is not a problem. After 6 weeks of age, stool count is no longer reliable because many breastfeeding babies have fewer stools, even when getting plenty of milk. For more details, see p. 214- "Other Signs of Milk Intake."

• •

If the baby needs to be supplemented, offer to discuss the feeding options available.

A variety of feeding methods are available for young babies, including spoon, cup, bowl, eyedropper, at-breast supplementer, feeding bottle, and others. Ask if the mother would like to discuss them. If so, see p. 811- "Alternative Feeding Methods" in Appendix B, and support the mother's choice. If the baby is older than 6 to 8 months, the mother may be able to give expressed milk in a cup. The best supplement is nearly always mother's milk. If that is not available, suggest the mother consult with her baby's healthcare provider. See also on p. 234- "When and How to Supplement."

Protect Mother's Milk Production

If a newborn is refusing the breast, encourage the mother to express her milk effectively at least eight times per day.

If a baby is not breastfeeding or breastfeeding well, milk expression can help a mother keep herself comfortable and establish or maintain her milk production. How often she needs to express and what method she uses will depend upon her situation. For a newborn who is not breastfeeding at all or breastfeeding ineffectively, expressing milk at least eight times per day is as often as her baby would be breastfeeding. Especially during the first 2 weeks postpartum, encourage the mother to express frequently to activate her prolactin receptors, which is vital to ample milk production in the long term (de Carvalho, 1983). For more specifics, see p. 394- "Hormone Levels and Receptors" and p. 466- "Establishing Full Milk Production After Birth."

If the baby is breastfeeding well at some feedings, tailor her expression plan to the need.

Each situation will be different and requires a different milk-expression plan. How often to suggest the mother express her milk will depend on her baby's age, the number of times per day he is feeding well, her milk production, and her baby's weight. Table 3.1 describes how much milk, on average, babies take per day and per feeding by age. Discuss the specifics of the mother's situation and help her calculate how much expressed milk her baby needs. Assure her that when breastfeeding is going well, her baby will likely be able to maintain her milk production without the need for milk expression.

Table 3.1. Milk Intake by Age

Baby's Age	Average Milk Per Feeding	Average Milk Per Day
First week (after Day 4)	1-2 oz. (30-60 mL)	10-20 oz. (300-600 mL)
Weeks 2 and 3	2-3 oz. (60-90 mL)	15-25 oz. (450-750 mL)
Months 1-6	3-4 oz. (90-160 mL)	25-35 oz. (750-1035 mL)

(Mohrbacher & Kendall-Tackett, 2005, pp. 99-100)

If the feeding difficulties started after the mother's milk production was well established, she may be able to express less often to maintain production.

The number of times per day the mother needs to express to maintain milk production depends on her breast storage capacity. For details, see p. 473-"Maintaining Full Milk Production."

FEEDING PROBLEMS IN THE EARLY WEEKS

Gathering Basic Information

Before making suggestions for a feeding problem, first try to determine the cause(s).

Determining the cause(s) will help determine the strategy that will be most effective. Babies with a medical problem—such as ear infection or thrush—may need diagnosis and treatment. If distractibility is the primary cause, minimizing distractions may be the best approach. For the baby who's teething, comfort measures may help. If a mother is engorged, the first step may be to use Reverse Pressure Softening (see Appendix A, "Techniques") before putting baby to breast and breastfeeding more often. The baby who struggles with a fast milk flow may find a change to a laid-back breastfeeding position makes it easier for him to manage the milk flow.

Some situations require time, patience, and specialized information, such as a poor fit between mother's nipple size and baby's mouth or feeding problems caused by prematurity, unusual oral anatomy, pain from birth injuries, reflux disease, breathing problems, neurological issues, sensory processing problems, or other health issues.

In some cases, such as when mother or baby is emotionally upset, tincture of time and some common-sense suggestions may be all that are needed. Occasionally, an allergy, hypersensitivity, or intolerance to a food, drug, perfume, or other product may be the trigger. In this case, experimentation with diet or products may bring improvement. In a few cases, the cause of the feeding problem may never be determined.

When an obvious issue is identified, it can be tempting to assume that addressing it will lead to settled breastfeeding. But sometimes more than one factor is at work. When a strategy is tried and improvement is seen, be sure the baby is truly breastfeeding well before assuming the problem is completely resolved. More detective work may be needed.

Ask questions in a calm, relaxed manner and affirm the mother for what she is doing right.

Asking questions in a calm, relaxed manner rather than in quick succession will help put the mother at ease. Try to word sensitive questions as tactfully as possible. Make sure the mother knows that not all of the factors discussed will cause breastfeeding problems. Individual differences in mothers and babies result in a wide range of reactions to the same factor. For example, a baby who easily coordinates sucking, swallowing, and breathing may be able to cope well with his mother's overabundant milk production, while another baby who is not as well-coordinated may find his mother's milk flow overwhelming and refuse the breast. One baby may breastfeed well no matter what foods his mother eats, while another baby may be sensitive to foods in his mother's diet. One baby is easygoing and resilient, while another baby fusses or refuses the breast whenever household stress runs high.

The intensity of a baby's response may also vary with the same factor, causing one baby to fuss at the breast and another baby to refuse the breast altogether. To make the mother less likely to blame herself for the breastfeeding problem, emphasize these individual differences, which also explain why many mothers notice breastfeeding differences from one child to the next. There are general breastfeeding dynamics at work, but there are no hard-and-fast rules.

Ask questions in a calm, relaxed manner rather than in quick succession.

Because a mother whose baby is struggling with breastfeeding likely feels vulnerable, be sure to affirm her for what she is doing right and for her efforts to overcome her problem.

Ask the baby's age now, his age when the breastfeeding difficulties started, and at what point in the breastfeeding the problem starts.

Knowing at what age the breastfeeding problem started provides a good starting point and valuable clues to the causes(s) of the problem. See Table 3.2 for an overview of feeding problems starting at birth and Table 3.3 for an overview of feeding problems that start from Day 2 to 5. Knowing when during the breastfeeding the problem starts may also help in determining the cause.

Problem starts before milk ejection. Consider:

- Positioning issues causing discomfort or shallow breastfeeding
- Shallow breastfeeding caused by positioning issues or taut breast tissue
- Pain from a birth injury, medical procedure, or other cause
- Unusual oral anatomy in the baby

- Health problems, such as prematurity, respiratory issues, sensory processing problems or neurological impairment

Problem starts at milk ejection. If the baby coughs or gasps when the mother's milk ejects, he may have problems coping with her milk flow. In this case, suggest the mother try feeding in a semi-reclined position with baby tummy down on her body. Other contributing factors could be overabundant milk production, unusual oral anatomy, breathing problems, sensory processing problems, or neurological impairment.

Problem starts later in the feeding. If the baby gets fussier and fussier as the feeding goes on, the baby may simply need to burp or pass a stool. Consider the need to burp when the baby gulps loudly as he breastfeeds, which may indicate he's swallowing air. Babies who swallow incorrectly also have more difficulty as the feeding progresses and their airway becomes wetter. Babies with neurological, cardiac, or respiratory issues fatigue easily and perform more poorly as the feeding goes on.

Table 3.2. Factors Contributing to Feeding Problems That Start at Birth

Less-Than-Optimal Breastfeeding Dynamics

- Postpartum practices that interfere with inborn feeding behaviors (see "Rhythms" chapter), such as labor medications and mother-baby separation
- Positioning issues and/or shallow breastfeeding (latch)
- Poor fit (large nipple/small mouth)

Baby Factors

- Pain from birth injuries
- Breast aversion from rough suctioning or rough handling at breast
- Unusual oral anatomy
- Sensory processing problems
- Neurological impairment
- Health problems (i.e., cardiac defect, Down syndrome, illness, etc.)

Mother Factors

- Taut breast tissue
- Unusual nipple or breast anatomy

Table 3.3. Factors Contributing to Feeding Problems That Start on Days 2-5

Baby Factors

- Inability to cope with increased milk flow due to oral anatomy, such as tongue tie, breathing problems, or other health issues
- Pain from circumcision or any other medical procedure

Mother Factors

- Newly taut breast tissue from edema (due to excess IV fluids), breast fullness from increased milk production, and/or engorgement
- Delay in milk production, baby is stressed by hunger (weight loss ≥10%)
- Fast milk flow from overabundant milk production, which overwhelms baby

Mother-Baby Dynamics

Positioning

Ask the mother what feeding positions she uses.

Breastfeeding can be more challenging in the early weeks if a mother sits upright or lies on her side because gravity pulls the baby's body away from hers. This is not an issue for the older baby who has more coordination and head-and-neck control. A newborn, however, needs much more help in these positions. His mother must keep his body pressed against hers and keep him well-aligned to the breast. When a first-time mother is unfamiliar with the help a newborn needs in these positions, this can lead to shallow breastfeeding, breast refusal, and other feeding problems (Colson, 2008; Dewey, Nommsen-Rivers, Heinig, & Cohen, 2003). U.K. research has found that when a mother leans back into a semi-reclined feeding position (at a 15° to 64° angle) and places her baby tummy down on her body for support, this more effectively triggers baby's inborn feeding behaviors and makes early breastfeeding easier (Colson, Meek, & Hawdon, 2008).

A semi-reclined feeding position may help a mother who is having feeding problems.

Suggest any mother having feeding problems try a semi-reclined feeding position and experiment by reclining at different angles and positioning her baby on her body at different angles to her breast until they find their own best fit. Some babies take the breast more easily if they are first allowed to lie for a few minutes on their mother's body in a position similar to the one they assumed in the womb (Colson, 2005). Ideally, in any position, the mother should have enough body support so that her neck and shoulders are relaxed and she can maintain the position comfortably for at least an hour. For more details, see Chapter 1, "Basic Breastfeeding Dynamics."

Ask the mother if she has nipple pain or trauma.

Nipple pain and trauma may indicate:

- Baby is breastfeeding shallowly, which may be due to positioning issues or baby's inability to draw mother's taut breast tissue deeply into his mouth.

- Baby is not moving his tongue normally during breastfeeding, due to unusual anatomy, such as a short frenulum (tongue tie), or "superficial nipple sucking" from early use of bottles and pacifiers (Righard, 1998).

Postpartum Practices

For early feeding problems, ask the mother about her birth and early breastfeeding experiences.

Interventions, such as medications during labor and delivery, aggressive suctioning after birth, the use of bottles and pacifiers, and separation of mother and baby after birth can contribute to breastfeeding difficulties in some babies. For details, see p. 55- "Birth Practices and Breastfeeding."

• •

Ask the mother if her baby has been fed by bottle or used a pacifier.

In some—but not all—cases, the use of artificial nipples can affect breastfeeding. In one Swedish study, early use of bottles and pacifiers was associated with a type of ineffective breastfeeding the researchers called "superficial nipple sucking" in 73% of the babies given artificial nipples as compared with 30% of those babies who were not (Righard, 1998). One U.S. study found that 30% of mothers whose babies received bottles in the hospital reported severe breastfeeding problems compared with 14% of those whose babies did not receive bottles (Cronenwett et al., 1992).

Pacifier or bottle use can have a negative impact on breastfeeding.

In *The Breastfeeding Atlas,* U.S. lactation consultants Barbara Wilson-Clay and Kay Hoover suggest the mother's anatomy may also play a role in a baby's response to a bottle teat or pacifier. The authors wrote: "If women have erectile nipples with good elasticity, their babies may not be vulnerable...." (Wilson-Clay & Hoover, 2008, p. 41). In other words, bottles or pacifiers may pose a greater risk of feeding problems in babies whose mothers have flat or inverted nipples. They suggest the fast flow of the bottle and the firm teat provide a "supernormal stimulus" in the baby's mouth, which may lead to feeding problems, especially for mothers with nonprotruding nipples.

The way a baby is fed by bottle may also be a factor in his response. One U.S. lactation consultant reported that if a baby is given a bottle in a similar way that he is put to breast (lips touched first, nipple inserted only after baby opens wide, etc.), bottle-feeding may not be as likely to cause feeding problems, and in some cases may even be used as a "tool to reinforce breastfeeding" (Kassing, 2002).

Poor Fit

Does one or both of the mother's nipples seem to be too large for the baby?

The term "poor fit" is used to describe a mother with very large nipples (wide and/or long) whose baby has a very small mouth. No matter how good their breastfeeding dynamics, in some cases, the baby may be able to take only the nipple in his mouth, which can lead to nipple pain and/or slow milk flow. This is considered a "mother-baby dynamics" issue because if the same mother had a larger baby with a larger mouth, breastfeeding might go smoothly. For more details, see p. 132, the later section "Large Nipples."

Baby Factors

Sleepy Baby

Ask the mother to describe her baby's wake and sleep patterns.

During the first few weeks of life, some babies spend so much time sleeping that their mothers find it difficult to breastfeed at least eight times each day. If so, suggest the following strategies:

- **Make sure baby is not too warm**. Unwrap the baby or dress in lighter clothes; an overheated baby is a sleepy baby.
- **Keep baby tummy down against mother's semi-reclined body** as much as possible, either skin-to-skin or clothed, to trigger baby's inborn feeding behaviors.s**Cluster or bunch feedings together** during baby's naturally occurring alert times.
- **Guide baby onto the breast when he is in a light sleep.** Don't wait until baby is wide awake to feed; help him onto the breast when baby moves (eyes moving under eyelids, mouth or hand movements, etc.).

U.K. research found that newborns—even late preterm newborns—can breastfeed effectively while in a light sleep. Some babies even take the breast better and feed more effectively in this state (Colson, DeRooy, & Hawdon, 2003).

Babies can feed effectively while in light sleep.

Newborns move in and out of sleep often. A long sleep stretch of up to 4 to 5 hours is not a cause for concern. Make sure the parents know that breastfed babies do not typically feed at regular intervals (Benson, 2001) and that there is no advantage to doing so. Suggest the mother count the number of feedings over a 24-hour period without worrying about the length of the intervals between feedings. Most newborns breastfeed 8 to 12 times per day (Bystrova et al., 2007; Hill, Aldag, Chatterton, & Zinaman, 2005).

• •

Ask the mother about her baby's weight and diaper output.

If a baby is not getting enough milk, eventually he will lose energy, start sleeping more, and be difficult to rouse. Be sure to rule out this cause of sleepiness by asking about baby's weight and diaper output. Although wet and soiled diapers are not a completely reliable gauge of milk intake (Nommsen-Rivers et al., 2008), this information can provide a clue to milk intake. By Day 4, four stools at least the size of a U.S. quarter (2.5 cm) per day is average (Shrago et al., 2006).

A baby who is well fed may also be sleepy, but his weight gain will be average or above and he will have good diaper output. For more details about diaper output and weight gain, see p. 215- "Other Signs of Milk Intake."

• •

Ask the mother if her baby's sleepiness began after her breasts felt firmer.

Taut breast tissue can be naturally occurring or it may be caused temporarily by increasing milk production or excess IV fluids given during labor (Cotterman, 2004). Breast firmness from excess IV fluids may occur within a day after delivery and may prolong breast engorgement for as long as 10 to 14 days (Gonik & Cotton, 1984).

If the baby's sleepiness started after the mother's breast became firm and taut between Days 2 and 5, it may be because the baby is unable to draw the firmer breast tissue deeply into his mouth (which triggers active suckling), and he may need help in the form of Reverse Pressure Softening or breast shaping. For details, see the later section "Taut Breast Tissue" and Appendix A, "Techniques."

Ask the mother if the baby goes to the breast and then quickly falls asleep.

The most common cause of babies falling asleep quickly during feedings is shallow breastfeeding. Active suckling is triggered by a combination of the feel of the breast deep in the baby's mouth and good milk flow. When a baby takes the breast shallowly, both of these triggers may be missing. Helping the baby take the breast deeper in his mouth is often all that's needed to turn a sleepy baby into an actively suckling baby. For strategies to achieve deeper breastfeeding, see Chapter 1, "Basic Breastfeeding Dynamics" and Appendix A, "Techniques."

U.K. research has found what appear to be instinctive responses in mothers during feedings that encourage more active suckling at the breast, such as stroking their baby's body and feet (Colson et al., 2008). Semi-reclined, laid-back feeding positions give mothers either one or both hands free, making it easier for them to interact with their babies at feedings.

Combining breast compression with deeper breastfeeding is another effective strategy to speed milk flow and stimulate active suckling. For details on breast compression, see Appendix A, "Techniques."

Ask the mother about her labor and birth and whether her baby is jaundiced or ill.

A difficult labor and delivery can exhaust a baby, and pain medications the mother receives during labor can sedate him, decreasing baby's alertness and making him appear less interested in breastfeeding. For details on the research on the link between some labor medications and a baby's ability to breastfeed, see p. 55- "Birth Practices and Breastfeeding."

A baby who is severely jaundiced or ill may be less alert. For details, see the chapter "Hypoglycemia and Jaundice." Ask the mother when the baby was last seen by his healthcare provider and whether he has any health issues.

Baby Stressed by Hunger

Ask the mother to describe how she and her baby breastfeed—how many feedings per day, how much time is spent at each breast—and her baby's birthweight and weight now.

If the mother breastfeeds by the clock, limiting number of feedings or limiting feeding length, and her baby's weight gain is borderline or lower than expected, her baby may not be getting enough milk and may feel stressed. When a baby is stressed by hunger, this can contribute to feeding problems, such as extreme sleepiness (see previous section), fussiness at the breast, and breast refusal. Babies feed better when they are well-nourished.

If this is an issue, the first priority is to feed the baby, either with expressed mother's milk or, if not available, substitutes recommended by the baby's healthcare provider. Next, it is important to get to the root cause of the baby's low milk intake, which could be due to low milk production in the mother (see p. 408- "Low Milk Production" or the baby's inability to breastfeed effectively (see p. 223- "Ineffective Suckling"), or both. If baby's weight gain is normal or high, consider other causes.

The first priority is to feed the baby with either expressed breastmilk or a breastmilk substitute.

Ask if either mother or baby has been diagnosed with any health problems and if either of them is taking any medications.

A variety of health problems in the mother can affect her early milk production, such as Type 1 diabetes, gestational ovarian theca lutein cysts, and hypothyroidism (which can cause low milk production at any stage of breastfeeding), as can some medications. For more details, see p. 410- Table 10.2. A baby's feeding effectiveness can also be affected by health problems, such as cardiac disease, cleft palate, Down syndrome, illness, and others (see the chapter "Health Issues—Baby").

Baby Injured or in Pain

Ask if the baby was born in an unusual position (i.e., breech, posterior, etc.) or if he suffered any birth injuries.

A long and difficult labor is stressful for both mother and baby, and may leave baby sore or uncomfortable in some or all feeding positions. If forceps were used, the baby may be bruised or have a headache or hematoma. The pain of a dislocated hip or a broken clavicle can decrease a baby's interest in feeding. Ask if the baby has been carefully examined by a healthcare professional to rule out pain or injury, especially if the baby also seems fussy much of the time.

Babies who are in pain may have difficulties breastfeeding.

If the baby has a painful physical condition that is causing difficult feedings, encourage the mother to experiment with different positions until she finds one that is more comfortable for them both. Suggest she also ask the baby's healthcare provider about giving the baby pain medication. If a comfortable feeding position cannot be found and the baby is unwilling to breastfeed, suggest the mother express her milk for the baby until the injuries have healed enough to breastfeed comfortably. For strategies for establishing full milk production with milk expression, see p. 466- "Establishing Full Milk Production after Birth."

If the baby is a boy, ask if he has been circumcised.

The pain of circumcision causes breastfeeding problems in some babies. After this procedure, a baby may have trouble settling at the breast, may refuse the breast, or may shut down and be unresponsive. If this may be the cause, suggest the mother ask her baby's healthcare provider to recommend pain medication for the baby while he recovers.

Ask if the baby keeps his head turned to one side and if her baby's lower jaw looks tilted.

U.S. research estimates that 10% of babies under 8 weeks old prefer to hold their heads to one side (Boere-Boonekamp & van der Linden-Kuiper, 2001). In some cases, this may be a sign of torticollis, from the Latin words meaning "twisted neck," which can be caused by a confined position in the womb. When a baby's neck muscles are pulled to one side, this pulls the baby's lower jaw and affects jaw development in utero, which may give it an asymmetrical look. In some cases, the baby also may be in pain (Mojab, 2007).

One U.S. article described 11 babies with asymmetrical lower jaws, whose lower gumlines looked tilted to one side rather than parallel (Wall & Glass, 2006). Ten of the 11 mothers had labor and birth complications. All had breastfeeding problems, including the babies having difficulty taking the breast, nipple pain, and ineffective feeding. Nine of the 11 babies needed supplementation. The authors suggested that feeding problems may be the first symptoms in babies with undiagnosed torticollis.

For babies with this condition, encourage the mother to experiment with different feeding positions until she finds one most comfortable for her and her baby.

They may find that the positions that work for them are very different at each breast. In some cases, the mother may need to position the baby in the same way on both breasts, simply sliding baby's body over as needed. An occupational or physical therapist can recommend therapeutic exercises to help improve the baby's range of motion.

• •

If the baby has hip dysplasia and wears a brace or cast, finding a comfortable breastfeeding position can be challenging.

Hip dysplasia occurs when a baby's hip socket did not form correctly, requiring a brace or cast to keep the thigh bone pressed into the hip socket. For this baby, unusual stress on the hip should be avoided, which makes positioning at the breast more challenging because a brace or cast may make it impossible for a s(Figure 3.1) or semi-reclined straddle position may make breastfeeding more comfortable. The mother may also find it helpful to use a pillow for support between the baby's legs (Marmet & Shell, 2008).

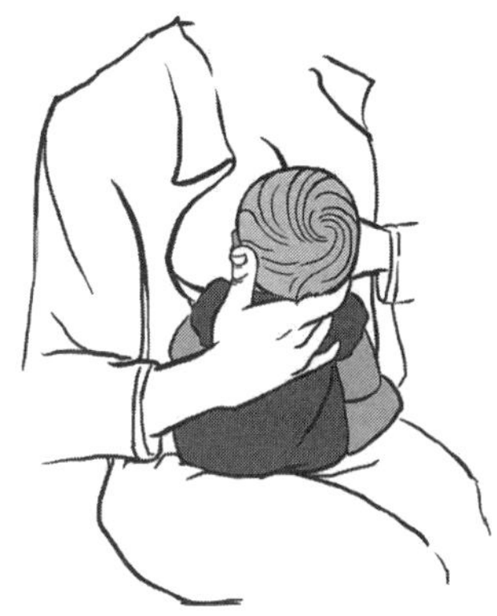

Figure 3.1. An upright straddle feeding position

©Anna Mohrbacher, used with permission

Inconsistent or Ineffective Breastfeeding

Ask the mother if during breastfeeding she can hear her baby swallow and ask about other signs of feeding effectiveness.

If a baby is not gaining weight well (or losing weight) and it is clear that he is only feeding effectively at some feedings, discuss some of the signs the mother can look for that indicate effective breastfeeding, such as the outward signs of deep breastfeeding (wide jaw angle, wiggling movement near baby's ears), swallowing sounds, increasing relaxation, and baby coming off the breast satisfied. If needed, share the following signs of possible ineffective breastfeeding:

- **No swallowing heard.** At milk ejection, most babies swallow after every one or two suckles, swallowing less and less often as the feeding progresses. Some babies breastfeed effectively, but swallow too quietly to be heard. In this case, the baby will be gaining weight well and have good diaper output.
- **Baby never seems satisfied**. The mother may say he breastfeeds "all the time."
- **Shallow breastfeeding.** When the baby breastfeeds shallowly, with the nipple in the front of his mouth (instead of farther back in the "comfort zone"), the angle of baby's jaws will appear narrow. Shallow

breastfeeding can cause slow milk flow, less milk intake, and/or difficulty staying on the breast.

- **Coughing or choking at the breast**. This can occur with very fast milk flow and also with uncoordinated sucking and swallowing or respiratory problems.
- **Low or high muscle tone.** "Floppy" babies with low tone include those with Down syndrome and other neurological impairments. Babies with high tone may be in the high-normal range or also be neurologically impaired. High-tone babies may arch away at the breast, especially if upright feeding positions are used. For breastfeeding strategies for high- and low-tone babies, see p. 309- "More Strategies for Babies with High/ Low Tone."
- **A clicking sound** at the breast usually indicates suction is being broken. If baby is gaining weight well, this is not a problem.
- **Cheek dimpling** during feedings indicates the baby's mouth is empty and can occur with or without loss of suction. Again, if the baby is gaining weight well, this is not a problem.
- **Nipple pain or trauma** can be due to shallow breastfeeding, unusual tongue movements, or anatomical variations, such as tongue tie.
- **Unrelieved breast fullness or recurring mastitis** can be due to ineffective milk removal.

If the mother can't hear her baby swallow at all, the baby's audible swallowing stops early in the feeding, or he falls asleep quickly, suggest the mother increase active breastfeeding by helping him take the breast deeper and use breast compression (for details, see Appendix A, "Techniques.") for a faster milk flow. If these don't improve breastfeeding effectiveness, try to determine possible underlying causes (see Table 3.2).

Ask the mother if the baby goes to the breast and then quickly falls asleep.

See previous section, "Sleepy Baby."

Tongue, Palate, and Other Oral Issues

Tongue issues

The tongue plays an integral part in effective breastfeeding, and baby's tongue movements are affected by both anatomy and experience.

All physical aspects of the tongue—length, symmetry, tone, frenulum—affect feeding. To suckle and swallow effectively, a baby must be able to:

- **Extend his tongue past his lower gums** to help cushion the breast for comfortable breastfeeding
- **Lift the front of his tongue to the roof of his mouth** (see Figure 3.2) to keep the breast in place
- **Lower the back of his tongue** to create the vacuum that removes the milk from the breast (Geddes, Kent, Mitoulas, & Hartmann, 2008)
- **Form a groove with his tongue** to keep the breast in place and collect the milk for easier swallowing

How much these tongue movements are restricted will determine whether or not the baby can breastfeed effectively. The ability to move the tongue from side to side (called lateralization) does not usually affect breastfeeding (Genna, 2008a), but it is important when a baby eats solid foods (Hiiemae & Palmer, 2003).

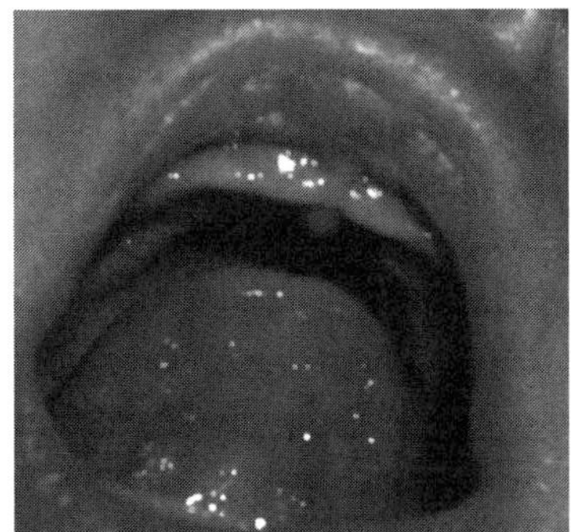

Figure 3.2. Normal tongue elevation

©2010 Catherine Watson Genna, BS, IBCLC, used with permission

How the baby chooses to move his tongue also plays a role in feedings and can be influenced by his experiences. Some babies develop an aversion to anything entering their mouths after being roughly aspirated after birth or shoved roughly to the breast. When this happens, they may use their tongue to block entry to their mouth, causing feeding problems.

• •

Ask the mother if anyone in their family is tongue-tied.

The frenulum is the string-like membrane that attaches the tongue to the floor of the mouth. A short frenulum, called tongue tie or ankyloglossia, may run in families. One U.S. study of 88 tongue-tied babies with breastfeeding problems noted a positive family history for tongue tie in 21% of the babies identified (Ballard, Auer, & Khoury, 2002). Most studies report a tongue tie incidence of 3% to 5%, with more boys affected than girls (Ballard et al., 2002; Messner, Lalakea, Aby, Macmahon, & Bair, 2000; Ricke, Baker, Madlon-Kay, & DeFor, 2005).

Also ask about a family history of speech therapy, orthodontia, and sleep apnea, which can occur with undiagnosed tongue tie (Coryllos, 2008).

• •

Tongue tie may or may not cause breastfeeding problems.

One U.S. study found that 25% of the tongue-tied babies had trouble breastfeeding (Messner et al., 2000). Literature reviews report the most common breastfeeding problems associated with tongue tie are difficulty taking or staying on the breast, nipple pain and trauma, inadequate milk intake, and continuous feedings (Hall & Renfrew, 2005; Segal, Stephenson, Dawes, & Feldman, 2007). One U.K. study of 215 tongue-tied babies *with breastfeeding problems* found (Griffiths, 2004):

- 88% had difficulty taking the breast.
- 77% of the mothers had nipple pain or trauma.
- 72% fed continuously while awake due to inadequate milk intake.
- 52% experienced all three of these symptoms.

If a short frenulum causes breastfeeding problems, they are usually obvious when breastfeeding begins. One U.S. study of 88 tongue-tied babies with breastfeeding problems reported that all the problems were apparent during their hospital stay (Ballard et al., 2002). Another U.S. study found that tongue-tied babies were three times more likely to be exclusively bottle-fed at 1 week compared with a matched control group of babies who were not tongue-tied (Ricke et al., 2005).

An Australian study of 24 tongue-tied babies having feeding problems used ultrasound to examine what occurred inside these babies' mouths during breastfeeding (Geddes, Langton et al., 2008). The researchers found that the babies fell into two groups. One group had difficulty staying on the breast and took the breast shallowly, compressing the end of the mother's nipple. The second group stayed on the breast and took the breast deeper, compressing the base of the nipple. The feeding dynamics of both groups caused nipple pain and slowed milk flow.

Ask the mother if she hears a clicking sound during breastfeeding or if her baby has trouble staying on the breast.

Both difficulty staying on the breast and a clicking sound during breastfeeding are signs a baby is unable to maintain suction at the breast and may not be taking milk effectively. Any baby who repeatedly breaks the suction during breastfeeding should be checked for a short frenulum. However, if a clicking baby is gaining weight well, otherwise feeding normally, and breastfeeding is comfortable for the mother, this is not necessarily a problem.

Ask the mother if the baby can extend his tongue past his lower gum, which is a sign of one of the four types of tongue tie.

Many feeding problems previously lumped into the category of "sucking problems" are now understood to be caused by newly identified types of tongue tie. If the baby's frenulum is short and attaches near the tongue tip and baby's gums, it may restrict the tongue and prevent it from making any of the necessary movements described in the first point of this section. The most commonly recognized type of short frenulum (type 1) pulls on the tongue tip, making it look heart-shaped rather than rounded and often prevents the baby from extending his tongue past the lower gumline.

Many feeding problems previously called "sucking problems" are now identified as types of tongue-tie.

In recent years, four distinct types of tongue tie have been identified, and many do not cause this heart-shaped appearance (Genna, 2008a). Tongue tie type is determined by where the frenulum attaches to the tongue and to the floor of the baby's mouth:

- **Type 1**. Frenulum is attached near the tip of the tongue and on or near the gumline (Figure 3.3).
- **Type 2**. Frenulum is attached 2-4 mm behind tongue tip and just behind the gumline (Figure 3.4).
- **Type 3**. Frenulum is attached to the middle of the tongue and in the middle of the floor of baby's mouth (Figure 3.5).
- **Type 4**. Frenulum is attached behind the mucous membrane of the floor of the mouth, which can make the tongue look short (Figure 3.6).

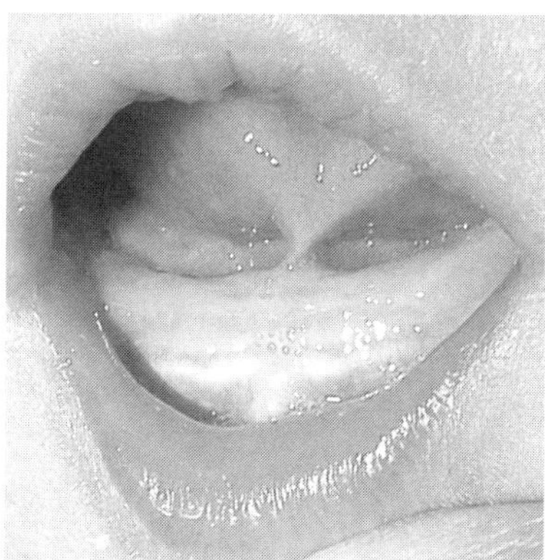

Figure 3.3. Type 1 tongue tie

©2010 Catherine Watson Genna, BS, IBCLC, used with permission

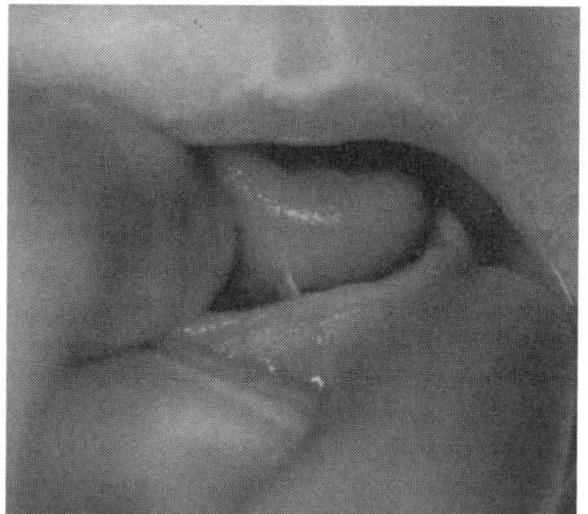

Figure 3.4. Type 2 tongue tie

©2010 Catherine Watson Genna, BS, IBCLC, used with permission

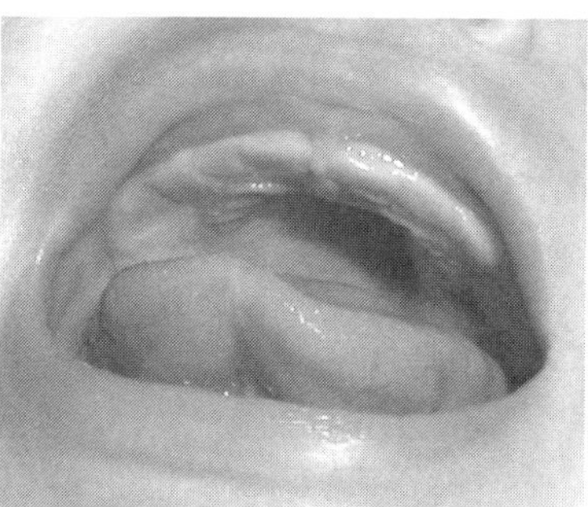

Figure 3.5. Type 3 tongue tie

©2010 Catherine Watson Genna, BS, IBCLC, used with permission

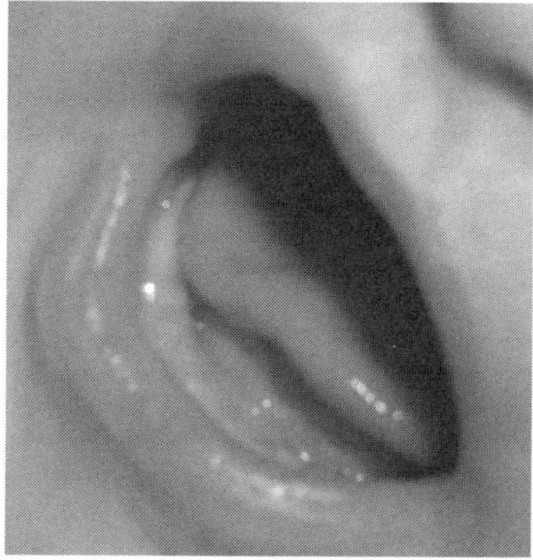

Figure 3.6. Type 4 tongue tie

©2010 Catherine Watson Genna, BS, IBCLC, used with permission

Type 3 and 4 are sometimes referred to as posterior tongue ties. Signs of posterior tongue ties include the tongue tip appearing curled down, the inability to lift the tongue to the roof of the mouth when baby opens wide, tongue twisting, a raised tongue tip while the back of the tongue appears flat, the back of the tongue looking like it's pulled down, and the tongue looking asymmetrical when raised (Genna, 2008a).

The location of the frenulum can affect the baby's ability to breastfeed, but other factors are important, too, such as the thickness, length, and stretchiness of the frenulum. The frenulum in types 1 and 2 tongue ties are usually thin and elastic, whereas in types 3 and 4, they're usually thicker and more fibrous (Genna, 2008a). One U.S. study found that 75% of the babies who had a very thick frenulum had breastfeeding problems (Messner et al., 2000).

U.S. authors Diana West and Lisa Marasco wrote about a technique they called the "Murphy Maneuver," after U.S. pediatrician James Murphy, who described how to feel for tongue tie in a baby's mouth. If the baby is willing, this can be done by "pushing your little finger to the base of the tongue on one side and sweeping it across to the other side to see what you can feel. If you feel little or no resistance more than a small 'speed bump,' then most likely there is no problem" (West & Marasco, 2009, p. 92). However, if it feels like a "tree trunk," a "fence," or a "piano wire" (when pushing it causes the tongue to curve downward and crease down the middle), these are types of short frenula that often (but not always) cause breastfeeding problems.

In many cases of tongue tie, improving breastfeeding technique will improve the comfort and effectiveness of breastfeeding.

Another factor affecting breastfeeding is the consistency of the floor of the baby's mouth, as a loose mouth floor can sometimes help compensate for a short frenulum by allowing greater tongue movement. Another important factor is the tautness or looseness of the mother's breast tissue. The same baby might do well if his mother's breast tissue is soft and pliable, but struggle if her breast becomes firm or taut.

• •

A good first strategy for a tongue tied baby having breastfeeding problems is to help him take the breast deeper in his mouth and more off-center.

In many cases of tongue tie, improving breastfeeding technique can help increase breastfeeding comfort and effectiveness. To take advantage of gravity, suggest the mother use a semi-reclined feeding position and allow the baby to take an active role in going to the breast by first triggering baby's inborn feeding behaviors. For details, see Chapter 1.

To take the breast deeply, the baby's tongue needs to be down while going onto the breast. This can be challenging because with some tongue ties, opening wide may cause the baby's tongue to retract or pull down. By allowing the baby to take his time when going to the breast and triggering inborn feeding behaviors first, a baby may be better able to organize his movements as he takes the breast.

Shaping the breast may also help the baby get a better grasp. For details, see "Breast Shaping" in Appendix A, "Techniques." If the mother is helping the baby onto the breast, encourage her to align the baby nose to nipple, so his lower jaw is as far from the nipple as possible. For details, see "Asymmetric Latch" in the "Techniques" appendix.

If effectiveness and comfort do not improve after adjusting breastfeeding technique, suggest the mother consider having her baby's frenulum clipped. This procedure, called a frenotomy, is simple, can be done in a doctor's or dentist's office, involves no stitches, and is usually done without anesthesia. Because there are few nerves and blood vessels in the frenulum, it involves little discomfort or bleeding.

If feedings are still painful or ineffective, even with better breastfeeding dynamics, discuss having the frenulum clipped.

In one U.K. study of 215 tongue-tied babies who underwent frenotomies, 18% slept through the procedure, 22% who were awake did not cry, and 60% who were crying cried more after the procedure (Griffiths, 2004). Of the babies who cried more, 44% cried for less than 5 seconds, 85% cried for less than 10 seconds, and only two babies cried for more than 1 minute. After their frenotomy, 38% had no bleeding, 52% had a few drops of blood, and 9% had a "small amount" of blood (equal to about a 1-inch or 6.25 cm area on a paper towel).

In cases where improved technique does not help, a frenotomy may be neccessary.

When looking for a healthcare provider to do a frenotomy, suggest the mother ask if they know the techniques used to identify and treat type 3 and 4 tongue ties, as they differ from those used for type 1 and 2. U.S. physician Elizabeth Coryllos provides a detailed explanation of what healthcare providers need to know to recognize and clip the posterior or "hidden" tongue ties in Chapter 9 of the book *Supporting Sucking Skills in Breastfeeding Infants* edited by Catherine Watson Genna (Coryllos, 2008).

Published in 1992, the Assessment Tool for Lingual Frenulum Function (ATLFF) was developed by Alison Hazelbaker as a way to systematically determine whether a baby would benefit from a frenotomy (Hazelbaker, 1992). This tool assigns a score to different aspects of the appearance and function of the baby's frenulum, with the function score more heavily weighted than the appearance score. In recent years, some controversy has arisen about this tool's reliability. Some found it very reliable (Amir, James, & Donath, 2006) and others found it missed many babies who would benefit from a frenotomy (Ricke et al., 2005).

One review of the research on tongue tie concluded: "The diagnosis should rest primarily on observation and analysis of feeding difficulties rather than the static appearance of the tongue" (Hall & Renfrew, 2005, p. 1215). In other words, a tongue tie alone is not reason enough to consider a frenotomy. Only if the tongue tie also causes feeding problems should it be considered.

Because performing frenotomies has fallen out of favor, a mother may have to search for a healthcare professional willing to do it. One U.S. study found that 90% of pediatricians and 70% of ear-nose-and-throat specialists believe that tongue tie rarely causes feeding problems (Messner & Lalakea, 2000). If the baby's pediatrician is unwilling to perform the frenotomy or to refer the mother to someone who will, suggest she ask breastfeeding specialists in her area if they know of healthcare providers, such as pediatricians, family practice doctors, oral surgeons, dentists, ear-nose-and-throat specialists, and general surgeons, who perform them.

After the frenulum is clipped, improvement can be expected either immediately or within a week or two.

In one Israeli study, babies received either 1) a sham procedure, then breastfed, then had an actual frenotony, and then breastfed again or 2) had an actual frenotomy, breastfed, and then had a sham procedure and breastfed again (Dollberg, Botzer, Grunis, & Mimouni, 2006). Mothers and healthcare personnel caring for the baby were blinded to what order these procedures occurred. There was a significant difference in pain scores after frenotomy, but not after the sham procedure. A U.K. study found that breastfeeding improved in 54 of the 57 babies (95%) who underwent frenotomies (Hogan, Westcott, & Griffiths, 2005). Of the 29 tongue-tied babies in the control group (who received only intensive lactation help for the first 48 hours), only one (3%) improved. Of the 57 babies who had a frenotomy, 79% of the mothers reported immediate improvement, 16% within 48 hours.

In a Canadian study of 27 tongue-tied babies with breastfeeding problems who received frenotomies, 92% of the mothers reported being pain-free after the procedure, as well as long-term, and 88% said they thought the frenotomy had helped (Srinivasan, Dobrich, Mitnick, & Feldman, 2006). An Israeli study of 25 tongue-tied babies also found a significant decrease in mothers' pain scores after frenotomy (Dollberg et al., 2006).

In an Australian study of 24 tongue-tied babies (Geddes, Langton et al., 2008), 7 days after frenotomy all 24 babies took the breast more easily, took more milk (mean feed of 51 g increased to 69 g), and the mothers reported significantly increased comfort (mean pain score of 4 of 10 reduced to 0.5). One review of the literature noted that "all studies showed an improvement in recorded outcomes after frenotomy" (Segal et al., 2007, p. 1030).

In *The Breastfeeding Atlas*, U.S. authors Barbara Wilson-Clay and Kay Hoover suggest "the longer a baby waits to have the frenotomy, the longer the period of rehabilitation" (Wilson-Clay & Hoover, 2008, p. 145).

If there are no plans to clip a baby's tongue and feeding problems continue, suggest the mother express her milk and try tongue exercises.

If the baby is not breastfeeding effectively or the mother is in so much pain she cannot breastfeed at all feedings, offer to help a mother tailor a milk-expression plan to maintain her milk production and provide milk for her baby.

If for whatever reason a frenotomy is not an option, suggest the mother try doing tongue exercises with her baby to encourage more normal tongue movements during feeding. Although tongue exercises may not be as effective as a frenotomy, they may help improve a baby's breastfeeding effectiveness over time. See Appendix A, "Techniques," for two exercises to try.

A nipple shield may help any baby with tongue issues breastfeed more effectively.

If breastfeeding is still painful or ineffective after helping the baby take the breast deeper, suggest the mother try using a silicone nipple shield at the breast. The layer of silicone over the mother's breast may make breastfeeding more comfortable. The nipple shield may also help the baby stay attached more consistently and trigger the right stimulation for more effective suckling (Wilson-Clay & Hoover, 2008, p. 15). See Appendix B, "Tools and Products" for details on choosing, fitting, and applying a nipple shield.

One U.K. study reported that 44% (95) of the mothers of its 215 tongue-tied babies tried a nipple shield with professional guidance, and it helped 41% (39) of these, or 18% of the mothers overall (Griffiths, 2004).

For the baby with a large or low-tone tongue, suggest the mother first trigger her baby's inborn feeding behaviors and allow him time to take the breast on his own.

If the baby with a large or low-tone tongue also has Down syndrome, see this section in the chapter, "Health Issues—Baby." Whatever the cause, using the feeding dynamics described in Chapter 1 will make breastfeeding easier for the baby. If he needs encouragement to keep his tongue down while taking the breast, see the tongue exercises described in Appendix A, "Techniques."

Unusual Palates

Unusual palates—high, bubble, grooved—sometimes cause feeding difficulties.

In a baby, the average (or "reference") palate is smooth and sloping. When given a finger pad side up to suck, an average baby will draw it back about 1.5 inches (3.75 cm)—near where his soft and hard palates meet—and the length of the finger will stay in contact with the palate. With a bubble palate, rather than the finger touching the entire palate, a gap (or bubble) can be felt above the finger, which may be shallow, deep, round, or oval. With a grooved palate, a thin groove runs along the length of the palate, which may cause a baby to have trouble maintaining suction at the breast.

An average palate slopes upward about 0.25 inches (0.5 cm). A high palate may cause broken suction and a clicking sound during breastfeeding. In some cases, a baby with a high or bubble palate may resist taking the breast deeply in his mouth because he is not used to having the highest part of his palate touched, and this may stimulate a gag reflex. In this case, it may help over several days to gradually help a baby adjust to normal touch on his palate by making it a pleasant game to first touch his lips, wait for an open mouth, and then gently slide a clean finger with a closely trimmed nail back along his hard palate—pad side up—stopping just before the gag reflex is triggered. By making this a happy time and gradually moving the finger further back, it can help a baby get used to this feel and overcome this sensitivity (Genna, 2008a, p. 200).

Suggest any baby with an unusual palate be checked for tongue tie.

Experienced clinicians have noticed an association between unusual palates and tongue tie. This may be because, as the baby's palate develops, it is "almost as malleable as softened wax" (Palmer, 1998, p. 96) and can be molded by tongue movements, pacifier/dummy, and bottle use, and anything else that comes in regular contact with it. For example, babies who are intubated for long periods may form grooves—or high, narrow arches—in their palates (Wilson-Clay & Hoover, 2008, p. 16; Wolf & Glass, 1992, p. 122).

Depending on size and location, a cleft—or opening—in the baby's palate can undermine effective breastfeeding.

An opening in the baby's palate can make it difficult or impossible for the baby to generate suction, which is key to transferring milk from the breast (Geddes, Kent et al., 2008). A cleft lip alone is usually less of a challenge. For details, see "Cleft Lip and/or Palate" in the chapter "Health Issues—Baby."

Other Oral Issues

A tight labial frenulum sometimes causes feeding problems.

The labial frenulum is the membrane that connects the upper lip with the gumline. One case report documented the experience of a baby who was unable to breastfeed effectively until his labial frenulum was clipped at 18 weeks of age (Wiessinger & Miller, 1995). The thick, fibrous membrane had previously prevented him from flanging back his lips during feedings, which had compromised his milk intake. In *The Breastfeeding Atlas*, a tight labial frenulum is also mentioned as being responsible for orthodontia later in life to close the gap between the top front teeth (Wilson-Clay & Hoover, 2008, p. 154).

Babies with receding chins and short tongues may find breastfeeding easier in a laid-back breastfeeding position because gravity helps pull the tongue forward.

A baby's natural feeding position is tummy down (prone) on a stable surface (Colson et al., 2008). Babies with receding chins and short tongues may find this position especially helpful because gravity helps to bring the tongue forward (Marmet & Shell, 2008). In some babies, such as those with Pierre-Robin sequence, a receding chin may be one of several issues that affect breastfeeding (Genna, 2008a).

Respiratory Issues

Ask the mother if her baby often coughs or chokes at the breast and/or makes a high-pitched "squeaky" sound.

A young baby who struggles to keep up with his mother's fast milk flow may cough or choke at the breast (see next point). If a high-pitched squeaky sound known as stridor occurs during breastfeeding or at other times, this may be a sign that the baby has a narrowed airway and is one sign of breathing problems, such as laryngomalacia (narrowing of the upper airway), tracheomalacia (narrowing of the lower airway), vocal cord paralysis, or other respiratory issues.

For effective breastfeeding, a baby needs to coordinate suckling, swallowing, and breathing. A baby with an airway malformation or instability usually breathes faster (more breaths per minute) to get the oxygen needed. Faster breathing means less time to swallow. And when a baby has to choose between breathing and eating, breathing always wins.

Baby's weight gain can help distinguish milk-flow issues from breathing issues.

When a respiratory issue compromises a baby's ability to breastfeed, this can lead to ineffective breastfeeding, struggling at the breast (coughing and gasping), and breast refusal. When babies struggle with milk flow, some assume this means the mother has overabundant milk production or "hyperlactation" (Livingstone, 1996) or "overactive let-down" (Andrusiak & Larose-Kuzenko, 1987). But babies with respiratory issues often gain weight slowly, even becoming failure-to-thrive, whereas babies of mothers with overabundant milk production usually gain weight faster than average, well above 2 pounds (900 grams) per month.

Babies with breathing problems are at higher risk for reflux disease and may benefit from treatment.

The increased airway pressure these babies generate puts them at higher risk for gastroesophageal reflux disease (GERD) (Bibi et al., 2001), which can cause painful feedings, further complicating breastfeeding. When a baby has a respiratory issue, suggest the mother have her baby evaluated by their healthcare provider for GERD, and if found, consider treatment. For more details about GERD, see p. 287- "Reflux Disease (GERD)."

Patience and positioning adjustments can make breastfeeding easier for babies with breathing problems.

Although all babies benefit when their mothers breastfeed in semi-reclined positions, these prone positions are particularly helpful in babies with breathing problems because they have more control over milk flow. Another important positioning point for these babies is to be sure their head can tilt back slightly, which extends their airway and reduces respiratory distress (Genna, 2008a). This can be done no matter what position is used by sliding the baby's body a little in the direction of his feet.

Prone feeding positions give babies with feeding problems more control over milk flow.

No matter what position is used, suggest the mother make sure her baby can release the breast whenever needed to take a break. (Avoid holding baby's head to breast.) Some of these babies are more comfortable feeding for long periods at a leisurely pace, while others prefer to feed often for a short time.

If needed, the mother can express milk and supplement.

If a baby breastfeeds ineffectively, the mother may need to safeguard her milk production by expressing milk and supplementing him with it. Due to difficulties with milk flow, if she needs to supplement, suggest she consider a specialized feeding device, such as a Haberman Feeder set to the slowest flow setting, as this may be easiest for the baby to manage.

Sensory Processing Issues

Feeding problems may be the first sign of a sensory processing issue.

Sensory processing, sometimes called sensory integration, is how we organize and interpret the information we receive from our senses. People with good sensory processing can focus on important sensory input—like the cars when crossing a street—and disregard the unimportant—like the feeling of clothing on the skin. When a baby over-responds to sensory stimulation, he may react intensely to normal touch by arching away or screaming when put down. Or a baby may be unusually unresponsive. A baby may over-respond to some senses and under-respond to others. Sensory processing issues can manifest in many ways:

- Little or no response when the baby takes the breast, even if he is on deeply
- Long feedings
- Inconsistent feedings, breastfeeding well at one feeding, but not at the next
- Gagging when the baby takes the breast deeply enough
- Ineffective breastfeeding from misreading of sensory cues in his mouth
- Intense frustration at the breast when feedings don't go well

If sensory processing issues are suspected, parents can have their child's sensory processing evaluated by an occupational or physical therapist certified in sensory processing.

Feeding strategies will vary based on whether the baby tends to over-respond or under-respond to sensory stimulation.

Most babies with sensory processing issues will breastfeed more effectively if feedings are started before they get too hungry. Babies who over-respond to stimulation may breastfeed better when (Genna, 2008b):

- Before feedings, place baby on a blanket, gather up the corners, and gently swing baby from head to foot until he relaxes and flexes his muscles (blanket swing).
- During feedings, movement is kept to a minimum (mother in a stable semi-reclined position with baby lying tummy down on her body, baby in a snug sling, swaddled, lying on a firm pillow, or side-lying on a firm surface).
- Deep touch is used rather than light touch.
- Light and sound are kept low.
- If the baby gags easily at the breast, allow the baby to take a more active role in taking the breast.

Resources for Parents

Books

Stock, C. (2006). *The out-of-sync child: Recognizing and coping with sensory integration dysfunction*. Karnowitz. Perigree.

Biel, L. & Peske, N. (2005). *Raising a sensory smart child: The definitive handbook for helping your child with sensory integration issues*. Penguin.

Websites

Sensory Processing Foundation
www.spdfoundation.net

Sensory Processing Disorder Resource Center
http://www.sensory-processing-disorder.com/

Sensory Nation
www.sensorynation.com

Online group for parents

Yahoo group AP_sensory

Babies who have low muscle tone and under-respond to stimulation may breastfeed better (if not hypersensitive to touch) when:

- Before feedings, their mother gently massages their face, mouth, tongue, and palate and/or the mother holds them upright against her chest and bounces up and down on the balls of her feet.
- They are swaddled for feedings with arms and legs flexed.

Skin-to-skin contact helps calm and comfort some of these babies. Some babies may be so ineffective at feedings that they do not gain weight well and need to be supplemented.

Neurological Impairment

A baby may be neurologically impaired due to immaturity or physical problems, such as a brain bleed, seizures, or one of many syndromes, such as Prader-Willi, Williams, and others. When a baby's brain or nervous system is affected, it can compromise his ability to organize his movements and feed effectively, leading to feeding problems (Genna, Fram, & Sandora, 2008; Radzyminski, 2005). However, with practice and patience, many of these babies can learn to breastfeed.

Babies with a neurological impairment often have either high or low muscle tone, which may make feedings difficult.

Typically, neurological impairment leads to either high or low muscle tone. Babies with high tone may arch their bodies, over-respond to stimulation, and bite or clench at the breast. Babies with low muscle tone tend to under-respond to feeding triggers. Both high- and low-tone babies may have trouble coordinating suckling, swallowing, and breathing. For details and strategies, see p. 306- "Neurological Impairment."

Mother Issues

Birth-Related Pain or Psychological Trauma

A traumatic birth can affect how a mother experiences breastfeeding.

One New Zealand study of 52 women (Beck & Watson, 2008) found that after a traumatic birth the mothers reacted either very positively or very negatively to breastfeeding. Mothers in the positive group felt a strong determination to breastfeed to "make up" for the birth experience to their baby or to themselves or to prove themselves as a mother. Mothers who reacted negatively to breastfeeding considered their breasts as "one more thing to be violated," felt the need take a time-out to heal mentally, perceived breastfeeding as another painful ordeal, experienced flashbacks from the birth that intruded on breastfeeding, or felt a "disturbing detachment" from their baby. The researchers suggested that traumatized mothers may need ongoing one-on-one support to establish breastfeeding.

Mothers may experience psychological trauma, or symptoms of trauma, as a result of their births.

Some of the mothers in this study also experienced insufficient milk production. Other research has also found an association between stressful birth and delay in milk increase. For more details, see p. 409- "Delayed Milk Increase After Birth."

• •

After a cesarean section, suggest comfortable feeding positions that do not put pressure on a mother's incision.

U.K. midwife and researcher Suzanne Colson described how a semi-reclined "Biological Nurturing" (BN) position can be used by mothers after a cesarean birth:

> "In the first postnatal hours, many mothers are afraid that any body contact with the baby near the recent surgical site will be painful.... [M]others in comfortable semi-reclined or flat-lying BN postures can either use an over-the-shoulder position with baby...or...transverse... with the baby's body draped across her upper torso. Trying different lies often helps a worried mother to breastfeed almost immediately, thus avoiding any direct friction with her fresh wound" (Colson, 2005, pp. 29-30).

To get a sense of the positioning possibilities, Colson suggests thinking of the breast as a 360 degree circle and the baby being positioned anywhere around the circle. For more details and illustrations of possible positions, see Chapter 1, "Basic Breastfeeding Dynamics."

If the mother prefers to sit upright, she can avoid any contact with her incision by holding her baby at her side (sometimes referred to as the "football" or "rugby" hold). A mother lying on her side can roll up a towel or blanket to protect her incision while she breastfeeds lying down, although that will prevent close body contact with her baby, which triggers inborn feeding behaviors.

Breast and Nipple Challenges

Taut Breast Tissue

Ask the mother if her ankles are swollen, and if so, ask if she has breast swelling, too.

Within the first day or two after birth—even before a mother's milk increases—IV fluids received during labor can cause breast swelling that can make feedings difficult. Some report seeing an increase in the incidence of breast swelling (edema):

> Over the years, I have observed a rising incidence of severe edema in the postpartum breast, sometimes making it nearly impossible to soften the areola by hand expression, causing unnecessary postpartum and neonatal problems, despite optimal management of early breastfeeding (Cotterman, 2004, p. 227).

Feeding problems can occur when the increased tautness of the breast tissue flattens the nipple and makes it difficult for the baby to draw the breast deeply into his mouth. To understand this dynamic, imagine trying to suck a firm beach ball or soccer ball into the back of the mouth. When breast tissue is taut, it can lead to frustration at the breast.

Breast swelling or edema can lead to breastfeeding problems.

In some cases, laboring mothers receive more IV fluids than ordered by their doctor (Gonik & Cotton, 1984). Also, one type of commonly used IV fluid (crystalloid) both adds to the body's fluid load and reduces the ability to process excess fluid, extending the amount of time it takes for swelling to resolve. See the next point for strategies.

When a mother has taut breast tissue, suggest she start by using Reverse Pressure Softening and breast shaping.

If the mother's areola has become taut, swollen, or engorged, encourage her first to try Reverse Pressure Softening to move any swelling further back into her breast, softening her areola and making it easier for the baby draw the breast deeper into his mouth. This technique, along with breast shaping, is often enough to make feedings easier. For details on these techniques, see Appendix A, "Techniques."

If Reverse Pressure Softening is not enough to soften the mother's breast and the mother's milk has increased (usually sometime between Day 2 and 5), another approach is to express enough milk to soften the areola. Hand expression is the first choice because its use of positive pressure on the areola is less likely than the negative pressure (vacuum) of a pump to cause more areolar swelling (Cotterman, 2004). Assure the mother that removing milk will not make her engorgement worse. Removing milk will help decrease her engorgement. For details, see p. 677- "Engorgement."

Another strategy to help the baby draw the breast farther back in his mouth is breast shaping. For details, see p. 802- "Breast Shaping." Also, suggest she try breastfeeding in a semi-reclined position, which gives the baby more control and enhances baby's inborn feeding behaviors. These positions may use gravity to help draw the swelling away from the areola.

Ask the mother if her breasts feel full or engorged and how often the baby has been breastfeeding.

Between the 2nd and 5th day after birth, normal breast fullness may become engorgement. This is more likely if the baby has not been breastfeeding often or long. Engorgement can cause feeding problems if fullness makes breast tissue taut. When this happens, some babies will refuse the breast. Others may try to breastfeed shallowly. If the tautness of the areola causes the baby to take only the nipple, it can make breastfeeding painful for the mother and reduce the milk flow, further aggravating the engorgement.

If the mother becomes severely engorged despite frequent breastfeeding, this may be a sign the baby is not breastfeeding effectively. If so, suggest the baby be checked for unusual oral anatomy and any other health problems. Also, encourage the mother to express her milk to relieve engorgement, safeguard her milk production, and provide milk for her baby.

If a mother's breast tissue is naturally taut, suggest breast shaping.

Some mothers have breast tissue that is naturally taut. In this case, breast-shaping may be key to effective breastfeeding during the early learning period. Usually, as babies get older, stronger, and more coordinated, taut breast tissue is less of a challenge for them. For details on breast-shaping strategies, see p. 802- "Breast Shaping."

Nipple Shape and Size

Flat and Inverted Nipples

Ask if one or both of the mother's nipples is flat or inverted.

At first, most mothers find learning to breastfeed takes time and patience. If the mother has flat or inverted nipples and the baby has difficulty taking the breast, review the basic suggestions in Chapter 1 on p. 49- "Checklist" and those in the last section of this chapter. See also p. 663 for the section "Difficulties Associated with Flat or Inverted Nipples" in the chapter "Nipple Issues." Most important is patience and persistence. Assure the mother that with gentle persuasion and time her baby will likely master breastfeeding.

Flat or inverted nipples can lead to breastfeeding problems.

Research has found an association between flat and inverted nipples and early breastfeeding challenges. An Iranian study of first-time mothers examined the effect of "maternal breast variations" (including flat and inverted nipples and "abnormally large breasts") on weight gain during the first 7 days (Vazirinejad, Darakhshan, Esmaeili, & Hadadian, 2009). At 7 days of life, the mean weight of the babies whose mothers had one or more of these "breast variations" was below birthweight, whereas the mean weight among the babies whose mothers did not have a variation was above birthweight. A U.S. study of 328 mothers found an association between flat and inverted nipples and early breastfeeding problems (Dewey et al., 2003).

Although flat and inverted nipples can make the early learning period more challenging, protruding (everted) nipples are not a requirement for effective breastfeeding. Most babies are happy to suck on anything they can get into their mouth, including caregivers' arms, shoulders, and necks. In *The Breastfeeding Atlas* (2008), authors Wilson-Clay and Hoover suggest that the babies whose mothers have flat or inverted nipples may be more at risk for breastfeeding problems after experiencing the "supernormal stimulus" of bottles and pacifiers/dummies. Ultimately, what is most important is the baby feeling the stimulation of the breast deeply in his mouth (protruding nipple or not) to trigger active suckling.

Research from India found that using a suction device to draw out the mother's flat or inverted nipple before feeding may help resolve the feeding problem (Kesaree, Banapurmath, Banapurmath, & Shamanur, 1993). In this study, a makeshift suction device was used, which consisted of a syringe with one end cut off and the plunger inserted backwards for a smooth surface against the mother's breast, but several manufactured products made for this specific purpose are now available. (See Appendix B.)

Ask the mother if her nipples were flat before her baby was born.

In some cases, flat nipples may not be what they seem. IV fluids given during labor can cause breast tissue swelling (edema) that causes a mother's nipples to appear flat within a day or so after birth (Cotterman, 2004). In this case, the real feeding challenge is not "flat nipples," but taut breast tissue (see the previous section).

Large Nipples

Does one or both of the mother's nipples seem too large for the baby?

Sometimes called a "poor fit," this can happen when a mother with very large nipples (wide and/or long) gives birth to a baby with a very small mouth. No matter how good their breastfeeding dynamics, in some cases, the baby may fit only the nipple in his mouth, which can lead to nipple pain and/or slow milk flow. If a mother's long nipples extend far enough back to trigger her baby's gag reflex, feeding aversion may occur. In *The Breastfeeding Atlas* (2008), Wilson-Clay and Hoover suggested a mother's nipple texture may also play a role in a baby's ability to breastfeed, with "pliable" large nipples appearing easier to manage than "meaty" large nipples.

With a poor fit, the most reliable solution is tincture of time. Fortunately, newborns grow quickly, and it may take only a few weeks of growth before a baby can breastfeed well. Since the baby's "oral reach" (the distance from the lips to the area near his hard and soft palate junction) increases as he grows, babies will outgrow poor fit. If the mother establishes her milk production with milk expression, her baby can begin breastfeeding as soon as their fit issues are outgrown.

Breast Size and Nipple Placement

Ask the mother if she has large breasts, and if so, what breastfeeding positions she uses.

An Iranian study of first-time mothers examined the effect of "maternal breast variations" (including flat and inverted nipples and "abnormally large breasts") on weight gain during the first 7 days (Vazirinejad et al., 2009). At 7 days of life, the mean weight of the babies whose mothers had one or more of these "breast variations" was below birthweight, whereas the mean weight among the babies whose mothers did not have variations was above birthweight.

When a mother has large breasts and/or unusual nipple placement, creative positioning may help. Figure 3.7 illustrates one breastfeeding couple's solution. Begin by encouraging the mother to find a comfortable semi-reclined position in which she is well supported and place her baby tummy down on her body, allowing the baby's inborn feeding behaviors to be triggered before going to the breast. Breast support or shaping may also be helpful for some babies, but encourage the mother to start with the breast at its natural height first to see if the baby can get on the breast well. The less she has to lift and support, the easier breastfeeding will be.

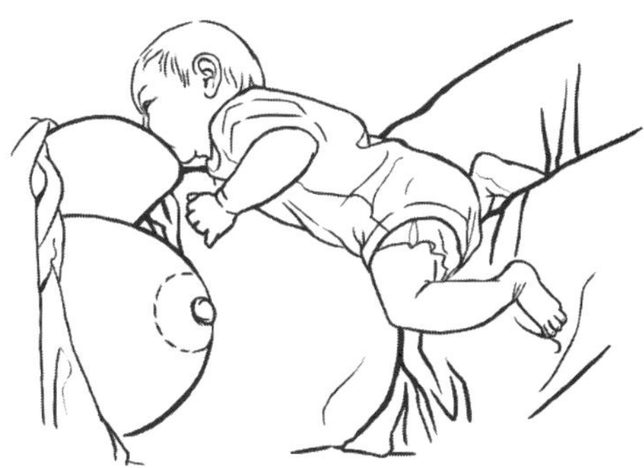

Figure 3.7. A laid-back feeding position for a mother with large breasts and nipples pointing down.

©2010 Anna Mohrbacher, used with permission

Milk Flow

Depending on the baby, either fast or slow milk flow may contribute to feeding problems.

Milk flow at either end of the spectrum can create breastfeeding challenges. At one end, a very fast milk flow, often linked to overabundant milk production, can be a struggle for a baby to manage. He may gulp, cough, and sputter at milk ejection, and go on and off the breast many times during each feeding to catch his breath. At the other end of the spectrum, slow milk flow may cause the baby who is stressed by hunger to become frustrated and struggle at feedings.

Overabundant Milk Production

If fast milk flow is a possible problem, ask about the baby's weight gain.

If the baby is coughing, gasping, and pulling off the breast at feedings, determine first if this is due to an overabundance of milk or other reasons. If he is gaining significantly more than 2 pounds (900 g) per month, it is likely that the mother has overabundant milk production. See p. 425 for other symptoms. In this case, the mother may also have discomfort from fullness between feedings or have a history of recurring mastitis. If overabundant milk production is the cause, suggest the mother take steps to slow her milk production. For details, see p. 427- "Strategies for Making Less Milk." If the baby's weight gain is not above average, consider other possible causes.

When a baby struggles with milk flow and is not gaining quickly, consider physical causes.

If a baby is having difficulty coping with the mother's milk flow and it is clear from baby's weight gain that she is producing, at best, an average amount of milk, suggest the mother have the baby's healthcare provider rule out any physical problems. The following factors, which are covered in more details in previous sections, are some that could contribute to a baby's inability to cope with average milk production:

- Feeding positions in which baby is below the breast and milk is flowing "downhill"
- Short frenulum or other unusual oral anatomy
- Pain or birth injury
- Respiratory issues
- Sensory processing issues
- Neurological issues (most babies would have obvious physical problems) or other health issues

To give the baby more control over milk flow, suggest the mother use a semi-reclined position with baby's head tilted slightly back and free to pull off as needed.

One common recommendation for problems coping with milk flow is to use a feeding position in which the baby breastfeeds "uphill," with his head and throat higher than the mother's nipple. Gravity gives the baby more control and his inborn feeding behaviors are more effectively triggered when he is supported tummy down on mother's body (Colson et al., 2008). When the baby takes the breast, suggest the mother be sure he tilts his head slightly back, rather than chin down or head turned to the side, as a slight head extension makes swallowing easier (Glover & Wiessinger, 2008).

The semi-reclined position gives babies more control over milk flow.

Because the baby may need to be on and off the breast to catch his breath, suggest the mother avoid holding his head to the breast, which could cause feeding aversion.

For babies struggling with milk flow, breastfeeding more often may make the flow more manageable.

Rather than postponing breastfeeding, which may be a mother's first impulse when her baby has feeding problems, feeding more often reduces the amount of milk in the breast at each feeding, making milk flow more manageable.

Some babies handle milk flow more easily when a nipple shield is used.

If the other suggestions have been tried without improvement, suggest a mother try using a thin, silicone nipple shield. The shield slows the milk flow, which may help her baby better cope with feedings while she is working on other strategies, such as slowing milk production. For details on nipple shield fit, application, and use, see the section "Nipple Shields" in Appendix B, "Tools and Products."

Low Milk Production

Slow milk flow can frustrate a hungry baby, which can cause feeding problems.

If a mother's milk production is low, see the chapter "Making Milk" for strategies to increase it, and if it is very low, see also the chapter "Relactation, Induced Lactation, and Emergencies." When a hungry baby goes to breast and there is very little milk, this can create frustration and feeding problems.

FEEDING PROBLEMS AFTER THE EARLY WEEKS

If the baby is more than a couple of weeks old and breastfeeding has been going well—mother was comfortable and baby was gaining weight as expected—it is less likely that many of the physical causes described in the previous section (birth injury, tongue tie, respiratory issues, sensory processing issues, neurological impairment, breast and nipple challenges, etc.) would suddenly cause problems now. An exception is some babies with mild tongue tie or respiratory problems, who may do well in the early weeks when the mother's milk production is ample, but as milk production adjusts downward and the baby is unable to feed effectively, problems may develop. This section describes possible causes of feeding challenges that start later.

When feeding problems start after several weeks of uneventful breastfeeding, unusual anatomy and conditions present at birth are unlikely to be the cause.

• •

The baby's age can provide clues to the cause of the problem. If a baby begins having feeding problems after the first couple of weeks, consider the causes listed in Table 3.4, which provides an overview of many possible causes and the ages at which they are most likely to appear.

Ask how old the baby was when the feeding problems started.

Table 3.4. Contributing Factors for Feeding Problems after the Early Weeks

Baby Issues

- Change in baby's suckling patterns from use of artificial nipples (Righard, 1998). Can occur when bottles or pacifiers are introduced. More likely in the baby younger than 1 month.
- Temperament. Some previously easygoing babies "wake up" at 2 to 3 weeks of age and become colicky.
- Illness, such as ear infection, cold, or others. Can happen at any age.
- Gastroesophageal reflux disease (GERD). Symptoms usually first appear after about 4 weeks or so.
- Hypersensitivity, intolerance, or allergy, causing discomfort, congestion, skin rash. Symptoms usually appear after about 3 to 4 weeks of age.
- Pain when held. May be caused by immunization, medical procedure, or injury. Can occur at any age.
- Candida (thrush). Can occur at any age.
- Teething. Usually occurs after about 3 to 4 months of age.
- Distractibility. Usually starts at around 3 months and increases over time.
- Reaction to a new product the mother is using, such as deodorant, detergents, etc.
- Nursing strike. Usually occurs after 2 months or so.

Mother Issues

- Overabundant or low milk production, causing fast or slow milk flow.
- Mastitis or other breast disease.
- Stress, overstimulation, or upset, such as household move, holidays, etc. Anything that delays or decreases breastfeeding, reducing milk production.

Ask when during the feeding the difficulty usually starts and what it is.

The symptoms may provide clues to the cause. Is the problem just at one breast or both? When during the feeding problems start can also provide clues.

Feeding problem starts before milk ejection. When a problem begins at the start of a feeding, consider:

- Positioning issues causing discomfort or frustration. Has the baby recently been immunized or is sore from an injury?
- Use of pacifiers/dummies or bottles. This can contribute to feeding problems in some babies (Righard, 1998).
- Breast or milk-flow issues. Is the mother's breast tissue taut from missed feedings? Is the baby sleeping longer at night and the mother's milk production slowed? Might she have mastitis?

Feeding problem starts at milk ejection. If the baby coughs or gags, this may be a sign the baby has problems coping with milk flow. If so, suggest the mother try adjusting her positioning, so baby's face is higher than her nipple. Discuss possible overabundant milk production or health problems in the baby.

Feeding problem starts later in the feeding. When baby starts fussing later, consider:

- The need to burp or pass a stool. Loud gulping indicates air being swallowed and regular burping may help. Babies often fuss before passing a stool.
- Low milk production. Is the baby's weight gain borderline or low?
- Overabundant milk production. Is the baby gaining much more than the average of 2 pounds (900 grams) per month?
- Gastroesophageal reflux disease (GERD). Babies with GERD fuss because feedings are painful. These symptoms usually occur after about 4 weeks of age.
- Hypersensitivity, intolerance, or allergy. Look for other symptoms, like rash or wheezing/congestion.

If the baby's weight gain has slowed and the fussiness increases the longer he feeds, suggest the mother ask her baby's healthcare provider to rule out allergy and/or reflux disease.

Ask the mother to describe how she and her baby breastfeed—feedings per day, time at each breast—and her baby's weight, at birth and now.

If the mother breastfeeds by the clock, limiting number of feedings or feeding length, and her baby's weight gain is borderline or questionable, her baby may not be getting enough milk and may be stressed.

Also ask if her baby is fed by bottle and if he takes a pacifier. If she answers yes, ask how often. Ask, too, if her baby is eating solid foods. Overuse of bottles, pacifiers, and solid foods can rapidly decrease the number of feedings at the breast and lower a mother's milk production, causing slow flow at the breast, which can lead to an unhappy baby. If the exclusively breastfeeding baby's weight gain is normal or high, consider other causes. Very fast weight gain may indicate overabundant milk production.

Ask the mother if she has nipple pain or has recently had mastitis.

Nipple pain after a period of comfortable breastfeeding can indicate shallow breastfeeding, candida (thrush), or teething (usually in a baby older than 3 or 4 months). Ask the mother if she has ever had nipple cracks or bleeding. If so, she is also at increased risk for an overgrowth of candida and bacterial infection.

If the mother recently had mastitis, her baby may be reacting to the slower milk flow in that breast or the salty taste. If so, assure her that her milk production will rebound after about a week of frequent feeding or expressing.

Baby Factors

Physical Causes

Ask the mother if the baby has nasal congestion.

When a baby with a stuffy nose closes his mouth around the breast, he may struggle to breathe. Although a sick baby almost always copes more easily with breastfeeding than with bottle-feeding, neither will be easy when his nose is blocked. Congestion can be caused by a cold or virus and can lead to an ear infection. Persistent congestion may be a symptom of allergy or illness. For breastfeeding strategies and more details, see p. 281- "Colds, Flu, Breathing Problems, and Ear Infections."

Ask the mother how much of the day her baby cries and at what age this started.

Colic is defined as crying at least 3 hours per day at least 3 days a week for at least 3 weeks (Wessel, Cobb, Jackson, Harris, & Detwiler, 1954). It often starts when a baby is about 2 to 3 weeks old and is estimated to affect between 8% to 40% of babies (Howard, Lanphear, Lanphear, Eberly, & Lawrence, 2006). Sometimes called "high-need," colicky babies may spend much of their first 3 months crying, both on and off the breast. The mother may describe her baby as demanding or intense and find it difficult to help him settle and breastfeed. Living with a colicky baby is stressful. Parents report the strategies that work best to comfort their babies (in order of effectiveness) are holding, breastfeeding, walking, and rocking (Howard et al., 2006). If the baby has trouble settling down to breastfeed, also suggest the following strategies:

Mothers often find that living with a colicky baby is stressful.

Before breastfeeding:

- Be sure baby is not too warm or too cold and that his clothing is not binding.
- To help calm baby, if needed, offer a clean, trimmed finger to suck on, pad side up.

During breastfeeding:

- Keep sound and lights low.
- Begin breastfeeding when baby is in a light sleep and not yet fully awake.
- Use a semi-reclined breastfeeding position with baby tummy down on mother's body, so gravity helps rather than hinders breastfeeding.
- Allow the baby to finish feeding on one breast before offering the other.

At other times:

- Devote as much time as possible to holding baby or wearing him in a soft baby carrier or sling.

What appears to be colic may be caused by health problems, such as reflux disease or allergy.

Because many babies with gastroesophageal reflux disease (GERD) cry for long periods, they may be mislabeled as having colic (Berkowitz, Naveh, & Berant, 1997; Gupta, 2007; Heine, Jordan, Lubitz, Meehan, & Catto-Smith, 2006; Miller-Loncar, Bigsby, High, Wallach, & Lester, 2004; Sicherer, 2003). A baby with reflux disease may breastfeed well for a few minutes and become more and more agitated as he continues to feed. If this might be the cause of a baby's "colic," suggest the mother ask her baby's healthcare provider to check for this health problem. For details, see p. 287- "Reflux Disease (GERD)."

Colic symptoms could be due to hypersensitivity, intolerance, allergy, or an overabundant milk supply.

What appears to be colic may also be a symptom of hypersensitivity, intolerance, or allergy (Hill, Roy et al., 2005), which is associated with GERD (Gupta, 2007; Sicherer, 2003). For details and strategies, see p. 517- "Is Baby Reacting to Something in Mother's Diet." One symptom of allergy or sensitivity is crying during or after feedings. Others include skin rashes, congestion or wheezing, gastrointestinal symptoms, and sleep problems. These types of reactions are more common when there is a family history of allergy. If one parent has allergies, the baby has a 20-40% risk of being allergic, and if both parents have allergies, the baby's risk increases to 50-80% (Ferreira & Seidman, 2007).

Colic-like symptoms can also occur when a mother has overabundant milk production (Livingstone, 1996; Woolridge & Fisher, 1988). If the baby has gained significantly more than 2 pounds (900 grams) per month, discuss this possibility with the mother and consider taking steps to slow the mother's milk production. For more details, see p. 427- "Strategies for Making Less Milk."

Ask the mother if the baby could be teething.

Sore gums from teething can make a baby unsettled at the breast. While teething, which usually occurs after about 3 to 4 months of age, a baby may breastfeed differently, bearing down on the breast or even making chewing movements because pressure can help ease gum discomfort. He may even refuse the breast when the pain is at its peak. For strategies, see p. 642- "Teething and Biting."

Ask if the baby has white patches in his mouth and if the mother has nipple pain.

The organism that causes oral thrush, *Candida albicans*, is a fungus that thrives in dark, moist places, such as the mother's nipple and the baby's mouth and diaper area. An overgrowth of candida in a baby's mouth, also known as thrush, can make his mouth painful. He may go to the breast eagerly, but pull away repeatedly from the pain.

To determine whether or not this may be a factor in baby's feeding difficulty, ask the mother if her baby has white patches in his mouth that when wiped off look red or bleed. Another possible sign is a red diaper rash, with or without raised dots. The mother may report nipple pain after a time of comfortable breastfeeding. For more details and treatment options, see p. 652- "Candida/ Thrush."

If the baby bumped his mouth and has a sore area inside, this could affect his feeding comfort. Also, any sores in the mouth, such as cold sores, could affect feedings.

Ask the mother to check inside the baby's mouth for anything unusual.

Babies sometimes resist feeding if a sensitive area is touched. This could be an injection site or a bruise. If so, suggest the mother try a different feeding position until the sore area heals.

Ask if the baby recently had an injection, a medical procedure, or was injured.

Each stage of development brings new skills that can distract a baby from breastfeeding and change his feeding behaviors. For breastfeeding strategies at different ages and stages, see p. 228 in "Other Breastfeeding Dynamics."

Ask if the baby has been distractible and if that might be contributing to his feeding problems.

Distractibility is part of baby's normal development and is not a sign he's ready to wean. For more details, see p. 184- last point in "The Role of Mother and Baby." If the mother is concerned because her baby is breastfeeding for such a short time, assure her that older babies can get a lot of milk from the breast quickly and her baby may only need to breastfeed for 5 to 10 minutes. His weight gain will tell the mother if shorter breastfeeding is a cause for concern.

Environmental Causes

Ask if the family has been under unusual stress lately or if there have been any major changes in the baby's routine.

Moving a household, family tensions, or the mother returning to work all have the potential to affect breastfeeding, especially in a sensitive baby. Even a positive stress, like holiday preparations, can sometimes affect a baby's willingness to feed.

Ask if the mother has been using any new products on her breasts or on her body.

Use of some nipple creams or ointments may change the taste, causing the baby to become unsettled during feeding or refuse to breastfeed. A sensitive baby may register his dislike for a new product, like a new deodorant, body lotion, or laundry detergent, by becoming unsettled at the breast or refusing to breastfeed. If this might be the cause, suggest the mother rinse her breasts with clear water before the next breastfeeding. If her deodorant is the cause, changing from a spray to a stick may be all that's needed.

Mother Factors

Milk Flow

With overabundant milk production, a baby may have trouble coping with his mother's milk flow and gain weight faster than average.

A mother has an overabundant milk production when she makes much more milk than her baby needs. As a result, her milk flow may be very fast and hard to manage. Some refer to the struggles babies have with milk flow as an "overactive let-down reflex" (Andrusiak & Larose-Kuzenko, 1987). The baby struggling with milk flow may:

- Swallow a lot of air from gulping during feeding
- Spit up regularly
- Pass a lot of gas

- Wake soon after falling asleep, may wake and act hungry, even if he just breastfed
- Be considered colicky
- Fuss during feedings, choking, sputtering, or arching away when the milk ejects
- Have regular or occasional explosive green or watery stools

Similar symptoms may also occur in the baby with colic, reflux disease, and allergies.

The baby may have a strong suck, strong muscle tone, and want to breastfeed often. Or he may refuse some feedings. Some mothers report that their baby's fussiness and refusal continues as the baby gets older. The mother may leak milk profusely during and between feedings, and her milk ejection may feel painful.

Over time, a baby who struggles with fast milk flow may develop other feeding problems.

As baby gets older, if fast milk flow continues to be an issue, some babies may:

- Start to become reluctant to breastfeed, even when obviously hungry
- Refuse to breastfeed to sleep, preferring instead fingers or thumb
- Use chewing or "biting" motions at the breast to avoid triggering fast milk flow
- Go on a nursing strike

Ask about the baby's weight gain, which may help determine the cause.

Before considering slowing a mother's milk production when a baby has trouble with milk flow, be sure that the baby is gaining much more than the average 2 pounds (900 grams) per month. For strategies for coping with fast milk flow and slowing overabundant milk production, see p. 425- "Overabundant Milk Production."

If the baby is sputtering and coughing when the mother's milk ejection occurs, but weight gain is not above average, see the earlier section on respiratory problems.

If a baby's weight gain is borderline or questionable, a baby's feeding difficulties could be related to low milk production and slow milk flow. The baby may be frustrated at the breast or stressed by hunger. If the baby's weight is average or above, consider other causes. To boost her milk production, see p. 413- "Strategies for Making More Milk."

Ask the mother if she has started menstruating recently.

Although it is unusual, some babies become unhappy at the breast or refuse to breastfeed when their mother's menstrual cycle begins. Two U.S. physicians wrote that according to some mothers "the infant will reject the breast for a day or so with each period" (Lawrence & Lawrence, 2005, p. 301).

Breast Health

Ask the mother if she has a lump, swelling, or any discomfort in one or both breasts.

One cause of difficult feedings is mastitis, which includes plugged ducts, infection, and abscess. Although mastitis usually occurs in one breast, in some cases, both breasts are affected. Some babies breastfeed reluctantly on the affected breast; others refuse it altogether.

During mastitis, milk flow in the affected breast is slowed (Fetherston, Lai, & Hartmann, 2006; Matheson, Aursnes, Horgen, Aabo, & Melby, 1988; Wambach, 2003). Also, sodium and chloride levels increase, giving the milk a saltier taste. And sugar levels (lactose and glucose) decrease, making the milk less sweet (Fetherston et al., 2006).

During mastitis, milk flow on the affected breast is slowed.

Assure the mother that if she treats her mastitis as recommended (see p. 685- "Mastitis Treatments", as her mastitis clears, her milk production will rebound and its original taste will return. To help her baby accept the affected breast again, suggest the mother follow the strategies in the last section and continue breastfeeding on the other breast. Also suggest she express her milk from the affected breast as often or more often than her baby had been breastfeeding, so the mastitis clears more quickly and the milk production in the affected breast returns to normal. Usually, within a week or so of the mastitis resolving, the taste of her milk should return to normal.

REFUSAL OF ONE OR BOTH BREASTS

When a baby refuses one or both breasts, the first step is to rule out medical issues.

If a baby refuses one or both breasts from birth, suggest the mother first ask the baby's healthcare provider to rule out medical reasons, such as torticollis, birth injury, unusual oral anatomy, and other illnesses and conditions.

When a baby begins refusing one or both breasts after a time of uneventful breastfeeding, ruling out a medical issue is also important. Nasal congestion, ear infections, reflux disease, and other health problems can lead to breast refusal. See Table 3.4 on p. 135 for a summary of possible causes after the newborn period.

Refusal of One Breast

If a newborn refuses one breast, ask if the mother's nipples differ in size or shape or one breast feels firmer.

Nipple differences. If one of a mother's nipples is more everted (protruding) or less inverted than the other, her baby may take one breast and refuse the other. The same can happen if the baby prefers the size or texture of one nipple over the other. To help her baby accept both, suggest the mother use a semi-reclined position and first trigger her baby's inborn feeding behaviors so that he has an active role in taking the breast. Another strategy is to use breast support and shaping to make it easier for her baby to take the refused breast deeper into his mouth. Helping the baby get a more asymmetric latch may also help. For details, see these sections in Appendix A, "Techniques." If one nipple is too large for her baby to handle, see the earlier section "Large Nipples" on p. 132.

Breast firmness. If one breast is consistently firmer than the other, the baby may find it more difficult to take it deeply and get frustrated. Suggest the mother start by using Reverse Pressure Softening to first soften that areola before offering that breast (see p. 795). Expressing just enough milk to soften the breast may also help. Suggest the mother try breast support and the breast shaping techniques described in the "Techniques" appendix. Softening the areola and helping the baby get on the breast deeper may solve this problem.

Ask the mother of a newborn what feeding positions she uses.

Some newborns feel discomfort when held in certain positions and may be willing to take the refused breast if a more comfortable feeding position is used. In an upright feeding position with the baby held in front, typically the baby's head is pointed one direction when on the right breast and the other direction when on the left breast. When using this type of position, suggest the mother try sliding the baby to the other breast in exactly the same body position (called the "slide-over position") to see if that makes a difference. Babies likely to refuse one breast when their position changes include those with torticollis (see p. 116) who may not be able to turn their head easily, those with a birth injury who may feel pain when pressure is applied in some positions, and those recently immunized. In some cases, a mother may be more coordinated on one side and breastfeeding may go more smoothly if she is able to use her dominant hand to help her baby.

Babies may take a refused breast if a more comfortable position is used.

Ask the mother if she's noticed differences in milk production or milk flow between breasts.

At any stage, it is common for rates of milk production to vary tremendously between breasts (Hill, Aldag, Zinaman, & Chatterton, 2007; Kent et al., 2006). Also, over time, a mother's rate of milk production may change. A case of mastitis, for example, may cause milk production in one breast to drastically decrease (see next point).

Baby prefers faster flow. In this case, suggest the mother stimulate her milk ejection before putting baby to the refused breast, so the baby won't have to wait.

Baby prefers slower flow. In this case, suggest the mother try using a semi-reclined feeding position at the refused breast, with her baby tummy down on her body. A prone position keeps a baby's torso against his mother's body and gravity gives him more control over milk flow, which may make that breast easier to manage. For more strategies, see p. 425- "Coping with Too Much Milk."

Ask the mother if the refused breast is very firm or if she has discomfort in it or feels a lump or swollen area.

Breast fullness and mastitis may cause a baby of any age to refuse one breast. Breast fullness can make the breast difficult to draw deeply into the baby's mouth. Mastitis can change the taste of the milk, making it saltier and slowing milk flow (see next point). If mastitis is a possibility (sore area or lump in one breast), see p. 681- "Mastitis."

Exclusive breastfeeding is possible using one breast, but the mother may want to first try to persuade the baby to take both.

Many mothers have exclusively breastfed twins, triplets, and even higher-order multiples, so most mothers can easily produce enough milk in one breast to satisfy a baby. However, the mother should expect that her baby may breastfeed more often if only one breast is used.

A worry some mothers have about one-sided breastfeeding is whether their breasts will ever be the same size again, as the used breast may become noticeably larger than the other. If so, assure the mother that after weaning her breasts should be about the same size as before she became pregnant. If they were the same size then, she can expect this again after breastfeeding ends.

If she wants to try to persuade the baby to breastfeed on the refused breast, suggest she express milk from the refused breast after every breastfeeding during her waking hours to establish or maintain good milk flow on that side while she works with her baby. Strategies to persuade the baby to take the refused breast include:

- Start breastfeeding on the preferred breast, and after her milk ejection, slide the baby over to the other breast without changing his body position.
- Offer the refused side after first stimulating her milk ejection.
- Experiment with different positions, starting with semi-reclined positions.
- Give the baby more help, such as breast shaping and support (for details, see Appendix A, "Techniques"), when taking the refused breast.
- Offer the refused breast when baby is in a light sleep and less aware.
- Try breastfeeding in a darkened room.
- Try moving the baby to the refused breast while walking or rocking to distract him.

If the mother is concerned about her baby's milk intake, suggest she monitor her baby's weight and diaper output.

See p. 205 for adequate weight gains for different ages. If her baby's weight gain is too low when he breastfeeds from one breast only and she doesn't have enough expressed or donor milk available to use as a supplement, she should consult her baby's healthcare provider for advice on choosing an appropriate supplement. See also the chapter "Making Milk" for strategies to increase milk production.

If a baby suddenly refuses one breast without obvious cause, suggest the mother see her healthcare provider to rule out a breast-related medical cause.

Several articles have suggested that sudden refusal of one breast for no apparent reason is a possible indicator of breast disease. One Saudi Arabian journal article reported that of eight mothers whose babies suddenly refused one breast, two had a breast abscess, two had an infected galactocele, and four had malignant breast cancer (Makanjuola, 1998). (For more details on these conditions, see the chapter "Breast Issues.") Two U.S. articles described cases of mothers with sudden, one-sided breast refusal who after weeks or months were eventually diagnosed with malignant breast cancer (Goldsmith, 1974; Saber, Dardik, Ibrahim, & Wolodiger, 1996). Encourage the mother to see her healthcare provider as soon as possible to rule out breast disease as the cause of the breast refusal.

Refusal of Both Breasts in the Early Weeks

Ask the baby's age and how long he has refused both breasts.

If the baby has refused the breast since birth, suggest the mother have the baby's healthcare provider rule out physical causes (see Table 3.2). If the breast refusal started between the 2nd and 5th day, consider engorgement or a delay in the mother's milk increasing, which may stress the baby (see Table 3.3). If the breast refusal started within the first month and the baby has received artificial nipples, consider that as a possible contributing factor (Righard, 1998).

Ask the mother if the baby was suctioned roughly at birth or if they have been struggling at the breast.

Some babies are roughly aspirated at birth or shoved roughly to the breast, overriding their inborn feeding behaviors. In some cases, mothers are so motivated to breastfeed that they spend time every day trying to get their babies to the breast while they are clearly upset. Some babies will go on to breastfed well after such experiences, but some may develop negative associations that cause breast refusal. If this is the case, suggest the mother devote some time to making the breast a pleasant place to be (for details, see the last section).

Try to determine what the baby is looking for at the breast that he is not finding.

Babies refusing the breast often do so because they are looking for something they cannot find, such as:

- The feel of the mother's body against their torso and chin to trigger their inborn feeding behaviors.
- The opportunity to go to the breast and take it in their own time.
- The feeling of the breast deep in their mouth.
- A faster milk flow or a slower, more manageable milk flow.
- A firm, protruding nipple (in babies who have been fed by bottle or given pacifiers).

In some cases, all that is needed to solve breast refusal is to improve technique. At a time when the baby is not too hungry, suggest the mother get into a comfortable, semi-reclined position with her breast accessible and put her baby tummy down on her body, triggering his inborn feeding behaviors, and letting the baby go to the breast in his own time.

Suggest the mother devote some time to making the breast a pleasant place to be.

If a baby takes the breast shallowly, he may not feel the sensation in the back of the mouth that triggers active sucking and become frustrated. In this case, a mother may need to take a more active role in helping the baby get farther onto the breast by using breast shaping and asymmetrical latch. If the baby's inability to feel the breast in the back of his mouth is related to the mother's engorgement, see the section "Taut Breast Tissue." For more strategies, see the last section in this chapter.

If a baby has received artificial nipples and is becoming frustrated with the mother's soft breast tissue, suggest she start by using breast shaping and support to help the baby feel the breast deeper in his mouth (see "Techniques" appendix). Sometimes dripping milk on the breast can help as well. In some cases, a thin, silicone nipple shield may be needed to help the baby transition to the breast. For using a nipple shield (style, fit, application, and weaning from the shield), see that section in Appendix B, "Tools and Products."

Nursing Strike

A nursing strike is most common after about 2 months of age, and sometimes, but not always, the cause can be determined.

The term "nursing strike" describes the baby who has been breastfeeding well and suddenly completely refuses the breast. Some mothers whose babies go "on strike" wonder if this is their baby's way of weaning. However, if the baby is younger than 1 year, this is unlikely, since babies this age have a physical need for mother's milk. Something else that distinguishes a nursing strike from a natural weaning is that the baby is usually unhappy about it. Typically, a nursing strike lasts 2 to 4 days, but it may last as long as 10 days and may require some ingenuity and careful analysis to find the cause and help the baby transition back to breastfeeding. Sometimes the cause is never determined.

But it is helpful to at least try to determine the cause. All previous possible causes of difficult breastfeeding should be considered. Individual babies respond to these factors differently, with some fussing at the breast, while others refuse the breast completely. The causes of a nursing strike fall into two general categories:

Physical causes:

- Ear infection, cold, or other illness
- Gastroesophageal reflux (GERD), which can make feedings painful
- Overabundant milk production, as a very fast milk flow can upset baby
- Hypersensitivity, intolerance, or allergy
- Pain when held from injury, medical procedure, or injection
- Mouth pain due to teething, thrush, or mouth injury
- Reaction to a product, such as deodorant, lotion, laundry detergent, etc.

Environmental causes:

- Stress, upset, overstimulation, or a chaotic home environment
- Breastfeeding on a strict schedule, timed feedings, or frequent interruptions
- Baby left to cry for long periods
- Major changes in baby's routine, like traveling, a household move, or mother returning to work
- Arguments with others or yelling while breastfeeding
- A strong reaction when the baby bites
- An unusually long separation of mother and baby

If the cause is found, it will reassure the mother and may influence which strategies are suggested. Even if the cause cannot be determined, suggest the strategies described in the last section, "Strategies for Settled Breastfeeding."

Suggest the mother safeguard breastfeeding by making sure her baby is well fed and her milk production is protected.

Suggest the mother express her milk as often as the baby was breastfeeding to avoid uncomfortable breast fullness and to maintain her milk production. She can give her baby her expressed milk using any method she chooses, which will depend in part on the baby's age. If a baby is at least 6 to 8 months old, feeding her milk in a cup has advantages, as it does not satisfy a baby's sucking urge like a bottle nipple/teat. Without a sucking outlet, the baby may be more motivated to go back to breastfeeding. A younger baby can be supplemented with a cup, spoon, eyedropper, or bowl. For details, see the section "Alternative Feeding Methods" in Appendix B, "Tools and Products." If she can avoid giving her baby artificial nipples, this may shorten the strike. If the baby had been taking a pacifier, suggest she discontinue it.

STRATEGIES TO ACHIEVE SETTLED BREASTFEEDING

Knowing the cause of the baby's feeding problem will affect the strategies used.

Knowing the cause of difficult feedings or breast refusal can help determine the best approach. For example, the baby with a medical problem, such as an ear infection or reflux disease, will need diagnosis and treatment. For environmental causes, minimizing distractions and creating a calmer setting may help. For the baby in pain, comfort measures and a tincture of time may be most important. But no matter what the cause, the basic strategies described in this section may also be helpful.

Before suggesting strategies, review with the mother basic breastfeeding dynamics.

Talk to the mother about what happens when she breastfeeds.

- Is baby calm?
- Are mother and baby looking into each other's eyes, touching, and talking?
- Are the baby's torso and hips well supported, in line, and pressed against mother's body? Are the baby's feet touching the mother or something else?
- Is gravity working for or against breastfeeding?
- Is the baby relaxed with no muscle tension on either side?
- Is baby's chin or cheek touching the breast?
- Is the baby's head tilted back slightly for easier swallowing?

Discuss the baby's alignment with the breast. If the mother is pushing on the back of baby's head or the baby must tuck his chin to take the breast, suggest she adjust how she's holding her baby, so he can tilt his head slightly back while taking the breast.

Time-tested approaches can help breastfeeding go more smoothly and persuade the baby who's "on strike" to accept the breast again.

Approaches the mother can use to decrease stress at feedings include:

- **Make sure the breast is a pleasant place to be**, not a battleground. If breastfeeding feels stressful, feed another way and instead give baby lots of cuddle time at the breast, including while asleep (Smillie, 2008).
- **Spend time touching and in skin-to-skin contact.** When not feeding, suggest the mother hold the baby and—if baby likes it—provide skin-to-skin contact, with baby's bare torso against her skin. This is soothing to both mother and baby, and the oxytocin released makes them more open to one another (Uvnas-Moberg, 2003). In a one-group, prospective exploratory study of 48 healthy, ethnically diverse mothers, four sessions of skin-to-skin contact while breastfeeding during the first 2 days was found to be a successful intervention (Chiu, Anderson, & Burkhammer, 2008). Despite having early breastfeeding problems, 81% of these mothers were still breastfeeding at a 1-month follow-up call. Time spent before breastfeeding in skin-to-skin contact has also been found to act as a stress-reliever and to lower blood pressure in mothers (Jonas et al., 2008).

- **Offer the breast while baby is in a light sleep or drowsy.** Some babies take the breast more easily when in a relaxed, sleepy state.
- **Use feeding positions baby likes best** and experiment, starting first with a semi-reclined position with baby tummy down and supported on mother's body.
- **Trigger a milk ejection before baby goes to breast** to give an instant reward or try first expressing a little milk onto baby's lips.
- **Try breast shaping or support.** Breast sandwich, nipple tilting, and other techniques may help the baby take the breast deeper to trigger active suckling. For details, see the "Techniques" appendix.
- **Try breastfeeding in motion**—walking or rocking.
- **Spend as much time as possible breastfeeding** at those times the baby is breastfeeding well.
- **Supplement if baby's weight gain slows or stops** to make sure the baby gets the milk he needs to feel calm and open to breastfeeding. For a choice of feeding methods, see "Alternative Feeding Methods" on p. 811 in the "Tools and Products" appendix.

• •

Tools and other strategies can help in some situations.

Drip expressed milk at the breast. If the baby goes to the breast, but won't stay there, ask a helper to use a spoon or eyedropper to drip expressed milk on the breast or in the corner of baby's mouth. Swallowing triggers suckling, which can get baby started breastfeeding. Give more milk if baby comes off.

Feed a little milk first. Some babies are more willing to try breastfeeding if they are not very hungry. Suggest the mother give her baby one-third to half a feeding, and then offer the breast. Another variation of this is called "bait and switch" in which the mother begins by bottle-feeding in a breastfeeding position and when her baby is actively sucking and swallowing, pulls out the bottle teat and offers her breast. Some babies will just keep suckling at the breast.

If using an upright feeding position, try a pillow for support. For a mother with a disability or one who prefers an upright feeding position, a pillow for support may make breastfeeding easier. Rarely, a baby may find close body contact too stimulating. In these rare cases, a baby may be more willing to take the breast if a firm pillow is used to provide good support while he takes the breast.

If the mother's nipples are flat or inverted, draw them out with a suction device before breastfeeding. Research from India found this an effective strategy for overcoming feeding problems in mothers with inverted nipples (Kesaree et al., 1993).

Try a thin, silicone nipple shield. In some situations nipple shields can be a useful tool to preserve breastfeeding. Consider this tool for the baby who's not taking the breast, the baby whose feeding problems may be caused by bottle and pacifier use, the baby with tongue tie or unusual tongue movements, the mother with inverted nipples, preterm babies who are not yet feeding effectively or able to stay on the breast. For details on use, fit, and application, see "Nipple Shields" on p. 835 in the "Tools and Products" appendix.

Try an at-breast supplementer. If slow milk flow is an issue, this type of device will provide flow at the breast and may help the baby accept the breast and keep breastfeeding. If slow flow is not the cause, this may not be a good choice, as taking the breast can be more challenging for some with the added element of the tubing of the at-breast supplementer (Borucki, 2005) For details, see "At-Breast Supplementers" on p. 815 in Appendix B, "Tools and Products."

REFERENCES

Amir, L. H., James, J. P., & Donath, S. M. (2006). Reliability of the Hazelbaker assessment tool for lingual frenulum function. *International Breastfeeding Journal, 1*(1), 3.

Andrusiak, F., & Larose-Kuzenko, M. (1987). *The effects of an overactive let-down reflex* (Vol. 13). Garden City Park, NY: Avery Publishing Group, Inc.

Ballard, J. L., Auer, C. E., & Khoury, J. C. (2002). Ankyloglossia: assessment, incidence, and effect of frenuloplasty on the breastfeeding dyad. *Pediatrics, 110*(5), e63.

Beck, C. T., & Watson, S. (2008). Impact of birth trauma on breast-feeding: a tale of two pathways. *Nursing Research, 57*(4), 228-236.

Benson, S. (2001). What is normal? A study of normal breastfeeding dyads during the first sixty hours of life. *Breastfeeding Review, 9*(1), 27-32.

Berkowitz, D., Naveh, Y., & Berant, M. (1997). "Infantile colic" as the sole manifestation of gastroesophageal reflux. *Journal of Pediatric Gastroenterology and Nutrition, 24*(2), 231-233.

Bibi, H., Khvolis, E., Shoseyov, D., Ohaly, M., Ben Dor, D., London, D., et al. (2001). The prevalence of gastroesophageal reflux in children with tracheomalacia and laryngomalacia. *Chest, 119*(2), 409-413.

Boere-Boonekamp, M. M., & van der Linden-Kuiper, L. L. (2001). Positional preference: prevalence in infants and follow-up after two years. *Pediatrics, 107*(2), 339-343.

Borucki, L. C. (2005). Breastfeeding mothers' experiences using a supplemental feeding tube device: finding an alternative. *Journal of Human Lactation, 21*(4), 429-438.

Bystrova, K., Matthiesen, A. S., Widstrom, A. M., Ransjo-Arvidson, A. B., Welles-Nystrom, B., Vorontsov, I., et al. (2007). The effect of Russian Maternity Home routines on breastfeeding and neonatal weight loss with special reference to swaddling. *Early Human Development, 83*(1), 29-39.

Chiu, S. H., Anderson, G. C., & Burkhammer, M. D. (2008). Skin-to-skin contact for culturally diverse women having breastfeeding difficulties during early postpartum. *Breastfeeding Medicine, 3*(4), 231-237.

Colson, S. (2005). Maternal breastfeeding positions: have we got it right? (2). *Practicing Midwife, 8*(11), 29-32.

Colson, S. (2008). *Biological Nurturing: laid-back breastfeeding*. Hythe, Kent, UK: The Nurturing Project.

Colson, S., DeRooy, L., & Hawdon, J. (2003). Biological Nurturing increases duration of breastfeeding for a vulnerable cohort. *MIDIRS Midwifery Digest, 13*(1), 92-97.

Colson, S. D., Meek, J. H., & Hawdon, J. M. (2008). Optimal positions for the release of primitive neonatal reflexes stimulating breastfeeding. *Early Human Development, 84*(7), 441-449.

Coryllos, E. V. (2008). Minimally invasive treatment for posterior tongue-tie (The hidden tongue-tie). In C. W. Genna (Ed.), *Supporting sucking skills in breastfeeding infants*. Boston, MA: Jones and Bartlett.

Cotterman, K. J. (2004). Reverse pressure softening: a simple tool to prepare areola for easier latching during engorgement. *Journal of Human Lactation, 20*(2), 227-237.

Cronenwett, L., Stukel, T., Kearney, M., Barrett, J., Covington, C., Del Monte, K., et al. (1992). Single daily bottle use in the early weeks postpartum and breast-feeding outcomes. *Pediatrics, 90*(5), 760-766.

de Carvalho, M., et al. (1983). Effect of frequent breast feeding on early milk production and infant weight gain. *Pediatrics, 72*, 307-311.

Dewey, K. G., Nommsen-Rivers, L. A., Heinig, M. J., & Cohen, R. J. (2003). Risk factors for suboptimal infant breastfeeding behavior, delayed onset of lactation, and excess neonatal weight loss. *Pediatrics, 112*(3 Pt 1), 607-619.

Dollberg, S., Botzer, E., Grunis, E., & Mimouni, F. B. (2006). Immediate nipple pain relief after frenotomy in breast-fed infants with ankyloglossia: a randomized, prospective study. *Journal of Pediatric Surgery, 41*(9), 1598-1600.

Ferreira, C. T., & Seidman, E. (2007). Food allergy: a practical update from the gastroenterological viewpoint. *Jornal de Pediatria, 83*(1), 7-20.

Fetherston, C. M., Lai, C. T., & Hartmann, P. E. (2006). Relationships between symptoms and changes in breast physiology during lactation mastitis. *Breastfeeding Medicine, 1*(3), 136-145.

Geddes, D. T., Kent, J. C., Mitoulas, L. R., & Hartmann, P. E. (2008). Tongue movement and intra-oral vacuum in breastfeeding infants. *Early Human Development, 84*(7), 471-477.

Geddes, D. T., Langton, D. B., Gollow, I., Jacobs, L. A., Hartmann, P. E., & Simmer, K. (2008). Frenulotomy for breastfeeding infants with ankyloglossia: effect on milk removal and sucking mechanism as imaged by ultrasound. *Pediatrics, 122*(1), e188-194.

Genna, C., Fram, J. L., & Sandora, L. (2008). Neurological issues and breastfeeding. In C. W. Genna (Ed.), *Supporting sucking skills in breastfeeding infants* (pp. 253-303). Boston, MA: Jones and Bartlett.

Genna, C. W. (2008a). The influence of anatomic and strucural issues on sucking skills. In C. W. Genna (Ed.), *Supporting sucking skills in breastfeeding infants*. Boston, MA: Jones and Bartlett.

Genna, C. W. (2008b). Sensory integration and breastfeeding. In C. W. Genna (Ed.), *Supporting sucking skills in breastfeeding infants* (pp. 235-252). Boston, MA: Jones and Bartlett.

Glover, R., & Wiessinger, D. (2008). The infant-mother breastfeeding conversation: Helping when they lose the thread. In C. W. Genna (Ed.), *Supporting sucking skills in breastfeeding infants* (pp. 97-129). Boston, MA: Jones and Bartlett.

Goldsmith, H. S. (1974). Milk-rejection sign of breast cancer. *American Journal of Surgery, 127*(3), 280-281.

Gonik, G., & Cotton, D. B. (1984). Peripartum colloid osmotic pressure changes influence of intravenous hydration. *American Journal of Obstetrics and Gynecology, 150*, 174-177.

Griffiths, D. M. (2004). Do tongue ties affect breastfeeding? *Journal of Human Lactation, 20*(4), 409-414.

Gupta, S. K. (2007). Update on infantile colic and management options. *Current Opinion in Investigational Drugs, 8*(11), 921-926.

Hall, D. M., & Renfrew, M. J. (2005). Tongue tie. *Archives of Disease in Childhood, 90*(12), 1211-1215.

Hazelbaker, A. (1992). *The assessment tool for lingual frenulum function (ATLFF): Use in a lactation consultant private practice*. Encino, CA: Lactation Institute.

Heine, R. G., Jordan, B., Lubitz, L., Meehan, M., & Catto-Smith, A. G. (2006). Clinical predictors of pathological gastro-oesophageal reflux in infants with persistent distress. *Journal of Paediatrics and Child Health, 42*(3), 134-139.

Hiiemae, K. M., & Palmer, J. B. (2003). Tongue movements in feeding and speech. *Critical Reviews in Oral Biology and Medicine, 14*(6), 413-429.

Hill, D. J., Roy, N., Heine, R. G., Hosking, C. S., Francis, D. E., Brown, J., et al. (2005). Effect of a low-allergen maternal diet on colic among breastfed infants: a randomized, controlled trial. *Pediatrics, 116*(5), e709-715.

Hill, P. D., Aldag, J. C., Chatterton, R. T., & Zinaman, M. (2005). Comparison of milk output between mothers of preterm and term infants: the first 6 weeks after birth. *Journal of Human Lactation, 21*(1), 22-30.

Hill, P. D., Aldag, J. C., Zinaman, M., & Chatterton, R. T., Jr. (2007). Comparison of milk output between breasts in pump-dependent mothers. *Journal of Human Lactation, 23*(4), 333-337.

Hogan, M., Westcott, C., & Griffiths, M. (2005). Randomized, controlled trial of division of tongue-tie in infants with feeding problems. *Journal of Paediatrics and Child Health, 41*(5-6), 246-250.

Howard, C. R., Lanphear, N., Lanphear, B. P., Eberly, S., & Lawrence, R. A. (2006). Parental responses to infant crying and colic: the effect on breastfeeding duration. *Breastfeed Med, 1*(3), 146-155.

Isabella, P. H., & Isabella, R. A. (1994). Correlates of successful breastfeeding: a study of social and personal factors. *Journal of Human Lactation, 10*(4), 257-264.

Jonas, W., Nissen, E., Ransjo-Arvidson, A. B., Wiklund, I., Henriksson, P., & Uvnas-Moberg, K. (2008). Short- and long-term decrease of blood pressure in women during breastfeeding. *Breastfeeding Medicine, 3*(2), 103-109.

Kassing, D. (2002). Bottle-feeding as a tool to reinforce breastfeeding. *Journal of Human Lactation, 18*(1), 56-60.

Kent, J. C., Mitoulas, L. R., Cregan, M. D., Ramsay, D. T., Doherty, D. A., & Hartmann, P. E. (2006). Volume and frequency of breastfeedings and fat content of breast milk throughout the day. *Pediatrics, 117*(3), e387-395.

Kesaree, N., Banapurmath, C. R., Banapurmath, S., & Shamanur, K. (1993). Treatment of inverted nipples using a disposable syringe. *Journal of Human Lactation, 9*(1), 27-29.

Lawrence, R. A., & Lawrence, R. M. (2005). *Breastfeeding: A guide for the medical profession*. Philadelphia, PA: Elsevier Mosby.

Livingstone, V. (1996). Too much of a good thing. Maternal and infant hyperlactation syndromes. *Canadian Family Physician, 42*, 89-99.

Makanjuola, D. (1998). A clinico-radiological correlation of breast diseases during lactation and the significance of unilateral failure of lactation. *West African Journal of Medicine, 17*(4), 217-223.

Marmet, C., & Shell, E. (2008). Therapeutic positioning for Breastfeeding. In C. W. Genna (Ed.), *Supporting Sucking Skills in Breastfeeding Infants* (pp. 305-325). Boston, MA: Jones and Bartlett.

Matheson, I., Aursnes, I., Horgen, M., Aabo, O., & Melby, K. (1988). Bacteriological findings and clinical symptoms in relation to clinical outcome in puerperal mastitis. *Acta Obstetricia et Gynecologica Scandinavica, 67*(8), 723-726.

Messner, A. H., & Lalakea, M. L. (2000). Ankyloglossia: controversies in management. *International Journal of Pediatric Otorhinolaryngology, 54*(2-3), 123-131.

Messner, A. H., Lalakea, M. L., Aby, J., Macmahon, J., & Bair, E. (2000). Ankyloglossia: incidence and associated feeding difficulties. *Archives of Otolaryngology -- Head and Neck Surgery, 126*(1), 36-39.

Miller-Loncar, C., Bigsby, R., High, P., Wallach, M., & Lester, B. (2004). Infant colic and feeding difficulties. *Archives of Disease in Childhood, 89*(10), 908-912.

Mohrbacher, N., & Kendall-Tackett, K. (2005). *Breastfeeding made simple: seven natural laws for nursing mothers*. Oakland, CA: New Harbinger Publications.

Mojab, C. G. (2007). Congenital torticollis in the nursling. *Journal of Human Lactation, 23*(1), 12.

Nommsen-Rivers, L. A., Heinig, M. J., Cohen, R. J., & Dewey, K. G. (2008). Newborn wet and soiled diaper counts and timing of onset of lactation as indicators of breastfeeding inadequacy. *Journal of Human Lactation, 24*(1), 27-33.

Palmer, B. (1998). The influence of breastfeeding on the development of the oral cavity: a commentary. *Journal of Human Lactation, 14*(2), 93-98.

Radzyminski, S. (2005). Neurobehavioral functioning and breastfeeding behavior in the newborn. *Journal of Obstetric, Gynecologic, and Neonatal Nursing, 34*(3), 335-341.

Rempel, L. A. (2004). Factors influencing the breastfeeding decisions of long-term breastfeeders. *Journal of Human Lactation, 20*(3), 306-318.

Ricke, L. A., Baker, N. J., Madlon-Kay, D. J., & DeFor, T. A. (2005). Newborn tongue-tie: prevalence and effect on breast-feeding. *Journal of the American Board of Family Practice, 18*(1), 1-7.

Righard, L. (1998). Are breastfeeding problems related to incorrect breastfeeding technique and the use of pacifiers and bottles? *Birth, 25*(1), 40-44.

Saber, A., Dardik, H., Ibrahim, I. M., & Wolodiger, F. (1996). The milk rejection sign: a natural tumor marker. *American Surgeon, 62*(12), 998-999.

Segal, L. M., Stephenson, R., Dawes, M., & Feldman, P. (2007). Prevalence, diagnosis, and treatment of ankyloglossia: methodologic review. *Canadian Family Physician, 53*(6), 1027-1033.

Shrago, L. C., Reifsnider, E., & Insel, K. (2006). The Neonatal Bowel Output Study: indicators of adequate breast milk intake in neonates. *Pediatric Nursing, 32*(3), 195-201.

Sicherer, S. H. (2003). Clinical aspects of gastrointestinal food allergy in childhood. *Pediatrics, 111*(6 Pt 3), 1609-1616.

Smillie, C. (2008). How infants learn to feed: A neurbehavioral model. In C. W. Genna (Ed.), *Supporting Sucking Skills in Breastfeeding Infants* (pp. 79-95). Boston, MA: Jones and Bartlett.

Srinivasan, A., Dobrich, C., Mitnick, H., & Feldman, P. (2006). Ankyloglossia in breastfeeding infants: the effect of frenotomy on maternal nipple pain and latch. *Breastfeeding Medicine, 1*(4), 216-224.

Taveras, E. M., Li, R., Grummer-Strawn, L., Richardson, M., Marshall, R., Rego, V.H., et al. (2004). Opinions and practices of clinicians associated with continuation of exclusive breastfeeding. *Pediatrics,* 113(4), e283-290.

Uvnas-Moberg, K. (2003). *The oxytocin factor: tapping the hormone of calm, love, and healing*. Cambridge, MA: Da Capo Press.

Vazirinejad, R., Darakhshan, S., Esmaeili, A., & Hadadian, S. (2009). The effect of maternal breast variations on neonatal weight gain in the first seven days of life. *International Breastfeeding Journal, 4*, 13.

Wall, V., & Glass, R. (2006). Mandibular asymmetry and breastfeeding problems: experience from 11 cases. *Journal of Human Lactation, 22*(3), 328-334.

Wambach, K. A. (2003). Lactation mastitis: a descriptive study of the experience. *Journal of Human Lactation, 19*(1), 24-34.

Wessel, M. A., Cobb, J. C., Jackson, E. B., Harris, G. S., Jr., & Detwiler, A. C. (1954). Paroxysmal fussing in infancy, sometimes called colic. *Pediatrics, 14*(5), 421-435.

West, D., & Marasco, L. (2009). *The breastfeeding mother's guide to making more milk*. New York, NY: McGraw Hill.

Wiessinger, D., & Miller, M. (1995). Breastfeeding difficulties as a result of tight lingual and labial frena: a case report. *Journal of Human Lactation, 11*(4), 313-316.

Wilson-Clay, B., & Hoover, K. (2008). *The breastfeeding atlas* (4th ed.). Manchaca, TX: LactNews Press.

Wolf, L., & Glass, R. (1992). *Feeding and swallowing disorders in infancy*. Tucson, AZ: Therapy Skill Builders.

Woolridge, M. W., & Fisher, C. (1988). Colic, "overfeeding", and symptoms of lactose malabsorption in the breast-fed baby: a possible artifact of feed management? *Lancet, 2*(8607), 382-384.

Solid Foods

Chapter

4

Starting solid foods is a part of the weaning process. This process begins when a baby takes any food other than mother's milk, and ends with the last breastfeeding. In some parts of the world, "weaning" refers to starting solid foods, which are referred to as "weaning foods." Recently, some have suggested changing these terms, with "weaning" generally agreed to mean the end of breastfeeding (Fewtrell et al., 2007). These organizations include the World Health Organization (WHO, 2001) and the American Academy of Pediatrics (AAP).

WHEN TO BEGIN SOLIDS

Many health organizations recommend exclusive breastfeeding for the first 6 months, with solids foods introduced at about 6 months, along with continued breastfeeding.

Not Too Early

Health outcomes

Starting solids before 6 months is associated with negative health outcomes.

Starting solids within the first 4 months of life was common practice in the U.S. and elsewhere for many years. However, research found that this practice is associated with an increased risk of atopic disease and other health problems.

Before 1997, the American Academy of Pediatrics (AAP) recommended that babies start eating solid foods between 4 and 6 months of age. But within the last decade, this recommendation has changed. The change began in 1997, when the AAP Section on Breastfeeding issued its revised policy statement, recommending delaying solids until 6 months of age (AAP, 1997).

In 2001, the World Health Organization published a report by its expert panel (WHO, 2001), which reviewed over 3,000 studies and concluded that starting solids before 6 months had health drawbacks for both mothers and babies:

- Babies are at greater risk of gastrointestinal infections and diarrhea in both developed and developing countries (Kramer, 2003).
- Mothers lose less weight and return to fertility sooner.

There was also some evidence that babies who are not exclusively breastfed for 6 months are at increased risk for delayed motor development (K. G. Dewey, Cohen, Brown, & Rivera, 2001). The WHO expert panel agreed that in most cases exclusive breastfeeding for 6 months results in normal growth and that the benefits of waiting until 6 months to start solid foods outweighed the risks (WHO, 2001).

Other authors agreed based on a reanalysis of studies in Brazil and Bangladesh, which concluded that breastfed infants in the first 6 months of life given solid foods died at a two- to three-fold higher rate from diarrhea and pneumonia compared with babies who were exclusively breastfed (R. E. Black & Victora, 2002).

This led to the following conclusion in one Cochrane Review article (Kramer & Kakuma, 2002):

> Infants who are exclusively breastfed for 6 months experience less morbidity from gastrointestinal infection than those who are mixed breastfed as of 3 or 4 months, and no deficits have been demonstrated in growth among infants from either developing or developed countries who are exclusively breastfed for 6 months or longer.

Studies published since the WHO expert panel review have also found an association between very early solids and an increased risk for allergy (Muraro et al., 2004) and celiac disease (Norris et al., 2005). Other more recent studies found that when babies who are at risk for developing type 1 diabetes mellitus start gluten-containing foods younger than 3 to 4 months of age, they are at increased risk of developing the autoantibodies associated with type 1 diabetes mellitus, which may increase their chances of developing this disease later in life (Norris et al., 2003; Rosenbauer, Herzig, Kaiser, & Giani, 2007; Ziegler, Schmid, Huber, Hummel, & Bonifacio, 2003).

Another reason to delay solid foods until 6 months is that babies are more developmentally ready, making it easier and more pleasant for everyone.

From a practical standpoint, the following developmental changes indicate increased readiness to start solid foods and are good reasons to wait until 6 months.

- **Tongue-thrust reflex fades** between 4 and 6 months of age. Until this happens, babies push out their tongue when their mouth is touched, so little food is swallowed and feedings are frustrating and messy.
- **Baby can sit up and reach for foods.** At 6 months, a baby is able to take a more active role in feeding himself because he can sit up alone, reach for foods, and put them in his mouth.
- **Eruption of teeth.** Teething encourages chewing and makes it easier for a baby to break down his food for easier swallowing.

Talking with Parents

Many parents are eager to give their baby solid foods.

Many parents—especially first-time parents—look forward to giving their baby solid foods. When their baby starts solids, many parents feel "proud" and consider it a "big achievement" (Anderson et al., 2001; Danowski & Gargiula, 2002). For the exclusively breastfed baby, solid foods may be the first time others become involved in baby's feeding, which can be an exciting time for the whole family. Parents' eagerness to start solids can sometimes lead them to start earlier than is recommended (Gijsbers, Mesters, Andre Knottnerus, Legtenberg, & van Schayck, 2005).

Parents' willingness to delay solid foods until 6 months varies by area and cultural beliefs.

In some parts of the world, the vast majority of parents start solids at the recommended age. Examples include Sweden (Brekke, Ludvigsson, van Odijk, & Ludvigsson, 2005; Mikkelsen, Rinne-Ljungqvist, Borres, & van Odijk, 2007), the Netherlands (Gijsbers et al., 2005), and many developing countries (Sellen, 2001).

However, in other parts of the world, many parents start solid foods earlier than recommended, some even before 4 months. Examples include the U.S. (Briefel, Reidy, Karwe, & Devaney, 2004; Crocetti, Dudas, & Krugman, 2004; Danowski & Gargiula, 2002; Heinig, 2006), the U.K. (Alder et al., 2004; Anderson et al., 2001; Savage, Reilly, Edwards, & Durnin, 1998; Sloan, Gildea, Stewart,

Sneddon, & Iwaniec, 2008), Brazil (Wayland, 2004), Australia (Donath & Amir, 2005; Walker, Conn, Davies, & Moore, 2006), and some developing countries (Marriott, Campbell, Hirsch, & Wilson, 2007).

Many mothers are influenced by cultural beliefs and advice from others to start solids early, thinking their babies will cry less and sleep more.

Family and friends are major influencers of new parents on what foods to give and when to give them (Alder et al., 2004; Crocetti et al., 2004; Gijsbers et al., 2005). Research also has found that many mothers start solids early because they believe infant crying is a sign of hunger and that giving solids will help "settle" their baby (Crocetti et al., 2004; Danowski & Gargiula, 2002).

The belief that solids will help their babies sleep better is another reason mothers give for early introduction of solids, which is often reinforced by family and friends (M. M. Black, Siegel, Abel, & Bentley, 2001; Crocetti et al., 2004; Danowski & Gargiula, 2002; Heinig et al., 2006). In one Scottish study, many mothers reported believing that milk alone was not enough to satisfy their babies and that solids were needed to help babies sleep through the night (Savage et al., 1998). Although research has found no association between solid foods and babies sleeping through the night, this belief is still strong in many places (Keane, 1988; Macknin, Medendorp, & Maier, 1989).

A common reason U.K. mothers give for early introduction of solids is rapid infant weight gain, which they interpret as meaning their baby "needs" other foods (Savage et al., 1998; Wright, Parkinson, & Drewett, 2004). Some baby food manufacturers encourage this belief by advising parents to start solids based on weight rather than age.

In cultures where overweight babies are considered "healthier," introducing solid foods may be considered necessary to insure babies "get enough." If these beliefs cause mothers to override their babies' signs of fullness and continue to feed, they may increase the risk of childhood obesity.

If a mother has already started solids early, before giving information, ask her open-ended questions about why she made that choice, then affirm her feelings.

When a mother who gives solids early expresses any of the reasons described in the previous point, first affirm her feelings (her desire for a "settled" and healthy baby, her need for sleep). One study reported that many of the low-income women interviewed disregarded recommendations given by healthcare providers and public health staff because they thought those giving advice did not understand the situations they faced (Heinig et al., 2006). By affirming the mother and asking open-ended questions about her situation, she is more likely to be receptive and feel understood.

Strategies that are effective in delaying the early introduction of solid foods address cultural beliefs and family dynamics, as well as provide health information.

If a family's culture does not value breastfeeding or its cultural beliefs run counter to recommended practices, it may be difficult to convince parents that delaying solid foods for 6 months is wise or practical (Alder et al., 2004; Anderson et al., 2001; Crocetti et al., 2004; Danowski & Gargiula, 2002; Heinig et al., 2006; Horodynski et al., 2007; Savage et al., 1998; Sloan et al., 2008; Wayland, 2004).

One U.S. study examined the behavior of single, low-income, African-American teen mothers, one of the American ethnic groups least likely to both breastfeed and delay solid foods until 6 months (M. M. Black et al., 2001). The strategies used in this study effectively helped these mothers delay solid foods longer. Early introduction of solid foods is common in this ethnic group in part because of the following cultural beliefs (Crocetti et al., 2004; Horodynski et al., 2007):

- Heavy babies are healthier.
- Solid foods reduce infant crying.
- Solid foods help babies sleep through the night.

The teen mothers in this study lived with their own mothers, who also held these beliefs. Within many African-American communities, mothers tend to give greater credibility to their mothers' advice than advice given by healthcare professionals (Horodynski et al., 2007).

In one of the two study groups, teen mothers were given the usual health recommendations about the appropriate age to start solids. In the other group, teen mothers received this information along with the following interventions to help counteract their cultural beliefs.

- At their first home visit, they were shown a video featuring successful African-American teen mothers sharing information on how to distinguish baby's feeding cues from other needs. It also showed nonfood strategies for managing babies' behavior. Segments included teen mothers talking about ways to avoid conflicts with their own mother and how to achieve good feeding practices at home, school, and at day care.
- The home visitors who showed the video were college-educated African- American mothers with good communication skills. They were about 10 years older than the teen mothers and were chosen to be role models and mentors.

The teen mothers who received these interventions were four times more likely to delay solid foods than the teen mothers who were simply given the health recommendations.

To improve practices, another study suggests targeting grandmothers, as well as mothers, in African-American communities (Horodynski et al., 2007).

• •

Mothers may be more likely to follow recommendations if the health risks of early solids are stressed, rather than the health benefits of delaying solids.

One study that examined strategies to delay introduction of solid foods found that African-American mothers were much more likely to delay solids until the recommended age if the risks to their baby's health from early solids was emphasized, rather than the health benefits of waiting (Horodynski et al., 2007).

• •

To delay solids until the recommended age, mothers need to know which behaviors are age-appropriate and nonfood strategies for meeting their babies' needs.

Although many mothers say they start solid foods early in response to their babies' "cues," in most cases before a baby is 6 months old, giving solid foods is not the best response (Anderson et al., 2001; M. M. Black et al., 2001; Crocetti et al., 2004; Heinig et al., 2006; Wright et al., 2004). Many mothers misinterpret normal infant behaviors or other needs as "hunger for solids."

Suggest the mother consider other responses, such as breastfeeding when a baby fusses, holding and playing with her baby, or wearing her baby in a soft baby carrier as she does her chores. Mothers need to know that night-waking is common in babies younger than 6 months and not necessarily a problem to be solved. For mothers struggling with fatigue, discuss strategies for meeting her baby's needs at night that maximize her sleep, such as keeping baby near her for night feedings (Gartner et al., 2005). Attending mother support group meetings may also be helpful, as she can hear a wide range of strategies from other mothers.

• •

Some mothers may continue to give solids if they feel they have "lost control" over baby's feedings.

In one study, some mothers reported that when other people gave their baby solid foods or infant formula, they felt that they "must" continue giving the solids or formula because they had lost control of their baby's feeding (Heinig et al., 2006). In this case, help the mother understand that even if the baby has received solids, it is possible to return to exclusive breastfeeding.

Not Too Late

Delaying solid foods longer than 7 months, especially foods containing gluten, does not seem to be beneficial and may have risks.

Some mothers delay solid foods longer than 6 months in the hopes that this will provide their babies with greater protection from allergy. However, one review of the literature concluded that delaying solids foods past 6 months does not offer significant protection (Greer, Sicherer, & Burks, 2008).

Based on another review of the literature, an upper age limit of 26 weeks for starting solids was recommended in a position paper by a European health organization (Agostoni et al., 2008). This upper age limit was suggested because some research has found that when solid foods are delayed longer than 7 months, especially foods containing gluten (a type of protein found in wheat, rye, and barley), there may be an increased incidence of Type 1 diabetes, allergy, and celiac disease. In other words, there may be a critical window between 6 and 7 months in babies susceptible to these health problems during which it is best to offer small to moderate amounts of gluten-containing solid foods, such as strips of toasted wheat or rye bread or cereals made from wheat, rye, or barley.

Delaying solids past 6 months increases the risk of allergy and chronic disease.

Type 1 diabetes mellitus. When babies at risk for developing Type 1 diabetes mellitus start gluten-containing foods after 7 months of age, one U.S. study found an increased risk of developing the autoantibodies associated with this disease (Norris et al., 2003). This long-term study followed 1,183 of these at-risk children for 9 months to 9 years. Although others have not yet replicated these results, Norris and colleagues acknowledge that this "window of exposure" would be easy to miss in studies using only one age cutoff (for example, before or after 6 months (Ziegler et al., 2003). The Norris study also found that if these foods were introduced while the child was still breastfeeding, the risk of developing these autoantibodies was reduced independent of the age of exposure.

Wheat allergy. Another U.S. study followed 1,612 children from birth to a mean age of 4.7 years (Poole et al., 2006). Children were chosen who either had a family history of allergy or whose blood test revealed a susceptibility to allergy. The study found that children who were started on wheat cereal at 7 months of age or older had a four times higher risk of developing a wheat allergy than children who were started on wheat cereal earlier than 7 months.

Celiac disease. This disease, which can be life-threatening, is an allergy to gluten. The increased risk of developing celiac disease first came to light when Swedish health authorities began advising parents to delay giving babies foods with gluten until after 7 months. As a result, a fourfold increase in cases of celiac disease occurred in Sweden (Ivarsson et al., 2000). After this recommendation was reversed and Swedish babies again received gluten-containing foods before 7 months, the incidence of celiac disease decreased to previous levels.

Later, another study that followed 627 children with celiac disease and 1,254 without found an association between celiac disease and the amount of gluten-containing foods received when solids were started (Ivarsson, Hernell, Stenlund, & Persson, 2002). The risk of developing celiac disease was reduced when babies received smaller amounts of the gluten-containing foods and further reduced if the babies were still breastfeeding when these foods were started. The risk was reduced even more when the babies continued to breastfeed after starting the gluten-containing foods.

• •

If a 6-month-old baby rejects solid foods, suggest the mother try again in a few days with a different food.

For more, see the next section, "Strategies for Giving Solids."

Iron

Most babies begin to need solid foods at around 6 months of age, when their iron stores from birth begin to run low.

The AAP's Section on Breastfeeding (Gartner et al., 2005, p. 499) recommends "...foods rich in iron should be introduced gradually."

Research indicates that full-term babies born at average weight or more to well-nourished mothers have enough iron stores to last through their first 6 to 9 months of life (K.G. Dewey, 2007; Raj, Faridi, Rusia, & Singh, 2008). The iron in human milk is much better absorbed than iron from other sources, up to 50% absorption from human milk (Griffin & Abrams, 2001) compared with 4% absorption from infant formula (Lawrence, 2005, p. 143). This is due, at least in part, to the vitamin C and lactose in human milk, which enhance iron absorption. But because the amount of iron in human milk is low, breastfed babies need iron from other sources, beginning around 6 to 9 months of age. For this reason, some suggest introducing foods early on that are naturally high in iron, such as meats (Krebs et al., 2006).

One Swedish study found that as babies mature, their ability to absorb iron increases (Domellof, Lonnerdal, Abrams, & Hernell, 2002). Between 6 and 9 months of age, developmental changes appear to enhance a baby's ability to absorb iron, but only when on a low-iron diet. Breastfed babies who received iron supplements that were added to their mother's expressed milk and fed by bottle absorbed a much smaller percentage of the iron than babies who received no iron supplements (17% vs. 37%). The researchers wrote:

> ...this observation supports the theory that the dietary regulation of iron absorption is immature in the 6-month-old infant and is subject to developmental changes between 8 and 9 months of age...This might prove to be a valuable compensatory mechanism in partially breastfed infants with low-iron diets and might explain why we found no correlation between complementary food iron intake and iron status in 9-month-old Swedish infants (Domellof, Lonnerdal, Abrams et al., 2002, p. 203).

The effects of too little iron are well known. Too little iron can cause iron deficiency in babies, as well as anemia, which are associated with developmental delays and neurological problems (Lozoff & Georgieff, 2006). If iron levels are too low for too long, it is not always possible to reverse these problems by giving iron supplements (Lozoff et al., 2006). Some research indicates that boys may be at a greater risk of iron deficiency than girls (Domellof, Lonnerdal, Dewey et al., 2002).

Healthy iron levels are important, as both too much and too little iron are associated with developmental delays and other negative outcomes.

Too much iron has been linked to slower growth, neurodevelopmental delays, and an increased incidence of some diseases One study examined growth and health outcomes among 101 Swedish and 131 Honduran babies (Dewey et al., 2002; Domellof, Cohen, Rivera, Hernell, & Lonnerdal, 2002). It found that when iron-sufficient babies received extra iron, their growth in length and head circumference was significantly less. The researchers concluded that while routine iron supplements provided benefits to babies who were iron deficient, they presented risks for babies who were not.

One 2008 study that followed 494 Chilean babies for 10 years found that feeding babies who are iron-sufficient a high-iron (12 mg/L ferrous sulfate) versus a low-iron infant formula (2.3 mg/L ferrous sulfate) from 6 to 18 months of age resulted in neurodevelopmental delays (Kerr, 2008). The babies who received the high-iron formula had significantly lower IQ scores (by an average of 11 points) at 10 years of age.

Too much iron has also been linked to an increased incidence of malaria (Oppenheimer et al., 1986) and severe sepsis (Barry & Reeve, 1977). When iron is present in the baby's digestive tract—which is not normally the case—it enhances the growth of disease-causing bacteria.

Supplementing these babies with iron can result in too-high iron levels, the risks of which are described in detail in the previous point.

Routine iron supplements are not recommended for babies with normal iron levels.

For babies needing extra iron for any reason, the American Academy of Pediatrics recommends giving iron supplements while continuing full breastfeeding (Gartner et al., 2005). In areas where pregnant mothers suffer from iron deficiencies, rather than starting solids early, the World Health Organization recommends finding ways to help mothers meet their own nutritional needs during pregnancy (WHO, 2001).

Low birthweight and preterm babies and those born to iron-deficient mothers may have low iron stores at birth and need iron supplementation before 6 months.

With some nutrients, such as vitamin D, a mother can boost the levels in her milk by taking a supplement, but that is not the case with iron (Griffin & Abrams, 2001; Hopkinson, 2007; Vuori, Makinen, Kara, & Kuitunen, 1980; Zavaleta et al., 1995). Iron-deficient mothers have the same amount of iron in their milk as mothers with healthy iron levels (Hopkinson, 2007).

The amount of iron in a mother's milk is not affected by her iron status.

If there is concern about a baby's iron levels, the baby's healthcare provider can check the levels with a simple blood test.

This blood test can usually be performed in the healthcare provider's office. In recent years, research has examined and redefined healthy iron levels in breastfed babies at 4, 6, and 9 months of age (Domellof, Dewey, Lonnerdal, Cohen, & Hernell, 2002). According to this study, healthy hemoglobin levels in breastfed babies are ≥10.5 g/dL at 4 and 6 months and ≥10.0 g/dL at 9 months.

STRATEGIES FOR GIVING SOLIDS

How solid foods are introduced is as important as what foods are given.

As with breastfeeding, introducing solid foods tends to go more smoothly if the baby perceives it as a positive experience. When meals are a happy, social time and baby's needs and preferences are respected, he is more likely to accept the foods that are offered (Pelto, Levitt, & Thairu, 2003). Encourage parents to approach feeding time with patience, encouragement, and eye contact and not to be too concerned about how much food the baby takes. In some cultures, little attention is paid to how much a baby eats, unless the baby is sick or is refusing to eat (Engle & Zeitlin, 1996).

Meal times should be a happy, social time.

Giving the baby more control over the feeding makes mealtimes more positive and results in more food eaten.

One U.K. study found that when less pressure is used on babies to eat solids, less mealtime negativity is observed at 1 year of age (Farrow & Blissett, 2006). When mothers used more controlling strategies at mealtimes and were less sensitive to their babies' cues, the babies behaved more negatively at mealtimes at 1 year. Continued breastfeeding was also associated with less controlling behavior at mealtimes, perhaps because breastfeeding itself teaches mothers to give their babies more control over their feedings. Longer breastfeeding duration was also associated with less restrictive child-feeding behaviors at 1 year (Taveras et al., 2004).

Giving greater control to the child also results in more food eaten. Breastfeeding through the first year was associated with more calories consumed at 18 months (Fisher, Birch, Smiciklas-Wright, & Picciano, 2000).

To avoid overfeeding or underfeeding, beginning at about 6 months, suggest parents take a "baby-led" approach to feeding solid foods.

Just as breastfeeding is a part of the relationship between a mother and a baby, so too is their time together at family mealtimes. Responsive feeding of any type involves learning and respecting baby's hunger and satiety cues (Pelto et al., 2003).

One easy way to accomplish this is to include the baby at family mealtimes and allow the baby to take the lead in feeding himself. Some call this a "baby-led" approach to starting solid foods or "baby-led weaning" (Gill, 2007; Rapley, 2006). This means allowing a baby to feed himself from the start. When using this approach, the adult decides when baby eats and what foods are offered. The baby decides whether to eat and how much food to take. This approach assumes that the baby is old enough to sit up by himself, reach for and grab the food, and bring it to his mouth on his own.

At around 6 months, most babies can handle semi-solid and some finger foods by themselves. There is no need for all of a baby's foods to be pureed or given by spoon. By 8 months, most babies can easily manage many finger foods. Family foods can be used, as long that they are not too highly seasoned or contain added salt and sugar (Dewey & Brown, 2003).

There are advantages to offering firmer, rather than pureed, foods from the start. Some research indicates that feeding babies only smooth, pureed foods after 10 months of age increases the risk for feeding difficulties later (Northstone, Emmett, & Nethersole, 2001).

To most easily manage the inevitable mess, many parents dress their babies down to their diapers, use large bibs, and/or use drop cloths or plastic sheets on the floor to catch spills.

At about 6 months, suggest mothers continue frequent breastfeeding while offering small meals, increasing the number of daily meals as baby grows.

Continued frequent breastfeeding is important because even babies older than 1 year of age receive necessary nutrients from mother's milk. Breastfed babies 1 to 2 years old getting average amounts of mother's milk receive 35% to 40% of their energy intake from it (K. G. Dewey & Brown, 2003). Mother's milk is an important source of fatty acids and other key nutrients, such as vitamin A, calcium, and riboflavin (PAHO/WHO, 2001).

Begin at 6 months by including baby at family mealtimes two or three times per day. As baby gets older, suggest parents increase the number of meals and snacks, allowing baby to eat as much as desired at each sitting (Table 4.1).

Table 4.1. Recommended Number of Daily Meals by Age

Baby's Age	# Meals/Snacks Per Day
6 to 8 months	2 to 3
9 to 11 months	3 to 4
12 to 24 months	3 to 4 meals, 1 to 2 snacks

(PAHO/WHO, 2001)

If a 6-month-old baby rejects solid foods, suggest the mother try again in a few days with a different food.

Not all babies are ready to begin solids at the same age, and the family table should never become a battleground. Some children who are prone to food allergies or intolerances may reject solids until they are a little older. If the exclusively breastfeeding baby has adequate iron levels and a steady weight gain, these are good indicators that he is thriving. Even so, encourage parents to continue to regularly offer different foods until the baby begins to show an interest in them.

As a baby takes more solid foods, he takes less mother's milk.

At first, solid foods do not boost a baby's overall intake. Rather, solids take the place of mother's milk in a baby's diet (Cohen, Brown, Canahuati, Rivera, & Dewey, 1994). Intake of mother's milk decreases as soon as the first day after babies begin eating solid foods (Islam, Peerson, Ahmed, Dewey, & Brown, 2006). This is a normal stage of breastfeeding, ideally with the baby controlling the overall amount of food and milk he consumes.

SPECIFIC FOODS

Babies grow quickly, so a variety of nutrient-dense foods are recommended.

Specific food choices for babies vary greatly around the world. For this reason, the World Health Organization does not give a list of specific foods, but recommends offering babies a variety of nutritious foods to increase the likelihood that babies will receive the nutrients they need (PAHO/WHO, 2001).

Although specific diets vary across cultures, a high percentage include milk products, fruits and vegetables, and meat, poultry or fish.

The WHO Multicentre Growth Reference Study (the research used to create the growth charts based on breastfeeding babies) found that the babies at its six international sites (Brazil, Ghana, India, Norway, Oman, and the U.S.) had some aspects of their diets in common. Although the specific foods varied, the diets were nutrient dense, with more than 75% of children receiving milk products and fruits/vegetables and 50% to 95% receiving meat, poultry, or fish (Complementary feeding in the WHO Multicentre Growth Reference Study, 2006).

One U.S. study found that meat, which is high in iron, worked well as an early solid food (Krebs et al., 2006). Examples of nutritious foods by texture that can be given before 12 months include:

Soft and Semi-Soft Foods

- Tender, ground poultry or meat
- Cooked vegetables, such as sweet potato, yam, parsnip, carrot, or white potato
- Tofu
- Ripe fruit, such as banana, peaches, mangos, avocados
- Cooked cereal, including wheat, rice, oat, and barley
- Cooked egg yolks
- Grated apples or applesauce

Finger Foods

- Finger-sized slices of toasted or untoasted whole-grain leavened or unleavened breads or crackers
- Tofu cut into slivers
- Fresh or frozen peas
- Soft, ripe, fresh fruit, such as peaches, pears, mangos, etc. cut into slivers
- Tender, cooked, thin slivers of poultry or meat
- Cooked egg yolks cut into slivers or bite-sized pieces

In the U.S., some recommend delaying eggs (especially egg whites) until 12 months. Egg yolks are a good source of iron, and research has found the risk of allergy very low when only the yolks are given (Makrides, Hawkes, Neumann, & Gibson, 2002).

When starting a new food, allow 2 to 3 days before adding another new food.

This gives parents time to notice if the baby has any allergic reactions to the new food (AAP, 2007; Agostoni et al., 2008), such as:

- Diarrhea
- Rash
- Vomiting

If the baby has any of these reactions, suggest the parents stop that food for now and give the baby a couple of months to mature before trying it again. Once a baby has consumed a food without a reaction for 2 to 3 days, this food can then be served with other foods that have been tried or with a single new food.

Tell the mother to expect changes in baby's stools after solids are started.

Often babies on solids have less frequent stools that smell stronger and are darker in color than they had while exclusively breastfeeding. The mother may also see bits of undigested food in her baby's stools.

Babies are more likely to accept foods their mothers consumed regularly during pregnancy and breastfeeding.

During pregnancy and breastfeeding, all mammal young are exposed to the flavors of the foods their mothers eat through amniotic fluid and their mother's milk. This helps babies recognize safe foods when they are ready to expand their diet to non-milk foods (Forestell & Mennella, 2007; Mennella, 2007; J. A. Mennella, Jagnow, & Beauchamp, 2001).

Several studies indicate that when mothers eat a food regularly during pregnancy and breastfeeding, their babies are more likely to accept it later as a solid food. In one U.S. study, mothers drank either carrot juice or water 4 days per week for 3 weeks during pregnancy (Mennella et al., 2001). When carrots were introduced later as a solid food, the babies' enjoyment of them was rated higher by the mothers who drank the carrot juice than by the mothers who drank the water.

Suggest avoid adding salt to baby's foods.

This recommendation (Agostoni et al., 2008) is based on a study that followed babies for 15 years and found that babies may be more sensitive to salt intake than adults and that salt intake during infancy may lead to high blood pressure later in life (Geleijnse et al., 1997).

Unpasteurized honey is not recommended during a baby's first 12 months.

To help establish healthy eating habits, unsweetened foods are preferred for babies 6 to 12 months old. Because cases of botulism have been reported in babies younger than 1 year who received unpasteurized honey, the American Academy of Pediatrics and other health organizations recommend avoiding unpasteurized honey until a baby is at least 12 months of age (AAP, 2006; Agostoni et al., 2008).

Foods that can cause choking are not recommended until 3 years of age.

If a food can easily get lodged in a baby's throat and cause choking, it is recommended to wait until the baby is 3 years old before offering it. Examples include:

- Nuts
- Grapes
- Popcorn
- Hot dogs
- Raw carrots

Many health organizations no longer recommend delaying potentially allergenic foods after the first year of life.

In the past, the American Academy of Pediatrics suggested that parents wait to introduce potentially allergic foods, such as wheat, eggs, fish, peanuts, and other nuts, to babies with a family history of allergy (Committee on, 2000; Meek, 2002). However, in 2008 this recommendation changed based on a review of the literature that concluded there is no evidence that delaying highly allergic foods longer than 1 year has a protective effect against allergies (Greer et al., 2008). This is consistent with the recommendations of other international health organizations (Agostoni et al., 2008; Halken & Host, 2001).

A baby on a restricted vegetarian diet may need vitamin supplements or fortified foods.

When a baby starts solids, some of the recommended foods include meat, poultry, fish, and eggs (K. G. Dewey & Brown, 2003; PAHO/WHO, 2001). If a family on a vegan diet chooses not to give their baby these foods, suggest the baby be offered dairy products (Agostoni et al., 2008).

Depending upon the family's diet, the baby may also need vitamin/mineral supplements or fortified foods containing iron, zinc, and vitamin B_{12}. A vegan or macrobiotic diet containing little or no meat or dairy can lead to nutritional deficiencies and is not recommended for babies (Agostoni et al., 2008). Dutch babies fed on a macrobiotic diet deficient in protein, vitamin B_{12}, vitamin D, calcium, and riboflavin experienced retarded growth, muscle wasting, and delayed motor development (Dagnelie & van Staveren, 1994).

BEVERAGES

After around 8 to 9 months, many babies begin to enjoy drinking from a cup.

As babies develop better muscle control, many enjoy taking a drink from a cup. This could be any time after 8 or 9 months or so (Agostoni et al., 2008). Nutrient-rich drinks that could be offered in a cup include:

- Expressed mother's milk
- Home-cooked broths or thin soups without added salt or spices

Other drinks that could be given in a cup in small amounts include:

- Water
- Unsweetened fruit and vegetable juices

Cow's milk has been found to cause intestinal bleeding in babies younger than 9 months (Agostoni et al., 2008), which can result in lower iron status (Griffin & Abrams, 2001). Because cow's milk is also a poor source of iron, giving it as a substitute for mother's milk or infant formula has been associated with iron deficiency in babies (Agostoni et al., 2008; Gunnarsson, Thorsdottir, & Palsson, 2004; Thorsdottir, Gunnarsson, Atladottir, Michaelsen, & Palsson, 2003).

Cow's milk is not recommended in significant amounts until twelve months of age, but other dairy products can be given earlier.

For these reasons, most recommend cow's milk not be given to babies younger than twelve months as their main drink (Agostoni et al., 2008). However, in Canada, Sweden, and Denmark, cow's milk is considered an acceptable drink after 9 or 10 months. Some processed dairy products, such as cheese and yogurt, are recommended after 6 months.

In some countries, babies are commonly given fruit juice to drink. Fruit juice provides some nutrition, but far less than mother's milk or whole fruit. Also, fruit juice fills up a baby, making him less interested in breastfeeding and in other foods. For these reasons, when a baby is given too much fruit juice, it puts him at increased risk of both extremes of malnutrition—failure to thrive (Smith & Lifshitz, 1994) and obesity (Dennison, Rockwell, & Baker, 1997)—as well as short stature (Dennison et al., 1997). Fruit juice consumption has also been linked to gastrointestinal problems, such as diarrhea, abdominal pain, and bloating (AAP, 2001).

Fruit juice should only be given to babies older than 6 months and limited to no more than 4 to 6 ounces (120 to 180 ml) per day.

In 2001, the American Academy of Pediatrics Committee on Nutrition (AAP, 2001) reviewed the research and published the following recommendations on fruit juice intake in babies and young children:

- Fruit juice should not be given to babies younger than 6 months of age.
- Only pasteurized fruit juice should be given, and daily intake of juice should be no more than 4 to 6 ounces (120 to 180 ml).
- Whole fruits are preferred over fruit juice.
- Juice should be limited to mealtimes, and babies should not be given containers of juice to drink from throughout the day or at bedtime.
- Ask about fruit juice consumption whenever a child has malnutrition, chronic diarrhea, abdominal pain and bloating, or dental caries.

In some cultures, teas are commonly given to babies. Both teas and coffees are not recommended because they interfere with iron absorption (PAHO/WHO, 2001). Teas, coffees, and sodas are best avoided completely because they have low nutritional value and can decrease a baby's interest in nutritious foods during a time when he is growing quickly. Also, some contain caffeine, which can decrease appetite and disrupt sleep. Soda consumption in early life has also been associated with overweight and dental caries (Ismail, Sohn, Lim, & Willem, 2009; Warner, Harley, Bradman, Vargas, & Eskenazi, 2006).

Other drinks, such as tea, coffees, and sodas, are not recommended for babies.

RESOURCES FOR PARENTS

Websites

http://whqlibdoc.who.int/paho/2004/a85622.pdf

http://www.llli.org/NB/NBsolids.html

Videos/DVDs

Rapley, G. (2006). *I can feed myself: A baby-led approach to introducing solid foods* (U.S.) and *Baby-led weaning* (U.K.). 17 minutes. Available in the U.S. at www.platypusmedia.com and in the U.K. at http://www.babyfriendly.org.uk/items/resource_detail.asp?item=422.

La Leche League of Great Britain. (2007). *Starting solids*. 14 minutes. Available at http://www.lllgbbooks.co.uk/go_shopping/videos_and_dvds/

Books

Rapley, G. and Murkett, T. (2008). *Baby-led weaning: Helping your baby to love good food.* London: Vermillion Press.

REFERENCES

AAP. (1997). Breastfeeding and the use of human milk. American Academy of Pediatrics. Work Group on Breastfeeding. Pediatrics, 100(6), 1035-1039.

AAP. (2001). American Academy of Pediatrics: The use and misuse of fruit juice in pediatrics. Pediatrics, 107(5), 1210-1213.

AAP. (2007, March 2007). Starting Solid Foods. Retrieved 4/4/08, from http://www.aap.org/publiced/BR_Solids.htm.

AAP. (2009). Prevention of disease from potentially contaminated food products. In L. K. Pickering, C. J. Baker, D. W. Kimberlin & S. S. Long (Eds.), Red Book: 2009 Report of the Committee on Infecious Diseases (28th ed., pp. 857-859). Elk Grove Village, IL: American Academy of Pediatrics.

Agostoni, C., Decsi, T., Fewtrell, M., Goulet, O., Kolacek, S., Koletzko, B., et al. (2008a). Complementary feeding: a commentary by the ESPGHAN Committee on Nutrition. J Pediatr Gastroenterol Nutr, 46(1), 99-110.

Agostoni, C., Decsi, T., Fewtrell, M., Goulet, O., Kolacek, S., Koletzko, B., et al. (2008b). Complementary feeding: a commentary by the ESPGHAN Committee on Nutrition. Journal of Pediatric Gastroenterology and Nutrition, 46(1), 99-110.

Alder, E. M., Williams, F. L., Anderson, A. S., Forsyth, S., Florey Cdu, V., & van der Velde, P. (2004). What influences the timing of the introduction of solid food to infants? British Journal of Nutrition, 92(3), 527-531.

Anderson, A. S., Guthrie, C. A., Alder, E. M., Forsyth, S., Howie, P. W., & Williams, F. L. (2001). Rattling the plate--reasons and rationales for early weaning. Health Education Research, 16(4), 471-479.

Barry, D. M., & Reeve, A. W. (1977). Increased incidence of gram-negative neonatal sepsis with intramuscula iron administration. Pediatrics, 60(6), 908-912.

Black, M. M., Siegel, E. H., Abel, Y., & Bentley, M. E. (2001). Home and videotape intervention delays early complementary feeding among adolescent mothers. Pediatrics, 107(5), E67.

Black, R. E., & Victora, C. G. (2002). Optimal duration of exclusive breast feeding in low income countries. British Medical Journal, 325(7375), 1252-1253.

Brekke, H. K., Ludvigsson, J. F., van Odijk, J., & Ludvigsson, J. (2005). Breastfeeding and introduction of solid foods in Swedish infants: the All Babies in Southeast Sweden study. British Journal of Nutrition, 94(3), 377-382.

Briefel, R. R., Reidy, K., Karwe, V., & Devaney, B. (2004). Feeding infants and toddlers study: Improvements needed in meeting infant feeding recommendations. Journal of the American Dietetic Association, 104(1 Suppl 1), s31-37.

Cohen, R. J., Brown, K. H., Canahuati, J., Rivera, L. L., & Dewey, K. G. (1994). Effects of age of introduction of complementary foods on infant breast milk intake, total energy intake, and growth: a randomised intervention study in Honduras. Lancet, 344(8918), 288-293.

Committee on, N. (2000). Hypoallergenic Infant Formulas. Pediatrics, 106(2), 346-349.

Complementary feeding in the WHO Multicentre Growth Reference Study. (2006). Acta Paediatrica Supplement, 450, 27-37.

Crocetti, M., Dudas, R., & Krugman, S. (2004). Parental beliefs and practices regarding early introduction of solid foods to their children. Clinical Pediatrics, 43(6), 541-547.

Dagnelie, P. C., & van Staveren, W. A. (1994). Macrobiotic nutrition and child health: results of a population-based, mixed-longitudinal cohort study in The Netherlands. American Journal of Clinical Nutrition, 59(5 Suppl), 1187S-1196S.

Danowski, L., & Gargiula, L. (2002). Selections from current literature. Attitudes and practices regarding the introduction of solid foods to infants. Family Practice, 19(6), 698-702.

Dennison, B. A., Rockwell, H. L., & Baker, S. L. (1997). Excess fruit juice consumption by preschool-aged children is associated with short stature and obesity. Pediatrics, 99(1), 15-22.

Dewey, K. G. (2007). Nutrition, growth, and complementary feeding of the breastfed infant. In T. W. Hale & P. Hartmann (Eds.), Hale & Hartmann's Textbook of Human Lactation (pp. 415-423). Amarillo, TX: Hale Publishing.

Dewey, K. G., & Brown, K. H. (2003). Update on technical issues concerning complementary feeding of young children in developing countries and implications for intervention programs. Food and Nutrition Bulletin, 24(1), 5-28.

Dewey, K. G., Cohen, R. J., Brown, K. H., & Rivera, L. L. (2001). Effects of exclusive breastfeeding for four versus six months on maternal nutritional status and infant motor development: results of two randomized trials in Honduras. Journal of Nutrition, 131(2), 262-267.

Dewey, K. G., Domellof, M., Cohen, R. J., Landa Rivera, L., Hernell, O., & Lonnerdal, B. (2002). Iron supplementation affects growth and morbidity of breast-fed infants: results of a randomized trial in Sweden and Honduras. Journal of Nutrition, 132(11), 3249-3255.

Domellof, M., Dewey, K. G., Lonnerdal, B., Cohen, R. J., & Hernell, O. (2002). The diagnostic criteria for iron deficiency in infants should be reevaluated. Journal of Nutrition, 132(12), 3680-3686.

Domellof, M., Lonnerdal, B., Abrams, S. A., & Hernell, O. (2002). Iron absorption in breast-fed infants: effects of age, iron status, iron supplements, and complementary foods. American Journal of Clinical Nutrition, 76(1), 198-204.

Domellof, M., Lonnerdal, B., Dewey, K. G., Cohen, R. J., Rivera, L. L., & Hernell, O. (2002). Sex differences in iron status during infancy. Pediatrics, 110(3), 545-552.

Donath, S. M., & Amir, L. H. (2005). Breastfeeding and the introduction of solids in Australian infants: data from the 2001 National Health Survey. Australian and New Zealand Journal of Public Health, 29(2), 171-175.

Engle, P. L., & Zeitlin, M. (1996). Active feeding behavior compensates for low interest in food among young Nicaraguan children. Journal of Nutrition, 126(7), 1808-1816.

Farrow, C., & Blissett, J. (2006). Breast-feeding, maternal feeding practices and mealtime negativity at one year. Appetite, 46(1), 49-56.

Fewtrell, M. S., Morgan, J. B., Duggan, C., Gunnlaugsson, G., Hibberd, P. L., Lucas, A., et al. (2007). Optimal duration of exclusive breastfeeding: what is the evidence to support current recommendations? American Journal of Clinical Nutrition, 85(2), 635S-638S.

Fisher, J. O., Birch, L. L., Smiciklas-Wright, H., & Picciano, M. F. (2000). Breast-feeding through the first year predicts maternal control in feeding and subsequent toddler energy intakes. Journal of the American Dietetic Association, 100(6), 641-646.

Forestell, C. A., & Mennella, J. A. (2007). Early determinants of fruit and vegetable acceptance. Pediatrics, 120(6), 1247-1254.

Gartner, L. M., Morton, J., Lawrence, R. A., Naylor, A. J., O'Hare, D., Schanler, R. J., et al. (2005). Breastfeeding and the use of human milk. Pediatrics, 115(2), 496-506.

Geleijnse, J. M., Hofman, A., Witteman, J. C., Hazebroek, A. A., Valkenburg, H. A., & Grobbee, D. E. (1997). Long-term effects of neonatal sodium restriction on blood pressure. Hypertension, 29(4), 913-917.

Gijsbers, B., Mesters, I., Andre Knottnerus, J., Legtenberg, A. H., & van Schayck, C. P. (2005). Factors influencing breastfeeding practices and postponement of solid food to prevent allergic disease in high-risk children: results from an explorative study. Patient Education and Counseling, 57(1), 15-21.

Gill, S. (Writer) (2007). Starting Solids [DVD]. In D. McFarlane (Producer). United Kingdom: AquaMan Design.

Greer, F. R., Sicherer, S. H., & Burks, A. W. (2008). Effects of early nutritional interventions on the development of atopic disease in infants and children: the role of maternal dietary restriction, breastfeeding, timing of introduction of complementary foods, and hydrolyzed formulas. Pediatrics, 121(1), 183-191.

Griffin, I. J., & Abrams, S. A. (2001). Iron and breastfeeding. Pediatric Clinics of North America, 48(2), 401-413.

Gunnarsson, B. S., Thorsdottir, I., & Palsson, G. (2004). Iron status in 2-year-old Icelandic children and associations with dietary intake and growth. European Journal of Clinical Nutrition, 58(6), 901-906.

Halken, S., & Host, A. (2001). Prevention. Current Opinions on Allergy and Clinical Immunology, 1(3), 229-236.

Heinig, M. J. (2006). The ones that got away: when breastfeeding mothers wean their infants despite our efforts. Journal of Human Lactation, 22(4), 385-386.

Heinig, M. J., Follett, J. R., Ishii, K. D., Kavanagh-Prochaska, K., Cohen, R., & Panchula, J. (2006). Barriers to compliance with infant-feeding recommendations among low-income women. Journal of Human Lactation, 22(1), 27-38.

Hopkinson, J. (2007). Nutrition in Lactation. In T. W. Hale & P. Hartmann (Eds.), Hale & Hartmann's Textbook of Human Lactation (pp. 381-382). Amarillo, TX: Hale Publishing.

Horodynski, M., Olson, B., Arndt, M. J., Brophy-Herb, H., Shirer, K., & Shemanski, R. (2007). Low-income mothers' decisions regarding when and why to introduce solid foods to their infants: influencing factors. Journal of Community Health Nursing, 24(2), 101-118.

Islam, M. M., Peerson, J. M., Ahmed, T., Dewey, K. G., & Brown, K. H. (2006). Effects of varied energy density of complementary foods on breast-milk intakes and total energy consumption by healthy, breastfed Bangladeshi children. American Journal of Clinical Nutrition, 83(4), 851-858.

Ismail, A. I., Sohn, W., Lim, S., & Willem, J. M. (2009). Predictors of dental caries progression in primary teeth. Journal of Dental Research, 88(3), 270-275.

Ivarsson, A., Hernell, O., Stenlund, H., & Persson, L. A. (2002). Breast-feeding protects against celiac disease. American Journal of Clinical Nutrition, 75(5), 914-921.

Ivarsson, A., Persson, L. A., Nystrom, L., Ascher, H., Cavell, B., Danielsson, L., et al. (2000). Epidemic of coeliac disease in Swedish children. Acta Paediatrica, 89(2), 165-171.

Keane, V., et al. (1988). Do solids help baby sleep through the night? American Journal of Diseases of Children, 142, 404-405.

Kerr, M. (2008, May 12). Neurodevelopmental delays associated with iron-fortified formula for healthy infants. Retrieved June 10, 2008, from www.medscape.com/viewarticle/57363.

Kramer, M. S., & Kakuma, R. (2002). Optimal duration of exclusive breastfeeding. Cochrane Database of Systematic Reviews(1), CD003517 003510.001002/14651858.CD14003517.

Krebs, N. F., Westcott, J. E., Butler, N., Robinson, C., Bell, M., & Hambidge, K. M. (2006). Meat as a first complementary food for breastfed infants: feasibility and impact on zinc intake and status. Journal of Pediatric Gastroenterology and Nutrition, 42(2), 207-214.

Lawrence, R. A., & Lawrence, R. M. (2005). Breastfeeding: A guide for the medical profession. Philadelphia, PA: Elsevier Mosby.

Lozoff, B., Beard, J., Connor, J., Barbara, F., Georgieff, M., & Schallert, T. (2006). Long-lasting neural and behavioral effects of iron deficiency in infancy. Nutrition Reviews, 64(5 Pt 2), S34-43; discussion S72-91.

Lozoff, B., & Georgieff, M. K. (2006). Iron deficiency and brain development. Seminars in Pediatric Neurology, 13(3), 158-165.

Macknin, M. L., Medendorp, S. V., & Maier, M. C. (1989). Infant sleep and bedtime cereal. American Journal of Diseases of Children, 143(9), 1066-1068.

Makrides, M., Hawkes, J. S., Neumann, M. A., & Gibson, R. A. (2002). Nutritional effect of including egg yolk in the weaning diet of breast-fed and formula-fed infants: a randomized controlled trial. American Journal of Clinical Nutrition, 75(6), 1084-1092.

Marriott, B. M., Campbell, L., Hirsch, E., & Wilson, D. (2007). Preliminary data from demographic and health surveys on infant feeding in 20 developing countries. Journal of Nutrition, 137(2), 518S-523S.

Meek, J. Y. (2002). New Mother's Guide to Breastfeeding. New York, New York: Bantam Books.

Mennella, J. A. (2007). Chemical senses and the development of flavor preferences in humans. In T. W. Hale & P. Hartmann (Eds.), Hale & Hartmann's Textbook of Human Lactation (pp. 403-413). Amarillo, TX: Hale Publishing.

Mennella, J. A., Jagnow, C. P., & Beauchamp, G. K. (2001). Prenatal and postnatal flavor learning by human infants. Pediatrics, 107(6), E88.

Mikkelsen, A., Rinne-Ljungqvist, L., Borres, M. P., & van Odijk, J. (2007). Do parents follow breastfeeding and weaning recommendations given by pediatric nurses? A study with emphasis on introduction of cow's milk protein in allergy risk families. Journal of Pediatric Health Care, 21(4), 238-244.

Muraro, A., Dreborg, S., Halken, S., Host, A., Niggemann, B., Aalberse, R., et al. (2004). Dietary prevention of allergic diseases in infants and small children. Part III: Critical review of published peer-reviewed observational and interventional studies and final recommendations. Pediatric Allergy and Immunology, 15(4), 291-307.

Norris, J. M., Barriga, K., Hoffenberg, E. J., Taki, I., Miao, D., Haas, J. E., et al. (2005). Risk of celiac disease autoimmunity and timing of gluten introduction in the diet of infants at increased risk of disease. Journal of the American Medical Association, 293(19), 2343-2351.

Norris, J. M., Barriga, K., Klingensmith, G., Hoffman, M., Eisenbarth, G. S., Erlich, H. A., et al. (2003). Timing of initial cereal exposure in infancy and risk of islet autoimmunity. Journal of the American Medical Association, 290(13), 1713-1720.

Northstone, K., Emmett, P., & Nethersole, F. (2001). The effect of age of introduction to lumpy solids on foods eaten and reported feeding difficulties at 6 and 15 months. Journal of Human Nutrition and Dietetics, 14(1), 43-54.

Oppenheimer, S. J., Gibson, F. D., Macfarlane, S. B., Moody, J. B., Harrison, C., Spencer, A., et al. (1986). Iron supplementation increases prevalence and effects of malaria: report on clinical studies in Papua New Guinea. Transactions of the Royal Society of Tropical Medicine and Hygiene, 80(4), 603-612.

PAHO/WHO. (2001). Guiding Principles for Complementary Feeding of the Breastfed Child. Retrieved 3/21/08. from http://whqlibdoc.who.int/paho/2004/a85622.pdf.

Pelto, G. H., Levitt, E., & Thairu, L. (2003). Improving feeding practices: current patterns, common constraints, and the design of interventions. Food and Nutrition Bulletin, 24(1), 45-82.

Poole, J. A., Barriga, K., Leung, D. Y., Hoffman, M., Eisenbarth, G. S., Rewers, M., et al. (2006). Timing of initial exposure to cereal grains and the risk of wheat allergy. Pediatrics, 117(6), 2175-2182.

Raj, S., Faridi, M., Rusia, U., & Singh, O. (2008). A prospective study of iron status in exclusively breastfed term infants up to 6 months of age. International Breastfeeding Journal, 3, 3.

Rapley, G. (2006). Baby-led weaning. In V. H. Moran & F. Dykes (Eds.), Baby-led weaning in maternal and infant nutrition and nurture: Controversies and challenges. London: Quay Books.

Rosenbauer, J., Herzig, P., Kaiser, P., & Giani, G. (2007). Early nutrition and risk of Type 1 diabetes mellitus--a nationwide case-control study in preschool children. Experimental and Clinical Endocrinology and Diabetes, 115(8), 502-508.

Savage, S. A., Reilly, J. J., Edwards, C. A., & Durnin, J. V. (1998). Weaning practice in the Glasgow Longitudinal Infant Growth Study. Archives of Disease in Childhood, 79(2), 153-156.

Sellen, D. W. (2001). Comparison of infant feeding patterns reported for nonindustrial populations with current recommendations. Journal of Nutrition, 131(10), 2707-2715.

Sloan, S., Gildea, A., Stewart, M., Sneddon, H., & Iwaniec, D. (2008). Early weaning is related to weight and rate of weight gain in infancy. Child: care, health and development, 34(1), 59-64.

Smith, M. M., & Lifshitz, F. (1994). Excess fruit juice consumption as a contributing factor in nonorganic failure to thrive. Pediatrics, 93(3), 438-443.

Taveras, E. M., Scanlon, K. S., Birch, L., Rifas-Shiman, S. L., Rich-Edwards, J. W., & Gillman, M. W. (2004). Association of Breastfeeding With Maternal Control of Infant Feeding at Age 1 Year. Pediatrics, 114(5), e577-583.

Thorsdottir, I., Gunnarsson, B. S., Atladottir, H., Michaelsen, K. F., & Palsson, G. (2003). Iron status at 12 months of age -- effects of body size, growth and diet in a population with high birth weight. European Journal of Clinical Nutrition, 57(4), 505-513.

Vuori, E., Makinen, S. M., Kara, R., & Kuitunen, P. (1980). The effects of the dietary intakes of copper, iron, manganese, and zinc on the trace element content of human milk. American Journal of Clinical Nutrition, 33(2), 227-231.

Walker, R. B., Conn, J. A., Davies, M. J., & Moore, V. M. (2006). Mothers' views on feeding infants around the time of weaning. Public Health Nutr, 9(6), 707-713.

Warner, M. L., Harley, K., Bradman, A., Vargas, G., & Eskenazi, B. (2006). Soda consumption and overweight status of 2-year-old Mexican-American children in california. Obesity (Silver Spring), 14(11), 1966-1974.

Wayland, C. (2004). Breastfeeding patterns in Rio Branco, Acre, Brazil: a survey of reasons for weaning. Cadernos de Saude Publica, 20(6), 1757-1761.

WHO. (2001). Optimal Duration of Exclusive Breastfeeding: Report of an expert consultation. Retrieved 3/21/08. from http://www.who.int/nutrition/publications/optimal_duration_of_exc_bfeeding_report_eng.pdf.

Wright, C. M., Parkinson, K. N., & Drewett, R. F. (2004). Why are babies weaned early? Data from a prospective population based cohort study. Archives of Disease in Childhood, 89(9), 813-816.

Zavaleta, N., Nombera, J., Rojas, R. et al. (1995). Iron and lactoferrin in milk of anemic mothers given iron supplements. Nutrition Research, 15, 681-690.

Ziegler, A. G., Schmid, S., Huber, D., Hummel, M., & Bonifacio, E. (2003). Early infant feeding and risk of developing type 1 diabetes-associated autoantibodies. Journal of the American Medical Association, 290(13), 1721-1728.

Weaning from the Breast

Chapter

5

In this chapter, weaning is defined as the end of breastfeeding, but it is far more than that. Depending on the cultural beliefs, weaning may be considered a time of withdrawal or deprivation, or alternatively, a time of growth and new maturity. But in every culture, weaning is always a time of transition as the child adjusts to new sources of nourishment and comfort and new ways of exploring the world. Weaning is not an act but a process that begins when a baby takes any food other than at the breast and ends with the last breastfeeding. In some parts of the world, "weaning" refers to starting solid foods, which are referred to as "weaning foods." In these areas, some have suggested changing this definition, with "weaning" generally agreed to mean the end of breastfeeding (Fewtrell et al., 2007).

Weaning has different meanings and implications in different cultures.

RECOMMENDATIONS

In its 2005 policy statement (Gartner et al., 2005, pp. 499, 500), the American Academy of Pediatrics wrote:

> Breastfeeding should be continued for at least the first year of life and beyond for as long as mutually desired by mother and child...There is no upper limit to the duration of breastfeeding and no evidence of psychologic or developmental harm from breastfeeding into the 3rd year of life or longer.

Health organizations recommend exclusive breastfeeding for 6 months and continued breastfeeding with other foods until at least 1 to 2 years of age.

During the first year of life, early weaning is associated with greater incidence of acute illnesses, such as respiratory and ear infections, diarrhea, other gastrointestinal problems, and even death. Using child-mortality statistics from UNICEF, a U.K. article estimated that if 90% of women worldwide breastfed, 1.3 million child deaths per year could be prevented (Jones, Steketee, Black, Bhutta, & Morris, 2003). A U.S. article estimated that if all U.S. babies breastfed, annually it would prevent or delay the deaths of 720 children between the ages of 1 and 12 months (Chen & Rogan, 2004). Recent reviews of the research have found that even in developed countries, not breastfeeding is associated with significantly worse health outcomes for mothers and babies (Ip et al., 2007; Ip, Chung, Raman, Trikalinos, & Lau, 2009).

One year was also recommended as the minimum age of weaning by the AAP because the negative health outcomes associated with breastfeeding for less than a year can last a lifetime (Hanson, 2004). Children never breastfed or those breastfed for less than 12 months are at greater risk for diabetes mellitus (Type 1 and Type 2), lymphoma, Hodgkins disease, overweight and obesity, and celiac disease and other inflammatory bowel disorders (Ip et al., 2007; Ip et al., 2009). This list continues to grow, along with our understanding of the biological mechanisms responsible.

The World Health Organization recommends continued breastfeeding for up to 2 years of age or beyond (PAHO/WHO, 2001). In developing areas of the world, the health risks of early weaning are greater due to sanitation problems, unreliable food and water supplies, and lack of available healthcare, but these recommendations are meant to apply to all babies in all areas. Research has found that weaned children between 16 and 36 months have more types of illness, longer duration of illness, and require more medical care than breastfeeding children the same age (Gulick, 1986). Also, weaned children between 12 and 36 months were 3.5 times more likely to die than those still breastfeeding (Molbak, 1994). No matter where a child lives, weaning before age 2 is associated with greater incidence of illness and death.

THE DECISION TO WEAN

A mother who asks for information on weaning may feel vulnerable to criticism. Affirm her and answer her questions.

Many mothers consider breastfeeding and weaning a central part of their relationship with their child and their expectations of themselves as mothers (Hauck & Irurita, 2002). For this reason, when discussing breastfeeding and weaning, the mother may feel vulnerable to criticism and worry about not meeting others' expectations.

When a mother asks about weaning, first it is important to affirm her and allay her fear of criticism. Once the mother's concerns about being negatively judged are laid to rest, answer her specific questions, so she knows you are willing to help her wean. Once she has the information she wants about weaning, in the interest of knowing all her options, ask her if she is interested in hearing about other alternatives as well.

The mother may have mixed feelings about weaning. Help her explore her feelings and expectations by asking her open-ended questions.

In cultures where early weaning is common, pressure from others may influence a mother to consider weaning and create expectations for weaning that cannot be met. To get a sense of how the mother feels about breastfeeding and her expectations, ask her some open-ended questions, such as:

- "How do you think weaning will change your life"?
- "Are there others in your life with strong opinions about breastfeeding and weaning"?
- "Describe your relationship with your baby."
- "What are your feelings about weaning"?

In some cultures, mothers may feel pressured to wean early.

If a mother's expectations of weaning are unrealistic, affirm her and then share relevant information.

Some mothers have expectations for weaning that are unlikely to be met. For example, a mother may think weaning will make her baby more independent or decrease his night-waking. If the mother's expectations are unlikely to be met, affirm her underlying need and share the information you have. For example:

- "It's hard to be a good mother when you feel exhausted much of the time. But weaning may not help you get more rest. Research has found that weaned babies do not sleep longer than babies still breastfeeding" (Yilmaz, Gurakan, Cakir, & Tezcan, 2002). Would you like to talk about other ways to get more rest, or do you have other reasons you'd like to wean now"?
- "Your mother feels strongly that you should wean because breastfeeding is too stressful for you. You are a good daughter to want to be responsive to her feelings. However, there is research your mother might not know about that indicates bottle-feeding is more stressful for mothers than breastfeeding" (Mezzacappa & Katlin, 2002).

Cultural Expectations

Every breastfeeding child eventually weans. However, in different parts of the world, weaning may be viewed very differently. The word "wean" is derived from a word meaning "satisfaction" or "fulfillment." During much of human history and in many parts of the world, weaning is considered a natural stage of growth, a sign that the child had had his fill and is ready to move away from his mother into the wider world.

Depending on cultural norms, weaning may be seen as a positive and natural stage of growth or something a mother does to a child against his wishes.

However, in the U.S. and some other Western countries, weaning is not seen as a process to be celebrated or a naturally occurring stage of growth. Weaning is seen as a time of deprivation and unhappiness, something that a mother does to a child against his wishes. In cultures where babies tend to wean young, some mothers are cautioned to be sure their babies are weaned by a certain age or their babies will breastfeed "forever." But this does not reflect the broader human experience.

• •

According to cultural anthropologists, the average age of weaning internationally is between 3 and 4 years of age (Dettwyler, 1995). In 1967, anthropologist Margaret Mead and early breastfeeding researcher Niles Newton published an article describing weaning practices of 64 traditional societies (Mead & Newton, 1967). Among these societies, the average weaning age was 3 years, and only one weaned their children as early as 6 months.

When viewed cross-culturally, the average age of weaning is between 3 and 4 years.

History tells us that in most times and places it was common practice to breastfeed for years. The Koran recommends breastfeeding until age 2, and the custom of the Egyptian Pharaohs in Moses' time was to breastfeed for 3 years. Until the 20th century, children in both China and Japan breastfed until age 4 or 5. Even in England and the U.S., historical writings tell us that not so long ago 2 to 4 years of breastfeeding was typical. In 1725, authors of child-care texts clearly disapproved of 4-year-olds breastfeeding, which implies there were more than a few of them around. By 1850, breastfeeding for 11 months was recommended and breastfeeding for 2 years was criticized (Bumgarner, 2000).

• •

Anthropologist Katherine Dettwyler used the same criteria for humans that biologists use to determine the natural age of weaning in other mammals to predict the natural age of weaning for humans without the influence of culture (Dettwyler, 1995). These criteria (followed by the equivalent age for humans) include:

Without the influence of culture, the "natural" age of weaning is estimated to be between 2.5 and 7 years.

- Age at tripling-quadrupling birthweight (2 to 3 years)
- Age when one-third of adult weight is reached (4 to 7 years)
- Age at eruption of permanent teeth (5.5 to 6 years)
- Gestational length (our nearest relative, the chimpanzee weans at about 6 times its gestational length; which for humans would be 4.5 yrs.)

As a result, Dettwyler concluded that from a biological perspective the natural age of weaning for humans is between 2.5 and 7 years.

The Mother's Perspective

Individual mothers can have very different feelings about breastfeeding and weaning.

Feelings about breastfeeding vary greatly among mothers and can also vary in the same mother over time. One qualitative Australian study of 25 mothers explored the breastfeeding experience by interviewing these mothers prenatally and several times during the first 6 months postpartum (Schmied & Barclay, 1999).

In Australia, where breastfeeding has become the cultural norm, all of the study mothers considered breastfeeding crucial to their relationship with their baby, and most considered it a part of good mothering (Scott, Binns, Oddy, & Graham, 2006). Most were committed to persevering in order "to achieve their identity as a breastfeeding mother."

But not all mothers felt the same way about breastfeeding. For example, while some mothers enjoyed their breastfeeding baby's dependence on them, others found this difficult and emotionally overwhelming and sought time away from their babies. Although 8 of the 25 mothers (32%) found breastfeeding intimate and pleasurable, 9 (nearly 40%) had mixed feelings and another 8 (32%) experienced "searing pain" during the early weeks and months, and at times considered it "agonizing," "horrendous," and "violent." Rather than feeling in harmony with their babies, as other study mothers did, these mothers at times felt alienated from their babies. Some of these mothers blamed themselves; others blamed their babies. Some also reported feeling restricted from activities they used to enjoy and felt they had to "put their lives on hold."

Mothers' decisions about when to wean may be due to breastfeeding problems or deeper issues.

Some of the study mothers weaned early. Others who had early breastfeeding problems continued breastfeeding and eventually enjoyed a connected and intimate breastfeeding relationship with their babies. But all considered breastfeeding central to their experience of motherhood. Of these mothers, 20 of the 25 continued to breastfeed at 3 months and 18 of the 25 were breastfeeding at 6 months.

• • • • • • • • • • • • • • • • • • • •

A mother's decision to wean may be influenced more by her overall feelings about breastfeeding than by a specific breastfeeding problem.

When mothers are asked why they chose to wean, many cite specific breastfeeding problems, such as worries about milk supply or nipple pain. However, breastfeeding is a complex social behavior, and there are often deeper issues that affect a mother's decisions.

One Canadian study of 80 women who had breastfed a baby for 9 months noted that at every stage of breastfeeding the less control the mothers felt they had over breastfeeding, the weaker their intentions to continue breastfeeding were and the earlier they weaned (Rempel, 2004). This perceived control included three variables: breastfeeding ease, mothers' perception that they could breastfeed as long as they wanted, and mothers' confidence. Even at 9 months, the mothers cited biting and maintaining their milk production as key issues they faced, and these variables affected whether they weaned their babies then. The mothers also perceived their support decreasing the longer they breastfed, which also influenced their weaning decisions. The author suggested that for women to breastfeed for at least a year, social norms need to change and mothers need to receive support and encouragement for longer breastfeeding. Understanding how breastfeeding works and the adjustment mothers can make to it as needed may be the key to women's comfort with longer breastfeeding.

In one U.S. study, the decision to wean was more strongly associated with a lack of support and difficult adjustment to pregnancy and motherhood than to breastfeeding problems (Isabella & Isabella, 1994). Another U.S. study that interviewed 52 mothers from the U.S. and Canada found that many were surprised by the discomfort they experienced during early breastfeeding, but if they perceived the discomfort as temporary and had support, they were more likely to keep breastfeeding (Kelleher, 2006).

In one Australian study, researchers used the Maternal Breastfeeding Evaluation Scale (Leff, Gagne, & Jefferis, 1994; Leff, Jefferis, & Gagne, 1994) to rate breastfeeding satisfaction based on answers to a series of questions about her adjustment to motherhood, her baby's satisfaction, and her feelings about her lifestyle (Cooke, Sheehan, & Schmied, 2003).

The 215 study mothers were surveyed before birth and postpartum at 2 weeks, 6 weeks, and 3 months to rate their breastfeeding satisfaction and determine the relationship between their perceived breastfeeding problems and the decision to wean. At 2 and 6 weeks, almost 50% of the mothers reported having breastfeeding problems, such as painful nipples or worries about milk production. By 3 months, the percentage of mothers reporting problems decreased to 28%.

The researchers found the decision to wean was more closely related to the mothers' overall level of breastfeeding satisfaction than to specific problems. For example, more than half the mothers reported having painful nipples during the first 2 weeks, but less than one-third thought it made breastfeeding difficult and at no time did this significantly affect the mothers' decision to wean.

Mothers who reported engorgement and leaking milk were actually less likely to wean than other mothers. This may be because they perceived engorgement and leaking as indicating abundant milk production, which increased their breastfeeding satisfaction.

• •

Unrealistic expectations can lead to worries about milk production, which can lead to decreased self-esteem and enjoyment of breastfeeding, which can lead to weaning.

In one U.S. study, the most common breastfeeding problem its 215 mothers cited at 2 weeks, 6 weeks, and 3 months was their perception their babies were not satisfied by their milk, but only one-third of the mothers said this made breastfeeding difficult (Isabella & Isabella, 1994). This study rated the mother's overall satisfaction with breastfeeding based in part on their baby's satisfaction. The mothers' perception that their babies were unsettled or that their time at the breast was too long or too short lowered their baby's satisfaction score, which also lowered their overall breastfeeding satisfaction score.

Worries about milk supply is the most common reason women give for weaning.

Unrealistic expectations of how long a baby should stay satisfied after breastfeeding can affect a mother's perception of her ability to nurture her baby, a factor closely linked to a mother's enjoyment of breastfeeding and her breastfeeding satisfaction. According to many studies, "worries about milk supply" is the most common reason women give for weaning (Ahluwalia, Morrow, & Hsia, 2005; Cooke et al., 2003; Dennis, 2002; Heath, Tuttle, Simons, Cleghorn, & Parnell, 2002; Taveras et al., 2003). It is also possible that some of these mothers may have had legitimate milk production issues based on poor breastfeeding practices in the hospital or bad advice, which is rampant in many Western areas. But there is often more going on below the surface. One researcher wrote:

> ...the most prevalent reason for discontinuing or supplementing breastfeeding has been insufficient milk. Yet it appears unlikely that many women truly experience insufficient milk...Thus, the rationale for discontinuing breastfeeding is a convoluted interplay of factors (Dennis, 2002, p. 14).

Or, as other researchers wrote:

> Breastfeeding is a complex social behavior, and maternal perceptions of successful breastfeeding are not fully explained by the presence or absence of breastfeeding problems (Cooke et al., 2003, p. 145).

The decision to wean may occur in several phases.

One Australian study examined the perspectives of 33 breastfeeding mothers as they made the decision to wean and afterwards. The researchers noted the distinct changes in perspective and attitude that occurred as the mother made the decision to wean (Hauck & Irurita, 2002).

- **Shifting Focus.** Triggered by the conflicting expectations of others, the mothers described how first their tolerance for this conflict was exceeded, and then how they took charge by deciding what was important to them and making their decision on that basis.
- **Selective Focusing.** After making their decision, the mothers chose to focus only on those who agreed with their decision and avoided or ignored the rest.
- **Confirming Focus.** After weaning, the mothers sought affirmation for their decision by first assessing the impact on their child and then by acknowledging what breastfeeding had meant to them.

The Influence of Others

Timing of weaning is influenced by others and the presence or absence of social support.

Support from others appears to be a crucial ingredient for longer-term breastfeeding. Conversely, lack of support can lead to weaning. In one Brazilian study of the factors that led to weaning, researchers noted two issues mentioned by all 24 of the mothers surveyed: "the loneliness/isolation" the mothers experienced and their need for support for breastfeeding to succeed (Ramos & Almeida, 2003).

Social support is essential for longer breastfeeding.

In cultures where early weaning is the norm, the longer mothers breastfeed, in general the less support they receive from others (Kendall-Tackett & Sugarman, 1995; Rempel, 2004). Withdrawal of support is associated with the decision to wean (Rempel, 2004). Mothers in two Canadian studies reported that previously supportive people began to withdraw their support when their babies were 9 to 12 months old (Rempel, 2004; Williams & Morse, 1989). One Canadian study noted that those close to the mothers most strongly influenced their decision to wean, particularly when after having been supportive before, they began making negative comments (Williams & Morse, 1989).

An Australia study examined 33 mothers' weaning experiences and noted that the mothers' expectations of breastfeeding and weaning were influenced mostly by experts, their past experience, their current experience, the experience of others, and partner's input (Hauck & Irurita, 2003). These mothers evaluated their breastfeeding efforts based on their own expectations and those of their significant others, some of which were expressed openly and some of which were expressed as advice or as comments.

A Japanese article noted that many early weanings in Japan occur as a result of negative comments made about breastfeeding by family members during visits to the mother's home after childbirth (Haku, 2007).

In two reviews of the literature, the authors concluded that fathers strongly influenced both initiation and duration of breastfeeding (Bar-Yam & Darby, 1997; Raj & Plichta, 1998). Others who influence mothers' decision to wean included friends, lactation consultants, and healthcare professionals (Raj & Plichta, 1998).

Where breastfeeding is not the cultural norm, lack of support contributes to early weaning, especially among vulnerable mothers.

In countries like the U.S., breastfeeding initiation and duration rates are lowest among mothers who are young, single, and less educated (Ryan & Zhou, 2006). Barriers women face include minimal breastfeeding help from the healthcare system, lack of money to pay for breastfeeding help, and lack of information. To prevent premature weaning, broad social support for breastfeeding from all those in contact with new mothers must be in place (Forste & Hoffmann, 2008). In countries such as Sweden and Australia, where all new mothers routinely receive this type of support, breastfeeding initiation and duration rates no longer vary by ethnicity, income, and education (Scott, Binns, Graham, & Oddy, 2006).

Lack of breastfeeding help and encouragement by a mother's healthcare provider is associated with weaning during the early months.

One U.S. study found that women whose healthcare providers encouraged breastfeeding were about half as likely to wean by 12 weeks postpartum as those whose healthcare providers did not encourage breastfeeding (Taveras et al., 2003). Another U.S. study found that mothers are more likely to wean if their healthcare provider recommended formula or didn't think his or her opinion mattered (Taveras et al., 2004). A French study found a longer duration of breastfeeding and more exclusive breastfeeding among mothers whose primary-care physician attended a 5-hour breastfeeding training program and provided one routine, preventive outpatient visit within 2 weeks after birth (Labarere et al., 2005).

Some mothers are told by others to wean for reasons that are ill-informed.

In parts of the world where early weaning is common, mothers may be advised to wean for any number of unnecessary reasons, including returning to work, taking a medication compatible with breastfeeding, mastitis, illness, and pregnancy. Some mothers are told to wean for baby-related reasons, such as colic, reflux, slow weight gain, eruption of teeth, illness, preterm birth, and chronic illness. When a mother asks about weaning for questionable reasons, ask if she would be interested in more information.

The influence of others seems to be greatest during early motherhood.

As mothers become more experienced, they may be less influenced by others. In one U.S. study of mothers who breastfed long-term, the authors wrote:

> Comments from our subjects illustrate that support is most *influential* in modifying parenting practices and beliefs during the initial stages of mothering (but we hasten to add that it is *important* at all stages). As women gain confidence, they are more likely to make their own decisions and less likely to be influenced—one way or the other—by

opinions of others. Indeed, the women in this sample indicated that both positive and negative reactions were more likely to influence their *feelings* than their behavior (Kendall-Tackett & Sugarman, 1995, p. 183).

WEANING DYNAMICS

The Role of Mother and Baby

Even when mothers do not actively encourage weaning, children will outgrow breastfeeding on their own.

Babies are born hardwired to breastfeed, but children outgrow breastfeeding as they mature and their need for mother's milk decreases. However, just as children get their first tooth, learn to walk, and learn to use the toilet at different ages, children also outgrow breastfeeding at different ages. Factors that may influence the age of weaning include allergies, strength of sucking urge, emotional temperament, and many others.

Weaning may be driven mostly by mother, mostly by baby, or it may be a mutual process.

When weaning is perceived by a mother as being a mutual process, her emotional adjustment may be easier (Hauck & Irurita, 2002). But weaning is not always mutual. In some cases, the child may decide to wean before the mother feels ready. Then the mother may feel a greater sense of loss. If the mother weans before the child is ready, she may worry about her child's emotional and physical adjustment to this transition.

Where early weaning is common, many mothers misread normal infant behaviors as signs their babies are ready to wean.

Due to their biological need for mother's milk, babies younger than 12 months are unlikely to be developmentally ready to wean. However, where early weaning is the cultural norm, many mothers encourage weaning without realizing it by regularly substituting bottles and pacifiers/dummies for breastfeeding. When the baby shifts his interest from the breast to the breast substitute, many mothers think the baby has "weaned himself."

Weaning can also happen inadvertently when parents misinterpret normal infant behavior as signs their baby is ready to wean. In one Canadian study, 96% of the 80 mothers who weaned their babies between 9 and 12 months said they did so because they were convinced their babies were "ready to wean" by the following behaviors (Rempel, 2004):

- Asking to breastfeed less often
- Shorter breastfeeding sessions
- More distractibility while breastfeeding

All of these behaviors are part of normal growth and development at this age and are not signs of weaning readiness. A baby who "weans himself" before 12 months should be considered on a nursing strike, a solvable breastfeeding problem described on p. 144- "Nursing Strike."

Weaning Basics

When a mother weans a baby younger than 1 year, suggest she first consult her baby's healthcare provider about what food should be substituted for her milk.

Before 1 year, some type of infant formula will most likely be recommended as a substitute for breastfeeding, as other milks, such as cow's milk, are not recommended in most parts of the world until after 1 year (Agostoni et al., 2008).

• •

The feeding method chosen will depend upon the baby's age and where the family lives.

In Western cultures, where sanitation is good, if a mother is not breastfeeding, she is most likely to feed a younger baby with infant feeding bottles. If the baby is older than 6 to 8 months or so and is drinking well from a cup, he may be able to forego the bottle and wean directly to a cup, so there is no need to wean again from a bottle later.

In parts of the world where sanitation is poor, infant feeding bottles are not recommended (PAHO/WHO, 2001). In these areas, safer feeding methods include easy-to-clean containers without crevices, such as small cups with straight sides or spoons. Also, because powdered infant formula is not sterile, it is not recommended for babies younger than 4 weeks.

• •

The child's age and readiness to wean, as well as the approach used, will affect how easy or difficult it is for mother and child.

A sudden weaning is often painful for a mother and difficult for a child. But there are also gentle, loving, and gradual ways to wean. Weaning gradually--with consideration for the feelings and preferences of both mother and child—can make weaning a positive experience, even when a child has not yet outgrown breastfeeding on his own.

Approaches to Weaning

Weaning tends to fall into several general categories: gradual, partial, and abrupt.

Although mothers have access to much information and advice on how to wean, there is limited research on how mothers actually wean.

In a Canadian study, which is one of the few about weaning, 90 first-time mothers were asked to describe their weaning experiences (Williams & Morse, 1989). Their babies were weaned between 6 weeks and 20 months old, with a median age at weaning of about 9.5 months. As in some other studies, this study's authors did not include those who weaned earlier than 6 weeks because full breastfeeding had not yet been established (Hauck & Irurita, 2002).

Weaning fell into three general categories: gradual, with the process taking 1 to 8 weeks; minimal breastfeeding (or partial weaning), a two-stage process starting with a gradual partial weaning over 6 to 8 weeks with continued breastfeeding once or twice a day for a while before full weaning occurred; and sudden or "cold turkey" weaning, which was started and ended within 1 day. Most of the study mothers chose the first two gradual approaches:

- Gradual weaning (42%)
- Partial weaning, or "minimal breastfeeding" (49%)
- Sudden weaning or "cold turkey" (9%)

The younger the baby was when weaning happened, the more likely he was to be weaned suddenly.

The most common reason given for weaning (41%) was returning to work. Other reasons included:

- It was time (11%)
- Baby lost interest (10%)
- Mother wanted more freedom (9%)
- Pressure from others (9%)
- To have another baby (7%)
- Teeth (5%)
- Illness in mother or baby (4%)
- Mother tired (2%)
- Disliked breastfeeding (2%)

In another U.S. study, all of the 222 mothers weaned before their babies were 5 months old and weaning approaches were defined differently (Neighbors, Gillespie, Schwartz, & Foxman, 2003). A weaning was considered "gradual" if it took 4 or more days, and "all at once" if the last breastfeeding occurred within 3 days of when weaning began. Using these definitions:

- 67% weaned gradually
- 33% weaned all at once

Half of these mothers weaned within 7 days. The older the baby, the more likely the mother was to choose a gradual approach:

- 0-5 weeks of age—67% weaned ≤3 days
- 21-25 weeks of age—26% weaned ≤3 days

The more gradual weaning was associated with returning to work. Women weaning quickly were more likely to be experiencing pain.

Another U.S. study looked at weaning an older child (Sugarman & Kendall-Tackett, 1995). In this study, average age of weaning was 2.5 to 3.0 years of age. The 179 mothers who responded to the survey belonged to La Leche League and lived in a culture generally unsupportive of breastfeeding after a year.

- More than half of the mothers (56%) reported that their youngest child weaned gradually, with 53% describing the weaning as "child-led."
- Only about 13% considered the weaning sudden.

Nearly a quarter of these mothers encouraged weaning by talking to their child about it.

Gradual Weaning

A gradual weaning has physical and emotional advantages for mother and baby.

A gradual weaning allows a mother to avoid painful breast fullness and reduces the risk of mastitis. By cutting back on breastfeeding gradually and expressing a small amount of milk whenever she feels fullness, a mother can slow her milk production comfortably.

A gradual weaning also gives a mother some time before her milk is gone to be sure her baby tolerates well whatever food she substitutes for her milk. This may be especially important for a younger baby, who may be more vulnerable to allergies, but it can also be important for some very sensitive older babies and children.

From an emotional standpoint, a gradual weaning allows a baby more time to adjust to the loss of the closeness breastfeeding provides.

Gradual Weaning from Birth to 12 Months

For a gradual weaning of a younger baby, suggest the mother allow at least 3 days for her milk production to decrease each time she drops a breastfeeding.

Before a baby is old enough to have strong preferences about his daily routine, weaning usually involves substituting a feeding of infant formula for a breastfeeding. During a gradual weaning, it may takes about 2 to 3 weeks for the mother to comfortably go from exclusive breastfeeding to completely weaned. To help her accomplish this, suggest she:

Gradual weaning takes about 2 to 3 weeks to accomplish.

- Note the times each day she usually breastfeeds.
- Pick one daily breastfeeding (leave the first morning breastfeeding for last) and instead feed the substitute food by the chosen method.
- Allow at least 3 days before dropping another breastfeeding to give her milk production time to decrease comfortably and gradually.

NOTE: If at any time her breasts feel full, suggest she express her milk to comfort or allow the baby to breastfeed for a short time. Be sure she knows to pay attention to her body cues, expressing milk to comfort whenever needed. (For more details, see last section.)

• •

During weaning, suggest the child receive extra focused attention and cuddling.

To help offset the emotional loss of the closeness of breastfeeding, suggest during weaning that the child receive extra focused attention and skin-to-skin contact either from the mother or from someone else. This might include holding, rocking, cuddling, reading stories, or any other activity the child enjoys.

• •

Tell the mother to expect her child to seek other sucking outlets and decide which one she prefers.

Because children have a strong urge to suckle until they outgrow breastfeeding, they may find another outlet, such as thumbsucking, during or after weaning. If a mother prefers her child use a bottle or pacifier/dummy, suggest she be prepared to offer this instead.

Gradual Weaning After 12 Months

For weaning to be a positive experience for the child older than 1 year, suggest the mother respect his preferences.

A child a year or older usually has strong preferences about breastfeeding, as he will about all aspects of his daily routine. But even so, weaning can still be a gradual and positive experience. To accomplish this, first allow plenty of time. It may take several weeks to wean, depending on how many times a day he has been breastfeeding. It will also be helpful for a mother to consider his temperament and opinions, and factor them into her strategies.

Suggest the mother try different weaning strategies and use those that work best with her child.

Every child is different and what works for one may not work well for another. When a mother chooses to wean, suggest she experiment with the following approaches and see which one most effectively reduces her child's desire to breastfeed.

Don't offer, don't refuse. This approach, popularized by La Leche League International, refers to breastfeeding when the child asks but not offering the breast when he doesn't ask. When used with other strategies, this can speed the process.

Offer regular meals, snacks, and drinks to minimize his hunger and thirst and age-appropriate fun activities to avoid breastfeeding out of boredom.

Change daily routines. Think about the times and places he asks to breastfeed and how to change their routine, so he will be reminded less often. For example, if he usually asks to breastfeed when the mother sits in a certain chair, suggest she avoid sitting in that chair.

Get her partner involved. If the child usually breastfeeds upon waking in the morning, suggest the mother ask her partner to get him up and make his breakfast. Her partner can also help him get back to sleep when he wakes at night and can plan special daytime outings.

A variety of strategies can help with the weaning process.

Anticipate and offer substitutes and distractions. Be sure the mother knows to offer substitutes *before* the child asks to breastfeed, because once he has asked, he will likely feel rejected and upset if a substitute is offered. As an example, right before a usual breastfeeding time offer a special snack and drink and then take him to a favorite place, such as a playground as a distraction. Some children breastfeed more often at home with nothing to do and breastfeed less often when out and distracted. With this type of child, spend as much of the day as possible out of the house. Some children breastfeed more often when out of the house and in new surroundings. With this type of child, stay home more and keep distractions to a minimum.

Postpone. This works for a child who breastfeeds at irregular times and places and is old enough to accept waiting. If postponing leaves the child feeling as though the mother is keeping him at arm's length, he may become even more determined to breastfeed. If so, use other strategies.

Shorten the length of breastfeedings. This is most effective with children older than 2 years and is a good beginning to the weaning process.

Bargaining can work well with the older child. A child who is close to outgrowing breastfeeding may give up breastfeeding earlier by mutual agreement. But most children younger than 3 are not mature enough to understand the meaning of a promise.

Adjust the weaning plan as needed based on the child's reactions and preferences. Pick and choose among these strategies based on the child's reactions. One child may be unhappy with postponing, but do well with distraction and substitution. Also, certain breastfeedings may be more important to the child than others. If so, suggest the mother continue those until the end and allow her child to give them up last. If he clings to his bedtime breastfeeding, for example, she can continue those for a while longer.

Be flexible when unusual situations arise. If the child is ill, allow him to breastfeed more often for comfort. Tell the mother she can go back to weaning after he is feeling better.

When to slow down. Even at the same age, some children will be more ready to wean than others. If the child becomes upset and cries or insists upon breastfeeding even when the mother tries to distract or comfort him in others ways, this may mean that weaning is going too fast or that different strategies would be better. Other signs that weaning may be moving too fast are changes or regressions in behavior, such as stuttering, night-waking, an increase in clinginess, a new or increased fear of separation, biting (if he has never bitten before), stomach upsets, and constipation.

Some mothers choose a type of gradual weaning called "natural weaning," which involves allowing the child to outgrow breastfeeding on his own.

Even in the U.S., where at this writing about 80% of babies are weaned by 1 year, some mothers allow their children to wean according to their own internal timetable. Some choose it because it feels right to them. Some choose it because it allows their child to grow at his own pace. And some choose it because it is the least work.

Where early weaning is the norm, some assume that breastfeeding past 1 year is an act of martyrdom, but mothers report that in many ways breastfeeding a toddler makes their lives easier (Buckley, 1992; Kendall-Tackett & Sugarman, 1995). The relaxing breastfeeding hormones help mothers keep their tempers, even when under duress, and breastfeeding makes naptimes and bedtimes easy and ends tantrums quickly.

Natural weaning is usually gradual, although an occasional child may wean earlier and more abruptly than his mother expects. More commonly, though, the mother's milk production reduces slowly and comfortably without any thought or effort as the child's attention becomes more focused on the world around him and less on his mother.

One advantage of natural weaning is that a mother never has to deal with an unhappy child resisting her efforts to wean or weaning again from the bottle later. As one mother said, "I wouldn't think of limiting or ending the breastfeeding relationship any more than I would think of limiting or ending my love for my children. Gradual weaning allowed us both to grow into other ways of expressing our love" (Kendall-Tackett & Sugarman, 1995, p. 181). Many women who wean naturally report that the process was so gradual that they are not even sure when their child's last breastfeeding happened.

The age that natural weaning occurs will vary from child to child.

Children mature at different rates. They learn to walk, talk, and get their first tooth at different ages, and the same is true for weaning. One child may wean at 1 or 2 years, while another may be avidly breastfeeding at age 3. A child with a strong sucking urge, an intense need for closeness, or an unrecognized allergy or other physical problem may breastfeed longer than others. As mentioned previously, breast refusal before 1 year should be considered a nursing strike rather than a natural weaning because at that age the baby still had a biological need for mother's milk.

Where early weaning is common, many mothers find the biggest challenge of natural weaning is coping with others' opinions as their children get older.

The older the child, the more challenging this can sometimes become (Kendall-Tackett & Sugarman, 1995; Williams & Morse, 1989). Yet, in spite of this, some mothers feel that the positives outweigh the negatives.

One way mothers handle the social challenges is to keep breastfeeding private, which is possible because an older child does not usually breastfeed as often as a young baby. Time-tested strategies for avoiding breastfeeding in less-than-friendly places include:

- Setting limits on where and when the child can breastfeed.
- Bringing snacks, drinks, toys, and/or books to distract the child when out.
- Choosing a "code word" for breastfeeding that won't be obvious to others.
- Finding private places to breastfeed away from home, such as fitting rooms or "mothers' lounges" at the mall.
- Carefully choosing clothing. Two-piece outfits allow mothers to breastfeed more easily. So do cover-ups, like ponchos or shawls.

Keeping breastfeeding private can help mothers cope with negative opinions of others.

Mothers who breastfeed longer than their cultural norm find this easier if they have support. Mother-to-mother breastfeeding groups, like La Leche League, Nursing Mother's Council, and the Australian Breastfeeding Association, are places mothers can meet other mothers who value breastfeeding at all ages. The baby cafes available in some countries are another way mothers can gather, share stories, and give and get support.

Partial Weaning

A partial weaning can be an alternative to total weaning for some employed mothers and those feeling overwhelmed by breastfeeding.

Some employed mothers consider a full weaning when they are unable to breastfeed or express their milk at work. In this case, a partial weaning can allow a mother to breastfeed at home, while staying comfortable at work. In some cases, a partial weaning can also be an alternative to a full weaning for the mother who feels overwhelmed by breastfeeding. For example, some mothers with a history of abuse find the intimate contact of breastfeeding difficult. More limited breastfeeding may make it possible for a mother in this situation to continue. For more details, see p. 756- "Past Sexual Abuse, Assault, or Childhood Trauma."

A Canadian study found one factor that led some mothers to breastfeed longer was their discovery that they could cut back on the number of daily feedings and continue breastfeeding in a more limited way (Williams & Morse, 1989). These included employed mothers returning to work, as well as mothers who wanted to spend more time away from their babies.

A partial weaning involves eliminating some breastfeedings while continuing others.

A partial weaning usually occurs in several steps. First, suggest the mother consider what the baby will be fed instead of her milk.

- If her baby is younger than a year, suggest she talk to her baby's healthcare provider about what to feed at the missed breastfeedings.

- If the baby is older than a year, family foods and other milks can be substituted for breastfeeding.

To begin, suggest the mother notice her usual breastfeeding times and decide which feedings she wants to drop. If she will be away from her baby for part of the day, suggest she start with a feeding during the hours she'll be away (except for the first morning feeding, when she will likely feel full already). When she drops that breastfeeding, suggest she continue to give the replacement food at this same feeding every day.

Before dropping another feeding, suggest she give her body at least 3 days for her milk production to adjust downward. If at any time her breasts feel full, suggest she express just enough milk to stay comfortable, which will cause her milk production to slow gradually, while avoiding pain and health risks.

When she reaches her desired level of breastfeeding and no longer feels breast fullness between feedings, she has achieved a partial weaning. The mother can keep breastfeeding at this level for as long as she wishes.

Abrupt Weaning

An abrupt weaning is usually most physically and emotionally difficult for mother and baby.

Mothers who find breastfeeding painful are more likely to wean abruptly, perhaps to eliminate the cause of their pain as quickly as possible (Neighbors et al., 2003). Weaning abruptly leads to overly full breasts, which can cause intense breast pain and, as a result, may lead to mastitis. Because breastfeeding provides both emotional as well as physical closeness, an abrupt weaning may be a more difficult emotional adjustment for the baby than a gradual weaning.

During an abrupt weaning, suggest the baby receive extra focused attention and touching.

To help offset the emotional loss of the closeness of breastfeeding, as with any type of weaning, suggest during weaning that the baby receive extra focused attention and skin-to-skin contact. Depending on the age of the child, this might involve talking, cuddling, reading stories, rocking, doing art projects together, or any other age-appropriate behavior that the child enjoys.

If a mother asks about comfort measures for an abrupt weaning, ask if she has time for a more gradual weaning.

Abrupt weaning is the only approach some mothers know. It may be a relief to learn that weaning can be done gradually and comfortably. If a sudden weaning can't be avoided, help the mother make it as comfortable as possible by reviewing the comfort measures in the next section.

If a baby younger than 1 year abruptly refuses the breast, consider it a nursing strike rather than a natural weaning.

A baby younger than 1 year has a physical need for mother's milk. This makes it highly unlikely that breast refusal at this age is due to natural weaning. Most babies who wean naturally do so gradually over a period of weeks and months, but some children do wean quickly. If this happens, help the mother reduce her milk production comfortably. In a baby older than 12 months, one way to tell a natural weaning from a nursing strike is the baby's reaction. If the baby seems upset with the change, it is most likely a nursing strike. If the child seems content, it is probably a natural weaning. In most cases, a nursing strike can be overcome and breastfeeding resumed. For details on overcoming a nursing strike, see p. 144- "Nursing Strike."

Comfort Measures During Weaning

The more gradual the weaning, the less comfort measures will be needed.

One U.S. study described the comfort measured used by 222 women who weaned before their babies were 6 months old, including breast-binding, ice packs, milk expression, and over-the-counter pain medications (Neighbors et al., 2003). Women who took 4 days or longer to wean used these comfort measures less often than women who weaned within 3 days.

Breast-binding was once recommended during weaning, but this practice—which was never studied—has fallen out of favor.

Unfortunately, there is little evidence available to help determine the best comfort measures for mothers who do not breastfeed after birth or mothers who wean after establishing breastfeeding (McGee, 1992). Practices such as breast-binding and cold compresses have been used, but there is no research to indicate the effectiveness of these strategies and which are best.

"Dry-up" medication is no longer recommended to suppress milk production.

In years past, mothers were routinely given bromocriptine (Parlodel), a prolactin suppressor, as "dry-up" medication to suppress milk production either after birth or during weaning. However, serious side effects were reported, including stroke, seizure, even death, and the U.S. Food and Drug Administration withdrew its clearance for this use (FDA, 1994; Hale, 2008).

Expressing milk while weaning can increase a mother's comfort and reduce health risks.

Whether a mother weans gradually or abruptly, she can use milk expression to stay comfortable. One milk-expression strategy is called "express to comfort," which means expressing just enough milk to stay comfortable any time the mother feels breast fullness. When using this strategy, rather than expressing milk long enough to drain her breasts well, suggest the mother stop when her breasts feel more comfortable.

Another milk-expression strategy sometimes recommended during weaning (especially for mothers with a hardened area in her breast [blocked duct] that won't go away) is to fully drain the breasts and then go for longer and longer stretches without breastfeeding or expressing (S. Burger, personal communication, November 18, 2009).

Encourage the mother to use whichever strategy works best for her.

A variety of other comfort measures are recommended in the popular literature and used by mothers during weaning.

The book for parents, *How Weaning Happens,* describes some of the most commonly used (but not necessarily researched) comfort measures:

> Ice packs wrapped in cloth and applied to the breasts may help diminish swelling. Taking a warm shower will help ease engorgement and cause the milk to flow. Wearing a comfortable supportive bra (maybe even a size larger) may help. The mother should drink to thirst, but may find that it helps to restrict salt intake (Bengson, 1999, p. 74).

Another book for parents, *The Nursing Mother's Guide to Weaning,* offers three other comfort measures intended to relieve the swelling and engorgement that can occur with a quick weaning:

- Wear chilled cabbage leaves inside the bra, replacing them every 4 to 8 hours with fresh chilled leaves.
- For no more than 1 week, every day drink 3 cups (750 mL) of sage tea, made by steeping 1½ teaspoons (6 mL) dry sage leaves in a pint of freshly boiled water for 10 minutes.
- Take two 100 mg vitamin B_6 (pyridoxine) pills 3 times a day for the first day, and one tablet daily thereafter; possible side effects include nausea, vomiting, diarrhea, and dark yellow-colored urine (Huggins, 2007).

Mother's Physical and Emotional Changes with Weaning

Some mothers have no physical or emotional symptoms during weaning, others do.

In one study of 222 U.S. mothers who weaned their babies before 6 months, many physical and emotional changes were reported (Neighbors et al., 2003). This study divided the mothers into two groups, those who weaned their baby within 3 days and those whose weaning took 4 days or longer. Any weaning taking less than a week is more abrupt than gradual, but even so, the incidence of symptoms varied by the time taken to wean (Table 5.1). The mothers who weaned within 3 days were more than twice as likely to have been previously suffering from nipple pain, which may explain why a larger percentage of these mothers felt "happier overall" after weaning. An Australian study found that nipple pain can contribute to anxiety and depression, but most mothers' mood improved after their nipple pain resolved (Amir, 1997).

Table 5.1. Symptoms Mothers (%) Reported after Weaning

Symptom	Weaned ≤3 days (N=86)	Weaned ≥4 days (N=136)
No symptoms	36	26
Increased energy	15	13
Decreased energy	5	14
Feeling happier overall	23	9
Feeling sadder overall	10	14
Increase in weight	24	28
Decrease in weight	15	15
Change in hair texture or shine	10	24
Increased appetite	4	16
Decreased appetite	13	13
Other	6	9

(Neighbors et al., 2003)

If a mother's menstrual cycles have not returned before weaning, she should expect them to return—along with her fertility—after weaning.

If a mother weans before her menstrual cycles have returned she should expect weaning to trigger a return to menstruation and fertility. A woman's menses can be suppressed by the hormones released by frequent breastfeeding (Labbok, 2007). During weaning, as the number of breastfeedings per day decreases and eventually stops, a mother will begin ovulating and her menses will resume. For more details, see p. 491- "Before the Menses Resume."

After weaning occurs, many mothers experience some feelings of loss and sadness.

Even when weaning is a positive experience for mother and child, it is still a kind of "letting go," which can lead to feelings of loss and sadness. Some mothers describe weaning as the loss of a special bond that can "never be recaptured with that child again" (Hauck & Irurita, 2002).

The baby's age at weaning can affect the intensity of a mother's sadness. In one U.S. study, researchers found that 65% of the women who weaned at 3 months or younger wished they had breastfed longer and that more than half of the women who weaned at 4 to 6 months were sorry they had weaned their babies so young (Rogers, Morris, & Taper, 1987). One author (Bumgarner, 2000) received letters from hundreds of mothers describing their feelings about weaning and noted that those who most consistently described feelings of loss and regret were those who weaned babies younger than 2 years of age.

Weaning is a "letting go", which can cause feeling of loss and sadness.

When nursing continues past 2 or 3, mothers much less frequently describe weaning in the same mixed terms. It seems that a time comes in the growth of the mother-child relationship when it is easier for both to move on and leave baby things behind (Bumgarner, 2000, p. 288).

Another U.S. study of mothers who weaned before 6 months found that gradual weaning was positively associated with sadness from birth to 5 weeks (Neighbors et al., 2003). It also found that mothers who weaned had less sadness when the baby was 21 to 25 weeks old. One Australian study found that mothers who did not feel ready to wean experienced a longer period of emotional adjustment before they reached acceptance (Hauck & Irurita, 2002).

RESOURCES FOR PARENTS

Websites

http://www.llli.org/NB/NBweaning.html

http://www.kellymom.com/bf/weaning/index.html

Books

Bengsen, D. (1999). *How weaning happens.* Schaumburg IL: La Leche League International.

Bumgarner, N.J. (2000). *Mothering your nursing toddler.* Schaumburg IL: La Leche League International.

Huggins, K. & Ziedrich, L. (2007). *The nursing mother's guide to weaning.* Revised edition. Boston, MA: Harvard Commons Press.

Mohrbacher, N. & Kendall-Tackett, K. (2010). *Breastfeeding made simple: Seven natural laws for nursing mothers, 2nd Edition.* Oakland CA: New Harbinger Publications.

REFERENCES

Agostoni, C., Decsi, T., Fewtrell, M., Goulet, O., Kolacek, S., Koletzko, B., et al. (2008). Complementary feeding: a commentary by the ESPGHAN Committee on Nutrition. *Journal of Pediatric Gastroenterology and Nutrition, 46*(1), 99-110.

Ahluwalia, I. B., Morrow, B., & Hsia, J. (2005). Why do women stop breastfeeding? Findings from the Pregnancy Risk Assessment and Monitoring System. *Pediatrics, 116*(6), 1408-1412.

Amir, L. H. (1997). Psychological aspects of nipple pain in lactating women. *Breastfeeding Review, 5*(1), 29-32.

Bar-Yam, N. B., & Darby, L. (1997). Fathers and breastfeeding: a review of the literature. *Journal of Human Lactation, 13*(1), 45-50.

Bengson, D. (1999). *How weaning happens*. Schaumburg, IL: La Leche League International.

Buckley, K. M. (1992). Beliefs and practices related to extended breastfeeding among La Leche League mothers. *The Journal of Perinatal Education, 1*(2), 45-53.

Bumgarner, N. J. (2000). *Mothering your nursing toddler*. Schaumburg, IL: La Leche League International.

Chen, A., & Rogan, W. J. (2004). Breastfeeding and the risk of postneonatal death in the United States. *Pediatrics, 113*(5), e435-439.

Cooke, M., Sheehan, A., & Schmied, V. (2003). A description of the relationship between breastfeeding experiences, breastfeeding satisfaction, and weaning in the first 3 months after birth. *Journal of Human Lactation, 19*(2), 145-156.

Dennis, C. L. (2002). Breastfeeding initiation and duration: a 1990-2000 literature review. *Journal of Obstetric, Gynecologic, and Neonatal Nursing, 31*(1), 12-32.

Dettwyler, K. A. (1995). A time to wean: The hominid bluprint for the natural age of weaning in modern human populations. In P. Stuart-Macadam & K. A. Dettwyler (Eds.), *Breastfeeding: Biocultural perspectives* (pp. 39-73). New York, NY: Aldine de Gruyter.

FDA. (1994). Bromocriptine indication widthrawn. *FDA Med Bulletin, 24*(2), 2.

Fewtrell, M. S., Morgan, J. B., Duggan, C., Gunnlaugsson, G., Hibberd, P. L., Lucas, A., et al. (2007). Optimal duration of exclusive breastfeeding: what is the evidence to support current recommendations? *American Journal of Clinical Nutrition, 85*(2), 635S-638S.

Forste, R., & Hoffmann, J. P. (2008). Are US mothers meeting the Healthy People 2010 Breastfeeding Targets for initiation, duration, and exclusivity? The 2003 and 2004 National Immunization Surveys. *Journal of Human Lactation, 24*(3), 278-288.

Gartner, L. M., Morton, J., Lawrence, R. A., Naylor, A. J., O'Hare, D., Schanler, R. J., et al. (2005). Breastfeeding and the use of human milk. *Pediatrics, 115*(2), 496-506.

Gulick, E. (1986). The effects of breastfeeding on toddler health. *Pediatric Nursing, 12*, 51-54.

Haku, M. (2007). Breastfeeding: factors associated with the continuation of breastfeeding, the current situation in Japan, and recommendations for further research. *Journal of Medical Investigation, 54*(3-4), 224-234.

Hale, T. W. (2008). Bromocriptine mesylate. In *Medications and mothers' milk* (Vol. 13, pp. 122-123). Amarillo TX: Hale Publishing.

Hanson, L. A. (2004). *Immunobiology of human milk*. Amarillo, TX: Pharmasoft Publishing.

Hauck, Y. L., & Irurita, V. F. (2002). Constructing compatibility: managing breast-feeding and weaning from the mother's perspective. *Qualitative Health Research, 12*(7), 897-914.

Hauck, Y. L., & Irurita, V. F. (2003). Incompatible expectations: the dilemma of breastfeeding mothers. *Health Care for Women International, 24*(1), 62-78.

Heath, A. L., Tuttle, C. R., Simons, M. S., Cleghorn, C. L., & Parnell, W. R. (2002). A longitudinal study of breastfeeding and weaning practices during the first year of life in Dunedin, New Zealand. *Journal of the American Dietetic Association, 102*(7), 937-943.

Huggins, K. & Ziedrich, L. (2007). *The nursing mother's guide to weaning* (Revised edition ed.). Boston, MA: Harvard Commons Press.

Ip, S., Chung, M., Raman, G., Chew, P., Magula, N., DeVine, D., et al. (2007). Breastfeeding and maternal and infant health outcomes in developed countries. *Evidence Report/ Technology Assessment (Full Rep),* (153), 1-186.

Ip, S., Chung, M., Raman, G., Trikalinos, T. A., & Lau, J. (2009). A summary of the Agency for Healthcare Research and Quality's evidence report on breastfeeding in developed countries. *Breastfeeding Medicine, 4 Suppl 1,* S17-30.

Isabella, P. H., & Isabella, R. A. (1994). Correlates of successful breastfeeding: a study of social and personal factors. *Journal of Human Lactation, 10*(4), 257-264.

Jones, G., Steketee, R. W., Black, R. E., Bhutta, Z. A., & Morris, S. S. (2003). How many child deaths can we prevent this year? *Lancet, 362*(9377), 65-71.

Kelleher, C. M. (2006). The physical challenges of early breastfeeding. *Social Science and Medicine, 63*(10), 2727-2738.

Kendall-Tackett, K. A., & Sugarman, M. (1995). The social consequences of long-term breastfeeding. *Journal of Human Lactation, 11*(3), 179-183.

Labarere, J., Gelbert-Baudino, N., Ayral, A. S., Duc, C., Berchotteau, M., Bouchon, N., et al. (2005). Efficacy of breastfeeding support provided by trained clinicians during an early, routine, preventive visit: a prospective, randomized, open trial of 226 mother-infant pairs. *Pediatrics, 115*(2), e139-146.

Labbok, M. (2007). Breastfeeding, birth spacing, and family planning. In T. W. Hale & P. Hartmann(Eds.), *Hale & Hartmann's textbook of human lactation* (pp. 305-318). Amarillo, TX: Hale Publishing.

Leff, E. W., Gagne, M. P., & Jefferis, S. C. (1994). Maternal perceptions of successful breastfeeding. *Journal of Human Lactation, 10*(2), 99-104.

Leff, E. W., Jefferis, S. C., & Gagne, M. P. (1994). The development of the Maternal Breastfeeding Evaluation Scale. *Journal of Human Lactation, 10*(2), 105-111.

McGee, M. L. (1992). Abrupt weaning: is breast-binding effective? *Journal of Human Lactation, 8*(3), 126.

Mead, M., & Newton, N. (1967). Cultural patterns of perinatal behavior. In S. Richardson & A. Guttmacher (Eds.), *Childbearing: Its social and psychological aspects.* Baltimore, MD: Willliams & Wilkins.

Mezzacappa, E. S., & Katlin, E. S. (2002). Breast-feeding is associated with reduced perceived stress and negative mood in mothers. *Health Psychology, 21*(2), 187-193.

Molbak, K. (1994). Prolonged breastfeeding, diarrhoeal disease, and survival of children. *BMJ, 308,* 1403-1406.

Neighbors, K. A., Gillespie, B., Schwartz, K., & Foxman, B. (2003). Weaning practices among breastfeeding women who weaned prior to six months postpartum. *Journal of Human Lactation, 19*(4), 374-380; quiz 381-375, 448.

PAHO/WHO. (2001). *Guiding principles for complementary feeding of the breastfed child.* Retrieved. from http://whqlibdoc.who.int/paho/2004/a85622.pdf.

Raj, V. K., & Plichta, S. B. (1998). The role of social support in breastfeeding promotion: a literature review. *Journal of Human Lactation, 14*(1), 41-45.

Ramos, C. V., & Almeida, J. A. (2003). [Maternal allegations for weaning: qualitative study]. *Jornal de Pediatria, 79*(5), 385-390.

Rempel, L. A. (2004). Factors influencing the breastfeeding decisions of long-term breastfeeders. *Journal of Human Lactation, 20*(3), 306-318.

Rogers, C. S., Morris, S., & Taper, L. J. (1987). Weaning from the breast: influences on maternal decisions. *Pediatric Nursing, 13*(5), 341-345.

Ryan, A. S., & Zhou, W. (2006). Lower breastfeeding rates persist among the Special Supplemental Nutrition Program for Women, Infants, and Children participants, 1978-2003. *Pediatrics, 117*(4), 1136-1146.

Schmied, V., & Barclay, L. (1999). Connection and pleasure, disruption and distress: women's experience of breastfeeding. *Journal of Human Lactation, 15*(4), 325-334.

Scott, J. A., Binns, C. W., Graham, K. I., & Oddy, W. H. (2006). Temporal changes in the determinants of breastfeeding initiation. *Birth, 33*(1), 37-45.

Scott, J. A., Binns, C. W., Oddy, W. H., & Graham, K. I. (2006). Predictors of breastfeeding duration: evidence from a cohort study. *Pediatrics, 117*(4), e646-655.

Sugarman, M., & Kendall-Tackett, K. A. (1995). Weaning ages in a sample of American women who practice extended breastfeeding. *Clinical Pediatrics, 34*(12), 642-647.

Taveras, E. M., Capra, A. M., Braveman, P. A., Jensvold, N. G., Escobar, G. J., & Lieu, T. A. (2003). Clinician support and psychosocial risk factors associated with breastfeeding discontinuation. *Pediatrics, 112*(1 Pt 1), 108-115.

Taveras, E. M., Scanlon, K. S., Birch, L., Rifas-Shiman, S. L., Rich-Edwards, J. W., & Gillman, M. W. (2004). Association of breastfeeding with maternal control of infant feeding at age 1 year. *Pediatrics, 114*(5), e577-583.

Williams, K. M., & Morse, J. M. (1989). Weaning patterns of first-time mothers. *MCN; American Journal of Maternal Child Nursing, 14*(3), 188-192.

Yilmaz, G., Gurakan, B., Cakir, B., & Tezcan, S. (2002). Factors influencing sleeping pattern of infants. *Turkish Journal of Pediatrics, 44*(2), 128-133.

Weight Gain and Growth

Chapter 6

NORMAL GROWTH

Ages and Stages

Weight Loss After Birth

While in utero, the baby floats in amniotic fluid. After birth, he naturally loses weight as he sheds the excess fluids in his tissues and passes the meconium stools from his intestines. Weight loss occurs in both formula-fed and breastfed newborns, but those exclusively formula-fed lose less weight than those exclusively breastfed.

Most newborns lose weight after birth no matter how they are fed, which may be beneficial over the long term.

In one Canadian study, researchers audited the charts of 812 newborns born in six hospitals (Martens & Romphf, 2007). At 2 days of age, when not yet at their lowest weight, the formula-fed newborns lost an average of 2.5% of their birthweight, while exclusively breastfed babies lost an average of 5.5%. Because U.S. research has found that formula-fed babies who gain more weight during their first week are at greater risk of overweight and other health problems later in life (Stettler et al., 2005), the Canadian researchers cautioned against overfeeding formula-fed babies in the hospital. Due to the "metabolic programming" that occurs during the first week, they suggested formula-fed newborns receive no more formula at each feeding than a baby receives at the breast, 10 to 30 mL at most. For more details, see the last point in the next section.

Exclusively breastfed infants lose more weight after birth than those who are formula fed.

• •

In a Canadian literature review on weight loss after birth in breastfed babies, the range of normal weight loss was 3.2% to 8.3% (Noel-Weiss, Courant, & Woodend, 2008). The mean weight loss was 5.7% to 6.6%, and the standard deviation was 2%. This standard deviation is important because it means that many babies who lose more than the average should still be considered in the normal range.

The average weight loss of a breastfed baby after birth is 5% to 7%, with the lowest weight occurring on Day 3 or 4.

• •

Although a baby's weight loss can occur for reasons other than low milk intake (see next point), the American Academy of Pediatrics recommended:

> Weight loss in the infant of greater than 7% from birthweight indicates possible breastfeeding problems and requires more intensive evaluation of breastfeeding and possible intervention to correct problems and improve milk production and transfer (Gartner et al., 2005, p. 499).

If a baby loses more than 7% of his birthweight or continues to lose weight after Day 4, breastfeeding dynamics should be evaluated.

According to the Academy of Breastfeeding Medicine:

> Weight loss in excess of 7% may be an indication of inadequate milk transfer or low milk production. Although weight loss in the range of 8-10% may be within normal limits, if all else is going well and the physical exam is normal, it is an indication for careful assessment and possible breastfeeding assistance (ABM, 2009, p. 176).

Evaluate breastfeeding dynamics if a baby loses more than 7% of his birthweight.

Even if the baby's weight loss is due to other causes, making sure breastfeeding is going well is always wise. One U.S. study found that when mothers received regular breastfeeding guidance very few babies lost more than 7% of their birthweight (DeMarzo, Seacat, & Neifert, 1991).

• •

Factors other than milk intake affect weight loss after birth.

The authors of a Canadian review of the literature suggest a 7% weight loss not be used as a cut-off for determining when to supplement a newborn because a greater weight loss does not necessarily mean a baby is at risk (Noel-Weiss et al., 2008). Weight loss is affected by many factors unrelated to milk intake, such as birth experiences, birthing practices, and hospital routines. For example, mothers who receive IV fluids during labor pass along some of these extra fluids to their babies in utero, elevating their birthweight and causing greater weight loss after birth, as these extra fluids are shed (Dahlenburg, Burnell, & Braybrook, 1980).

Babies with a greater weight loss are not necessarily at risk.

Other Canadian research found a greater weight loss associated with the use of epidurals for pain relief during labor, most likely due at least in part to extra fluids mother and baby receive (Martens & Romphf, 2007). In this same study, other factors associated with percentage of weight loss after birth included:

- **Birthweight**—Heavier babies lost more weight.
- **Cesarean birth**—Babies born surgically lost more weight.
- **Gestational age**—Babies born earlier lost more weight.
- **Gender**—Baby girls lost more weight than baby boys.

Because birth practices vary from place to place, country of birth also appears to affect weight loss. When comparing their own research to two previous studies U.S. scientists noticed that a higher percentage of babies born in the U.S. lost more than 10% of their birthweight compared with babies born in other countries (Nommsen-Rivers & Dewey, 2009). Seven to 10% of newborns in both Italy and Peru lost more than 10% of their birthweight (Manganaro, Mami, Marrone, Marseglia, & Gemelli, 2001; Matias, Nommsen-Rivers, & Creed-Kanashiro, 2009). But among U.S. babies, 16% and 18% lost more than 10% of birthweight, and these U.S. statistics were consistent even among mothers in different ethnic and socioeconomic groups (Dewey, Nommsen-Rivers, Heinig, & Cohen, 2003; Dewey, Nommsen, & Cohen, 2009). The authors suggested that greater weight loss among U.S. babies may be more common in part because "Childbirth is a highly medicalized event in the United States, and this type of birth setting may contribute to additional challenges to successfully establishing lactation" (Nommsen-Rivers & Dewey, 2009, pp. S47-S48).

The day babies reach their lowest weight also varied among studies and from place to place. One Scottish study of 971 newborns found that on average both formula-fed and breastfed babies reached their lowest weight at 2.7 days of age (Macdonald, Ross, Grant, & Young, 2003). An Italian study (see next point) found that babies born vaginally reached their lowest weight on Day 3 or 4, but those born by cesarean section reached their low weight on Day 4 or 5 (Manganaro et al., 2001).

If a baby loses more than 10% of birthweight, breastfeeding should be evaluated and the baby should be checked for jaundice and dehydration.

In all cases, a weight loss of more than 10% of birthweight is a red flag to evaluate breastfeeding. If feeding problems are not overcome quickly or if the baby shows signs of dehydration, supplements may be needed. In an Italian prospective study of 686 full-term babies born over a 6-month period at one hospital, 7.7% (53) of the exclusively breastfed babies lost more than 10% of their birthweight (Manganaro et al., 2001). In 74% of these babies, poor milk transfer was found to be the cause, and after providing breastfeeding help, weight improved. In 26% of these babies, delayed milk production was the cause, which can sometimes be a side effect of less-than-optimal breastfeeding (for details, see the chapter "Making Milk"). The researchers recommended all babies be scheduled for a routine weight check at 5 days of age to prevent dehydration.

In some cases, dehydration can lead to hypernatremia, or elevated blood sodium levels, which may require hospitalization to balance the baby's electrolytes in order to prevent seizures and other serious health problems (Caglar, Ozer, & Altugan, 2006). When babies become dehydrated or hypernatremic, mothers are more likely to give up on breastfeeding (Harding, Cairns, Gupta, & Cowan, 2001; Oddie, Richmond, & Coulthard, 2001).

Most breastfed babies begin gaining weight by about Day 4 and regain their birthweight by about Day 10 to 14.

The Scottish study of 971 babies described in a previous point (Macdonald et al., 2003) found that the median time to regain birthweight among breastfeeding babies was 8.3 days of life (Macdonald et al., 2003). Formula-fed babies, in contrast, were back up to their birthweight by a median of 6.5 days of life. A Canadian review of the literature found in the 11 studies it reviewed, most of the breastfed babies had regained their birthweight by 2 weeks (Noel-Weiss et al., 2008).

The earlier a breastfeeding problem is corrected, the faster it is usually resolved. The more weight a baby loses after birth, the longer it may take for him to regain it. Babies who are ill or born preterm may take longer to regain their birthweight than healthy, full-term babies.

If a baby has not regained birthweight by 10 days to 2 weeks, this is another red flag to take a closer look at how breastfeeding is going and make any needed adjustments. To boost weight gain, a good first step is to help the baby take the breast deeper. Suggest the mother try breastfeeding more often or for longer periods and use breast compression (see "Techniques" appendix) to increase both fat content and milk intake (Stutte, 1988).

Growth from Birth to 12 Months

When a breastfed baby starts gaining weight on about Day 3 or 4, an average weight gain is about 8 ounces (245 g) per week.

Weight gain after birth should always be measured from the lowest weight, which is usually on the 3rd or 4th day. But weight checks done around this time can be confusing. For example, if a baby is weighed on Day 2 while he is still losing weight and again on Day 4, his weight may be lower on Day 4 than on Day 2, and it may appear that he is still losing. But that may not be the case. He may have reached his lowest weight on Day 3, and then started to gain, but not yet reached his Day 2 level. Another weight check is needed for an accurate gauge of how the baby is doing. If a baby is still losing weight after Day 5, breastfeeding should be closely evaluated.

Average weight gain for the first 2 to 3 months is about 8 ounces (245 g) per week, with boys gaining slightly faster than girls. See Appendix D (p. 859) for the World Health Organization's charts on weight gain in exclusively breastfeeding boys and girls. As with other measurements, the 50th percentile is considered average, and some babies will be above it and some below it. If a baby is gaining weight at well below the 50th percentile, this is a sign breastfeeding needs closer attention. For example, a weight gain of 4.5 ounces (133 g) per week during the first 3 months is at the 1st percentile for a breastfeeding girl (Tables 6.1 and 6.2). See the later section "Slow Weight Gain" for strategies for increasing weight gain. Gaining more weight gain than average is not a problem (see the last section in this chapter, "Rapid Weight Gain").

Between 3 and 12 months, weight gain gradually slows.

Babies grow rapidly during the first 3 months of life, with growth slowing during months 3 through 12. Slowing growth is normal. If a baby kept growing at his newborn rate, he would be a giant by adulthood. See Table 6.1 and 6.2 for weight gains by month for boys and girls from birth to 12 months broken down into percentiles (WHO, 2006). The average breastfed baby doubles his birthweight by 5 to 6 months of age. When growth charts based on growth data from formula-fed babies are used (see next section), between 3 and 6 months of age, a breastfed baby's weight may appear to be faltering. Growth charts based on normal growth in breastfeeding babies are available from the World Health Organization free and online at: http://www.who.int/childgrowth/standards/en/. Some samples of these charts can be found in Appendix D. For more details, see the next section, "Growth Charts."

During the second 6 months of life, healthy, thriving babies average a monthly growth in length of 0.5 inch (1.27 cm) and head circumference of about 0.25 inch (64 mm). At 12 months, the average breastfed baby weighs about 2.5 times his birthweight, has increased in length by 50%, and has increased head circumference by 33%.

Growth in length and head circumference is an important sign of healthy growth.

Weight gain is not the only important measure of a baby's growth because weight gain also includes any increase in tissue fluids and fat. During the first 6 months of life, healthy, thriving babies average a monthly growth in length of about 1 inch (2.5 cm) and head circumference of about 0.5 inch (1.27 cm). No differences in adult height have been found between those fed in infancy by breast or bottle (Li, Manor, & Power, 2004; Martin, Smith, Mangtani, Frankel, & Gunnell, 2002; Victora, Barros, Lima, Horta, & Wells, 2003).

U.S. research found that babies do not grow consistently in length and head circumference (Lampl, Veldhuis, & Johnson, 1992). Length and head circumference stay static 90% to 95% of the time, with measurable bursts of growth occurring during the remaining 5% to 10%.

Table 6.1. WHO Monthly Weight Chart for Girls—Birth to 12 Months

1-month weight increments (g) GIRLS
Birth to 12 months (percentiles)

World Health Organization

Interval	1st	3rd	5th	15th	25th	50th	75th	85th	95th	97th	99th
0 - 4 wks	280	388	446	602	697	879	1068	1171	1348	1418	1551
4 wks - 2 mo	410	519	578	734	829	1011	1198	1301	1476	1545	1677
2 - 3 mo	233	321	369	494	571	718	869	952	1094	1150	1256
3 - 4 mo	133	214	259	376	448	585	726	804	937	990	1090
4 - 5 mo	51	130	172	286	355	489	627	703	833	885	983
5 - 6 mo	-24	52	93	203	271	401	537	611	739	790	886
6 - 7 mo	-79	-4	37	146	214	344	480	555	684	734	832
7 - 8 mo	-119	-44	-2	109	178	311	450	526	659	711	811
8 - 9 mo	-155	-81	-40	70	139	273	412	489	623	675	776
9 - 10 mo	-184	-110	-70	41	110	245	385	464	598	652	754
10 - 11 mo	-206	-131	-89	24	95	233	378	459	598	653	759
11 - 12 mo	-222	-145	-102	15	88	232	383	467	612	670	781

WHO Growth Velocity Standards

From http://www.who.int/childgrowth/standards/w_velocity/en/index.html
(28.35 grams = 1 ounce)

Table 6.2. WHO Monthly Weight Chart for Boys—Birth to 12 Months

1-month weight increments (g) BOYS
Birth to 12 months (percentiles)

World Health Organization

Interval	1st	3rd	5th	15th	25th	50th	75th	85th	95th	97th	99th
0 - 4 wks	182	369	460	681	805	1023	1229	1336	1509	1575	1697
4 wks - 2 mo	528	648	713	886	992	1196	1408	1524	1724	1803	1955
2 - 3 mo	307	397	446	577	658	815	980	1071	1228	1290	1410
3 - 4 mo	160	241	285	403	476	617	764	845	985	1041	1147
4 - 5 mo	70	150	194	311	383	522	666	746	883	937	1041
5 - 6 mo	-17	61	103	217	287	422	563	640	773	826	927
6 - 7 mo	-76	0	42	154	223	357	496	573	706	758	859
7 - 8 mo	-118	-43	-1	111	181	316	457	535	671	724	827
8 - 9 mo	-153	-77	-36	77	148	285	429	508	646	701	806
9 - 10 mo	-183	-108	-66	48	120	259	405	486	627	683	790
10 - 11 mo	-209	-132	-89	27	100	243	394	478	623	680	791
11 - 12 mo	-229	-150	-106	15	91	239	397	484	635	695	811

WHO Growth Velocity Standards

From http://www.who.int/childgrowth/standards/w_velocity/en/index.html
(28.35 grams = 1 ounce; to convert to ounces, divide grams by 28.35)

Formula-fed babies gain significantly more weight than breastfed babies between 3 and 12 months of age and have more negative health outcomes.

In addition to gaining more weight between 3 and 12 months of age, babies fed non-human milks also experience a greater incidence of infection, allergy, asthma, and many other illnesses (Ip, Chung, Raman, Trikalinos, & Lau, 2009). See the last section "Rapid Weight Gain" for details on the association between formula-feeding and obesity.

The greater milk intake in formula-fed babies and the higher protein levels in formula (Koletzko et al., 2009) are two factors that contribute to formula-fed babies' greater weight gain. But there are many others (Dewey, 2003):

- The bottle flows more consistently, giving formula-fed babies less control over their milk intake, which may contribute to an overfeeding habit from birth.
- Families who choose to formula-feed tend to also choose other less healthy behaviors and attitudes that lead to unhealthy feeding dynamics.
- Babies fed formula don't receive the components of mother's milk that contribute to better use of food nutrients and healthier metabolic programming.

Formula-fed babies may also be more likely to be fed by the clock rather than on cue, with less regard for their hunger and satiety.

Higher protein and greater intake contribute to greater weight gain in formula-fed infants.

Milk intake. One reason babies fed non-human milks gain more weight between 3 and 12 months than breastfed babies is that they consume much more milk. On average, babies fed formula consume 15% more milk at 3 months, 23% more at 6 months, 20% more at 9 months, and 18% more at 12 months (Heinig, Nommsen, Peerson, Lonnerdal, & Dewey, 1993). But because breastfed babies leave milk in the breast after feedings, researchers concluded that limited milk availability is not the reason they take less milk (Dewey, Heinig, Nommsen, & Lonnerdal, 1991b). Researchers noted that breastfed babies continued to gain less weight even after solid foods were started, and if availability of food was the reason, they could have consumed more solids to make up for the difference, but they didn't (Dewey, Heinig, Nommsen, & Lonnerdal, 1991a).

Eating habits. Differences in milk flow between breast and bottle may be another reason bottle-fed babies consume more milk and gain more weight. Due to an inborn reflex, during the first 3 to 4 months of life, swallowing milk automatically triggers suckling (Wolf & Glass, 1992). When babies outgrow this reflex, feeding becomes a fully voluntary activity. Because milk flows more consistently from the bottle than the breast (which has a natural ebb and flow of milk due to milk ejections), babies tend to consume more milk from the bottle at a feeding. Before reflexive suckling is outgrown, babies fed by bottle are at greater risk of overfeeding, which can cause unhealthy feeding patterns that last a lifetime. One large, prospective randomized, controlled trial (16,755 babies in Belarus) compared volume of milk per feeding in formula-fed and breastfed babies (Kramer et al., 2004). At each feeding the formula-fed babies took 49% more milk at 1 month, 57% more at 3 months, and 71% more at 5 months. Mothers' behaviors also influenced milk intake. Babies whose mothers encouraged them to finish the bottle were heavier than other babies. Babies also took more formula at feedings when their mothers offered bottles containing more than 6 ounces (177 mL).

Family behaviors and attitudes. Families who value health and fitness are more likely to breastfeed, but there is more to it. As described above, breastfeeding encourages healthy eating habits by giving the baby more control over how much milk he consumes. But the baby is not the only one who learns from this experience. As the breastfed baby grows and thrives, his mother learns to trust her baby to take the milk he needs, and this trust extends to solid foods at family meals. Whatever foods the baby eats, an important aspect of healthy parenting (and a lesson taught by breastfeeding) is responsive feeding, which means learning and respecting baby's hunger and satiety cues (Pelto, Levitt, & Thairu, 2003). One U.K. study found that between 6 and 12 months of age breastfeeding mothers put less pressure on their babies to eat solid foods and were more sensitive to their baby's cues, which were associated with less mealtime negativity at 1 year (Farrow & Blissett, 2006). U.S. research found that longer breastfeeding duration was associated with less restrictive child-feeding behaviors by parents at 1 year (Taveras et al., 2004).

Nutrient use and metabolic programming. Another reason for differences in milk intake may be the differences in how mother's milk and formula are metabolized by the baby. Formula-fed babies appear to use the nutrients in formula less efficiently, so they may require more milk to meet their nutritional needs. For example, one U.S. study concluded that "formula-fed infants are almost twofold less efficient than breastfed infants in their utilization of dietary nitrogen…" (Motil, Sheng, Montandon, & Wong, 1997, p. 15).

Formula has a different effect on a baby's metabolism than mother's milk. U.K. research has found that at 6 days of age formula-fed newborns had a more prolonged insulin response than breastfed babies, which U.S. research has found is associated with more fatty tissue, greater weight gain, and obesity (Lucas, Boyes, Bloom, & Aynsley-Green, 1981; Odeleye, de Courten, Pettitt, & Ravussin, 1997). Another preliminary U.S. study on babies 5 months old also found that those fed formula had elevated insulin levels (Dewey, Nommsen-Rivers, & Lonnerdal, 2004). This mechanism may also explain in part the association between formula-feeding and increased risk of Type 2 diabetes later in life (Young et al., 2002). Formula is also missing hormones, such as leptin and adiponectin, which help babies regulate appetite and energy metabolism (Li, Fein, & Grummer-Strawn, 2008). Higher leptin levels in mother's milk have been associated with lower body mass index (BMI) in their babies at 3 to 4 weeks of age (Doneray, Orbak, & Yildiz, 2009).

Due in part to differences in calories consumed while asleep (sleeping metabolism), formula-fed babies need more calories from food than breastfed babies to function and grow: 7% more at 3 months and 9% more at 6 months (Butte, Wong, Hopkinson, Heinz et al., 2000).

Another aspect of metabolic programming that may affect later weight gain was suggested by the U.S. researchers who monitored the weight gain and health outcomes of 653 people formula-fed during infancy for 2 to 3 decades (Stettler et al., 2005). These researchers found that greater weight gain during the first 8 days of life was associated with increased incidence of overweight 20 to 30 years later. They concluded that the first 8 days may be a "critical period" during which human physiology is programmed. This means that during this critical period breastfed babies' greater weight loss after birth and slower return to birthweight may help activate a healthier metabolic program, which reduces the risk of overweight and obesity during childhood and beyond.

Growth After 12 Months

At 12 months, babies fed non-human milks are typically heavier than breastfed babies, but by 24 months there is no difference in growth.

U.S. research on normal growth in healthy babies found that at 12 months breastfed babies were on average a little less than 1.5 lbs. (600-650 g) lighter than formula-fed babies (Dewey, Heinig, Nommsen, Peerson, & Lonnerdal, 1992). However, this was not an advantage, as the breastfed babies have been found to have better health outcomes, no matter where they live (Ip et al., 2009). By 24 months, any differences in weight gain and growth between breastfed and formula-fed babies have disappeared (Butte, Wong, Hopkinson, Smith, & Ellis, 2000; Dewey et al., 1992). No differences in height have been found in adulthood between those breastfeed or formula-fed as infants (Dewey, 2009b).

After 12 months, breastfeeding is still an important source of a baby's nourishment.

Breastfeeding is still important after 12 months.

Continued, frequent breastfeeding after 12 months provides babies with necessary nutrients. Breastfed babies 1 to 2 years old, consuming an average volume of mother's milk, receive 35% to 40% of their energy intake (Dewey & Brown, 2003), and it provides an important source of fatty acids and other key nutrients, such as vitamin A, calcium, and riboflavin (PAHO/WHO., 2001).

In developing areas, babies who breastfeed after 12 months grow better in length.

Research in developing countries has found that when babies older than a year continue to breastfeed and other confounding factors are eliminated, they grow faster in length than their weaned counterparts (Onyango, Esrey, & Kramer, 1999; Simondon, Simondon, Costes, Delaunay, & Diallo, 2001).

Growth Charts

Growth charts can be helpful, but they can also be confusing. In some cases, their misuse can undermine breastfeeding.

Growth charts can be a useful tool to understand how one baby's growth compares to the growth of other babies the same age, but they can also confuse parents and put the focus in the wrong place.

Growth charts plot a baby's growth on a series of percentile lines. An average child will be at the 50th percentile for weight and length. For weight, what this actually means is that out of 100 children, 49 will weigh less and 50 will weigh more. A weight that falls at a higher percentile is not "good" and a weight that falls at a lower percentile is not "bad." By definition, there will be healthy children at every percentile. Some will be chunky and some will be petite, but their percentile does not necessarily reflect their overall health or growth.

The child at the 5th percentile is not necessarily growing poorly and the child at the 95th percentile is not necessarily growing well. That's because growth can only be evaluated over time, and the evaluation will only be accurate when the chart itself is based on breastfeeding norms (see next point). For example, a preterm baby born very small will likely fall on a low percentile for weight and height at first, even when he is growing and gaining weight well, although his growth should eventually catch up to others born full-term. Also, a baby's large birthweight may be due more to the influence of the mother during the pregnancy, such as her blood sugar levels, weight gain, and height. After birth, a large baby may "regress to the mean" by falling in percentiles at first as his growth adjusts to his genetic potential (L. Nommsen-Rivers, personal communication, January 29, 2010).

One point on a baby's growth chart should never be considered in isolation. More important is how this one point compares to the other points on the chart.

To accurately evaluate a baby's growth, the answers to the following questions are needed:

- Is the baby gaining weight at a healthy pace?
- Is he growing normally in length and head circumference?

The baby's growth pattern over days, weeks, and months is what provides an accurate picture of how breastfeeding is going. If a baby is growing consistently and well, his actual percentile is irrelevant. However, if over time his percentile drops, this is a red flag to take a closer look (see next section).

One U.K. study examined through multiple interviews at well-baby checkups mothers' and healthcare providers' understanding of growth charts (Sachs, Dykes, & Carter, 2006). The researchers found that many mothers worried about their baby's weight gain between checkups and that both mothers and healthcare providers considered the 50th percentile a goal to be achieved. When babies fell below the 50th percentile, rather than focusing on optimizing breastfeeding, healthcare providers often recommended the mothers give their babies formula and solid foods to try to boost baby's weight gain to reach this percentile. In their conclusion, the researchers recommended more training for healthcare providers on assessing growth patterns of breastfeeding babies and more training on how to provide mothers with information that supports rather than undermines breastfeeding.

• •

Between 3 and 12 months of age, a baby's percentile on the growth chart will vary depending on whether the chart is based on breastfeeding norms.

Some growth charts are based on data on the growth of mostly formula-fed babies, who have different growth patterns than breastfed babies (for details on these differences see the last point in the previous section). For example, the 1977 National Center for Health Statistics (NCHS) growth charts used for many years in the U.S. were based on data from a study conducted in one Ohio town. The data used to create these charts had limitations, including a lack of ethnic diversity, data collection at infrequent, 3-month intervals, sample-size problems, and few breastfed babies (Dewey, 2009a).

Unfortunately, the U.S. Centers for Disease Control (CDC) charts that replaced them in 2000 also included few breastfed babies. The overrepresentation of formula-feeding babies in these studies was a problem because babies fed by breast and bottle gain weight differently from 3 to 12 months. When these charts were used, many exclusively breastfed babies who were gaining normally were thought to be faltering.

It wasn't until 2006 that the World Health Organization (WHO) released growth charts that accurately reflected the normal growth of the breastfed baby. This process began in 1997, when WHO began its ambitious Multicentre Growth Reference Study (WHO, 2006). This study's goal was to define optimal growth in six culturally and ethnically diverse countries (Brazil, Ghana, India, Norway, Oman, and the U.S.) over a 6-year period. About 8,500 children—including about 300 newborns—participated in the study. The mothers of these babies followed healthy practices by breastfeeding exclusively, not smoking, and adding appropriate solid foods to their babies' diet at the recommended age.

Researchers found that no matter where these mothers and children lived, and no matter what their ethnic background, average growth was nearly identical in all six countries. The charts developed from this research for children aged 0-60 months are free and downloadable online at: http://www.who.int/childgrowth/

standards/en/ and include weight for age, weight for length, weight for height, length/height for age, body mass index, and motor development milestones.

The WHO growth charts reflect norms for breastfeeding babies.

These WHO growth charts reflect breastfeeding norms and differ from the previous CDC growth charts in the following ways: from birth to 6 months more babies are heavier and from 6 to 12 months more babies are lighter (Dewey, 2009a). Previously used growth charts were a reflection of how mostly formula-fed children grew in a particular time and place. In contrast, the data used to create the WHO growth charts were compiled internationally among families using optimal feeding practices, making them a benchmark of how all children should grow. They are a standard that can be used to judge childhood growth anywhere in the world.

SLOW WEIGHT GAIN

When a baby is gaining weight slowly, be prepared to listen to and acknowledge the mother's feelings, which may be intense.

When a baby is not gaining well, a mother's feelings may run high. She may be frustrated and upset. She may be worried about her ability to care for her baby. She may feel anxious about her baby's health. She may feel guilty, wondering if her baby's slow weight gain is her fault or if she has not provided good care. She may feel like a failure.

Giving the mother an outlet to express her worries, fears, and doubts may make it easier for her to discuss and evaluate her situation. Assure her there is a reason for the slow weight gain and the odds are good that she'll be able to overcome this problem.

Gathering Basic Information

Before making suggestions, first determine the cause(s) of the slow weight gain.

When a baby does not gain well on mother's milk alone, everyone becomes concerned. Something needs to be done, but inappropriate actions can lead to premature weaning. Finding the cause(s) will help determine the best course of action. The cause of slow weight gain usually involves one or more of the following three areas:

- **Breastfeeding dynamics.** Is the baby on the breast deeply? Is the baby breastfeeding at least eight times each day and staying on the breast until done?
- **Baby's anatomy and health.** Is the baby breastfeeding ineffectively due to unusual anatomy or a health problem? Or is a health problem causing slow weight gain despite a healthy milk intake?
- **Mother's anatomy, health, and milk production.** Is the mother producing as much milk as her baby needs?

The strategies chosen to improve the baby's weight gain would depend on which of these areas are contributing to the problem. If breastfeeding dynamics are the main issue, which is most common, an adjustment in feeding pattern or achieving deeper breastfeeding is needed. If the baby has a medical problem, he may need diagnosis and treatment. Unusual anatomy, such as tongue tie, may require assessment and possibly a medical procedure. If the mother's milk production is low, the cause needs to be determined and production boosted.

To find the cause(s), some detective work is in order. The answers to the questions in the following sections will provide information that can help get to the root of the problem. Some basic questions should be asked of all mothers of slow-gaining babies, but some may not be necessary to explore with all mothers.

Ask questions in a calm, relaxed manner and affirm the mother for what she is doing right.

To gather the needed information, listen carefully, take notes, and ask questions calmly to help put the mother at ease. Be aware that some areas may be sensitive, so try to word questions tactfully. Because the mother may be worried that her baby's slow weight gain is her "fault," emphasize that every mother and baby is different and there are no hard-and-fast rules. Some basic breastfeeding dynamics are good to know (such as drained breasts make milk faster and full breasts make milk slower), but not all babies respond in the same way. One baby may breastfeed five times a day and gain weight well (although this is rare), while another may need to breastfeed every hour or two to gain weight well. The mother of a slow-gaining baby may feel vulnerable, and her family or friends may be criticizing her for her efforts to breastfeed. Be sure to affirm her for whatever she is doing right and for seeking help.

The mother's answers should guide the conversation.

During the course of the discussion, the mother's answers to certain questions may give clues to the cause of her baby's slow weight gain. When that happens, stop and talk more about this area to allow her to expand on her answer and to clarify her understanding of breastfeeding and her individual circumstances. If the reasons for the baby's slow weight gain are not obvious after these first three sections, continue to the others. The most common cause of slow weight gain is breastfeeding dynamics, which includes shallow breastfeeding and not breastfeeding often or long enough. Breastfeeding more often may not help the baby on the breast shallowly, for example, so pay careful attention to the mother's answers.

Be sure the baby is being regularly evaluated by a healthcare provider.

In all cases of slow weight gain, the baby should be seen regularly by his healthcare provider to rule out health problems. Although most cases of slow weight gain are not caused by physical problems, this is a possibility that needs to be considered.

If the baby's healthcare provider recommends supplementing the baby with formula and the mother wants to try other alternatives first, encourage her to contact him/her to discuss this. (See also Appendix C,"Working with Healthcare Professionals.")

Weight Gain and Loss

How much weight has the baby gained since birth, and how close is his weight gain to the normal range?

Ask the mother for the following information:

- Her baby's age
- The baby's current weight
- The baby's birthweight and gestational age at birth (preterm or full-term)
- The baby's lowest weight after birth
- His age and weights at each of his weight checks

If available, a baby's weight gain should be calculated from its lowest point. For example:

- Birthweight: 7 lbs., 13 ounces (3544 g)
- Lowest weight (age 4 days): 7 lbs., 0 ounces (3175 g)
- Current weight (age 5 weeks): 8 lbs., 13 ounces (3997 g)

Some might mistakenly think this baby girl is gaining slowly because she is only 1 lb. (454 g) over her birthweight at 5 weeks. But when the weight gain is calculated from the lowest point after birth, her weight gain for the last 4 weeks was actually 1 lb., 13 ounces (29 ounces or 823 g). She is not gaining slowly. She is gaining 7.3 ounces (206 g) per week, which is very close to an average weight gain for a girl. The 50th percentile of weight gain from birth to 4 weeks is 879 grams or 220 grams (7.75 ounces) per week (see p. 205- Table 6.1).

When a baby is born with an elevated birthweight, this can affect perception of weight gain later. For example, IV fluids given to the mother during labor can be absorbed by the baby's tissues in utero, boosting his birthweight and causing greater weight loss after birth as these extra fluids are shed (Dahlenburg et al., 1980). Birthweight may also be elevated in babies born to mothers with Type 1, Type 2, or gestational diabetes. In these babies, growth after birth is usually slower than average as the baby sheds the excess fluids and fat laid down in utero as a result of their mothers' abnormal blood sugar levels.

Growth usually slows with age (see first section), so what is considered slow weight gain will vary by age and stage.

If a baby's weight gain is close to the normal range (in a baby girl younger than 3 months, this is at least about 7 to 8 ounces (198-237 g) per week or about 28 g per day), the mother and the baby's healthcare provider will probably be more open to improving breastfeeding dynamics first, rather than insisting the baby be supplemented right away. To have the energy needed to feed effectively, a baby who is continuing to lose weight or is far from a healthy weight gain will need to be supplemented (see later section "When and How To Give Supplements").

Was the baby's weight an issue from birth, or did the baby gain well at first?

If a baby continues to lose weight after Day 4 or 5 or weight gain is low from the beginning, focus on baby's suckling effectiveness and mother's milk production (see later sections). If the baby's weight loss was in the normal range and baby regained his birthweight by 2 weeks, slow weight gain must have started after that. In this case, focus on breastfeeding dynamics, baby's health, and mother's milk production. Because a baby needs more milk per day over the first 5 weeks or so of life (see the later section "When and How to Supplement"), a mother whose milk production is limited by breast surgery or underdeveloped breast tissue, for example, may make enough milk for her baby to gain weight well during the first few weeks, but weight gain may falter after that.

Was the same scale used for each of the weight checks, was the baby's clothing the same when he was weighed, and when was the scale last calibrated?

Many parents and healthcare providers have assumed at one weight check that a baby was gaining slowly only to discover the problem was actually the scale or differences in how the baby was dressed when he was weighed. Before assuming the baby's weight is the problem, suggest the baby be weighed again using the same scale and wearing the same clothing as before. If the baby wears a diaper/nappy during weight checks, the difference between one that's dry or full also affects the results.

A healthy weight gain is the most reliable indicator of adequate milk intake, but some babies take adequate milk at the breast, yet still gain slowly.

When an exclusively breastfeeding baby has a healthy weight gain and is growing normally, it is safe to assume he is getting the milk he needs at the breast. However, it is possible for a baby to be taking adequate milk at the breast, but still gain weight slowly. That's because there is more to weight gain than milk intake alone.

In addition to consuming enough milk, a baby must also be able to digest the milk, and it must meet his energy needs. Babies with congenital heart disease, for example, usually gain weight slowly no matter how they are fed because they take more breathes per minute than a healthy baby in order to maintain adequate oxygen levels and circulation (Clemente, Barnes, Shinebourne, & Stein, 2001). (For more details, see p. 224 for the later section, "Slow Weight Gain with Good Milk Intake" and the chapter "Health Issues—Baby"). Other genetic conditions and metabolic, endocrine, and digestive disorders may also require treatment or interventions for normal growth, despite good milk intake.

How much has the baby grown in length and head circumference?

Growth in length and head circumference is also an important aspect of normal development. During the first 6 months, growth in length averages about 1 inch (2.54 centimeters) per month and head circumference about 0.5 inch (1.27 centimeters) per month. Growth in head circumference indicates brain growth.

What has the baby's healthcare provider said about the baby's overall health?

The baby's health is an important factor when considering weight gain. If the baby had been ill, for example, it is common for weight gain to slow or even stop for a time. Illness can affect a baby's feeding effectiveness and his appetite.

Illness can slow a baby's weight gain.

If the baby seems to be otherwise developing well and appears healthy and alert, this means there is probably time to fine-tune breastfeeding to increase baby's weight gain before supplements are needed.

Is the diagnosis slow weight gain or failure-to-thrive?

The difference between slow weight gain and failure to thrive is one of degree and definition. The diagnosis of failure to thrive, in addition to indicating the baby is seriously underweight, may also imply abuse or neglect (Walker, 2006). A baby identified as failure to thrive is at risk for malnutrition and immediate intervention is needed. Failure to thrive usually involves feeding problems, continued weight loss after the first week, not reaching birthweight by 3 weeks of age, and depending on birthweight, a weight below the 10th percentile on the growth charts by 1 month of age (Lawrence & Lawrence, 2005). The baby may grow little in length or head circumference, pass concentrated urine and few stools, and have symptoms of malnutrition or dehydration, such as lethargy and a sunken fontanel. A baby older than one month with failure to thrive, in addition to most of the previous symptoms, is usually below the 3rd percentile in weight, has fallen at least two standard deviations on the growth chart by 8 weeks, and may be delayed in reaching developmental milestones. In some cases, failure to thrive is due to health problems, such as infection, birth or heart defects, malabsorption, endocrine problems, or other chronic diseases. In some cases, the baby may be otherwise healthy and simply have feeding problems (Tolia, 1995). One U.S. report of 38 babies with failure to thrive found that underlying illness was the cause in half of those diagnosed after 1 month of age (Lukefahr, 1990).

A slow-gaining baby, on the other hand, usually feeds well and often has pale urine and the expected number of stools, appears alert and active, is developing normally, has good skin and muscle tone, and is gaining weight, just gaining slower than average. For this baby, it may be possible to make adjustments to breastfeeding before supplementing.

Other Signs of Milk Intake

How long during feedings can the mother hear baby swallowing?

How effectively a baby suckles is an important determinant of milk intake, and swallowing sounds can provide clues to effectiveness. When babies swallow, it is usually loud enough to be heard. After milk ejection, most babies swallow after every or every other suckle with occasional pauses. As breastfeeding continues, milk flow slows, and as the baby's hunger is satisfied, there is usually more time between swallows and more suckles to swallows. If the baby suckles many times before swallowing right after milk ejection, this is one possible sign of ineffective suckling.

• •

Are there any other indicators the baby is breastfeeding ineffectively?

Other signs of ineffective breastfeeding include:

- **No swallowing heard.** But there are exceptions. Some babies breastfeed effectively, but swallow too quietly to be heard. If so, the baby will be gaining weight well.
- **Baby never seems satisfied**. The mother may say he breastfeeds "all the time."
- **Shallow breastfeeding.** When the baby breastfeeds with the nipple in the front of his mouth (instead of in the "comfort zone" near where his hard and soft palates meet), this can contribute to slower milk flow, less milk intake, and/or difficulty staying on the breast.
- **Choking at the breast** can occur with very fast milk flow and also with uncoordinated suckling and swallowing or respiratory problems.
- **Low or high muscle tone.** "Floppy" babies with low tone include those with Down syndrome and other neurological impairments. Babies with high tone may arch away at the breast, especially if upright feeding positions are used. For breastfeeding strategies, see p. 309 in the chapter "Health Issues—Baby."
- **Cheek dimpling or a clicking sound** at the breast indicates suction is being broken. If baby is gaining weight well, this is not a problem.
- **Nipple pain or trauma** can be due to shallow breastfeeding, unusual tongue movements, or anatomical variations, such as tongue tie.
- **Unrelieved breast fullness or recurring mastitis** due to ineffective milk removal.

If the mother can't hear her baby swallow at all, the baby's audible swallowing stops early in the feeding, or he falls asleep quickly, suggest the mother help keep him actively breastfeeding longer by first helping him take the breast deeper and then using breast compression (see p. 804 in Appendix A, "Techniques") for a faster milk flow.

• •

Scales are available in some areas that can measure babies' milk intake at the breast.

Weighing the baby before and after a breastfeeding with a very accurate baby scale (to 2 g) can determine a baby's milk intake at the breast at that feeding, assuming baby's clothing remains the same at both weights (Meier et al., 1994). These scales are available in many hospitals, at many lactation offices, and in some areas they can be rented for home use at pump rental companies. However, milk intake at one feeding does not necessarily reflect a baby's daily milk intake because feeding volumes can vary by baby's appetite, how deeply he takes the breast, and other factors. But confirmed good milk intake at the breast can rule out ineffective suckling at that feeding. Good milk intake would be at least 2 ounces (59 mL) within 10 to 15 minutes of breastfeeding after the first 2 weeks of life. See the later section, "When and How to Supplement" for average feeding volumes during the first month. If a test-weighing is done, ask the mother if that feeding seemed typical to her.

• •

Diaper output is not a reliable indicator of milk intake in the breastfeeding baby.

During the first day or two of life, daily diaper output is typically one to two wet diapers and stools. After that, some health organizations suggest breastfeeding parents track daily diaper output to estimate milk intake. According to the American Academy of Pediatrics, parents should look for the following (Gartner et al., 2005):

- By Days 3 to 5—3-5 wet diapers and 3-4 stools
- By Day 5 to 7—4-6 wet diapers and 3-4 stools

According to the International Lactation Consultant Association, signs of effective breastfeeding are at least three stools per day after Day 1 and at least six wet diapers per day by Day 4 (ILCA, 2005). The Academy of Breastfeeding Medicine considers indicators of adequate mother's milk intake to be yellow stools by Day 5 and three to four stools per day by the 4th day of life (ABM, 2007).

Two U.S. studies examined whether diaper output accurately reflects adequate milk intake. Both found that there was much room for error. One study of 73 exclusively breastfeeding mother-baby couples monitored the babies' weight loss and gain, breastfeeding patterns, and diaper output for the first 14 days (Shrago, Reifsnider, & Insel, 2006). The researchers found that more stools during the first 5 days were associated with positive infant outcomes. More stools during the first 14 days were associated with the lowest weight loss and early transition to yellow stools. (Mean number of stools per day was four, but some babies had as many as eight.) The first day of yellow stools was a significant predictor of percentage of weight loss (the earlier the babies' stools turned yellow, the less weight was lost). The average number of daily stools was not an accurate predictor of initial weight loss, but the more stools passed during the entire 14-day study period, the earlier birthweight was regained.

Because some newborns breastfed ineffectively, number of daily feedings at the breast were not related to initial weight loss, start of weight gain, regaining of birthweight, or weight at Day 14. (Mean number of daily feedings at the breast was 8.5, with a range of 6 to 11.) In fact, the researchers considered unusually frequent feeding with low stool output a red flag to check baby's weight, as the study baby who breastfed the most times per day had the poorest weight outcomes. They found that frequent feedings with good stool output was a sign of effective breastfeeding, but frequent feedings without much stooling should be considered a red flag of breastfeeding ineffectiveness.

The second U.S. study followed 242 exclusively breastfeeding mother-baby couples, also for the first 14 days of life. These researchers found that "diaper output measures, when applied in the home setting, show too much overlap between infants with adequate versus inadequate breastmilk intake to serve as stand-alone indicators of breastfeeding adequacy" (Nommsen-Rivers, Heinig, Cohen, & Dewey, 2008, p. 32). The most reliable predictor of poor milk intake was fewer than four stools on Day 4, but only when paired with the mothers' perception that her milk had not yet increased. But even when both of these criteria were true, there were many false positives, meaning that many of these babies' weight was in the normal range.

Diaper output is at best a rough indicator of milk intake.

So at best, diaper output can be considered a rough indicator of milk intake. While it can be helpful to track diaper output on a daily basis between regular weight checks, diaper output alone cannot substitute for an accurate weight. Regular weight checks during the first weeks are vital to identifying breastfeeding babies at risk of low milk intake.

Also, diaper output patterns change over time. Four stools per day are average during the early weeks, but after 6 weeks of age stooling frequency often decreases, sometimes dramatically. Some breastfed babies older than 6 weeks may go as a long as a week between stools, which is not a cause for concern from a breastfeeding perspective as long as the baby is gaining weight well.

Consistently green stools may indicate an overabundant milk production (see p. 425- "Overabundant Milk Production") or that the baby is sensitive to a substance he is taking (such as a medication) or a substance passed to the baby through the milk from the mother's diet. Mucus or blood in the stools may also be a sign of sensitivity or allergy. For more details, see p. 517- "Is Baby Reacting to Something in Mother's Diet" in the chapter "Nutrition, Exercise, and Lifestyle Issues."

• •

If the baby's diaper output is low after Day 5 and his stools have not yet turned yellow, is he alert and is his skin resilient?

Normally by Day 5, most breastfed babies have at least five to six wet diapers per day and their stools have changed color from black or greenish to yellow and seedy (Shrago et al., 2006). If not, suggest the mother have the baby's healthcare provider check his weight. As described in the first section, most babies have reached their low weight by Day 5 at the latest and then begin gaining weight (Macdonald et al., 2003).

If after Day 3 or 4, the baby still has two or fewer wet diapers per day, suggest the mother be alert to the warning signs of dehydration, which indicate the baby needs more fluids immediately:

- The baby acts lethargic and may have a weak cry.
- The baby's skin becomes less resilient (after pinched, it stays pinched-looking).
- The baby looks very yellow.
- The baby's eyes and mouth seem dry.

- The baby's fontanel (soft spot) looks sunken.
- The baby has a fever.

If the mother notices any of these symptoms, suggest she contact her baby's healthcare provider without delay.

A baby's temperament and sleep patterns are not reliable indicators of milk intake.

Many mothers mistakenly assume that wakefulness, irritability, and fussiness are signs that their baby is not getting enough milk. Swedish research of 51 mothers revealed that many breastfeeding mothers go through periods when they are convinced their milk production is low, even though their babies are gaining well and their milk intake is comparable to other babies (Hillervik-Lindquist, Hofvander, & Sjolin, 1991).

Two studies, however, found that even when breastfeeding is going well, breastfed babies initially tend to be fussier than their formula-fed counterparts (di Pietro, Larson, & Porges, 1987; Lucas & St James-Roberts, 1998). As long as an irritable and wakeful baby is able to breastfeed effectively (which she will know for certain from his weight gain), assure the mother that this behavior is not necessarily a sign of low milk intake. Placid and undemanding babies who do not feed often enough are actually at higher risk of slow weight gain.

Basic Breastfeeding Dynamics

How many times each day does the baby breastfeed?

To gain weight and thrive, most newborns breastfeed at least eight times every 24 hours (Gartner et al., 2005). If the slow-gaining baby has been breastfeeding fewer than eight times each day, ask the mother if she is breastfeeding by the clock—feeding at set intervals, limiting number of feedings, or limiting feeding length. If she says yes, ask her why. Some books and parenting programs recommend strict feeding schedules (Ezzo & Bucknam, 2006). If a mother believes strongly in scheduled feedings (for either secular or religious reasons), she may not be open to breastfeeding her baby on cue because (without evidence) these authors equate frequent feedings with discipline problems later in life. When faced with a slow-gaining baby, however, even some mothers who believe strongly in feeding schedules may be willing to schedule feedings closer together and increase the number of feedings per day.

Babies should breastfeed at least 8 times per day.

Some mothers breastfeed fewer than eight times per day because the baby is sleepy or doesn't show feeding cues more often. In this case, suggest the mother start by taking an active role in initiating breastfeeding, rather than waiting for the baby to indicate a need. For example, if her baby only shows feeding cues six times a day, suggest she initiate breastfeeding at least 10 or 12 times per day.

How long does a breastfeeding usually take, does the baby take both breasts, and who usually ends the feeding, mother or baby?

Breastfeeding rhythm varies tremendously from place to place. U.S. researcher Kathleen Kennedy described how a "breastfeeding" means something very different to mothers in different cultures (Kennedy, 2010). A Western mother, for example, may consider a "breastfeeding" a lengthy, ritualized activity that may involve changing the baby's diaper, making herself a drink, turning off her phone, settling into a certain chair, and then putting her baby to breast for an extended time. A mother in a developing country, in contrast, may keep her baby on her body, putting him to breast at the slightest cue for just a few minutes 15 to 20 times each day. These two babies may get about the same amount of milk in 24 hours, but there are immense cultural differences between their breastfeeding patterns. Be aware of these cultural differences when discussing breastfeeding dynamics.

Finish the first breast first. It is helpful to know whether the mother or baby decides when the baby is finished on the first breast. One recommended strategy is called "finish the first breast first," which means the baby determines the length of the feeding and feeds on the first breast until he comes off on his own, and then the second breast is offered. If the baby still wants to breastfeed after taking the second breast, the baby can go back to the first breast again.

Some mothers have been erroneously told to limit breastfeeding to a set number of minutes per breast to avoid nipple pain or because the baby gets all the milk he needs within a short time. But U.S. research has found that limiting time at the breast does not prevent nipple pain (Carvalho, Robertson, & Klaus, 1984). (Helping the baby take the breast deeply is a better strategy.) Ending feedings after a set number of minutes per breast is counterproductive for most babies because some are fast feeders and some are slow feeders. For the same reason adults' plates are not removed from the dinner table after a set time, breastfeeding by the clock does not allow for individual differences in feeding pace.

Mothers should not limit breastfeeding sessions to a set number of minutes.

There are also additional reasons important to weight gain for letting the baby set the feeding pace. One is that the milk's fat content increases during the breastfeeding. Limiting length of feedings can decrease the fat and calories the baby receives from the milk, which can slow weight gain. Suggest the mother expect most feedings at first to take 10 to 20 minutes per breast or longer. If the baby is gaining weight well on shorter feedings, a shorter time is fine. Breast compression may be used to help keep the baby active as needed (see p. 804 in Appendix A, "Techniques" for a description of this technique).

One breast or more? Australian research on 71 healthy breastfeeding babies 1 to 6 months old found that at some feedings babies took one breast, at some feedings both breasts (called a "paired breastfeed"), and at some feedings babies took both breasts, and then fed again from the first breast (called a "clustered breastfeed") (Kent et al., 2006). To increase milk intake in a slow-gaining baby, suggest the mother encourage the baby to take both breasts at least once at each feeding, and twice if possible, following the baby's lead. On average babies take only about 70% of the milk in the breast before coming off, so there is still milk in the breast if the baby takes it again at that feeding (Kent, 2007).

• •

Does the baby go to the breast and quickly fall asleep or does the mother have nipple pain?

Nipple pain and falling asleep quickly at the breast can both be signs of a shallow latch. See Chapter 1, "Basic Breastfeeding Dynamics," and Appendix A, "Techniques," for strategies for achieving deeper breastfeeding that can increase milk intake at feedings. Helping the baby take the nipple deeper in his mouth can help make breastfeeding more effective and more comfortable.

Nipple pain may also be a sign of unusual anatomy in the baby or the mother. When a baby is tongue tied, for example, his limited tongue movements may cause painful breastfeeding and reduced milk intake (see later sections "Baby's Anatomy and Health" and "Breast/Nipple Issues").

What is the baby's sleep/wake pattern, and how long is the baby's longest sleep stretch?

If a baby sleeps so much that he does not wake to breastfeed at least eight times per day, the baby may be unusually placid, he may be overdressed and overheated, which can make him sleepy, or the mother may be using soothers that can suppress feeding cues (see the next point). Newborn jaundice can also cause sleepiness during the first few weeks of life. Suggest the mother rule out physical causes and try the following strategies:

- **Make sure baby is not too warm.** Unwrap the baby or dress in lighter clothes.
- **Breastfeed at least once during the night.** If a slow-gaining baby is sleeping longer than about 5 hours at night, suggest the mother rouse him for a feeding at least once during his longest sleep stretch.
- **"Cluster" or bunch feedings** during baby's naturally occurring alert periods, rather than waiting for a set interval to feed again.
- **Spend more time with baby tummy down on mother's semi-reclined body**, either skin-to-skin or clothed, to trigger baby's inborn feeding behaviors more often.
- **Guide baby onto the breast when he is in a light sleep.** Signs of light sleep include any movement, such as eyes moving under eyelids.

U.K. research has found that newborns—even late preterm babies—can breastfeed effectively when drowsy and in light sleep (Colson, DeRooy, & Hawdon, 2003). Encourage the mother to take advantage of that to add more daily feedings. Some babies go to the breast more easily and feed more effectively when drowsy or asleep.

Newborns move in and out of sleep often. A long sleep stretch of up to 4 to 5 hours is not a cause for concern. When discussing their breastfeeding rhythm, make sure the mother knows that breastfed babies do not usually feed at regular intervals (Benson, 2001). Rather than focusing on maintaining regular feeding intervals, suggest she focus instead on the total number of feedings every 24 hours, which is more important in terms of overall milk intake in an effectively breastfeeding baby. In a slow-gaining baby younger than 6 months, suggest a target goal of at least 10 to 12 feedings per day.

Is the mother regularly swaddling the baby for long periods or using a soother, such as a pacifier or a baby swing?

For the slow-gaining baby, suggest the mother avoid using products and techniques that mask baby's feeding cues or decrease a baby's interest in feeding.

Pacifier/dummy use decreases number of feedings per day. One U.S. prospective study found that at 2 weeks mothers using pacifiers breastfed on average eight times per day compared with nine times per day when the pacifier was not used (Howard et al., 1999). An Australian prospective cohort study of 556 mothers and babies found that mothers using pacifiers breastfed on average 6.9 times per day at 6 weeks compared with 7.4 feedings per day among those not using a pacifier (Binns & Scott, 2002). A Swedish descriptive, longitudinal, prospective study of 506 mothers and babies found that at 2, 4, 6, 8, and 10 weeks, babies taking pacifiers breastfed fewer times per day than those who did not (Aarts, Hornell, Kylberg, Hofvander, & Gebre-Medhin, 1999). Fewer feedings per day mean less daily milk intake.

Swaddled babies sleep more. U.S. research has found that swaddled babies arouse less and sleep longer (Franco et al., 2005). More time asleep can mean less breastfeeding, which can contribute to slow weight gain.

Is the baby consuming anything other than mother's milk at the breast?

Ask the mother specifically if the baby is receiving water, juice, formula, or solid foods. Also ask if her baby receives expressed milk, and if so, how it is fed. Although formula provides calories, if formula feeds replace breastfeeding, this delays or reduces the time baby spends at the breast, which can potentially decrease mother's milk production by decreasing breast stimulation. Some studies have found that using feeding bottles during the early weeks can interfere with the baby's ability to suckle effectively at the breast (Righard, 1998).

If the baby is fed low-calorie solid foods in large amounts earlier than recommended—before 6 months of age—this reduces the volume of mother's milk baby takes at the breast (Cohen, Brown, Canahuati, Rivera, & Dewey, 1994; Islam, Peerson, Ahmed, Dewey, & Brown, 2006). Feeding cereal to babies 3 to 6 months old has been associated with lower weight gain (Kramer et al., 2004).

Babies should only receive breastmilk for the first 6 months.

Water and juice are not recommended for breastfed babies younger than 6 months (Gartner et al., 2005). They make babies feel full, but do not provide the nutrients needed for healthy weight gain and growth. For the younger baby, suggest the mother gradually replace other foods or liquids with more frequent breastfeeding. If the baby is not breastfeeding effectively or the supplements are a substantial part of his intake, caution the mother to eliminate the supplements gradually, with the baby's weight carefully monitored by his healthcare provider as she increases time spent breastfeeding.

Supplements can decrease a mother's milk supply and/or slow weight gain.

If the baby is older than 6 months and receiving water or juice, suggest the mother replace these with her milk, if her milk production allows, or other, higher-calorie drinks, such as nutritious soups. For the baby older than 12 months, other milks are an option. Regular water or fruit juice supplements can reduce baby's caloric intake, causing weight gain to slow (Smith & Lifshitz, 1994).

Is the mother using a nipple shield?

If the mother is using a nipple shield, ask her why. These thin, silicone nipples have holes in the tip for milk flow at the breast. They are sometimes recommended for babies who suckle ineffectively (Genna, 2008). If this is the reason for the shield's use and her baby is gaining slowly, the shield may not be improving breastfeeding effectiveness enough and the baby may need to be supplemented. If the baby is not getting enough milk through the shield to gain weight normally, suggest the mother express her milk after breastfeeding to safeguard her milk production. Effective breastfeeding with a nipple shield also depends on fit, application, and how the baby takes the breast. For details, see p. 835 in Appendix B, "Tools and Products."

Causes of Slow Weight Gain in the First 6 Weeks

Slow weight gain may be due to a combination of factors.

Often there is more than one cause of slow weight gain. As information is gathered, it wouldn't be unusual for there to be more than one dynamic at work. See Table 6.3 for a summary of many of the causes of slow weight gain in a baby younger than 6 weeks.

Other Breastfeeding Dynamics

How did the birth and early breastfeeding go?

Excess weight loss and slow weight gain during the first 6 weeks can sometimes begin with birth and early breastfeeding. Questions to ask include:

- Was the birth difficult? Was it a vaginal or cesarean birth? Was the labor medicated or unmedicated? If medicated, what drugs were used?
- Was there more than usual blood loss? If so, how much?
- Did either mother or baby suffer any birth-related injuries or receive treatment for any health problems?
- How often did the baby breastfeed after birth and how much were they separated?
- How did early breastfeeding go?
- Was the baby supplemented in the hospital? If so, what was he fed, how much, and with what feeding method?
- Was the mother engorged or was the baby jaundiced?

When mothers and babies get off to a slow breastfeeding start due to birth-related difficulties, health problems, hospital practices, or other factors, this can lead to less effective breastfeeding in the baby and delayed milk increase in the mother, both of which can contribute to greater weight loss and lead to early slow weight gain (Dewey et al., 2003).

A difficult birth or medications during labor and delivery can reduce a baby's breastfeeding effectiveness at first (see p. 55). Early separation after birth can also affect weight gain and loss (Bystrova, Matthiesen et al., 2007). Supplements can delay or replace breastfeeding, slowing the increase in milk production. If baby or mother is in pain from birth-related injuries, this can delay or compromise feedings. Babies are sometimes born with broken bones, torticollis (see p. 116- "Baby Injured or in Pain"), or hematomas (large bruises). Engorgement in the mother and exaggerated jaundice in the newborn can also lead to less effective early breastfeeding. Excess maternal blood loss can lead to delayed or inhibited milk production (see later section, "Mother's Health and Milk Production" and the chapter, "Making Milk."). Babies can also develop feeding aversion when handled roughly at the breast or when roughly aspirated after birth.

• •

Can the baby fit more than the just nipple in his mouth during breastfeeding?

"Poor fit" is another aspect of breastfeeding dynamics that can affect early weight gain. This term describes a mother with very large nipples (wide and/or long) and a baby with a very small mouth, which is most common among small and preterm newborns. No matter how they adjust their positioning and no matter how deeply the baby takes the breast, in some cases, the baby's mouth may only accommodate the nipple, which can lead to nipple pain and/or slow milk flow. For strategies, see p. 113- "Poor Fit."

Table 6.3. Factors That Can Cause Slow Weight Gain during the First 6 Weeks

Breastfeeding Dynamics

- Shallow latch—Can decrease milk transfer and/or cause nipple pain and may be due to positioning issues or poor fit (large nipple, small mouth)
- Too little active suckling time at the breast—Scheduled, limited, or infrequent feedings, sleepy baby (overdressed?), overuse of swaddling or soothers (pacifier/dummy, swing), depression
- Less-than-optimal early breastfeeding due to birth or hospital practices—Separation, medications, rough suctioning or rough handling at breast
- Feeding low-calorie liquids or solid foods (water, juice, cereal, etc.)—Which can delay or replace breastfeeding

Baby Factors

- Temperament—Placid/sleepy baby or difficult to settle for feedings
- Anatomy or health issues that can cause ineffective suckling—Unusual oral anatomy (tongue tie, cleft palate, etc.), illness, preterm birth, birth injury (hematoma, broken bone, torticollis), respiratory problems, sensory processing problems, neurological impairment (high/low tone)
- Health issues that can cause slow weight gain with healthy milk intake—Cardiac defect, cystic fibrosis (baby tastes salty), metabolic disorders, other disorders

Mother's Anatomy, Health, and Milk Production

- Breast/Nipple Issues—Breast surgery or injury (severed milk ducts or nerve damage preventing milk ejection), inadequate glandular tissue (hypoplastic breasts), unusual nipple anatomy or nipple piercing (may decrease or prevent milk transfer)
- Birth-related Issues—Delayed breastfeeding, postpartum hemorrhage, retained placenta
- Health and Medication Issues—Serious illness, drugs/herbs that decrease milk production or are incompatible with breastfeeding, obesity (may delay milk increase), thyroid, pituitary, or hormonal problems, birth injury that makes breastfeeding painful, polycystic ovary syndrome (PCOS)

Baby's Anatomy and Health

Has the baby been ill? If so, do his symptoms include nasal congestion, vomiting, or diarrhea?

Illness, such as a cold, the flu, or other virus, can affect a baby's appetite and compromise his weight gain. Because not all sick babies run a fever or have the symptoms common in an ill older child, any baby gaining weight slowly should be checked by his healthcare provider for illness. Ear and urinary tract infections can cause slow weight gain, so routine ear check and urinalysis should be done to rule out these easily treated illnesses.

Nasal congestion in the baby can reduce milk intake because when given a choice between breathing and feeding, babies always choose breathing. Struggles with breathing during feedings may be due to a cold, another illness, allergy, inflammation of the mouth or throat from rough suctioning or intubation after birth, spasms, or physical abnormalities of the mouth or throat, such as tracheomalacia and laryngomalacia (softened cartilage that blocks the trachea or larynx) (Genna, 2008; Walker, 2006). Any baby who consistently struggles with breathing at feedings or who makes high-pitched, squeaky sounds (called "stridor") while breastfeeding, should be checked by his healthcare provider to determine the cause. While the baby is not breastfeeding well, suggest the mother use milk expression to safeguard her milk production.

Vomiting and diarrhea can also slow a baby's weight gain because the milk may not stay down long enough to be digested and nutrients are not well-absorbed when the milk rushes quickly through the baby's digestive tract during diarrhea. For more details, see p. 282- "Diarrhea and Vomiting."

Ineffective Suckling

A baby who suckles ineffectively may breastfeed "all the time," yet gain weight slowly.

If a baby is breastfeeding long and often, but is still gaining weight slowly, this may be a sign of ineffective suckling. He may have many wet diapers but few stools because he is getting some of the first rush of milk at milk ejection, but is not suckling effectively enough to trigger more milk ejections and reach the fatty hindmilk. Some types of ineffective suckling may cause nipple pain or trauma, while others do not. In the early weeks, the mother may have regular breast fullness and recurring mastitis because her baby is not draining her breasts well. For a more complete list of symptoms, see the point about ineffective breastfeeding in the previous section.

• •

Has the baby been checked by a lactation consultant or another healthcare provider for unusual mouth, tongue, and jaw anatomy?

Effective breastfeeding requires a good fit between the mother's and baby's anatomy. In some cases, unusual anatomy of the baby's mouth, tongue, or jaw can contribute to ineffective breastfeeding. Examples include cleft lip, tongue tie, large tongue, high or bubble palate, cleft palate (including submucous clefts), tight labial frenulum (the membrane that connects the lip to the gums), and receding chin (micronathia).

Unusual anatomy of the baby's mouth, tongue or jaw can contribute to ineffective breastfeeding.

If an anatomical variation in the baby is the cause of ineffective breastfeeding, this will most likely cause breastfeeding issues right from birth. One U.S. study of 88 tongue-tied babies with breastfeeding problems reported that all the problems were apparent during their hospital stay (Ballard, Auer, & Khoury, 2002). But anatomical variations, like tongue tie, do not always cause ineffective breastfeeding or other feeding problems. One U.S. study found that only 25% of its tongue-tied babies had difficulty breastfeeding (Messner, Lalakea, Aby, Macmahon, & Bair, 2000). Another factor that can affect whether the baby with an anatomical variation has trouble breastfeeding is the tautness or looseness of the mother's breast tissue. For example, a tongue-tied baby might breastfeed well when his mother's breast tissue is soft and pliable, but struggle when his mother's breast tissue is firm or taut. For more details, see p. 118- "Tongue, Palate, and Other Oral Issues."

• •

Has the baby been diagnosed with a neurological impairment or other health issue?

Babies with sensory processing issues or a neurological impairment may have high or low muscle tone, which can also reduce suckling effectiveness and cause inconsistent feedings (some effective, some ineffective). For more details and breastfeeding strategies, see p. 306 for the section "Neurological Impairment" in the chapter, "Health Issues—Baby" and p. 127 for "Sensory Processing Issues" in the chapter "Challenges at the Breast."

Was the baby born full-term?

Prematurity can affect a baby's suckling effectiveness. Depending on how early the preterm baby was born and his health, he may or may not be ready to breastfeed exclusively without supplements. For strategies to help make the transition to exclusive breastfeeding without compromising a preterm baby's weight gain, see p. 359- "Transitioning to Full Breastfeeding."

Slow Weight Gain with Good Milk Intake

Does the baby taste salty? Has he been checked for heart or metabolic problems?

By weighing a baby before and after breastfeeding with a very accurate baby scale (to 2 g), a baby's milk intake at the breast can be accurately determined (Meier et al., 1994). When the scale reveals that a slow-gaining baby is clearly taking enough milk at the breast, keep in mind there is more to weight gain than milk intake alone.

In addition to consuming enough milk, a baby must also be able to digest the milk and it must meet his energy needs. Babies with congenital heart disease, for example, usually gain weight slowly no matter how they are fed because their hearts beat faster and they take more breaths per minute than a healthy baby in order to maintain adequate oxygen levels and circulation (Clemente et al., 2001). Another example is babies with the genetic disease cystic fibrosis, many of whom also gain weight slowly, despite effective breastfeeding and excellent milk intake, because they cannot fully digest the milk. Their body produces a thick, gluey mucus that blocks their digestive enzymes from leaving the pancreas. For normal weight gain, many of these babies need to receive special enzymes before feedings to aid in digestion. The first sign of this condition is often slow weight gain and salty tasting skin. For more details, see p. 301- "Cystic Fibrosis." Other conditions may also require treatment or other interventions for normal growth, despite good milk intake. Examples include congenital hypothyroidism, kidney disease, intestinal malabsorption or obstruction, parasites, neuromuscular disease, and hypoadrenalism. A baby gaining weight slowly despite excellent milk intake should be carefully evaluated by his healthcare provider.

Mother's Anatomy, Health, and Milk Production

Breast and Nipple Issues

Does the mother have flat or inverted nipples or unusually large breasts?

Because unusual nipple or breast anatomy may make it more challenging for a newborn to take the breast and achieve deep breastfeeding, it may also affect milk transfer and weight gain. Flat or inverted nipples were associated with delayed milk increase in one U.S. study (Dewey et al., 2003). An Iranian study of first-time mothers examined the effect of "maternal breast variations" (including flat and inverted nipples and "abnormally large breasts") on weight gain during the first 7 days (Vazirinejad, Darakhshan, Esmaeili, & Hadadian, 2009). At 7 days of life, the mean weight of the babies whose mothers had one or more of these "breast variations" was below birthweight, whereas the mean weight among the babies whose mothers did not have breast variations was above birthweight.

Some types of breast surgery or injury, such as breast reduction surgery, put a mother at increased risk of inadequate milk production. A surgical incision near the areola may damage milk ducts and cause nerve damage, which may inhibit milk ejection and compromise milk transfer. For details, see p. 706- "Breast Surgery or Injury."

Does the mother have a history of breast surgery, injury, or nipple piercing?

Breast surgery or injury can increase risk of low milk production.

Although there are several case reports of mothers who successfully breastfed after a nipple piercing (Lee, 1995; Wilson-Clay & Hoover, 2008), there are also case reports of mothers whose complications from the piercing caused milk duct obstruction, which resulted in minimal milk transfer during breastfeeding and milk expression (Garbin, Deacon, Rowan, Hartmann, & Geddes, 2009). For more details, including questions to ask the mother, see p. 665- "Nipple Piercing."

Are the mother's breasts symmetrical in size and shape and did she did have breast growth during pregnancy?

In some unusual cases, a mother's breasts may be incapable of producing enough milk to fully sustain her baby because her milk-producing glands did not fully develop. Also known as "insufficient glandular tissue" or "hypoplastic breasts," according to one estimate, this occurs in about 1 in 1000 mothers (Powers, 1999). Some mothers with this condition have bulbous areolae or unusually shaped breasts because some of the normal glandular tissue is missing. One U.S. prospective study of 34 mothers found the mothers who were unable to produce enough milk had widely spaced breasts (more than 1.5 inches or about 4 cm apart), had large differences in breast size, or had tubular or cone-shaped breasts, rather than rounded breasts (Huggins, Petok, & Mireles, 2000). When the breasts are felt, there may be some obvious patches of glandular tissue in a mostly soft breast (Wilson-Clay & Hoover, 2008).

Many of the study mothers with low milk production noticed no breast changes during pregnancy or breast fullness after birth. But it is important never to assume from a mother's breast shape or lack of breast changes during or after pregnancy that she will not be able to produce enough milk. One Australian study found that breast tissue growth continues during breastfeeding throughout the first month postpartum (Cox, Kent, Casey, Owens, & Hartmann, 1999). However, these symptoms should be considered a red flag to monitor mother and baby closely after birth. For more details, see p. 703- "Underdeveloped Breasts."

Birth-Related Issues

Did the mother lose more blood than usual after birth?

Mothers who suffer severe blood loss (more than 500 cc of blood) after birth are at greater risk of insufficient milk production (Willis & Livingstone, 1995). In severe cases, extreme blood loss can cause pituitary damage, known as Sheehan syndrome, which can completely inhibit milk production and fertility (Schrager & Sabo, 2001). For details, see p. 413- "Delayed Milk Increase After Birth."

A severe loss of blood should never be assumed to reduce milk production. However, this is another red flag to monitor mother and baby closely in the early weeks. With time and sufficient breast stimulation, many of these mothers achieve ample milk production.

Could some fragments of the mother's placenta have been retained after birth?

Was the mother's placenta delivered intact after birth? Did her healthcare provider use forceps to remove the placenta? Has she had postpartum bleeding longer than 6 weeks? The hormonal cascade of events that leads to an increase in milk production after birth begins with the separation of the placenta from the uterus. If placental fragments are retained after birth, her body may continue to inhibit milk production as if she is still pregnant. In this case, removing the fragment will trigger the hormonal changes needed for greater milk production to occur.

Mother's Health and Medications

Has the mother been ill?

Although most illnesses will not affect breastfeeding or milk production, if the mother has been seriously ill, she may have been separated from her baby and breast stimulation reduced, causing a decrease in milk production. In some extreme cases, severe dehydration or life-threatening illness may cause a decrease in milk production.

Is the mother taking any herbal preparations or prescribed, over-the-counter, or recreational drugs?

Although most medications are compatible with breastfeeding, certain drugs (such as some diuretics and the over-the-counter decongestant pseudoephedrine) have been associated with a decrease in milk production (Aljazaf et al., 2003). Other drugs may inhibit milk ejection or affect the baby, sedating the baby or making him jittery. Ask the mother if she has talked to her healthcare provider about taking this drug while breastfeeding. Also ask the mother specifically if she is using hormonal contraception, as some mothers receive injectables, such as Depo-Provera soon after birth and may not remember that or connect it with breastfeeding (Halderman & Nelson, 2002). For details, see next section.

If a mother takes a drug that is contraindicated during breastfeeding, even a temporary weaning may cause a decrease in mother's milk production. For the latest information on the effects of drugs on milk production, see the current edition of *Medications and Mother's Milk* by Thomas W. Hale (Amarillo, TX: Hale Publishing).

Some herbs, such as sage and peppermint (in amounts greater than what a mother would usually consume), have been associated with decreased milk production, so ask the mother if she has been taking any herbal preparations and if so which ones. A resource on the effects of herbs on milk production is *The Nursing Mother's Herbal* by Sheila Humphrey (Humphrey, 2003).

Does the mother have a history of Type-1 diabetes or pituitary, thyroid, or hormonal problems?

Some research has found that women with Type-1 diabetes have a delay in increase of milk production after birth. For more details, see p. 759- "Type 1 (Insulin-Dependent) Diabetes Mellitus."

Regarding hormonal problems, depending on the hormone involved and whether it is too high or too low, a hormonal imbalance may cause too much milk, too little milk, or inhibit milk ejection. One U.S. article describes the postpartum breastfeeding experiences of two women with gestational ovarian theca lutein cysts who had abnormally high testosterone levels that delayed initiation of milk production (Hoover, Barbalinardo, & Platia, 2002). After producing very little milk for 3 weeks with good breast stimulation, their testosterone fell to more normal levels and their milk production finally increased.

Polycystic ovary syndrome (PCOS) is another condition that is a risk factor for inadequate milk production. Although some women with PCOS produce abundant milk, some do not. One U.S. article describes the breastfeeding experiences of three women with PCOS, all three of whom produced little milk, despite expert help and the use of many strategies to increase milk production (Marasco, Marmet, & Shell, 2000). Other hormonal and endocrine problems, such as hypo- and hyperthyroidism, have also been linked to low milk production or lactation failure. For more details, see p. 409- "Delayed Milk Increase After Birth."

• •

Is the mother in the normal weight range for her height?

Obesity has been associated with increased risk of a delay in milk increase after birth and decreased prolactin response to baby's suckling (Chapman & Perez-Escamilla, 1999; Hilson, Rasmussen, & Kjolhede, 2004; Rasmussen & Kjolhede, 2004). However, this may or may not be entirely due to the biological effects of obesity. U.S. research has found that heavier women with a body mass index (BMI) higher than 26 are less likely to put their newborns to the breast within the first 2 hours after birth (Kugyelka, Rasmussen, & Frongillo, 2004) , which has also been associated with a delay in milk increase (Bystrova, Widstrom et al., 2007). The higher the mothers' BMI, the less likely they were to breastfeed early. Until more information is available, consider obesity another red flag to closely monitor mother and baby after birth. For more details, see p. 526- "Obesity."

• •

What is the mother's emotional state?

Depression has been found to influence a mother's interactions with her baby, which could affect how many times each day a mother breastfeeds and baby's weight gain. For more details, see p. 751- "Depression and Mental Health."

Causes of Slow Weight Gain After 6 Weeks

If a baby gained weight well at first, start by discussing the basics.

If the baby's weight loss was in the normal range and baby regained his birthweight by 2 weeks, the slow weight gain must have started after that. Begin with the "Gathering Basic Information" section to understand the baby's previous weight loss and weight gain patterns, other signs of milk intake, and basic breastfeeding dynamics. In most cases, the cause(s) of the slow weight gain will be found there.

But if not, explore the other possibilities in the previous section, as well as those listed in Table 6.2. Because a baby's milk needs increase over the first 5 weeks or so of life (see the later section "When and How to Supplement"), a mother whose milk production is limited by breast surgery or underdeveloped breast tissue, for example, may make enough milk for her baby to gain weight well during the first few weeks, but weight gain may falter after that.

Other Breastfeeding Dynamics

Have the baby's breastfeeding or sleep patterns changed during the last month or so?

Most Western cultures put a high value on babies sleeping for long stretches at night. Many parenting books include strategies to increase the length of babies' nighttime sleep stretch (Ezzo & Bucknam, 2006; Ferber, 2006). If a mother has a large breast storage capacity (see p. 399- "Breast Storage Capacity"), long sleep stretches of 7 to 8 hours or more may not compromise her rate of milk production. But if a mother has an average or small breast storage capacity, these longer night stretches may slow both her milk production and her baby's weight gain.

Slow weight gain after 6 weeks can be caused by a variety of mother and baby factors including distractibility, stress, and changes in sleep patterns.

If weight gain slowed within a couple of weeks after the baby began sleeping for longer stretches at night, suggest the mother either wake the baby to breastfeed at least once during the night (which will be necessary for the mother with an average or small breast storage capacity) or breastfeed more often during the day so that the baby receives more milk.

• •

What foods or drinks is the baby consuming other than mother's milk at the breast?

See p. 217- "Basic Breastfeeding Dynamics." Low-calorie foods and drinks can replace breastfeeding and cause slow weight gain. Babies who receive only mother's milk well into the second half of their first year may slow down in weight gain. If this is the situation, suggest the mother offer solid foods (see chapter "Solid Foods").

• •

Has the mother become less available for breastfeeding or are there any unusual stresses in the household?

Changes that cause significant upheavals in family routines, such as the mother returning to work or school, a household move, marital problems, holidays, or even an especially hectic week or two, can decrease breastfeeding frequency and slow a mother's milk production.

When a mother is under stress, this may slow or inhibit her milk ejection, so the baby takes less milk at the breast. Or with more demands on a mother's time and energy, she may breastfeed less often or for a shorter time. Stress can also affect a mother's feelings about breastfeeding and her responsiveness to her baby's cues.

If the mother has been under unusual stress, encourage her to rest when she can and ask for help from her partner, friends, and relatives, or if they aren't available to consider hiring help. If that's not an option financially, suggest she check into trading time with another mother. If her milk ejection seems to be slow, suggest she try using the laid-back breastfeeding positions described in Chapter 1 to help her relax while breastfeeding.

• •

Has the baby been more distracted at feedings lately?

A baby's rate of weight gain normally slows after 3 months of age (see p. 205- Table 6.1), so it is important to gauge an exclusively breastfeeding baby's weight gain on growth charts based on data from breastfeeding babies (see earlier section "Growth Charts."). Normal developmental changes in behavior often affect breastfeeding dynamics, which may affect weight gain. Each stage of development brings new distractions:

Two to 4 months of age. With greater awareness of his surroundings, a baby may pause and come off the breast more often before finishing. Suggest the mother offer the breast several times before assuming baby is done. If needed, she can breastfeed in a quiet or darkened area where there are fewer distractions.

Four to 6 months of age. Teething can make a baby's gums sore, which can lead to fussiness during breastfeeding or chewing on his hands afterwards, which some mothers misinterpret as a sign the baby is not getting enough milk. Be sure the mother is aware these behaviors indicate teething and suggest she offer the baby something cold or hard to chew on to numb his gums before breastfeeding, such as a cold, wet washcloth or a refrigerated or frozen teething toy. At this age, many babies also become more sensitive to raised voices, which may interrupt breastfeeding.

Six to 12 months of age. Babies this age are usually easily distracted while breastfeeding. It may help to darken the room and reduce noise. Some 9- to 12-month-olds become so involved in crawling and walking they forget to breastfeed. Suggest the mother encourage nighttime breastfeeding to help offset missed feedings during the day.

• •

Is the baby using a pacifier/dummy or sucking on his fingers or thumb?

Other sucking outlets can reduce time at the breast and contribute to slow weight gain. Suggest the mother of a slow-gaining baby who is spending significant time every day sucking on a pacifier/dummy, fingers, or thumb to offer the breast instead when he wants to suck. More breastfeeding may be all that's needed to increase baby's weight gain. If an older baby prefers to suck on his thumb or fingers rather than be confined to his mother's lap, suggest she eliminate the pacifier and encourage more night feedings.

Baby's Health

Low Milk Intake

Has the baby been ill?

An illness can slow baby's weight gain by decreasing baby's appetite or the time the milk spends in the baby's gut (i.e., vomiting and diarrhea). For more details, see p. 282- "Diarrhea and Vomiting."

• •

If the baby is older than 6 months, has he had blood checks to rule out iron deficiency anemia?

This blood test is usually part of most well-baby checks after 6 months. Iron deficiency anemia can contribute to slow weight gain (Dewey et al., 2002).

• •

Does the baby seem unhappy or in pain during breastfeeding?

Transient pain during breastfeeding can be caused by pain at a recent immunization site when baby is held. But regular pain related to feeding may be caused by the following health problems, both of which can also contribute to slow weight gain, as the baby reduces milk intake to avoid pain.

Reflux disease. Irritability during feedings can be a sign of reflux disease, which is sometimes mistaken for colic. When the washing back of the baby's acidic stomach contents into the esophagus causes damage to its lining, normal gastroesophageal reflux (GER) becomes gastroesophageal reflux disease (GERD). A baby with GERD may have respiratory problems (congestion, coughing, wheezing, bronchitis, pneumonia), inflammation of the esophagus, and pain during feedings. When in pain, baby may limit milk intake, leading to slow weight gain and failure to thrive (Semeniuk & Kaczmarski, 2008). Common symptoms include frequent hiccups, sleep problems day and night, back arching and head turning, crying and irritability, and feeding aversion and refusal. For more details, see p. 287- "Reflux Disease (GERD)."

Allergy, Sensitivity, or Intolerance. When a breastfeeding baby is allergic or sensitive to a food in his mother's diet or something in the environment, symptoms can include gastrointestinal problems, such as vomiting, diarrhea, blood or mucus in stools; skin problems, such as eczema, dermatitis, hives, rash, dry skin; respiratory problems, such as congestion, runny nose, wheezing, coughing; crying during or after feedings; and difficulty going to sleep and staying asleep. Pain, vomiting, and diarrhea can lead to slow weight gain. For more details, see p. 517- "Is Baby Reacting to Something in Mother's Diet?"

Slow Weight Gain with Good Milk Intake

The baby's or mother's health can also slow weight gain.

For details, see p. 224 in this chapter. Depending on their severity, symptoms of conditions that cause slow weight gain with good milk intake, such as cardiac issues and cystic fibrosis, may first appear after 6 weeks.

Mother's Milk Production

Breast and Nipple Issues

The effects of breast surgery, injury, inadequate glandular tissue, or nipple piercing on milk production may not be obvious until after the first few weeks.

Mothers whose breast and nipple issues cause reduced milk production may produce enough milk for good weight gain during the first few weeks, but as her baby's need for milk increases and her milk production "maxes out," weight gain slows. For more details, see the chapter "Breast Issues."

Mother's Health and Medications

Has the mother had an acute or chronic illness?

Although most acute illnesses will not affect breastfeeding or milk production, if the mother has been seriously ill, she may have been separated from her baby and have reduced breast stimulation, causing a decrease in milk production. In some extreme cases, severe dehydration or life-threatening illness may decrease milk production.

Chronic illnesses, such as diabetes, thyroid problems, congestive heart failure, hormonal imbalances, and anemia, especially if untreated, can affect a mother's milk production. With untreated diseases, especially hypothyroidism, treatment may increase milk production. In one U.S. study, anemia was associated with low milk production (Henly et al., 1995). Anemia can also increase feelings of fatigue and susceptibility to infection (Fetherston, 1998). If the mother has a history of any of these health problems, suggest she see her healthcare provider for blood tests to rule out these and other health issues as contributing factors. (For details, see the chapter "Health Issues—Mother.")

• •

When asking the mother if she takes herbal preparations or any prescribed medications, be sure to ask specifically about hormonal contraceptives.

Illnesses, such as asthma, allergies, depression, hypertension, insomnia, migraine headaches, autoimmune diseases, and heart problems, may require a mother to take medications that can affect milk production (see previous section). But after 6 weeks, another medication that may affect milk production that becomes a more likely possibility is hormonal contraception.

Be sure to ask the mother specifically about hormonal contraception, as some mothers may not remember to mention it, especially if they are using a patch, injectables, or hormonal IUDs, which release hormones continuously without action by the mother. Combined oral contraceptives that contain estrogen and progesterone are not recommended before the baby is 6 months old because they have been found to decrease milk production (Koetsawang, 1987; Labbok, 2007; WHO, 2004). Research on progestin-only hormonal contraception, such as the mini-pill, implants, and injectables, have not found a significant effect on milk production or infant weight gain when given after the first 3 days (Halderman & Nelson, 2002; Hannon et al., 1997), but anecdotal reports indicate that some mothers do have a drop in milk production when progestin-only methods are used. For more details, see p. 500- "Progestin-Only Methods."

Could the mother be pregnant?

The hormones that maintain a pregnancy also cause milk production to decrease. Most mothers (60% to 65%) report a significant decrease in milk during the 4th or 5th month of pregnancy (Moscone & Moore, 1993; Newton & Theotokatos, 1979). If the baby is younger than 12 months, this naturally occurring decrease in milk production could compromise his nutritional needs. If weight gain slows, supplements may be needed.

Does the mother have a history of gastric bypass surgery or is she on a restricted diet?

Mothers on vegetarian diets with no animal products (such as vegan and macrobiotic diets) and mothers with a history of gastric bypass surgery are at greater risk for vitamin B_{12} deficiency. Because vitamin B_{12} deficient mothers produce milk low in vitamin B_{12}, their breastfeeding babies are also at risk of vitamin B_{12} deficiency, which can cause slow weight gain. Symptoms of vitamin B_{12} deficiency in the baby often develop before symptoms in the mother, appearing within the first few months of life or going unrecognized until later. One of the first symptoms is lack of interest in feeding, which can lead to slow weight gain, failure to thrive, and eventually neurological problems. Although the mother may have no symptoms, tests on her blood or milk can detect this deficiency.

Mother's B_{12} deficiency can cause slow weight gain.

To avoid vitamin deficiencies after gastric bypass surgery and in mothers who are vegan, vitamin B_{12} and other nutritional supplements are recommended. Ask any mother with this history or who is on a restricted diet if she is taking supplements. If a mother on a restricted diet does not want to consume animal products or take vitamin supplements, another option is eating fortified soy products. For more details, see p. 516 in "Nutrition, Exercise, and Lifestyle Issues."

Increasing Weight Gain

In some situations, interventions to boost weight gain should be started immediately.

One U.S. author describes when immediate action should be taken (Powers, 2001):

- A newborn younger than 2 weeks who is more than 10% below birthweight
- Any newborn who has not regained birthweight by 2 weeks of age
- A baby whose stools have not turned yellow by 7 days of age
- A baby with no urine output for 24 hours
- Any baby with clinical signs of dehydration (see p. 216 "Other Signs of Milk Intake.")

- A baby between 2 weeks and 3 months old gaining less than 20 g per day
- A baby with a lack of weight gain, significant jaundice, or unexplained weight loss at any age

Evaluating and improving breastfeeding dynamics is one possible intervention that can be tried first when the mother's milk production is good enough and the baby's suckling is effective. The baby's condition and weight would determine whether supplements might also be needed.

While a mother is working to increase her baby's weight gain, suggest she keep a written record of number of feedings and stools.

An "input/output" diary may be helpful in evaluating breastfeeding dynamics, and it doesn't have to be complicated. Over a several-day period, suggest the mother divide a blank piece of paper (a different section or sheet for each day) into two columns:

- Number of breastfeedings
- Number of stools (if the baby is younger than 6 weeks)

By marking a line in the appropriate column for every feeding at least 5 minutes long and every stool the diameter of a U.S. quarter (2.5 cm) or larger, this will provide a quick, daily count of feedings and stools. Counting wet diapers may be unnecessary because baby's stools are formed from the fatty hindmilk, which the baby receives after the watery foremilk. This means when a baby younger than 6 weeks has at least four stools of this size per day, he has also by default received enough fluids. Although stools are not a reliable stand-alone indicator of milk intake, they can be used as a general gauge between weight checks in the baby younger than 6 weeks (Nommsen-Rivers et al., 2008).

A baby younger than 6 weeks should have at least four stools per day the size of a U.S. quarter (2.5 cm).

Strategies for increasing weight gain should be based on the cause(s) of the slow weight gain.

Not all slow weight gain is due to low milk production, although low milk production can be a side effect of not breastfeeding often enough, long enough, or effectively enough.

See Tables 6.3 and 6.4 for a synopsis of the cause(s) of slow weight gain before and after 6 weeks, and tailor the interventions to the cause(s). Although in most cases strategies will include improving breastfeeding dynamics (see next point), there are many unrelated strategies that may be instrumental to increasing a baby's weight gain, such as a frenotomy (tongue clipping) in a tongue-tied baby, vitamin B_{12} or iron supplements for a deficient baby, replacement thyroid hormones for a mother with hypothyroidism, and medical treatment for a baby with reflux disease, ear infection, or other illness. In some cases, such as a very preterm baby or a newborn in pain from a birth injury, patience may also be important.

Table 6.4. Factors That Can Cause Slow Weight Gain after 6 Weeks

Breastfeeding Dynamics

- Too little active suckling time at the breast—Scheduled, limited, or infrequent feedings, longer nighttime sleep stretch or sleep training (depending on mother's breast storage capacity), overuse of swaddling or soothers (pacifier/dummy or swing)
- Feeding baby low-calorie liquids or solid foods (water, juice, cereal, etc.)—Which can delay or replace breastfeeding

Baby's Health

- Issues that can reduce baby's milk intake—Illness, allergy, reflux disease
- Issues that can cause slow weight gain with healthy milk intake—Cardiac defect, cystic fibrosis (baby tastes salty), metabolic disorder, other disorders

Mother's Anatomy, Health, Milk Production/Transfer Issues

- Health or Medication Issues—Serious illness, drugs that decrease milk production or are incompatible with breastfeeding, hormonal, thyroid, or pituitary problems, pregnancy, polycystic ovary syndrome, vitamin B_{12} deficiency from gastric bypass surgery or a restricted diet
- Breast/Nipple Issues—Nipple piercing, breast surgery, injury, or inadequate glandular tissue (hypoplastic breasts), effect on weight gain may not be obvious until baby needs full milk production to gain weight at about 5 weeks of age

Suggest the mother start by using optimal breastfeeding dynamics, increasing feedings, and taking steps to boost her milk production.

Make sure the baby is taking the breast deeply. Shallow breastfeeding can reduce the milk flow and may (but not always) cause a mother nipple pain. Try laid-back breastfeeding positions in which gravity helps pull the baby onto the breast farther. If need be, the mother can help the baby achieve deeper breastfeeding by using an asymmetric latch and breast shaping as described in Appendix A, "Techniques." See also Chapter 1.

Breastfeed more. If the baby is suckling effectively (the mother hears a swallow after every suckle or two for at least 5 minutes of active breastfeeding), suggest the mother increase the number of feedings. If the baby is younger than 6 months old, the baby's healthcare provider does not consider him at immediate risk, and the baby was breastfeeding fewer than eight times per day, suggest she spend the next several days increasing the number of feedings. To do this, suggest the mother keep her baby tummy down on her semi-reclined body as much as possible to trigger feeding behaviors and guide her baby to the breast while he's in a light sleep. By substantially increasing the number of feedings each day, the mother may find her milk production noticeably increases.

Finish the first breast first, offer both breasts, and use breast compression as needed. Offer both breasts more than once for as long as the baby will breastfeed. Leave the baby on the first breast while the baby is suckling actively. Whenever possible, wait until the baby comes off the breast on his own before offering the other breast. But if the baby does not suckle actively (just lightly mouthing the breast without swallowing) or falls asleep quickly, use breast compression to keep him active longer and increase the milk's fat content (Stutte, 1988). For a description, see Appendix A, "Techniques."

Keep all suckling at the breast and avoid the use of soothers. As mentioned on p. 219- "Basic Breastfeeding Dynamics", pacifiers/dummies reduce the number of feedings and can contribute to ineffective suckling.

When possible, give baby only mother's milk or breastfeed first. Avoid water and juice. If the baby has been fed more than 2 to 3 ounces (59 to 89 mL) of formula per day, it should not be discontinued suddenly. Instead, it should be reduced gradually as the mother's milk production increases. Suggest the mother ask the baby's healthcare provider to monitor baby's weight as supplements are being decreased. If the baby is between 6 and 12 months old, high-calorie solids should be offered after breastfeeding rather than before.

Consider other strategies to boost milk production. See p. 419- "Strategies for Making More Milk" for a description of galactogogues (milk-enhancing herbs and medications) that the mother can discuss with her healthcare provider in light of her and her baby's health and history. Expressing milk after or between feedings can also help increase milk production because drained breasts make milk faster. As many times per day as practical, encourage the mother to express her milk until 2 minutes after the last drop of milk. (For more details, see p. 475- "When Milk Production Needs a Boost.")

If a nipple shield is used, be sure it's used correctly. If the baby is not taking the breast deeply enough, he may be suckling only on the firm tip of the shield rather than the softer brim, which can mean a slower milk flow. For details on application, fit, use and weaning from the shield, see p. 835- "Nipple Shields."

Accept all offers of help. Having a slow-gaining baby is stressful. Encourage the mother to keep up her energy and boost her mood by taking good care of herself. The food she eats and the fluids she drinks are unlikely to affect her milk production, except under extreme conditions, but skipping meals and losing sleep can add to her stress and reduce her ability to cope. Accepting help from others may make this intense time easier.

When and How to Supplement

If the baby is not at risk, increasing weight gain, even if minimal, indicates the strategy is working and that supplements are not yet needed.

As the mother improves her breastfeeding dynamics (see previous section), suggest she contact her baby's healthcare provider and ask for her baby's weight to be checked regularly for a week or two to assess their progress.

With more frequent and more effective breastfeeding, the mother may notice slow improvement at first, but as long as the baby's weight gain is increasing and the baby is not at risk, it makes sense to allow more time. For example, a 6-week-old baby had been gaining 3 ounces (85 g) per week, and after his mother began breastfeeding more often and using breast compression, his weight gain increased to 4 ounces (113 g) per week. Suggest the mother continue with what's she's doing for another week. By then her baby's weight gain may reach the normal range. As long as the baby's weight is improving, patience is warranted. If her baby's healthcare provider insists on supplementing despite an improvement in weight gain, suggest the mother consider getting a second opinion. However, if despite all her efforts, her baby's weight stays the same or even decreases and it is clear low milk intake is the cause of her baby's slow gain (see next point), supplements should be given.

Before starting supplements, be sure the baby's slow weight gain is due to low milk intake.

As mentioned on p. 224- "Slow Weight Gain with Good Milk Intake", some babies gain slowly despite good milk intake due to health problems, such as a cardiac defect, genetic disease, metabolic disorder, malabsorption, intestinal blockage, parasites, or other condition that increases their energy needs or prevents them from fully metabolizing the milk. Unless the baby's condition is dire, before starting supplements, be sure these causes are ruled out by the baby's healthcare provider. If one of these conditions is the cause, supplements will not improve weight gain and will undermine breastfeeding.

Rule out baby's health problems as the cause of slow weight gain before starting supplements.

A baby's milk intake at the breast can be measured with an accurate electronic scale.

In some parts of the world, baby scales accurate to 2 g are available in hospitals, lactation offices, and for home rental and can be used to measure milk intake at the breast by weighing babies before and after breastfeeding (Meier et al., 1994). These can sometimes be useful in determining the cause of the slow weight gain and in monitoring the baby's weight. For more details, see p. 842- "Scales for Test-Weighing."

If supplements are needed and the mother finds this upsetting, discuss her feelings and be sure she knows they may help the baby breastfeed more effectively.

Supplements are sometimes necessary, especially when a baby is stressed by hunger. But this can generate strong feelings in some mothers. If the mother's feelings of competence were shaken by her baby's slow weight gain, she may see the need to supplement as proof positive of her inadequacy as a mother. In this case, acknowledge her feelings and assure her that supplementation can be a way to help get breastfeeding back on track, rather than a sign of failure. When a baby's weight gain is well below borderline, being stressed by hunger can cause extreme sleepiness, ineffective or difficult feedings, and even breast refusal. Assure the mother that babies feed better when they are well-nourished. If it is clear the mother's milk production will not increase enough to fully meet her baby's needs, see the points on p. 413- "Strategies for Making More Milk" and p. 424- "Strategies for Supplementing That Enhance Milk-Making."

Discuss the mother's choice of feeding methods for the supplement.

For the baby older than 6 or 8 months of age, a cup is the logical first choice for giving extra milk, as the baby will be old enough to drink from it and it will not satisfy his need to suckle, so it is less likely than a bottle to decrease his desire to take the breast.

However, if a younger baby needs to be supplemented, discuss with the mother her choices (at-breast supplementer, cup, feeding syringe, eyedropper, bottle), describing their advantages and disadvantages. (For details, see p. 811 "Alternative Feeding Methods" in Appendix B "Tools and Products".) If the mother is open to using it, an at-breast supplementer can decrease her time spent feeding (she won't have to feed again after breastfeeding), and in some cases, it may help improve her baby's effectiveness by giving positive reinforcement at the breast.

The first choice of a supplement is almost always expressed mother's milk.

If low milk intake has been confirmed, the first priority is to feed the baby. According to the World Health Organization, in order of healthiest to least healthy, the best feeding choices for the baby younger than 6 months are:

- Breastfeeding
- Expressed mother's milk
- Donor human milk
- Non-human milks, such as infant formula

With a confirmed low milk supply, the first priority is to feed the baby.

Exceptions include babies with the metabolic disorders galactosemia and PKU, who require special formulas due to their inability to metabolize mother's milk (for details, see these sections in the chapter, "Health Issues—Baby"). For the baby older than 6 months, high-calorie solid foods are also an option. Suggest the mother consult her baby's healthcare provider about a choice of supplement.

If the mother's milk production allows, suggest she provide her expressed milk as her baby's supplement. If the problem is her baby's effectiveness at the breast and she is making more than enough milk, she may also want to consider providing her high-fat, high-calorie hindmilk as a supplement. She can do this by expressing milk right after the baby breastfeeds. When she expresses milk at other times, another way is to set aside the milk she expresses during the first few minutes (storing it for later use) and use the milk she expresses afterward (called "hindmilk feeding") as the supplement. For details on choosing an expression method, see p. 453- "Choosing a Method." If needed, offer to discuss how she might fit milk expression into her daily routine.

If by choice or necessity the mother supplements with formula, make sure she knows to follow her baby's healthcare provider's recommendations and not to either dilute it or make it too strong, which could be harmful to the baby.

The volume of milk a baby needs per day to gain weight will vary by age and by baby.

During the first 5 weeks of life, as newborns grow larger and heavier, they gradually need more and more milk per day to grow and thrive (Neville et al., 1988). Table 6.5 shows average milk intake per feeding and per day for the first 6 months of life. For a starting point on the amount of supplememnt needed, see Table B.2 on p. 818. But not all babies are average, and milk intake can vary greatly from one baby to another. An Australian study of 71 healthy, thriving, exclusively breastfed 1- to 6-month-old babies found their daily milk intakes varied by baby almost threefold, from 15.5 to 43 ounces (440 to 1220 g) per day (Kent et al., 2006).

Table 6.5. Milk Intake by Age

Baby's Age	Average Milk Volume Per Feeding	Average Milk Intake Per Day
First week (after Day 4)	1-2 oz. (30-59 mL)	10-20 oz. (300-600 mL)
Weeks 2 and 3	2-3 oz. (59-89 mL)	15-25 oz. (450-750 mL)
Months 1-6	3-5 oz. (89-148 mL)	25-35 oz. (750-1035 mL)

(Mohrbacher & Kendall-Tackett, 2005, pp. 99-100)

What this means in practical terms is that the amount of milk needed for a baby to begin gaining weight will vary. However, it is not necessary to know a baby's exact milk-intake needs, because if a baby's weight gain or loss is low enough to be of concern, he should be given as much extra milk as he will take whenever a supplement is given (see next point). With supplementing (as with breastfeeding), it is best to let the baby set the pace.

Usually, babies who have been seriously underfed will start by taking small amounts of supplement. But within a day or two as their stomachs expand, they will begin taking more and more milk and their weight gain will increase markedly. If after receiving regular supplements the baby is still not gaining weight, suggest the mother have the baby checked again by his healthcare provider for health problems.

If a baby's weight gain is close to borderline, knowing average milk intakes can be helpful, especially if an accurate baby scale can be used to determine the baby's actual daily milk intake. For example, knowing that a 6-week-old takes on average 25 to 35 ounces (750-1035 mL) per day and feeds eight times per day, this means an average feeding is 3 to 4 ounces (89-118 mL). So if a baby is only taking 2 ounces (59 mL) at each of his eight feedings, this gives a general idea of how much extra milk he will eventually need per day (9 to 19 ounces or 266-562 mL) to gain weight consistently. Some babies will need less and others will need more. After beginning supplementation, suggest the mother have the baby's weight checked at least weekly to be sure his weight gain is in the normal range. If not, increase the supplement.

• •

Depending on the baby's breastfeeding effectiveness and the mother's milk production, the baby may not need a supplement after every breastfeeding.

Supplementation should be tailored to each situation. But the following general principles may be helpful when determining a plan.

Supplement only during waking hours. To make this process easier for the mother, supplements are usually restricted to her normal waking hours. During her sleeping hours, suggest she breastfeed exclusively. If the baby needs a lot of supplements, they may be given after (or during, if an at-breast supplementer is used) every waking breastfeeding.

More or less often. If a baby's weight gain is close to borderline, the baby may not need to be supplemented after every waking breastfeeding. Every other feeding or even less often may be enough. One approach is to offer supplements two to five times per day, so the baby does not come to expect a supplement after every feeding. This might work well if a baby is feeding effectively and the mother's milk production is not too low. How many times per day the supplement should be given depends on how much the baby is gaining, with less supplement given for a borderline weight gain and more supplement given if a baby is at risk or if the weight gain is very low. Any plan should be started with the idea that it may need to be adjusted to better meet mother and baby's needs.

Smaller rather than larger volumes. In general, it is better for breastfeeding dynamics for the baby to be given smaller volumes of the supplement more often, rather than a large volume (4 ounces or more [118 mL]) once or twice a day. For this reason when formula is needed, some clinicians recommend smaller amounts of high-calorie formula as a supplement (C. Wagner, personal communication, February 15, 2010). A baby who receives too much supplement at once may skip one or more breastfeedings, which can decrease a mother's breast stimulation.

Supplementation plans should be tailored to each individual baby.

Time of day. The best overall strategy will depend on the circumstances. For example, if the baby feeds effectively and the mother's milk production is low, depending on how much milk she produces daily, she may be able to provide full feedings early in the day and give supplements only in the afternoon and evening, to coincide with her milk production's natural ebb and flow.

Effect of feeding method. Whether the supplement is given during or after the breastfeeding will affect the strategy. For example, if an at-breast supplementer is used, the tubing may be clamped shut to prevent milk flow early in the feeding while the baby is suckling actively and taking milk well directly from the breast. As the baby swallows less often or begins to doze, the tubing could then be opened to allow the supplement to flow, stimulating longer breastfeeding and more milk production. If the baby is not supplemented at the breast and is suckling effectively, breastfeeding first and giving the supplement afterward will usually be a good strategy. However, in some cases, a baby may breastfeed better if he's had some milk first and feels stronger. Encourage the mother to experiment to see what works best for her and her baby.

• •

When it is time to wean from the supplement, suggest the mother do it gradually as her milk production and/or baby's effectiveness improves.

When the breastfeeding dynamics are improving and it is time to begin reducing the supplements, the first step is to make arrangements to carefully monitor the baby's weight during this process. The mother can either rent a very accurate baby scale (to 2 g) for home use and do regular weight checks at home or arrange to have the baby's weight monitored regularly by his healthcare provider. Then suggest the mother:

- **Decrease the supplement gradually.** Set reasonable goals for decreasing the supplement and increasing breastfeeding. Unless the baby is obviously ready to discontinue the supplement faster, suggest the mother decrease the supplement by about 2 ounces (59 mL) every other day while increasing time at the breast.
- **Begin by eliminating supplements at the first morning breastfeeding.** Many babies breastfeed best at this time, probably due to faster milk flow.

- **Make sure the baby is continuing to gain weight well.** During this process, monitor the baby's weight gain at least once or twice per week using the same scale. If the baby's weight gain drops to below 5 to 6 ounces (142-177 g) per week, reintroduce that supplement. The baby needs adequate milk to suckle effectively.
- **Expect it may take time before baby is exclusively breastfeeding.** Reassurance and support will make it easier for the mother to be patient.

In some cases, a mother may not be able to produce enough milk to exclusively breastfeed.

Sometimes even dedicated breastfeeding mothers are unable to produce enough milk for their babies. The chapter "Making Milk" describes physical issues that can compromise a mother's milk production, such as breast surgery, postpartum hemorrhage, hormonal disorders, inadequate glandular tissue, and others. Sometimes the reason is never found.

If after the cause for the slow weight gain is determined and it becomes clear that exclusive breastfeeding is not an option for this mother and baby, it may help her come to terms with her disappointment if someone helps her understand what happened, sort through her feelings, and acknowledge her disappointment (Williams, 2002). See also p. 424.

Feeling like a breastfeeding failure can be a huge blow to a mother's self-esteem and providing emotional support is vital. Applaud the mother's efforts and assure her that even though her baby needs supplements she is still a good mother. Also ask her how her partner, her family, and others in her social network feel about breastfeeding and supplementation, as their opinions will affect the mother. Let her know that it is possible to supplement her baby at the breast so that they can continue to share that closeness. If she prefers a bottle, she can continue to comfort her baby at the breast, even if she is producing little milk. Also during bottle-feedings, she can still look into her baby's eyes and give skin-to-skin contact so that feedings remain a time of closeness with her baby.

RAPID WEIGHT GAIN

If an exclusively breastfeeding mother is concerned that her baby is overweight, ask about his weight and discuss obesity-prevention strategies.

Weight can be a very emotional subject for mothers, especially for those who are overweight or obese. If the mother of a rapidly gaining breastfeeding baby is concerned about future obesity, begin by asking for some basic information, such as the baby's age and whether he is exclusively breastfeeding. If not, ask what other foods he consumes and how much per day. Also ask for his current weight, his birthweight, and his weight at each of his weight checks.

In a breastfeeding baby, rapid weight gain is normal during the first few months, however, during months 6 to 12, breastfed babies lose more body fat than formula-fed babies, so tell the mother to expect her baby will slim down then (Dewey, Heinig, Nommsen, Peerson, & Lonnerdal, 1993).

Whether a mother's milk-fat content is high or low, doesn't matter, as the baby adjusts his milk intake accordingly. Babies whose mothers make higher-fat milk take less milk per day and those whose mothers make lower-fat milk take more milk per day (Dewey, 2003; Nommsen, Lovelady, Heinig, Lonnerdal, & Dewey, 1991; Perez-Escamilla et al., 1995).

Be sure the mother knows that a baby in the 95th percentile on the growth charts is not necessarily overweight. Most of these babies are also longer than average, and it is the weight-for-length ratio that determines overweight (Hopkinson, 2003). Weight-for-length growth charts are on p. 863 and available free online from the World Health Organization at: http://www.who.int/childgrowth/standards/en/.

During the first year of life, a baby's healthcare provider will typically notice and comment when a baby is seriously overweight. Overweight babies often find it difficult to roll over and crawl. Ask the mother what the healthcare provider has said about the baby's weight and how her baby is doing with these developmental milestones to determine if her baby is indeed overweight or if her concerns are a reflection of her own body image issues.

Although breastfeeding has been found to reduce the risk of overweight and obesity (see next point), one of the strongest predictors of overweight and obesity in children is having overweight or obese parents (Butte, 2009; Hawkins, Cole, & Law, 2009; Panagiotakos et al., 2008). If the mother is overweight or obese, suggest she be proactive about helping her child develop healthy eating habits and exercise regularly. If the mother is very concerned about her baby's weight, suggest she consider seeing a dietitian or nutritionist to discuss strategies to minimize her baby's chances of become an overweight child or adult.

Attempting to slow a baby's weight gain by limiting time at the breast is not a good strategy because the young child is growing rapidly and needs the nutrients in mother's milk for normal development.

• •

Breastfeeding is associated with a 20% to 30% reduced risk of childhood obesity.

Many studies and meta-analyses have found early breastfeeding reduces the risk of obesity in childhood, adolescence, and adulthood, even within families (Arenz, Ruckerl, Koletzko, & von Kries, 2004; Gillman et al., 2006; Grummer-Strawn & Mei, 2004; Ip et al., 2007; Ip et al., 2009). This association is most obvious in research that measures the effect of breastfeeding duration and exclusivity and when the children are followed for at least 6 to 15 years (Dewey, 2009b).

Although other factors, such as parental overweight, have a greater effect on a baby's risk for overweight and obesity (see previous point), the effect of breastfeeding is significant.

Be sure the mother knows that greater intensity and duration of breastfeeding have been associated with decreased risk of overweight. This was the finding of two U.S. studies that compared weight gain in babies fed by breast and bottle, along with the effects of mothers' attempts to coax their babies to finish the bottle and regular emptying of the bottle by the baby. One found that for every 3 months the babies breastfed, their body mass index (BMI) score decreased by 0.045 (Taveras et al., 2006). Mothers who regularly coaxed their babies to finish the bottle increased their babies' odds of becoming overweight by 13%. But this study found that future risk of overweight was only partly explained by feeding mechanics. The other study concluded that when less than 80% of babies' daily milk intake was mother's milk, babies were twice as likely to become overweight between 6 and 12 months as those who received more than 80% mother's milk each day (Li et al., 2008). In this second study, babies who often emptied their bottles were 69% more likely than those who rarely emptied their bottles to be overweight between 6 to 12 months.

Several studies have found rapid weight gain during the first 4 months of life to be a significant risk factor for later overweight or obesity (Baird et al., 2005; Dennison, Edmunds, Stratton, & Pruzek, 2006; Ong & Loos, 2006; Stettler, Zemel, Kumanyika, & Stallings, 2002). Unfortunately, these studies did not examine the effects of infant feeding (breast or bottle) on later weight, so it is not known whether later overweight and obesity were more common among formula-fed babies (Dewey, 2009b). For reasons formula-feeding contributes to greater weight gain, see p. 206- "Growth from Birth to 12 Months."

• •

If the baby is eating solid foods, discuss feeding strategies and food choices that may affect weight gain.

Solid foods and weight gain before 6 months. Both babies and mothers have better health outcomes when solid foods are delayed until 6 months (see p. 155- "Not Too Early"). But rapid weight gain is a common reason for early introduction of solids among U.K. mothers, who consider this an indication their baby "needs" other foods (Savage, Reilly, Edwards, & Durnin, 1998; Wright, Parkinson, & Drewett, 2004).

Mothers' concerns that their babies are not getting enough to eat may cause them to override their babies' satiety cues.

In cultures that believe overweight babies are "healthier," parents may consider introducing solid foods early necessary, so their babies "get enough." If this belief causes mothers to consistently override their babies' signs of fullness and give more food, this can set up unhealthy feeding habits that increase the risk of childhood obesity later.

Ask the mother what solids she's been feeding her baby and how often. Also ask her why she decided to start solids early. Although feeding cereal to babies 3 to 6 months old has been associated with lower weights (Kramer et al., 2004), giving large amounts of high-calorie solids may contribute to rapid weight gain. If solids have been a substantial part of the baby's diet and the mother wants to reduce or eliminate them, encourage her to reduce them gradually and breastfeed more often to boost her milk production and fill the gap.

Solid foods and weight gain after 6 months. Food choices can affect a baby's weight gain. If the baby is gaining weight very rapidly, suggest the mother avoid high-calorie solids (like egg yolks and avocados and "empty calories", such as sweetened foods and drinks) and offer a greater variety of fresh fruits and vegetables. Suggest the mother also breastfeed first, before giving solids. Encourage her to think of her milk as her baby's primary food during his first year and solids as a supplement to breastfeeding. Greater intensity and duration of breastfeeding have been associated with lower weight gain between 3 and 12 months (Li et al., 2008; Taveras et al., 2006).

VACCINES AND VITAMIN/MINERAL SUPPLEMENTS

Vaccines

The same immunization schedule is used for all babies, breastfed or not. Vaccines seem to enhance a baby's immune response to immunization.

Although not all mothers choose to have their babies immunized, vaccines are recommended on the same timetable in both breastfed and formula-fed babies (AAP, 2009). Breastfeeding does not need to be delayed before, during, or after immunization.

Research in Sweden, Canada, and elsewhere has found that some immunizations produce a more active immune response and, therefore, offer more protection from disease in breastfed babies as compared with formula-fed babies (Pabst & Spady, 1990; Pabst et al., 1997; Silfverdal, Ekholm, & Bodin, 2007).

Some components of mother's milk appear to increase the effectiveness of vaccines in some babies. One U.S. 12-month, controlled, randomized, and blinded multisite feeding trial divided its 311 babies into two groups fed different infant formulas and one group who breastfed (Pickering et al., 1998). The breastfed babies had significantly greater antibody response to the polio vaccine than the formula-fed babies.

Breastfeeding has been found to provide effective pain relief during immunizations.

One of the most difficult aspects of immunizations for many mothers is seeing their baby in pain. Breastfeeding during immunizations is an effective way to soothe babies and reduce pain. A Canadian review of 23 studies concluded that breastfeeding was associated with reduced pain during immunizations and recommended it be suggested in clinical practice (Shah, Taddio, & Rieder, 2009). Other studies published since this review have confirmed this effect (Dilli, Kucuk, & Dallar, 2009).

Vitamin Supplements

Daily vitamin D supplements are now recommended for all exclusively breastfed babies.

Vitamin D is not actually a vitamin; it's a hormone made by the body when the skin is exposed to the ultraviolet rays of the sun. Only about 10% of our vitamin D intake comes from the food we eat (Wagner, Taylor, & Hollis, 2008). When early humans spent their daylight hours working outdoors with their skin exposed, this guaranteed healthy vitamin D blood levels. With the lifestyle changes that occurred as people moved to northern climates and wore more clothing, by the 17th century, vitamin D deficiency and rickets had become a major health problem. In the 1800s, scientists discovered that lack of sunlight exposure was the cause of rickets and began to recommend fish-liver oils to prevent and treat it. In the 1920s, vitamin D was formally identified, and in the 1930s, milk fortified with vitamin D began to be sold. For a time, rickets was virtually eliminated. However, over the past decades as people began spending more time indoors and using sunscreen when outside, the incidence of rickets increased. Also, among some cultures, religious beliefs require women to cover themselves completely when away from home. As a result, researchers have turned their focus to vitamin D intake recommendations, incidence of vitamin D deficiency, and the effects of vitamin D levels on overall health.

Scientists question current recommended daily allowances of vitamin D. When analyzing current recommendations for vitamin D intake, scientists thought it curious that the same daily allowance (400 IU) was recommended for a tiny preterm baby, an older child, and an adult (Hollis & Wagner, 2004a). As they investigated further, they found the less-than-scientific basis for this recommendation. The amount of vitamin D recommended—400 IU—equals the amount in the traditional cod-liver-oil treatment for rickets. Yet U.K. research found that 400 IU per day was not enough to increase vitamin D levels in pregnant mothers (Cockburn et al., 1980), and that at 400 IU per day blood vitamin D levels often decreased during the winter months (Vieth, Cole, Hawker, Trang, & Rubin, 2001). Research done worldwide has found vitamin D deficiency to be widespread among pregnant women:

- 8% of light-skinned women and 59%-84% of dark-skinned women in the Netherlands (van der Meer et al., 2006)
- 18% in the U.K. (Javaid et al., 2006)
- 42% in northern India (Sachan et al., 2005)
- 61% in New Zealand (Judkins & Eagleton, 2006)
- 80% in Iran (Bassir et al., 2001)

The current recommendation of 400 IU of vitamin D per day is not sufficient to increase vitamin D levels in pregnant women.

When babies are born to vitamin-D deficient mothers, they are at increased risk of vitamin D deficiency, which has been associated with a greater incidence of health issues, such as cardiovascular problems, Type 1 and 2 diabetes, many types of cancer, and autoimmune diseases, such as lupus and multiple sclerosis (Wagner et al., 2008).

When a mother breastfeeds, her blood vitamin D level determines the level of vitamin D in her milk. In recent years, the number of reported cases of rickets and vitamin D deficiency among exclusively breastfed babies worldwide has increased (Beck-Nielsen, Jensen, Gram, Brixen, & Brock-Jacobsen, 2009; Bener, Al-Ali, & Hoffmann, 2009; Girish & Subramaniam, 2008; Lazol, Cakan, & Kamat, 2008; Ward, Gaboury, Ladhani, & Zlotkin, 2007; Weisberg, Scanlon, Li, & Cogswell, 2004; Wondale, Shiferaw, & Lulseged, 2005). As more mothers become vitamin D deficient, so do their breastfed babies.

Risk factors for vitamin D deficiency. Women and babies with dark skin are at greater risk of vitamin D deficiency because darker skin pigmentation acts as a natural filter of ultraviolet light, so they require more sunlight exposure for the body to make vitamin D. Other risk factors for vitamin D deficiency include spending little time outdoors, keeping the skin covered with clothing or sunscreen while outside, and living in areas with heavy air pollution or little sunlight for parts of the year. In temperate climates with cold winters that keep people indoors more, vitamin D levels among people with lighter skin are higher during the summer and lower during the winter (Ziegler, Hollis, Nelson, & Jeter, 2006). The recommendation for mothers and babies to avoid exposure to sunlight to prevent sun damage and skin cancer also contributes to greater risk of vitamin D deficiency (AAP, 1999).

As a result of widespread vitamin D deficiencies among mothers and increasing reports of rickets among exclusively breastfeeding babies, in 2008 the American Academy of Pediatrics recommended all exclusively breastfed babies be supplemented with 400 IU of vitamin D (1 drop) each day, starting within the first 2 months of life and continuing through adolescence (Wagner & Greer, 2008). Some companies make a liquid vitamin supplement with only vitamin D. Because infant formula already contains extra vitamin D, giving a vitamin D supplement is not recommended for any baby receiving more than 500 mL (17 ounces) of formula per day.

Some exclusively breastfeeding mothers may worry about giving their baby vitamin D due to concerns about altering their baby's gut flora or triggering allergies. One preliminary Swedish study of 206 babies found an association with vitamin D intake during the first year of life and increased risk of allergy independent of family history (Back, Blomquist, Hernell, & Stenberg, 2009). A U.S. study found that early vitamin use was associated with a higher risk of allergy among exclusively formula-fed African-American babies (Milner, Stein, McCarter, & Moon, 2004).

• •

An alternative to supplementing the breastfeeding baby with vitamin D is supplementing the mother.

When only the baby is supplemented with vitamin D, there is still the mother's vitamin D status to consider. Vitamin D deficiency in mothers has been associated with depression (Murphy & Wagner, 2008), as well as the same health problems associated with vitamin D deficiency in the baby mentioned in the previous point.

Several U.S. studies have examined how much extra vitamin D would be needed each day to raise a mother's blood levels into the normal range and increase the levels in her milk to fully meet her breastfed baby's vitamin D needs. If a mother takes only her daily prenatal vitamin (which contain 400 IU), her vitamin D levels may actually decrease over time (Hollis & Wagner, 2004a). Finnish research found that neither 1,000 IU nor 2,000 IU per day were enough to bring either the mother's or baby's vitamin D levels into the range of those who live in sun-rich environments (Ala-Houhala, 1985; Ala-Houhala, Koskinen, Terho, Koivula, & Visakorpi, 1986). Two U.S. pilot studies examined the effects of 4,000 and 6,400 IU per day and found that taking 6,400 IU per day for 90 days was enough to bring both a mother's blood and milk vitamin D up to recommended levels (Hollis & Wagner, 2004b; Wagner, Hulsey, Fanning, Ebeling, & Hollis, 2006). Taking 6,400 IU each day would increase a mother's milk vitamin D levels enough to eliminate the need to supplement her breastfeeding baby.

At this writing, larger studies are being conducted with diverse populations to confirm that these larger doses of vitamin D are safe and effective. Although previous research has found that even vitamin D intake as high as 10,000 IU per day does not produce blood levels higher than the levels found in people working outside in sunny climates (Heaney, Davies, Chen, Holick, & Barger-Lux, 2003; Vieth, 1999; Vieth, Chan, & MacFarlane, 2001). Until the results of these larger studies are in, the recommendation stands to supplement the breastfeeding baby directly with 400 IU of vitamin D per day (Wagner & Greer, 2008).

As mentioned previously, mothers at risk of a vitamin B_{12} deficiency include those on a restricted diet without animal protein (such as a vegan or macrobiotic diet) and those with a history of gastric bypass or other bariatric surgery. Other women at risk are those with Crohn's disease and other malabsorption disorders. Because vitamin B_{12} deficient mothers produce milk low in vitamin B_{12}, their breastfeeding babies are also at risk of vitamin B_{12} deficiency. Symptoms of vitamin B_{12} deficiency in the baby often develop before symptoms in the mother, appearing within the first few months of life or going unrecognized until later. These symptoms include lack of interest in feeding, slow weight gain, failure to thrive, and eventually neurological problems. Although the mother may have no symptoms, a blood test can detect this deficiency. In this case, both mother and baby may need to receive vitamin B_{12} supplements. For more details, see p. 523- "The Vegetarian Mother."

Vitamin B_{12} supplements are recommended for breastfeeding babies whose mothers are vitamin B_{12} deficient.

Mineral Supplements

Iron Supplements

Healthy iron levels are important for normal development, but routine iron supplements can be detrimental in babies with normal iron levels.

Babies born full term to well-nourished mothers usually have enough iron stores to last through their first 6 to 9 months of life (Dewey, 2007; Raj, Faridi, Rusia, & Singh, 2008). The iron in human milk is much better absorbed than iron from other sources, (50% compared to 4% from formula) (Griffin & Abrams, 2001; Lawrence & Lawrence, 2005). But because the amount of iron in human milk is low, breastfed babies need iron from solid foods starting after 6 months of age.

When a baby's blood iron levels are too low, this puts him at risk for iron deficiency and anemia, which are associated with developmental delays and neurological problems (Lozoff & Georgieff, 2006). If iron levels stay too low for too long, these problems may be irreversible.

If there is concern about a baby's iron levels, a simple blood test to measure the baby's iron status can usually be done in a healthcare office or clinic. According to U.S. research, healthy hemoglobin levels in breastfed babies are ≥10.5 g/dL at 4 and 6 months and ≥10.0 g/dL at 9 months (Domellof, Dewey, Lonnerdal, Cohen, & Hernell, 2002).

Routine iron supplements for babies are not recommended unless a baby has been found to be iron deficient because too-high iron levels have also been found to be detrimental. High iron levels have been linked to slower growth, neurodevelopmental delays, lower IQ, decreased growth in length and head circumference, and an increased incidence of some diseases (Barry & Reeve, 1977; Dewey et al., 2002; Kerr, 2008). For more details, please see p. 160- "Iron."

Babies born preterm or at low birthweight to iron-deficient mothers may need extra iron before 6 months.

When a baby is born with low iron stores, such as some preterm, low-birth-weight babies, and babies born to iron-deficient mothers, their iron stores may run low before 6 months. The American Academy of Pediatrics recommends that any breastfeeding baby needing iron supplements receive them while continuing full breastfeeding (Gartner et al., 2005).

Fluoride

Fluoride supplements are not recommended for the breastfeeding baby younger than 6 months.

Fluoride supplementation in babies younger than 6 months has been associated with a permanent discoloration of the teeth called fluorosis. As a result, both the American Academy of Pediatrics and the U.S. Centers for Disease Control and Prevention recommend against fluoride supplements before 6 months (CDC, 2001; Gartner et al., 2005). Fluoride supplements are only recommended in babies older than 6 months when local drinking water contains less than 0.3 ppm of fluoride.

RESOURCES FOR PARENTS

Websites

http://www.who.int/childgrowth/standards/en/ World Health Organization growth charts based on breastfeeding norms.

REFERENCES

AAP. (1999). Ultraviolet light: a hazard to children. American Academy of Pediatrics. Committee on Environmental Health. *Pediatrics, 104*(2 Pt 1), 328-333.

AAP. (2009). Active immunization. In L. K. Pickering, C. J. Baker, D. W. Kimberlin & S. S. Long (Eds.), *Red Book: 2009 report of the Committee on Infecious Diseases* (28th ed.). Elk Grove Village, IL: American Academy of Pediatrics.

Aarts, C., Hornell, A., Kylberg, E., Hofvander, Y., & Gebre-Medhin, M. (1999). Breastfeeding patterns in relation to thumb sucking and pacifier use. *Pediatrics, 104*(4), e50.

ABM. (2007). ABM Clinical Protocol #2 (2007 revision): Guidelines for hospital discharge of the breastfeeding term newborn and mother: "the going home protocol". *Breastfeeding Medicine, 2*(3), 158-165.

ABM. (2009). ABM clinical protocol #3: Hospital guidelines for the use of supplementary feedings in the healthy term breastfed neonate, revised 2009. *Breastfeeding Medicine, 4*(3), 175-182.

Ala-Houhala, M. (1985). 25-Hydroxyvitamin D levels during breast-feeding with or without maternal or infantile supplementation of vitamin D. *Journal of Pediatric Gastroenterology and Nutrition, 4*(2), 220-226.

Ala-Houhala, M., Koskinen, T., Terho, A., Koivula, T., & Visakorpi, J. (1986). Maternal compared with infant vitamin D supplementation. *Archives of Disease in Childhood, 61*(12), 1159-1163.

Aljazaf, K., Hale, T. W., Ilett, K. F., Hartmann, P. E., Mitoulas, L. R., Kristensen, J. H., et al. (2003). Pseudoephedrine: effects on milk production in women and estimation of infant exposure via breastmilk. *British Journal of Clinical Pharmacology, 56*(1), 18-24.

Arenz, S., Ruckerl, R., Koletzko, B., & von Kries, R. (2004). Breast-feeding and childhood obesity--a systematic review. *International Journal of Obesity and Related Metabolic Disorders, 28*(10), 1247-1256.

Back, O., Blomquist, H. K., Hernell, O., & Stenberg, B. (2009). Does vitamin D intake during infancy promote the development of atopic allergy? *Acta Dermato-Venereologica, 89*(1), 28-32.

Baird, J., Fisher, D., Lucas, P., Kleijnen, J., Roberts, H., & Law, C. (2005). Being big or growing fast: systematic review of size and growth in infancy and later obesity. *British Medical Journal, 331*(7522), 929.

Ballard, J. L., Auer, C. E., & Khoury, J. C. (2002). Ankyloglossia: assessment, incidence, and effect of frenuloplasty on the breastfeeding dyad. *Pediatrics, 110*(5), e63.

Barry, D. M., & Reeve, A. W. (1977). Increased incidence of gram-negative neonatal sepsis with intramuscula iron administration. *Pediatrics, 60*(6), 908-912.

Bassir, M., Laborie, S., Lapillonne, A., Claris, O., Chappuis, M. C., & Salle, B. L. (2001). Vitamin D deficiency in Iranian mothers and their neonates: a pilot study. *Acta Paediatrica, 90*(5), 577-579.

Beck-Nielsen, S. S., Jensen, T. K., Gram, J., Brixen, K., & Brock-Jacobsen, B. (2009). Nutritional rickets in Denmark: a retrospective review of children's medical records from 1985 to 2005. *European Journal of Pediatrics, 168*(8), 941-949.

Bener, A., Al-Ali, M., & Hoffmann, G. F. (2009). High prevalence of vitamin D deficiency in young children in a highly sunny humid country: a global health problem. *Minerva Pediatrica, 61*(1), 15-22.

Benson, S. (2001). What is normal? A study of normal breastfeeding dyads during the first sixty hours of life. *Breastfeeding Review, 9*(1), 27-32.

Binns, C. W., & Scott, J. A. (2002). Using pacifiers: what are breastfeeding mothers doing? *Breastfeeding Review, 10*(2), 21-25.

Butte, N. F. (2009). Impact of infant feeding practices on childhood obesity. *Journal of Nutrition, 139*(2), 412S-416S.

Butte, N. F., Wong, W. W., Hopkinson, J. M., Heinz, C. J., Mehta, N. R., & Smith, E. O. (2000). Energy requirements derived from total energy expenditure and energy deposition during the first 2 y of life. *American Journal of Clinical Nutrition, 72*(6), 1558-1569.

Butte, N. F., Wong, W. W., Hopkinson, J. M., Smith, E. O., & Ellis, K. J. (2000). Infant feeding mode affects early growth and body composition. *Pediatrics, 106*(6), 1355-1366.

Bystrova, K., Matthiesen, A. S., Widstrom, A. M., Ransjo-Arvidson, A. B., Welles-Nystrom, B., Vorontsov, I., et al. (2007). The effect of Russian Maternity Home routines on breastfeeding and neonatal weight loss with special reference to swaddling. *Early Human Development, 83*(1), 29-39.

Bystrova, K., Widstrom, A. M., Matthiesen, A. S., Ransjo-Arvidson, A. B., Welles-Nystrom, B., Vorontsov, I., et al. (2007). Early lactation performance in primiparous and multiparous women in relation to different maternity home practices. A randomised trial in St. Petersburg. *International Breastfeeding Journal, 2*, 9.

Caglar, M. K., Ozer, I., & Altugan, F. S. (2006). Risk factors for excess weight loss and hypernatremia in exclusively breast-fed infants. *Brazilian Journal of Medical and Biological Research, 39*(4), 539-544.

Carvalho, M., Robertson, S., & Klaus, M. H. (1984). Does the duration and frequency of early breastfeeding affect nipple pain? *Birth, 11*(2), 81-84.

CDC. (2001). Recommendations for using fluoride to prevent and control dental caries in the United States. Centers for Disease Control and Prevention. *MMWR Recommendations and Reports, 50*(RR-14), 1-42.

Chapman, D. J., & Perez-Escamilla, R. (1999). Identification of risk factors for delayed onset of lactation. *Journal of the American Dietetic Association, 99*(4), 450-454; quiz 455-456.

Clemente, C., Barnes, J., Shinebourne, E., & Stein, A. (2001). Are infant behavioural feeding difficulties associated with congenital heart disease? *Child: Care, Health and Development, 27*(1), 47-59.

Cockburn, F., Belton, N. R., Purvis, R. J., Giles, M. M., Brown, J. K., Turner, T. L., et al. (1980). Maternal vitamin D intake and mineral metabolism in mothers and their newborn infants. *British Medical Journal, 281*(6232), 11-14.

Cohen, R. J., Brown, K. H., Canahuati, J., Rivera, L. L., & Dewey, K. G. (1994). Effects of age of introduction of complementary foods on infant breast milk intake, total energy intake, and growth: a randomised intervention study in Honduras. *Lancet, 344*(8918), 288-293.

Colson, S., DeRooy, L., Hawdon, J. (2003). Biological Nurturing increases duration of breastfeeding for a vulnerable cohort. *MIDIRS Midwifery Digest, 13*(1), 92-97.

Cox, D. B., Kent, J. C., Casey, T. M., Owens, R. A., & Hartmann, P. E. (1999). Breast growth and the urinary excretion of lactose during human pregnancy and early lactation: endocrine relationships. *Experimental Physiology, 84*(2), 421-434.

Dahlenburg, G. W., Burnell, R. H., & Braybrook, R. (1980). The relation between cord serum sodium levels in newborn infants and maternal intravenous therapy during labour. *British Journal of Obstetrics and Gynaecology, 87*(6), 519-522.

DeMarzo, S., Seacat, J., & Neifert, M. (1991). Initial weight loss and return to birthweight criteria for breast-fed infants: Challenging the 'rules of thumb'. *American Journal of Diseases of Children, 145*(4), 402.

Dennison, B. A., Edmunds, L. S., Stratton, H. H., & Pruzek, R. M. (2006). Rapid infant weight gain predicts childhood overweight. *Obesity (Silver Spring), 14*(3), 491-499.

Dewey, K. G. (2003). Is breastfeeding protective against child obesity? *Journal of Human Lactation, 19*(1), 9-18.

Dewey, K. G. (2007). Nutrition, growth, and complementary feeding of the breastfed infant. In T. W. a. H. Hale, P. (Ed.), *Hale & Hartmann's textbook of human lactation* (pp. 415-423). Amarillo, TX: Hale Publishing.

Dewey, K. G. (2009a). Infant feeding and growth. *Advances in Experimental Medicine and Biology, 639*, 57-66.

Dewey, K. G. (2009b). Infant feeding and growth. In G. Goldberg, A. Prentice, P. A., S. Filteau & K. Simondon (Eds.), *Breast-feeding: Early influences on later health* (pp. 57-66). New York, NY: Springer.

Dewey, K. G., & Brown, K. H. (2003). Update on technical issues concerning complementary feeding of young children in developing countries and implications for intervention programs. *Food and Nutrition Bulletin, 24*(1), 5-28.

Dewey, K. G., Domellof, M., Cohen, R. J., Landa Rivera, L., Hernell, O., & Lonnerdal, B. (2002). Iron supplementation affects growth and morbidity of breast-fed infants: results of a randomized trial in Sweden and Honduras. *Journal of Nutrition, 132*(11), 3249-3255.

Dewey, K. G., Heinig, M. J., Nommsen, L. A., & Lonnerdal, B. (1991a). Adequacy of energy intake among breast-fed infants in the DARLING study: relationships to growth velocity, morbidity, and activity levels. Davis Area Research on Lactation, Infant Nutrition and Growth. *Journal of Pediatrics, 119*(4), 538-547.

Dewey, K. G., Heinig, M. J., Nommsen, L. A., & Lonnerdal, B. (1991b). Maternal versus infant factors related to breast milk intake and residual milk volume: the DARLING study. *Pediatrics, 87*(6), 829-837.

Dewey, K. G., Heinig, M. J., Nommsen, L. A., Peerson, J. M., & Lonnerdal, B. (1992). Growth of breast-fed and formula-fed infants from 0 to 18 months: the DARLING Study. *Pediatrics, 89*(6 Pt 1), 1035-1041.

Dewey, K. G., Heinig, M. J., Nommsen, L. A., Peerson, J. M., & Lonnerdal, B. (1993). Breast-fed infants are leaner than formula-fed infants at 1 y of age: the DARLING study. *American Journal of Clinical Nutrition, 57*(2), 140-145.

Dewey, K. G., Nommsen-Rivers, L. A., Heinig, M. J., & Cohen, R. J. (2003). Risk factors for suboptimal infant breastfeeding behavior, delayed onset of lactation, and excess neonatal weight loss. *Pediatrics, 112*(3 Pt 1), 607-619.

Dewey, K. G., Nommsen-Rivers, L. A., & Lonnerdal, B. (2004). Plasma insulin and insulin-releasing amino acid (IRAA) concentrations are higher in formula-fed than in breastfed infants at 5 mo. of age. [abstract]. *Experimental Biology 2004*.

Dewey, K. G., Nommsen, L. A., & Cohen, R. J. (2009). Delayed lactogenesis and excess neonatal weight loss are common across ethnic and socioeconimic categories of primiparous women in northern California. *FASEB Journal, 23*, 344.347 [meeting abstract].

di Pietro, J. A., Larson, S. K., & Porges, S. W. (1987). Behavioral and heart rate pattern differences between breast-fed and bottle-fed neonates. *Developmental Psychology, 23*(4), 467-474.

Dilli, D., Kucuk, I. G., & Dallar, Y. (2009). Interventions to reduce pain during vaccination in infancy. *Journal of Pediatrics, 154*(3), 385-390.

Domellof, M., Dewey, K. G., Lonnerdal, B., Cohen, R. J., & Hernell, O. (2002). The diagnostic criteria for iron deficiency in infants should be reevaluated. *Journal of Nutrition, 132*(12), 3680-3686.

Doneray, H., Orbak, Z., & Yildiz, L. (2009). The relationship between breast milk leptin and neonatal weight gain. *Acta Paediatrica, 98*(4), 643-647.

Ezzo, G., & Bucknam, R. (2006). *On becoming babywise*. Sisters, OR: Parent-Wise Solutions, Inc.

Farrow, C., & Blissett, J. (2006). Breast-feeding, maternal feeding practices and mealtime negativity at one year. *Appetite, 46*(1), 49-56.

Ferber, R. (2006). *Solve your child's sleep problems*. London, England: Dorling Kindersley.

Fetherston, C. (1998). Risk factors for lactation mastitis. *Journal of Human Lactation, 14*(2), 101-109.

Franco, P., Seret, N., Van Hees, J. N., Scaillet, S., Groswasser, J., & Kahn, A. (2005). Influence of swaddling on sleep and arousal characteristics of healthy infants. *Pediatrics, 115*(5), 1307-1311.

Garbin, C. P., Deacon, J. P., Rowan, M. K., Hartmann, P. E., & Geddes, D. T. (2009). Association of nipple piercing with abnormal milk production and breastfeeding. *Journal of the American Medical Association, 301*(24), 2550-2551.

Gartner, L. M., Morton, J., Lawrence, R. A., Naylor, A. J., O'Hare, D., Schanler, R. J., et al. (2005). Breastfeeding and the use of human milk. *Pediatrics, 115*(2), 496-506.

Genna, C. W. (2008). The influence of anatomic and strucural issues on sucking skills. In C. W. Genna (Ed.), *Supporting sucking skills in breastfeeding infants*. Boston, MA: Jones and Bartlett.

Gillman, M. W., Rifas-Shiman, S. L., Berkey, C. S., Frazier, A. L., Rockett, H. R., Camargo, C. A., Jr., et al. (2006). Breast-feeding and overweight in adolescence: within-family analysis [corrected]. *Epidemiology, 17*(1), 112-114.

Girish, M., & Subramaniam, G. (2008). Rickets in exclusively breast fed babies. *Indian Journal of Pediatrics, 75*(6), 641-643.

Griffin, I. J., & Abrams, S. A. (2001). Iron and breastfeeding. *Pediatric Clinics of North America, 48*(2), 401-413.

Grummer-Strawn, L. M., & Mei, Z. (2004). Does breastfeeding protect against pediatric overweight? Analysis of longitudinal data from the Centers for Disease Control and Prevention Pediatric Nutrition Surveillance System. *Pediatrics, 113*(2), e81-86.

Halderman, L. D., & Nelson, A. L. (2002). Impact of early postpartum administration of progestin-only hormonal contraceptives compared with nonhormonal contraceptives on short-term breast-feeding patterns. *American Journal of Obstetrics and Gynecology, 186*(6), 1250-1256; discussion 1256-1258.

Hannon, P. R., Duggan, A. K., Serwint, J. R., Vogelhut, J. W., Witter, F., & DeAngelis, C. (1997). The influence of medroxyprogesterone on the duration of breast-feeding in mothers in an urban community. *Archives of Pediatrics and Adolescent Medicine, 151*(5), 490-496.

Harding, D., Cairns, P., Gupta, S., & Cowan, F. (2001). Hypernatraemia: why bother weighing breast fed babies? *Archives of Disease in Childhood. Fetal and Neonatal Edition, 85*(2), F145.

Hawkins, S. S., Cole, T. J., & Law, C. (2009). An ecological systems approach to examining risk factors for early childhood overweight: findings from the UK Millennium Cohort Study. *Journal of Epidemiology and Community Health, 63*(2), 147-155.

Heaney, R. P., Davies, K. M., Chen, T. C., Holick, M. F., & Barger-Lux, M. J. (2003). Human serum 25-hydroxycholecalciferol response to extended oral dosing with cholecalciferol. *American Journal of Clinical Nutrition, 77*(1), 204-210.

Heinig, M. J., Nommsen, L. A., Peerson, J. M., Lonnerdal, B., & Dewey, K. G. (1993). Energy and protein intakes of breast-fed and formula-fed infants during the first year of life and their association with growth velocity: the DARLING Study. *American Journal of Clinical Nutrition, 58*(2), 152-161.

Henly, S. J., Anderson, C. M., Avery, M. D., Hills-Bonczyk, S. G., Potter, S., & Duckett, L. J. (1995). Anemia and insufficient milk in first-time mothers. *Birth, 22*(2), 86-92.

Hillervik-Lindquist, C., Hofvander, Y., & Sjolin, S. (1991). Studies on perceived breast milk insufficiency. III. Consequences for breast milk consumption and growth. *Acta Paediatrica Scandinavica, 80*(3), 297-303.

Hilson, J. A., Rasmussen, K. M., & Kjolhede, C. L. (2004). High prepregnant body mass index is associated with poor lactation outcomes among white, rural women independent of psychosocial and demographic correlates. *Journal of Human Lactation, 20*(1), 18-29.

Hollis, B. W., & Wagner, C. L. (2004a). Assessment of dietary vitamin D requirements during pregnancy and lactation. *American Journal of Clinical Nutrition, 79*(5), 717-726.

Hollis, B. W., & Wagner, C. L. (2004b). Vitamin D requirements during lactation: high-dose maternal supplementation as therapy to prevent hypovitaminosis D for both the mother and the nursing infant. *American Journal of Clinical Nutrition, 80*(6 Suppl), 1752S-1758S.

Hoover, K. L., Barbalinardo, L. H., & Platia, M. P. (2002). Delayed lactogenesis II secondary to gestational ovarian theca lutein cysts in two normal singleton pregnancies. *Journal of Human Lactation, 18*(3), 264-268.

Hopkinson, J. M. (2003). Is it possible for a breastfed baby to be overweight? *Journal of Human Lactation, 19*(2), 189-190.

Howard, C. R., Howard, F. M., Lanphear, B., deBlieck, E. A., Eberly, S., & Lawrence, R. A. (1999). The effects of early pacifier use on breastfeeding duration. *Pediatrics, 103*(3), E33.

Huggins, K. E., Petok, E. S., & Mireles, O. (2000). Markers of lactation insufficiency: A study of 34 mothers. In *Current issues in clinical lactation*. Boston, MA: Jones and Bartlett.

Humphrey, S. (2003). *The nursing mother's herbal.* Minneapolis, MN: Fairview Press.

ILCA. (2005). *Clinical guidelines for the establishment of exclusive breastfeeding*. Raleigh, NC: International Lactation Consultant Association.

Ip, S., Chung, M., Raman, G., Chew, P., Magula, N., DeVine, D., et al. (2007). Breastfeeding and maternal and infant health outcomes in developed countries. *Evidence Report - Technology Assessment (Full Report)*(153), 1-186.

Ip, S., Chung, M., Raman, G., Trikalinos, T. A., & Lau, J. (2009). A summary of the Agency for Healthcare Research and Quality's evidence report on breastfeeding in developed countries. *Breastfeeding Medicine, 4 Suppl 1*, S17-30.

Islam, M. M., Peerson, J. M., Ahmed, T., Dewey, K. G., & Brown, K. H. (2006). Effects of varied energy density of complementary foods on breast-milk intakes and total energy consumption by healthy, breastfed Bangladeshi children. *American Journal of Clinical Nutrition, 83*(4), 851-858.

Javaid, M. K., Crozier, S. R., Harvey, N. C., Gale, C. R., Dennison, E. M., Boucher, B. J., et al. (2006). Maternal vitamin D status during pregnancy and childhood bone mass at age 9 years: a longitudinal study. *Lancet, 367*(9504), 36-43.

Judkins, A., & Eagleton, C. (2006). Vitamin D deficiency in pregnant New Zealand women. *New Zealand Medical Journal, 119*(1241), U2144.

Kennedy, K. I. (2010). Fertility, sexuality, and contraception during lactation. In J. Riordan & K. Wambach (Eds.), *Breastfeeding and human lactation* (4th ed., pp. 705-736). Boston, MA: Jones and Bartlett.

Kent, J. C. (2007). How breastfeeding works. *Journal of Midwifery & Women's Health, 52*(6), 564-570.

Kent, J. C., Mitoulas, L. R., Cregan, M. D., Ramsay, D. T., Doherty, D. A., & Hartmann, P. E. (2006). Volume and frequency of breastfeedings and fat content of breast milk throughout the day. *Pediatrics, 117*(3), e387-395.

Kerr, M. (2008, May 12). Neurodevelopmental delays associated with iron-fortified formula for healthy infants. Retrieved June 10, 2008, from www.medscape.com/viewarticle/57363

Koetsawang, S. (1987). The effects of contraceptive methods on the quality and quantity of breastmilk. *International Journal of Gynaecology and Obstetrics, 25(suppl)*, 115-128.

Koletzko, B., von Kries, R., Closa, R., Escribano, J., Scaglioni, S., Giovannini, M., et al. (2009). Lower protein in infant formula is associated with lower weight up to age 2 y: a randomized clinical trial. *American Journal of Clinical Nutrition, 89*(6), 1836-1845.

Kramer, M. S., Guo, T., Platt, R. W., Vanilovich, I., Sevkovskaya, Z., Dzikovich, I., et al. (2004). Feeding effects on growth during infancy. *Journal of Pediatrics, 145*(5), 600-605.

Kugyelka, J. G., Rasmussen, K. M., & Frongillo, E. A. (2004). Maternal obesity is negatively associated with breastfeeding success among Hispanic but not Black women. *Journal of Nutrition, 134*(7), 1746-1753.

Labbok, M. H. (2007). Breastfeeding, birth spacing, and family planning. In T. W. Hale & P. F. Hartmann (Eds.), *Hale & Hartmann's textbook of human lactation* (pp. 305-318). Amarillo, TX: Hale Publishing.

Lampl, M., Veldhuis, J. D., & Johnson, M. L. (1992). Saltation and stasis: a model of human growth. *Science, 258*(5083), 801-803.

Lawrence, R. A., & Lawrence, R. M. (2005). *Breastfeeding: A guide for the medical profession* (6th ed.). Philadelphia, PA: Elsevier Mosby.

Lazol, J. P., Cakan, N., & Kamat, D. (2008). 10-year case review of nutritional rickets in Children's Hospital of Michigan. *Clinical Pediatrics, 47*(4), 379-384.

Lee, N. (1995). More on pierced nipples. *Journal of Human Lactation, 11*(2), 89.

Li, L., Manor, O., & Power, C. (2004). Early environment and child-to-adult growth trajectories in the 1958 British birth cohort. *American Journal of Clinical Nutrition, 80*(1), 185-192.

Li, R., Fein, S. B., & Grummer-Strawn, L. M. (2008). Association of breastfeeding intensity and bottle-emptying behaviors at early infancy with infants' risk for excess weight at late infancy. *Pediatrics, 122 Suppl 2*, S77-84.

Lozoff, B., & Georgieff, M. K. (2006). Iron deficiency and brain development. *Seminars in Pediatric Neurology, 13*(3), 158-165.

Lucas, A., Boyes, S., Bloom, S. R., & Aynsley-Green, A. (1981). Metabolic and endocrine responses to a milk feed in six-day-old term infants: differences between breast and cow's milk formula feeding. *Acta Paediatrica Scandinavica, 70*(2), 195-200.

Lucas, A., & St James-Roberts, I. (1998). Crying, fussing and colic behaviour in breast- and bottle-fed infants. *Early Human Development, 53*(1), 9-18.

Lukefahr, J. L. (1990). Underlying illness associated with failure to thrive in breastfed infants. *Clinical Pediatrics, 29*(8), 468-470.

Macdonald, P. D., Ross, S. R., Grant, L., & Young, D. (2003). Neonatal weight loss in breast and formula fed infants. *Archives of Disease in Childhood. Fetal and Neonatal Edition, 88*(6), F472-476.

Manganaro, R., Mami, C., Marrone, T., Marseglia, L., & Gemelli, M. (2001). Incidence of dehydration and hypernatremia in exclusively breast-fed infants. *Journal of Pediatrics, 139*(5), 673-675.

Marasco, L., Marmet, C., & Shell, E. (2000). Polycystic ovary syndrome: a connection to insufficient milk supply? *Journal of Human Lactation, 16*(2), 143-148.

Martens, P. J., & Romphf, L. (2007). Factors associated with newborn in-hospital weight loss: comparisons by feeding method, demographics, and birthing procedures. *Journal of Human Lactation, 23*(3), 233-241, quiz 242-235.

Martin, R. M., Smith, G. D., Mangtani, P., Frankel, S., & Gunnell, D. (2002). Association between breast feeding and growth: the Boyd-Orr cohort study. *Archives of Disease in Childhood. Fetal and Neonatal Edition, 87*(3), F193-201.

Matias, S. L., Nommsen-Rivers, L. A., & Creed-Kanashiro, H. (2009). Risk factors for early lactation problems among Peruvian primiparous mothers. *Maternal and Child Nutrition*(Epub June 24).

Meier, P. P., Engstrom, J. L., Crichton, C. L., Clark, D. R., Williams, M. M., & Mangurten, H. H. (1994). A new scale for in-home test-weighing for mothers of preterm and high risk infants. *Journal of Human Lactation, 10*(3), 163-168.

Messner, A. H., Lalakea, M. L., Aby, J., Macmahon, J., & Bair, E. (2000). Ankyloglossia: incidence and associated feeding difficulties. *Archives of Otolaryngology -- Head and Neck Surgery, 126*(1), 36-39.

Milner, J. D., Stein, D. M., McCarter, R., & Moon, R. Y. (2004). Early infant multivitamin supplementation is associated with increased risk for food allergy and asthma. *Pediatrics, 114*(1), 27-32.

Mohrbacher, N., & Kendall-Tackett, K. (2005). *Breastfeeding made simple: Seven natural laws for nursing mothers*. Oakland, CA: New Harbinger Publications.

Moscone, S. R., & Moore, M. J. (1993). Breastfeeding during pregnancy. *Journal of Human Lactation, 9*(2), 83-88.

Motil, K. J., Sheng, H. P., Montandon, C. M., & Wong, W. W. (1997). Human milk protein does not limit growth of breast-fed infants. *Journal of Pediatric Gastroenterology and Nutrition, 24*(1), 10-17.

Murphy, P. K., & Wagner, C. L. (2008). Vitamin D and mood disorders among women: an integrative review. *Journal of Midwifery & Women's Health, 53*(5), 440-446.

Neville, M. C., Keller, R., Seacat, J., Lutes, V., Neifert, M., Casey, C., et al. (1988). Studies in human lactation: milk volumes in lactating women during the onset of lactation and full lactation. *American Journal of Clinical Nutrition, 48*(6), 1375-1386.

Newton, N., & Theotokatos, M. (1979). Breastfeeding during pregnancy in 503 women: Does a psychobiological weaning mechanism exist in humans? *Emotion & Reproduction, 20B*, 845-849.

Noel-Weiss, J., Courant, G., & Woodend, A. K. (2008). Physiological weight loss in the breastfed neonate: A systematic review. *Open Medicine, 2*(3), E11-22.

Nommsen-Rivers, L. A., & Dewey, K. G. (2009). Growth of breastfed infants. *Breastfeeding Medicine, 4 Suppl 1*, S45-49.

Nommsen-Rivers, L. A., Heinig, M. J., Cohen, R. J., & Dewey, K. G. (2008). Newborn wet and soiled diaper counts and timing of onset of lactation as indicators of breastfeeding inadequacy. *Journal of Human Lactation, 24*(1), 27-33.

Nommsen, L. A., Lovelady, C. A., Heinig, M. J., Lonnerdal, B., & Dewey, K. G. (1991). Determinants of energy, protein, lipid, and lactose concentrations in human milk during the first 12 mo of lactation: the DARLING Study. *American Journal of Clinical Nutrition, 53*(2), 457-465.

Oddie, S., Richmond, S., & Coulthard, M. (2001). Hypernatraemic dehydration and breast feeding: a population study. *Archives of Disease in Childhood, 85*(4), 318-320.

Odeleye, O. E., de Courten, M., Pettitt, D. J., & Ravussin, E. (1997). Fasting hyperinsulinemia is a predictor of increased body weight gain and obesity in Pima Indian children. *Diabetes, 46*(8), 1341-1345.

Ong, K. K., & Loos, R. J. (2006). Rapid infancy weight gain and subsequent obesity: systematic reviews and hopeful suggestions. *Acta Paediatrica, 95*(8), 904-908.

Onyango, A. W., Esrey, S. A., & Kramer, M. S. (1999). Continued breastfeeding and child growth in the second year of life: a prospective cohort study in western Kenya. *Lancet, 354*(9195), 2041-2045.

Pabst, H. F., & Spady, D. W. (1990). Effect of breast-feeding on antibody response to conjugate vaccine. *Lancet, 336*(8710), 269-270.

Pabst, H. F., Spady, D. W., Pilarski, L. M., Carson, M. M., Beeler, J. A., & Krezolek, M. P. (1997). Differential modulation of the immune response by breast- or formula-feeding of infants. *Acta Paediatrica, 86*(12), 1291-1297.

PAHO/WHO. (2001). *Guiding principles for complementary feeding of the breastfed child*. Retrieved March 21, 2008 from http://whqlibdoc.who.int/paho/2004/a85622.pdf.

Panagiotakos, D. B., Papadimitriou, A., Anthracopoulos, M. B., Konstantinidou, M., Antonogeorgos, G., Fretzayas, A., et al. (2008). Birthweight, breast-feeding, parental weight and prevalence of obesity in schoolchildren aged 10-12 years, in Greece; the Physical Activity, Nutrition and Allergies in Children Examined in Athens (PANACEA) study. *Pediatrics International, 50*(4), 563-568.

Pelto, G. H., Levitt, E., & Thairu, L. (2003). Improving feeding practices: current patterns, common constraints, and the design of interventions. *Food and Nutrition Bulletin, 24*(1), 45-82.

Perez-Escamilla, R., Cohen, R. J., Brown, K. H., Rivera, L. L., Canahuati, J., & Dewey, K. G. (1995). Maternal anthropometric status and lactation performance in a low-income Honduran population: evidence for the role of infants. *American Journal of Clinical Nutrition, 61*(3), 528-534.

Pickering, L. K., Granoff, D. M., Erickson, J. R., Masor, M. L., Cordle, C. T., Schaller, J. P., et al. (1998). Modulation of the immune system by human milk and infant formula containing nucleotides. *Pediatrics, 101*(2), 242-249.

Powers, N. G. (1999). Slow weight gain and low milk supply in the breastfeeding dyad. *Clinics in Perinatology, 26*(2), 399-430.

Powers, N. G. (2001). How to assess slow growth in the breastfed infant. Birth to 3 months. *Pediatric Clinics of North America, 48*(2), 345-363.

Raj, S., Faridi, M., Rusia, U., & Singh, O. (2008). A prospective study of iron status in exclusively breastfed term infants up to 6 months of age. *International Breastfeeding Journal, 3*, 3.

Rasmussen, K. M., & Kjolhede, C. L. (2004). Prepregnant overweight and obesity diminish the prolactin response to suckling in the first week postpartum. *Pediatrics, 113*(5), e465-471.

Righard, L. (1998). Are breastfeeding problems related to incorrect breastfeeding technique and the use of pacifiers and bottles? *Birth, 25*(1), 40-44.

Sachan, A., Gupta, R., Das, V., Agarwal, A., Awasthi, P. K., & Bhatia, V. (2005). High prevalence of vitamin D deficiency among pregnant women and their newborns in northern India. *American Journal of Clinical Nutrition, 81*(5), 1060-1064.

Sachs, M., Dykes, F., & Carter, B. (2006). Feeding by numbers: an ethnographic study of how breastfeeding women understand their babies' weight charts. *International Breastfeeding Journal, 1*, 29.

Savage, S. A., Reilly, J. J., Edwards, C. A., & Durnin, J. V. (1998). Weaning practice in the Glasgow Longitudinal Infant Growth Study. *Archives of Disease in Childhood, 79*(2), 153-156.

Schrager, S., & Sabo, L. (2001). Sheehan syndrome: a rare complication of postpartum hemorrhage. *Journal of the American Board of Family Practice, 14*(5), 389-391.

Semeniuk, J., & Kaczmarski, M. (2008). Acid gastroesophageal reflux and intensity of symptoms in children with gastroesophageal reflux disease. Comparison of primary gastroesophageal reflux and gastroesophageal reflux secondary to food allergy. *Advances in Medical Sciences, 53*(2), 293-299.

Shah, V., Taddio, A., & Rieder, M. J. (2009). Effectiveness and tolerability of pharmacologic and combined interventions for reducing injection pain during routine childhood immunizations: systematic review and meta-analyses. *Clinical Therapeutics, 31 Suppl 2*, S104-151.

Shrago, L. C., Reifsnider, E., & Insel, K. (2006). The Neonatal Bowel Output Study: indicators of adequate breast milk intake in neonates. *Pediatric Nursing, 32*(3), 195-201.

Silfverdal, S. A., Ekholm, L., & Bodin, L. (2007). Breastfeeding enhances the antibody response to Hib and Pneumococcal serotype 6B and 14 after vaccination with conjugate vaccines. *Vaccine, 25*(8), 1497-1502.

Simondon, K. B., Simondon, F., Costes, R., Delaunay, V., & Diallo, A. (2001). Breast-feeding is associated with improved growth in length, but not weight, in rural Senegalese toddlers. *American Journal of Clinical Nutrition, 73*(5), 959-967.

Smith, M. M., & Lifshitz, F. (1994). Excess fruit juice consumption as a contributing factor in nonorganic failure to thrive. *Pediatrics, 93*(3), 438-443.

Stettler, N., Stallings, V. A., Troxel, A. B., Zhao, J., Schinnar, R., Nelson, S. E., et al. (2005). Weight gain in the first week of life and overweight in adulthood: a cohort study of European American subjects fed infant formula. *Circulation, 111*(15), 1897-1903.

Stettler, N., Zemel, B. S., Kumanyika, S., & Stallings, V. A. (2002). Infant weight gain and childhood overweight status in a multicenter, cohort study. *Pediatrics, 109*(2), 194-199.

Stutte, P. (1988). The effects of breast massage on volume and fat content of human milk. *Genesis, 10*(2), 22-25.

Taveras, E. M., Rifas-Shiman, S. L., Scanlon, K. S., Grummer-Strawn, L. M., Sherry, B., & Gillman, M. W. (2006). To what extent is the protective effect of breastfeeding on future overweight explained by decreased maternal feeding restriction? *Pediatrics, 118*(6), 2341-2348.

Taveras, E. M., Scanlon, K. S., Birch, L., Rifas-Shiman, S. L., Rich-Edwards, J. W., & Gillman, M. W. (2004). Association of breastfeeding with maternal control of infant feeding at age 1 year. *Pediatrics, 114*(5), e577-583.

Tolia, V. (1995). Very early onset nonorganic failure to thrive in infants. *Journal of Pediatric Gastroenterology and Nutrition, 20*(1), 73-80.

van der Meer, I. M., Karamali, N. S., Boeke, A. J., Lips, P., Middelkoop, B. J., Verhoeven, I., et al. (2006). High prevalence of vitamin D deficiency in pregnant non-Western women in The Hague, Netherlands. *American Journal of Clinical Nutrition, 84*(2), 350-353; quiz 468-359.

Vazirinejad, R., Darakhshan, S., Esmaeili, A., & Hadadian, S. (2009). The effect of maternal breast variations on neonatal weight gain in the first seven days of life. *International Breastfeeding Journal, 4*, 13.

Victora, C. G., Barros, F., Lima, R. C., Horta, B. L., & Wells, J. (2003). Anthropometry and body composition of 18 year old men according to duration of breast feeding: birth cohort study from Brazil. *British Medical Journal, 327*(7420), 901.

Vieth, R. (1999). Vitamin D supplementation, 25-hydroxyvitamin D concentrations, and safety. *American Journal of Clinical Nutrition, 69*(5), 842-856.

Vieth, R., Chan, P. C., & MacFarlane, G. D. (2001). Efficacy and safety of vitamin D3 intake exceeding the lowest observed adverse effect level. *American Journal of Clinical Nutrition, 73*(2), 288-294.

Vieth, R., Cole, D. E., Hawker, G. A., Trang, H. M., & Rubin, L. A. (2001). Wintertime vitamin D insufficiency is common in young Canadian women, and their vitamin D intake does not prevent it. *European Journal of Clinical Nutrition, 55*(12), 1091-1097.

Wagner, C. L., & Greer, F. R. (2008). Prevention of rickets and vitamin D deficiency in infants, children, and adolescents. *Pediatrics, 122*(5), 1142-1152.

Wagner, C. L., Hulsey, T. C., Fanning, D., Ebeling, M., & Hollis, B. W. (2006). High-dose vitamin D3 supplementation in a cohort of breastfeeding mothers and their infants: a 6-month follow-up pilot study. *Breastfeeding Medicine, 1*(2), 59-70.

Wagner, C. L., Taylor, S. N., & Hollis, B. W. (2008). Does vitamin D make the world go 'round'? *Breastfeeding Medicine, 3*(4), 239-250.

Walker, M. (2006). *Breastfeeding management for the clinician: Using the evidence*. Boston, MA: Jones and Bartlett.

Ward, L. M., Gaboury, I., Ladhani, M., & Zlotkin, S. (2007). Vitamin D-deficiency rickets among children in Canada. *Canadian Medical Association Journal, 177*(2), 161-166.

Weisberg, P., Scanlon, K. S., Li, R., & Cogswell, M. E. (2004). Nutritional rickets among children in the United States: review of cases reported between 1986 and 2003. *American Journal of Clinical Nutrition, 80*(6 Suppl), 1697S-1705S.

WHO. (2004). *Selected practice recommendations for contraceptive use* (2nd ed.). Geneva, Switzerland: WHO Reproductive Health Research Division.

WHO. (2006). Breastfeeding in the WHO Multicentre Growth Reference Study. *Acta Paediatrica. Supplement, 450*, 16-26.

Williams, N. (2002). Supporting the mother coming to terms with persistent insufficient milk supply: the role of the lactation consultant. *Journal of Human Lactation, 18*(3), 262-263.

Willis, C. E., & Livingstone, V. (1995). Infant insufficient milk syndrome associated with maternal postpartum hemorrhage. *Journal of Human Lactation, 11*(2), 123-126.

Wilson-Clay, B., & Hoover, K. (2008). *The breastfeeding atlas* (4th ed.). Manchaca, TX: LactNews Press.

Wolf, L. S., & Glass, R. P. (1992). *Feeding and swallowing disorders in infancy*. Tucson, AZ: Therapy Skill Builders.

Wondale, Y., Shiferaw, F., & Lulseged, S. (2005). A systematic review of nutritional rickets in Ethiopia: status and prospects. *Ethiopian Medical Journal, 43*(3), 203-210.

Wright, C. M., Parkinson, K. N., & Drewett, R. F. (2004). Why are babies weaned early? Data from a prospective population based cohort study. *Archives of Disease in Childhood, 89*(9), 813-816.

Young, T. K., Martens, P. J., Taback, S. P., Sellers, E. A., Dean, H. J., Cheang, M., et al. (2002). Type 2 diabetes mellitus in children: prenatal and early infancy risk factors among native canadians. *Archives of Pediatrics and Adolescent Medicine, 156*(7), 651-655.

Ziegler, E. E., Hollis, B. W., Nelson, S. E., & Jeter, J. M. (2006). Vitamin D deficiency in breastfed infants in Iowa. *Pediatrics, 118*(2), 603-610.

Hypoglycemia and Newborn Jaundice

Chapter 7

HYPOGLYCEMIA

Glucose, one type of sugar, is the baby's primary brain fuel. While in utero, the baby stores glucose in the form of glycogen in his liver and some muscles. After delivery, when the umbilical cord is cut and he no longer receives glucose from his mother, hormones are released that help him use his glycogen stores for brain fuel while he adapts to life on the outside. About 70% of a baby's brain glucose needs are met this way, with the other 30% coming from alternative fuels (see next point) (Walker, 2006).

A newborn's blood sugar levels normally drop after birth and then rise again as he adapts to life outside the womb.

In a healthy newborn, blood sugar levels are usually at their lowest at about 1 to 2 hours after birth. They begin to rise, independent of feeding, within 2 to 4 hours and continue rising for the first 96 hours after birth (Hawdon, Ward Platt, & Aynsley-Green, 1992; WHO, 1997; Wight & Marinelli, 2006). No short- or long-term benefits have been found to testing and treating newborns for this normal dip in blood-sugar levels during the first hours after birth (Wight & Marinelli, 2006).

By 12 hours after birth, the baby's glycogen stores are gone, milk feeding and fat stores provide needed glucose.

By 12 hours after birth, a newborn's glycogen stores are gone, and milk feedings and fat stores provide a baby with the glucose his brain needs (Hagedorn & Gardner, 1999).

• •

For many reasons, breastfeeding within the first 2 hours after birth is important to both mother and baby, but this first feeding appears to have little effect on baby's blood sugar levels (Sweet, Hadden, & Halliday, 1999). So from a blood-sugar perspective, if the first breastfeeding is delayed, the baby will not benefit from being fed a supplement. In fact, U.K. research indicates that giving formula can make a newborn's blood sugar problems worse by compromising his ability to use alternative brain fuels (de Rooy & Hawdon, 2002; Hawdon & Williams, 2000; Hawdon, Ward Platt, & Aynsley-Green, 1992).

The exclusively breastfed baby can access alternative brain fuels more effectively than babies fed formula.

As part of a newborn's natural adaptation from womb to world, in addition to using his glycogen stores for brain fuel, he can access other fuel sources, such as ketone bodies and lactate. Giving formula, however, has been found to suppress a baby's ability to use ketone bodies for fuel. The more formula he consumes, the less he can access this alternative fuel, potentially worsening his blood-sugar problems.

Full-term, healthy, exclusively breastfeeding babies are not considered to be at risk for hypoglycemia, in part because they have greater access to these alternative fuels. Routine blood-sugar testing is not recommended (Cornblath et al., 2000; Eidelman, 2001; Wight, 2006), even when a healthy newborn without symptoms goes as long as 8 hours without breastfeeding (Hawdon, Ward Platt, & Aynsley-Green, 1992). In fact, researchers recommend against routine blood-sugar testing, even for babies born large-for-gestational-age, as long as they have no symptoms or other risk factors for hypoglycemia (see next point) (de Rooy & Hawdon, 2002).

Hypoglycemia can cause symptoms and serious health problems in at-risk babies.

Symptoms of hypoglycemia include tremors, irritability, jitteriness, a high-pitched cry, irregular breathing, low body temperature, and refusal to feed, as well as low muscle tone, lethargy, and seizures. Unfortunately, some of the symptoms, such as jitteriness, can be difficult to distinguish from normal newborn behavior (D'Harlingue & Durand, 1993). One Israeli study of 102 newborns identified as jittery found that 80% stopped acting jittery when they suckled on the clinician's finger, leading to the recommendation that this be tried before a blood test for hypoglycemia is done (Linder et al., 1989; Nicholl, 2003). Putting baby to the breast is an even better alternative.

Some situations and conditions that put a newborn at risk for hypoglycemia include preterm birth, small-for-gestation age, sepsis (blood infection), Rh disease, respiratory distress, high bilirubin levels (see next section), inborn errors of metabolism, a diabetic mother, congestive heart failure, and cold stress (Walker, 2006). Tests exists that can identify which small-for-gestational-age babies are at risk for hypoglycemia (Hawdon, Ward Platt, McPhail, Cameron, & Walkinshaw, 1992).

The normal and temporary dip in blood sugar after birth that occurs in most mammal species is distinctly different from the prolonged, severe, and untreated hypoglycemia that can cause brain damage and lead to vision problems, neuromotor retardation, epilepsy, cerebral palsy, and in rare cases, death (Hawdon, 1999; Inder, 2008; Per, Kumandas, Coskun, Gumus, & Oztop, 2008; Wight, 2006).

Unfortunately, there is no generally agreed upon definition for hypoglycemia, and many common testing methods are inaccurate.

What blood-sugar levels indicate hypoglycemia? This varies among healthcare providers and in different parts of the world. One common guideline is less than 40 mg/dL or 2.2 mmol/L (whole blood glucose level lower than 35 mg/dL or 1.9 mmol/L). But U.S. research found that when this guideline was used, more than 20% of healthy term newborns with normal blood-sugar levels were misidentified as hypoglycemic (Sexson, 1984). Even so, in many U.S. hospitals, even higher levels, such as 50 mg/dL (2.8 mmol/L), are now being used without factoring in the naturally lower blood-glucose levels in breastfed newborns (DePuy, Coassolo, Som, & Smulian, 2009).

No matter what the level used, there are problems with defining hypoglycemia as one blood-glucose level for all newborns. One blood-glucose level does not reflect the many factors that determine the effect of that level on an individual baby, such as his gestational age, his health, where he is on the normal blood-sugar curve after birth, and his symptoms or lack of symptoms. For this reason, some researchers have suggested instead that thresholds be used that take these influencing factors into account (Cornblath et al., 2000) (see Table 7.1).

Another factor that can contribute to overtreatment of hypoglycemia is the variations in how blood sugar is measured. For example, when whole blood is tested, the results are 10% to 15% lower than when plasma is tested. Also, common methods of measuring blood sugar levels have been found to be inaccurate. The American Academy of Pediatrics and World Health Organization recommends against the use of Dextrostix reagent strips or Chemstrips for testing hypoglycemia due to their proven inaccuracies (AAP, 1993; WHO, 1997). In one U.S. study, one of the bedside machines used to test newborns' blood-sugar levels was found to accurately identify hypoglycemia only 76% of the time (Meloy, Miller, Chandrasekaran, Summitt, & Gutcher, 1999).

Table 7.1. When to Treat Hypoglycemia

Baby's status	Baby's age in hours	Glucose levels indicating need for treatment
No symptoms Born 34-40 weeks Healthy Taking milk feedings No risk factors	≤24 hours >24 hours	<30-35 mg/dL <40-50 mg/dL
Symptoms	Any age	<45 mg/dL
Illness or birth-related issues Low birthweight Preterm Respiratory distress or failure Sepsis (blood infection)	≤24 hours >24 hours	<45-50 mg/dL <40-50 mg/dL
At risk Diabetic mother Glucose IV in labor (Sexson, 1984) Sepsis Small-for-gestational age Oxygen deprivation Metabolic disorder Endocrine disorder	Any age	<36 mg/dL
Low blood-glucose levels <20-25 mg/dL	Any age	Start IV glucose treatment and monitor

Adapted from (Cornblath & Ichord, 2000; Walker, 2006)

Postpartum practices, such as skin-to-skin contact and frequent breastfeeding, can reduce a newborn's risk of hypoglycemia.

Separation of mother and baby leads to lower infant body temperature (Bystrova et al., 2007), one risk factor for hypoglycemia. Skin-to-skin contact has been found to be more effective than incubators at maintaining newborn body temperature, even among preterm babies (Bergman, Linley, & Fawcus, 2004). One Swedish study found that babies separated from their mothers cried 10 times more, had elevated cortisol (a stress hormone), and blood-sugar levels, on average, 10 mg/dL lower than babies kept in skin-to-skin contact (Christensson et al., 1992). Specific postpartum practices that can reduce the risk of hypoglycemia include:

Mother-baby separation can increase the risk of hypoglycemia.

- In the hours after birth, keep mother and baby in skin-to-skin contact and together day and night (Bystrova et al., 2007; Suman, Udani, & Nanavati, 2008).
- Encourage frequent body contact to trigger inborn breastfeeding behaviors and early and frequent feedings (Colson, DeRooy, & Hawdon, 2003).
- Respond quickly to a baby's earliest signs of hunger before crying starts. The stress of crying decreases blood-sugar levels (Christensson et al., 1992).
- If baby is not breastfeeding, every 2 hours or so, suggest the mother express a little colostrum into a spoon and feed it to the baby (Walker, 2006).

Colostrum, either directly from the breast or expressed and fed, enhances a newborn's ability to use alternative brain fuels and improves gut function, allowing nutrients to be absorbed more quickly. One U.S. study found that at-risk babies of mothers with gestational diabetes who breastfed in the delivery room were significantly less likely to develop hypoglycemia (10%) than babies whose first breastfeeding was later (28%) (Chertok, Raz, Shoham, Haddad, & Wiznitzer, 2009). One U.K. study of full-term, healthy babies with no risk factors found that with frequent breastfeeding, even those with very low blood sugar levels at 1 hour developed no symptoms of hypoglycemia (Hoseth, Joergensen, Ebbesen, & Moeller, 2000). Making sure baby is feeding well at the breast is also vital, as some newborns discharged from the hospital not breastfeeding well became hypoglycemic later (Moore & Perlman, 1999).

IV glucose therapy is the recommended treatment for hypoglycemia with continued breastfeeding.

If hypoglycemia is confirmed, IV glucose therapy is recommended rather than glucose water feeding (Eidelman, 2001; Wight & Marinelli, 2006). A baby can breastfeed during IV glucose therapy if he will go to breast (Wight, 2006). Reassure the mother that her milk had nothing to do with her baby's hypoglycemia, and if needed, provide information on how to best keep breastfeeding and milk production on track, either through frequent breastfeeding (if the baby is feeding effectively) or frequent milk expression (for details, see the chapter "Milk Expression and Storage").

NEWBORN JAUNDICE

Jaundice Basics

In utero babies have extra red blood cells to transport the oxygen they receive from their mother. After a baby is born and breathing air, however, these extra red blood cells are no longer needed and are broken down and eliminated. Bilirubin, a yellow pigment, is a byproduct of the breakdown of these extra red blood cells. Jaundice occurs as bilirubin accumulates in baby's blood and enters the skin, muscles, and mucous membranes, giving the baby a yellow tinge. Jaundice is more common among newborns than older children and adults for several reasons:

Most newborns become visibly jaundiced during the first week of life.

- Newborns make more bilirubin as extra red blood cells are broken down.
- Newborns process bilirubin more slowly because their liver is immature.
- Newborns absorb bilirubin more easily through their gut.

During the first week of life, more than 60% of newborns become visibly jaundiced, and among breastfeeding babies, bilirubin levels can remain elevated for as long as 15 weeks (Gartner, 2007; Gourley, Kreamer, Cohnen, & Kosorok, 1999; Maruo, Nishizawa, Sato, Sawa, & Shimada, 2000).

• •

At first, bilirubin is insoluble. Before it can leave the body, it is first bound to water-soluble proteins in the blood and processed or "conjugated" by the liver, where bile takes it to the intestines and it is excreted from the baby's body in the stool.

Bilirubin leaves the body in the stools and colostrum has a laxative effect.

Frequent breastfeeding in the first 6 days lowers bilirubin levels.

Breastfeeding early and often encourages earlier passage of the bilirubin-rich meconium stools that are in the baby's intestines at birth. Because a newborn reabsorbs bilirubin so easily through his gut, if the meconium is not passed, this bilirubin may reenter the baby's bloodstream and cause blood bilirubin levels to rise. One Japanese study of 140 healthy, full-term babies found an association between the number of times the babies breastfed in the first 24 hours, meconium passage, and bilirubin levels on Day 6 (Yamauchi & Yamanouchi, 1990). On the first day of life, the fewer times the babies breastfed, the less meconium was passed, and the more babies on Day 6 had bilirubin levels higher than 14 mg/dL:

- 28.1% who fed two or fewer times
- 24.5% who fed three to four times
- 15.2% who fed five to six times
- 11.8% who fed seven to eight times
- 0% of those who fed nine more times

The babies' milk intake was also significantly associated with the number of feedings in the first 24 hours. By Day 2, the babies who breastfed 7 to 11 times their first day consumed 86% more milk than the babies who breastfed fewer than seven times during their first day. So, one way to help keep bilirubin levels moderate is to encourage frequent breastfeeding, especially during the first day of life (see Chapter 2).

• •

Moderately elevated bilirubin levels may be beneficial to newborns.

As long as bilirubin levels stay moderate, elevated levels may play an important role in protecting newborn health (McDonagh, 1990; Sedlak & Snyder, 2004). During the early weeks of life, bilirubin acts as an antioxidant while other antioxidants are absent, which can reduce the levels of free radicals that can cause injury in at-risk babies (Baranano, Rao, Ferris, & Snyder, 2002). One Dutch study found that bilirubin reduced free-radical levels in 18 preterm babies (van Zoeren-Grobben et al., 1994), while two U.S. studies found that higher bilirubin levels were associated with fewer health problems related to free-radical injury in preterm babies, such as necrotizing enterocolitis and retinopathy of prematurity (Hegyi, Goldie, & Hiatt, 1994; Heyman, Ohlsson, & Girschek, 1989).

Other research has found an association in adults between higher bilirubin levels and lower incidence of coronary heart disease and death from cancer (Djousse et al., 2001; Temme, Zhang, Schouten, & Kesteloot, 2001).

• •

The baby may have an underlying health problem if he becomes visibly jaundiced during the first 24 hours or it quickly becomes severe.

Although mild to moderate jaundice is common and possibly beneficial in the breastfed baby, this normal or "physiological jaundice" takes several days to occur and is not usually visible until the 2nd to 5th day of life. When jaundice becomes visible within the first 24 hours, this is what some call "pathological jaundice" because it is likely due to an underlying physical issue that may require treatment. Another indication of this is bilirubin levels rising faster than 5 mg/dL (85 μmmol/L) per day and higher than 17 mg/dL (290 μmol/L) in a full-term baby. (See the later point for details on bilirubin levels in a preterm baby.) Possible underlying causes include a variety of diseases or conditions that:

- Cause increased red blood cell breakdown
- Interfere with bilirubin processing in the liver
- Increase reabsorption of bilirubin by the gut

Jaundice in the first 24 hours may indicate an underlying health problem.

Examples include sepsis (blood infection), liver disease, rubella, Rh or ABO incompatibility, inborn errors of metabolism, congenital thyroid deficiency, serious bruising or cephalohematoma, and intestinal obstruction or defect. One more common condition is the blood disorder G6PD deficiency, which occurs in 11% to 13% of African Americans and is more commonly found among those from Mediterranean and southeast Asian countries (Kaplan, Herschel, Hammerman, Hoyer, & Stevenson, 2004).

With early and severe jaundice from these causes, breastfeeding can and should continue, with only rare exceptions. Some tests can pinpoint treatable causes, such as identifying blood and Rh type, direct antibody (Coombs) test, complete blood count, and red blood cell smear, as well as both a total bilirubin and a direct-reacting fraction (Gartner, 2007). But underlying causes cannot always be found (there are more than 50 known red blood cell enzyme deficiencies), so some suggest once the usual causes have been ruled out to focus on keeping bilirubin levels within safe levels (Maisels, 2006) (see next section).

Jaundice is not usually visible to the eye until bilirubin levels reach at least 4 mg/dL (68 µmmol/L). As bilirubin levels rise, the yellow color spreads from the head to the chest (about 10 mg/dL [170 µmmol/L]) to the abdomen and finally (usually when levels reach more than 15 mg/dL [255 µmol/L]) to the palms and soles of the feet (Walker, 2006). Although the color of the baby's body can provide a general indication of the severity of jaundice, research has found that bilirubin levels cannot be reliably gauged by skin color alone, as room lighting and racial differences affect perception of skin tone (Holland & Blick, 2009; Mishra et al., 2009)

As a baby's bilirubin levels rise, the yellow skin color spreads from the head down.

In most newborns, jaundice is temporary, resolves on its own, and does not require treatment (Jangaard, Fell, Dodds, & Allen, 2008; Maisels & Kring, 2006). Bilirubin levels in the full-term, healthy baby usually peak between the 3rd and 5th days of life at less than 12 mg/dl (204 µmol/L), and rarely go higher than 15 mg/dl (255 µmol/L) (Jangaard et al., 2008; Newman et al., 1999).

Most newborn jaundice does not require treatment.

Prolonged jaundice after the first 2 weeks of life was once thought to be a separate and distinct type of jaundice ("late-onset" or "breastmilk jaundice") that affected only a small percentage of breastfeeding babies. However, this is now recognized as an extension of normal newborn jaundice, and bilirubin can remain in the moderate range for many weeks, especially among babies who had higher bilirubin levels earlier.

Even after the first 2 weeks, jaundice is common among breastfeeding babies.

Bilirubin levels can remain elevated for many weeks.

By 2 to 3 weeks of age, newborns fed nonhuman milks have adult bilirubin levels of less than1.3 to 1.5 mg/dL (22 to 26 µmol/L). But at 2 to 3 weeks of age:

- One-third of breastfed babies are visibly jaundiced, with bilirubin levels above 5 mg/dL (85 µmol/L).
- One-third of breastfed babies still have elevated bilirubin levels of between 1.5 and 5 mg/dL (26 to 85 µmol/L), even though their jaundice is not visible.

In healthy, term babies, as long as bilirubin levels stay below 20 mg/dL (340 µmol/L) and are not rising rapidly, this prolonged jaundice will eventually clear without treatment within about 15 weeks (Gartner, 2007; Gourley et al., 1999). Sometimes a temporary weaning is recommended in this situation, but as long as bilirubin levels stay moderate, this is neither beneficial nor necessary. As two U.S. researchers wrote: "Breastfeeding should not be interrupted, even in the more severe cases of jaundice, either to make a diagnosis of breastmilk jaundice or for fear of kernicterus unless the serum bilirubin concentration is 20 mg/dL [340 mg/dL] or higher or rising rapidly. The proven benefits of breastfeeding far outweigh any theoretical advantage of reducing mild to moderate levels of jaundice" (Gartner & Lee, 1999, p. 441). If a baby's healthcare provider recommends temporary weaning and the mother is unhappy with this, see suggestions in Appendix C on p. 853 "Working with Healthcare Professionals."

Some suspect that the babies with prolonged elevated bilirubin at higher levels may have inherited conditions that affect bilirubin processing or blood disorders that have not yet been identified (Maruo et al., 2000). Iranian research has found an association between prolonged jaundice and urinary tract infection, so suggest this possible cause be ruled out (Pashapour, Nikibahksh, & Golmohammadlou, 2007).

With few exceptions, once a baby's bilirubin levels have reached their peak and begun to decline, they are unlikely to rise again.

Whether a baby's bilirubin levels plateau and decline naturally or whether this occurs with treatment (see later section), once the bilirubin levels have peaked and begun to decline, in most cases, they are unlikely to increase again. One exception is babies with some inherited hemolytic disorders, such as G6PD deficiency and Spherocytosis. Also, a slight rebound in bilirubin levels is common after phototherapy is stopped or when the baby begins breastfeeding again after a temporary interruption. Any rebound should be slight, but should be closely followed.

Monitoring Bilirubin Levels

Monitoring newborn jaundice is vital because, although rare, high bilirubin levels can cause severe health problems.

Very high bilirubin levels are rare in full-term, healthy babies. One Canadian prospective study of 56,019 mostly white babies born at least 35 weeks gestation found that only 0.6% had total serum bilirubin levels of ≥19 milligrams of bilirubin per deciliter of blood (or mg/dL) (325 μmol/L) (Jangaard et al., 2008). Race also plays a role. One study found that Chinese babies were at a 64% higher risk of jaundice compared to non-Chinese babies (Huang, Tai, Wong, Lee, & Yong, 2009), which is generally true for all babies of Asian origin.

For bilirubin to be excreted in the stool, it must first be processed by the liver, or "conjugated" (also known as bound or direct), a form that is harmless to the newborn. It is the unprocessed bilirubin—the "unconjugated" (free or indirect) bilirubin—that poses a risk because this form can be reabsorbed by the intestines, spread to other parts of the body via the bloodstream, and if levels get too high (≥30 mg/dL [510 μmol/L]), can cause brain damage. Because the newborn's gut is sterile, conjugated (bound) bilirubin is more easily transformed to unconjugated (free) bilirubin in the gut, which then returns to the liver for reprocessing.

Bilirubin levels that are higher than 25 mg/dL can cause severe health problems such as bilirubin enchephatopathy and kernicterus.

Although bilirubin may be beneficial if kept at moderate levels, when at the rare times it exceeds 25 mg/dL (425 μmol/L), it may cross the blood-brain barrier, causing a condition known as bilirubin encephalopathy. The early symptoms of bilirubin encephalopathy include lethargy and feeding refusal and can eventually progress to a high-pitched cry and neurological symptoms, such as seizures, arching back of the head and spine, and even fever (Gartner, 2007). If not treated promptly, the baby may develop kernicterus, or permanent neurological damage, which can cause lifelong problems, such as cerebral palsy, hearing loss, developmental delays, paralysis, mental retardation, and even death.

Although not all newborns with bilirubin levels higher than 25 mg/dL (425 μmol/L) develop kernicterus, treatment should be started before kernicterus becomes a risk (Newman, Liljestrand, & Escobar, 2003). In one U.S. study of 51,387 babies, bilirubin levels reached 30 mg/dL in only 1 in 10,000 (Newman et al., 1999). In the large Canadian study mentioned previously, not one of its 56,019 babies developed kernicterus. One expert estimates the incidence of kernicterus to be between 1 in 100,000 and 1 in 1,000,000 newborns (Ip, Lau et al., 2004).

Bilirubin levels can be measured with a blood test or by less invasive methods.

Observing the spread of yellow skin tone from the head down gives a general indication of bilirubin levels, but it is not reliable enough to determine when a baby needs treatment. Not long ago, bilirubin levels could only be confirmed through painful blood tests that often needed to be done repeatedly.

Today the less-invasive transcutaneous bilirubinometry is often used to provide an initial bilirubin screening by gently pressing an instrument against the baby's skin that reflects light through the skin to the underlying tissues and back into the instrument to calculate the intensity of the skin's yellow color. Research has found these instruments to be more reliable than the eye alone in gauging the severity of the baby's jaundice, and they are often used first, so blood is drawn only from babies in need of medical follow-up (Holland & Blick, 2009; Jangaard, Curtis, & Goldbloom, 2006; Thayyil & Marriott, 2005; Varvarigou et al., 2009).

It is recommended that all healthcare institutions routinely screen every newborn for jaundice before discharge.

To prevent dangerously high bilirubin levels, hospitals are asked to screen all newborns at hospital discharge (AAP, 2004; Johnson & Bhutani, 1998). This screening often involves a combination of checking babies' skin color visually, determining any risk factors, and/or using one or more of the methods for checking bilirubin levels described in the previous point (Keren et al., 2005; Maisels, Deridder, Kring, & Balasubramaniam, 2009). Some large hospital systems have successfully implemented screening strategies that have reduced both the number of newborns who developed dangerously high bilirubin levels and the rate of rehospitalizations for jaundice (Eggert, Wiedmeier, Wilson, & Christensen, 2006).

Close follow-up with a healthcare provider after discharge is strongly recommended.

Another way to prevent babies from developing dangerously high bilirubin levels is to arrange for early follow-up after hospital discharge. The American Academy of Pediatrics recommends that all babies be seen by a healthcare provider between 3 and 5 days of age (Gartner et al., 2005). If the healthcare provider discovers that a newborn is not breastfeeding well at this visit, the mother and baby can be referred for skilled breastfeeding help. Babies born at less than 38 weeks gestation are considered at higher risk and require even closer monitoring (AAP, 2004; Sarici et al., 2004).

Jaundice Treatments

When newborn jaundice is diagnosed, it can be upsetting, put breastfeeding at risk, and change a mother's behaviors and attitudes.

A mother whose baby needs treatment for jaundice may feel worried, anxious, and upset, depending in part on her familiarity with newborn jaundice, how well it is explained, and whether its dangers are overemphasized. If she is given a medical explanation while she is upset, she will probably forget many of the specifics. If so, suggest she contact her baby's healthcare provider to discuss it again when she is feeling calmer. Even something as simple as the healthcare provider encouraging the mother to breastfeed has been found to greatly influence her decisions (Willis, Hannon, & Scrimshaw, 2002). Offer the mother moral support with comments like, "You have obviously put a lot of thought into making the best decision for your baby," or "You are wise to find out more about your options."

If treatment for jaundice involves separation, feeding formula, or temporary weaning, this can increase a mother's anxiety and affect her feelings about breastfeeding. If she is discouraged from spending time with or breastfeeding her baby, she may wonder whether her milk might be causing the jaundice or if it has any value to her baby (Hannon, Willis, & Scrimshaw, 2001). If getting her baby back to the breast is a challenge, this adds to her stress and worry.

Treatments for jaundice and how they are handled, can increase a mother's anxiety and her feelings about breastfeeding.

No negative long-term health effects have been associated with mild to moderate newborn jaundice (Ip, Chung et al., 2004). But even so, treating jaundice can affect mothers' behavior and attitudes. U.S. research found that after the jaundice resolved, many of these mothers considered their baby at-risk or "vulnerable." One U.S. study of 209 mothers found that 1 month after hospital discharge, mothers whose babies had been jaundiced were more likely to have stopped breastfeeding (42% versus 19%), even though more mothers of jaundiced babies started breastfeeding at birth (79% versus 61%) (Kemper, Forsyth, & McCarthy, 1989). Both the jaundiced and non-jaundiced babies had similar numbers of health problems, but the mothers of the jaundiced babies were more likely to take their baby to well-baby checkups and more than twice as likely to take the baby to his healthcare provider for a sick visit (not counting bilirubin checks) or to the hospital emergency room.

Another U.S. study followed mothers of initially jaundiced and non-jaundiced babies at 6 months (Kemper, Forsyth, & McCarthy, 1990). The mothers whose babies were jaundiced had more feeding problems, were less likely to be breastfeeding, and were more likely to have tried a special formula. They were also more likely to consider their baby's minor illnesses as serious and to have made at least one trip to the emergency room with their child. The authors concluded that jaundice treatments have adverse effects on breastfeeding and may affect a mother's relationship with her baby.

• •

When the baby's bilirubin levels decline after treatment, they are unlikely to go up again by much.

Once a baby's bilirubin levels have peaked, leveled off, and begun to decline, they are unlikely to go up again. The exception is a slight rebound that is common after phototherapy or when the baby begins breastfeeding again after a temporary weaning. If this rebound occurs, the rise in bilirubin is usually slight.

Optimizing Breastfeeding

Effective breastfeeding does not increase a baby's risk for severe jaundice, but inadequate milk intake does.

Over the years, some studies have found breastfeeding to be a risk factor for severe jaundice (Dahms et al., 1973; Schneider, 1986). While it is true that breastfeeding newborns have naturally higher bilirubin levels than non-breastfeeding babies, most research that has linked breastfeeding and severe jaundice did not provide specifics on breastfeeding and postpartum practices, such as number and length of feedings, whether mothers and babies were separated or together, and whether newborns received water or formula supplements. In studies in which babies breastfed within an hour after birth, roomed-in, breastfed on cue at least 10 times per day, and no supplements were given, jaundice was equally likely to occur in both breastfed and non-breastfed babies (Bertini, Dani, Tronchin, & Rubaltelli, 2001; Gartner & Herschel, 2001; Huang et al., 2009).

In the American Academy of Pediatrics' practice guidelines, the first of its 10 key elements is "Promote and support successful breastfeeding," and exclusive breastfeeding is considered a risk factor for severe jaundice only if it is "not going well and weight loss is excessive" (AAP, 2004, pp. 298, 301).

Newborn jaundice is the most common reason babies are readmitted to the hospital after discharge, in part because breastfeeding and postpartum practices are often less-than-optimal and many of these babies did not breastfeed well initially (Brown et al., 1999; Tyler & Hellings, 2005). As in adults, when babies are deprived of adequate nourishment, bilirubin levels rise. Some call this "starvation jaundice." A U.S. expert wrote:

Breastfeeding at least 10 to 12 times per day can help prevent and resolve jaundice.

> This is not normal, however, and is a reflection of inadequate breastfeeding practices in most Western medical settings where infants are born. These deficiencies in breastfeeding practices include delays in initiation, insufficient frequency of suckling, poor positioning, and truncation of feeding sessions. Several studies have demonstrated that a breastfeeding frequency of approximately 10 to 12 sessions per day starting on the 1st day of life results in the lowest serum bilirubin concentrations on the 3rd day of life and prevents early starvation jaundice in normal infants (Gartner, 2007, p. 261).

Strategies for encouraging early and frequent breastfeeding include:

- Skin-to-skin contact within the first few hours after birth
- Keeping baby unswaddled tummy down on mother's body as much as possible in the early days to trigger inborn feeding behaviors

See chapter 2, "Breastfeeding Rhythms" for more details. Optimal breastfeeding helps to prevent high bilirubin levels during the first week of life, which also helps prevent prolonged jaundice at higher levels later (Gartner, 2007).

A baby's weight loss after birth and color of stools can be used as indicators of early breastfeeding effectiveness.

Since a maximum average weight loss of about 6% of birthweight occurs by Day 3 in unsupplemented breastfed newborns, a weight loss of more than 7% to 10% or continued weight loss after Day 4 puts a baby at risk for jaundice and indicates the need for skilled breastfeeding help (AAP, 2004; Gartner, 2007). According to the practice guidelines of the American Academy of Pediatrics, by the 4th day of life, each day a newborn should have four to six thoroughly wet diapers and three to four yellow stools. Dark, meconium stools on Day 4 are a red flag to take a closer look at breastfeeding.

By Day 4, dark meconium stools are a red flag.

To increase milk intake at feedings, suggest the mother breastfeed more often each day and use breast compression.

The first step in increasing milk intake is to breastfeed more often (Gartner, 2007). Be sure the baby feels the mother's body against his torso so that his feeding behaviors are activated (see chapter 1). If a baby is swaddled in a separate bed, this can suppress feeding behaviors and decrease overall number of feedings (Bystrova et al., 2007).

If the baby takes the breast but does not breastfeed actively, suggest the mother try breast compression, which is described on p. 804 in the "Techniques" appendix. A variation of this is called "alternate breast massage." Both use pressure to stimulate faster milk flow at the breast, keep the baby active and interested for longer, and increase the fat content of the milk (Stutte, 1988).

If high bilirubin levels make the baby lethargic, suggest laid-back positions to trigger feeding behaviors.

Some severely jaundiced babies appear sleepy or disinterested in breastfeeding. Rather than waiting until the baby is awake to feed, encourage the mother to lean back into a comfortable, well-supported, semi-reclining position and lay her baby on her body tummy down (see Chapter 1). The feel of her body against his will trigger inborn feeding behaviors. Suggest she help guide her baby to the breast even while asleep, which can stimulate active breastfeeding (Colson et al., 2003).

If despite the mother's efforts the baby is unresponsive and not breastfeeding actively, strongly encourage her to begin expressing her milk. The baby's milk intake is important to resolving the jaundice and the stimulation of milk expression is vital for the mother's milk production. If the mother must initiate milk production mostly with milk expression, see the strategies described on p. 466 in the chapter, "Milk Expression and Storage."

Discuss feeding methods with the mother. Her milk can be fed using an at-breast supplementer, which also stimulates milk production, or it can be fed by spoon, cup, eyedropper, feeding syringe, or bottle. For details on the pros and cons of each method, see Table B1 on p. 814 in Appendix B, "Tools and Products."

Feeding Formula

Expressed mother's milk and donor milk are the first and second choices if the baby needs more milk than he can take at the breast.

When bilirubin levels rise high enough to be of concern in a full-term, healthy baby, it is usually because the baby has not been getting enough milk for one or more of the following reasons:

- Too little time spent breastfeeding effectively, either too few feedings or too little time actively breastfeeding each time
- Breastfeeding ineffectively because the baby is tongue-tied, has an unusual palate, or other infant factors (see the chapter "Challenges at the Breast")
- Low milk production, possibly related to lack of stimulation (above)

One U.S. study found that as many as 22% of 3-day-old newborns did not breastfeed optimally (Dewey, Nommsen-Rivers, Heinig, & Cohen, 2003).

Whatever the reason for insufficient milk intake, the baby still needs to be fed. When considering a supplement, the first choice is the mother's own expressed milk. If the mother cannot express as much milk as the baby will take, the second choice, if available, is donor human milk (Herschel, 2003).

Elemental formula is the third choice for supplementing a jaundiced baby.

When a jaundiced baby needs a supplement and mother's own milk and donor human milk are not available, elemental (casein–hydrolysate) formulas are recommended over other infant formulas for two reasons:

- They reduce bilirubin levels faster than other formulas because they contain an ingredient that prevents bilirubin in the baby's intestine from being reabsorbed (Gourley et al., 1999).
- They are less likely to sensitize at-risk newborns to allergy and diabetes.

If the baby is fed formula, let the mother know that this is temporary and suggest she work on increasing her milk production by expressing her milk and breastfeeding frequently until she is making enough milk to meet her baby's need. Suggest she also consider using an at-breast supplementer to increase breast stimulation when the formula is given.

• •

Formula may be recommended as a supplement to breastfeeding or as a temporary replacement for breastfeeding.

When high bilirubin levels are primarily due to lack of milk intake, even before the baby's bilirubin reaches the level at which phototherapy is recommended (see next section), some healthcare providers suggest formula supplements or interrupting breastfeeding temporarily and feeding only formula. Although no short- or long-term ill effects have been associated with phototherapy (Ip, Chung et al., 2004), it can be a costly treatment and lengthen hospital stay, so some healthcare providers consider this as a more cost-effective alternative.

Depending on the baby's bilirubin levels, giving formula supplements while breastfeeding may be recommended as a 12-hour trial or a 24-hour interruption of breastfeeding with or without phototherapy, which may be extended to 48 hours if the baby's bilirubin levels have not decreased significantly.

Breastfeeding should be continued, if at all possible during treatment for jaundice.

In its practice guidelines, the American Academy of Pediatrics wrote: "In breastfed infants who require phototherapy, the AAP recommends that if possible, breastfeeding should be continued. It is also an option to interrupt temporarily breastfeeding and substitute formula. This can reduce bilirubin levels and/or enhance the efficacy of phototherapy" (AAP, 2004, p. 303). If the baby's healthcare provider recommends the baby be given formula and the mother wants to explore other alternatives, see p. 853 in Appendix C, "Working with Healthcare Professionals" for strategies.

A temporary weaning puts breastfeeding at risk. Whether a mother interrupts breastfeeding for 12, 24, or 48 hours, suggest she express her milk to stay comfortable and to establish or maintain her milk production. For strategies to maintain milk production with milk expression, see the chapter "Milk Expression and Storage." Also, be sure the mother understands the value of her milk and the reasons for the interruption. Many mothers of jaundiced babies assume that formula is recommended because their milk is "bad" for their baby, which can lead to feelings of guilt and undermine continued breastfeeding (Hannon et al., 2001; Willis et al., 2002).

Phototherapy

Phototherapy uses special fluorescent or spot lights to lower bilirubin levels faster.

During phototherapy, the baby is typically laid nearly naked with his eyes covered under a white, blue, or green fluorescent light (called "bili-lights"). This light is absorbed by the bilirubin under baby's skin, changing it to a water-soluble form that allows the baby to eliminate it without needing to first process it in the liver. Phototherapy can be used for all types of jaundice and is sometimes used along with other treatments. Phototherapy is a relatively safe procedure that has been found to have fewer side effects than alternatives like exchange transfusions (see next section) (Ip, Chung et al., 2004).

The bilirubin level at which phototherapy should be started depends on the baby's age and his risk factors.

As with hypoglycemia, one level (of bilirubin or blood sugar) does not reflect the many factors that determine the effect of that level on an individual baby. With a jaundiced newborn, some of the factors that affect when phototherapy should begin include the baby's gestational age, how soon after birth his jaundice appeared, how fast his bilirubin levels are rising, the compatibility of his blood type with his mother, any bruising, a sibling with a history of jaundice, and his race.

The American Academy of Pediatrics' practice guidelines for starting phototherapy on hospitalized newborns at least 35 weeks gestation first divide newborns by risk into three groups (AAP, 2004)(Table 7.2):

- Lower risk (≥38 weeks at birth and healthy)
- Medium risk (≥38 weeks at birth with risk factors or 35 to 35 6/7 weeks at birth and healthy)
- Higher risk (35 to 35 6/7 weeks at birth with risk factors)

They define major risk factors as:

- Bilirubin levels in the high-risk zone (if 3 days or older >16 mg/dl)
- Jaundice visible during the first 24 hours
- Blood group incompatibility or other hemolytic disease
- An older sibling who received phototherapy
- Significant bruising or cephalohematoma
- Exclusive breastfeeding with feeding problems and/or weight loss ≥12%
- East Asian race

Along with the baby's bilirubin level, the rate at which it is rising is also important. A rise of more than 0.5 mg/dL (8.5 μmol/L) per hour puts the baby at increased risk.

Table 7.2. Bilirubin Levels at which Phototherapy is Recommended in Babies Born ≥35 Weeks

Baby's Age in Hours	**Lower Risk**	**Medium Risk**	**Higher Risk**
24 Hours	12 mg/dL (204 μmol/L)	10 mg/dL (170 μmol/L)	8 mg/dL (136 μmol/L)
48 Hours	15 mg/dL (255 μmol/L)	13 mg/dL (221 μmol/L)	11 mg/dL (187 μmol/L)
72 Hours	17 mg/dL (289 μmol/L)	15 mg/dL (255 μmol/L)	13 mg/dL (221 μmol/L)
96 Hours	20 mg/dL (340 μmol/L)	17 mg/dL (289 μmol/L)	14 mg/dL (238 μmol/L)
5 Days or Older	21 mg/dL (357 μmol/L)	18 mg/dL (306 μmol/L)	15 mg/dL (255 μmol/L)

Adapted from (AAP, 2004)

Maximum allowable bilirubin levels are lower in babies born earlier than 35 weeks.

A preterm baby is at greater risk of brain injury at lower bilirubin levels because his immature liver is less effective at processing bilirubin and his blood-brain barrier is less effective at blocking it. Adding illness (such as infection, oxygen deprivation, and acidosis) to prematurity increases the risk of injury at lower levels. Safe bilirubin levels for the preemie are determined individually based on the baby's gestational age, weight, and health.

Premature infants are at higher risk for problems caused by elevated bilirubin levels.

If mother and baby are separated during phototherapy, discuss other options.

Suggest the mother ask about the following alternatives to separation during phototherapy. In some hospitals, babies are given phototherapy in the nursery, but mothers are welcome to sit near the baby and breastfeed whenever he shows feeding cues. In other hospitals, the bili-lights are set up in the mother's room to make it easier for her to breastfeed the baby under the lights or to take the baby out from under the lights to breastfeed when he is ready (Kovach, 2002). The baby doesn't have to be under the lights continuously for phototherapy to be effective. In some areas, phototherapy units are available for home or hospital use that consist of fiberoptic blankets that can be wrapped around the baby, so the mother can breastfeed while the baby receives treatment without the need for eye patches.

Breastfeeding often during phototherapy can help meet the baby's need for extra fluids.

Babies lose more water than usual through their skin and stools during phototherapy. Frequent breastfeeding can help offset this increased water loss. Be sure the mother knows that a baby's stools become looser during phototherapy as the bilirubin in the stools increases.

In some cases, formula may be recommended as a supplement or a replacement for breastfeeding during phototherapy.

See the previous section "Feeding Formula" for more details. U.S. research has found that replacing breastfeeding with formula during phototherapy brings down bilirubin levels faster than continuing to breastfeed during phototherapy (Martinez et al., 1993). However, there are no short- or long-term negative health outcomes associated with mild to moderate jaundice, and this strategy has the potential to undermine breastfeeding, so this recommendation only makes sense if bilirubin levels are high enough to be of real concern (Ip, Chung et al., 2004).

Exchange Transfusions

If a baby's bilirubin levels are dangerously high or he has neurological symptoms, an exchange transfusion is recommended.

If a baby is at or near dangerously high bilirubin levels (see Table 7.3) or is having symptoms of neurological injury, an exchange transfusion is the fastest way to bring down bilirubin levels. During an exchange transfusion, small amounts of the baby's blood are continuously replaced with donor blood. Because safe bilirubin levels are lower in sick or very preterm babies, exchange transfusions may be recommended at lower levels in these at-risk babies.

Exchange transfusions are used less today than in years past due to the use of RhoGAM to prevent severe jaundice from Rh incompatibility. There are more health risks associated with exchange transfusions than phototherapy, so phototherapy is routinely used first to prevent the need for this procedure (AAP, 2004).

Breastfeeding can continue before and after exchange transfusions.

The baby should continue to be breastfed because withholding feedings can increase bilirubin levels (Gartner, 2007).

Table 7.3. Bilirubin Levels at Which Exchange Transfusions are Recommended in Babies Born ≥35 Weeks

Baby's Age in Hours	Lower Risk	Medium Risk	Higher Risk
24 Hours	19 mg/dL (323 μmol/L)	17 mg/dL (289 μmol/L)	15 mg/dL (255 μmol/L)
48 Hours	22 mg/dL (374 μmol/L)	19 mg/dL (323 μmol/L)	17 mg/dL (289 μmol/L)
72 Hours	24 mg/dL (408 μmol/L)	21 mg/dL (357 μmol/L)	18 mg/dL (306 μmol/L)
96 Hours or Older	25 mg/dL (425 μmol/L)	22 mg/dL (374 μmol/L)	19 mg/dL (323 μmol/L)

Adapted from (AAP, 2004)

Other Jaundice Treatments

Some medications can bring down bilirubin levels.

The drug tin-mesoporphyrin has been found to be an effective treatment for jaundice by preventing hemoglobin from being converted to bilirubin (Kappas, Drummond, Munson, & Marshall, 2001; Martinez, Garcia, Otheguy, Drummond, & Kappas, 1999; Suresh, Martin, & Soll, 2003). At this writing, this drug has not yet been approved for use in the U.S. by the Food and Drug Administration (FDA) because the safety of this treatment has not been determined.

Other drugs have been used occasionally to treat jaundice. One example is the anti-seizure medication Phenobarbital, but it takes about 6 days before it significantly lowers bilirubin levels. Cholestyramine has also been used during phototherapy, but it has not been found to be very effective (L. Gartner, personal communication, January 10, 2010).

What to Avoid

Some drugs or other treatments given to mother or baby can increase the risk of injury from jaundice.

Aspirin, other salicylates, ibruprofen, and certain sulfa drugs can increase the risk of injury from jaundice by preventing bilirubin from binding to the protein in the baby's blood (Gartner, 2007; Zecca et al., 2009). Other drugs and treatments that can have this same effect include the antibiotic sulfisoxazole (Gantrisin), benzyl alcohol, and its byproduct, benzoic acid, a preservative in some IV fluids. When a newborn is jaundiced, these treatments should be avoided and, if needed, a substitute found.

Because only 2% of a baby's bilirubin is excreted in his urine and 98% in his stools, glucose or plain water supplements do not prevent jaundice or bring down a newborn's bilirubin levels. In fact, one U.S. study found that water supplements were associated with higher bilirubin levels (Nicoll, Ginsburg, & Tripp, 1982). This may be because water supplements leave the baby feeling full without stimulating meconium passage or providing nourishment. Another U.S. study found that babies fed large volumes of glucose water during their first 3 days took less milk per feeding by the 4th day and were more likely than the babies not fed glucose water to be jaundiced (Kuhr & Paneth, 1982). U.K. research found plain water supplements had no effect on bilirubin levels (de Carvalho, Hall, & Harvey, 1981). As a result, health organizations in both the U.S. and Canada recommend against giving plain or glucose water supplements to newborns (AAP, 2004; CPS, 2007).

Glucose or plain water supplements do not prevent jaundice and may even increase bilirubin levels, so they should be avoided.

In years past, some mothers were advised to undress their baby to their diaper and lay him near a window because, like phototherapy, indirect sunlight could help bring down bilirubin levels. However, unlike phototherapy, it is impossible to gauge the amount of light the baby receives and its effect on his bilirubin levels, so this is not a reliable jaundice treatment. Also, direct sunlight on a newborn can cause a dangerous increase in body temperature and burn his skin. To prevent bilirubin levels from going dangerously high, a jaundiced baby should be promptly seen and evaluated by a healthcare provider.

Putting the baby in indirect sunlight is no longer recommended to treat jaundice.

REFERENCES

AAP. (1993). American Academy of Pediatrics Committee on Fetus and Newborn: Routine evaluation of blood pressure, hematocrit, and glucose in newborns. *Pediatrics, 92*(3), 474-476.

AAP. (2004). Management of hyperbilirubinemia in the newborn infant 35 or more weeks of gestation. *Pediatrics, 114*(1), 297-316.

Baranano, D. E., Rao, M., Ferris, C. D., & Snyder, S. H. (2002). Biliverdin reductase: a major physiologic cytoprotectant. *Proceedings of the National Academy of Sciences of the United States of America, 99*(25), 16093-16098.

Bergman, N. J., Linley, L. L., & Fawcus, S. R. (2004). Randomized controlled trial of skin-to-skin contact from birth versus conventional incubator for physiological stabilization in 1200- to 2199-gram newborns. *Acta Paediatrica, 93*(6), 779-785.

Bertini, G., Dani, C., Tronchin, M., & Rubaltelli, F. F. (2001). Is breastfeeding really favoring early neonatal jaundice? *Pediatrics, 107*(3), E41.

Brown, A. K., Damus, K., Kim, M. H., King, K., Harper, R., Campbell, D., et al. (1999). Factors relating to readmission of term and near-term neonates in the first two weeks of life. Early Discharge Survey Group of the Health Professional Advisory Board of the Greater New York Chapter of the March of Dimes. *Journal of Perinatal Medicine, 27*(4), 263-275.

Bystrova, K., Matthiesen, A. S., Widstrom, A. M., Ransjo-Arvidson, A. B., Welles-Nystrom, B., Vorontsov, I., et al. (2007). The effect of Russian Maternity Home routines on breastfeeding and neonatal weight loss with special reference to swaddling. *Early Human Development, 83*(1), 29-39.

Chertok, I. R., Raz, I., Shoham, I., Haddad, H., & Wiznitzer, A. (2009). Effects of early breastfeeding on neonatal glucose levels of term infants born to women with gestational diabetes. *Journal of Human Nutrition and Dietetics, 22*(2), 166-169.

Christensson, K., Siles, C., Moreno, L., Belaustequi, A., De La Fuente, P., Lagercrantz, H., et al. (1992). Temperature, metabolic adaptation and crying in healthy full-term newborns cared for skin-to-skin or in a cot. *Acta Paediatrica, 81*(6-7), 488-493.

Colson, S., DeRooy, L., & Hawdon, J. (2003). Biological Nurturing increases duration of breastfeeding for a vulnerable cohort. *MIDIRS Midwifery Digest, 13*(1), 92-97.

Cornblath, M., Hawdon, J. M., Williams, A. F., Aynsley-Green, A., Ward-Platt, M. P., Schwartz, R., et al. (2000). Controversies regarding definition of neonatal hypoglycemia: suggested operational thresholds. *Pediatrics, 105*(5), 1141-1145.

Cornblath, M., & Ichord, R. (2000). Hypoglycemia in the neonate. *Seminars in Perinatology, 24*(2), 136-149.

CPS. (2007). Guidelines for detection, management and prevention of hyperbilirubinemia in term and late preterm newborn infants (35 or more weeks' gestation) - Summary. *Paediatrics & Child Health, 12*(5), 401-418.

D'Harlingue, A. E., & Durand, D. J. (1993). Recognition, Stabilization and transport of the high-risk newborn. In *Care of the High Risk Neonate* (pp. 62-85). Philadelphia, PA: Saunders.

Dahms, B. B., Krauss, A. N., Gartner, L. M., Klain, D. B., Soodalter, J., & Auld, P. A. (1973). Breast feeding and serum bilirubin values during the first 4 days of life. *Journal of Pediatrics, 83*(6), 1049-1054.

de Carvalho, M., Hall, M., & Harvey, D. (1981). Effects of water supplementation on physiological jaundice in breast-fed babies. *Archives of Disease in Childhood, 56*(7), 568-569.

de Rooy, L., & Hawdon, J. (2002). Nutritional factors that affect the postnatal metabolic adaptation of full-term small- and large-for-gestational-age infants. *Pediatrics, 109*(3), E42.

DePuy, A. M., Coassolo, K. M., Som, D. A., & Smulian, J. C. (2009). Neonatal hypoglycemia in term, nondiabetic pregnancies. *American Journal of Obstetrics and Gynecology, 200*(5), e45-51.

Dewey, K. G., Nommsen-Rivers, L. A., Heinig, M. J., & Cohen, R. J. (2003). Risk factors for suboptimal infant breastfeeding behavior, delayed onset of lactation, and excess neonatal weight loss. *Pediatrics, 112*(3 Pt 1), 607-619.

Djousse, L., Levy, D., Cupples, L. A., Evans, J. C., D'Agostino, R. B., & Ellison, R. C. (2001). Total serum bilirubin and risk of cardiovascular disease in the Framingham offspring study. *American Journal of Cardiology, 87*(10), 1196-1200; A1194, 1197.

Eggert, L. D., Wiedmeier, S. E., Wilson, J., & Christensen, R. D. (2006). The effect of instituting a prehospital-discharge newborn bilirubin screening program in an 18-hospital health system. *Pediatrics, 117*(5), e855-862.

Eidelman, A. I. (2001). Hypoglycemia and the breastfed neonate. *Pediatric Clinics of North America, 48*(2), 377-387.

Gartner, L. M. (2007). Hyperbilirubinemia and breastfeeding. In T. W. Hale & P. E. Hartmann (Eds.), *Hale & Hartmann's Textbook of Human Lactation* (pp. 255-270). Amarillo, TX: Hale Publishing.

Gartner, L. M., & Herschel, M. (2001). Jaundice and breastfeeding. *Pediatric Clinics of North America, 48*(2), 389-399.

Gartner, L. M., & Lee, K. S. (1999). Jaundice in the breastfed infant. *Clinics in Perinatology, 26*(2), 431-445, vii.

Gartner, L. M., Morton, J., Lawrence, R. A., Naylor, A. J., O'Hare, D., Schanler, R. J., et al. (2005). Breastfeeding and the use of human milk. *Pediatrics, 115*(2), 496-506.

Gourley, G. R., Kreamer, B., Cohnen, M., & Kosorok, M. R. (1999). Neonatal jaundice and diet. *Archives of Pediatrics and Adolescent Medicine, 153*(2), 184-188.

Hagedorn, M. I. E., & Gardner, S. L. (1999). Hypoglycemia: in the newborn, part 1: Pathophysiology and nursing management. *Mother Baby J, 4*, 15-21.

Hannon, P. R., Willis, S. K., & Scrimshaw, S. C. (2001). Persistence of maternal concerns surrounding neonatal jaundice: an exploratory study. *Archives of Pediatrics and Adolescent Medicine, 155*(12), 1357-1363.

Hawdon, J., & Williams, A. F. (2000). Formula supplements given to healthy breastfed preterm babies inhibit postatal metabolic adaptation: Results of a randomised controlled trial. [abstract]. *Archives of Disease in Childhood, 82*(suppl 1).

Hawdon, J. M. (1999). Hypoglycaemia and the neonatal brain. *European Journal of Pediatrics, 158 Suppl 1*, S9-S12.

Hawdon, J. M., Ward Platt, M. P., & Aynsley-Green, A. (1992). Patterns of metabolic adaptation for preterm and term infants in the first neonatal week. *Archives of Disease in Childhood, 67*(4 Spec No), 357-365.

Hawdon, J. M., Ward Platt, M. P., McPhail, S., Cameron, H., & Walkinshaw, S. A. (1992). Prediction of impaired metabolic adaptation by antenatal Doppler studies in small for gestational age fetuses. *Archives of Disease in Childhood, 67*(7 Spec No), 789-792.

Hegyi, T., Goldie, E., & Hiatt, M. (1994). The protective role of bilirubin in oxygen-radical diseases of the preterm infant. *Journal of Perinatology, 14*(4), 296-300.

Herschel, M. (2003). *Jaundice and Breastfeeding: Independent Study Module #12*. Schaumburg, IL: La Leche League International.

Heyman, E., Ohlsson, A., & Girschek, P. (1989). Retinopathy of prematurity and bilirubin. *New England Journal of Medicine, 320*(4), 256.

Holland, L., & Blick, K. (2009). Implementing and validating transcutaneous bilirubinometry for neonates. *American Journal of Clinical Pathology, 132*(4), 555-561.

Hoseth, E., Joergensen, A., Ebbesen, F., & Moeller, M. (2000). Blood glucose levels in a population of healthy, breast fed, term infants of appropriate size for gestational age. *Archives of Disease in Childhood. Fetal and Neonatal Edition, 83*(2), F117-119.

Huang, A., Tai, B. C., Wong, L. Y., Lee, J., & Yong, E. L. (2009). Differential risk for early breastfeeding jaundice in a multi-ethnic Asian cohort. *Annals of the Academy of Medicine, Singapore, 38*(3), 217-224.

Inder, T. (2008). How low can I go? The impact of hypoglycemia on the immature brain. *Pediatrics, 122*(2), 440-441.

Ip, S., Chung, M., Kulig, J., O'Brien, R., Sege, R., Glicken, S., et al. (2004). An evidence-based review of important issues concerning neonatal hyperbilirubinemia. *Pediatrics, 114*(1), e130-153.

Ip, S., Lau, J., Chung, M., Kulig, J., Sege, R., Glicken, S., et al. (2004). Hyperbilirubinemia and kernicterus: 50 years later. *Pediatrics, 114*(1), 263-264.

Jangaard, K., Curtis, H., & Goldbloom, R. (2006). Estimation of bilirubin using BiliChektrade mark, a transcutaneous bilirubin measurement device: Effects of gestational age and use of phototherapy. *Paediatrics & Child Health, 11*(2), 79-83.

Jangaard, K. A., Fell, D. B., Dodds, L., & Allen, A. C. (2008). Outcomes in a population of healthy term and near-term infants with serum bilirubin levels of >or=325 micromol/L (>or=19 mg/dL) who were born in Nova Scotia, Canada, between 1994 and 2000. *Pediatrics, 122*(1), 119-124.

Johnson, L., & Bhutani, V. K. (1998). Guidelines for management of the jaundiced term and near-term infant. *Clinics in Perinatology, 25*(3), 555-574, viii.

Kaplan, M., Herschel, M., Hammerman, C., Hoyer, J. D., & Stevenson, D. K. (2004). Hyperbilirubinemia among African American, glucose-6-phosphate dehydrogenase-deficient neonates. *Pediatrics, 114*(2), e213-219.

Kappas, A., Drummond, G. S., Munson, D. P., & Marshall, J. R. (2001). Sn-Mesoporphyrin interdiction of severe hyperbilirubinemia in Jehovah's Witness newborns as an alternative to exchange transfusion. *Pediatrics, 108*(6), 1374-1377.

Kemper, K., Forsyth, B., & McCarthy, P. (1989). Jaundice, terminating breast-feeding, and the vulnerable child. *Pediatrics, 84*(5), 773-778.

Kemper, K. J., Forsyth, B. W., & McCarthy, P. L. (1990). Persistent perceptions of vulnerability following neonatal jaundice. *American Journal of Diseases of Children, 144*(2), 238-241.

Keren, R., Bhutani, V. K., Luan, X., Nihtianova, S., Cnaan, A., & Schwartz, J. S. (2005). Identifying newborns at risk of significant hyperbilirubinaemia: a comparison of two recommended approaches. *Archives of Disease in Childhood, 90*(4), 415-421.

Kovach, A. C. (2002). A 5-year follow-up study of hospital breastfeeding policies in the Philadelphia area: a comparison with the ten steps. *Journal of Human Lactation, 18*(2), 144-154.

Kuhr, M., & Paneth, N. (1982). Feeding practices and early neonatal jaundice. *Journal of Pediatric Gastroenterology and Nutrition, 1*(4), 485-488.

Linder, N., Moser, A. M., Asli, I., Gale, R., Livoff, A., & Tamir, I. (1989). Suckling stimulation test for neonatal tremor. *Archives of Disease in Childhood, 64*(1 Spec No), 44-46.

Maisels, M. J. (2006). What's in a name? Physiologic and pathologic jaundice: the conundrum of defining normal bilirubin levels in the newborn. *Pediatrics, 118*(2), 805-807.

Maisels, M. J., Deridder, J. M., Kring, E. A., & Balasubramaniam, M. (2009). Routine transcutaneous bilirubin measurements combined with clinical risk factors improve the prediction of subsequent hyperbilirubinemia. *Journal of Perinatology, 29*(9), 612-617.

Maisels, M. J., & Kring, E. (2006). Transcutaneous bilirubin levels in the first 96 hours in a normal newborn population of > or = 35 weeks' gestation. *Pediatrics, 117*(4), 1169-1173.

Martinez, J. C., Garcia, H. O., Otheguy, L. E., Drummond, G. S., & Kappas, A. (1999). Control of severe hyperbilirubinemia in full-term newborns with the inhibitor of bilirubin production Sn-mesoporphyrin. *Pediatrics, 103*(1), 1-5.

Martinez, J. C., Maisels, M. J., Otheguy, L., Garcia, H., Savorani, M., Mogni, B., et al. (1993). Hyperbilirubinemia in the breast-fed newborn: a controlled trial of four interventions. *Pediatrics, 91*(2), 470-473.

Maruo, Y., Nishizawa, K., Sato, H., Sawa, H., & Shimada, M. (2000). Prolonged unconjugated hyperbilirubinemia associated with breast milk and mutations of the bilirubin uridine diphosphate- glucuronosyltransferase gene. *Pediatrics, 106*(5), E59.

McDonagh, A. F. (1990). Is bilirubin good for you? *Clinics in Perinatology, 17*, 359-369.

Meloy, L., Miller, G., Chandrasekaran, M. H., Summitt, C., & Gutcher, G. (1999). Accuracy of glucose reflectance testing for detecting hypoglycemia in term newborns. *Clinical Pediatrics, 38*(12), 717-724.

Mishra, S., Chawla, D., Agarwal, R., Deorari, A. K., Paul, V. K., & Bhutani, V. K. (2009). Transcutaneous bilirubinometry reduces the need for blood sampling in neonates with visible jaundice. *Acta Paediatrica.*

Moore, A. M., & Perlman, M. (1999). Symptomatic hypoglycemia in otherwise healthy, breastfed term newborns. *Pediatrics, 103*(4 Pt 1), 837-839.

Newman, T. B., Escobar, G. J., Gonzales, V. M., Armstrong, M. A., Gardner, M. N., & Folck, B. F. (1999). Frequency of neonatal bilirubin testing and hyperbilirubinemia in a large health maintenance organization. *Pediatrics, 104*(5 Pt 2), 1198-1203.

Newman, T. B., Liljestrand, P., & Escobar, G. J. (2003). Infants with bilirubin levels of 30 mg/dL or more in a large managed care organization. *Pediatrics, 111*(6 Pt 1), 1303-1311.

Nicholl, R. (2003). What is the normal range of blood glucose concentrations in healthy term newborns? *Archives of Disease in Childhood, 88*(3), 238-239.

Nicoll, A., Ginsburg, R., & Tripp, J. H. (1982). Supplementary feeding and jaundice in newborns. *Acta Paediatrica Scandinavica, 71*(5), 759-761.

Pashapour, N., Nikibahksh, A. A., & Golmohammadlou, S. (2007). Urinary tract infection in term neonates with prolonged jaundice. *Urology Journal, 4*(2), 91-94; discussion 94.

Per, H., Kumandas, S., Coskun, A., Gumus, H., & Oztop, D. (2008). Neurologic sequelae of neonatal hypoglycemia in Kayseri, Turkey. *Journal of Child Neurology, 23*(12), 1406-1412.

Sarici, S. U., Serdar, M. A., Korkmaz, A., Erdem, G., Oran, O., Tekinalp, G., et al. (2004). Incidence, course, and prediction of hyperbilirubinemia in near-term and term newborns. *Pediatrics, 113*(4), 775-780.

Schneider, A. P., 2nd. (1986). Breast milk jaundice in the newborn. A real entity. *Journal of the American Medical Association, 255*(23), 3270-3274.

Sedlak, T. W., & Snyder, S. H. (2004). Bilirubin benefits: cellular protection by a biliverdin reductase antioxidant cycle. *Pediatrics, 113*(6), 1776-1782.

Sexson, W. R. (1984). Incidence of neonatal hypoglycemia: a matter of definition. *Journal of Pediatrics, 105*(1), 149-150.

Stutte, P. (1988). the effects of breast massage on volume and fat content of human milk. *Genesis, 10*(2), 22-25.

Suman, R. P., Udani, R., & Nanavati, R. (2008). Kangaroo mother care for low birth weight infants: a randomized controlled trial. *Indian Pediatrics, 45*(1), 17-23.

Suresh, G. K., Martin, C. L., & Soll, R. F. (2003). Metalloporphyrins for treatment of unconjugated hyperbilirubinemia in neonates. *Cochrane Database of Systematic Reviews*(2), CD004207.

Sweet, D. G., Hadden, D., & Halliday, H. L. (1999). The effect of early feeding on the neonatal blood glucose level at 1-hour of age. *Early Human Development, 55*(1), 63-66.

Temme, E. H., Zhang, J., Schouten, E. G., & Kesteloot, H. (2001). Serum bilirubin and 10-year mortality risk in a Belgian population. *Cancer Causes and Control, 12*(10), 887-894.

Thayyil, S., & Marriott, L. (2005). Can transcutaneous bilirubinometry reduce the need for serum bilirubin estimations in term and near term infants? *Archives of Disease in Childhood, 90*(12), 1311-1312.

Tyler, M., & Hellings, P. (2005). Feeding method and rehospitalization in newborns less than 1 month of age. *Journal of Obstetric, Gynecologic, and Neonatal Nursing, 34*(1), 70-79.

van Zoeren-Grobben, D., Lindeman, J. H., Houdkamp, E., Brand, R., Schrijver, J., & Berger, H. M. (1994). Postnatal changes in plasma chain-breaking antioxidants in healthy preterm infants fed formula and/or human milk. *American Journal of Clinical Nutrition, 60*(6), 900-906.

Varvarigou, A., Fouzas, S., Skylogianni, E., Mantagou, L., Bougioukou, D., & Mantagos, S. (2009). Transcutaneous bilirubin nomogram for prediction of significant neonatal hyperbilirubinemia. *Pediatrics, 124*(4), 1052-1059.

Walker, M. (2006). *Breastfeeding Management for the Clinician: Using the Evidence*. Boston, MA: Jones and Bartlett.

WHO (1997). Hypoglycaemia of the newborn: Review of the literature. *Journal*. Retrieved from http://whqlibdoc.who.int/hq/1997/WHO_CHD_97.1.pdf

Wight, N., & Marinelli, K. A. (2006). ABM clinical protocol #1: guidelines for glucose monitoring and treatment of hypoglycemia in breastfed neonates. *Breastfeeding Medicine, 1*(3), 178-184.

Wight, N. E. (2006). Hypoglycemia in breastfed neonates. *Breastfeeding Medicine, 1*(4), 253-262.

Willis, S. K., Hannon, P. R., & Scrimshaw, S. C. (2002). The impact of the maternal experience with a jaundiced newborn on the breastfeeding relationship. *Journal of Family Practice, 51*(5), 465.

Yamauchi, Y., & Yamanouchi, I. (1990). Breast-feeding frequency during the first 24 hours after birth in full-term neonates. *Pediatrics, 86*(2), 171-175.

Zecca, E., Romagnoli, C., De Carolis, M. P., Costa, S., Marra, R., & De Luca, D. (2009). Does Ibuprofen increase neonatal hyperbilirubinemia? *Pediatrics, 124*(2), 480-484.

Health Issues—Baby

Chapter

8

ILLNESS IN THE BREASTFEEDING BABY

The mother may be concerned about how her baby's illness will affect breastfeeding.

When talking to the mother of a sick child, ask her how she's coping and what her baby's healthcare provider has recommended. Continued breastfeeding is almost always the best option, because it comforts a sick baby and helps him recover faster by supplying antibodies specific to his illness.

Colds, Flu, Breathing Problems, and Ear Infections

When a baby with nasal congestion struggles with breathing while breastfeeding, give the mother some basic strategies to make feedings easier.

A baby with a cold or the flu usually feeds more easily from the breast because he can better coordinate suckling, swallowing, and breathing than with a fast-flowing bottle (Lawrence & Lawrence, 2005). But if breastfeeding becomes challenging when a baby's nose is clogged, the following basic strategies may help:

- Before breastfeeding, keep the baby upright (in arms or in a sling or carrier) so that his sinuses can drain.
- If the baby's healthcare provider recommends it, use a soft, rubber-bulb syringe to gently clear his nose.
- Breastfeed in an upright position that allows baby's sinuses to continue to drain.
- Breastfeed more often, as frequent feedings are often easier to manage.
- Breastfeed where the air is moist; use a cool-mist vaporizer or breastfeed in the bathroom with the shower running.
- Contact the baby's healthcare provider for other suggestions for easing baby's symptoms and ways to prevent the spread of illness.

A baby with a cold, the flu or an ear infection usually feeds more easily from the breast, but may need some modifications that will make breastfeeding easier.

If during an ear infection or while congested the baby refuses the breast, suggest the mother express her milk and feed it by spoon or cup.

Babies sometimes refuse the breast when they are so congested they cannot breathe when they create an air seal at the breast or if an ear infection causes intense pain when they suckle. If the baby won't or can't breastfeed, suggest the mother express her milk as often as her baby had been breastfeeding and offer him expressed milk in a spoon or cup, offering the breast every hour or so. This insures the baby will get the fluids he needs and will help keep the mother comfortable and prevent mastitis. Assure the mother that when the baby can breathe through his nose again or the ear infection subsides, he should return to breastfeeding.

A baby with chronic congestion or trouble breathing at the breast for other reasons should be evaluated by a healthcare provider.

Chronic congestion can be a sign of allergy, gastroesophageal reflux disease (see later section), or other physical problems. Breathing always comes before eating, so if breathing is difficult while at the breast, a baby will usually pull on and off and may gain weight slowly.

Struggles with breathing during feedings may be due to inflammation in the mouth or throat from rough suctioning or intubation after birth, spasms, or physical abnormalities of the mouth or throat, such as choanal atresia (a blockage between the nose and pharynx), tracheomalacia, and laryngomalacia (softened cartilage that narrows the trachea or larynx) (Genna, 2008a; Walker, 2006). Any baby who consistently struggles with breathing at feedings or who makes high-pitched, squeaky sounds (called "stridor") while breastfeeding, should be checked by his healthcare provider to determine and treat the cause.

Diarrhea and Vomiting

Nearly all breastfed babies with diarrhea and/or vomiting will recover faster if they keep breastfeeding.

If a baby takes anything by mouth, it should be mother's milk, in part because it is absorbed so quickly that some fluids and nutrients will be retained (Heyman, 2006).

Although it is rarely necessary, when diarrhea and/or vomiting are severe, the baby's doctor may recommend supplementing the baby with an oral electrolyte solution, such as Pedialyte, or oral rehydration therapy (ORT) in addition to breastfeeding. If the baby has lost enough fluid to be severely dehydrated, the doctor may recommend giving fluids intravenously while continuing to breastfeed.

Breastfeeding may need to be discontinued only in the very rare cases where diarrhea and vomiting are symptoms of a metabolic disorder, such as galactosemia (see later section). The baby born with galactosemia lacks the liver enzyme needed to fully metabolize lactose, or milk sugar. If untreated, galactosemia causes vomiting, weight loss, cataracts, liver disease, and eventually mental retardation, which is why U.S. newborns are routinely screened for it (Kaye et al., 2006). Metabolic disorders usually become obvious within a baby's first weeks.

• •

When a gastrointestinal illness causes diarrhea and/or vomiting, suggest the mother be alert to signs of dehydration.

When a breastfeeding baby contracts an illness that causes vomiting and/or diarrhea, it usually passes within a few days. But if prolonged, it can cause more serious problems. Diarrhea occurs when the lining of the intestine becomes inflamed and irritated. Nutrients pass too quickly through the body and fluid is leaked. Either diarrhea alone or diarrhea with vomiting can cause the baby's body to lose water and salt, which may lead to dehydration and eventually to shock.

Any time a mothers sees any of the following signs of dehydration, encourage her to contact her baby's healthcare provider right away:

- Listlessness, lethargy, and/or sleeping through feedings
- Weak cry
- Baby's skin loses its resiliency (when pinched, it no longer bounces back)
- Dry mouth and eyes
- Fewer tears
- Fewer wet diapers ($\leq$2 in 24 hours)
- Baby's fontanel (soft spot) appears sunken or depressed
- Fever

Dehydration can be prevented by feeding the baby frequently, so he gets enough fluids.

Diarrhea

Not all frequent and loose stools are diarrhea. A baby's first stool, called meconium, is greenish black and sticky. Usually by about the 3rd or 4th day of life, the stools turn yellow, yellow-green, or tan and appear loose and unformed, resembling split pea soup. Occasional green stools are also not uncommon. Because of the beneficial bacterial in the exclusively breastfed baby's intestine, the odor is usually mild and inoffensive.

Diarrhea differs from normal breastfed stools in frequency, consistency, and/or smell.

On one end of the spectrum, some breastfed babies pass frequent stools, sometimes after every feeding. Typically, babies younger than 6 weeks old have at least 3 to 4 stools each day (Shrago, Reifsnider, & Insel, 2006). After 6 weeks of age, some breastfed babies stool less often—as infrequently as once a week—but more profusely. As long as the baby is gaining weight well, fewer stools a day are not a cause for concern.

Diarrhea is less common among breastfeeding babies, but when it occurs it may be caused by gastrointestinal illness or as a side effect of a food or medication. The difference between normal stools and diarrhea include:

- More stools, as many as 12 to 16 per day.
- Watery stools, often with few "curds".
- A stronger, more offensive smell.

• •

Some healthcare providers recommend mothers with fussy babies or babies with diarrhea wean to formula because they have "lactose intolerance," but this is counter to current recommendations, and many babies switched to lactose-free formulas do not improve (Heyman, 2006).

Diarrhea lasting for weeks after an illness is usually due to temporary lactose intolerance, and continued breastfeeding is recommended.

Lactose is a sugar abundant in human milk. The enzyme lactase, which is produced in the small intestine, processes lactose by breaking it down into glucose and galactose. Lactose intolerance usually refers to the reactions (bloating, gas, abdominal pain, diarrhea, nausea) that occur when a lack of lactase leaves lactose unprocessed in the gut.

Babies with temporary lactose intolerance should continue breastfeeding.

Some types of lactose intolerance occur only in older children and adults; others occur only in babies. The four main types include:

- **Primary lactase deficiency** is the most common. It does not affect young babies but occurs later in life in about 70% of the world's population (with the exception of those of northern European ancestry). Lactase production gradually decreases as early as age 3 or as late as adulthood. *When a mother has this type, her baby will not become lactose intolerant until he is older.* It does not cause diarrhea in babies.
- **Congenital lactase deficiency** (hypolactasia) is very rare and becomes obvious shortly after birth, causing dehydration, illness, and lack of weight gain (Savilahti, Launiala, & Kuitunen, 1983). Like babies with the metabolic disorder galactosemia, the few babies with this condition cannot be safely breastfed.
- **Developmental lactase deficiency** describes the temporarily lower level of lactase production common in preterm babies younger than 34 weeks gestation.

- **Secondary lactase deficiency**, which is most common in babies, is a temporary condition caused by damage to the lining of the small intestine from infection, celiac disease, other illness, or medication.

This last type is a temporary condition that usually occurs in a baby or toddler after a gastrointestinal illness, when gut damage temporarily slows or stops the production of lactase. While this damage is healing, diarrhea continues for 2 to 4 weeks (sometimes referred to as "nuisance diarrhea"), and then resolves on its own. When the diarrhea does not immediately resolve, many mothers are told to switch their breastfed babies to formula. However, the American Academy of Pediatrics (AAP) currently recommends continued breastfeeding both during infectious illness with diarrhea and after, as long as the baby has no more than mild dehydration. The AAP wrote: "Breastfed infants should be continued on human milk in all cases" (Heyman, 2006, p. 1284). The AAP also concluded that except in severely malnourished formula-fed babies, low-lactose and lactose-free formulas have no clinical advantages.

Other possible causes of "nuisance diarrhea" from intestinal damage include treatment with antibiotics, solid foods that irritate the lining of the child's gut, and more than 4 ounces (118 mL) of fruit juice per day (AAP, 2001; Smith & Lifshitz, 1994).

• •

Green watery stools without symptoms of illness may be a sign the baby is sensitive to a food or drug.

If the baby seems otherwise healthy, green stools may simply be a normal variation or may indicate a sensitivity to a food or drug the baby consumed directly or a sensitivity to something the mother ingested that passed into her milk. Two U.S. physicians wrote in their book for medical professionals: "Occasionally, an infant will have diarrhea or an intestinal upset because of something in the mother's diet. It is usually self-limited, and the best treatment is to continue to nurse at the breast. If the mother has been taking a laxative that is absorbed or has been eating laxative foods, such as fruits in excess, she should adjust her diet" (Lawrence & Lawrence, 2005, p. 521). See also, "Is Baby Reacting to Something in Mother's Diet?" on p. 517 in the chapter "Nutrition, Exercise, and Other Lifestyle Issues."

• •

A foremilk-hindmilk imbalance has been suggested as a possible cause for some cases of green, watery stools with other symptoms.

One theory proposed by two U.K. researchers to explain green, watery stools is referred to as "foremilk-hindmilk imbalance" (Woolridge & Fisher, 1988). In their 1988 article, they described case reports of irritable, slow-gaining babies with gas and frequent, sometimes green, watery stools, whose symptoms resolved when the mothers changed their breastfeeding rhythm by allowing the baby to "finish the first breast first," rather than switching breasts after a set 10-minute period. The researchers suggested that in mothers with abundant milk production, switching breasts before the baby reached the fattier hindmilk could have overloaded the baby's small intestine with more lactose from the low-fat foremilk than it could absorb, causing their symptoms. These results have not been replicated. Ideally babies should come off the first breast when finished, rather than after a set time. If a baby has these symptoms and the mother has been feeding by the clock, suggest she try this approach. There is no need for most mothers to be concerned about this because research has found that breastfeeding babies using a wide variety of feeding rhythms easily access the right balance of foremilk and hindmilk (Kent et al., 2006).

Interruption of breastfeeding during diarrhea is not usually beneficial.

When a baby's illness includes vomiting or diarrhea, the standard advice was once to interrupt breastfeeding and feed instead an oral electrolyte solution, such as Pedialyte, or other oral rehydration therapy (ORT). But research found that temporary weaning was associated with more negative health outcomes than continuing to breastfeed, in part because mother's milk is so easily and rapidly digested (Lawrence, 2005; Litman, Wu, & Quinlivan, 1994). Even in cases of rotavirus, in its *Red Book*, the American Academy of Pediatrics wrote: "Breastfeeding is associated with milder disease and should be continued" (AAP, 2009, p. 576). Discontinuing breastfeeding when an ill baby has diarrhea has been found to double the risk of increased severity and death (Clemens et al., 1988; Mahalanabis, Alam, Rahman, & Hasnat, 1991).

Babies with diarrhea should continue breastfeeding.

In developing countries where diarrhea is a serious health problem responsible for the deaths of millions of infants and small children, studies have found that babies return to health faster when they continue to breastfeed, with exclusively breastfed babies recovering faster than mixed-fed or formula-fed babies (Brown, 1994). To improve health outcomes in babies with diarrhea, in India, Bangladesh, and other developing countries, many non-breastfeeding mothers are helped to relactate during their babies' hospital stay (Haider, Kabir, Fuchs, & Habte, 2000).

If the baby's healthcare provider recommends temporary weaning and the mother would like to explore other options, suggest she tell her baby's healthcare provider she wants to continue breastfeeding and ask if he or she would be willing to look over some references with her, such as those listed in this section. If the healthcare provider is not open to that option, suggest the mother seek a second opinion. For more strategies, see p. 853 in Appendix C, "Working with Health Professionals."

Vomiting

When a mother says her baby is vomiting, rule out the possibility that the baby is not ill but "spitting up" after feedings.

If a baby is simply bringing up some milk after a breastfeeding, otherwise known as "spitting up," he would have no other symptoms of illness. Although most use the term "vomit" to describe a more forceful ejection of milk, some even refer to a dribble of milk in the corner of the baby's mouth that way. In Western cultures where longer breastfeeding intervals are the cultural norm, more than half of the babies spit up at least once a day during their first 3 months of life, with spitting up peaking at 4 to 5 months (Hegar et al., 2009; Nelson, Chen, Syniar, & Christoffel, 1997). Even if a baby appears to be spitting up a lot of milk, what's more important is how he is growing and gaining and whether he seems generally happy when held or whether he's irritable and fussy most of the time. Borderline or slow weight gain and a generally unhappy temperament could be a sign of gastroesophageal reflux disease (see next section). If he is gaining weight well, seems content when held, and has a good diaper output, assure the mother there is no cause for concern.

If a baby who wasn't spitting up starts, it may be due to a sensitivity to a food or drug.

If there are no other signs of illness, vomiting that starts after weeks or months of uneventful breastfeeding may be a sign of a sensitivity to a food or drug he is receiving directly or through his mother's milk. Depending on the type of reaction (IgA mediated or non-IgA mediated), spitting up could occur as quickly as right after the exposure or as long as 48 hours later (Heine, 2008). For details, see the section "Is Baby Reacting to Something in Mother's Diet?" on p. 517 in the "Nutrition" chapter.

If a baby projectile vomits at least once a day, suggest the mother have him checked for pyloric stenosis.

Regular projectile vomiting is a symptom of pyloric stenosis, an overgrowth of the muscular tube between the stomach and duodenum, which makes it harder for milk to move through it. In a baby with pyloric stenosis, the milk does not move easily from the baby's stomach into his intestines, which can limit the nutrients the baby receives.

Symptoms of pyloric stenosis usually appear between 2 and 6 weeks of age. The cause of projectile vomiting—often the first symptom—is the contraction of the baby's stomach muscles, which forces the milk up his throat and out his mouth, sometimes as far as several feet away. At first this may happen only occasionally, but usually it occurs more and more over time until the baby projectile vomits after every feeding, which can lead to weight loss and dehydration. Projectile vomiting is not always due to pyloric stenosis, but if it happens at least once a day, suggest the mother have the baby's healthcare provider rule it out.

Projectile vomiting may be caused by pyloric stenosis.

The treatment for pyloric stenosis is to first evaluate the baby for dehydration and, if needed, restore his electrolyte balance, and then perform a simple surgery called a pyloromyotomy, the most common surgery of the early months (Ohshiro & Puri, 1998). The mother may need to express her milk during the surgery, but if it is uncomplicated, the baby should be able to breastfeed after he recovers from the anesthesia. Early feedings post-surgery have been associated with decreased hospital stay and reduced stress on the family (Carpenter et al., 1999; Garza, Morash, Dzakovic, Mondschein, & Jaksic, 2002; Puapong, Kahng, Ko, & Applebaum, 2002).

If an obviously sick baby vomits after every breastfeeding, share strategies that can help keep the baby hydrated and decrease the vomiting.

When a baby has a gastrointestinal illness, the mother may worry that because he vomits after every breastfeeding he's not keeping enough milk down and is at risk of becoming dehydrated. Suggest the mother try reducing the vomiting by expressing most of her milk before the baby breastfeeds and offering a less-full breast. This allows the baby to take a little milk while being comforted at the breast. Offering a less-full breast more often provides the fluids the baby needs in small doses and keeps vomiting to a minimum until he can handle larger feedings again.

If the baby is 6 months or older, suggest the mother offer ice chips or water from a spoon. Ice goes down slowly and can distract a miserable baby, so the baby's stomach stays emptier longer. Also share with the mother the symptoms of dehydration in the previous section "Vomiting and Diarrhea," so she'll know the red flags. See also the information on the value of continued breastfeeding.

Reflux Disease (GERD)

During the first months of life, the sphincter between a baby's esophagus and stomach has low muscle tone and relaxes often (Omari et al., 2002). In an average baby, several times each day his stomach contents wash back into his esophagus, also known as gastroesophageal reflux (GER). Spitting up occurs when the stomach contents make it all the way up the esophagus and out the mouth. Spitting up occurs in up to 70% of babies and peaks around 4 to 5 months of age, occurring less and less often as the digestive system matures (Campanozzi et al., 2009; Nelson et al., 1997). By 12 months, only about 4% of babies still spit up.

A baby with gastroesophageal reflux disease (GERD) may or may not spit up, but he may have pain, feeding problems, and other symptoms.

When a baby is growing, thriving, and feeding normally, spitting up is a temporary inconvenience. But when GER causes damage to the lining of the esophagus, normal GER becomes gastroesophageal reflux disease (GERD). A baby with GERD may spit up or he may not, because damage to the esophagus can occur even if the stomach contents don't make it all the way to the mouth. GERD can cause health issues, such as respiratory problems (congestion, coughing, wheezing, bronchitis, pneumonia), apnea, esophageal narrowing or stricture, anemia, failure to thrive, and esophagitis, or inflammation of the esophagus, which can cause pain during and after feedings (Semeniuk & Kaczmarski, 2008). GERD can cause behaviors that can be upsetting to both babies and parents:

- Frequent hiccups
- Sleep problems day and night (Ghaem et al., 1998)
- Back arching and head turning (Frankel, Shalaby, & Orenstein, 2006)
- Crying and irritability
- Feeding aversion, which sometimes leads to feeding refusal (Heine, 2008)

GERD can cause a wide range of health problems in babies and be stressful for mothers as well.

GERD has proved to be the cause of many puzzling feeding problems and behaviors that are sometimes given the all-purpose label "colic." In one Belgian study of 60 irritable babies 1 to 6 months old who had not responded to mothers' elimination of cow's milk, 66% had test results indicating GERD and 43% had esophagitis (Vandenplas, Badriul, Verghote, Hauser, & Kaufman, 2004). One Israeli study confirmed GERD in 16 of 26 babies (62%) thought to have colic; within 2 weeks of treatment with GERD medication, all 16 babies were colic-free (Berkowitz, Naveh, & Berant, 1997). One Belgian study of 700 infants and young children with feeding problems diagnosed 33% with GERD (Rommel, De Meyer, Feenstra, & Veereman-Wauters, 2003). The esophageal damage caused by GERD may lead to other physical problems, such as vocal cord swelling, which can contribute to swallowing and breathing difficulties (Mercado-Deane et al., 2001).

Allergy to cow's milk protein may also play a role in the development of GERD in some babies, as can cause tissue irritation along the gastrointestinal tract (Salvatore & Vandenplas, 2002). Early exposure to formula (sometimes without the mother's knowledge) can sensitize a baby to cow's milk protein, which can cause a reaction later to either formula or dairy in the mother's diet (de Boissieu, Matarazzo, Rocchiccioli, & Dupont, 1997; Hill, Heine, Cameron, Francis, & Bines, 1999; Host, Husby, & Osterballe, 1988).

Western baby-care and feeding practices may contribute to GERD.

The "misalignment of culture and biology" may play a role in GERD in infants. One Australian author suggests that in addition to better diagnostic techniques, some aspects of western culture may contribute to increasing reports of GERD (Douglas, 2005):

- **Longer intervals between feedings** contribute to esophageal damage, because the milk still in the stomach during the first hour or two after feeding buffers the baby's stomach contents making them less acidic (Grant & Cochran, 2001; Mitchell, McClure, & Tubman, 2001). With longer feeding intervals, there is more time each day when the stomach is emptier and its contents are more acidic and, therefore, more likely to cause damage if they wash back into the esophagus.
- **Carrying babies in infant seats** puts their torso and legs at a 60° angle, which increases episodes of reflux (Carroll, Garrison, & Christakis, 2002).
- **Use of infant formula**. Babies on formula have more reflux episodes each day and continue to reflux longer (Campanozzi et al., 2009; Hegar et al., 2009). In some babies, formula use can also trigger sensitivity to cow's milk protein, a contributor to reflux disease (Salvatore & Vandenplas, 2002).
- **Encouraging babies to sleep for long stretches at night** means longer periods of empty stomachs with higher-acid contents. Also, babies in a sound sleep may not clear their esophagus as often.

Weaning can make reflux worse.

When a baby is miserable much of the time and struggles at the breast or has other symptoms of reflux, this can demoralize even the most dedicated breastfeeding mother. A mother in this situation may wonder if weaning will make her life easier and if breastfeeding is the problem. She may wonder if her baby is fussy because she doesn't have enough milk or because her baby doesn't like breastfeeding. Her baby's healthcare providers may encourage her to wean under the mistaken assumption that switching to formula will help.

Weaning usually does not improve GERD.

Unfortunately, many mothers do not discover until their baby is already weaned that giving formula can actually make his discomfort worse. One Australian study that compared 37 breastfed and 37 formula-fed babies with reflux discovered that the episodes of reflux were shorter among the breastfed babies (Heacock, Jeffery, Baker, & Page, 1992). A questionnaire completed by Italian pediatricians from the records of 313 children aged 1 to 12 months who spit up found that breastfed babies stop spitting up earlier than babies fed formula (Campanozzi et al., 2009). A prospective Belgian study of 130 babies followed for 1 year concluded that exclusively breastfed babies spit up less than breastfed babies who also received formula (Hegar et al., 2009).

Some basic strategies can help minimize the effects of reflux while baby is being evaluated by his healthcare provider.

If reflux is suspected, in addition to seeing her baby's healthcare provider, a mother can try some basic strategies to help keep her baby more comfortable.

Use positioning to minimize reflux. Gravity can affect the backflow of the baby's stomach contents into the esophagus, so suggest the mother use positions to hold, feed, change, and sleep that discourage reflux. Suggest she use gravity in her baby's favor by:

- After feedings keep baby upright for 20 to 30 minutes, either in arms or in an upright baby carrier (Vartabedian, 2007).
- At diaper changes, avoid lifting baby's legs; instead roll him on his left side to wipe.
- Breastfeed with baby's head higher than bottom at about a 45° angle. The mother can lean back with the baby's body tummy down on hers (see next point) or sit upright and hold him with his bottom in her lap or on a pillow (Wolf & Glass, 1992).
- When baby is awake and horizontal, lay him on his left side or on his tummy (prone). The baby's esophagus connects to the stomach near his back, and lying tummy down triggers less reflux than back-lying (supine) (Ewer, James, & Tobin, 1999).
- Avoid putting baby in a car seat except when riding in the car, as this position increases reflux (Carroll et al., 2002).

Eliminate cow's milk and dairy from her diet. An exclusively breastfeeding mother can rule in or out allergy to cow's milk protein, a secondary cause of reflux disease, by avoiding all forms of cow's milk protein, including milk, yogurt, ice cream, cheese, and butter, and all other sources of casein and whey (Heine, Jordan, Lubitz, Meehan, & Catto-Smith, 2006). It may take several weeks to notice improvement (Salvatore & Vandenplas, 2002). If formula is given, suggest the mother use a hypoallergenic type.

Feed often. A baby needs a certain volume of milk every 24 hours to grow and thrive (on average 25 oz. [750 mL]). Taking less milk more often means less milk in the stomach to wash back into the esophagus and less time with an empty high-acid-content stomach. One author noted that in the pediatric gastroenterology office where she worked, many mothers of babies with reflux had overabundant milk production (Boekel, 2000). She reported that many of these mothers regularly coaxed their babies to breastfeed longer because although they seemed finished after 5 to 10 minutes, the mothers worried they had not breastfed "long enough." As in an adult, an overly full stomach may worsen GERD symptoms.

• •

Thickening feeds decreases spitting up, but has not been found to reduce other symptoms.

Parents of babies with GERD are often advised to add cereal or starch to "thicken feeds." Thickeners may be added to formula or a breastfeeding mother may be asked to give her baby cereal before breastfeeding. (The enzymes in human milk digest thickeners, so adding them to expressed milk won't thicken it.)

A Cochrane Review article on this practice concluded that "...[T]here is no current evidence to support or refute the use of feed thickeners in treating newborn babies with gastroesophageal reflux" (Huang, Tai, Wong, Lee, & Yong, 2009). Other reviews have also concluded that the research is mixed (McPherson, Wright, & Bell, 2005). Although in some studies thickeners decreased episodes of spit up, there is no evidence that thickeners prevent reflux or decrease other GERD symptoms (Wenzl et al., 2003).

One drawback to using thickeners is that when these starches are regurgitated, they may irritate the baby's tissues, especially if aspirated into his lungs (Orenstein,

Shalaby, & Putnam, 1992). Early solids also have the potential to sensitize an already sensitive baby to allergy (Poole et al., 2006).

Although babies "outgrow" reflux, lack of treatment may cause later health problems.

Spitting up is outgrown as the sphincter between stomach and esophagus lengthens with age and increases in muscle tone. But when normal reflux becomes reflux disease, weight gain and growth can slow, pain can lead to feeding aversion, and damage to the esophagus may put babies at risk later in life. One U.S. study followed 100 babies diagnosed with GERD that led to esophageal damage, or esophagitis (Orenstein, Shalaby, Kelsey, & Frankel, 2006). These babies were divided into four treatment groups (19 received a placebo) and followed until 12 months of age. The symptoms of the babies in the placebo group eventually resolved, but at 12 months their esophagus still had abnormalities, which the researchers concluded increased these babies' risk later in life for GERD and even more potentially serious health problems, such as esophageal stricture, precancerous conditions, and in rare cases esophageal cancer (Gold, 2006).

The most common GERD treatment for babies is prescription medication. If a baby receives medication, be sure the mother knows that the dose of the drug or combination of drugs will probably need to be adjusted as baby grows, because it is determined by the baby's weight, which changes quickly. If a drug treatment worked well for a while and the baby's symptoms return, suggest the mother talk to the baby's doctor about the possibility of adjusting the dose. The sooner GERD is diagnosed and treated, the less likely it will become severe. In severe cases, if a baby continues to lose weight, surgery may be recommended.

CHRONIC CONDITIONS IN THE BREASTFEEDING BABY

Parents of babies with chronic health problems may have conflicting feelings and have trouble remembering information.

When a baby is born with special needs, the parents may have mixed emotions, including helplessness, anger, disappointment, and guilt, which may be ongoing. They may need time to grieve the healthy baby they expected before they can accept the baby in their arms. If the baby is diagnosed later, they may worry that something they did may have caused their baby's health problems. A mother with strong feelings may find it difficult to remember information. Rather than just providing information verbally, it may be more helpful to give it to her in writing and go over it with her several different times.

If the mother has breastfeeding problems, she may blame herself and see it as a reflection of her own inadequacy as a mother. Or she may interpret normal baby behavior, such as fussiness, as a symptom of her baby's physical problem. When talking to the mother:

- Encourage her to talk about her feelings and acknowledge them, which will make it easier for her to think through her situation more clearly.
- Suggest she plan to take 1 day at a time, and watch her baby's responses to best determine what will work for them.

- Ask the normal questions any new parents are asked—who the baby looks like and how he responds to those around him.
- Discuss the availability of a support group, if one exists.

Cardiac Issues

The baby with a cardiac issue may gain weight slowly.

Heart problems at birth are referred to as congenital heart disease, which includes defects of the heart and major blood vessels. Cardiac issues may occur alone or with Down syndrome, Turner syndrome, or other syndromes (Frommelt, 2004). Babies with cardiac issues usually gain weight slowly no matter how they are fed because they use more energy than a healthy baby. To maintain adequate oxygen levels and circulation, they take more breaths each minute and their hearts beat faster. Adequate weekly weight gain in a healthy newborn is at least 5 oz. (142 g), but because of their increased energy needs, even with good milk intake, many babies with heart disease gain less weight or even lose weight (Clemente, Barnes, Shinebourne, & Stein, 2001).

For the baby with a cardiac issue, breastfeeding is easier and results in better health outcomes than bottle-feeding formula.

Some mothers are discouraged from breastfeeding when their baby has a cardiac issue due to the misconception that bottle-feeding is "easier" than breastfeeding (Lambert & Watters, 1998). However, research has found the opposite to be true. As with preterm babies, oxygen saturation was found to be higher during breastfeeding among both preterm babies and babies with congenital heart issues (Marino, O'Brien, & LoRe, 1995). Research on preterm babies found that coordinating sucking, swallowing, and breathing, which is a major challenge for babies with cardiac issues, was easier at the breast than during bottle-feeding (Meier, 1988; Meier & Anderson, 1987).

Differences between mother's milk and formula may also affect the energy a baby must expend. One U.S. study of healthy 2-day-old babies found that the breastfed newborns had more energy-efficient heart rhythms, lower heart rates, and expended less energy overall than non-breastfed babies, even though the breastfed babies spent less time sleeping than their bottle-fed counterparts (Zeskind & Goff, 1992). The researchers suggested that formula may have a sedating effect that decreases behavioral organization.

In a U.S. study of 45 babies with congenital heart disease, the severity of the babies' cardiac issue was found to be unrelated to their ability to breastfeed (Combs & Marino, 1993). In the "breastfed" group, the researchers included babies who received even a little mother's milk. Even so, the differences between these two groups were significant. The breastfed babies had shorter hospital stays and weighed more than those who were exclusively formula-fed. The researchers attributed the slower weight gain of the non-breastfed babies to lower oxygen levels from breathing interruptions during bottle-feeding.

Practical strategies may make it easier to breastfeed the baby with cardiac issues.

Mothers of babies with cardiac problems face many breastfeeding challenges. They are often separated from their babies, who may need to fast before procedures. Mothers receive inconsistent breastfeeding support from healthcare providers (Barbas & Kelleher, 2004). They feel anxious about feeding and wonder if their baby is satisfied after coming off the breast or just worn out (Lobo, 1992). Mothers also report concerns about lack of adequate weight gain, breathlessness, and fatigue during breastfeeding, unrelated to the severity of their baby's cardiac issue (Clemente et al., 2001). Suggest the mother experiment with the following practical tips to see if any are helpful to her and her baby (Walker, 2006):

- Try upright feeding positions, such as the laid-back positions described in Chapter 1, that allow the baby's head to tilt back slightly for easier swallowing and breathing.
- Use breast compression (see p. 804) to help the baby get more hindmilk more quickly.
- Feed often—A baby with less stamina may do better with smaller, more frequent feedings.
- Stop breastfeeding if the baby becomes short of breath, his lips turn blue, or he looks pale or tired.
- If the baby's breastfeeding effectiveness is questionable, express milk after feedings to safeguard milk production.
- If the baby is not feeding well, try the Dancer Hand position for more support (see p. 805 in the "Techniques" appendix) or a nipple shield (see p. 835 in the appendix "Tools and Products").
- During procedures, as needed, request a place to express milk, food and drink, a place to rest, and equipment, such as a breast pump, refrigerator, or cleaning supplies.

Exclusive breastfeeding is possible for some babies with cardiac problems; others need to be supplemented.

Depending on the severity of the cardiac issue, some babies with cardiac defects can breastfeed exclusively. One U.S. study found that lactation support resulted in improved breastfeeding outcomes among these mothers and babies (Barbas & Kelleher, 2004).

If the baby gains too little weight while exclusively breastfeeding, other strategies may help boost weight gain (Walker, 2006):

If a baby with cardiac issues gains too little weight, mothers may need to use extra strategies to boost their supply.

- Use breast compression (alternate breast massage) while breastfeeding to increase the fat content of the milk (Stutte, 1988). (See appendix "Techniques.)
- Give the baby high-calorie hindmilk as a supplement, with an at-breast supplementer or another feeding method. (See p. 811 in the appendix "Tools and Products.")
- Add calorie-rich supplements to mother's milk.
- Feed high-calorie hindmilk that provides 28 to 30 calories per oz. [30 mL].
- Breastfeed during the day and feed baby with a continuous feeding pump at night (Imms, 2001).

To provide her hindmilk, suggest the mother express milk after breastfeeding. If the mother is exclusively expressing, suggest she set aside the milk she gets during the first few minutes, and then collect the milk for feeding that she expresses after that.

Whatever supplement is used, the mother and her baby's healthcare provider need to discuss how often and how much supplement should be given. Depending on the baby's weight gain and his breastfeeding effectiveness, the mother may supplement the baby after every feeding, after every other feeding, or less often.

The need for a supplement causes some mothers to question the value of their milk, their milk production, even their adequacy as a mother. Assure the mother that her milk provides her baby with live cells important to his health that are not available elsewhere. Emphasize that her baby's cardiac issues mean he needs extra nutrients that cannot necessarily be provided simply by increasing his milk intake.

Practice at the breast, medication, and/or surgery may help the baby with a cardiac issue improve his feeding effectiveness.

Depending on the severity of the cardiac problem, a baby's feeding effectiveness may be improved with practice at the breast, with prescribed medication, or if the problem is severe, with surgery (Jadcherla, Vijayapal, & Leuthner, 2009). One case report describes a baby born with hypoplastic left heart syndrome who breastfed effectively after heart transplant surgery at 30 days of age (Owens, 2002).

Cleft Lip and Cleft Palate

A cleft (or opening) of the lip or palate is one of the most common birth defects and is correctible by surgery.

Incidence of cleft defects varies around the world. Between 1 and 3 babies in 1,000 are born with a cleft lip and/or palate, which can occur together or separately. About 20% of these babies are born with a cleft lip only, 30% with a cleft palate only, and 50% with both conditions (Reilly, Reid, & Skeat, 2007).

Even before surgical correction, by using some simple strategies (see next section), most babies with a cleft lip can breastfeed normally. With a cleft of the hard palate, however, most babies cannot. The more mother's milk these babies receive, the more normal their development and health outcomes. One Finnish study found that human milk intake for less than 3 months was associated with poorer school performance among 10-year-old children born with cleft defects (Erkkila, Isotalo, Pulkkinen, & Haapanen, 2005).

Breastfeeding insures that mothers spend time looking at their babies.

But time at the breast is also important to these babies. Efforts to breastfeed promote better mouth, tongue, and jaw development. And time at the breast also enhances the mother-baby relationship, which may be at risk if an obvious birth defect, such as a cleft lip, causes a mother to consciously or unconsciously avoid face-to-face contact with her baby. Even when a baby gets very little milk at the breast, this experience may be important to them. Some mothers say that the only time their babies look "normal" to them is during breastfeeding, while the baby's facial defect is obscured by the breast (Wilson-Clay & Hoover, 2008). Breastfeeding also assures that mother and baby spend time cuddling in skin-to-skin contact, which is calming, comforting, and nourishes their intimate bond.

Encourage the mother of a baby with a cleft defect to breastfeed early and often after birth.

When a baby has a cleft lip or palate, early breastfeeding provides the opportunity for the baby to learn to take the breast when it is still soft and pliable. Early practice at the breast also makes it easier for the baby undergoing early cleft-lip repair to return to breastfeeding afterwards. Early skin-to-skin contact also encourages normal interactions between mother and baby, which can be comforting to a mother adjusting emotionally to such an obvious birth defect.

Cleft Lip Only

The baby with a cleft lip can usually breastfeed effectively, but will need help forming a seal at the breast, so he can generate the suction required.

A cleft lip may be either incomplete or complete (all the way up into the baby's nasal cavity), on one side (unilateral), or both (bilateral). It occurs during in utero development when parts of the baby's upper lip do not fuse. Babies with a cleft lip are at much greater risk of also having a submucous cleft palate (see later section on p. 300) than other babies, so suggest the mother have him checked for this condition, too (Gosain, Conley, Santoro, & Denny, 1999).

During early breastfeeding, suggest the mother experiment with different feeding positions and use her thumb or breast tissue to fill in the defect and help her baby form a seal on the breast. This seal is important because to breastfeed effectively, the baby needs to generate suction inside his mouth, which is impossible unless he first creates an air seal (Geddes, Kent, Mitoulas, & Hartmann, 2008). The location and size of the baby's cleft will affect which feeding position or sealing strategy works best. Some mothers pull up breast tissue between two fingers and press it into the cleft (Wilson-Clay & Hoover, 2008). With a unilateral (one-sided) cleft lip, some mothers position their nipple to one side of the baby's cleft and use their thumb or a finger to fill the space. If the baby also has an alveolar ridge defect (incomplete development of the bony ridge under the gums), suggest she try using her thumb to fill that, too.

In one Australian study of 40 2-week-old bottle-fed babies with cleft lip only (8), cleft palate only (22), and cleft lip and palate (10), all the babies in the cleft lip only group were able to generate suction (Reid, Reilly, & Kilpatrick, 2007).

• •

Breastfeeding may be easier than bottle-feeding for the baby with a cleft lip and intact palate.

For many babies with cleft defects, feedings can be time-consuming, especially during the early learning period. But let the mother know that the breast may be easier for her baby to manage than the bottle because her breast tissue is more flexible than an artificial nipple/teat and the breast can mold itself more easily to compensate for any lip or mouth abnormalities (Reilly et al., 2007).

Research has found that babies with only a cleft lip have far fewer feeding problems than those with cleft palates. A Brazilian study of 31 babies with cleft lip or cleft palate found that those with a cleft lip had a rate of exclusive breastfeeding during the first year of life that was higher than those with a cleft palate, and even higher than the babies in the general population without cleft defects (Garcez & Giugliani, 2005). The researchers concluded that cleft lip is compatible with successful breastfeeding. Another Brazilian study of 881 children with cleft defects also found higher breastfeeding rates among babies with only a cleft lip and found that these babies had better weight gain and growth than the babies with a cleft palate (Montagnoli, Barbieri, Bettiol, Marques, & de Souza, 2005).

• •

Surgery to correct a cleft lip may be done as early as 48 hours after birth or as late as 2 to 3 months.

It was once believed that cleft-lip surgery should be delayed until the baby was at least 10 weeks old and weighed at least 10 pounds (4.5 kg), but research has found no drawbacks to early repair and no differences in outcomes (Weatherley-White, Kuehn, Mirrett, Gilman, & Weatherley-White, 1987).

With cleft lip repair, breastfeeding may be interrupted for only a few hours. If the interruption is longer, suggest the mother express her milk to maintain her milk production. Research has found that after surgery the baby's stitches are not at risk of being disturbed, even if the baby begins breastfeeding again as he leaves the recovery room (Cohen, Marschall, & Schafer, 1992; Darzi, Chowdri, & Bhat, 1996; Weatherley-White et al., 1987). In one Indian study of 40 babies, unrestricted breastfeeding after cleft-lip surgery was also associated with greater weight gain 6 weeks later (Darzi et al., 1996).

If the mother wants to breastfeed her baby immediately after surgery, suggest she make these arrangements in advance with the baby's surgeon. If the surgeon is uncomfortable with this, suggest the mother share these study citations with him/her. If the surgeon has no personal experience with early breastfeeding after surgery, he/she may be more comfortable with it if a nurse stays on hand to observe the baby for signs of damage to the stitches. If the mother is not happy with the surgeon's response, encourage her to get a second opinion.

Cleft Palate With or Without Cleft Lip

A cleft can occur in the hard palate, the soft palate, or both, and its location and size will affect the baby's ability to feed effectively.

A cleft palate occurs when parts of the baby's palate do not fuse in utero, leaving an opening in the roof of his mouth. The baby may have a cleft of the soft palate, which is comprised of soft muscle covered with mucous membrane and located near the back of the baby's mouth. Or the baby's cleft may include both the soft and hard palates. It is unusual for a cleft to be located only in the hard palate, which is comprised of bone covered with mucous membrane and located near the front of the baby's mouth.

The muscles of the soft palate are used for swallowing, so a large cleft of the soft palate can have a major impact on the baby's ability to feed by breast or bottle. Another type of cleft is called a "submucous cleft," which is an opening of muscle or bone beneath the intact skin that is invisible to the eye (see later section on p. 300).

A U.K. study of 344 individuals with cleft palates (without cleft lip or submucous clefts) found that 28% of clefts were not detected on the first day of life and five were not detected until after 1 year (Habel, Elhadi, Sommerlad, & Powell, 2006). The researchers suggested that all newborns' mouths be checked for clefts, using a light and a tongue depressor.

A cleft palate can also be one feature of a genetic syndrome, such as Pierre-Robin syndrome. Up to 13% of cleft-affected babies have other birth defects (Walker, 2006). One Australian study of 62 babies with clefts rated their feeding skills at 2 weeks, 3 months, and 14 months, and found that babies with clefts that were part of a syndrome were 15 times more likely to have poor feeding skills (Reid, Kilpatrick, & Reilly, 2006). A U.K. study of 147 babies with clefts found that 100% of those with Pierre-Robin syndrome were failure-to-thrive (Pandya & Boorman, 2001).

Hard and Soft Palate Clefts

To feed effectively, a baby needs a firm surface to compress the nipple and the ability to generate suction inside his mouth.

For several reasons, an opening in the roof of a baby's mouth makes feeding challenging.

- It prevents the baby from creating an air seal to keep breast or bottle in place.
- It may make it impossible for the baby to generate suction in his mouth, which is needed to draw milk from breast or bottle (Geddes et al., 2008; Reid et al., 2007).

- It allows milk in the baby's mouth to flow into his nasal cavity, where it can irritate tissues or enter the airway.
- Depending on the size of the cleft, there may be no firm surface against which the baby can compress a nipple/teat.
- The baby may keep his tongue mostly in the cleft and when he does move it forward, its movements may be uncoordinated rather than smooth.

Due to these dynamics, the mother may need to spend most of her baby's waking hours feeding him, especially during his first few weeks. Whether fed by breast or bottle, a baby with a cleft palate may take up to two or three times longer to feed than a baby without a cleft defect. The mother will need to try different strategies to help make feedings go more smoothly (see the following sections).

• •

A few babies with a cleft palate may eventually exclusively breastfeed, but the vast majority will need to be supplemented by other methods.

Because some individual mothers and breastfeeding counselors published reports of babies able to breastfeed exclusively in spite of their cleft palate, for many years the assumption in the breastfeeding literature was that with good technique and dedication full breastfeeding was possible for all but a few severe cases (Danner, 1992; Danner & Wilson-Clay, 1986; Grady, 1983). However, after more experience and research, exclusive breastfeeding now appears to be an elusive goal for all but a few babies with very small cleft palates, and even in these cases, it may not be possible for the first few months.

One U.K. study found that only 4% of its 50 cleft-affected babies had normal oral-motor feeding skills during their first month (Masarei et al., 2007). A combination of many factors may make it possible for a few of these babies to breastfeed effectively: a malleable breast, a healthy milk production, and a cleft of the right size and location. The mother must also be willing through trial and error to determine the positions, techniques, and devices that allow the baby to keep the breast far enough back in his mouth to transfer milk with compression and keep the milk flowing down his throat rather than into his nasal cavity. Even with all of these factors present, it may take months before these babies can breastfeed without also needing supplements. For most, exclusive breastfeeding won't be possible until they've recovered from corrective surgery.

Only a small percentage of babies with cleft palates can exclusively breastfeed, but breastfeeding may still be important to them.

Regarding the location and severity of the baby's cleft, if the cleft is small and the mother can plug it with her breast tissue, this may allow the baby to seal his mouth and provide the suction needed to keep the breast in place and the milk flowing in the right direction. One U.K. study compared 50 babies with clefts (some breastfeeding, some bottle-feeding) with 20 babies without clefts and found that the location and severity of the cleft made a significant difference in the babies' suckling efficiency (Masarei et al., 2007). While the suckling of all the babies without clefts was rated as normal, only 2 were rated as normal among the 50 babies with either a complete cleft lip and cleft palate or a cleft of the soft palate and at least two-thirds of the hard palate. Of the others in the cleft group who received a rating, all suckled markedly faster (average 109 sucks per minute versus 75 sucks per minute, indicating less milk transfer) and were rated as either disorganized or dysfunctional feeders.

In a U.S. study of 143 babies with cleft defects, the researchers found that a baby was more likely to breastfeed effectively if he could do two things: 1) generate at least some suction and 2) move the tongue appropriately against the nipple

(Clarren, Anderson, & Wolf, 1987). If a baby with a cleft palate could do both of these things, breastfeeding was more likely to go well. When one or both were impossible, effective breastfeeding was unlikely.

From birth, to establish and maintain her milk production for the baby with a cleft palate, encourage the mother to safeguard her milk production by expressing milk.

Because the vast majority of babies with a cleft palate cannot stimulate full milk production by breastfeeding alone, encourage the mother to safeguard her milk production by using the same milk-expression strategies as the mother whose baby cannot breastfeed. For details, see p. 466 in the chapter, "Milk Expression and Storage."

Make sure she knows that milk expression can allow her to provide her baby with exclusive mother's milk feedings, even if he cannot breastfeed effectively. Providing milk for her baby will contribute to better health for both of them (Ip, Chung, Raman, Trikalinos, & Lau, 2009). There are several drawbacks specific to these babies from using human-milk substitutes:

- **More ear infections**. With an intact palate, the muscles of the palate open the ear tubes during swallowing to equalize air pressure. A cleft interferes with this process, leaving fluid in the middle ear that can become infected. In both U.S. and Swedish studies, babies with cleft palates who were fed formula developed more ear infections than those receiving some human milk (Aniansson, Svensson, Becker, & Ingvarsson, 2002; Paradise, Elster, & Tan, 1994).
- **Greater irritation of sensitive nasal membranes**. With every swallow milk leaks through the cleft into baby's nose. As a natural body fluid, mother's milk is less irritating than formula to the baby's sensitive tissues (Wilson-Clay & Hoover, 2008).

If the mother wants to breastfeed a baby with a cleft palate, discuss goals and strategies.

If exclusive mother's milk feeding is the mother's goal, suggest she focus primarily on milk expression to establish and maintain her milk production. Even without much milk intake, the act of breastfeeding promotes normal development of his mouth, tongue, and facial muscles. Suggest she also think of breastfeeding as one way to enjoy a closeness and connection with her baby and provide comfort. Breastfeeding may be more comforting to her baby than an artificial nipple because the baby also receives skin-to-skin contact, which releases the calming hormone oxytocin, and because her breast is more flexible than a silicone nipple and more easily molds to the baby's lips and mouth (Uvnas-Moberg, 2003).

Depending upon the type and location of the baby's cleft, breastfeeding may be soothing to them both or it may be difficult.

Every mother-baby couple is unique, and the way they breastfeed will be unique as well. With time and practice, a few mothers have eventually been able to exclusively breastfeed a baby with a cleft palate, although most supplemented their babies during the learning period. As mentioned, it is best to start breastfeeding right after birth, while the breast is soft and pliable, to give the baby practice before the breast becomes fuller.

Feeding positions. When choosing a breastfeeding position, comfort is most important. Suggest the mother first try the laid-back, semi-reclining positions described in Chapter 1 (see Figure 8.2). These positions have the advantage of keeping the baby's head higher than the breast, which can lessen milk flow into the nose and ear tubes (Reilly et al., 2007). These positions also use gravity to help rather than hinder breastfeeding (Colson, Meek, & Hawdon, 2008). Because the baby's weight rests on the mother's well-supported body, this is less strain for her as well. Another upright option, which may work better for babies with a cleft on both sides (bilateral), is to position baby to sit in mother's lap and straddle her body (Figure 8.1).

Firm breast/soft breast. One mother of a baby with a cleft of the soft palate experimented with different positions at different times, keeping careful track of what worked to find an effective approach that worked consistently (Grady, 1983). She found that her baby breastfed best when her breast was firm and full.

Breast support. When this same mother held the breast firmly in the baby's mouth, the baby was able to use her gums and tongue to transfer milk. But because suction was broken whenever the nipple reached the cleft, the mother's nipple dropped back to the front of the baby's mouth. The baby was finally able to breastfeed effectively when the mother held her nipple firmly in the back of the baby's mouth by using the "scissors hold" and pressed the baby's head into her breast. Another dynamic helpful to milk production was that this baby was a twin. The other twin had an intact palate and could breastfeed normally.

Jaw and chin support. Some of these babies need support to hold their jaw and chin steady while breastfeeding. If the baby's cheeks appear to collapse inward as the baby breastfeeds, try the Dancer Hand position to provide jaw support (for details see p. 805 in the "Techniques" appendix). As the baby grows and gets more practice at the breast, his muscle tone will improve, and he may need chin support with only her index finger.

At-breast supplementers. An at-breast supplementer can be used to provide the cleft-affected baby with an experience similar to normal breastfeeding. At this writing, all commercially manufactured at-breast supplementers provide milk flow only when a baby generates suction inside his mouth, which these babies cannot do. However, some suggest that gravity can be used to speed milk flow for these babies by attaching these supplementers to an object much higher than the baby (Wilson-Clay & Hoover, 2008). Another option is to create an at-breast supplementer that allows the feeder to actively deliver milk to the baby ("suction not required" type), using either a 5 French feeding tube, a butterfly catheter, a port, and a syringe full of milk with the needle removed (Genna, 2008a). In the book *Selecting and Using Breastfeeding Tools,* U.S. lactation consultant Catherine Watson Genna describes easy ways to modify two commercial at-breast supplementers made by different manufacturers to give the feeder more control over milk flow and better meet these babies' feeding needs (Genna, 2009). By carefully timing the milk flow with the baby's suckling, a baby may receive at least a partial feeding at breast.

Patience. Tell the mother to expect that finding a good fit for her and her baby takes time and patience. Encourage her to seek help and support during this time.

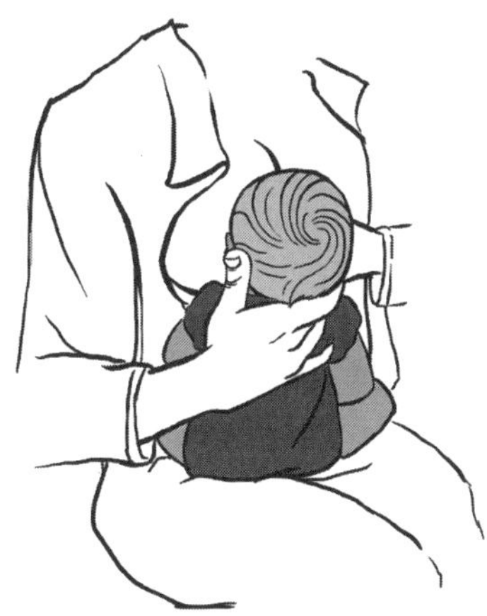

Figure 8.1. Baby straddling mother to breastfeed

©Anna Mohrbacher, used with permission

Without feeding help, the baby with a cleft palate is at risk for failure-to-thrive and inadequate weight gain and growth (Gopinath & Muda, 2005; Montagnoli et al., 2005). Some older studies indicate that babies with cleft palates gain weight slowly no matter how they are fed (Avedian & Ruberg, 1980), but a more recent review of the literature found that using a combination of the strategies below improved weight gain and growth (Reid, 2004).

Some interventions may help increase weight gain and make feedings easier for the baby with a cleft palate.

Education and support. Providing parents of cleft-affected babies with education and ongoing counseling is one intervention, when combined with others, that has been found to improve weight gain and growth (Reid, 2004). One Danish study of 115 babies with clefts found that when counseling was started at birth by trained health professionals, these babies grew at the same rate as Danish babies without clefts, although they received human milk for a shorter time (Smedegaard, Marxen, Moes, Glassou, & Scientsan, 2008). A Brazilian study of 26 babies with clefts found that when education was not consistently given to parents, weight gain and growth suffered (Amstalden-Mendes, Magna, & Gil-da-Silva-Lopes, 2007).

Some adaptive equipment may be necessary when feeding babies with cleft palates.

Specially designed feeding bottles and nipples. Feeding bottles are available that allow the baby with a cleft palate to use compression rather than suction to draw out the milk (Turner et al., 2001). Some nipples are made with special cuts to send the milk past the cleft and into baby's throat. Other bottles designed for these babies allow the feeder to squeeze them to generate milk flow as baby suckles (Mizuno, Ueda, Kani, & Kawamura, 2002). Although the research on these "assisted feeding" devices is weak, one review concluded that some babies with clefts appear to feed faster and gain more weight when they are used (Reid, 2004). A Cochrane review article concluded that while squeezable bottles seem easier to use, the evidence of a difference in outcomes among bottle types is weak (Glenny et al., 2004). As when breastfeeding, an upright position while bottle-feeding prevents milk flow through baby's nose.

Palatal obturators. These plastic plates are fitted to the baby's mouth and sometimes used before corrective surgery to keep the cleft in the baby's hard palate from closing improperly. They don't allow the baby to create suction inside his mouth, but they do provide a firm surface on which baby can press breast or bottle nipple with his tongue during feedings. Although some studies have found them helpful in shortening feeding times (Turner et al., 2001), reviews of the literature concluded they provide no significant feeding benefit (Glenny et al., 2004; Reid, 2004). If the breastfeeding baby is fitted with an obturator, suggest the mother request one with a smooth surface to reduce friction on her nipple.

Cleft palate repair may be done as early as 2 weeks and as late as 18 months.

Repair of the cleft palate is usually scheduled sometime during the baby's 1st or 2nd year, after the face and mouth have grown more mature, but before the baby has begun to do much talking. Timing and method of surgery varies from one treatment center to another (Wilson-Clay & Hoover, 2008).

After cleft palate repair, breastfeeding may be uncomfortable for the baby because his mouth feels sore. With a newly structured palate, suckling—even if not too painful—will feel different to him, and this new sensation may be unsettling. For some babies, feeling the mother's nipple in his mouth may be comforting. But sometime within a few weeks of the surgery, as breastfeeding becomes easier, he may begin breastfeeding with more enthusiasm than before. In one case report from Australia, a 7-month-old baby who had never directly breastfed was able to breastfeed exclusively after his cleft-palate repair (Crossman, 1998). If the mother uses milk expression to maintain her milk production, she will have ample milk when her baby comes to the breast.

Submucous Cleft

If milk flows through a baby's nose and feedings usually last for more than 40 minutes, he should be checked for a submucous cleft.

A submucous cleft is an opening of muscle or bone beneath the intact skin that is invisible to the eye. A submucous cleft is 150 to 600 times more likely among babies with a cleft lip than in the general population (Gosain et al., 1999).

Depending on which muscles are missing, some babies with a submucous cleft can generate suction inside their mouth, but even so, the cleft alters the muscles of the soft palate, which affects swallowing. As a result, many babies with this condition have feeding problems, such as prolonged (more than 40 minutes), ineffective feedings and regular milk flow through the nose. In one U.K. study, 48% of those with confirmed submucous clefts had feeding problems (Moss, Jones, & Pigott, 1990). This condition was also associated with chronic middle ear infections and speech problems later.

Upright breastfeeding positions can give baby more control over milk flow.

One U.S. author wrote that many babies with submucous clefts seem to feed better on the breast than on the bottle (Genna, 2008a). Using the upright breastfeeding positions described in the previous section can give a baby who finds swallowing difficult more control over milk flow and reduce milk flow through the nose. Some of these babies develop more feeding problems as their head grows, which widens the gap in the muscles of the soft palate and makes feedings more challenging (Walker, 2006).

Cystic Fibrosis

Cystic fibrosis is a genetic disease that causes the baby to secrete a thick, gluey mucus that clogs the bronchial tubes, interfering with breathing, and blocks digestive enzymes from leaving the pancreas, causing incomplete digestion. This mucus also blocks the sweat glands, which causes the baby's sweat and skin to taste salty.

The first indication a baby has cystic fibrosis may be slow weight gain and a salty taste to his skin.

There are more than 1,000 mutations of the gene responsible for cystic fibrosis, which means the disease may be mild or severe. Cases range from those detectable only through laboratory tests to those that are life-threatening. Depending on the severity, a baby with cystic fibrosis may have breathing problems and regular respiratory infections, and he may look thin, pale, and undernourished.

The first clue that a baby has cystic fibrosis may be the baby's salty taste, which the mother may notice when she kisses him. Or it may be a puzzling slow weight gain in a baby who vigorously breastfeeds and has many wet diapers and stools. Slow weight gain is due to incomplete digestion of food and is unrelated to the baby's milk intake.

• •

Babies with cystic fibrosis who do not breastfeed have poorer health outcomes and earlier onset of symptoms than those who breastfeed.

Breastfeeding has been promoted among U.S. cystic fibrosis centers because exclusive formula feeding has been associated with an increased incidence of respiratory infections and slow growth (Luder, Kattan, Tanzer-Torres, & Bonforte, 1990). In 2002, the U.S. Cystic Fibrosis Foundation stated, "Breastfeeding is recommended for most infants [with cystic fibrosis] as the primary source of nutrition for the first year of life" (Borowitz, Baker, & Stallings, 2002, p. 250). Research has found several downsides to less-than-exclusive breastfeeding in the baby with cystic fibrosis:

- **Less weight gain and shorter height.** In an Australian study of 65 babies with cystic fibrosis, those who did not exclusively breastfeed gained less weight and were not as tall as those who received only mother's milk (Holliday et al., 1991).
- **More severe disease and earlier onset of symptoms.** A U.S. retrospective survey of 863 people with cystic fibrosis found that any formula intake during the first 6 months of life was associated with a more severe form of the disease (based on treatment with IV antibiotics during the previous 2 years) and a trend toward earlier onset of symptoms and poorer lung function (Parker, O'Sullivan, Shea, Regan, & Freedman, 2004).
- **More infections and greater decline in lung function.** In an Italian retrospective study of 146 people with cystic fibrosis, weaning before 4 months was associated with more infections during the first 3 years of life and a greater decline in lung function (Colombo et al., 2007).

• •

Some breastfeeding babies with cystic fibrosis grow better and stay healthier when given medications, digestive enzymes, and/or nutritional supplements.

In about half of the babies with cystic fibrosis, excess mucous blocks the flow of digestive enzymes from the pancreas and replacement enzymes are needed to grow and gain weight appropriately (Koletzko & Reinhardt, 2001). These enzymes can be dissolved in soft foods and given by spoon before breastfeeding. Some of these babies also need extra vitamins, minerals, and salt, especially in hot weather (Gaskin & Waters, 1994; Krebs et al., 2000).

To prevent respiratory infections, the mother may be advised to keep the baby upright as much as possible and to use aerosols, antibiotics, and/or give the baby an expectorant.

Down Syndrome

Some babies with Down syndrome need time and practice to breastfeed effectively, but this learning process promotes better health and development.

Down syndrome is a genetic birth defect caused by the presence of an extra chromosome that causes developmental delays. Even so, these babies can lead positive and productive lives with love, care, and support.

Rates of breastfeeding among babies with Down syndrome vary from country to country. In the Netherlands, babies born with Down syndrome are breastfed at the same rate as other babies (Hopman et al., 1998). Not so in Italy, where a study compared 550 babies with Down syndrome to a group of control children (Pisacane et al., 2003). Those with Down syndrome were more likely to not have breastfed (57% vs. 15%). Among those whose babies did not go to the special-care nursery at birth, the reasons given for not breastfeeding included depression, perceived insufficient milk, and suckling difficulties.

Babies with Down syndrome who breastfeed have better health outcomes than babies who don't.

In some babies with Down syndrome, breastfeeding is more challenging during the early weeks, but as with any other baby, those who exclusively breastfeed are more likely to enjoy better health. Babies with Down syndrome have a greater incidence of respiratory tract infections and heart and bowel problems, and mother's milk contains components that contribute to normal immune system development. A Mexican study found that babies with Down syndrome who were not breastfed had more infections and rehospitalizations during the first year and a greater incidence of childhood leukemia later in life (Flores-Lujano et al., 2009). In addition to better health outcomes, breastfeeding strengthens facial muscle tone, promoting mouth and tongue coordination, which is often a challenge for these babies.

When a baby is born with this genetic defect, the skin-to-skin contact that comes with breastfeeding provides physical stimulation that promotes better neurodevelopment. The physical contact and hormones released during breastfeeding also enhance the emotional attachment between mother and baby during the vulnerable time that the mother adjusts emotionally to the birth of a special-need baby. As the mother helps her baby learn to breastfeed, it also hones her mothering skills. Her encouragement and responsiveness to her baby's cues are the same skills she will need as he grows to help him maximize his potential.

• •

Low muscle tone and health problems contribute to early breastfeeding challenges in many babies with Down syndrome.

Due to low muscle tone, many babies with Down syndrome are "floppy" and, at first, cannot breastfeed effectively. A low-tone baby may need extra help in finding, taking, and staying on the breast, especially in upright or side-lying positions. Be sure the mother knows that her baby's muscle tone and suckling will improve with time and practice.

During the early weeks, suggest the mother allow extra time for feedings. A baby with low muscle tone may have difficulty cupping his tongue around the breast, and when a baby's tongue stays flat, milk slides to the sides of the mouth rather than being swallowed, requiring extra effort for less milk. A Japanese study of bottle-feeding babies with Down syndrome found that ineffective breastfeeding was only partly due to low tone in the mouth, lips, and jaw. Another factor was their uncoordinated tongue movements. Only with time and maturity were they able to master the wave-like coordinated tongue motions needed for effective feeding (Mizuno & Ueda, 2001b).

But not all babies with Down syndrome have difficulty breastfeeding. In a U.K. study of 59 breastfed babies with Down syndrome, their mothers reported that at birth 52% had no trouble breastfeeding effectively (Aumonier & Cunningham, 1983). Within the first week, 7% more were suckling well. At 1 week of age, 14% more breastfed effectively. For the remaining 27%, it took longer than 1 week to learn to breastfeed effectively.

Admission to the special-care nursery also affects breastfeeding outcomes in these babies. In the Italian study of 550 babies with Down syndrome mentioned previously, 44% were admitted to the special-care nursery at birth, and of those, only 30% breastfed, with illness given as the main reason by the mothers for not breastfeeding (Pisacane et al., 2003).

• •

If the baby is in the special-care nursery or can't yet breastfeed, offer to provide the mother with information on milk expression and strategies for transitioning to the breast.

If due to the respiratory infections and heart and bowel problems common in these babies, the baby needs special care, let the mother know she can still use milk expression to provide her milk for her baby. For details, see the chapter, "Milk Expression and Storage."

When a baby is fed by mouth, health outcomes are better when he is fed mother's milk. If a baby is tube-fed at first, he can begin to go to the breast even before transitioning off the tube (Genna, Fram, & Sandora, 2008). If extra help is needed in taking the breast, see "More Strategies for Babies with High/Low Tone" on p. 309 under "Neurological Impairment."

When the baby begins taking the breast, suggest the mother think of these first feedings at the breast as practice sessions and focus on enjoying their time together, rather than how much milk he takes. Tell her that she and her baby will have many opportunities to breastfeed and not to worry if it takes some time for him to catch on.

• •

If the baby seems sleepy most of the time, encourage the mother to keep him on her body as much as possible to trigger feeding behaviors.

Many babies with Down syndrome are sleepy during the first few weeks and can be difficult to rouse for feeding. If so, suggest the mother:

- Lean back and lay her baby on her body as much of the day as possible, which provides the stimulation needed to trigger feeding behaviors (Colson, DeRooy, & Hawdon, 2003).
- Move the baby to the breast whenever he goes from a deep sleep to a light sleep, such as when he begins to squirm, when his eyes move under his eyelids, or when his mouth moves.
- Keep the baby skin-to-skin as much as possible, so the mother will know from her baby's movements and changes in breathing when he might be willing to feed.

In laid-back breastfeeding positions, gravity gives a low-tone baby who coughs at the breast more control over milk flow.

Low muscle tone can leave a baby's airway unprotected during swallowing, which causes the gulping and coughing common among babies with Down syndrome. In this case, breastfeeding often goes more smoothly when the baby feeds in positions that keep his head higher than the mother's nipple. See Figure 8.2 and Chapter 1 for illustrations of laid-back breastfeeding positions.

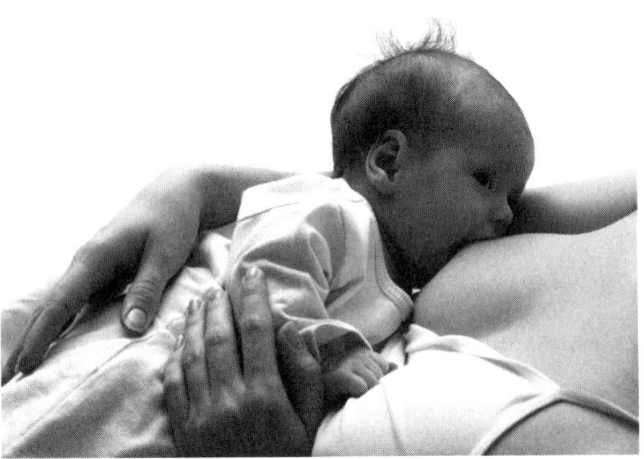

Figure 8.2. A laid-back breastfeeding position.

A low-tone, protruding tongue can make taking the breast more challenging.

For suggestions on ways to increase mouth and tongue tone before breastfeeding and techniques and tools that can be used during feeding, see the section "More Strategies for Babies with High/Low Tone" on p. 309.

If the baby gains weight slowly, supplements may be needed.

If despite the mother's efforts the baby does not breastfeed effectively or often enough, supplements—ideally mother's milk—may be needed, as gaining weight means gaining strength as well.

A baby who does not gain at least 5 oz. (142 g) per week, despite good milk intake probably has a health problem, such as a heart defect. A baby with a heart defect may use extra energy and calories just to maintain adequate circulation (see the section "Cardiac Issues" on p. 291). One U.K. study found that among babies with Down syndrome, the more severe the heart defect, the less effectively the baby breastfed (Aumonier & Cunningham, 1983).

One way a mother can increase her baby's calorie intake is by giving her own high-calorie hindmilk as a supplement. She can provide this fattier milk by first expressing milk for a few minutes, then switching containers and continuing to express. The milk she expresses into the second container can be stored as the supplement.

Breastfeeding the baby with Down syndrome sometimes can be challenging, but assure the mother that with patience and persistence, as the baby grows, gets stronger, and increases in muscle tone, feedings will go more smoothly.

Galactosemia

Lactose, or milk sugar, is broken down by a baby's liver enzymes into glucose and galactose, which is then further broken down. Galactosemia is a rare (1 in 60,000), inherited metabolic disorder in which the liver does not produce the enzyme that metabolizes galactose, causing it to accumulate in the baby's system. Too much galactose usually becomes apparent on about the 3rd day of life as jaundice, enlarged liver, vomiting, and lethargy. If treatment is not begun soon, it can progress to failure-to-thrive, liver and kidney damage, convulsions, and mental retardation. Human milk is high in lactose, so with classic galactosemia, breastfeeding is contraindicated and the baby must be fed galactose-free formula.

Breastfeeding is contraindicated when a baby has classic galactosemia, but blood tests produce many false-positive results.

In the U.S., newborns are routinely screened for galactosemia during the first week of life (Kaye et al., 2006). But because the liver enzyme the blood test is designed to detect is sensitive to heat, babies who do not have this disorder sometimes test positive for it, especially during the summer months when blood samples are not always kept cool.

Blood tests for galactosemia sometimes yield false-positive results.

If the baby tests positive for galactosemia, suggest the mother first ask her baby's healthcare provider to evaluate the baby for symptoms and arrange for another blood test as soon as possible. By being proactive with the healthcare provider and the testing facility, a mother may get the second test results faster. For example, the mother can ask the baby's healthcare provider to call the testing facility and request special handling of the test. Overnight delivery is an option, or if the mother is within driving distance of the testing facility, she may be able to arrange for someone she trusts to drive her baby's blood sample there. After the sample reaches the testing facility, results should be available within a day or two.

After evaluating the baby's health, the baby's healthcare provider can advise the mother whether she should begin feeding him a special galactose-free formula until the second test results are received. If so, encourage the mother to express her milk to maintain her milk production until she receives the results. If her baby has classic galactosemia, breastfeeding is contraindicated. In this case, offer to talk to the mother about her feelings and provide strategies for reducing her milk production gradually and comfortably.

If the baby has a milder form of galactosemia, partial or full breastfeeding may be possible.

The term galactosemia covers more than 100 mutations of this disorder. Duarte galactosemia is one type in which the baby may produce varying levels of the liver enzyme needed to break down galactose. Depending on the combination of genes the baby inherited, he may produce 75%, 50%, or 25%-50% of the enzyme needed to metabolize galactose (Walker, 2006). A blood test can determine the baby's enzyme level. Some of these babies may be able to partially or exclusively breastfeed. Suggest before a mother stops expressing her milk that she discuss this possibility with her baby's healthcare provider.

Neurological Impairment

A neurological impairment can affect a baby's ability to breastfeed.

Many babies with a neurological impairment have obvious and serious issues. The baby may have a brain bleed (most common in preterm babies) or have seizures. The baby may have an abnormal brain structure caused by a birth defect, such as macrocephaly (a very large head) or microcephaly (a very small head). Some neurological impairments are caused by the mother's substance abuse during pregnancy, such as fetal alcohol spectrum disorders. Other possible causes of neurological impairment are hydrocephaly, autism spectrum disorders, and genetic neurological conditions associated with syndromes such as Prader-Willi, Williams, Kabuki, Phelan-McDermid, and others. When a baby's brain or nervous system is affected by injury or abnormal development, it may compromise his ability to organize his movements and feed effectively, as well as his ability to learn and stay alert (Genna et al., 2008; Radzyminski, 2005).

Even if challenging at first, breastfeeding should be encouraged.

But even if breastfeeding does not come easily to this baby, suggest the mother think of it as a normal behavior to be encouraged, like walking and talking. Unless the baby has a degenerative neurological disorder, with patience, persistence, and maturity, he will become stronger and more coordinated, which makes breastfeeding easier. Time spent learning to breastfeed helps improve a baby's neuro-muscular coordination. Finnish researchers found that unlike sucking on a pacifier, the baby's autonomic nervous system responds uniquely to breastfeeding and concluded: "We consider this response an essential part of the overall psychophysiological maturation of infants" (Lappi et al., 2007, p. 546). In addition, the baby receives via his mother's milk countless components not found in human-milk substitutes that promote the normal development of his immune and digestive systems.

The feelings of closeness associated with breastfeeding also may be important to this family. If the baby is not as responsive to his parents as other babies, this puts their relationship at risk (Clark & Seifer, 1983; Clark & Seifer, 1985). The hormones released by breastfeeding and the regular skin-to-skin contact can help strengthen their attachment and help the mother experience her baby as a person first and a child with a disability second.

If the baby's neurological problem is so severe that it is impossible for him to breastfeed, emphasize to the mother the value of her milk and offer to provide details on how to establish full milk production through milk expression. For details, see p. 466 in the chapter "Milk Expression and Storage."

Encourage the mother to seek out healthcare providers supportive of breastfeeding and early intervention programs to prevent or minimize developmental delay.

Feeding problems are sometimes the first sign of a neurological impairment (Mizuno & Ueda, 2005). In parts of the world where breastfeeding is not the norm, some healthcare providers are willing to overlook a breastfeeding problem if a baby can be bottle-fed—even if poorly—rather than seeking the cause. Although some feeding problems are temporary, a neurological impairment may be missed, along with the opportunity for early intervention.

Ideally, when a baby has a breastfeeding problem, the cause will be found, so that if it is due to a neurological impairment, the baby can be referred for help. Early intervention programs can be found online with the keywords "early intervention" along with the country or area name. Usually local lactation consultants know individuals, such as breastfeeding-knowledgeable occupational therapists and speech-and-language pathologists, or agencies that provide skilled help. Let the mother know that early intervention can help resolve a mild problem quickly and that it does not necessarily mean the baby will need long-term therapy. For a baby with a severe neurodevelopmental impairment, however, early intervention can be vital to the timely development of pre-feeding skills that will allow him to eventually transition to the breast (Morris & Klein, 2001).

Even when a neurological impairment affects a baby's ability to coordinate suckling, swallowing, and breathing, with practice and patience, many of these babies can learn to breastfeed, and some can learn to feed effectively. The act of bottle-feeding differs fundamentally from breastfeeding, and research has found that babies with feeding problems experience higher stress responses and lower oxygen levels when bottle-fed than when breastfed (Meier, 1988; Meier & Anderson, 1987; Mizuno & Ueda, 2006). So a baby's ability to bottle-feed should not be used to determine whether a baby is able to breastfeed.

If in severe cases the baby needs to be tube-fed, mother's milk should be the first choice. Japanese research has found that even in babies tube-fed for months, feeding competence can improve with maturity and practice at the breast (Mizuno & Ueda, 2001a). Breastfeeding can often begin even before tube-feeding ends (Genna et al., 2008).

• •

Babies with a neurological impairment often have either high or low muscle tone, which can contribute to feeding problems.

Typically, a baby with a neurological impairment has either high or low muscle tone, although some babies have high muscle tone in their body and low muscle tone in their mouth, and vice versa. Babies with high tone may arch their bodies, over-respond to stimulation, and bite or clench at the breast. They are often fussy during feedings. Babies with low muscle tone tend to under-respond to feeding triggers. Both high- and low-tone babies may have trouble coordinating suckling, swallowing, and breathing, and they may take very little milk, even after long periods at the breast. The following two sections describe strategies that can help babies achieve a "middle tone" during feedings that enhances both their feeling of well-being and their breastfeeding effectiveness.

High Muscle Tone

A baby with high muscle tone tends to over-respond to sensory stimulation.

Suggest the mother keep the feeding environment quiet and dim to avoid overstimulation. Most babies with high muscle tone breastfeed more effectively if feedings start before they get too hungry. This baby may have an unusually sensitive mouth, which can cause gagging during feedings. He may arch his body or hyperextend his head. He may clench his jaw muscles or tense his tongue, causing bunching, humping, or retraction.

• •

Strategies used before and during breastfeeding may help increase milk intake in high-tone babies.

When trying the following strategies, suggest the mother of the high-tone baby use only those that work well with her baby and discontinue any that the baby doesn't like or that seems to cause problems (Genna, 2008b):

- Before feedings, hold him in the "colic hold" (see Figure 8.3) or gently swing from head to foot in a blanket gathered up at the corners (blanket swing) until he relaxes and flexes.

- During feedings, avoid movement, such as rocking or swaying, and try a stable semi-reclining position with baby lying tummy down on her body, in a snug sling, swaddled, lying on a firm pillow, or side-lying on a firm surface.
- Use deep, firm touch rather than light touch.
- Keep light and sound low.

If the baby gags easily at the breast, suggest the mother encourage her baby to take a more active role in taking the breast (see Chapter 1).

Skin-to-skin contact helps calm and comfort some of these babies. If the baby is so ineffective at feedings that he is not gaining weight adequately, he will need to be supplemented (see later section).

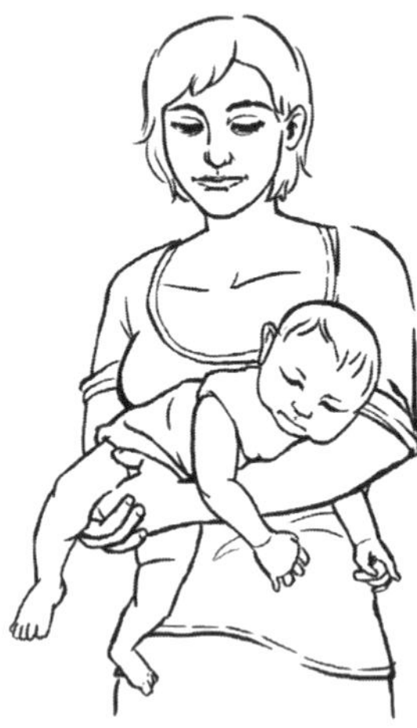

Figure 8.3. The "Colic Hold"

©Anna Mohrbacher, used with permission

Low Muscle Tone

A baby with low muscle tone tends to under-respond to sensory stimulation and may breastfeed ineffectively.

When a neurologically impaired baby with low oral muscle tone is at the breast, he may suckle weakly and dribble milk out of the sides of his mouth. When not at the breast, his mouth may stay open and his tongue protrude. Reflux disease is also common among these babies due to low-tone sphincter muscles that keep food down (Genna et al., 2008).

Strategies used before and during breastfeeding may help increase milk intake in low-tone babies.

When trying the following strategies, suggest the mother of the low-tone baby use only those that work well with her baby and discontinue any that the baby doesn't like or seems to cause problems (Genna, 2008b):

- **Increase muscle tone before feedings** by sitting baby on her knee and bouncing or leaning him forward and backward in a non-rhythmic way. If milk has been dribbling out of baby's mouth during feedings, try firmly patting the baby's lips before putting him to breast (Wolf & Glass, 1992).

- **Experiment with feeding positions.** Try first more upright positions, starting with semi-reclining, laid-back positions (see Figure 8.2 and Chapter 1), which provide the full-body support helpful to low-tone babies. One Japanese study found that compromised babies fed best when positioned tummy down (Mizuno, Inoue, & Takeuchi, 2000). Or try swaddling the baby with hips and knees flexed, hands positioned near mid-body, and shoulders slightly forward.
- **Encourage the baby to take an active role in going onto the breast,** using the baby's inborn feeding behaviors to trigger a wide open mouth and gravity to help the baby take the breast deeply and maintain a stable position (see Chapter 1).
- **Experiment with the baby's head position.** In neurologically normal babies, breastfeeding with the head slightly tilted back makes swallowing and breathing easier, but some babies with a neurological impairment or anatomical abnormality find swallowing easier with their chin tucked slightly toward their chest (Genna et al., 2008). Encourage the mother to do what works well for her baby.
- **Try the Dancer Hand position to support the baby's jaw** if an upright or side-lying position is used and the baby has trouble staying on the breast or if the baby uses wide jaw movements during feedings (see p. 805 in the "Techniques" appendix).
- **Apply gentle pressure with her fingertip under the baby's chin** if the baby's tongue movements are weak. The mother can do this by gently pressing upward, with her fingertip on the soft tissue behind her baby's jawbone, with a forward movement.

More Strategies for Babies with High/Low Tone

Even if the mother is at full milk production, the baby with a neurological impairment may be unable to exclusively breastfeed.

A baby may breastfeed ineffectively when his neurological impairment causes unusual piston-like tongue movements, wide jaw excursions, low or non-existent vacuum, uncoordinated suckling due to breathing or swallowing problems, and/or other deviations from the norm (Mizuno & Ueda, 2005). The mother may express plenty of milk for her baby, but her baby may be unable to take enough milk at the breast. Some of these babies take only 10% to 60% of the milk their mothers can express (Genna et al., 2008).

If the high-tone or low-tone baby cannot yet exclusively breastfeed, suggest the mother try a nipple shield.

Until the baby is exclusively breastfeeding, suggest the mother try using a silicone nipple shield at the breast to see if that improves her baby's effectiveness. The firmer nipple shield may be able to push past the tensed tongue of the high-tone baby and the protruding tongue of the low-tone baby to provide the right stimulation for more effective suckling. For the low-tone baby, the firmer feel of the shield may trigger a stronger sensory response.

Because milk flows through the holes in the shield's tip, if the baby's milk intake increases with use of the shield, the need to supplement may be reduced or eliminated. More milk intake also provides the baby with positive reinforcement at the breast. To be effective, the shield must be a good fit for both mother and baby. For details on how to choose, fit, apply, use, and wean from a nipple shield, see the "Tools and Products" appendix.

If the baby is unable to stimulate milk flow through the shield, suggest the mother try filling the tip of the shield with expressed milk (either by expressing milk into it or inserting milk with a curved-tip syringe). Getting milk in this way provides the baby with positive reinforcement at the breast, which may lead to more interest and effort (Genna et al., 2008).

Until the baby is able to take full feedings at the breast with the shield, the mother will need to express her milk after feedings to establish or maintain her milk production. If the shield does not improve her baby's milk intake or help in any other way, suggest she discontinue it.

If the baby feeds better with a faster milk flow, breast compression or an at-breast supplement may promote more effective breastfeeding.

No matter what the baby's neurological issue, he will feed best when the milk flow is fast enough to keep him interested and active, but not so fast that it overwhelms him. The baby's specific issues will determine which milk flow is right for him. For example, a baby with breathing or swallowing problems (dysphagia) may be easily overwhelmed and do best with a very slow milk flow, whereas a baby with low tone who needs more sensory stimulation to stay active at the breast may feed better with a faster flow. Except for the times a baby needs a little squirt of milk to "jumpstart" suckling, ideally the baby should control the milk flow, either through his own efforts or the feeder should coordinate the milk delivered to the baby with his suckling efforts (Genna et al., 2008). Unless a baby's efforts affect the milk flow, a feeding method will not promote more effective breastfeeding.

For a baby who feeds better with a faster milk flow, the mother can experiment with breast compression (see p. 804 in the appendix "Techniques") or an at-breast supplementer, which uses a thin tube at the mother's breast to deliver the supplement to the baby during breastfeeding. The baby's natural response to a swallow is to suckle. Some babies learn a more effective suckling pattern when the steady milk flow from the tube stimulates more active and consistent suckling and swallowing. When a baby suckles more vigorously, he also takes more milk directly from the breast and stimulates the mother's milk production.

Two types of at-breast supplementers, "suction required" and "suction not required," can be used At this writing all manufactured feeding-tube devices require suction, which means the baby must actively suck the milk through its thin tubing from the container. Makeshift at-breast supplementers that do not require suction can be created using a periodontal syringe or a syringe attached by a port to thin tubing. These "suction not required" devices allow the feeder to push the milk to the baby. Depending on the baby's issue, one or the other may be a more effective tool. For more details, see p. 815- "The Two Types of At-Breast Supplementers."

An at-breast supplementer may not improve a baby's breastfeeding if the baby learns to take the milk "like a straw" from the supplementer tube without suckling vigorously. In this case, it may help to make the end of the tube flush with the nipple, rather than extending it past the nipple (which is usually recommended). But if this doesn't help, the at-breast supplementer may not be the right tool. In some cases, the baby may do better if the at-breast supplementer is used with a nipple shield to provide both a faster milk flow and a firmer feel. In some cases, a different strategy, such as finger-feeding or oral exercises, may be more effective.

Mouth and tongue exercises may help, but should be tailored to address the baby's issues.

Some babies become more organized when oral exercises are used, and some become more disorganized. There is a wide range of possible tongue and mouth exercises (such as "Walking Back on the Tongue" on p. 806), but choosing an oral exercise should be done by someone familiar with the underlying cause of the baby's problem and the techniques that best address it (Genna et al., 2008). Unless the person providing skilled breastfeeding help is trained in oral-motor evaluation and therapy, she/he should consider referring the mother and baby to someone with this training, especially if the baby has difficulty feeding at breast and bottle. See the "Resources" section at the end of this chapter for websites to locate local people trained in oral-motor evaluation and therapy. Because many in these fields were trained using bottle-feeding norms, ask if they are familiar with the breastfeeding baby.

Tongue exercises can help a baby with a disorganized suck become more organized.

Mouth and tongue exercise should always be enjoyable for everyone. The baby should be actively involved and because his mouth is a private space, the baby should be the one to decide if others can enter it and for how long (Genna et al., 2008). Signs of stress in a baby with a neurological impairment may be subtle, so it is important to model sensitivity to the baby's responses. To avoid overstimulation, in some cases, these exercises may be best timed before the baby shows feeding cues or when switching breasts.

When helping a mother plan her day, base the amount of time the baby spends at the breast on effectiveness and the baby's interest.

If a baby is ineffective at the breast, most mothers appreciate some guidance in structuring their day to maximize their milk production, while keeping the rest of their life manageable. How much time a baby should spend at the breast will depend on how effectively he takes milk. If he is taking little or no milk at the breast, suggest the mother put him to the breast for "practice" whenever he seems interested and alert, rather than using a fixed schedule. Then she can focus most of her "feeding time" on expressing milk and feeding her baby.

On the other hand, if the baby takes most of his milk at the breast, regular breastfeeding time is important. In this case, less time should be spent on milk expression and more time on efforts to maximize the baby's effectiveness at the breast. In these cases, use of a nipple shield and/or at-breast supplementer may increase milk taken at the breast, which reduces the need to supplement after feedings.

As the baby's breastfeeding improves, the mother can gradually supplement less.

There are many ways to gradually reduce the amount of supplements the baby receives. If an at-breast supplementer is used, the flow can be slowed by raising the container, the tube can be kinked to stop flow for part of the breastfeeding, or it can be used at gradually fewer feedings during the day. Usually the first breastfeeding in the morning (or whenever the mother's breasts are fullest) is the first feeding to stop supplementing.

If other feeding methods are used, less supplement can be given at each feeding or supplements can be gradually given fewer and fewer times each day.

PKU

Because false positives are common with blood tests for PKU, any baby testing positive should be retested.

Phenylketonuria (PKU) is a rare metabolic disorder (1 in 14,000) in which the baby lacks the liver enzyme needed to break down the essential amino acid phenylalanine, an ingredient of both human milk and most formulas. If untreated, this amino acid accumulates in the blood, causing brain damage. Treatment consists of a lifelong diet of low-phenylalinine foods (Purnell, 2001).

During the first week of life, U.S. newborns are routinely screened for this disorder (Kaye et al., 2006). For results of the PKU test to be accurate, the baby must have consumed phenylalanine (be breastfeeding well) and be at least 24 hours old. Babies do not need to be fed formula before being tested for PKU.

False positives are common with the PKU test. But because exclusive breastfeeding can lead to permanent neurological damage in a baby with PKU, if a baby's test results are positive, encourage the mother to have the baby retested to confirm the diagnosis. Sometimes several retests are needed before PKU can be ruled out, during which time she can express her milk to safeguard her milk production. To speed this process, first suggest the mother ask her baby's healthcare provider to do another blood test as soon as possible. By being proactive with the healthcare provider and the testing facility, a mother may get the second test results faster. For example, the mother can ask the baby's healthcare provider to call the testing facility and request special handling of the test. Overnight delivery is an option, or if the mother is within driving distance of the testing facility, she may be able to arrange for someone she trusts to drive her baby's blood sample there. After the sample reaches the testing facility, results should be available within a day or two.

Exclusive breastfeeding is contraindicated in PKU, but partial breastfeeding is possible.

Partial breastfeeding can continue in the baby with PKU, with the addition of special formula supplements to maintain safe phenylalanine blood levels.

A baby with PKU has to balance his need for protein with the risk of receiving too much phenylalanine. Continued partial breastfeeding works because the baby with PKU needs some phenylalanine for normal growth. So in addition to being fed a special low-phenylalanine or phenylalanine-free formula, the baby also needs protein in his diet.

There are several reasons to consider continuing to breastfeed the baby with PKU. Because human milk is lower in phenylalanine than regular formula, less of the expensive low-phenylalanine formula is needed, saving the parents significant cost. Mother's milk also provides better nourishment and live cells that protect the baby from illness.

Throughout his life, the baby with PKU must be carefully monitored to avoid unsafe phenylalanine blood levels. After diagnosis, breastfeeding is usually interrupted for a few days to bring the baby's blood levels down to normal, during which time the mother can express her milk to safeguard her milk production. After this, breastfeeding can be combined with special formula in several ways. All of the following strategies have been used successfully:

- Alternate all-breast with all-formula feedings, allowing baby to take as much of each as desired (van Rijn et al., 2003).
- At each feeding, first give the baby a predetermined amount of special formula (65% of the baby's 24-hour milk intake divided by number

of feedings) and then breastfeed unrestrictedly (Motzfeldt, Lilje, & Nylander, 1999).

- At each feeding give the baby first a predetermined amount of mother's milk, followed by as much special formula as the baby will take (Ahring et al., 2009).
- Feed the baby a bottle of special formula every 3 hours and breastfeed as desired during the intervals between (Kanufre et al., 2007).
- Estimate the baby's total daily milk intake by age and calculate the volume of formula needed to maintain safe phenylalinine blood levels. Give the baby this volume of formula every 24 hours (however is most convenient). Schedule biweekly blood tests to monitor baby's blood levels and make adjustments as needed (Greve, Wheeler, Green-Burgeson, & Zorn, 1994).

Some of these feeding routines are simpler than others. The researchers who studied the last routine above concluded that even though more time was needed while establishing breastfeeding to monitor blood levels and assess weight gain, "eventually breastfeeding decreases the need for complicated formula mixtures and can make overall management easier" (Greve et al., 1994, p. 308).

At this writing, most European countries recommend breastfeeding the baby with PKU, with different countries recommending different feeding routines. The first routine listed above is recommended in the Netherlands, the second in Belgium, Denmark, Norway, Poland, and the U.K., and the third in Germany (Ahring et al., 2009).

• •

Newborns with PKU who were formula-fed before diagnosis lose more IQ points than those who were breastfed before diagnosis.

Because formula contains more phenylalanine than human milk, babies formula-fed before PKU diagnosis have higher phenylalanine blood levels, which can affect brain function. One Italian study found that children exclusively formula fed before PKU diagnosis (occurring before 6 weeks of age) scored an average of 14 points lower on intelligence tests during elementary school than the children breastfed before diagnosis. The researchers wrote that breastfeeding may offer a "positive nutritional benefit on later childhood neurodevelopmental performance," partly due to human milk's lower phenylalanine levels before diagnosis and partly because it is higher than most formulas in long-chain polyunsaturated fatty acids, which enhance neural functioning (Riva et al., 1996, p. 58).

HOSPITALIZATION OF THE BREASTFEEDING BABY

While Baby Is Hospitalized

Be prepared to talk about the mother's feelings while gathering information.

A baby's hospitalization is stressful for a mother. She may feel vulnerable and badly shaken. She may also be struggling with guilt. Be prepared to offer support during this difficult time.

As the mother describes her situation, try to gather the following information:

- The baby's age.
- How much he was breastfeeding before the hospitalization (partial/exclusive?).
- The reason the baby was hospitalized.
- About how long the baby may be in the hospital.
- How far she lives from the hospital and her transportation options.
- Her other responsibilities (employment/other children and their ages).

• •

Ask the mother what the baby's healthcare provider has told her about breastfeeding and how much time each day she can spend with her baby.

Is the baby being fed by mouth? If the baby can't yet feed by mouth, make sure she has the information she needs about milk expression (see next point), so she can safeguard her milk production, keep herself comfortable, and provide the milk her baby will need later. If the baby can take anything by mouth, her milk is the best first choice because it will be most easily digested and provides immunities to illness that can help a sick baby get well faster and provide protection from other illnesses the baby may be exposed to in the hospital. If the mother has been discouraged from breastfeeding, encourage her to discuss her wishes and work with those caring for her baby to find a mutually acceptable solution. For more, see the appendix, "Working with Health Professionals."

How much time each day can she spend with her baby? If the hospital is far from home, suggest the mother ask if her baby can be transferred to a hospital closer to home after his condition has stabilized. Discuss the mother's other responsibilities and help her brainstorm ways she can spend as much time as possible at the hospital (take sick or vacation time from work/arrange childcare for other children).

Can she room-in with her baby? This will depend on several factors: the baby's condition, the hospital's policy, and the mother's other responsibilities. Breastfeeding will be easier if the mother can stay with her baby day and night and breastfeed without restrictions, but circumstances (such as other children at home/job responsibilities) may interfere. Some hospitals encourage parents to stay with their children and help care for them, but even if the hospital doesn't usually allow 24-hour rooming-in, they may if the mother requests it. If the baby's healthcare provider is supportive, the mother can ask him or her to write orders for unlimited access. Suggest she get all special orders in writing and have them with her.

If the baby is not yet breastfeeding or they cannot be together, ask the mother about her breastfeeding goals and help her plan ahead.

Ask the mother if she wants to provide her milk for her baby when he can feed by mouth for those feedings she can't be with him. If she does, offer to discuss the practical details. For example, talk about a typical day and discuss the times and places she can express her milk. For details, see the chapter "Milk Expression and Storage."

If her baby will be given formula at missed feedings, be sure she knows:

1. Depending on her milk production, she may need to express milk just to keep herself comfortable and prevent mastitis.
2. If her baby had been exclusively breastfeeding and she wants to resume this after her baby is discharged, to maintain her milk production she should consider expressing milk as many times per day as her baby was breastfeeding or if she was exclusively breastfeeding, at least six times per day.

A drop in milk production during stressful times is not unusual.

Some mothers report that during a stressful time they "lost their milk." Let the mother know that when under unusual stress a temporary drop in milk production or a delay in milk ejection is common (Chatterton et al., 2000). Encourage her to use relaxation techniques and to keep breastfeeding or expressing her milk. Let her know that with time and regular breast stimulation her milk production will return to what it was.

The stress associated with the baby's hospitalization may cause a mother's milk production to drop.

Offer suggestions that may help make her baby's hospital stay easier.

Attention to details can sometimes make a difficult situation easier to cope with.

Environment

- If the baby is in a semi-private room, request the bed farthest from the door for more privacy and less traffic.
- Look into the possibility of a private room.

The mother's comfort

- If a large part of her day is spent at the hospital, bring drinks and snacks or ask about receiving hospital meals.
- Bring extra pillows or cushions from home for added comfort.
- Wear comfortable shoes and clothes that make breastfeeding easy.

Medical equipment and procedures

- If the baby is on an IV, ask for longer tubing for more freedom of movement while breastfeeding.
- If the baby needs an oxygen tent, can she breastfeed inside it?
- If painful procedures must be done, ask if topical anesthetics can be used to numb the site and multiple procedures be done at once, rather than spreading them out over the course of the day (Batton, Barrington, & Wallman, 2006).
- Breastfeed during painful procedures to reduce the baby's pain (see next point).

Breastfeeding is a potent pain-reliever, which can help speed baby's recovery.

Helping to reduce a baby's pain is always a kindness, but pain-relief can also be an important aspect of a faster recovery. In their joint policy statement on pain management in newborns, the American Academy of Pediatrics and the Canadian Paediatric Society explain that better pain management improves health outcomes after surgery by "minimizing the endocrine and metabolic responses" to pain (Batton et al., 2006). It was once thought that newborns did not feel pain and that their pain didn't matter because they wouldn't remember it later. But research has clearly demonstrated that pain is felt by preterm babies and newborns and has profound negative physical effects (Bartocci, Bergqvist, Lagercrantz, & Anand, 2006).

Breastfeeding is more effective in relieving pain than holding, swaddling, and sucking on a pacifier.

When a baby undergoes a painful medical procedure, research has found that breastfeeding reduces a baby's pain more effectively than holding, swaddling, or suckling on a pacifier (Abdulkader, Freer, Fleetwood-Walker, & McIntosh, 2007; Phillips, Chantry, & Gallagher, 2005; Uga et al., 2008). This difference may be due to body responses unique to breastfeeding. Finnish research found that unlike sucking on a pacifier, breastfeeding produces measurable changes in a baby's autonomic nervous system, which were reflected as changes in heart rate variability (Lappi et al., 2007). A Cochrane Review article concluded that compared to swaddling and sucking on a pacifier, babies breastfed during painful procedures had lower heart rates and spent less time crying (Shah, Aliwalas, & Shah, 2006). Other effective pain-reducers include skin-to-skin contact (Gray, Watt, & Blass, 2000), feeding mother's milk (an option when the mother isn't available) (Bucher, Baumgartner, Bucher, Seiler, & Fauchere, 2000), and giving sugar water (Carbajal, Veerapen, Couderc, Jugie, & Ville, 2003; Efe & Savaser, 2007).

Three potent non-drug pain relievers that can be used to comfort a baby in pain are skin-to-skin contact, a sweet taste, and suckling at the breast, and breastfeeding provides all three. Although much research exists on the effectiveness of breastfeeding in reducing babies' pain, many healthcare providers have not yet changed their practices to reflect this understanding (Gray, Trotter, Langbridge, & Doherty, 2006). Encourage the mother to suggest breastfeeding for her baby's pain relief if it hasn't yet been suggested to her.

A baby's usual breastfeeding rhythms may change during illness or injury.

Some babies want to breastfeed more often—sometimes almost constantly—when very sick or injured. Other babies, such as those who are lethargic from infection or other illness, may be less interested in breastfeeding. If a baby loses interest in the breast, suggest the mother consider expressing her milk to keep herself comfortable and to maintain her milk production until her baby is feeling better. A lethargic baby can be fed his mother's milk by tube (known as gavage feeding) if necessary.

Coping with Surgery

Suggest the mother ask how close to surgery her child can breastfeed and how soon after surgery breastfeeding can resume.

One of the most stressful aspects of surgery on a breastfeeding child is the period before the surgery when all food and drink stops, so that his stomach will be empty during the procedure. Described as "preoperative fasting" or being "NPO," this practice is meant to decrease the risk of the child's stomach contents entering his lungs (aspiration) during and after surgery.

In recent years, the length of time recommended for preoperative fasting has decreased, from "no food or drink after midnight" to much shorter periods, which vary by food, depending on how quickly it leaves the stomach. During the years this issue was being debated, one aspect that sometimes led to inconsistencies was disagreement about which food category human milk fell into, which affected fasting time. In 1999, when 44 U.S. hospitals were surveyed, their responses were varied, with some considering human milk a clear liquid (23%), somewhere between a clear liquid and formula (36%), a solid (34%), and the same as formula (7%) (Ferrari, Rooney, & Rockoff, 1999).

However, consensus appears to have been reached. A Cochrane Review of the research stated: "...clear liquids up to a few hours before surgery did not increase the risk of regurgitation during or after surgery. Indeed there is added benefit of a more comfortable preoperative experience..." (Brady, Kinn, O'Rourke, Randhawa, & Stuart, 2005). U.S. researchers wrote: "...after nearly 15 years of practice worldwide, the relative safety and benefits of [the following guidelines]...are well established" (Cook-Sather & Litman, 2006):

Human milk may be offered up to 3 hours before surgery.

- Light meal: 6 hours
- Formula: 4 hours
- Human milk: 3 hours
- Clear liquids: 2 hours

Encourage the mother to talk to her baby's surgeon and anesthesiologist before the day of the surgery to reach an agreement on the fasting time. During those difficult 3 hours before surgery, one possible option is to ask about breastfeeding the baby for comfort on a pre-pumped breast up to 2 hours before the surgery (Lawrence & Lawrence, 2005). Help her plan strategies for comforting and distracting her baby while breastfeeding is restricted.

After surgery, some mothers are able to arrange to breastfeed in the recovery room, which can be comforting to both mother and baby. Suggest the mother talk to her baby's healthcare provider about this possibility. Whenever the baby is ready to take feedings by mouth, breastfeeding should resume.

• •

Discuss with the mother possible milk-expression strategies based on how long breastfeeding will be restricted and her baby's need for milk.

Because some mothers find that stress temporarily decreases their milk production or delays their milk ejection, depending on her child's age and need for milk, the mother may want to express some extra milk to tide them over. If the mother has advance notice of at least several days before her baby's surgery, she may want to express and store extra milk in case she expresses less milk than usual before and after the surgery.

RESOURCES FOR PARENTS

Cleft Lip and/or Palate

Books

Genna, C. (2009). *Selecting and using breastfeeding tools: improving care and outcomes*. Amarillo, TX: Hale Publishing.

Websites

www.aboutfaceinternational.org – For parents of cleft-affected children internationally

www.clapa.com – The U.K. Cleft Lip & Palate Association

www.acpa-cpf.org – The American Cleft-Palate-Craniofacial Association which has a 24-hour support line for U.S. parents at 1-800-24-CLEFT

www.smiletrain.org –This organization raises funds to provide free cleft surgery for low-income families internationally

Cystic Fibrosis

http://www.cff.org/ – The Cystic Fibrosis Foundation is a U.S. nonprofit donor-supported organization that exists to improve the quality of life for those with the disease.

GERD

Books

Vartabedian, B. (2007). *Colic solved: The essential guide to infant reflux and the care of your crying, difficult-to-soothe baby*. New York, NY: Ballantine Books.

Websites

www.reflux.org – Pediatric/Adolescent Gastroesophageal Reflux Association (PAGER),

A US organization that provides information and support to families whose children have reflux. They offer brochures, hold monthly meetings, and publish a monthly newsletter.

Handouts/Tearsheets

Kombol, P. (2009). Soothing your breastfed baby with reflux. *Journal of Human Lactation, 25*(2), 237-238.

Down Syndrome

Websites

http://www.imdsa.org/ – The Inernational Mosaic Down Syndrome Association

www.ndss.org – The U.S. National Down Syndrome Society

http://www.ndsccenter.org/ – The U.S. National Down Syndrome Congress

Neurologically Impaired Baby

Books for Professionals

Genna, C.W., Fram, J. L., & Sandora, L. (2008). Neurological issues and breastfeeding. In C. W. Genna (Ed.), *Supporting sucking skills in breastfeeding infants* (pp. 253-303). Boston, MA: Jones and Bartlett.

Websites

www.nichcy.org –The U.S. National Information Centre for Children and Youth with Disabilities

www.asha.org – The U.S. website of the American Speech and Hearing Association, where parents can find a US speech pathologist trained in assessing and treating feeding problems

www.ndta.org/ – The U.S. website of the Neuro-Developmental Treatment Association, where parents can find a therapist who uses a neuro-developmental (whole child) approach

REFERENCES

AAP. (2009). Summaries of infectious diseases. In L. K. Pickering, C. J. Baker, D. W. Kimberlin & S. S. Long (Eds.), *Red Book: 2009 Report of the Committee on Infecious Diseases* (28th ed.). Elk Grove Village, IL: American Academy of Pediatrics.

Abdulkader, H. M., Freer, Y., Fleetwood-Walker, S. M., & McIntosh, N. (2007). Effect of suckling on the peripheral sensitivity of full-term newborn infants. *Archives of Disease in Childhood. Fetal and Neonatal Edition, 92*(2), F130-131.

Ahring, K., Belanger-Quintana, A., Dokoupil, K., Gokmen Ozel, H., Lammardo, A. M., MacDonald, A., et al. (2009). Dietary management practices in phenylketonuria across European centres. *Clinical Nutrition, 28*(3), 231-236.

Amstalden-Mendes, L. G., Magna, L. A., & Gil-da-Silva-Lopes, V. L. (2007). Neonatal care of infants with cleft lip and/or palate: feeding orientation and evolution of weight gain in a nonspecialized Brazilian hospital. *Cleft Palate-Craniofacial Journal, 44*(3), 329-334.

Aniansson, G., Svensson, H., Becker, M., & Ingvarsson, L. (2002). Otitis media and feeding with breast milk of children with cleft palate. *Scandinavian Journal of Plastic and Reconstructive Surgery and Hand Surgery, 36*(1), 9-15.

Aumonier, M. E., & Cunningham, C. C. (1983). Breast feeding in infants with Down's syndrome. *Child: Care, Health and Development, 9*(5), 247-255.

Avedian, L. V., & Ruberg, R. L. (1980). Impaired weight gain in cleft palate infants. *Cleft Palate Journal, 17*(1), 24-26.

Barbas, K. H., & Kelleher, D. K. (2004). Breastfeeding success among infants with congenital heart disease. *Pediatric Nursing, 30*(4), 285-289.

Bartocci, M., Bergqvist, L. L., Lagercrantz, H., & Anand, K. J. (2006). Pain activates cortical areas in the preterm newborn brain. *Pain, 122*(1-2), 109-117.

Batton, D. G., Barrington, K. J., & Wallman, C. (2006). Prevention and management of pain in the neonate: an update. *Pediatrics, 118*(5), 2231-2241.

Berkowitz, D., Naveh, Y., & Berant, M. (1997). "Infantile colic" as the sole manifestation of gastroesophageal reflux. *Journal of Pediatric Gastroenterology and Nutrition, 24*(2), 231-233.

Boekel, S. (2000). *Gastro-esophageal Reflux Disease (GERD) and the Breastfeeding Baby*. Raleigh, NC: International Lactation Consultant Association.

Borowitz, D., Baker, R. D., & Stallings, V. (2002). Consensus report on nutrition for pediatric patients with cystic fibrosis. *Journal of Pediatric Gastroenterology and Nutrition, 35*(3), 246-259.

Brady, M., Kinn, S., O'Rourke, K., Randhawa, N., & Stuart, P. (2005). Preoperative fasting for preventing perioperative complications in children. *Cochrane Database of Systematic Reviews*(2), CD005285.

Brown, K. H. (1994). Dietary management of acute diarrheal disease: contemporary scientific issues. *Journal of Nutrition, 124*(8 Suppl), 1455S-1460S.

Bucher, H. U., Baumgartner, R., Bucher, N., Seiler, M., & Fauchere, J. C. (2000). Artificial sweetener reduces nociceptive reaction in term newborn infants. *Early Human Development, 59*(1), 51-60.

Campanozzi, A., Boccia, G., Pensabene, L., Panetta, F., Marseglia, A., Strisciuglio, P., et al. (2009). Prevalence and natural history of gastroesophageal reflux: pediatric prospective survey. *Pediatrics, 123*(3), 779-783.

Carbajal, R., Veerapen, S., Couderc, S., Jugie, M., & Ville, Y. (2003). Analgesic effect of breast feeding in term neonates: randomised controlled trial. *BMJ, 326*(7379), 13.

Carpenter, R. O., Schaffer, R. L., Maeso, C. E., Sasan, F., Nuchtern, J. G., Jaksic, T., et al. (1999). Postoperative ad lib feeding for hypertrophic pyloric stenosis. *Journal of Pediatric Surgery, 34*(6), 959-961.

Carroll, A. E., Garrison, M. M., & Christakis, D. A. (2002). A systematic review of nonpharmacological and nonsurgical therapies for gastroesophageal reflux in infants. *Archives of Pediatrics and Adolescent Medicine, 156*(2), 109-113.

Chatterton, R. T., Jr., Hill, P. D., Aldag, J. C., Hodges, K. R., Belknap, S. M., & Zinaman, M. J. (2000). Relation of plasma oxytocin and prolactin concentrations to milk production in mothers of preterm infants: influence of stress. *Journal of Clinical Endocrinology and Metabolism, 85*(10), 3661-3668.

Clark, G., & Seifer, R. (1983). Facilitating mother-infant communication: A treatment model for high-risk and developmentally-delayed infants. *Infant Mental Health Journal, 4*(2), 67-81.

Clark, G., & Seifer, R. (1985). Assessment of parents' interactions with their developmentally delayed infants. *Infant Mental Health Journal, 6*(4), 214-225.

Clarren, S. K., Anderson, B., & Wolf, L. S. (1987). Feeding infants with cleft lip, cleft palate, or cleft lip and palate. *Cleft Palate Journal, 24*(3), 244-249.

Clemens, J. D., Harris, J. R., Sack, D. A., Huda, M. N., Chowdhury, S., Ali, M., et al. (1988). Discontinuation of breast-feeding during episodes of diarrhoea in rural Bangladeshi children. *Transactions of the Royal Society of Tropical Medicine and Hygiene, 82*(5), 779-783.

Clemente, C., Barnes, J., Shinebourne, E., & Stein, A. (2001). Are infant behavioural feeding difficulties associated with congenital heart disease? *Child: Care, Health and Development, 27*(1), 47-59.

Cohen, M., Marschall, M. A., & Schafer, M. E. (1992). Immediate unrestricted feeding of infants following cleft lip and palate repair. *Journal of Craniofacial Surgery, 3*(1), 30-32.

Colombo, C., Costantini, D., Zazzeron, L., Faelli, N., Russo, M. C., Ghisleni, D., et al. (2007). Benefits of breastfeeding in cystic fibrosis: a single-centre follow-up survey. *Acta Paediatrica, 96*(8), 1228-1232.

Colson, S., DeRooy, L., & Hawdon, J. (2003). Biological Nurturing increases duration of breastfeeding for a vulnerable cohort. *MIDIRS Midwifery Digest, 13*(1), 92-97.

Colson, S. D., Meek, J. H., & Hawdon, J. M. (2008). Optimal positions for the release of primitive neonatal reflexes stimulating breastfeeding. *Early Human Development, 84*(7), 441-449.

Combs, V. L., & Marino, B. L. (1993). A comparison of growth patterns in breast and bottle-fed infants with congenital heart disease. *Pediatric Nursing, 19*(2), 175-179.

Cook-Sather, S. D., & Litman, R. S. (2006). Modern fasting guidelines in children. *Best Pract Res Clin Anaesthesiol, 20*(3), 471-481.

Crossman, K. (1998). Breastfeeding a baby with a cleft palate: a case report. *Journal of Human Lactation, 14*(1), 47-50.

Danner, S. C. (1992). Breastfeeding the infant with a cleft defect. *NAACOGS Clinical Issues in Perinatal and Womens Health Nursing, 3*(4), 634-639.

Danner, S. C., & Wilson-Clay, B. (1986). Breastfeeding the Infant with a Cleft Lip/Palate. In *Lactation Conultant Series Unit 10*. Franklin Park, IL: La Leche League International.

Darzi, M. A., Chowdri, N. A., & Bhat, A. N. (1996). Breast feeding or spoon feeding after cleft lip repair: a prospective, randomised study. *British Journal of Plastic Surgery, 49*(1), 24-26.

de Boissieu, D., Matarazzo, P., Rocchiccioli, F., & Dupont, C. (1997). Multiple food allergy: a possible diagnosis in breastfed infants. *Acta Paediatrica, 86*(10), 1042-1046.

Douglas, P. S. (2005). Excessive crying and gastro-oesophageal reflux disease in infants: misalignment of biology and culture. *Medical Hypotheses, 64*(5), 887-898.

Efe, E., & Savaser, S. (2007). The effect of two different methods used during peripheral venous blood collection on pain reduction in neonates. *Agri, 19*(2), 49-56.

Erkkila, A. T., Isotalo, E., Pulkkinen, J., & Haapanen, M. L. (2005). Association between school performance, breast milk intake and fatty acid profile of serum lipids in ten-year-old cleft children. *Journal of Craniofacial Surgery, 16*(5), 764-769.

Ewer, A. K., James, M. E., & Tobin, J. M. (1999). Prone and left lateral positioning reduce gastro-oesophageal reflux in preterm infants. *Archives of Disease in Childhood. Fetal and Neonatal Edition, 81*(3), F201-205.

Ferrari, L. R., Rooney, F. M., & Rockoff, M. A. (1999). Preoperative fasting practices in pediatrics. *Anesthesiology, 90*(4), 978-980.

Flores-Lujano, J., Perez-Saldivar, M. L., Fuentes-Panana, E. M., Gorodezky, C., Bernaldez-Rios, R., Del Campo-Martinez, M. A., et al. (2009). Breastfeeding and early infection in the aetiology of childhood leukaemia in Down syndrome. *British Journal of Cancer, 101*(5), 860-864.

Frankel, E. A., Shalaby, T. M., & Orenstein, S. R. (2006). Sandifer syndrome posturing: relation to abdominal wall contractions, gastroesophageal reflux, and fundoplication. *Digestive Diseases and Sciences, 51*(4), 635-640.

Frommelt, M. A. (2004). Differential diagnosis and approach to a heart murmur in term infants. *Pediatric Clinics of North America, 51*(4), 1023-1032, x.

Garcez, L. W., & Giugliani, E. R. (2005). Population-based study on the practice of breastfeeding in children born with cleft lip and palate. *Cleft Palate-Craniofacial Journal, 42*(6), 687-693.

Garza, J. J., Morash, D., Dzakovic, A., Mondschein, J. K., & Jaksic, T. (2002). Ad libitum feeding decreases hospital stay for neonates after pyloromyotomy. *Journal of Pediatric Surgery, 37*(3), 493-495.

Gaskin, K. J., & Waters, D. L. (1994). Nutritional management of infants with cystic fibrosis. *Journal of Paediatrics and Child Health, 30*(1), 1-2.

Geddes, D. T., Kent, J. C., Mitoulas, L. R., & Hartmann, P. E. (2008). Tongue movement and intra-oral vacuum in breastfeeding infants. *Early Human Development, 84*(7), 471-477.

Genna, C. (2009). *Selecting and Using Breastfeeding Tools: Improving Care and Outcomes*. Amarillo, TX: Hale Publishing.

Genna, C. W. (2008a). The influence of anatomic and strucural issues on sucking skills. In C. W. Genna (Ed.), *Supporting Sucking Skills in Breastfeeding Infants*. Boston, MA: Jones and Bartlett.

Genna, C. W. (2008b). Sensory integration and breastfeeding. In C. W. Genna (Ed.), *Supporting Sucking Skills in Breastfeeding Infants* (pp. 235-252). Boston, MA: Jones and Bartlett.

Genna, C. W., Fram, J. L., & Sandora, L. (2008). Neurological issues and breastfeeding. In C. W. Genna (Ed.), *Supporting Sucking Skills in Breastfeeding Infants* (pp. 253-303). Boston, MA: Jones and Bartlett.

Ghaem, M., Armstrong, K. L., Trocki, O., Cleghorn, G. J., Patrick, M. K., & Shepherd, R. W. (1998). The sleep patterns of infants and young children with gastro-oesophageal reflux. *Journal of Paediatrics and Child Health, 34*(2), 160-163.

Glenny, A. M., Hooper, L., Shaw, W. C., Reilly, S., Kasem, S., & Reid, J. (2004). Feeding interventions for growth and development in infants with cleft lip, cleft palate or cleft lip and palate. *Cochrane Database of Systematic Reviews*(3), CD003315.

Gold, B. D. (2006). Is gastroesophageal reflux disease really a life-long disease: do babies who regurgitate grow up to be adults with GERD complications? *American Journal of Gastroenterology, 101*(3), 641-644.

Gopinath, V. K., & Muda, W. A. (2005). Assessment of growth and feeding practices in children with cleft lip and palate. *Southeast Asian Journal of Tropical Medicine and Public Health, 36*(1), 254-258.

Gosain, A. K., Conley, S. F., Santoro, T. D., & Denny, A. D. (1999). A prospective evaluation of the prevalence of submucous cleft palate in patients with isolated cleft lip versus controls. *Plastic and Reconstructive Surgery, 103*(7), 1857-1863.

Grady, E. (1983). *Nursing my baby with a cleft o the soft palate*. Franklin Park, IL: La Leche League International.

Grant, L., & Cochran, D. (2001). Acid versus non-acid reflux. *Journal of Pediatrics, 139*(3), 470.

Gray, L., Watt, L., & Blass, E. M. (2000). Skin-to-skin contact is analgesic in healthy newborns. *Pediatrics, 105*(1), e14.

Gray, P. H., Trotter, J. A., Langbridge, P., & Doherty, C. V. (2006). Pain relief for neonates in Australian hospitals: a need to improve evidence-based practice. *Journal of Paediatrics and Child Health, 42*(1-2), 10-13.

Greve, L. C., Wheeler, M. D., Green-Burgeson, D. K., & Zorn, E. M. (1994). Breast-feeding in the management of the newborn with phenylketonuria: a practical approach to dietary therapy. *Journal of the American Dietetic Association, 94*(3), 305-309.

Habel, A., Elhadi, N., Sommerlad, B., & Powell, J. (2006). Delayed detection of cleft palate: an audit of newborn examination. *Archives of Disease in Childhood, 91*(3), 238-240.

Haider, R., Kabir, I., Fuchs, G. J., & Habte, D. (2000). Neonatal diarrhea in a diarrhea treatment center in Bangladesh: clinical presentation, breastfeeding management and outcome. *Indian Pediatrics, 37*(1), 37-43.

Heacock, H. J., Jeffery, H. E., Baker, J. L., & Page, M. (1992). Influence of breast versus formula milk on physiological gastroesophageal reflux in healthy, newborn infants. *Journal of Pediatric Gastroenterology and Nutrition, 14*(1), 41-46.

Hegar, B., Dewanti, N. R., Kadim, M., Alatas, S., Firmansyah, A., & Vandenplas, Y. (2009). Natural evolution of regurgitation in healthy infants. *Acta Paediatrica, 98*(7), 1189-1193.

Heine, R. G. (2008). Allergic gastrointestinal motility disorders in infancy and early childhood. *Pediatric Allergy and Immunology, 19*(5), 383-391.

Heine, R. G., Jordan, B., Lubitz, L., Meehan, M., & Catto-Smith, A. G. (2006). Clinical predictors of pathological gastro-oesophageal reflux in infants with persistent distress. *Journal of Paediatrics and Child Health, 42*(3), 134-139.

Heyman, M. B. (2006). Lactose intolerance in infants, children, and adolescents. *Pediatrics, 118*(3), 1279-1286.

Hill, D. J., Heine, R. G., Cameron, D. J., Francis, D. E., & Bines, J. E. (1999). The natural history of intolerance to soy and extensively hydrolyzed formula in infants with multiple food protein intolerance. *Journal of Pediatrics, 135*(1), 118-121.

Holliday, K. E., Allen, J. R., Waters, D. L., Gruca, M. A., Thompson, S. M., & Gaskin, K. J. (1991). Growth of human milk-fed and formula-fed infants with cystic fibrosis. *Journal of Pediatrics, 118*(1), 77-79.

Hopman, E., Csizmadia, C. G., Bastiani, W. F., Engels, Q. M., de Graaf, E. A., le Cessie, S., et al. (1998). Eating habits of young children with Down syndrome in The Netherlands: adequate nutrient intakes but delayed introduction of solid food. *Journal of the American Dietetic Association, 98*(7), 790-794.

Host, A., Husby, S., & Osterballe, O. (1988). A prospective study of cow's milk allergy in exclusively breast-fed infants. Incidence, pathogenetic role of early inadvertent exposure to cow's milk formula, and characterization of bovine milk protein in human milk. *Acta Paediatrica Scandinavica, 77*(5), 663-670.

Huang, A., Tai, B. C., Wong, L. Y., Lee, J., & Yong, E. L. (2009). Differential risk for early breastfeeding jaundice in a multi-ethnic Asian cohort. *Annals of the Academy of Medicine, Singapore, 38*(3), 217-224.

Imms, C. (2001). Feeding the infant with congenital heart disease: an occupational performance challenge. *American Journal of Occupational Therapy, 55*(3), 277-284.

Ip, S., Chung, M., Raman, G., Trikalinos, T. A., & Lau, J. (2009). A summary of the Agency for Healthcare Research and Quality's evidence report on breastfeeding in developed countries. *Breastfeed Med, 4 Suppl 1*, S17-30.

Jadcherla, S. R., Vijayapal, A. S., & Leuthner, S. (2009). Feeding abilities in neonates with congenital heart disease: a retrospective study. *Journal of Perinatology, 29*(2), 112-118.

Kanufre, V. C., Starling, A. L., Leao, E., Aguiar, M. J., Santos, J. S., Soares, R. D., et al. (2007). Breastfeeding in the treatment of children with phenylketonuria. *Jornal de Pediatria, 83*(5), 447-452.

Kaye, C. I., Accurso, F., La Franchi, S., Lane, P. A., Northrup, H., Pang, S., et al. (2006). Introduction to the newborn screening fact sheets. *Pediatrics, 118*(3), 1304-1312.

Kent, J. C., Mitoulas, L. R., Cregan, M. D., Ramsay, D. T., Doherty, D. A., & Hartmann, P. E. (2006). Volume and frequency of breastfeedings and fat content of breast milk throughout the day. *Pediatrics, 117*(3), e387-395.

Koletzko, S., & Reinhardt, D. (2001). Nutritional challenges of infants with cystic fibrosis. *Early Human Development, 65 Suppl*, S53-61.

Krebs, N. F., Westcott, J. E., Arnold, T. D., Kluger, B. M., Accurso, F. J., Miller, L. V., et al. (2000). Abnormalities in zinc homeostasis in young infants with cystic fibrosis. *Pediatric Research, 48*(2), 256-261.

Lambert, J. M., & Watters, N. E. (1998). Breastfeeding the infant/child with a cardiac defect: an informal survey. *Journal of Human Lactation, 14*(2), 151-155.

Lappi, H., Valkonen-Korhonen, M., Georgiadis, S., Tarvainen, M. P., Tarkka, I. M., Karjalainen, P. A., et al. (2007). Effects of nutritive and non-nutritive sucking on infant heart rate variability during the first 6 months of life. *Infant Behavior and Development, 30*(4), 546-556.

Lawrence, R. A. (2005). Lactation support when the infant will require general anesthesia: assisting the breastfeeding dyad in remaining content through the preoperative fasting period. *Journal of Human Lactation, 21*(3), 355-357.

Lawrence, R. A., & Lawrence, R. M. (2005). *Breastfeeding: A Guide for the Medical Profession* (6th ed.). Philadelphia, PA: Elsevier Mosby.

Litman, R. S., Wu, C. L., & Quinlivan, J. K. (1994). Gastric volume and pH in infants fed clear liquids and breast milk prior to surgery. *Anesthesia and Analgesia, 79*(3), 482-485.

Lobo, M. L. (1992). Parent-infant interaction during feeding when the infant has congenital heart disease. *Journal of Pediatric Nursing, 7*(2), 97-105.

Luder, E., Kattan, M., Tanzer-Torres, G., & Bonforte, R. J. (1990). Current recommendations for breast-feeding in cystic fibrosis centers. *American Journal of Diseases of Children, 144*(10), 1153-1156.

Mahalanabis, D., Alam, A. N., Rahman, N., & Hasnat, A. (1991). Prognostic indicators and risk factors for increased duration of acute diarrhoea and for persistent diarrhoea in children. *International Journal of Epidemiology, 20*(4), 1064-1072.

Marino, B. L., O'Brien, P., & LoRe, H. (1995). Oxygen saturations during breast and bottle feedings in infants with congenital heart disease. *Journal of Pediatric Nursing, 10*(6), 360-364.

Masarei, A. G., Sell, D., Habel, A., Mars, M., Sommerlad, B. C., & Wade, A. (2007). The nature of feeding in infants with unrepaired cleft lip and/or palate compared with healthy noncleft infants. *Cleft Palate-Craniofacial Journal, 44*(3), 321-328.

McPherson, V., Wright, S. T., & Bell, A. D. (2005). Clinical inquiries. What is the best treatment for gastroesophageal reflux and vomiting in infants? *Journal of Family Practice, 54*(4), 372-375.

Meier, P. (1988). Bottle- and breast-feeding: effects on transcutaneous oxygen pressure and temperature in preterm infants. *Nursing Research, 37*(1), 36-41.

Meier, P., & Anderson, G. C. (1987). Responses of small preterm infants to bottle- and breast-feeding. *MCN; American Journal of Maternal Child Nursing, 12*(2), 97-105.

Mercado-Deane, M. G., Burton, E. M., Harlow, S. A., Glover, A. S., Deane, D. A., Guill, M. F., et al. (2001). Swallowing dysfunction in infants less than 1 year of age. *Pediatric Radiology, 31*(6), 423-428.

Mitchell, D. J., McClure, B. G., & Tubman, T. R. (2001). Simultaneous monitoring of gastric and oesophageal pH reveals limitations of conventional oesophageal pH monitoring in milk fed infants. *Archives of Disease in Childhood, 84*(3), 273-276.

Mizuno, K., Inoue, M., & Takeuchi, T. (2000). The effects of body positioning on sucking behaviour in sick neonates. *European Journal of Pediatrics, 159*(11), 827-831.

Mizuno, K., & Ueda, A. (2001a). Development of sucking behavior in infants who have not been fed for 2 months after birth. *Pediatrics International, 43*(3), 251-255.

Mizuno, K., & Ueda, A. (2001b). Development of sucking behavior in infants with Down's syndrome. *Acta Paediatrica, 90*(12), 1384-1388.

Mizuno, K., & Ueda, A. (2005). Neonatal feeding performance as a predictor of neurodevelopmental outcome at 18 months. *Developmental Medicine and Child Neurology, 47*(5), 299-304.

Mizuno, K., & Ueda, A. (2006). Changes in sucking performance from nonnutritive sucking to nutritive sucking during breast- and bottle-feeding. *Pediatric Research, 59*(5), 728-731.

Mizuno, K., Ueda, A., Kani, K., & Kawamura, H. (2002). Feeding behaviour of infants with cleft lip and palate. *Acta Paediatrica, 91*(11), 1227-1232.

Montagnoli, L. C., Barbieri, M. A., Bettiol, H., Marques, I. L., & de Souza, L. (2005). Growth impairment of children with different types of lip and palate clefts in the first 2 years of life: a cross-sectional study. *Jornal de Pediatria, 81*(6), 461-465.

Morris, S., & Klein, M. (2001). *Pre-feeding Skills*. Tucson, AZ: Therapy Skill Builders.

Moss, A. L., Jones, K., & Pigott, R. W. (1990). Submucous cleft palate in the differential diagnosis of feeding difficulties. *Archives of Disease in Childhood, 65*(2), 182-184.

Motzfeldt, K., Lilje, R., & Nylander, G. (1999). Breastfeeding in phenylketonuria. *Acta Paediatrica. Supplement, 88*(432), 25-27.

Nelson, S. P., Chen, E. H., Syniar, G. M., & Christoffel, K. K. (1997). Prevalence of symptoms of gastroesophageal reflux during infancy. A pediatric practice-based survey. Pediatric Practice Research Group. *Archives of Pediatrics and Adolescent Medicine, 151*(6), 569-572.

Ohshiro, K., & Puri, P. (1998). Pathogenesis of infantile hypertrophic pyloric stenosis: recent progress. *Pediatric Surgery International, 13*(4), 243-252.

Omari, T. I., Barnett, C. P., Benninga, M. A., Lontis, R., Goodchild, L., Haslam, R. R., et al. (2002). Mechanisms of gastro-oesophageal reflux in preterm and term infants with reflux disease. *Gut, 51*(4), 475-479.

Orenstein, S. R., Shalaby, T. M., Kelsey, S. F., & Frankel, E. (2006). Natural history of infant reflux esophagitis: symptoms and morphometric histology during one year without pharmacotherapy. *American Journal of Gastroenterology, 101*(3), 628-640.

Orenstein, S. R., Shalaby, T. M., & Putnam, P. E. (1992). Thickened feedings as a cause of increased coughing when used as therapy for gastroesophageal reflux in infants. *Journal of Pediatrics, 121*(6), 913-915.

Owens, B. (2002). Breastfeeding an infant after heart transplant surgery. *Journal of Human Lactation, 18*(1), 53-55.

Pandya, A. N., & Boorman, J. G. (2001). Failure to thrive in babies with cleft lip and palate. *British Journal of Plastic Surgery, 54*(6), 471-475.

Paradise, J. L., Elster, B. A., & Tan, L. (1994). Evidence in infants with cleft palate that breast milk protects against otitis media. *Pediatrics, 94*(6 Pt 1), 853-860.

Parker, E. M., O'Sullivan, B. P., Shea, J. C., Regan, M. M., & Freedman, S. D. (2004). Survey of breast-feeding practices and outcomes in the cystic fibrosis population. *Pediatric Pulmonology, 37*(4), 362-367.

Phillips, R. M., Chantry, C. J., & Gallagher, M. P. (2005). Analgesic effects of breast-feeding or pacifier use with maternal holding in term infants. *Ambulatory Pediatrics, 5*(6), 359-364.

Pisacane, A., Toscano, E., Pirri, I., Continisio, P., Andria, G., Zoli, B., et al. (2003). Down syndrome and breastfeeding. *Acta Paediatrica, 92*(12), 1479-1481.

Poole, J. A., Barriga, K., Leung, D. Y., Hoffman, M., Eisenbarth, G. S., Rewers, M., et al. (2006). Timing of initial exposure to cereal grains and the risk of wheat allergy. *Pediatrics, 117*(6), 2175-2182.

Puapong, D., Kahng, D., Ko, A., & Applebaum, H. (2002). Ad libitum feeding: safely improving the cost-effectiveness of pyloromyotomy. *Journal of Pediatric Surgery, 37*(12), 1667-1668.

Purnell, H. (2001). Phenylketonuria and maternal phenylketonuria. *Breastfeeding Review, 9*(2), 19-21.

Radzyminski, S. (2005). Neurobehavioral functioning and breastfeeding behavior in the newborn. *Journal of Obstetric, Gynecologic, and Neonatal Nursing, 34*(3), 335-341.

Reid, J. (2004). A review of feeding interventions for infants with cleft palate. *Cleft Palate-Craniofacial Journal, 41*(3), 268-278.

Reid, J., Kilpatrick, N., & Reilly, S. (2006). A prospective, longitudinal study of feeding skills in a cohort of babies with cleft conditions. *Cleft Palate-Craniofacial Journal, 43*(6), 702-709.

Reid, J., Reilly, S., & Kilpatrick, N. (2007). Sucking performance of babies with cleft conditions. *Cleft Palate-Craniofacial Journal, 44*(3), 312-320.

Reilly, S., Reid, J., & Skeat, J. (2007). ABM Clinical Protocol #17: Guidelines for breastfeeding infants with cleft lip, cleft palate, or cleft lip and palate. *Breastfeeding Medicine, 2*(4), 243-250.

Riva, E., Agostoni, C., Biasucci, G., Trojan, S., Luotti, D., Fiori, L., et al. (1996). Early breastfeeding is linked to higher intelligence quotient scores in dietary treated phenylketonuric children. *Acta Paediatrica, 85*(1), 56-58.

Rommel, N., De Meyer, A. M., Feenstra, L., & Veereman-Wauters, G. (2003). The complexity of feeding problems in 700 infants and young children presenting to a tertiary care institution. *Journal of Pediatric Gastroenterology and Nutrition, 37*(1), 75-84.

Salvatore, S., & Vandenplas, Y. (2002). Gastroesophageal reflux and cow milk allergy: is there a link? *Pediatrics, 110*(5), 972-984.

Savilahti, E., Launiala, K., & Kuitunen, P. (1983). Congenital lactase deficiency. A clinical study on 16 patients. *Archives of Disease in Childhood, 58*(4), 246-252.

Semeniuk, J., & Kaczmarski, M. (2008). Acid gastroesophageal reflux and intensity of symptoms in children with gastroesophageal reflux disease. Comparison of primary gastroesophageal reflux and gastroesophageal reflux secondary to food allergy. *Advances in Medical Sciences, 53*(2), 293-299.

Shah, P. S., Aliwalas, L. I., & Shah, V. (2006). Breastfeeding or breast milk for procedural pain in neonates. *Cochrane Database of Systematic Reviews, 3*, CD004950.

Shrago, L. C., Reifsnider, E., & Insel, K. (2006). The Neonatal Bowel Output Study: indicators of adequate breast milk intake in neonates. *Pediatric Nursing, 32*(3), 195-201.

Smedegaard, L., Marxen, D., Moes, J., Glassou, E. N., & Scientsan, C. (2008). Hospitalization, breast-milk feeding, and growth in infants with cleft palate and cleft lip and palate born in Denmark. *Cleft Palate-Craniofacial Journal, 45*(6), 628-632.

Stutte, P. (1988). the effects of breast massage on volume and fat content of human milk. *Genesis, 10*(2), 22-25.

Turner, L., Jacobsen, C., Humenczuk, M., Singhal, V. K., Moore, D., & Bell, H. (2001). The effects of lactation education and a prosthetic obturator appliance on feeding efficiency in infants with cleft lip and palate. *Cleft Palate-Craniofacial Journal, 38*(5), 519-524.

Uga, E., Candriella, M., Perino, A., Alloni, V., Angilella, G., Trada, M., et al. (2008). Heel lance in newborn during breastfeeding: an evaluation of analgesic effect of this procedure. *Italian Journal of Pediatrics, 34*(1), 3.

Uvnas-Moberg, K. (2003). *The Oxytocin Factor: Tapping the Hormone of Calm, Love, and Healing*. Cambridge, MA: Da Capo Press.

van Rijn, M., Bekhof, J., Dijkstra, T., Smit, P. G., Moddermam, P., & van Spronsen, F. J. (2003). A different approach to breast-feeding of the infant with phenylketonuria. *European Journal of Pediatrics, 162*(5), 323-326.

Vandenplas, Y., Badriul, H., Verghote, M., Hauser, B., & Kaufman, L. (2004). Oesophageal pH monitoring and reflux oesophagitis in irritable infants. *European Journal of Pediatrics, 163*(6), 300-304.

Vartabedian, B. (2007). *Colic Solved: The Essential Guide to Infant Reflux and the Care of Your Crying, Difficult-to-Soothe Baby*. New York, NY: Ballantine Books.

Walker, M. (2006). *Breastfeeding Management for the Clinician: Using the Evidence*. Boston, MA: Jones and Bartlett.

Weatherley-White, R. C., Kuehn, D. P., Mirrett, P., Gilman, J. I., & Weatherley-White, C. C. (1987). Early repair and breast-feeding for infants with cleft lip. *Plastic and Reconstructive Surgery, 79*(6), 879-887.

Wenzl, T. G., Schneider, S., Scheele, F., Silny, J., Heimann, G., & Skopnik, H. (2003). Effects of thickened feeding on gastroesophageal reflux in infants: a placebo-controlled crossover study using intraluminal impedance. *Pediatrics, 111*(4 Pt 1), e355-359.

Wilson-Clay, B., & Hoover, K. (2008). *The Breastfeeding Atlas* (4th ed.). Manchaca, TX: LactNews Press.

Wolf, L. S., & Glass, R. P. (1992). *Feeding and Swallowing Disorders in Infancy*. Tucson, AZ: Therapy Skill Builders.

Woolridge, M. W., & Fisher, C. (1988). Colic, "overfeeding", and symptoms of lactose malabsorption in the breast-fed baby: a possible artifact of feed management? *Lancet, 2*(8607), 382-384.

Zeskind, P. S., & Goff, D. M. (1992). Rhythmic organization of heart rate in breast-fed and bottle-fed newborn infants. *Early Development and Parenting, 1*(2), 79-87.

The Preterm Baby

Chapter 9

A baby is considered preterm when born at least 3 weeks before his due date. This covers a broad spectrum of gestational ages, breastfeeding abilities, and health issues, from tiny, fragile infants born months early to healthy, robust late preterm babies.

A baby is considered preterm when born earlier than 37 weeks gestation.

FEELINGS ABOUT BREASTFEEDING

Grieving the Expected Birth

After a preterm birth, a mother's grief may affect her ability to process and remember information.

Before a mother can come to terms with her preterm birth, she may need to mourn the loss of the healthy full-term baby and normal pregnancy she expected. This is especially true if her baby was born very preterm or has health problems. Her initial reactions may include shock and denial or worry and anxiety. It is not unusual for mothers to experience a lack of maternal feelings. During a mother's early stages of grief, she may not be able to accept and understand information unless it is repeated several times and given in written form.

Once the initial shock passes and the reality of her baby's condition sinks in, other intense feelings may surface. She may refuse to believe her baby's medical caregivers and search for a specialist who will solve her baby's problems. She may be overly optimistic or overly pessimistic. If her baby has serious health problems, she may feel anger, guilt, or depression. Anger may be directed at the hospital staff or the baby's healthcare provider. The mother may have feelings of helplessness, loss of control, and isolation. She may have crying bouts and develop physical symptoms, such as insomnia, eating problems, or fatigue.

Encourage the mother to express her feelings and let her know that these feelings are normal. The mother and her partner may be in different stages of grief, impairing their ability to communicate with and comfort each other. Congratulate her for what she is doing for her baby, such as providing her milk and any contact with her baby. Touch is comforting to both mother and baby and can help reduce anxiety. Encourage skin-to-skin contact as soon as the baby can be taken out of the incubator. Suggest the mother ask if her healthcare facility has a support group for parents with babies in the special-care nursery. Contact with others with similar experiences can be comforting and provide realistic expectations and practical information (Meier, Engstrom, Mingolelli, Miracle, & Kiesling, 2004). U.S. research found that ongoing peer support significantly increased breastfeeding duration among low-income mothers of preterm babies (Merewood et al., 2006).

Skin-to-skin contact can ease anxiety for both mother and baby.

Giving birth prematurely may affect a mother's feelings about breastfeeding.

Many mothers perceive a preterm birth as traumatic, which may affect their intention to breastfeed. One internet study surveyed 52 women worldwide who had experienced traumatic births. Some (49) felt that their birth trauma gave them a stronger motivation to breastfeed, while others (3) said it influenced their decision not to breastfeed (Beck & Watson, 2008). Those who wanted to breastfeed felt it could help them "make up" for the birth or prove themselves as a mother. One mother said, "I had failed in my first task as a mother, to carry her to term. I had lost so much because of her premature birth that I was going to be damned to hell before I was going to give up on nursing her, especially before it even started" (Beck & Watson, 2008, p. 233).

On the negative side, some of these mothers felt they needed a time-out to heal mentally, perceived breastfeeding as a painful ordeal, experienced flashbacks from birth that intruded on breastfeeding, or felt a "disturbing detachment" from their baby. One mother said, "I was sick of everyone grabbing my breasts like they didn't even belong to me. My breasts were just another thing to be taken away and violated." The researchers concluded it is important to ask mothers before touching their breasts and that after a traumatic birth one-on-one support to establish breastfeeding should be offered. Swedish research on mothers with babies in the NICU also found that mothers reacted negatively when their breasts were touched without asking and that a more effective way to teach hand expression and putting baby to breast was to demonstrate with breast models and dolls, rather than touching mother and baby directly (Weimers, Svensson, Dumas, Naver, & Wahlberg, 2006).

If a mother has mixed or negative feelings about breastfeeding, emphasize that the first few weeks are the most critical for a baby's health and to approach breastfeeding or milk expression as a temporary commitment. Assure her that even if she decides to quit after a week or two, her baby will receive protection from infection. Explain that it is much easier to stop breastfeeding or expressing milk than it is to start later.

• •

Ask the mother about her breastfeeding goals.

Not all mothers want to establish full milk production and exclusively breastfeed their preterm baby after discharge. However, all mothers of preemies should be encouraged to provide the milk their babies need during their hospital stay. (See later section "What Parents Need to Know.")

If a mother's goal is to express her milk short-term, encourage her to do so at whatever level of milk expression will meet her baby's short-term needs and that she finds acceptable. Also assure her that she will be able to discontinue expressing whenever she wants without experiencing pain, as long as she does it gradually. To help her formulate a plan, see "Milk Expression Strategies" on p. 466 in the chapter "Milk Expression and Storage."

What Parents Need to Know

Even if a mother did not intend to breastfeed, she needs to know the importance of her milk to her preterm baby's health.

Because preterm babies have significantly better health outcomes when they receive their mother's milk (see later section" Health Risks of Non-Human Milks"), parents need to be told the importance of their milk to their baby. But where breastfeeding is not the cultural norm, many healthcare providers hesitate to ask mothers to provide expressed milk for fear of putting pressure on them during a crisis or making them feel "guilty."

One U.S. study examined this dynamic among 21 women, 76% were African American or Latina and 62% were low-income. All had decided during pregnancy not to breastfeed, but when they delivered a preterm baby, hospital staff asked them to provide their milk and explained why it was important to their baby from a medical standpoint. When asked if they felt pressured or coerced, the mothers all said no. Two of these mothers were transferred from another hospital, which had given them no encouragement to breastfeed or express milk.

Rather than feeling pressured, both mothers were unhappy that the staff at the first hospital hadn't told them the importance of their milk to their babies. One said, "I think they must have a fake license, I can't imagine doctors and nurses do not tell mothers that there is a difference when a baby is fed their mother's milk" (Miracle, Meier, & Bennett, 2004, p. 695).

Another larger U.S. study examined the effects of providing lactation counseling to mothers of very-low-birthweight preterm babies (Sisk, Lovelady, Dillard, & Gruber, 2006). Among its 196 mothers, 115 had intended to breastfeed and 81 had not. After being told the importance of their milk to their babies, 100% of the mothers intending to breastfeed began expressing their milk, as did 85% of those who had not. Those with a prior intention to breastfeed provided more milk for a longer time, but all the mothers surveyed reported they were glad they did and study questionnaires found no increase of stress or anxiety among either group. A U.K. study of 44 mothers of diverse ethnic backgrounds also found that due to their baby's vulnerability, some mothers who had not intended to breastfeed provided their milk (Jaeger, Lawson, & Filteau, 1997). For suggestions on how to present this information to parents, see "Sharing the Science on Human Milk Feedings with Mothers of Very-Low-Birth-Weight Infants" (Rodriguez, Miracle, & Meier, 2005).

• •

Even if donor milk is available, parents need to know that babies' health outcomes are better when mother's own milk is given.

Donor milk consists of pooled milk mostly from mothers of term babies. While this is a better choice for preterm babies than formula (see later section), a mother's own milk is better suited to her baby's needs. For example, her preterm colostrum is higher in components that protect her baby from infection, such as anti-infectives, anti-inflammatories, growth factors, and others (Dvorak, Fituch, Williams, Hurst, & Schanler, 2003; Kunz, Rudloff, Baier, Klein, & Strobel, 2000; Magne et al., 2006; Mathur, Dwarkadas, Sharma, Saha, & Jain, 1990). Her preterm milk is also higher in protein, sodium, chloride, iron, and fatty acids than term milk (Kovacs, Funke, Marosvolgyi, Burus, & Decsi, 2005; Lemons, Moye, Hall, & Simmons, 1982; Schanler & Atkinson, 1999). The preterm baby needs more of these nutrients than the term baby.

• •

Mothers also need to know that mixed emotions about expressing their milk are normal.

One Australian longitudinal study of 17 mother and fathers of very-low-birth-weight preterm babies found that mothers had mixed emotions about milk expression, considering it a symbol of both their connection to their baby and their disconnection from their baby while others provided primary care (Sweet, 2008).

Expressing milk is a learned skill that is psychological as well as physical, and the mother's emotions influence how much milk she expresses. Some mothers feel odd, awkward about expressing their milk. Some feel discouraged if they may need to express for a while. If the mother mentions any of these feelings, assure her they are common.

• •

Offer the mother suggestions for making her wishes clear and working with her baby's healthcare team.

Encourage a mother to be clear about her breastfeeding goals and find the healthcare professionals most supportive of breastfeeding for moral support and help. For more suggestions on tactful ways to bring up concerns and questions, see the appendix on p. 853 "Working with Healthcare Professionals."

THE MOTHER'S ROLE IN HER BABY'S CARE

Taking an active role in her baby's care can decrease a mother's feelings of helplessness and help her process her grief more easily.

Building a Relationship

After a preterm birth, a mother may need to work at developing a relationship with her baby.

Love between a mother and baby does not always happen automatically, especially when they are separated after birth. Feelings develop and are reinforced through touch, behaviors, and cues, and it may take extra effort to develop a relationship with a preterm baby and for the mother to "feel" like a mother.

Other reasons, too, can make forming a close relationship with a preemie more difficult. For example, if the baby's life is at risk, the mother may be afraid to feel close to her baby for fear of making her vulnerable to a greater trauma if he should die. Once the mother feels sure her baby will live, it may be easier for her to let her feelings for him grow. Also, depending on how early her baby was born, the mother may find her baby's appearance upsetting. A very preterm baby is thin, with little fat under translucent skin, and has a protruding abdomen and low muscle tone. Seeing her baby surrounded by medical paraphernalia, with tubes and wires coming from his body, can also be upsetting.

Cultivating a relationship involves two people who are open and responsive to one another, but depending on his condition and his environment, a preemie may be unresponsive. In a bright, noisy, and busy NICU, for example, many preemies spend much of their time sleeping to protect themselves from overstimulation. Some hospitals are changing their intensive-care nurseries to reduce the stimulation preterm babies receive by combining medical procedures to minimize disruptions, draping blankets over incubators to reduce glare, providing tactile boundaries for the babies, and holding and positioning them in special ways. If her baby seems "shut down" much of the time, suggest she request these approaches be tried. Even for very preterm babies, encourage skin-to-skin contact as soon and as much as possible, as it enhances a mother's interactions with her baby and helps establish breastfeeding (see next section).

Encourage the mother to spend as much time as possible with her baby and try other ways to feel closer to him.

In addition to touching and holding her baby as much as possible (see next section), other strategies for feeling closer include:

- Name the baby and use his name when talking about him and to him.
- Take an active role in her baby's care (see next point).
- Share her goals, feelings, observations, and suggestions with the hospital staff.
- If they are apart, leave a recording of her voice and a family photo for the baby.

- Take photos of the baby and keep a journal or album to record his progress.

In Sweden, where breastfeeding is the norm, many NICUs consider parents their preterm baby's primary caregivers and encourage them to be active in all aspects of their baby's care. The healthcare providers teach parents to do routine medical procedures and support them as they learn (Nyqvist & Engvall, 2009). There parents receive automatic paid leave from work, and space is set aside for parents to move into the hospital to more easily be with their babies and care for them around the clock. They also promote early breastfeeding as a developmental skill to be facilitated. As a result, many preterm babies are exclusively breastfeeding at much earlier gestational ages than they are in the U.S. (Nyqvist, 2008b; Nyqvist, Sjoden, & Ewald, 1999).

In some hospitals, parents are encouraged to take an active role in their babies' care.

At this writing, in most U.S. NICUs, mothers have a different role in their preterm babies' care and are seen primarily as providers of milk because it is widely believed that preterm babies are incapable of breastfeeding effectively (Meier, 2001). The goal is for the babies to gain enough weight to be discharged as soon as possible, and to accomplish this, bottle-feeding is often suggested. In some U.S. NICUs, expressed milk is valued as a "medicine" for the baby and mothers' efforts to express milk are considered a priority (Meier, 2003). In some of these hospitals, mothers take an active role in their baby's care by learning how to measure their milk's fat content via creamatocrit (Griffin, Meier, Bradford, Bigger, & Engstrom, 2000), by labeling their milk with color-coded stickers, so the baby is fed colostrum first, and by attending peer-support groups that give them the information and encouragement they need to express milk long-term (Meier et al., 2004). In the U.S., exclusive breastfeeding of preterm babies before discharge is unusual.

Skin-to-Skin Contact

Infant Stability

Skin-to-skin contact, originally called "kangaroo care," was introduced as a postpartum practice in 1979 in a hospital in Bogota, Colombia, where many preterm babies were born, but incubators were not always available. Death from infection was common—babies born at less than 1350 grams (3 lbs.) usually died—and abandonment of preterm babies by their mothers was a serious problem. In the years since, kangaroo care (which when practiced 8 to 24 hours per day is referred to as "kangaroo mother care") has been studied internationally and used widely (Ruiz-Pelaez, Charpak, & Cuervo, 2004).

Keeping preemies in skin-to-skin contact saves many lives around the world.

Skin-to-skin contact stabilizes premature babies' vital signs.

Wearing only a diaper and often a hat, the preemie is held skin-to-skin against his mother, between her breasts or cradled against her breast under a shirt or binder that is tight enough to support the baby in the kangaroo position. In this position, the baby is supported with arms and legs flexed, tummy down on the mother's chest, with his head turned sideways between her breasts. When held this way, the baby can look at his mother, respond to her voice, breastfeed at will (if breastfeeding has begun), or relax and sleep peacefully. Fathers can also take an active role in kangaroo care (Ludington-Hoe, Hashemi, Argote, Medellin, & Rey, 1992)

In Colombia, babies who were cared for this way and were in good condition were discharged early (sometimes within a day of birth) from the infectious environment of the hospital and had their progress regularly monitored at special clinics. Heat loss, a major concern with preemies, was avoided by keeping the unwrapped baby completely under the mother's clothing and skin-to-skin (Acolet, Sleath, & Whitelaw, 1989).

In rural Zimbabwe, a variation of kangaroo care—called kangaroo mother care—began in the early 1990s when Nils Bergman, a South African physician and researcher, began work at a missionary hospital there and found a high death rate among its babies born preterm due to the lack of high-tech care. After charting the survival outcomes using the previous practice of separating mothers and preterm babies at birth, he and Swedish nurse midwife Agneta Jurisoo began this new approach inspired by the work in Colombia. This involved keeping mothers and their preemies in skin-to-skin contact from birth for 23 hours per day by wrapping babies against their mothers' body. Mothers could move around by day and sleep by night at a 30 degree angle with their babies on their bodies. With this intervention, survival rates improved from 70% to 90% among babies born between 1500 g and 2000 g, and from 10% to 50% for babies born between 1000 g and 1500 g—an increase in survival of 400% among the smallest preemies (Bergman & Jurisoo, 1994).

From birth, these kangaroo-mother-care babies were given small feedings of mother's milk by nasogastric tube at 2-hour intervals. By Day 7 to 10, as they learned to breastfeed, they received full feeds of mother's milk by dropper or cup. Among this population, babies born earlier than 31 weeks gestation did not usually survive, but those who did typically regained birthweight by 1 week, gaining on average 30 g (1 oz) per day. Of those who stabilized during the first day, 98% survived.

• •

Separation from the mother causes physiological stress in the preemie, while skin-to-skin contact decreases instability and stress and promotes health and growth.

After the dramatic results of Nils Bergman's Zimbabwe study (previous point), he began to investigate the mechanisms responsible for the 400% increase in survival rates.

After reviewing the scientific literature, Bergman discovered that human newborns—like other mammals—have inborn physiological programming that is key to survival and growth, and separating them triggers physiological changes that stress a preemie and make him more vulnerable to illness and death (Bergman, 2008). In contrast, keeping preterm babies on their mother's body decreases physiological stress, normalizes heart rate and breathing, triggers behaviors that lead to breastfeeding, and elicits the nurturing behaviors in the mother that enhance their bond. For details, see "Togetherness, Separateness, and Infant Stability" in the chapter "Breastfeeding Rhythms: The First Days."

Bergman suggested that in parts of the world where separation of mother and baby is routine, what is currently considered the preemies' "normal ranges" of stress hormones, breathing, heart rate, growth, and temperature reflect only the norms during separation, and what is truly normal needs to be redefined based on a preemie's physiological norms while in skin-to-skin contact with his mother.

In some low-income countries, such as South Africa and India, the more extensive kangaroo mother care is practiced, which in addition to skin-to-skin contact includes support of exclusive breastfeeding whenever possible, early hospital discharge with baby kept in kangaroo position, and adequate follow-up (Cattaneo, Davanzo, Uxa, & Tamburlini, 1998). In affluent areas, skin-to-skin contact is usually encouraged on a limited basis (intermittent periods of a few hours or less each day) after the preterm baby's temperature, breathing, and heart rate have stabilized in an incubator. However, South African research indicates that preterm babies become more stable more quickly when held in skin-to-skin on their mother's body, rather than in an incubator (Bergman, Linley, & Fawcus, 2004). In this prospective, unblinded, randomized clinical trial of 34 preemies (1200-2199 g), 12 of the 13 babies cared for in incubators had readings outside the stability parameters, while only 3 of 18 babies kept in skin-to-skin contact did. Eight of the 13 incubator babies experienced hypothermia (low temperature); none of the 20 babies in skin-to-skin care did. The babies in the incubators had more temperature fluctuations and cardio-respiratory instability.

Encourage the mother to request early skin-to-skin contact, which can help stabilize a preterm baby more effectively than an incubator.

In some cases, skin-to-skin contact may need to be delayed (Nyqvist, 2004) if the baby:

- Is less than 27 weeks gestation or born at less than 1000 g.
- Is severely unstable.
- Has had recent surgery.
- Has a large wound or drainage.

Several studies have found that continuous skin-to-skin contact results in better weight gain among preterm babies, especially in developing countries, and even very limited periods of skin-to-skin contact can improve growth (Charpak, Ruiz-Pelaez, Figueroa de, & Charpak, 2001; Kambarami, Chidede, & Kowo, 1998; Rao, Udani, & Nanavati, 2008; Rojas et al., 2003). In a prospective randomized controlled trial done in a Malaysian NICU, with 146 babies weighing less than 1501 g, one group of babies received skin-to-skin contact just 1 hour per day, and the researchers found that these babies had a greater growth in head circumference (Boo & Jamli, 2007).

Skin-to-skin contact can improve a preterm baby's growth and the quality of his sleep, and reduce crying.

In a Japanese study of 19 preterm babies weighing less than 1600 g, the researchers found that 1 hour of skin-to-skin contact per day significantly increased the time the babies spent in quiet sleep (Begum et al., 2008). The authors concluded that skin-to-skin contact may contribute to the activation of central nervous system and brain function. A U.S. randomized controlled trial concluded that preterm babies who received skin-to-skin contact had "more mature sleep organization" (Ludington-Hoe, Johnson et al., 2006).

A Cochrane Review of 30 studies of 1925 participants concluded that babies who received skin-to-skin contact stayed warmer, cried less, and had better cardio-respiratory stability (Moore, Anderson, & Bergman, 2007). Other studies from developing countries have found that preterm babies who receive regular skin-to-skin contact go home sooner and have better developmental outcomes (Charpak, Ruiz-Pelaez, Figueroa de, & Charpak, 1997; Charpak et al., 2001).

Skin-to-skin contact relieves pain during painful procedures.

Painful procedures are a common part of many preterm babies' medical care. When pain causes crying, this elevates heart rate, blood pressure, and causes cerebral blood flow changes, putting these vulnerable babies at risk. Studies on preterm babies have found that preemies kept skin-to-skin during painful procedures have reduced stress responses, such as crying and abnormal heart rate (Cong, Ludington-Hoe, McCain, & Fu, 2009; Kostandy et al., 2008; Ludington-Hoe, Hosseini, & Torowicz, 2005). Researchers suggest that skin-to-skin contact be used as an analgesia to reduce risk during painful procedures.

Kangaroo care has been linked to decreased depression in mothers.

In a Brazilian study of 177 low-income mothers of preterm babies, 66 (37%) were rated as depressed. After participating in kangaroo mother care, the number of depressed mothers dropped to less than half, with only 30 (17%) of the mothers still rated as depressed. Individual cases have also been reported in which a mother's emotional state has improved after kangaroo care (Dombrowski, Anderson, Santori, & Burkhammer, 2001).

Skin-to-skin contact triggers the production of antibodies in mother's milk to organisms her baby's been exposed to in the NICU.

This dynamic is referred to as the "enteromammary pathway," and receiving these antibodies through mother's milk helps prevent the specific infection the preemie has been exposed to (Goldman, 2007). While health outcomes when donor milk is fed are better than when formula is given, this is one reason better health outcomes are associated with mother's own milk.

If a mother is unable to do kangaroo care with her baby, encourage her to find other ways to touch her baby, such as infant massage.

Although skin-to-skin contact is the first choice, it is not always possible. In this case, encourage the mother to sit beside her baby's incubator, look into his eyes, and stroke him. Knowing that someone loves him is important to his progress. One U.S. study found that mothers' depression and anxiety scores were lower after they gave their preemies massage therapy in the NICU (Feijo et al., 2006). Other U.S. studies have found that after infant massage, babies had increased temperature, better digestion, fewer stress behaviors, and grew better (Diego, Field, & Hernandez-Reif, 2008; Diego et al., 2007; Field et al., 2004; Hernandez-Reif, Diego, & Field, 2007).

Implications for Breastfeeding

Skin-to-skin contact promotes both breastfeeding competence and milk production.

As a mother holds her baby against her chest, the baby can look at her, respond to her voice, breastfeed at will (if breastfeeding has begun), or just relax and sleep peacefully. As her baby rests against her body, the mother learns her baby's feel, sounds, and responses. This close body contact triggers a baby's inborn breastfeeding behaviors (see Chapter 1). In one Swedish NICU, frequent and extended skin-to-skin contact was associated with earlier exclusive breastfeeding (Nyqvist, 2004). For more details, see the later section on p. 359, "Transitioning to Full Breastfeeding."

Her baby's touch also affects a mother hormonally. Even an hour per day of skin-to-skin contact has been found to increase expressed milk volumes (Hurst, Valentine, Renfro, Burns, & Ferlic, 1997).

Early preterm birth is associated with a shorter duration of breastfeeding, even in countries where breastfeeding is the norm (Akerstrom, Asplund, & Norman, 2007; Flacking, Nyqvist, Ewald, & Wallin, 2003). But skin-to-skin contact can help to partly offset this dynamic. After reviewing 30 studies and 1925 participants, a Cochrane Review article concluded that babies who receive skin-to-skin contact were more likely to be breastfed and to breastfeed longer (Moore et al., 2007). Many studies from around the world have found an association between skin-to-skin contact and increased incidence and duration of breastfeeding (Rao et al., 2008; Ruiz-Pelaez et al., 2004). In a randomized, controlled study that followed 66 preterm babies from birth through 18 months, one U.S. NICU found that early and unlimited skin-to-skin contact was associated with significantly greater breastfeeding exclusivity (between birth and 6 months) and duration (to 18 months) (Hake-Brooks & Anderson, 2008).

Early and extensive skin-to-skin contact has been found to increase breastfeeding duration and exclusivity.

BREASTFEEDING THE PRETERM BABY

When to Start Breastfeeding

Preterm babies were once thought to breastfeed ineffectively until they reached the full-term age of 40 weeks gestation (Meier, 2001). Although preemies breastfeed differently than full-term babies, they are not necessarily ineffective. With time and practice at the breast, most can feed as effectively as full-term babies.

Rather than thinking in terms of "readiness," breastfeeding should be considered a normal behavior to be facilitated.

As Swedish researcher Kerstin Hedberg Nyqvist wrote: "In settings where breastfeeding is considered the norm for infant and young child feeding, mothers and personnel in neonatal units strive for 'normalcy'" (Nyqvist, 2008a, p. 153). In her innovative Swedish NICU, gestational age and weight are not considered. Breastfeeding begins as soon as the baby has been weaned off the ventilator and continuous positive airway (CPAP), and has no severe instability. However, in settings like the U.S., decisions are often made based on bottle-feeding research—such as recommendations to have preterm babies begin with an "emptied" breast—and as a result breastfeeding suffers.

In the past, mothers of preterm babies were often told to delay breastfeeding until their baby reached a specific weight or gestational age, or until bottle-feeding was going well. These recommendations were based on the following commonly held, but incorrect, assumptions:

Preterm babies can breastfeed early because it is less stressful than bottle-feeding.

- Breastfeeding is too physically stressful for babies who weigh less than 1500 g (3.3 pounds).
- The ability to coordinate sucking, swallowing, and breathing does not occur until 34 to 35 weeks gestation.
- Babies should be bottle-fed before breastfeeding, because breastfeeding is more difficult.

Research proved these assumptions wrong. Two of the earliest studies to compare breastfeeding to bottle-feeding observed five preterm babies doing both, with each baby serving as his own control (Meier, 1988; Meier & Anderson, 1987). The babies were about 32 weeks gestation, weighed on average 1300 g (about 2.9 pounds), and were 20 to 50 days old before they began breastfeeding. Body temperature, breathing, heart rate, and transcutaneous oxygen pressure were used to measure stress. The researchers found that breastfeeding was less physically stressful than bottle-feeding, and the smaller the babies, the greater the difference. These early studies found that preterm babies can organize sucking, swallowing, and breathing more easily during breastfeeding than bottle-feeding, and that the ability to breastfeed develops well before the ability to bottle-feed. These babies were able to suck and swallow regularly and predictably while breastfeeding, but when given a bottle—presumably due to the faster flow—their sucking and swallowing patterns became disorganized.

Breastfeeding is less stressful for preterm babies than bottle feeding.

Other studies have also found that bottle-feeding causes oxygen desaturation and that a preterm baby's oxygen saturation levels remain higher during breastfeeding (Blaymore Bier et al., 1997; Chen, Wang, Chang, & Chi, 2000; Dowling, 1999).

• •

Preterm babies can begin taking the breast as early as 28 weeks postmenstrual age.

Inborn feeding behaviors are a part of an infant's survival skills and are present in all babies, not just those born healthy and full-term. Swedish studies confirm that some babies born earlier than 30 weeks gestation can make their way to the breast and suckle. In one Swedish study of 71 babies without serious illness who were born preterm at 26 to 35 weeks gestation, breastfeeding was begun as soon as the babies could breathe without a ventilator or continuous positive airway pressure (CPAP) (Nyqvist et al., 1999). The earliest breastfeeding took place at just under 28 weeks postmenstrual age (the baby's age counted from the first day of the last menstrual period). In another study of babies born between 26 and 31 weeks gestation, babies began breastfeeding at 29 weeks, and 12 out of 15 were able to exclusively breastfeed between 32 and 38 weeks. Among them was a baby girl born at 26 weeks with chronic lung disease who was discharged home with oxygen treatment via nasal prongs (Nyqvist, 2008b).

How to Start Breastfeeding

Although some recommend offering very small preterm babies an "emptied" breast for early feedings, this is based on bottle-feeding norms.

Those who recommend this approach (Hurst & Meier, 2005), cite research that found restricted milk flow made bottle-feeding more manageable for preterm babies (Lau, Sheena, Shulman, & Schanler, 1997). However, during breastfeeding, preterm babies have more control over milk flow (Nyqvist, 2008a). Other research cited to support starting with an emptied breast suggested this as a way to provide "non-nutritive sucking" at the breast as a substitute for a pacifier during tube-feeding (Narayanan, 1990), which was found to improve weight gain (Measel & Anderson, 1979). Swedish research, however, has found that even very tiny preemies can breastfeed well from a full breast without the need for this intermediate step (Nyqvist, 2008b; Nyqvist et al., 1999).

Creating a Supportive Environment

Let the mother know that early breastfeeding is a learning process.

Early feedings usually require time and patience. The mother may feel awkward and even frustrated at times. To help her have realistic expectations, tell her that it will probably take several breastfeeding sessions before the baby begins to take milk, but that with practice and patience he will learn. The baby may begin by simply licking or mouthing the nipple. Many preemies suckle in short bursts and fall asleep quickly. Assure the mother that it is okay if the baby does not take milk at the breast during these early breastfeeding sessions because, if needed, he will be fed milk afterwards.

Creating a supportive environment can make early breastfeeding easier.

Privacy for mother and baby is ideal, preferably a separate room with a door. If the baby is very preterm, he may be on a monitor, oxygen, and an IV. If so, the mother and baby may not be able to go to a private room. But a private area can be created, even in a busy NICU, by using a curtain, partition wall, or screen. If that is not possible, position the mother's chair so that her back is to the room.

Comfort. A comfortable chair with good support for the mother's back and arms that can recline is ideal. Extra pillows may be helpful in getting comfortable while breastfeeding. Suggest she choose clothing that allows the baby easy access to the breast. Make sure the baby is not too warm and does not get overheated, which can make him drowsy. Close contact with his mother's body will provide warmth, and a hat and a blanket over him may be all that's needed to maintain his temperature.

Sound and light. A calm, quiet environment helps to keep stimulation manageable for the baby, so encourage any others to talk quietly. Try to position mother and baby away from any flashing lights and, if possible, dim the room lights and protect the baby's eyes from any direct light.

Relaxed time together. Suggest the mother ask not to be rushed or interrupted. In a supportive environment, mother-baby body contact is relaxing and can reduce stress.

In the beginning, provide skilled breastfeeding help and support.

Encourage the mother to ask for skilled breastfeeding help throughout the first few feedings. This will help her gain confidence as she learns her baby's cues. During the first feedings, offer the mother practical suggestions on how she can help the baby take the breast deeply and show her positions they may find comfortable. Demonstrating these strategies with a doll has been found to be better accepted by mothers, rather than touching them or their babies (Weimers et al., 2006).

If her baby has had breathing or heartbeat irregularities (apnea, bradycardia, oxygen desaturation), suggest the mother ask for someone to monitor the baby during early breastfeeding. If the baby remains stable during the first few feedings, then the mother can be taught to observe her baby's breathing and skin color and can contact a healthcare provider if needed (Nyqvist, 2008a). It may help the mother to know that as part of an immature suckling pattern, when a very preterm baby begins to take the breast, he may hold his breath while suckling, which can cause a temporary drop in his oxygen levels. This is not a cause for concern and the oxygen levels return to normal quickly (K. H. Nyqvist, personal communication, October 6, 2009).

Helping Baby Take the Breast

Avoid stressful events or procedures right before breastfeeding.

Because preterm babies are so sensitive to stimulation, even washing, bathing, and a diaper change may be stressful (Morelius, Hellstrom-Westas, Carlen, Norman, & Nelson, 2006). Suggest if possible these and any medical procedures be done after breastfeeding.

To encourage breastfeeding, start with unrestricted skin-to-skin contact.

When mothers and babies spend time skin-to-skin with the baby under mother's clothing, the mother will quickly learn from her baby's movements when he is waking and ready to feed. She will also feel changes in his breathing, hear his sounds, see when his eyes are opening, and notice when he starts making sucking movements.

A period of unrestricted skin-to-skin contact before feedings among mothers of full-term babies has been found to be helpful in overcoming breastfeeding problems, even among culturally diverse mothers (Chiu, Anderson, & Burkhammer, 2008).

Laid-back breastfeeding positions are an easy way to provide good body support.

Many pictures of breastfeeding mothers and babies show the mother sitting upright with the baby held horizontally across her body, his head resting on her forearm. This position, sometimes called the "cradle hold," does not usually work well for small preemies. In this position, they tend to slide easily away from the breast and roll into a little ball, because they are not yet strong enough to maintain their position at the breast.

Good body and head support are vital for the preterm baby to get onto the breast well and feed effectively. This can happen in a number of ways. For example, the laid-back feeding positions described in Chapter 1 were used in one U.K. study of 11 late preterm babies (35 to 37 weeks gestation) and one small-for-gestational-age baby born at 38 weeks (Colson, 2003). Using these laid-back positions, mothers are semi-reclined with babies lying tummy down on their bodies (see Figure 9.1). The mother's body supports the baby's weight, and after they have taken the breast, gravity helps keep the breast deeply in baby's mouth.

One Japanese study examined the effect of the body position during feedings on 14 babies (some term, some preterm) who were having trouble maintaining oxygen levels during bottle-feedings (Mizuno, Inoue, & Takeuchi, 2000). The researchers found that the babies had better oxygenation, exerted more sucking pressure, and took more milk when they fed prone (tummy down).

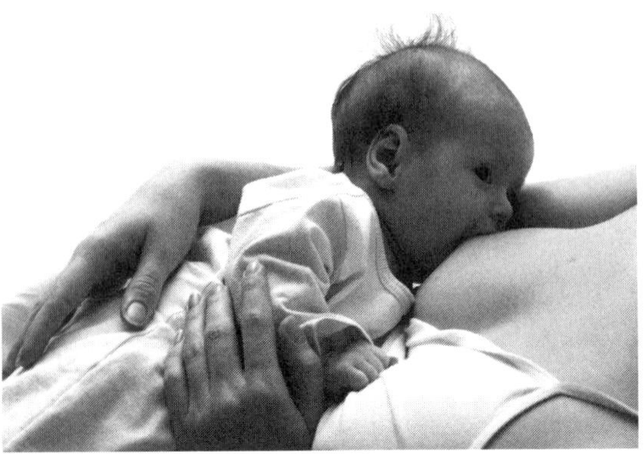

Figure 9.1. An example of a laid-back breastfeeding position.

In upright feeding positions, gravity works against rather than for with breastfeeding.

If upright feeding positions are used, a mother needs to work harder to provide her baby with body and head support. If the mother prefers an upright position or the laid-back positions do not work well for her or her baby, suggest she:

- Make sure she has good back, neck, and arm support.
- Hold the baby against her with his whole body facing hers.
- Help guide the baby to the breast by putting her palm on his back, with her thumb and index finger supporting the base of his head (see Figures 9.2 and 9.3).
- Align the baby nose to nipple, so that he can approach the breast chin first, with a wide open mouth and head slightly tilted back to make swallowing easier.
- Apply gentle pressure on the baby's shoulders as he takes the breast to ensure he takes a big mouthful, and throughout the feeding, so he stays on well.
- Consider putting a pillow or cushion under baby to support him at breast height.

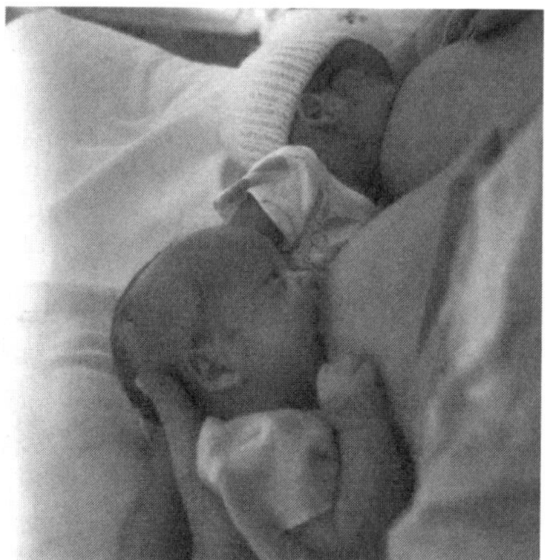

Figure 9.2. Preterm twins well supported in upright breastfeeding positions.

B. Wilson-Clay and K. Hoover, The Breastfeeding Atlas, 4th ed. 2008

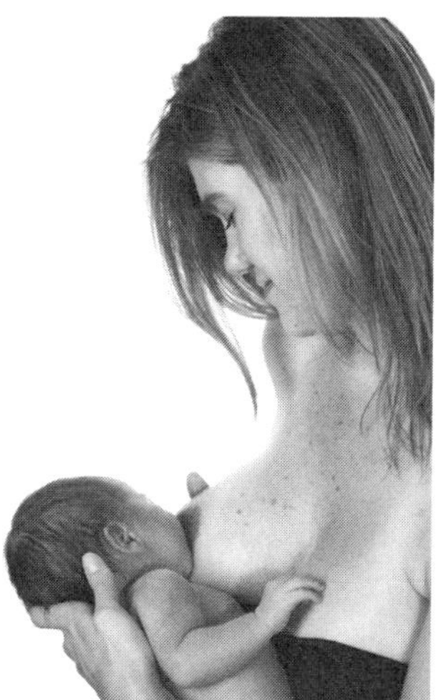

Figure 9.3. One possible upright feeding position for a preterm baby.

In upright feeding positions, it may help for the mother to support her breast.

Tiny babies sometimes have trouble staying on the breast. If this happens and the mother prefers to sit upright, suggest she support the weight of her breast, so it doesn't rest on the baby's chin. Depending on her breast size, it may help if she supports it throughout the feeding. If the baby needs more help, suggest the mother try the Dancer Hand position described on p. 805 in the appendix "Techniques" and see the later point on nipple shields.

After the mother finds a comfortable position, suggest she try to avoid too much movement or extra touching.

Because preterm babies are so sensitive to stimulation, the natural movements a mother makes during breastfeeding, like caressing, patting, tickling, and rocking, may overstimulate a preemie. At least until breastfeeding is well established, suggest the mother breastfeed with "still hands" (Nyqvist, 2008a).

It is not unusual for mothers to have a delay in milk ejection at first.

The first time a breastfeeding mother uses a breast pump, it often takes a couple of minutes for her milk ejection to occur and her milk to flow, because the feel of a pump is very different from the feel of her baby. The same can be true in reverse for the mother whose milk has been flowing well with the feel of the pump, but whose body is not yet conditioned to the feel of her baby at the breast.

When the mother who has been exclusively expressing her milk begins breastfeeding, it often takes a little longer for her milk ejection to occur. The baby may suck for several minutes and fall asleep before her milk starts to flow. Although this can be frustrating, assure the mother that her body will soon become conditioned to the feel of her baby at the breast, and her milk will flow more quickly. In the meantime, the best way to speed up the process is to spend some skin-to-skin time with her baby before breastfeeding. If this doesn't help, before putting baby to breast, suggest she stimulate milk ejection by using her breast pump (or hand-expression). Another alternative is to use the pump (or ask a helper to hold the pump) on the opposite breast after the baby takes the breast.

Help the mother learn to recognize the signs that her baby wants to continue breastfeeding and when he wants to stop.

Because of premies' sensitivity to stimulation, suggest the mother watch her baby's cues to determine which sounds and touches work best, so he does not get more stimulation than he can handle. Researcher and author Kerstin Hedberg Nyqvist describes "Cues of Approach" and "Cues of Avoidance" that can help interpret preterm babies needs during breastfeeding (Nyqvist, 2008a). "Cues of Approach" are signs the baby wants to continue breastfeeding and "Cues of Avoidance" indicate the baby wants to stop. These cues come from the work of Als and colleagues as part of the Newborn Individual Developmental Care and Assessment Program (NIDCAP), which was created to encourage care for preterm babies in harmony with their health and development (Als et al., 1994; Ross & Browne, 2002). These cues include physiological changes, movements, state changes, and ways of interacting, some of which are listed in Table 9.1.

Table 9.1. Preterm Babies' Cues During Breastfeeding

Cues of Approach	Cues of Avoidance
Changes in physiology	
Regular heartbeat and breathing Skin color unchanged Digestion stable Occasional startles or twitches	Fast, slow or irregular heartbeat/ breathing Skin color changes (pale, mottled, flushed) Spits up, gags, grunts while passing stool Hiccups, startles, tremors
Movements	
Stable muscle tone Shows signs of wanting more: Tucks himself closer to the breast Brings hands to face or mouth Smiles Mouths, licks, laps milk	Low tone in hands, arms, legs, trunk, face Flexes arms, legs, trunk and maintains this Shows tongue Extends arms/legs Arches head and/or trunk away or turns Spreads out fingers
State	
Stable sleep or alertness Deep sleep States easy to distinguish Oriented to mother with focused look Calm state changes Blocks stimuli easily	Light sleep Drowsy, movements with closed eyes Little alertness, fast shifting between states Looks glassy-eyed, tense, surprised, scared Difficult to calm, irritable, overactive Limited ability to shut out stimuli
Interactions	
Orients toward mother's face, voice Frowns Forms "oh" with lips Mimics facial expressions, coos	Looks away, stares in another direction Eyes "float" from side to side or roll Fusses, cries, becomes drowsy, closes eyes Yawns, sneezes

Adapted from (Nyqvist, 2008a)

Gauging Breastfeeding Effectiveness

Some simple signs indicate a baby is taking milk from the breast.

These signs include audible swallowing, milk around the baby's mouth, and fresh milk when the feeding tube is aspirated. In some NICUs, the appearance of these signs indicates it is time to begin regular test weighing (see next point).

One reliable way to measure milk intake at the breast is weighing baby before and after feedings with an accurate baby scale.

Knowing how much milk a baby takes at the breast can be important. It can prevent oversupplementation, which can delay the transition to full breastfeeding (Hurst, Meier, Engstrom, & Myatt, 2004). It can also prevent delays in initiating breastfeeding, as some healthcare providers are reluctant to allow early breastfeeding if they think they cannot accurately chart baby's intake. Knowing how well a baby is breastfeeding can also affect discharge plans, as feeding competence is usually one of the determining criteria (McCain, Gartside, Greenberg, & Lott, 2001; Nye, 2008).

One U.S. study found that neither mothers nor lactation consultants could accurately estimate preterm babies' milk intake at the breast using behaviors used to gauge milk intake in full-term healthy babies, such as audible swallowing and wide jaw movements (Meier, Engstrom, Fleming, Streeter, & Lawrence, 1996). U.S. research has found that one reliable way to gauge milk intake at the breast is by using a very accurate (to 2 g) baby scale for pre- and post-feed weights (Meier et al., 1994). Even when babies wear leads that connect them to other medical equipment, test-weighing has been found to be accurate (Haase, Barreira, Murphy, Mueller, & Rhodes, 2009). These scales are available in many hospitals, and in some areas, they can be rented for home use. However, if the mother finds test-weighing stressful or low milk intake leaves her feeling discouraged, as an alternative, she can reduce her baby's supplement gradually, while carefully monitoring his growth (Flacking et al., 2003).

Early Breastfeeding Rhythms

Once a preterm baby starts breastfeeding, ideally he should be encouraged to breastfeed often and without time restrictions.

Sometimes mothers are told to restrict breastfeeding to a specific number of feedings per day or a specific number of minutes. However, there is no evidence to support limited breastfeeding or cutting breastfeeding short. Suggest the mother ask that she and her baby be able to breastfeed as long as he wants and to expect that feeding time will vary a lot at first. A preterm baby usually has periods of rest and activity during breastfeeding, and restricting their time may substantially cut down on the milk he gets. If the baby falls asleep early in the feeding, suggest the mother continue holding him while he sleeps, keeping him close to the breast and offering the breast to him while he sleeps. Tube-feeding can ideally be done while baby is at the breast to provide him with positive reinforcement for his efforts.

There is no need to offer both breasts at a feeding unless the baby wants both.

At first, very tiny preemies may do better staying on one breast. Movement, repositioning, and taking the breast again may be too much stimulation. Just like a full-term baby, a preemie may get all the milk he needs from one breast, and it is better to feed well from one breast than to breastfeed less effectively on both. Encourage the mother to watch the baby's cues to avoid overtiring or stressing him.

If the baby is still awake and alert after the first breast and is interested, it is fine to offer the other breast.

At first, suggest she watch for feeding cues, and if possible, breastfeed at least every 2 hours or even more often.

Although in many countries, preterm babies are fed much less often, small babies can better handle smaller more frequent feedings, and this makes the transition to breastfeeding easier for the mother, because it is closer to a typical breastfeeding rhythm (Nyqvist, 2008a). In most cases, before a preterm baby is ready for exclusive breastfeeding, he will need to be supplemented (see next section). The amount given and the feeding pattern should be based on each baby's individual needs, so that he gets enough milk each day to gain weight well as he learns to breastfeed.

Once the baby is breastfeeding and taking milk, if the mother is not rooming in at the hospital, encourage her to work out a schedule with the hospital staff, so that she can breastfeed freely during the time she is with her baby. When the mother is not at the hospital, the nurses can feed the baby using other feeding methods (see next section).

If the baby is having trouble staying on the breast or not taking much milk, using a nipple shield may help.

Although it was once thought that nipple shields caused more problems than they solved, in some specific cases, they may be a useful tool. In one U.S. study of 34 preemies who were having trouble taking the breast, were slipping off the nipple during pauses, or were falling asleep quickly at the breast, these babies were able to take significantly more milk when the shield was used than when it wasn't (Meier et al., 2000). Milk transfer was greater for all 34 babies, with a mean increase of 14.4 ml or about half an ounce. With the shield, the babies were able to suck for longer bursts and stay awake longer at the breast. These preemies used the shield for a mean of 32.5 days (with a range of 2 to 171 days) out of a mean breastfeeding duration of 169.4 days (with a range of 14 to 365 days), so overall the mothers used the shield for about 24 percent of the time they breastfed. The researchers noted that the babies who had been unable to transfer milk without the shield used the shield longer than the babies who had been able to take milk from the breast alone. There was no association between the length of time the shield was used and duration of breastfeeding. The reasons the shield helps some preemies is not yet fully understood, but some think it helps to compensate for a preterm baby's weaker suction by maintaining the position of the breast back further in the baby's mouth (Hurst & Meier, 2005).

Nipple shields can be especially helpful for preterm infants.

The use of a nipple shield may make breastfeeding less stressful and time-consuming if it eliminates the need to supplement or shortens the time to exclusive breastfeeding. If a nipple shield helps increase milk intake at the breast, encourage the mother to use it for as long as needed. Preemies breastfeed better with the shield on average until they reach their full-term corrected age of about 40 weeks (Meier et al., 2000). For information on fitting, applying, and weaning from the shield, see "Nipple Shields" on p. 835 in the appendix "Tools and Products."

When using a nipple shield, the mother should plan to express her milk after most feedings to maintain her milk production until she is sure that her baby is draining her breasts effectively and taking full feedings with the shield. If she's not doing test-weights, suggest the mother look for milk in the tip of the shield after feedings and check for a decrease in breast fullness, as signs the baby is draining the breast.

Until the baby is exclusively breastfeeding, encourage the mother to continue milk expression.

If the baby is not yet breastfeeding effectively enough to get all his milk from the breast, to keep up her milk production, the mother will need to continue expressing her milk. Good milk production will improve milk flow, making breastfeeding easier for her baby.

Weight Gain And Supplementation

In most cases, after breastfeeding begins, the preterm baby will both breastfeed and receive supplements. While learning to breastfeed, the baby needs to be well fed.

How Should Preterm Babies Grow?

Optimal weight gain for preterm babies is not yet known.

Many suggest that preterm babies should gain and grow at about the same rate they would have in utero, but there is currently no evidence to support this goal. The focus on maintaining intrauterine growth rates began more than 40 years ago and originated from charts based on the growth patterns of the larger preterm babies of that time. However, because preemies today are being saved earlier and earlier, this information no longer makes sense as a guide (Bayes, Campoy, & Molina-Font, 1998).

Despite efforts to maintain intrauterine growth rates, U.S. research on 1660 preterm babies born from 500 to 1500 g found that on average this goal is not achieved (Ehrenkranz et al., 1999). Meeting this goal is challenging because a tiny preemie's immature digestive system is less able than a full-term baby's to absorb and digest food. Also, extra nutrients must be given in a digestible and absorbable form in just the right amounts, so the baby's kidneys and other organs are not stressed.

Developing guidelines for how much of each nutrient a very preterm baby needs is difficult because these babies vary so much in birthweight, gestational age, health, and nutritional status. In some studies done in India and Finland, babies fed their own mother's milk (either alone or mixed with donor milk) grew at intrauterine rates (Jarvenpaa, Raiha, Rassin, & Gaull, 1983; Ramasethu, Jeyaseelan, & Kirubakaran, 1993). Many tiny preemies fed mother's milk do not grow at intrauterine rates. In this case, some recommend supplementing mother's milk with fortifiers or with hindmilk to increase weight gains (see later section). However, even so, many tiny preemies still do not gain at intrauterine rates no matter what or how much they are fed, especially babies who are born small for gestational age (SGA) or who suffer from extrauterine growth retardation, and those with health problems (Stoll et al., 2004). The most important focus for any preterm baby is his long-term health outcomes, and some research indicates that faster weight gain may not always be in a tiny preemie's long-term best interests.

Gaining weight quickly may actually contribute to health problems later.

The term "nutritional programming" was coined to describe how early nutrition can affect health outcomes later in life. In full-term babies, for example, greater weight gain during the first week of life has been associated with adult obesity (Stettler et al., 2005). Other studies have found links between early nutrition and diabetes, high cholesterol, metabolic syndrome, and cardiovascular problems (Barker, 2003; Barker, 2005; Day et al., 2004; Eriksson, Forsen, Osmond, & Barker, 2003).

In preterm babies, there is evidence that faster weight gain at first may contribute later to a greater risk of cardiovascular disease, including high blood pressure (Singhal et al., 2007; Singhal, Cole, & Lucas, 2001). Other studies have found an association between preemies' early nutrition and the later development of hormonal disorders, allergy, and decreased bone mineralization (Kajantie et al., 2002; Lucas, 2005; Lucas, Brooke, Morley, Cole, & Bamford, 1990).

Adequate nourishment is vital to preventing jaundice and hypoglycemia, conditions to which preterm babies are more vulnerable.

Due to preterm babies' immaturity at birth, they are at greater risk for hypoglycemia and jaundice. Adequate nourishment helps prevent health complications from these conditions, especially with late preterm babies, who may look mature but not feed vigorously at birth (Meier, Furman, & Degenhardt, 2007; Sarici et al., 2004; Shapiro-Mendoza et al., 2008; Walker, 2008; Wang, Dorer, Fleming, & Catlin, 2004).

If the baby is gaining slowly and weight gain is a concern, ask about whether feedings can be increased in volume or frequency.

Acceptable weight is usually considered to be 15 to 30 g or 0.5 to 1 ounce per day. If the preterm baby's weight gain is slow enough to be of concern and the baby is not yet exclusively breastfeeding, suggest the mother first ask her baby's doctor if the baby might be ready to handle more milk per feeding, or if the same volume could be given more times per day. With rapid growth, sometimes feeding volumes are not increased quickly enough. One Australian study found that giving more milk to preemies born at less than 30 weeks gestation resulted in faster weight gain by 35 weeks, but there were no differences in overall growth or health outcomes at 1 year (Kuschel et al., 2000). See also the later section "Fortification and Hindmilk Feeding" on increasing the fat content of mother's milk and its fortification with protein or other nutrients.

If a mother is expressing her milk, ask how long she is expressing at each session.

Explain that the fat content of her milk increases the longer she expresses, and suggest that she continue expressing until her milk flow stops to get a higher fat content. In some hospitals, creamatocrits are done on mother's milk to measure its fat content, which varies from mother to mother (Griffin et al., 2000).

Milk delivery systems can also affect the fat a baby receives, which affects weight gain.

Systems that provide tiny preemies with continuous feedings have greater milk fat losses, because milk fat sticks to tubing. The longer the tubing between the milk and the baby, the more milk fat is lost. If the type of feeding system can't be changed, shortening the tubing may help cut down on fat loss. Feeding a baby intermittently reduces fat loss, but it may still be possible to improve milk fat received. When a syringe-and-pump system is used to tube feed, positioning the syringe upright has been found to decrease fat losses from 48% to 8% (Schanler

& Abrams, 1995). Some U.S. research has also found that mixing small amounts of lecithin with mother's milk reduced fat loss when milk is fed through these devices (Chan, Nohara, Chan, Curtis, & Chan, 2003).

Supplementing Breastfeeding

Milk Issues

A mother may feel upset if she is not expressing enough milk to meet her baby's needs or if she is told her milk needs to be fortified.

Too little mother's milk or its fortification may leave a mother feeling discouraged, depressed, and threatened. Even if she had wanted to breastfeed, this may instill doubts. A mother in this situation needs reassurance and support. See the later section "Risks of Non-Human Milks" for some of the many reasons any amount of her milk is important to her baby's health. Be sure she knows that some mother's milk is always better than none and that any fortification will be temporary.

Ensuring Adequate Milk Production

Be sure the mother knows what to expect at each stage of milk expression and how her actions affect her long-term goals.

For example, during the first few days after birth, be sure she knows that before her milk production increases, she may only express small amounts of colostrum. But no amount is too small to save for the baby, and the time and practice she devotes now will soon lead to much more milk later. See p. 466 in the chapter "Milk Expression and Storage."

Some mothers are advised to pump only as much milk as their preemie needs, which may be very little. However, this strategy can lead to low milk production later that may be difficult to increase (Hill, Aldag, Chatterton, & Zinaman, 2005a; Hill, Aldag, Chatterton, & Zinaman, 2005b). If a mother is finding it difficult to express milk often enough or if she is having other challenges, offer to brainstorm with her. If fitting in enough expressions is the problem, talk to her about her daily routine, emphasizing that the daily expression total is the top priority and the intervals between are not as important. For example, some mothers find their daily totals easier to meet if they express every hour for part of the day.

• •

Preterm birth affects milk volume, but frequency of expression affects volume more.

One small Australian study found that if a mother's preterm milk varied significantly in citrate, lactose, sodium, or protein content, she was more likely to have low milk production (Cregan, De Mello, Kershaw, McDougall, & Hartmann, 2002). Of the 22 mothers studied, in 82% at least one of these ingredients was off. It makes sense that a mother whose breast tissue has 40 weeks to develop during pregnancy might make more milk than a mother whose baby was born after only 30 weeks. However, another U.S. study that compared milk production in mothers of 98 term breastfeeding babies with 95 mothers exclusively expressing for preterm babies found that the baby's gestational age at birth only accounted for about 11% of the variance in milk production at Week 6, while frequency of milk expression accounted for 49% (Hill et al., 2005b).

• •

It is common for mother's milk production to fluctuate with her baby's condition.

When the mother is very worried about the baby's health or survival, milk ejection may be delayed or inhibited, decreasing the volume of milk she can express (Chatterton et al., 2000). Times of crisis may cause a temporary decrease in milk production. During this time, unsupportive comments from others may convince her to give up entirely unless she has a source of support. Assure her that this decrease is only temporary and her production will rebound as the baby's condition improves. It may also be comforting for her to talk to another mother who has had a similar experience.

One Canadian study found that babies who were exclusively human-milk-fed in Week 1 were more likely to eventually go to direct breastfeeding (Wooldridge & Hall, 2003). An adequate milk production at hospital discharge was also associated with moving to breastfeeding at home.

A healthy milk production is one factor associated with breastfeeding later.

Health Risks of Non-Human Milks

All babies—preterm included—are born expecting to receive the live cells and other unique components in their mother's milk. The preterm baby fed only infant formula is missing many ingredients essential for normal body function. For example, exclusive formula feeding of preterm babies is associated with slower maturation of a baby's brainstem (Amin, Merle, Orlando, Dalzell, & Guillet, 2000), as well as an increased incidence of many illnesses linked to immune system and digestive function.

Preterm babies who receive little or no mother's milk are at greater risk for many health problems, some life-threatening.

Infections. Immune factors in both colostrum and mature milk (macrophages, leukocytes, secretory IgA, and more) bind microbes and prevent them from entering the baby's delicate tissues. They kill microorganisms, block inflammation, and promote normal growth of the baby's thymus, an organ devoted solely to developing normal immune function.

A study of 212 very-low-birthweight babies admitted consecutively to a U.S. NICU over a 2-year period found that babies who were fed their mother's milk had a reduced incidence of infection (47% in the formula group vs. 29% in the mother's milk group) and sepsis or meningitis (33% in the formula group vs. 20% in the mother's milk group; (Hylander, Strobino, & Dhanireddy, 1998). Each infection cost on average $6,000 to $12,000 U.S. and increased the length of a baby's hospital stay by 4 to 7 days (Payne, Carpenter, Badger, Horbar, & Rogowski, 2004).

Human milk is essential in preventing illness in preterm babies.

A prospective study of all Norwegian babies born at less than 28 weeks gestation over a 2-year period found that the single biggest risk factor for late-onset septicemia (a life-threatening blood infection) was the number of days that passed before full human milk feedings began (Ronnestad et al., 2005).

Digestive Health and Inflammation. A newborn's digestive system is sterile and immature at birth and needs help to create the right environment for normal development and digestion. Colostrum and mature milk do this by encouraging the growth of good bacteria, which at the same time discourages the growth of harmful bacteria (Caicedo, Schanler, Li, & Neu, 2005). These good bacteria and other components of mother's milk also suppress gut inflammation, which can lead to necrotizing enterocolitis (see below) (Claud & Walker, 2008). Suppressing inflammation reduces the risk it will spread to other areas of the body, which can lead to neurodevelopmental problems later (Vohr et al., 2007; Vohr et al., 2006), chronic lung disease (Schanler, Lau, Hurst, & Smith, 2005), and vision problems (Hylander, Strobino, Pezzullo, & Dhanireddy, 2001).

Colostrum also seals the baby's gut to prevent harmful bacteria from sticking to it and penetrating. Growth factors in mother's milk speed the baby's gut maturation, help the intestinal mucous lining to grow and develop, and strengthen the baby's intestinal barrier (Taylor, Basile, Ebeling, & Wagner, 2009). Newborns secrete few digestive enzymes, and mother's milk provides most of those needed. Antioxidants in mother's milk prevent inflammation, and although refrigerating or freezing expressed milk reduces its antioxidant levels, they remain higher than those in formula (Aycicek, Erel, Kocyigit, Selek, & Demirkol, 2006; Ezaki, Ito, Suzuki, & Tamura, 2008; Hanna et al., 2004).

Necrotizing enterocolitis (NEC) is a life-threatening condition that occurs when part of the preterm baby's digestive tract dies. Because treatment is so costly—on average $73,000 U.S. per case when medically treated and $186,000 U.S. per case when surgery is needed (Bisquera, Cooper, & Berseth, 2002)—a U.S. government researcher estimated that a 9% increase in the number of babies receiving mother's milk could reduce U.S. healthcare costs by $3.1 billion due solely to NEC-related health issues (Weimer, 2001). Unfortunately, the health problems associated with NEC are not confined to infancy, as babies who develop NEC severe enough to require surgery are at greater risk for long-term growth delays and neurodevelopmental problems (Hintz et al., 2005). In a review of the literature, two U.S. scientists concluded that "use of human milk from the patient's own mother affords the most consistent protection from NEC" (Parish & Bhatia, 2008, p. S20). Two U.S. studies found that the more mother's milk a preterm baby receives, the less likely he is to contract NEC (Meinzen-Derr et al., 2009; Sisk, Lovelady, Dillard, Gruber, & O'Shea, 2007).

Feeding Tolerance. Preterm babies fed only formula take longer to tolerate tube-feedings and have more digestive problems. One U.S. study found that very-low-birthweight babies who received their mother's milk for more than 50% of their tube-feedings tolerated partial milk feedings 4½ days earlier and full milk feedings 5 days earlier than babies receiving only formula (Sisk, Lovelady, Gruber, Dillard, & O'Shea, 2008). And earlier feeding tolerance usually leads to earlier hospital discharge.

Long-term outcomes. Exclusive formula feeding of preterm babies has been associated with lower intelligence at age 7.5 to 8.0 years (Lucas, Morley, Cole, Lister, & Leeson-Payne, 1992), lower bone mineralization at age 20 (Fewtrell et al., 2009), and higher blood pressure during the teen years, which the researchers attribute to "programming of cardiovascular risk factor by early diet" (Singhal et al., 2001, p. 413).

The Use of Donor Milk

Mother's milk feedings lead to the best health outcomes, but donor human milk is a good second choice.

Depending on the country, the donor milk available from milk banks consists mainly of term mother's milk that is either pooled from many donors or comes from separate donors. In some countries, such as the U.S., all milk banks pasteurize donor milk before distribution. But in some countries, such as Norway, milk banks provide raw milk (Grovslien & Gronn, 2009). Pasteurizing reduces some of the protective components of human milk, but also kills any viruses and bacteria (Silvestre, Ruiz, Martinez-Costa, Plaza, & Lopez, 2008). All milk donors are carefully screened.

Because donor milk is mostly term milk, it is lower than preterm milk in many of the nutrients small preemies need. But even so, it still offers health advantages over formula. Both a meta-analysis of the research and a Cochrane Review concluded that preterm babies fed donor milk had significantly lower rates of NEC (see previous point). The Cochrane Review concluded that small preterm babies fed formula had a 2.5 times greater risk of NEC, as compared to those fed donor milk (Quigley, Henderson, Anthony, & McGuire, 2009). The meta-analysis concluded that preterm babies fed formula were 3.0 to 4.0 times more likely to develop NEC (McGuire & Anthony, 2003). Although using formula produced higher short-term growth compared with unfortified donor milk, no long-term benefits have been found with this faster growth. Both reviews suggested future research compare growth rates of preterm babies on formula and fortified—rather than unfortified—donor milk. Australian research is in progress on processing techniques that can make the fat content of donor milk more consistent, which may help improve weight gains (Czank, Simmer, & Hartmann, 2009). At this writing, some milk banks, such as the Mothers' Milk Bank in Austin, Texas, can provide donor milk at higher-than-average calorie counts. However, weight gain is not the only important measure of growth in a preterm baby. Weight gain can simply reflect a higher percentage of body fat, which is why growth in length is also important.

• •

Donor milk is more available to preterm babies in some parts of the world than others.

In some countries, such as Norway and Brazil, donor milk is routinely available to preterm babies when mother's milk is not (Grovslien & Gronn, 2009; Pimenteira Thomaz et al., 2008). In Brazil, there are more than 150 milk banks nationwide and donated milk is collected from mothers' homes by municipal workers. At this writing, North America has only 10 milk banks.

Fortification and Hindmilk Feeding

Very early and small preemies grow faster when extra protein and other nutrients are added to mother's milk.

Mothers of preterm babies produce milk higher in some nutrients, but within a month after birth, their preterm milk gradually becomes more like term milk, while their babies' need for extra nutrients remains high. Although some preterm babies grow and develop well when fed exclusively human milk (Jarvenpaa et al., 1983; Ramasethu et al., 1993), many recommend adding extra protein, calcium, phosphorus, and possibly other nutrients to mother's milk for extremely early and small preemies born at less than 34 weeks gestation or born at less than 1800 g (Wight, Morton, & Kim, 2008). A Cochrane Review concluded that adding fortification to mother's milk increased short-term weight gain and body growth, but found no long-term benefits (Kuschel & Harding, 2004). Another Canadian meta-analysis noted that although preemies receiving fortified human milk grew faster, "this benefit could not be weighted against the adverse consequences of elevated blood urea nitrogen levels and increased metabolic acidosis and neurodevelopmental abnormalities" (Premji, Fenton, & Sauve, 2006). A Swedish study found that although the babies who received fortifiers grew faster, there was also more illness in the fortified group and that exclusive breastfeeding led to later improvement in growth (Funkquist, Tuvemo, Jonsson, Serenius, & Hedberg-Nyqvist, 2006).

The term "lacto-engineering" sometimes refers to adding extra human-milk protein or fat to mother's milk. In one Finnish study of 44 preterm babies born at less than 1520 g, human milk protein culled from banked donor milk and added to mothers' milk significantly increased weight gain and growth in length (Rönnholm, Perheentupa, & Siimes, 1986). As of this writing, a commercial human milk-derived fortifier is being developed and researched (Chan, Lee, & Rechtman, 2007). One drawback of the cow's-milk-based fortifiers currently in use is the major and long-term change they cause in babies' gut flora (Rubaltelli, Biadaioli, Pecile, & Nicoletti, 1998). Thankfully, adding cow's-milk-based fortifiers to mother's milk does not appear to increase the risk of NEC (Schanler et al., 2005; Schanler, Shulman, & Lau, 1999).

Whether the fortifier is in powdered or liquid form may affect breastfeeding outcomes.

Cow's-milk-based fortifiers that can be added to the mother's expressed milk are available in both powdered and liquid forms. Powdered fortifiers are typically used when there is enough mother's milk to provide the needed liquid. Liquid fortifiers can be used to increase the volume of a feeding when mother's milk is in short supply. One Canadian study concluded that the choice of liquid or powdered fortifier affected breastfeeding outcomes. When powdered fortifier was used, the mothers expressed their milk for a longer time (Fenton, Tough, & Belik, 2000). The researchers suggested that the powdered fortifier gave mothers the impression that their babies received more mother's milk by volume than formula, which encouraged them to express longer. Conversely, the mothers whose milk was fortified with the liquid perceived their babies received more formula than expressed milk, which discouraged them from continuing to express.

Mothers were more likely to continue expressing when powdered fortifier was used.

Research has found benefits to tailoring fortification to preemies' individual needs.

Rather than giving every preterm baby of the same gestational age and weight the same amount of standard fortifier, researchers are examining how fortification can be tailored to the individual needs of each preemie. One U.S. study found that weight gain and growth were significantly better in preemies who received fortification adjusted to their nutritional needs (based on blood tests) rather than standard fortification (Arslanoglu, Moro, & Ziegler, 2006). To better provide the nutrients the preterm baby needs, in several countries both mother's milk and donor milk are analyzed routinely for protein, carbohydrates, and fat content (Polberger & Lonnerdal, 1993). A Japanese study recently tested a machine designed to be used at the bedside to analyze the nutritional content of mother's milk, which could help tailor fortification (Menjo et al., 2009). As these advances become commercially available, customizing mother's milk fortification may lead to better health outcomes.

Some slow-gaining preterm babies may benefit from receiving more hindmilk.

Another form of lacto-engineering, known as "hindmilk feeding," has been found to help some preemies improve slow weight gain. This may involve adding extra high-fat hindmilk to expressed milk or having mothers store the first milk expressed for future use, keeping the fattier milk at the end of the expression to feed their babies now, as hindmilk averages two to three times the fat content of foremilk and can boost the calories consumed. Of course, this strategy is practical only for mothers expressing more milk than their babies are taking. In one Canadian study, 82% of its 39 mothers expressed enough milk to provide hindmilk feedings for their preterm babies (Bishara, Dunn, Merko, & Darling, 2009). In some U.S. hospitals, the milk's fat content is measured by doing creamatocrits and making adjustments to mothers' expression routine, and the higher-fat milk is given to the baby for more fat and calories (Griffin et al., 2000). Some babies with high energy requirements benefit from this practice, but in addition to weight gain, growth in length is also important.

Hindmilk feeding has been used successfully to increase preterm weight gain in both developed and developing countries (Ogechi, William, & Fidelia, 2007;

Slusher et al., 2003; Valentine, Hurst, & Schanler, 1994). Foremilk and hindmilk contain about the same amount of protein, so if extra protein is recommended, hindmilk alone will not provide it (Valentine et al., 1994). In some cases, fortifiers may be used in combination with hindmilk feeding. One Canadian study found that because vitamins A and E are concentrated in fat, preterm babies receiving both hindmilk feeding and fortifiers may receive more than the recommended amounts of vitamins A and E (Bishara, Dunn, Merko, & Darling, 2008).

Milk Handling and Safety

Colostrum and mature milk should ideally be fed in the order they were expressed.

If the baby is not yet ready to take the breast, beginning tube-feeding with fresh or frozen colostrum helps prepare his gut for mature milk (Caicedo et al., 2005). In some NICUs, mother's milk containers are given color-coded labels to distinguish colostrum from mature milk, so colostrum can be given first (Meier, 2001). After all a mother's colostrum is given, suggest that for the first month, the mother's fresh or frozen mature milk be given in the order in which it was expressed.

• •

If formula is given, suggest giving it separately, rather than mixing it with mother's milk.

In some cases, mother's milk and donor milk are in short supply, so formula may be needed. One U.S. study recommended alternating feedings of human milk with feedings of formula, because mineral absorption was greater (Schanler & Abrams, 1995). Another U.S. study found that when cow's milk based formula is mixed with mother's milk, there is a 41-74% decrease in the anti-infection component lysozyme and a resulting increase in the growth of the bacteria E. coli, which can cause serious health problems.

• •

Guidelines for milk collection and storage for hospitalized babies have been simplified.

Many procedures used in years past to reduce bacterial contamination of mother's milk for hospitalized babies have been found to be ineffective and are no longer recommended, which has simplified this process. These now-unnecessary procedures include breast cleansing (other than routine daily hygiene), routine nipple lubrication before pumping, sterilizing pump parts after each use, discarding the first milk expressed, routine bacterial screening of the milk, and pasteurizing the mother's own milk. Some of these procedures, such as milk pasteurization, while unnecessary for the mother expressing milk for her own baby, may be recommended for donor milk.

The research-based guidelines used by many hospitals to set their protocols can be found in the publication of the Human Milk Banking Association of North America (HMBANA) "Best Practice for Expressing, Storing and Handling Human Milk in Hospitals, Home and Child Care Settings" (Jones & Tully, 2006). For more details, see p. 463 in the chapter "Expression and Storage of Human Milk." Although HMBANA's guidelines have been adopted by many hospitals, suggest the mother talk to her own hospital staff for specific instructions, which can vary among institutions.

If fortifier is added to mother's milk, it should be used within 24 hours.

U.S. studies have found that adding cow's-milk-based fortifiers to mother's milk did not affect bacteria counts, and even with the fortifier added, expressed milk continued to reduce bacteria levels for the first 72 hours (Santiago, Codipilly, Potak, & Schanler, 2005). Another study found that neither bacteria counts nor IgA levels in the milk were affected by adding cow's milk based fortifier, but the milk's osmolality increased with storage over time (Jocson, Mason, & Schanler, 1997). For that reason, a maximum storage time of 24 hours was suggested.

Mother's milk is not sterile and normal bacterial levels are not yet known, so routine screenings are not helpful.

Some hospitals culture expressed milk to check bacteria levels to be sure the milk is being collected in a safe and clean manner. Some bacteria in the milk is normal. Milk is usually judged acceptable if it does not contain certain disease-causing organisms and contains low levels of other types of bacteria, such as skin flora (Meier & Anderson, 1987). Currently, there are no accepted, research-based standards for "safe" milk, so the results of this testing are often inconclusive.

If there is concern about bacterial contamination of the milk, suggest the mother go over recommended hygiene.

The mother may be able to reduce her milk's bacterial levels by doing the following:

- Washing her hands well before touching pump parts and containers.
- After each use, washing the pump parts and containers according to instructions.
- Keeping her fingers away from the inside of her milk-storage containers.

Discarding the first milk expressed and cleaning the nipple before milk expression are not recommended (Jones & Tully, 2006).

Cytomegalovirus (CMV) and Other Maternal Illnesses

In some situations, CMV virus in mother's milk may put tiny preterm babies at low risk of serious illness.

Cytomegalovirus (CMV) is one of the five known herpes viruses that infect humans. By age 50, nearly all adults are CMV-infected, but few develop symptoms, such as fatigue, fever, swollen lymph glands, pneumonia, or liver or spleen defects.

If the mother is CMV-positive during pregnancy, the baby is exposed to both the virus and its antibodies in utero. The CMV virus and its antibodies are also shed into the milk of CMV-positive mothers (Schleiss, 2006). In full-term healthy babies, mother's milk acts like a vaccine, with more than two-thirds of the full-term babies of CMV-positive mothers testing positive themselves for CMV, but developing no symptoms.

However, although the risk is low (Schanler, 2005), some very preterm babies born CMV-negative at less than 1500 g (3 lbs. 5 oz.) have developed serious illness attributed to exposure to the virus through their CMV-positive mothers' milk (Buxmann et al., 2009; Miron et al., 2005; Neuberger et al., 2006). If a baby is born CMV-negative, this means he did not receive antibodies to the virus in utero. And being very preterm means that a baby's immune system is immature, making him more vulnerable to infections of all kinds (Bryant, Morley, Garland, & Curtis, 2002).

When there is a possibility of mother-baby CMV transmission, freezing milk can reduce risk and pasteurizing milk can eliminate it.

When a tiny preterm baby is CMV-negative and his mother is CMV-positive or her CMV status is unknown, there is no consensus about the best course of action (Wight et al., 2008), partly because the actual risk of serious illness is low (Miron et al., 2005).

Pasteurizing mother's milk (heating it to 63.5°C [145°F] for 30 minutes) kills the virus and eliminates the risk of infection, but it also destroys some of the milk's protective components. Heating mother's milk briefly at a high temperature (short-term pasteurization of 72°C [162°F] for 10-15 seconds) kills the CMV virus and also preserves more of the milk's protective components, but the equipment needed for this treatment is not yet commercially available (Maschmann, Hamprecht, Dietz, Jahn, & Speer, 2001).

Freezing mother's milk reduces virus levels, but does not completely kill it (Buxmann et al., 2009; Curtis et al., 2005; Forsgren, 2004; Maschmann et al., 2006). In each situation, the mother and healthcare provider must weigh the risk of active CMV disease with the risks associated with not giving mother's milk.

Few maternal illnesses would contraindicate feeding mother's milk to a preterm baby.

Illnesses that preclude feeding mother's milk to a preemie include HIV/AIDS (only in developed countries), HTLV 1 and 2, and active tuberculosis before treatment.

There are a few illnesses a mother could have that might temporarily require her to express and discard her milk. These include varicella-zoster, measles, and herpes sores on the breast that would touch the mother's hands or pump parts (Wight et al., 2008).

Mother's Diet and Medications

In most cases, a mother does not need to restrict her diet in any way, and her diet will not affect the quality of her milk.

The quality and quantity of a mother's milk production will not be affected by her diet unless it is very restricted, such during a famine or if she has an eating disorder (for details see p. 513- "Nutrition Basics"). A mother does not have to eat an ideal diet to produce good quality milk for her baby. If the mother eats poorly, though, she will have less energy, feel less able to cope, and have lower resistance to illness. This would be true even if she was not breastfeeding or expressing her milk.

Before taking any prescribed or over-the-counter medications, suggest the mother discuss this with her baby's healthcare provider.

A preterm baby is more vulnerable to drugs in mother's milk than a term baby because of his small size and immature ability to process and excrete them. For this reason, the baby's healthcare provider should evaluate any drug's compatibility in light of the baby's size and condition before the mother begins taking it.

However, even when a specific drug is problematic, a substitute compatible with continued breastfeeding and/or expressed milk feedings is likely available. (For details, see p. 729 in the chapter, "Health Issues—Mother.")

Suggest the mother talk to her baby's healthcare provider if she uses cigarettes, alcohol, and/or illegal drugs.

Alcohol, nicotine, and illegal drugs all pass into the mother's milk to some extent. Because a preterm baby is less able to process these substances than a healthy, full-term baby, it is vital that she discuss this with her baby's healthcare provider, even if she has an occasional cigarette or alcoholic drink. Illegal, recreational drugs may pose significant risk to both mother and baby.

Feeding Methods

Depending on a preterm baby's gestational age and condition, at first he may need to be fed intravenously or by tube.

If the baby is very small or ill, he may be fed a nutrient-rich solution via IV. When milk feedings begin, in some parts of the world—such as the U.S.—it may be given continuously by tube (Wight et al., 2008). However, in other parts of the world—such as Sweden—continuous feedings are not used and milk feedings are begun with small or larger amounts (called a "bolus") fed every couple of hours, often through a tube, called "gavage feeding." Suggest the mother put her baby skin-to-skin during these feedings, as it may help him digest the milk, increase the mother's milk production, and enhance her baby's breastfeeding (Hurst et al., 1997).

If a mother is asked for her preferences for supplementing her baby by mouth, discuss the options with her.

The previous section "When to Start Breastfeeding" described why breastfeeding is the best way to start oral feedings. However, most preterm babies who are moving from gavage (tube) feeding to oral feedings require more milk than they can yet get directly from the breast. If a supplement needs to be given along with breastfeeding, see p. 814 in the section "Alternative Feeding Methods" in the appendix "Tools and Products" for a complete list, along with the pros and cons of each. Some mothers have strong preferences about feeding methods, which should be honored.

Bottles are not ideal for preemies because their fast flow can cause heart rate and breathing irregularities.

Although the use of bottles is common in many developed countries, research has found that due to their fast flow, feeding preemies by bottle can cause breathing and heart irregularities, and oxygen desaturation (Blaymore Bier et al., 1997; Chen et al., 2000; Meier & Anderson, 1987; Poets, Langner, & Bohnhorst, 1997). Also some studies have found that supplementing with bottles may make the transition to the breast more difficult. As a result, some U.S. hospitals have developed protocols to transition preemies directly from tube-feeding to the breast, without the use of bottles and without increasing time to discharge (Bell, Geyer, & Jones, 1995; Stine, 1990). One U.S. randomized controlled trial found that babies who were supplemented only by nasogastric (NG) tube were 4.5 times more likely to be breastfeeding at hospital discharge and more than 9.0 times more likely to be exclusively breastfed than the babies who had been supplemented by bottle (Kliethermes, Cross, Lanese, Johnson, & Simon, 1999). At 3 months, the babies supplemented by NG tube were 3.0 times more likely to be breastfeeding and 3.0 times more likely to be fully breastfeeding than the preemies who were supplemented by bottle.

Cup-feeding is used routinely in some developed countries (Nyqvist, 2008a) because Brazilian research has found the feeding behaviors babies use while cup-feeding is closer to breastfeeding than other feeding methods (Gomes, Trezza, Murade, & Padovani, 2006). In parts of the developing world, cup-feeding is used where an unsafe water supply makes bottle-feeding dangerous (Bergman & Jurisoo, 1994). A cup-like device called a paladai is used traditionally in

India to supplement preterm babies (Aloysius & Hickson, 2007; Malhotra, Vishwambaran, Sundaram, & Narayanan, 1999). One early U.K. study on cup-feeding compared 85 preterm babies and found that babies could successfully feed by cup as young as 30 weeks gestation, earlier than they could bottle-feed (Lang, Lawrence, & Orme, 1994). More of the babies fed by cup were fully breastfeeding at hospital discharge than those fed by bottle (81% vs. 63%). During cup-feedings, the preemies maintained satisfactory heart rate, breathing, and oxygen levels, whereas during bottle-feeding, these were compromised (Blaymore Bier et al., 1997). A Brazilian study found that babies use the same mouth and facial muscles during cup-feeding and breastfeeding, but other muscles are used during bottle-feeding (Gomes et al., 2006). For more details on cup-feeding, see p. 823 in the appendix "Tools and Products."

Transitioning to Full Breastfeeding

Depending on how early a preterm baby was born, he may have several milestones between birth and full breastfeeding.

How long this transition takes will depend on the mother's milk production, the baby's health, and how much practice time the baby gets at the breast. Depending on how early the baby was born and the cultural norm, this may happen in the hospital or at home.

Kerstin Hedberg Nyqvist, a Swedish researcher who has extensively studied breastfeeding in the preterm baby, described seven milestones (Nyqvist, 2008a):

- Tube-feeding, skin-to-skin contact, and milk expression
- Breastfeeding begins
- Rooting, single sucks, short suckling bursts, long pauses, occasional milk intake
- Suckling bursts lengthen, stays on the breast longer, takes more milk more often, supplements are gradually reduced
- Milk intake increases, occasional larger volumes
- Variable milk volumes, immature suckling pattern, full breastfeeding possible with semi-demand feeding, mother ensuring baby gets minimum feedings per day (see later point)
- Vigorous, mature suckling pattern, long suckling bursts, breastfeeding on demand

The older or very healthy preterm baby may start at one of the later milestones.

Practice at the breast is the best way to improve breastfeeding effectiveness, so if the mother can, encourage her to offer the breast often.

Some have suggested that most preterm babies cannot feed effectively until they reach term age of 40 weeks gestation (Meier, 2001), but research has found that practice has a greater impact on breastfeeding effectiveness than gestational age. Although it is true that preterm babies have different suckling patterns than full-term babies, this does not necessarily make them less effective (Nyqvist, Farnstrand, Eeg-Olofsson, & Ewald, 2001). One Portuguese study compared the suckling patterns and milk intake of a group of 15 very-low-birth-weight babies (average gestational age 28 weeks) with those of a group of 25 full-term, healthy babies (Cunha, Barreiros, Goncalves, & Figueiredo, 2009). The researchers found that experience at the breast made a significant difference in breastfeeding effectiveness, while gestational age did not. Another U.S. study of 88 preterm babies also found that experience affected number of sucks, suckling bursts, and sucks per minute (Pickler, Best, Reyna, Gutcher, & Wetzel, 2006). Although illness, baby's alertness (state) at feedings, and maturity were also predictors, experience at the breast had the greatest effect.

In a setting in which preterm babies were given lots of time at the breast, two Swedish studies found that 85% of the babies were exclusively breastfeeding at 36 weeks gestation, with some fully breastfeeding as young as 32 weeks gestation (Nyqvist, 2008b; Nyqvist et al., 1999). In one of these studies, the median age of exclusive breastfeeding was 35 weeks (Nyqvist, 2008b). As early as 28 weeks gestation, babies were rooting at the breast and taking the nipple into their mouth. At an average of 30.6 weeks, these preemies began to take milk while breastfeeding. With regular practice at the breast, by 36 weeks, 57 of the 67 babies were exclusively breastfeeding (Nyqvist et al., 1999).

One Japanese study found that with practice even babies (some preterm) who had not been fed by mouth for 2 months quickly caught on and began suckling well. The researchers also found that sucking on a pacifier did not help improve feeding skills. They concluded that "oral feeding practice is necessary for the development of sucking behavior…" (Mizuno & Ueda, 2001, p. 251).

Health problems were associated with less effective breastfeeding, and these babies took longer to breastfeed exclusively than healthy preemies. Neurological issues, among others, can delay effective breastfeeding, which requires an intact and functioning central nervous system (Radzyminski, 2005). One Japanese study found that very-low-birthweight preterm babies with the respiratory problem bronchopulmonary dysplasia had more feeding problems than those without it (Mizuno et al., 2007). The more severe the breathing problem, the less sucking pressure the babies could generate, the fewer the babies' suckling bursts and swallows, and the lower their oxygen levels during feeding.

• •

Suggest the mother plan to be available to breastfeed at as many feedings as possible.

Giving preterm babies ample practice at the breast can be easy or difficult, depending on the cultural climate. In Sweden where breastfeeding is the norm, mothers are encouraged to stay at the hospital to feed and care for their preterm babies. With 1-year paid maternity leave, there is no financial pressure to return to work, even when a baby is hospitalized for months. In this breastfeeding-friendly environment, mothers are encouraged to breastfeed often with support from their healthcare providers. Learning their babies' feeding and sleeping rhythms before discharge makes this transition easier.

However, in countries like the U.S., where financial pressures force many mothers to return to work before their baby's hospital discharge, mothers' availability for feedings may be more limited and many are actively discouraged from breastfeeding early (Galtry, 2003). In situations like this, breastfeeding may be delayed, and at first the mother may breastfeed only once or twice a day, with other feedings given by tube, cup, or bottle. In this case, encourage the mother to do the best she can, perhaps devoting some of her days off to staying at the hospital and keeping her baby on her body for skin-to-skin contact and frequent feedings.

Also, encourage the mother to make sure the hospital staff knows when she will be at the hospital each day and post a sign on the baby's isolette as a reminder, so she won't arrive to find that the baby has just been fed. One Swedish study found that feeding the baby just before the mother's arrival felt "devastating" to some mothers and caused them to doubt their importance to their baby's care (Nyqvist, Sjoden, & Ewald, 1994).

• •

Tools can help make the mother more aware of her baby's breastfeeding behaviors and provide strategies for improving effectiveness.

A Swedish researcher developed and tested the Preterm Infant Breastfeeding Behavior Scale (PIBBS)(Table 9.2), which can be used by both mothers and professionals (Nyqvist, Rubertsson, Ewald, & Sjoden, 1996; Nyqvist et al., 1999). When using the PIBBS, mothers rate six aspects of each breastfeeding, with a higher score indicating greater breastfeeding competence.

Table 9.2. Preterm Infant Breastfeeding Behavior Scale (PIBBS)

Breastfeeding Behavior Observed					**Points awarded**
Rooting	1. No rooting	2. Some rooting	3. Obvious rooting		
Amount of breast in baby's mouth	1. Mouth just touched nipple	2. Part of the nipple in baby's mouth	3. Whole nipple in baby's mouth	4. Nipple and part of areola in baby's mouth	
Took the breast and stayed on	1. Did not stay on	2. Stayed on for <1 minute	Number of minutes baby stayed on		
Number of consecutive sucks	1. No activity at the breast	2. No suckling, only licked/tasted milk	3. Single suckles, occasional short bursts	4. 2 or more short suckling bursts >10 sucks	
Longest suckling burst	Maximum number of consecutive sucks before a pause				
Swallowing	1. Noticed no swallowing	2. Occasional swallowing	3. Repeated swallowing		
				Total points	

(Hedberg Nyqvist & Ewald, 1999; Nyqvist et al., 1996)

Based on her answers, the mother receives suggestions to improve breastfeeding effectiveness (Nyqvist, 2008a):

- **Rooting:** If no rooting, trigger it by touching baby's lips with her nipple or finger. Know that crying is a late hunger cue and touching the baby's cheek causes term babies to root, but may cause only restless movements in a preterm baby.
- **Amount of the breast in the baby's mouth.** If the baby is taking nothing, part of the nipple, or the nipple without any areola, follow the suggestions in the previous section "Helping Baby Take the Breast" to help baby get farther onto the breast.

- **Taking the breast and staying on.** If the baby does not stay on the breast or only stays on for a short time, if the mother is using an upright position and the baby does not stay on the breast, pull the baby's body closer.
- **Sucking**: If the baby does not start sucking or takes very long pauses while awake and breathing calmly, talk to the baby or touch his feet or palm.
- **Swallowing:** If no swallowing sounds are heard, the baby may be a quiet swallower, and this is not a reliable gauge of milk intake.

If these suggestions do not improve breastfeeding, suggest the mother try using a nipple shield (Meier et al., 2000).

As the baby becomes more adept at breastfeeding, some strategies can ease the transition to full breastfeeding.

From scheduled to semi-demand feedings. In innovative Swedish NICUs, as soon as test-weighing indicates that babies are taking about half the milk needed at a feeding, the 1- to 2-hour feeding schedule used at first is replaced with a "semi-demand" feeding plan (Nyqvist, 2008a). This involves offering the breast whenever the baby shows any interest and whenever it has been at least 3 hours since the baby last fed. If the baby is asleep, he is put to the breast with his mouth touching the nipple. Test-weighing is done at each feeding and milk volumes totaled. If the mother finds test-weighing stressful, the daily milk volumes given as a supplement are gradually reduced and the baby's weight gain is carefully monitored. The healthcare provider determines how much daily milk volume the baby needs by weight, and the mother and healthcare provider decide how any needed supplement is given and how often.

Once exclusive breastfeed is achieved, many mothers continue this semi-demand routine until the baby is more mature. Many Swedish babies go home at this semi-demand stage and make the transition to demand feedings there. Until the baby can self-regulate his feedings, mothers must remain vigilant about avoiding long intervals between feedings day and night and keep track of the number of daily feedings to make sure their baby gets enough.

From semi-demand to demand feedings. When the baby's sucking pattern becomes more mature—long, rhythmic suckling bursts interspersed with breathing—he has matured enough to regulate his own feedings and move to "demand" or "cue" feeding, where baby determines when to feed. Test-weighing is stopped, and for a time the baby is weighed every 1 to 3 days to make sure he is gaining weight well.

In a less-breastfeeding-friendly environment, ideally, as the baby becomes more adept at the breast, the mother will begin to breastfeed more times per day. Once all baby's feedings are by mouth, an individual plan can be made with help from baby's healthcare provider, including how much supplement to give and when based on baby's weight and breastfeeding skill. In one U.S. hospital, for example, if a 1700 gram baby needs 300 ml of milk in 24 hours, the baby's intake is monitored by test weighing to be sure the baby gets at least 100 ml (3.3 oz) every eight hours from all sources. By doing test-weights, the mother can see how much the baby takes at the breast and feed him on cue. At the end of each eight-hour period, if he has not yet taken 100 ml, he can be supplemented (Hurst & Meier, 2005). Thus baby begins to set the pace and practices at the breast even before he is fully breastfeeding, while the mother begins to learn her baby's cues.

If a mother feels anxious about breastfeeding, talk to her about her feelings and the advantages of breastfeeding over expressed-milk feeding.

Even when a mother's original goal was to breastfeed, spending weeks or months watching every feeding measured and recorded may increase her comfort with expressed-milk feeding. She may come to associate these feeding routines with her vulnerable baby's well-being and the thought of making a radical change may trigger anxiety. It can also change how a mother sees breastfeeding. As one Swedish researcher wrote:

> …mother-infant separation experienced by mothers of [low-birth-weight] infants, in combination with the strict feeding schedules and prescribed volumes of milk in exact milliliters in the hospital, creates an unnatural breastfeeding situation. Breastfeeding becomes mainly 'providing adequate nutrition,' not an expression of comfort, closeness and joy (Flacking et al., 2003, p. 162).

One U.S. study that analyzed mothers' breast pump use found that the 12 of its 236 mothers (5%) who exclusively pumped and bottle-fed long-term had preterm babies (Geraghty, Khoury, & Kalkwarf, 2005). In another U.S. study of 361 mothers and their very-low-birth-weight preterm babies, 60% started expressing milk, but only 27% did any direct breastfeeding (Smith, Durkin, Hinton, Bellinger, & Kuhn, 2003). Mothers who were more likely to go to direct breastfeeding were older and had health insurance, breastfeeding experience, and a shorter hospital stay (indicating a healthier baby). In contrast, one Swedish study reported that none of its 785 mothers were feeding their preterm babies expressed milk by bottle at hospital discharge (Akerstrom et al., 2007).

One U.S. researcher notes that many mothers lack the help and support needed to make the transition to the breast and that many others don't see the advantage of it to them or their baby (Buckley & Charles, 2006). Many ask the question, "Isn't my baby getting everything he needs from my pumped milk?" She suggests sharing with these mothers the benefits of breastfeeding and the drawbacks of expressed-milk feeding:

- Bottle-feeding stresses preemies, causing oxygen desaturation and heartbeat and breathing irregularities (Chen et al., 2000).
- Less skin-to-skin contact contributes to decreased milk volumes (Hurst et al., 1977).
- Some nutritional and immunological components are lost during milk storage, so the milk quality is lower.
- There is increased risk of dental problems and sleep apnea later in life as bottle-feeding causes malformation of baby's mouth and palate (Palmer, 1998).
- It is challenging to keep up milk production long-term.
- Pump fit issues and malfunction may cause possible breast trauma.
- There is a greater likelihood of going to formula earlier, putting both mother and baby at risk of health problems later in life.
- Breast pumps and formula are an added expense.
- There could be negative effects on mother's mood (Mezzacappa & Katlin, 2002) and feelings of contentment (Shepherd, Power, & Carter, 2000) associated with bottle-feeding.

- The extra time, work, and stress involved in expressing, bottle-feeding, and washing paraphernalia leads many mothers to abandon expressed-milk feeding long before their baby's 1-year birthday.

One U.S. study found that by the time the babies were 4 months old, 72% of the mothers who made the transition to direct breastfeeding were still breastfeeding, while only 10% of those who didn't were still expressing their milk (Smith et al., 2003).

• •

An important aspect of moving to breastfeeding is monitoring the baby's milk intake and weight gain.

A baby making this transition is at risk of inadequate milk intake, so a mother needs to know that her baby is getting enough milk. If while in the hospital the mother has access to its accurate electronic scale (to 2g) for test weights, suggest she use it to get a sense of how much milk her baby is taking at the breast and notice how he acts when fed at the breast compared to when he is fed in other ways. She can use this information to get a sense of outward signs that her baby has had a good feeding, such as acting relaxed and satisfied, audible swallowing, length of feeding, etc.

In one U.S. study in which babies were transitioned to the breast directly from NG tube feedings, a scale was not used. The amount and frequency of supplementation after breastfeeding was determined by how long the babies fed actively at the breast and if swallowing was heard (Kliethermes et al., 1999). If these signs were seen, no supplement was given. If a baby's breastfeeding was considered only fair—he took the breast but didn't keep up the sucking rhythm for very long and few swallows were heard—baby received half of a usual feeding via NG tube. If the baby rooted or licked the breast, but did not take the breast or suckle, he received a full feeding via NG tube. The babies made the transition to full breastfeeding gradually without using any other feeding method. However, research has found that it is impossible to gauge milk intake by observation alone (Meier et al., 1996). Baby's milk intake may be overestimated or underestimated. But what's ultimately most important is helping the mother meet her breastfeeding goal, rather than the time it takes to get there.

One U.S. study examined mothers' reactions to either using or not using a scale as they transitioned to breastfeeding (Hurst et al., 2004). All the mothers who used the scale found it either very or extremely helpful, and 75% of the mothers who didn't use the scale reported that it would have been somewhat to extremely helpful to them to know exactly how much milk their baby was taking at the breast. Another U.S. study found that there was no significant difference in confidence among mothers who transitioned to the breast using a scale for test-weighs and those who didn't (Hall, Shearer, Mogan, & Berkowitz, 2002).

Whether or not the mother uses a scale for test-weighing, frequent weight checks are important to be sure the baby is gaining at least a half-ounce or ounce per day (15 g to 30 g) (Wight et al., 2008).

• •

Until the baby is able to exclusively breastfeed on cue or "demand," the mother should plan to continue milk expression.

Until the exclusively breastfeeding preemie can self-regulate his milk intake at the breast without needing to be awakened or stimulated to feed often enough, suggest the mother continue expressing to keep up her milk production. Healthy milk production is an important aspect of effective breastfeeding, as faster flow keeps a baby more interested and active at the breast. If a mother's milk production slows and baby gets little milk during breastfeeding, encourage her to take steps to increase her milk production. For details see p. 475 in the chapter "Milk Expression and Storage." If a mother's milk production is low and the baby seems to lose interest easily, suggest the mother try an at-breast supplement to increase milk flow (see next point).

• •

If the baby has been supplemented by bottle and is having trouble breastfeeding well, suggest the mother make the bottle more like the breast.

One approach, known as "bait and switch," is to bottle-feed in a breastfeeding position, with the baby's cheek touching the exposed breast, and then as the baby is sucking and swallowing, quickly remove the bottle and put the baby to breast (Wilson-Clay & Hoover, 2008). Others suggest strategies for making bottle-feeding more like breastfeeding (Kassing, 2002). For example, when starting the feeding, touch the baby's lips with the bottle nipple/teat and wait until he opens wide. Then allow him to draw the bottle nipple well back into his mouth, rather than pushing it in. Hold the bottle horizontally rather than vertically, so the flow is not as fast, and hold the baby in a more upright position, rather than on his back. Suggest the mother avoid letting the baby take just the tip of the teat with a tightly closed mouth. The more similar taking the bottle can be made to breastfeeding, the easier this may make the transition to the breast.

When a baby appears to prefer the bottle, there is probably something he is looking for at the breast that is he is not finding—most likely the firm feeling of the teat or the faster flow of the bottle. If the mother can provide one or both of these at the breast, it may help. For example, a nipple shield will provide the baby with a firm feeling in his mouth and an at-breast supplementer can provide instant flow. (For details on these tools, see the appendix "Tools and Products.")

These tools can be used either individually or together to help the baby find what he is looking for and begin to form positive associations with the breast. If they are used together, this may be difficult for the mother to manage by herself. If so, encourage her to get help, as an extra pair of hands can make the process of getting the baby to breast easier. As baby learns, the mother can wean him from these transitional aids.

Most important is not to make the breast a battleground. If a baby is fussing or crying at the breast, suggest the mother stop and comfort him, so that the baby does not associate the breast with frustration and unhappiness. Relaxed skin-to-skin time at the breast will help the baby develop positive associations with the breast.

Going Home

Preparing for Discharge

Before hospital discharge, encourage the mother to get actively involved in her baby's care and check on any available post-discharge services.

The more time a mother can spend with her baby before discharge, the easier the transition to home will be. In some hospitals, parents are encouraged to room-in with their preemie and take over all his care before they go home. If that is an option, suggest the mother take advantage of it (ABM, 2004b). Also, if the mother has not yet been spending lots of time in skin-to-skin contact with her baby, suggest she start now to help bring them closer, to increase her confidence in their relationship, and to become familiar with her baby's sleep-wake rhythm.

Some hospitals provide parents with follow-up care after discharge; others do not. Encourage the mother to find out what services her hospital offers before discharge, so she will know what to expect and can make arrangements. One New Zealand study found that when good follow-up support was provided to mothers whose preterm babies were discharged fully breastfeeding, breastfeeding rates did not suffer, even when they were discharged earlier than routine (Gunn et al., 2000).

Mothers who've had little chance to care for their baby may find going home brings mixed emotions.

If a baby is not breastfeeding well and the mother has not cared for her baby during most of his hospitalization, she may experience a second crisis at hospital discharge that brings similar feelings as the birth. Even after the healthcare providers pronounce a baby healthy and growing well, earlier fears and difficulties tend to linger. It is common to feel helpless and apprehensive mixed with joy and happiness. The mother may feel overwhelmed that she will have to care for her special-need baby at home, while at the same time feel eager to be like a "normal" family and start enjoying her baby.

A mother may feel anxious about taking her baby home.

Suggest the mother arrange for household help.

If baby comes home before full breastfeeding is well established, she may have a lot to juggle at home. Some refer to this intense routine as "triple feeding"—breastfeeding, feeding expressed milk, and then expressing (Wight et al., 2008).

Although the mother may have had time to recover physically from childbirth before her baby comes home, no matter how well her baby is breastfeeding, the constant, 24-hour demands of caring for a small baby can be exhausting. Encourage her to plan her first week at home with her baby doing nothing but breastfeeding and caring for him. Many mothers who have been separated from their babies crave time alone with them. Also suggest, if at all possible, she consider getting household help from family or friends, or if not available, hire help to do laundry, cleaning, and cooking for at least the first week. Their homecoming may also be easier if the mother's partner can take time off to help and spend time together with their baby. Suggest the mother limit visitors who are not there to help and ask those who do come to not stay long.

If there are older children, suggest the mother consider making arrangements with relatives or friends to entertain them during the first week. One Swedish study found that for mothers of preterm babies, having older children was one risk factor for shorter breastfeeding duration (Flacking et al., 2003).

Breastfeeding Considerations

Mothers need to know how to tell that their baby is getting enough milk.

One U.S. descriptive study of 27 mothers of preterm babies reported that during the first few weeks at home, most mothers found feedings a struggle, and then gradually began to feel comfortable with their new routine (Reyna, Pickler, & Thompson, 2006). These mothers said it would have been helpful to be told how their baby's feedings would progress over time. Even mothers whose preemies breastfed well in the hospital report being worried about their baby's milk intake at home (Kavanaugh, Mead, Meier, & Mangurten, 1995).

The most reliable sign of good milk intake is a daily weight gain of at least half-an-ounce to an ounce (15 g to 30 g). One way to monitor the baby after discharge is to schedule frequent weight checks with the baby's healthcare provider, so the mother will know for sure how her baby is doing with their new routine. The American Academy of Pediatrics recommends pediatricians schedule a visit with any baby within 3 to 5 days of hospital discharge (Gartner et al., 2005). If her baby's weight gain is within the expected range, this will set her mind at ease.

Another way to monitor milk intake after discharge is for the mother to rent an accurate (to 2 g) electronic scale for short-term home use. This could be used either to monitor her baby's weight gain from day to day, or if she is concerned about intake at feedings, she can use it to do test weighs. This will give her an accurate measure of whether or not supplements are needed (Meier et al., 1994). Because parents consider their preemies vulnerable, if they feel anxious about his intake, the tendency is to oversupplement, rather than take a chance that he is not getting enough (Hurst et al., 2004). So for some mothers, having an accurate gauge of baby's milk intake at the breast can make the transition to breastfeeding faster and with fewer worries. Other mothers do fine without it (Hall et al., 2002). For more details, see p. 842.

• •

Encourage the mother to keep her baby on her body as much as possible and to take the lead with breastfeeding and seek out support.

Once mother and baby are home, she'll need to find a feeding strategy that works well for both of them. Depending on her baby's gestational age, her baby may not yet be ready for "demand" or "cue" feeding (see previous section). She may need to make sure breastfeeding happens more often than the baby actively demands. If a baby is sleepy, she can keep him on her body and offer the breast frequently, as preterm babies can breastfeed even when asleep (Colson, 2003; 2008). Tell the mother not to hesitate to wake him for frequent feedings as needed.

Even when breastfeeding has gone well in the hospital, many mothers of preemies have doubts and questions once they are home and breastfeeding. When a special program to support breastfeeding mothers of preemies was started in a U.S. hospital, the program team found that despite objective measures that the babies were breastfeeding well while in the hospital, detailed breastfeeding instructions to the mother before discharge, and telephone follow-up 48 hours after discharge, the mothers reported at least one major breastfeeding problem and serious concerns about their babies' intake (Kavanaugh et al., 1995). In hospitals without special breastfeeding support, worries about milk intake and milk production have also been found to be among the mothers' primary concerns after discharge (Hill, Hanson, & Mefford, 1994). Many hospitals have created peer support programs that have significantly increased breastfeeding duration (Meier et al., 2004; Merewood et al., 2006)

Suggest the mother create a comfortable breastfeeding area at home.

Especially at first, it may be helpful for the mother to find a private and comfortable place to breastfeed, away from activity and possible overstimulation, with plenty of pillows to support her and her baby. Suggestions from the previous section, "Putting the Baby to Breast," may be helpful in finding a comfortable and effective position and guiding the baby onto the breast. Also see Chapter 1, "Basic Breastfeeding Dynamics."

Suggest keeping baby nearby for night feedings.

Most health organizations recommend that for their first 6 months babies sleep in their parents' room at night, because it has been found to be protective for Sudden Infant Death Syndrome (Task Force on Sudden Infant Death, 2005). Many parents find breastfeeding easier at night when the baby is in their room, that their sleep is less disrupted, and they more easily rest during feedings. The baby might sleep in a crib, a bassinette, in a co-sleeper attached to their bed, or on the floor on a mattress or palette. If mother is not yet comfortable breastfeeding lying down, suggest that she lean back in bed to breastfeed, with extra pillows behind the mother's back and elbows, with the baby supported tummy down on her body.

When a night feeding is over, the mother can either return the baby to his own bed or keep him next to her, so she won't have to get out of bed for the next feeding. If the mother decides to keep her baby in bed with her, see the "Safe Sleep" recommendations on p. 93 in the chapter "Breastfeeding Rhythms."

In some cases, continued fortification of mother's milk is recommended after discharge.

For tiny preemies born at less than 1500 g (3.3 lbs.), the baby's healthcare provider may recommend the mother continue fortifying her milk after discharge at some feedings (ABM, 2004b). Before making this recommendation, ideally, a detailed nutritional assessment would be done first. Although tiny preemies fed mother's milk alone will eventually catch up in weight gain and growth, in some cases, this may take as long as 2 to 8 years. Also, preemies are born without the iron stores full-term babies have, so iron and other vitamins and minerals are often recommended.

To give fortified milk at home, at some feedings, the mother will use either an at-breast supplementer containing fortified milk or feed her baby her expressed milk mixed with fortifier using another feeding method. One Canadian study found that when mothers were provided with extensive breastfeeding support from a lactation consultant, this daily fortification did not shorten breastfeeding duration, despite the extra time and effort involved (O'Connor et al., 2008). Overall, the babies who did not receive the fortifier and self-regulated their milk intake at the breast took more milk daily overall. The babies who received fortified milk at half their daily feedings had grown longer at 12 weeks and those smallest at birth (≤1250 g) had larger head circumferences than those not receiving fortified milk. The researchers wrote: "The estimated energy intakes of infants in our study did not differ between feeding groups, suggesting that human milk-fed [low birthweight] infants are able to compensate to some degree for the energy and/or nutrient density of their feeding" (O'Connor et al., 2008, p. 773).

THE LATE PRETERM BABY

Once referred to as "near-term," babies born between 34 and 37 weeks gestation are now called "late preterm" to emphasize their vulnerability, which is not always obvious.

A late preterm baby may look healthy, but needs careful monitoring and may not yet be ready to set his own breastfeeding rhythm.

Although most babies born between 34 and 37 weeks are mature enough at birth to breathe on their own, the late-preterm baby should not treated like a full-term healthy baby. Due to his immaturity, he is at greater risk of low temperature, jaundice, hypoglycemia, apnea, and many other health problems (ABM, 2004a; Engle, Tomashek, & Wallman, 2007; Walker, 2009).

Depending on the late-preterm baby's gestational age at birth, his brain may be only 60 to 80% the size and maturity of the brain of a full-term baby (Kinney, 2006). This brain immaturity affects his arousal, sleep-wake cycles, breathing, and his ability to self-regulate feedings. Research has found prematurity to be significantly associated with suboptimal early breastfeeding (Dewey, Nommsen-Rivers, Heinig, & Cohen, 2003). Late-preterm babies are also four times more likely than term babies to have other medical problems (Wang et al., 2004)—which also affects breastfeeding—and after hospital discharge are more likely to be readmitted (Escobar, Clark, & Greene, 2006; Tomashek et al., 2006).

Swedish researcher Kerstin Hedberg Nyqvist describes seven breastfeeding milestones (see p. 359) that many preterm babies pass—beginning with tube-feeding and ending with exclusive breastfeeding (Nyqvist, 2008a). It is likely the late-preterm baby will begin further along this continuum than a younger preemie, but at birth he may not yet be ready to set his own feeding rhythm. At birth, many late-preterm babies have an immature suckling pattern and feed well at some feedings, but not at others. For many of these babies, full breastfeeding is possible with what Nyqvist described as "semi-demand feeding" (see p. 362). This means the mother takes charge of stimulating her baby to feed often enough each day. (See earlier section "Transitioning to Full Breastfeeding.")

The late-preterm baby will need careful monitoring to be sure he gets the milk he needs, and in some cases, he may need to be supplemented. To reduce the need for supplementation, suggest the mother spend as much time as possible with her baby on her body to help regulate his temperature and provide frequent feeding cues (see next point).

When a late preterm baby is kept on his mother's body, he can breastfeed more and feed even while asleep.

One small U.K. study of 12 babies (11 late-preterm and one small for gestational age) examined the effects of keeping babies tummy down on their mothers' semi-reclined bodies for extended periods during the first 3 days after birth, either skin-to-skin or lightly clothed (Colson, 2003). During the first 24 hours, the babies had a mean of 12 of these "biological nurturing episodes," which resulted in from 4 to 16 hours of close body contact and a mean total of 2 hours and 35 minutes of active breastfeeding. In some cases, the mothers moved the babies to the breast while the babies slept, and they fed well. At hospital discharge, all babies were exclusively breastfeeding, with 58% (seven) exclusively breastfed from birth. Five received supplements of mother's milk mixed with formula, 2 for borderline blood sugar levels during the first 2 days and three for jaundice on the 3rd or 4th day.

The long-term breastfeeding outcomes for these mothers and babies were much better than the U.K. norm, with 11 of the 12 mothers still breastfeeding at 4 months and more than half at 6 months, three of them exclusively. The researchers suggested that extensive early mother-baby body contact may be a factor, as it has been found to increase mothers' blood oxytocin levels and breastfeeding duration (Nissen et al., 1996).

PRETERM TWINS, TRIPLETS, AND MORE

Many multiples are born preterm, so during pregnancy suggest the mother prepare for this possibility.

Some ways she can prepare include:

- **Meet hospital staff and take an early breastfeeding class.** Suggest she be sure to meet the lactation consultants and those in the special care nursery and discuss options.
- **Learn about milk expression.** There's a good chance she'll need to know this, and it is much easier to learn new information before the babies are born than after.
- **Learn about skin-to-skin contact.** One preliminary U.S. study found that when preterm twins were held one on each breast that the breasts regulated temperature independently (Ludington-Hoe, Lewis et al., 2006). In other words, if the baby on the right breast was cool, its temperature rose to warm the baby; while if at the same time, the baby on the left breast was too warm, the temperature of that breast fell to cool him.
- **Plan to begin breastfeeding as soon as possible.** If her babies are healthy at birth, the mother can put them to breast right away. Make sure she knows that most mothers of multiples can produce enough milk for all their babies right from the beginning if the babies' breastfeed effectively. Many mothers have exclusively breastfed triplets, some quadruplets, and even quintuplets (Gromada, 2007; Gromada & Spangler, 1998).
- **Arrange for help at home**, for at least the first month, but ideally for the first 3 months.

If milk expression is needed to bring in full milk production, suggest she set as her goal 750 mL (25 oz.) per baby per day.

Suggest as a strategy she stay in Stage 2 (20 to 30 minute milk long expressions 8 to 10 times per day) for a longer time until she reaches this level of production. For details, see p. 466 in "Milk Expression Strategies".

If the mother notices that one of her babies is a more effective feeder, assure her this is common (Nyqvist, 2002). It may help for her to breastfeed two of her babies together, so the effective feeder can trigger milk ejection for the less effective baby.

It is not unusual for one baby to breastfeed more effectively than another or for the babies to be discharged at different times.

Some mothers of multiples find themselves bringing one baby home before the others are ready for discharge. This may mean breastfeeding at home and continuing to express milk for one or more babies in the hospital. Extra help at home can be invaluable during this hectic time. Once all the babies are home, one Swedish study found that after sharing a womb, sharing a sleep surface can help them keep their sleep cycles coordinated, so that both are awake and asleep at the same time (Nyqvist & Lutes, 1998).

RESOURCES FOR PROFESSIONALS

Websites

www.kangaroomothercare.com – Website of Dr. Nils Bergman, a researchers and proponent of skin-to-skin contact

Monographs

Walker, M. (2009). Breastfeeding the late preterm infant. *Clinics in Human Lactation 4.* Amarillo, TX: Hale Publishing.

Books

Nyqvist, K. (2008). Breastfeeding preterm infants. In C.W. Genna (Ed.), *Supporting sucking skills in breastfeeding infants.* Boston, MA: Jones and Bartlett, pp. 153-180.

Wight, N., Morton, J., & Kim, J. (2008). *Best medicine: Human milk in the NICU.* Amarillo, TX: Hale Publishing.

REFERENCES

ABM. (2004a). Protocol #10: Breastfeeding the near-term infant (35 to 37 weeks gestation). Retrieved July 12, 2009, from http://www.bfmed.org/Resources/Protocols.aspx

ABM. (2004b). Protocol #12: Transitioning the breastfeeding/breastmilk-fed premature infant from the neonatal intensive care unit to home. Retrieved July 12, 2009, from http://www.bfmed.org/Resources/Protocols.aspx

Acolet, D., Sleath, K., & Whitelaw, A. (1989). Oxygenation, heart rate and temperature in very low birthweight infants during skin-to-skin contact with their mothers. *Acta Paediatrica Scandinavica, 78*(2), 189-193.

Akerstrom, S., Asplund, I., & Norman, M. (2007). Successful breastfeeding after discharge of preterm and sick newborn infants. *Acta Paediatrica, 96*(10), 1450-1454.

Aloysius, A., & Hickson, M. (2007). Evaluation of paladai cup feeding in breast-fed preterm infants compared with bottle feeding. *Early Human Development, 83*(9), 619-621.

Als, H., Lawhon, G., Duffy, F. H., McAnulty, G. B., Gibes-Grossman, R., & Blickman, J. G. (1994). Individualized developmental care for the very low-birth-weight preterm infant. Medical and neurofunctional effects. *JAMA, 272*(11), 853-858.

Amin, S. B., Merle, K. S., Orlando, M. S., Dalzell, L. E., & Guillet, R. (2000). Brainstem maturation in premature infants as a function of enteral feeding type. *Pediatrics, 106*(2 Pt 1), 318-322.

Arslanoglu, S., Moro, G. E., & Ziegler, E. E. (2006). Adjustable fortification of human milk fed to preterm infants: does it make a difference? *Journal of Perinatology, 26*(10), 614-621.

Aycicek, A., Erel, O., Kocyigit, A., Selek, S., & Demirkol, M. R. (2006). Breast milk provides better antioxidant power than does formula. *Nutrition, 22*(6), 616-619.

Barker, D. J. (2003). Commentary: Developmental origins of raised serum cholesterol. *International Journal of Epidemiology, 32*(5), 876-877.

Barker, D. J. (2005). The developmental origins of insulin resistance. *Hormone Research, 64 Suppl 3*, 2-7.

Bayes, R., Campoy, C., & Molina-Font, J. A. (1998). Some current controversies on nutritional requirements of full-term and pre-term newborn infants. *Early Human Development, 53 Suppl*, S3-13.

Beck, C. T., & Watson, S. (2008). Impact of birth trauma on breast-feeding: a tale of two pathways. *Nurs Res, 57*(4), 228-236.

Begum, E. A., Bonno, M., Ohtani, N., Yamashita, S., Tanaka, S., Yamamoto, H., et al. (2008). Cerebral oxygenation responses during kangaroo care in low birth weight infants. *BMC Pediatr, 8*, 51.

Bell, E. H., Geyer, J., & Jones, L. (1995). A structured intervention improves breastfeeding success for ill or preterm infants. *MCN; American Journal of Maternal Child Nursing, 20*(6), 309-314.

Bergman, N. J. (2008). Breastfeeding and Perinatal Neuroscience. In C. W. Genna (Ed.), *Supporting Sucking Skills in Breastfeeding Infants* (pp. 43-78). Boston: Jones and Bartlett.

Bergman, N. J., & Jurisoo, L. A. (1994). The 'kangaroo-method' for treating low birth weight babies in a developing country. *Tropical Doctor, 24*(2), 57-60.

Bergman, N. J., Linley, L. L., & Fawcus, S. R. (2004). Randomized controlled trial of skin-to-skin contact from birth versus conventional incubator for physiological stabilization in 1200- to 2199-gram newborns. *Acta Paediatr, 93*(6), 779-785.

Bishara, R., Dunn, M. S., Merko, S. E., & Darling, P. (2008). Nutrient composition of hindmilk produced by mothers of very low birth weight infants born at less than 28 weeks' gestation. *Journal of Human Lactation, 24*(2), 159-167.

Bishara, R., Dunn, M. S., Merko, S. E., & Darling, P. (2009). Volume of Foremilk, Hindmilk, and Total Milk Produced by Mothers of Very Preterm Infants Born at Less Than 28 Weeks of Gestation. *Journal of Human Lactation.*

Bisquera, J. A., Cooper, T. R., & Berseth, C. L. (2002). Impact of necrotizing enterocolitis on length of stay and hospital charges in very low birth weight infants. *Pediatrics, 109*(3), 423-428.

Blaymore Bier, J. A., Ferguson, A. E., Morales, Y., Liebling, J. A., Oh, W., & Vohr, B. R. (1997). Breastfeeding infants who were extremely low birth weight. *Pediatrics, 100*(6), E3.

Boo, N. Y., & Jamli, F. M. (2007). Short duration of skin-to-skin contact: effects on growth and breastfeeding. *Journal of Paediatrics and Child Health, 43*(12), 831-836.

Bryant, P., Morley, C., Garland, S., & Curtis, N. (2002). Cytomegalovirus transmission from breast milk in premature babies: does it matter? *Archives of Disease in Childhood. Fetal and Neonatal Edition, 87*(2), F75-77.

Buckley, K. M., & Charles, G. E. (2006). Benefits and challenges of transitioning preterm infants to at-breast feedings. *Int Breastfeed J, 1*, 13.

Buxmann, H., Miljak, A., Fischer, D., Rabenau, H. F., Doerr, H. W., & Schloesser, R. L. (2009). Incidence and clinical outcome of cytomegalovirus transmission via breast milk in preterm infants </=31 weeks. *Acta Paediatrica, 98*(2), 270-276.

Caicedo, R. A., Schanler, R. J., Li, N., & Neu, J. (2005). The developing intestinal ecosystem: implications for the neonate. *Pediatric Research, 58*(4), 625-628.

Cattaneo, A., Davanzo, R., Uxa, F., & Tamburlini, G. (1998). Recommendations for the implementation of Kangaroo Mother Care for low birthweight infants. International Network on Kangaroo Mother Care. *Acta Paediatrica, 87*(4), 440-445.

Chan, G. M., Lee, M. L., & Rechtman, D. J. (2007). Effects of a human milk-derived human milk fortifier on the antibacterial actions of human milk. *Breastfeed Med, 2*(4), 205-208.

Chan, M. M., Nohara, M., Chan, B. R., Curtis, J., & Chan, G. M. (2003). Lecithin decreases human milk fat loss during enteral pumping. *Journal of Pediatric Gastroenterology and Nutrition, 36*(5), 613-615.

Charpak, N., Ruiz-Pelaez, J. G., Figueroa de, C. Z., & Charpak, Y. (1997). Kangaroo mother versus traditional care for newborn infants </=2000 grams: a randomized, controlled trial. *Pediatrics, 100*(4), 682-688.

Charpak, N., Ruiz-Pelaez, J. G., Figueroa de, C. Z., & Charpak, Y. (2001). A randomized, controlled trial of kangaroo mother care: results of follow-up at 1 year of corrected age. *Pediatrics, 108*(5), 1072-1079.

Chatterton, R. T., Jr., Hill, P. D., Aldag, J. C., Hodges, K. R., Belknap, S. M., & Zinaman, M. J. (2000). Relation of plasma oxytocin and prolactin concentrations to milk production in mothers of preterm infants: influence of stress. *Journal of Clinical Endocrinology and Metabolism, 85*(10), 3661-3668.

Chen, C. H., Wang, T. M., Chang, H. M., & Chi, C. S. (2000). The effect of breast- and bottle-feeding on oxygen saturation and body temperature in preterm infants. *Journal of Human Lactation, 16*(1), 21-27.

Chiu, S. H., Anderson, G. C., & Burkhammer, M. D. (2008). Skin-to-skin contact for culturally diverse women having breastfeeding difficulties during early postpartum. *Breastfeed Med, 3*(4), 231-237.

Claud, E. C., & Walker, W. A. (2008). Bacterial colonization, probiotics, and necrotizing enterocolitis. *Journal of Clinical Gastroenterology, 42 Suppl 2*, S46-52.

Colson, S. (Writer) (2008). Biological Nurturing: Laid-Back Breastfeeding. Hythe, Kent, UK: The Nurturing Project.

Colson, S., DeRooy, L., & Hawdon, J. (2003). Biological Nurturing increases duration of breastfeeding for a vulnerable cohort. *MIDIRS Midwifery Digest, 13*(1), 92-97.

Cong, X., Ludington-Hoe, S. M., McCain, G., & Fu, P. (2009). Kangaroo Care modifies preterm infant heart rate variability in response to heel stick pain: Pilot study. *Early Human Development*.

Cregan, M. D., De Mello, T. R., Kershaw, D., McDougall, K., & Hartmann, P. E. (2002). Initiation of lactation in women after preterm delivery. *Acta Obstetricia et Gynecologica Scandinavica, 81*(9), 870-877.

Cunha, M., Barreiros, J., Goncalves, I., & Figueiredo, H. (2009). Nutritive sucking pattern--from very low birth weight preterm to term newborn. *Early Human Development, 85*(2), 125-130.

Curtis, N., Chau, L., Garland, S., Tabrizi, S., Alexander, R., & Morley, C. J. (2005). Cytomegalovirus remains viable in naturally infected breast milk despite being frozen for 10 days. *Archives of Disease in Childhood. Fetal and Neonatal Edition, 90*(6), F529-530.

Czank, C., Simmer, K., & Hartmann, P. E. (2009). A method for standardizing the fat content of human milk for use in the neonatal intensive care unit. *Int Breastfeed J, 4*, 3.

Day, I. N., Chen, X. H., Gaunt, T. R., King, T. H., Voropanov, A., Ye, S., et al. (2004). Late life metabolic syndrome, early growth, and common polymorphism in the growth hormone and placental lactogen gene cluster. *Journal of Clinical Endocrinology and Metabolism, 89*(11), 5569-5576.

Dewey, K. G., Nommsen-Rivers, L. A., Heinig, M. J., & Cohen, R. J. (2003). Risk factors for suboptimal infant breastfeeding behavior, delayed onset of lactation, and excess neonatal weight loss. *Pediatrics, 112*(3 Pt 1), 607-619.

Diego, M. A., Field, T., & Hernandez-Reif, M. (2008). Temperature increases in preterm infants during massage therapy. *Infant Behav Dev, 31*(1), 149-152.

Diego, M. A., Field, T., Hernandez-Reif, M., Deeds, O., Ascencio, A., & Begert, G. (2007). Preterm infant massage elicits consistent increases in vagal activity and gastric motility that are associated with greater weight gain. *Acta Paediatrica, 96*(11), 1588-1591.

Dombrowski, M. A., Anderson, G. C., Santori, C., & Burkhammer, M. (2001). Kangaroo (skin-to-skin) care with a postpartum woman who felt depressed. *MCN; American Journal of Maternal Child Nursing, 26*(4), 214-216.

Dowling, D. A. (1999). Physiological responses of preterm infants to breast-feeding and bottle-feeding with the orthodontic nipple. *Nursing Research, 48*(2), 78-85.

Dvorak, B., Fituch, C. C., Williams, C. S., Hurst, N. M., & Schanler, R. J. (2003). Increased epidermal growth factor levels in human milk of mothers with extremely premature infants. *Pediatric Research, 54*(1), 15-19.

Ehrenkranz, R. A., Younes, N., Lemons, J. A., Fanaroff, A. A., Donovan, E. F., Wright, L. L., et al. (1999). Longitudinal growth of hospitalized very low birth weight infants. *Pediatrics, 104*(2 Pt 1), 280-289.

Engle, W. A., Tomashek, K. M., & Wallman, C. (2007). "Late-preterm" infants: a population at risk. *Pediatrics, 120*(6), 1390-1401.

Eriksson, J. G., Forsen, T. J., Osmond, C., & Barker, D. J. (2003). Pathways of infant and childhood growth that lead to type 2 diabetes. *Diabetes Care, 26*(11), 3006-3010.

Escobar, G. J., Clark, R. H., & Greene, J. D. (2006). Short-term outcomes of infants born at 35 and 36 weeks gestation: we need to ask more questions. *Seminars in Perinatology, 30*(1), 28-33.

Ezaki, S., Ito, T., Suzuki, K., & Tamura, M. (2008). Association between Total Antioxidant Capacity in Breast Milk and Postnatal Age in Days in Premature Infants. *J Clin Biochem Nutr, 42*(2), 133-137.

Feijo, L., Hernandez-Reif, M., Field, T., Burns, W., Valley-Gray, S., & Simco, E. (2006). Mothers' depressed mood and anxiety levels are reduced after massaging their preterm infants. *Infant Behav Dev, 29*(3), 476-480.

Fenton, T. R., Tough, S. C., & Belik, J. (2000). Breast milk supplementation for preterm infants: parental preferences and postdischarge lactation duration. *American Journal of Perinatology, 17*(6), 329-333.

Fewtrell, M. S., Williams, J. E., Singhal, A., Murgatroyd, P. R., Fuller, N., & Lucas, A. (2009). Early diet and peak bone mass: 20 year follow-up of a randomized trial of early diet in infants born preterm. *Bone, 45*(1), 142-149.

Field, T., Hernandez-Reif, M., Diego, M., Feijo, L., Vera, Y., & Gil, K. (2004). Massage therapy by parents improves early growth and development. *Infant Behav Dev, 27*, 435-442.

Flacking, R., Nyqvist, K. H., Ewald, U., & Wallin, L. (2003). Long-term duration of breastfeeding in Swedish low birth weight infants. *Journal of Human Lactation, 19*(2), 157-165.

Forsgren, M. (2004). Cytomegalovirus in breast milk: reassessment of pasteurization and freeze-thawing. *Pediatric Research, 56*(4), 526-528.

Funkquist, E. L., Tuvemo, T., Jonsson, B., Serenius, F., & Hedberg-Nyqvist, K. (2006). Growth and breastfeeding among low birth weight infants fed with or without protein enrichment of human milk. *Upsala Journal of Medical Sciences, 111*(1), 97-108.

Galtry, J. (2003). The impact on breastfeeding of labour market policy and practice in Ireland, Sweden, and the USA. *Social Science and Medicine, 57*(1), 167-177.

Gartner, L. M., Morton, J., Lawrence, R. A., Naylor, A. J., O'Hare, D., Schanler, R. J., et al. (2005). Breastfeeding and the use of human milk. *Pediatrics, 115*(2), 496-506.

Geraghty, S. R., Khoury, J. C., & Kalkwarf, H. J. (2005). Human milk pumping rates of mothers of singletons and mothers of multiples. *Journal of Human Lactation, 21*(4), 413-420.

Goldman, A. S. (2007). The immune system in human milk and the developing infant. *Breastfeed Med, 2*(4), 195-204.

Gomes, C. F., Trezza, E. M., Murade, E. C., & Padovani, C. R. (2006). Surface electromyography of facial muscles during natural and artificial feeding of infants. *Jornal de Pediatria, 82*(2), 103-109.

Griffin, T. L., Meier, P. P., Bradford, L. P., Bigger, H. R., & Engstrom, J. L. (2000). Mothers' performing creamatocrit measures in the NICU: accuracy, reactions, and cost. *Journal of Obstetric, Gynecologic, and Neonatal Nursing, 29*(3), 249-257.

Gromada, K. K. (2007). *Mothering Multiples: Breastfeeding & Caring for Twins or More!* (3rd ed.). Schaumburg, IL: La Leche League International.

Gromada, K. K., & Spangler, A. K. (1998). Breastfeeding twins and higher-order multiples. *Journal of Obstetric, Gynecologic, and Neonatal Nursing, 27*(4), 441-449.

Grovslien, A. H., & Gronn, M. (2009). Donor milk banking and breastfeeding in norway. *Journal of Human Lactation, 25*(2), 206-210.

Gunn, T. R., Thompson, J. M., Jackson, H., McKnight, S., Buckthought, G., & Gunn, A. J. (2000). Does early hospital discharge with home support of families with preterm infants affect breastfeeding success? A randomized trial. *Acta Paediatrica, 89*(11), 1358-1363.

Haase, B., Barreira, J., Murphy, P. K., Mueller, M., & Rhodes, J. (2009). The Development of an Accurate Test Weighing Technique for Preterm and High-Risk Hospitalized Infants. *Breastfeed Med.*

Hake-Brooks, S. J., & Anderson, G. C. (2008). Kangaroo care and breastfeeding of mother-preterm infant dyads 0-18 months: a randomized, controlled trial. *Neonatal Network, 27*(3), 151-159.

Hall, W. A., Shearer, K., Mogan, J., & Berkowitz, J. (2002). Weighing preterm infants before & after breastfeeding: does it increase maternal confidence and competence? *MCN; American Journal of Maternal Child Nursing, 27*(6), 318-326; quiz 327.

Hanna, N., Ahmed, K., Anwar, M., Petrova, A., Hiatt, M., & Hegyi, T. (2004). Effect of storage on breast milk antioxidant activity. *Archives of Disease in Childhood. Fetal and Neonatal Edition, 89*(6), F518-520.

Hedberg Nyqvist, K., & Ewald, U. (1999). Infant and maternal factors in the development of breastfeeding behaviour and breastfeeding outcome in preterm infants. *Acta Paediatrica, 88*(11), 1194-1203.

Hernandez-Reif, M., Diego, M., & Field, T. (2007). Preterm infants show reduced stress behaviors and activity after 5 days of massage therapy. *Infant Behav Dev, 30*(4), 557-561.

Hill, P. D., Aldag, J. C., Chatterton, R. T., & Zinaman, M. (2005a). Comparison of milk output between mothers of preterm and term infants: the first 6 weeks after birth. *Journal of Human Lactation, 21*(1), 22-30.

Hill, P. D., Aldag, J. C., Chatterton, R. T., & Zinaman, M. (2005b). Primary and secondary mediators' influence on milk output in lactating mothers of preterm and term infants. *Journal of Human Lactation, 21*(2), 138-150.

Hill, P. D., Hanson, K. S., & Mefford, A. L. (1994). Mothers of low birthweight infants: breastfeeding patterns and problems. *Journal of Human Lactation, 10*(3), 169-176.

Hintz, S. R., Kendrick, D. E., Stoll, B. J., Vohr, B. R., Fanaroff, A. A., Donovan, E. F., et al. (2005). Neurodevelopmental and growth outcomes of extremely low birth weight infants after necrotizing enterocolitis. *Pediatrics, 115*(3), 696-703.

Hurst, N. M., & Meier, P. P. (2005). Breastfeeding the Preterm Infant. In J. Riordan (Ed.), *Breastfeeding and Human Lactation* (3rd ed., pp. 367-406). Boston, MA: Jones and Bartlett.

Hurst, N. M., Meier, P. P., Engstrom, J. L., & Myatt, A. (2004). Mothers performing in-home measurement of milk intake during breastfeeding of their preterm infants: maternal reactions and feeding outcomes. *J Hum Lact, 20*(2), 178-187.

Hurst, N. M., Valentine, C. J., Renfro, L., Burns, P., & Ferlic, L. (1997). Skin-to-skin holding in the neonatal intensive care unit influences maternal milk volume. *Journal of Perinatology, 17*(3), 213-217.

Hylander, M. A., Strobino, D. M., & Dhanireddy, R. (1998). Human milk feedings and infection among very low birth weight infants. *Pediatrics, 102*(3), E38.

Hylander, M. A., Strobino, D. M., Pezzullo, J. C., & Dhanireddy, R. (2001). Association of human milk feedings with a reduction in retinopathy of prematurity among very low birthweight infants. *Journal of Perinatology, 21*(6), 356-362.

Jaeger, M. C., Lawson, M., & Filteau, S. (1997). The impact of prematurity and neonatal illness on the decision to breast-feed. *Journal of Advanced Nursing, 25*(4), 729-737.

Jarvenpaa, A. L., Raiha, N. C., Rassin, D. K., & Gaull, G. E. (1983). Preterm infants fed human milk attain intrauterine weight gain. *Acta Paediatrica Scandinavica, 72*(2), 239-243.

Jocson, M. A., Mason, E. O., & Schanler, R. J. (1997). The effects of nutrient fortification and varying storage conditions on host defense properties of human milk. *Pediatrics, 100*(2 Pt 1), 240-243.

Jones, F., & Tully, M. R. (2006). *Best Practices for Expressing, Storing and Handling Human Milk* (2nd ed.). Raleigh, NC: Human Milk Banking Association of North America.

Kajantie, E., Phillips, D. I., Andersson, S., Barker, D. J., Dunkel, L., Forsen, T., et al. (2002). Size at birth, gestational age and cortisol secretion in adult life: foetal programming of both hyper- and hypocortisolism? *Clinical Endocrinology, 57*(5), 635-641.

Kambarami, R. A., Chidede, O., & Kowo, D. T. (1998). Kangaroo care versus incubator care in the management of well preterm infants--a pilot study. *Annals of Tropical Paediatrics, 18*(2), 81-86.

Kassing, D. (2002). Bottle-feeding as a tool to reinforce breastfeeding. *Journal of Human Lactation, 18*(1), 56-60.

Kavanaugh, K., Mead, L., Meier, P., & Mangurten, H. H. (1995). Getting enough: mothers' concerns about breastfeeding a preterm infant after discharge. *Journal of Obstetric, Gynecologic, and Neonatal Nursing, 24*(1), 23-32.

Kinney, H. C. (2006). The near-term (late preterm) human brain and risk for periventricular leukomalacia: a review. *Seminars in Perinatology, 30*(2), 81-88.

Kliethermes, P. A., Cross, M. L., Lanese, M. G., Johnson, K. M., & Simon, S. D. (1999). Transitioning preterm infants with nasogastric tube supplementation: increased likelihood of breastfeeding. *Journal of Obstetric, Gynecologic, and Neonatal Nursing, 28*(3), 264-273.

Kostandy, R. R., Ludington-Hoe, S. M., Cong, X., Abouelfettoh, A., Bronson, C., Stankus, A., et al. (2008). Kangaroo Care (skin contact) reduces crying response to pain in preterm neonates: pilot results. *Pain Manag Nurs, 9*(2), 55-65.

Kovacs, A., Funke, S., Marosvolgyi, T., Burus, I., & Decsi, T. (2005). Fatty acids in early human milk after preterm and full-term delivery. *Journal of Pediatric Gastroenterology and Nutrition, 41*(4), 454-459.

Kunz, C., Rudloff, S., Baier, W., Klein, N., & Strobel, S. (2000). Oligosaccharides in human milk: structural, functional, and metabolic aspects. *Annual Review of Nutrition, 20*, 699-722.

Kuschel, C. A., Evans, N., Askie, L., Bredemeyer, S., Nash, J., & Polverino, J. (2000). A randomized trial of enteral feeding volumes in infants born before 30 weeks' gestation. *Journal of Paediatrics and Child Health, 36*(6), 581-586.

Kuschel, C. A., & Harding, J. E. (2004). Multicomponent fortified human milk for promoting growth in preterm infants. *Cochrane Database of Systematic Reviews, 1*, CD000343.

Lang, S., Lawrence, C. J., & Orme, R. L. (1994). Cup feeding: an alternative method of infant feeding. *Archives of Disease in Childhood, 71*(4), 365-369.

Lau, C., Sheena, H. R., Shulman, R. J., & Schanler, R. J. (1997). Oral feeding in low birth weight infants. *Journal of Pediatrics, 130*(4), 561-569.

Lemons, J. A., Moye, L., Hall, D., & Simmons, M. (1982). Differences in the composition of preterm and term human milk during early lactation. *Pediatric Research, 16*(2), 113-117.

Lucas, A. (2005). Long-term programming effects of early nutrition -- implications for the preterm infant. *Journal of Perinatology, 25 Suppl 2*, S2-6.

Lucas, A., Brooke, O. G., Morley, R., Cole, T. J., & Bamford, M. F. (1990). Early diet of preterm infants and development of allergic or atopic disease: randomised prospective study. *BMJ, 300*(6728), 837-840.

Lucas, A., Morley, R., Cole, T. J., Lister, G., & Leeson-Payne, C. (1992). Breast milk and subsequent intelligence quotient in children born preterm. *Lancet, 339*(8788), 261-264.

Ludington-Hoe, S. M., Hashemi, M. S., Argote, L. A., Medellin, G., & Rey, H. (1992). Selected physiologic measures and behavior during paternal skin contact with Colombian preterm infants. *Journal of Developmental Physiology, 18*(5), 223-232.

Ludington-Hoe, S. M., Hosseini, R., & Torowicz, D. L. (2005). Skin-to-skin contact (Kangaroo Care) analgesia for preterm infant heel stick. *AACN Clinical Issues, 16*(3), 373-387.

Ludington-Hoe, S. M., Johnson, M. W., Morgan, K., Lewis, T., Gutman, J., Wilson, P. D., et al. (2006). Neurophysiologic assessment of neonatal sleep organization: preliminary results of a randomized, controlled trial of skin contact with preterm infants. *Pediatrics, 117*(5), e909-923.

Ludington-Hoe, S. M., Lewis, T., Morgan, K., Cong, X., Anderson, L., & Reese, S. (2006). Breast and infant temperatures with twins during shared Kangaroo Care. *Journal of Obstetric, Gynecologic, and Neonatal Nursing, 35*(2), 223-231.

Magne, F., Abely, M., Boyer, F., Morville, P., Pochart, P., & Suau, A. (2006). Low species diversity and high interindividual variability in faeces of preterm infants as revealed by sequences of 16S rRNA genes and PCR-temporal temperature gradient gel electrophoresis profiles. *FEMS Microbiol Ecol, 57*(1), 128-138.

Malhotra, N., Vishwambaran, L., Sundaram, K. R., & Narayanan, I. (1999). A controlled trial of alternative methods of oral feeding in neonates. *Early Human Development, 54*(1), 29-38.

Maschmann, J., Hamprecht, K., Dietz, K., Jahn, G., & Speer, C. P. (2001). Cytomegalovirus infection of extremely low-birth weight infants via breast milk. *Clinical Infectious Diseases, 33*(12), 1998-2003.

Maschmann, J., Hamprecht, K., Weissbrich, B., Dietz, K., Jahn, G., & Speer, C. P. (2006). Freeze-thawing of breast milk does not prevent cytomegalovirus transmission to a preterm infant. *Archives of Disease in Childhood. Fetal and Neonatal Edition, 91*(4), F288-290.

Mathur, N. B., Dwarkadas, A. M., Sharma, V. K., Saha, K., & Jain, N. (1990). Anti-infective factors in preterm human colostrum. *Acta Paediatrica Scandinavica, 79*(11), 1039-1044.

McCain, G. C., Gartside, P. S., Greenberg, J. M., & Lott, J. W. (2001). A feeding protocol for healthy preterm infants that shortens time to oral feeding. *Journal of Pediatrics, 139*(3), 374-379.

McGuire, W., & Anthony, M. Y. (2003). Donor human milk versus formula for preventing necrotising enterocolitis in preterm infants: systematic review. *Archives of Disease in Childhood. Fetal and Neonatal Edition, 88*(1), F11-14.

Measel, C. P., & Anderson, G. C. (1979). Nonnutritive sucking during tube feedings: effect on clinical course in premature infants. *JOGN Nursing, 8*(5), 265-272.

Meier, P. (1988). Bottle- and breast-feeding: effects on transcutaneous oxygen pressure and temperature in preterm infants. *Nursing Research, 37*(1), 36-41.

Meier, P., & Anderson, G. C. (1987). Responses of small preterm infants to bottle- and breast-feeding. *MCN; American Journal of Maternal Child Nursing, 12*(2), 97-105.

Meier, P. P. (2001). Breastfeeding in the special care nursery: Prematures and infants with medical problems. In R. J. Schanler (Ed.), *Breastfeeding 2001: The Management of Breastfeeding* (Vol. 48, pp. 425-442). Philadelphia, PA: W.B. Saunders Company.

Meier, P. P. (2003). Supporting lactation in mothers with very low birth weight infants. *Pediatric Annals, 32*(5), 317-325.

Meier, P. P., Brown, L. P., Hurst, N. M., Spatz, D. L., Engstrom, J. L., Borucki, L. C., et al. (2000). Nipple shields for preterm infants: effect on milk transfer and duration of breastfeeding. *Journal of Human Lactation, 16*(2), 106-114; quiz 129-131.

Meier, P. P., Engstrom, J. L., Crichton, C. L., Clark, D. R., Williams, M. M., & Mangurten, H. H. (1994). A new scale for in-home test-weighing for mothers of preterm and high risk infants. *Journal of Human Lactation, 10*(3), 163-168.

Meier, P. P., Engstrom, J. L., Fleming, B. A., Streeter, P. L., & Lawrence, P. B. (1996). Estimating milk intake of hospitalized preterm infants who breastfeed. *Journal of Human Lactation, 12*(1), 21-26.

Meier, P. P., Engstrom, J. L., Mingolelli, S. S., Miracle, D. J., & Kiesling, S. (2004). The Rush Mothers' Milk Club: breastfeeding interventions for mothers with very-low-birth-weight infants. *Journal of Obstetric, Gynecologic, and Neonatal Nursing, 33*(2), 164-174.

Meier, P. P., Furman, L. M., & Degenhardt, M. (2007). Increased lactation risk for late preterm infants and mothers: evidence and management strategies to protect breastfeeding. *J Midwifery Womens Health, 52*(6), 579-587.

Meinzen-Derr, J., Poindexter, B., Wrage, L., Morrow, A. L., Stoll, B., & Donovan, E. F. (2009). Role of human milk in extremely low birth weight infants' risk of necrotizing enterocolitis or death. *Journal of Perinatology, 29*(1), 57-62.

Menjo, A., Mizuno, K., Murase, M., Nishida, Y., Taki, M., Itabashi, K., et al. (2009). Bedside analysis of human milk for adjustable nutrition strategy. *Acta Paediatrica, 98*(2), 380-384.

Merewood, A., Chamberlain, L. B., Cook, J. T., Philipp, B. L., Malone, K., & Bauchner, H. (2006). The effect of peer counselors on breastfeeding rates in the neonatal intensive care unit: results of a randomized controlled trial. *Archives of Pediatrics and Adolescent Medicine, 160*(7), 681-685.

Mezzacappa, E. S., & Katlin, E. S. (2002). Breast-feeding is associated with reduced perceived stress and negative mood in mothers. *Health Psychology, 21*(2), 187-193.

Miracle, D. J., Meier, P. P., & Bennett, P. A. (2004). Mothers' decisions to change from formula to mothers' milk for very-low-birth-weight infants. *Journal of Obstetric, Gynecologic, and Neonatal Nursing, 33*(6), 692-703.

Miron, D., Brosilow, S., Felszer, K., Reich, D., Halle, D., Wachtel, D., et al. (2005). Incidence and clinical manifestations of breast milk-acquired Cytomegalovirus infection in low birth weight infants. *Journal of Perinatology, 25*(5), 299-303.

Mizuno, K., Inoue, M., & Takeuchi, T. (2000). The effects of body positioning on sucking behaviour in sick neonates. *European Journal of Pediatrics, 159*(11), 827-831.

Mizuno, K., Nishida, Y., Taki, M., Hibino, S., Murase, M., Sakurai, M., et al. (2007). Infants with bronchopulmonary dysplasia suckle with weak pressures to maintain breathing during feeding. *Pediatrics, 120*(4), e1035-1042.

Mizuno, K., & Ueda, A. (2001). Development of sucking behavior in infants who have not been fed for 2 months after birth. *Pediatrics International, 43*(3), 251-255.

Moore, E. R., Anderson, G. C., & Bergman, N. J. (2007). Early skin-to-skin contact for mothers and their healthy newborn infants. *Cochrane Database of Systematic Reviews, 3*(10.1022/14651858.CD003519.pub2).

Morelius, E., Hellstrom-Westas, L., Carlen, C., Norman, E., & Nelson, N. (2006). Is a nappy change stressful to neonates? *Early Human Development, 82*(10), 669-676.

Narayanan, I. (1990). Sucking on the "emptied" breast--a better method of non-nutritive sucking than the use of a pacifier. *Indian Pediatrics, 27*(10), 1122-1124.

Neuberger, P., Hamprecht, K., Vochem, M., Maschmann, J., Speer, C. P., Jahn, G., et al. (2006). Case-control study of symptoms and neonatal outcome of human milk-transmitted cytomegalovirus infection in premature infants. *Journal of Pediatrics, 148*(3), 326-331.

Nissen, E., Uvnas-Moberg, K., Svensson, K., Stock, S., Widstrom, A. M., & Winberg, J. (1996). Different patterns of oxytocin, prolactin but not cortisol release during breastfeeding in women delivered by caesarean section or by the vaginal route. *Early Human Development, 45*(1-2), 103-118.

Nye, C. (2008). Transitioning premature infants from gavage to breast. *Neonatal Network, 27*(1), 7-13.

Nyqvist, K. H. (2002). Breast-feeding in preterm twins: Development of feeding behavior and milk intake during hospital stay and related caregiving practices. *Journal of Pediatric Nursing, 17*(4), 246-256.

Nyqvist, K. H. (2004). How can kangaroo mother care and high technology care be compatible? *Journal of Human Lactation, 20*(1), 72-74.

Nyqvist, K. H. (2008a). Breastfeeding preterm infants. In C. W. Genna (Ed.), *Supporting Sucking Skills in Breastfeeding Infants* (pp. 153-180). Boston, MA: Jones and Bartlett.

Nyqvist, K. H. (2008b). Early attainment of breastfeeding competence in very preterm infants. *Acta Paediatrica, 97*(6), 776-781.

Nyqvist, K. H., & Engvall, G. (2009). Parents as their infant's primary caregivers in a neonatal intensive care unit. *Journal of Pediatric Nursing, 24*(2), 153-163.

Nyqvist, K. H., Farnstrand, C., Eeg-Olofsson, K. E., & Ewald, U. (2001). Early oral behaviour in preterm infants during breastfeeding: an electromyographic study. *Acta Paediatrica, 90*(6), 658-663.

Nyqvist, K. H., & Lutes, L. M. (1998). Co-bedding twins: a developmentally supportive care strategy. *Journal of Obstetric, Gynecologic, and Neonatal Nursing, 27*(4), 450-456.

Nyqvist, K. H., Rubertsson, C., Ewald, U., & Sjoden, P. O. (1996). Development of the Preterm Infant Breastfeeding Behavior Scale (PIBBS): a study of nurse-mother agreement. *Journal of Human Lactation, 12*(3), 207-219.

Nyqvist, K. H., Sjoden, P. O., & Ewald, U. (1994). Mothers' advice about facilitating breastfeeding in a neonatal intensive care unit. *Journal of Human Lactation, 10*(4), 237-243.

Nyqvist, K. H., Sjoden, P. O., & Ewald, U. (1999). The development of preterm infants' breastfeeding behavior. *Early Human Development, 55*(3), 247-264.

O'Connor, D. L., Khan, S., Weishuhn, K., Vaughan, J., Jefferies, A., Campbell, D. M., et al. (2008). Growth and nutrient intakes of human milk-fed preterm infants provided with extra energy and nutrients after hospital discharge. *Pediatrics, 121*(4), 766-776.

Ogechi, A. A., William, O., & Fidelia, B. T. (2007). Hindmilk and weight gain in preterm very low-birthweight infants. *Pediatrics International, 49*(2), 156-160.

Palmer, B. (1998). The influence of breastfeeding on the development of the oral cavity: a commentary. *Journal of Human Lactation, 14*(2), 93-98.

Parish, A., & Bhatia, J. (2008). Feeding strategies in the ELBW infant. *Journal of Perinatology, 28 Suppl 1*, S18-20.

Payne, N. R., Carpenter, J. H., Badger, G. J., Horbar, J. D., & Rogowski, J. (2004). Marginal increase in cost and excess length of stay associated with nosocomial bloodstream infections in surviving very low birth weight infants. *Pediatrics, 114*(2), 348-355.

Pickler, R. H., Best, A. M., Reyna, B. A., Gutcher, G., & Wetzel, P. A. (2006). Predictors of nutritive sucking in preterm infants. *Journal of Perinatology, 26*(11), 693-699.

Pimenteira Thomaz, A. C., Maia Loureiro, L. V., da Silva Oliveira, T., Furtado Montenegro, N. C., Dantas Almeida Junior, E., Fernando Rodrigues Soriano, C., et al. (2008). The human milk donation experience: motives, influencing factors, and regular donation. *Journal of Human Lactation, 24*(1), 69-76.

Poets, C. F., Langner, M. U., & Bohnhorst, B. (1997). Effects of bottle feeding and two different methods of gavage feeding on oxygenation and breathing patterns in preterm infants. *Acta Paediatrica, 86*(4), 419-423.

Polberger, S., & Lonnerdal, B. (1993). Simple and rapid macronutrient analysis of human milk for individualized fortification: basis for improved nutritional management of very-low-birth-weight infants? *Journal of Pediatric Gastroenterology and Nutrition, 17*(3), 283-290.

Premji, S., Fenton, T., & Sauve, R. (2006). Does Amount of Protein in Formula Matter for Low-Birthweight Infants? A Cochrane Systematic Review. *JPEN. Journal of Parenteral and Enteral Nutrition, 30*(6), 507-514.

Quigley, M., Henderson, G., Anthony, M. Y., & McGuire, W. (2009). Formula milk versus donor breast milk for feeding preterm or low birth weight infants (Publication no. 10.1002/14651858.CD002971.pub2). Retrieved July 4, 2009, from John Wiley & Sons, Ltd.:

Radzyminski, S. (2005). Neurobehavioral functioning and breastfeeding behavior in the newborn. *J Obstet Gynecol Neonatal Nurs, 34*(3), 335-341.

Ramasethu, J., Jeyaseelan, L., & Kirubakaran, C. P. (1993). Weight gain in exclusively breastfed preterm infants. *Journal of Tropical Pediatrics, 39*(3), 152-159.

Rao, S., Udani, R., & Nanavati, R. (2008). Kangaroo Mother Care for low birth weight infants: A randomized controlled trial. *Indian Pediatrics, 45*, 17-23.

Reyna, B. A., Pickler, R. H., & Thompson, A. (2006). A descriptive study of mothers' experiences feeding their preterm infants after discharge. *Adv Neonatal Care,* 6(6), 333-340.

Rodriguez, N. A., Miracle, D. J., & Meier, P. P. (2005). Sharing the science on human milk feedings with mothers of very-low-birth-weight infants. *Journal of Obstetric, Gynecologic, and Neonatal Nursing, 34*(1), 109-119.

Rojas, M. A., Kaplan, M., Quevedo, M., Sherwonit, E., Foster, L. B., Ehrenkranz, R. A., et al. (2003). Somatic growth of preterm infants during skin-to-skin care versus traditional holding: a randomized, controlled trial. *Journal of Developmental and Behavioral Pediatrics, 24*(3), 163-168.

Ronnestad, A., Abrahamsen, T. G., Medbo, S., Reigstad, H., Lossius, K., Kaaresen, P. I., et al. (2005). Late-onset septicemia in a Norwegian national cohort of extremely premature infants receiving very early full human milk feeding. *Pediatrics, 115*(3), e269-276.

Ross, E. S., & Browne, J. V. (2002). Developmental progression of feeding skills: an approach to supporting feeding in preterm infants. *Semin Neonatol, 7*(6), 469-475.

Rubaltelli, F. F., Biadaioli, R., Pecile, P., & Nicoletti, P. (1998). Intestinal flora in breast- and bottle-fed infants. *Journal of Perinatal Medicine, 26*(3), 186-191.

Ruiz-Pelaez, J. G., Charpak, N., & Cuervo, L. G. (2004). Kangaroo Mother Care, an example to follow from developing countries. *BMJ, 329*(7475), 1179-1181.

Santiago, M. S., Codipilly, C. N., Potak, D. C., & Schanler, R. J. (2005). Effect of human milk fortifiers on bacterial growth in human milk. *Journal of Perinatology, 25*(10), 647-649.

Sarici, S. U., Serdar, M. A., Korkmaz, A., Erdem, G., Oran, O., Tekinalp, G., et al. (2004). Incidence, course, and prediction of hyperbilirubinemia in near-term and term newborns. *Pediatrics, 113*(4), 775-780.

Schanler, R. J. (2005). CMV acquisition in premature infants fed human milk: reason to worry? *Journal of Perinatology, 25*(5), 297-298.

Schanler, R. J., & Abrams, S. A. (1995). Postnatal attainment of intrauterine macromineral accretion rates in low birth weight infants fed fortified human milk. *Journal of Pediatrics, 126*(3), 441-447.

Schanler, R. J., & Atkinson, S. A. (1999). Effects of nutrients in human milk on the recipient premature infant. *Journal of Mammary Gland Biology and Neoplasia, 4*(3), 297-307.

Schanler, R. J., Lau, C., Hurst, N. M., & Smith, E. O. (2005). Randomized trial of donor human milk versus preterm formula as substitutes for mothers' own milk in the feeding of extremely premature infants. *Pediatrics, 116*(2), 400-406.

Schanler, R. J., Shulman, R. J., & Lau, C. (1999). Feeding strategies for premature infants: beneficial outcomes of feeding fortified human milk versus preterm formula. *Pediatrics, 103*(6 Pt 1), 1150-1157.

Schleiss, M. R. (2006). Acquisition of human cytomegalovirus infection in infants via breast milk: natural immunization or cause for concern? *Rev Med Virol, 16*(2), 73-82.

Shapiro-Mendoza, C. K., Tomashek, K. M., Kotelchuck, M., Barfield, W., Nannini, A., Weiss, J., et al. (2008). Effect of late-preterm birth and maternal medical conditions on newborn morbidity risk. *Pediatrics, 121*(2), e223-232.

Shepherd, C. K., Power, K. G., & Carter, H. (2000). Examining the correspondence of breastfeeding and bottle-feeding couples' infant feeding attitudes. *Journal of Advanced Nursing, 31*(3), 651-660.

Silvestre, D., Ruiz, P., Martinez-Costa, C., Plaza, A., & Lopez, M. C. (2008). Effect of pasteurization on the bactericidal capacity of human milk. *Journal of Human Lactation, 24*(4), 371-376.

Singhal, A., Cole, T. J., Fewtrell, M., Kennedy, K., Stephenson, T., Elias-Jones, A., et al. (2007). Promotion of faster weight gain in infants born small for gestational age: is there an adverse effect on later blood pressure? *Circulation, 115*(2), 213-220.

Singhal, A., Cole, T. J., & Lucas, A. (2001). Early nutrition in preterm infants and later blood pressure: two cohorts after randomised trials. *Lancet, 357*(9254), 413-419.

Sisk, P. M., Lovelady, C. A., Dillard, R. G., & Gruber, K. J. (2006). Lactation counseling for mothers of very low birth weight infants: effect on maternal anxiety and infant intake of human milk. *Pediatrics, 117*(1), e67-75.

Sisk, P. M., Lovelady, C. A., Dillard, R. G., Gruber, K. J., & O'Shea, T. M. (2007). Early human milk feeding is associated with a lower risk of necrotizing enterocolitis in very low birth weight infants. *Journal of Perinatology, 27*(7), 428-433.

Sisk, P. M., Lovelady, C. A., Gruber, K. J., Dillard, R. G., & O'Shea, T. M. (2008). Human milk consumption and full enteral feeding among infants who weigh </= 1250 grams. *Pediatrics, 121*(6), e1528-1533.

Slusher, T., Hampton, R., Bode-Thomas, F., Pam, S., Akor, F., & Meier, P. (2003). Promoting the exclusive feeding of own mother's milk through the use of hindmilk and increased maternal milk volume for hospitalized, low birth weight infants (< 1800 grams) in Nigeria: a feasibility study. *Journal of Human Lactation, 19*(2), 191-198.

Smith, M. M., Durkin, M., Hinton, V. J., Bellinger, D., & Kuhn, L. (2003). Initiation of breastfeeding among mothers of very low birth weight infants. *Pediatrics, 111*(6 Pt 1), 1337-1342.

Stettler, N., Stallings, V. A., Troxel, A. B., Zhao, J., Schinnar, R., Nelson, S. E., et al. (2005). Weight gain in the first week of life and overweight in adulthood: a cohort study of European American subjects fed infant formula. *Circulation, 111*(15), 1897-1903.

Stine, M. J. (1990). Breastfeeding the premature newborn: a protocol without bottles. *Journal of Human Lactation, 6*(4), 167-170.

Stoll, B. J., Hansen, N. I., Adams-Chapman, I., Fanaroff, A. A., Hintz, S. R., Vohr, B., et al. (2004). Neurodevelopmental and growth impairment among extremely low-birth-weight infants with neonatal infection. *JAMA, 292*(19), 2357-2365.

Sweet, L. (2008). Expressed breast milk as 'connection' and its influence on the construction of 'motherhood' for mothers of preterm infants: a qualitative study. *Int Breastfeed J, 3*, 30.

Task Force on Sudden Infant Death, S. (2005). The Changing Concept of Sudden Infant Death Syndrome: Diagnostic Coding Shifts, Controversies Regarding the Sleeping Environment, and New Variables to Consider in Reducing Risk. *Pediatrics, 116*(5), 1245-1255.

Taylor, S. N., Basile, L. A., Ebeling, M., & Wagner, C. L. (2009). Intestinal permeability in preterm infants by feeding type: mother's milk versus formula. *Breastfeed Med, 4*(1), 11-15.

Tomashek, K. M., Shapiro-Mendoza, C. K., Weiss, J., Kotelchuck, M., Barfield, W., Evans, S., et al. (2006). Early discharge among late preterm and term newborns and risk of neonatal morbidity. *Seminars in Perinatology, 30*(2), 61-68.

Valentine, C. J., Hurst, N. M., & Schanler, R. J. (1994). Hindmilk improves weight gain in low-birth-weight infants fed human milk. *Journal of Pediatric Gastroenterology and Nutrition, 18*(4), 474-477.

Vohr, B. R., Poindexter, B. B., Dusick, A. M., McKinley, L. T., Higgins, R. D., Langer, J. C., et al. (2007). Persistent beneficial effects of breast milk ingested in the neonatal intensive care unit on outcomes of extremely low birth weight infants at 30 months of age. *Pediatrics, 120*(4), e953-959.

Vohr, B. R., Poindexter, B. B., Dusick, A. M., McKinley, L. T., Wright, L. L., Langer, J. C., et al. (2006). Beneficial effects of breast milk in the neonatal intensive care unit on the developmental outcome of extremely low birth weight infants at 18 months of age. *Pediatrics, 118*(1), e115-123.

Walker, M. (2008). Breastfeeding the late preterm infant. *Journal of Obstetric, Gynecologic, and Neonatal Nursing, 37*(6), 692-701.

Walker, M. (2009). Breastfeeding the Late Preterm Infant. *Clinics in Human Lactation, 4*.

Wang, M. L., Dorer, D. J., Fleming, M. P., & Catlin, E. A. (2004). Clinical outcomes of near-term infants. *Pediatrics, 114*(2), 372-376.

Weimer, J. (2001). *The economic benefits of breastfeeding: A review and analysis*. Retrieved. from.

Weimers, L., Svensson, K., Dumas, L., Naver, L., & Wahlberg, V. (2006). Hands-on approach during breastfeeding support in a neonatal intensive care unit: a qualitative study of Swedish mothers' experiences. *Int Breastfeed J, 1*, 20.

Wight, N. E., Morton, J. A., & Kim, J. H. (2008). *Best Medicine: Human Milk in the NICU*. Amarillo, TX: Hale Publishing.

Wilson-Clay, B., & Hoover, K. (2008). *The Breastfeeding Atlas* (4th ed.). Manchaca, TX: LactNews Press.

Wooldridge, J., & Hall, W. A. (2003). Posthospitalization breastfeeding patterns of moderately preterm infants. *Journal of Perinatal and Neonatal Nursing, 17*(1), 50-64.

Making Milk

Chapter 10

BREAST ANATOMY

Breast development begins while a baby is still in the womb, but the breast doesn't become fully functional until lactation begins. The breast changes throughout the lifespan: during menstrual cycles, pregnancies, births, breastfeeding, weaning and menopause. When a woman goes through menopause, the gland begins to atrophy. The growth of the breasts during pregnancy and during the first month of breastfeeding is one indicator of functional breast tissue (Cox, Kent, Casey, Owens, & Hartmann, 1999, p. 568). A deeper understanding of the dynamics affecting breastfeeding starts with an awareness of breast anatomy.

A familiarity with breast anatomy increases understanding of some of the physical dynamics affecting breastfeeding.

Each part of breast anatomy falls into one of several basic categories:

- Glandular tissue, which makes milk and transports it to the nipple
- Connective (muscle) tissue, including Cooper's ligaments, which provides mechanical support to the breast
- Adipose (fatty) tissue, which provides protection from outside injury
- Nerves, which give the breast the sensitivity to touch needed for milk ejection
- Blood, which provides nourishment and the ingredients needed to make milk
- Lymph, which transports waste products away from the breast

The breast consists of several basic types of tissues and fluids.

Breast size is determined mostly by the amount of fatty tissue in the breast, which is unrelated to milk production. The proportion of glandular tissue to fatty tissue during lactation varies greatly among women, but on average, there is about twice as much glandular tissue as fatty tissue (63% vs. 37%), and they tend to be intermixed, rather than separated within the breast (Ramsay, Kent, Hartmann, & Hartmann, 2005). On average, about 70% of the glandular tissue is located within a 30 mm radius (a little over an inch) of the nipple. No relationship has yet been found between proportion of glandular to fatty tissue and breast storage capacity or volume of milk produced (Geddes, 2007).

About 70% of the glandular tissue of the breast is located within a 30 mm radius of the nipple.

The glandular or milk-making tissue is composed of the following components:

Alveoli are milk-making factories where cells called "lactocytes" draw the needed nutrients from the mother's blood. Resembling clusters of grapes, they are surrounded by a network of myoepithelial cells that squeeze the alveoli during milk ejection, pushing the milk into the ductules and on into the ducts (Berry, Thomas, Piper, & Cregan, 2007).

Duct and ductules are the small tubes that carry the milk from the alveoli to the nipple. The smaller ductules lead from the clusters of alveoli to the larger ducts, which join with other ducts before reaching the nipple. Ultrasound research has revealed that the branching of the major ducts is closer to the nipple than previously thought (Ramsay, Kent et al., 2005).

Our understanding of some aspects of breast anatomy has changed in recent years.

It was once thought that wider ducts were located under the areola and that faster milk flow only occurred during milk expression and breastfeeding, when these milk reservoirs (referred to then as "lactiferous sinuses" or "milk sinuses") were compressed. However, ultrasound research found the ducts in this area are the same diameter as ducts elsewhere in the breast, disproving the existence of these small milk reservoirs (Ramsay, Kent et al., 2005).

Recent research has demonstrated that there are no milk sinuses as previously thought.

At rest, the easily compressed milk ducts average 2 mm in diameter and increase in diameter during milk ejection by about 58% (Ramsay, Kent, Owens, & Hartmann, 2004). Some mothers' milk ducts are so close to the surface that expanded ducts can be seen on the surface of the unused breast when milk ejection occurs. Being easily compressible and close to the surface explains why consistent pressure on the breast may cause plugged or blocked ducts. Rather than radiating symmetrically from the nipple, as illustrated in many older breast diagrams, milk ducts appear more like tangled tree roots intermixed with the fatty tissue, which makes them difficult to avoid during breast surgery (see Figure 10.1).

Lobes and lobules are segments of the mammary gland. A lobule consists of a single branch of alveoli and milk ducts that deliver milk to a lobe, which leads to a single nipple pore. Until the 2000s, it was thought there were 15 to 20 lobes in a breast, but ultrasound research discovered most women have between 4 and 17 lobes per breast, with an average of 9 (Going & Moffat, 2004; Love & Barsky, 2004; Ramsay, Kent et al., 2005). Japanese research found that how deeply the baby takes the breast affects how evenly the breast is drained, with deep attachment draining the lobes more evenly and shallow attachment leaving some lobes well-drained and others full (Mizuno et al., 2008).

The nipple includes on its outer surface between 4 and 18 nipple openings (or pores) that measure, on average, 0.4 to 0.7 mm in diameter; these openings are connected to milk ducts that drain the lobes (Ramsay, Kent et al., 2005). A mother may have many more nipple pores that are not connected to functional ducts (Geddes, 2007; Going & Moffat, 2004; Love & Barsky, 2004). Another recent discovery that challenges previous assumptions is that very little fat is located under the skin near the nipple. The nipple and areola contain smooth muscle erectile tissue that contracts with stimulation, causing the nipple to firm and protrude. The nipple's flexibility allows it to stretch and conform to the inside of the baby's mouth during breastfeeding.

The areola, which can be pronounced "a RE ola" or "air e O la" (both are correct), is the darker pigmented area from which the nipple protrudes and where the Montgomery glands are located. Some have suggested that this darkened area may act as a "target" to help the baby find the nipple. The plural of areola is areolae.

Montgomery glands are a combination of sebaceous and mammary glands located on the areola that enlarge and become more prominent during pregnancy. Their number varies among women from 1 to 15 (Geddes, 2007). The fluid they secrete may serve several purposes:

- Protect the mother's skin from suckling friction
- Reduce bacteria counts by altering the pH of the skin
- Help the baby find the nipple after birth via the odor of their fluid (Doucet, Soussignan, Sagot, & Schaal, 2009)

Research of 64 French mothers found that having more Montgomery glands was associated with greater infant weight gain between birth and Day 3 (Schaal, Doucet, Sagot, Hertling, & Soussignan, 2006). Washing the nipples with soap or disinfecting fluids, including alcohol, can remove the fluids secreted by the Montgomery glands. Unless the mother has nipple trauma (see p. 650-"Preventing Infections"), a mother's usual bathing routine is all that's needed to keep the nipples clean and maintain this fluid's lubricating and anti-bacterial effects.

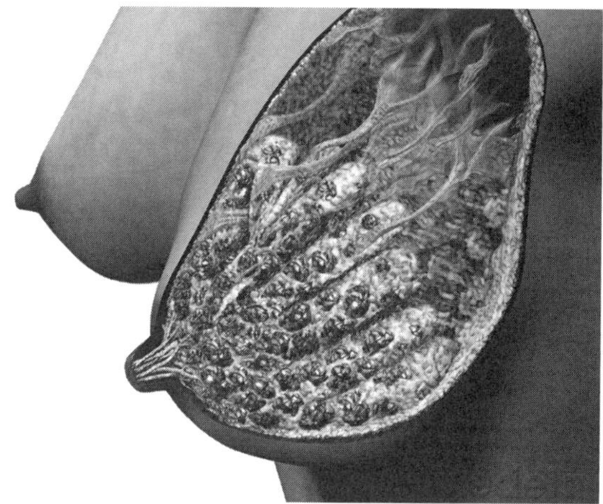

Figure 10.1. Illustration of fatty and glandular tissue inside the breast based on new research

Research indicates that breastfeeding does not cause a woman's breasts to sag.

Many women considering breast surgery attribute their loss of breast shape to breastfeeding (Rinker, Veneracion, & Walsh, 2008). Surveys done worldwide have found people of all ages believe that breastfeeding causes sagging breasts (Hull, Thapa, & Pratomo, 1990; McLennan, 2001; Pisacane & Continisio, 2004). On one popular U.S. website for new mothers, the question in its "ask the expert" section that generated the most responses was "How will breastfeeding change the appearance of my breasts?" (BabyCenter.com, 2007).

Three U.S. plastic surgeons examined whether breastfeeding is a risk factor for loss of breast shape ("breast ptosis") by doing a chart review and phone interviews with all 132 women seeking cosmetic breast surgery (breast implants or breast lifts) at one clinic between 1998 and 2006 (Rinker et al., 2008). Of the 91 women who had at least one term pregnancy, 58% had a history of breastfeeding. They found that a history of breastfeeding, number of children breastfed, how long each child breastfed, and how much weight was gained during pregnancy were not associated with loss of breast shape. Significant predictors of loss of breast shape included number of pregnancies, age, a history of smoking, larger pre-pregnancy bra cup size, and higher body mass index (BMI). Neither "any breastfeeding" nor duration of breastfeeding was an independent risk factor for loss of breast shape.

Italian researchers also concluded that breastfeeding does not alter breast shape after surveying 500 first-time mothers at three health centers in Italy (Pisacane & Continisio, 2004). Similar percentages of women who never breastfed reported breast changes as women who breastfed. The researchers concluded that changes in breast appearance occur as a result of pregnancy, not breastfeeding, and occur whether or not the mother breastfeeds.

MILK EJECTION (LET-DOWN OR MILK RELEASE)

Milk ejection is triggered by the release of the hormone oxytocin and is responsible for most of the milk flow during breastfeeding and milk expression.

During breastfeeding and milk expression, significant milk flow occurs only after milk ejection, sometimes referred to as "let-down." Without it, only the small amount of milk (0.1 to 10 mL) located in the ducts near the nipple can be accessed by the mother or baby, with most milk remaining in the breast (Ramsay et al., 2004; Ramsay, Mitoulas, Kent, Larsson, & Hartmann, 2005). Milk ejection occurs when the hormone oxytocin is released into the mother's bloodstream, which causes the band-like muscles around the milk-producing glands to squeeze and the milk ducts to shorten and dilate, pushing the milk out of the breast. Because its trigger is hormonal, milk ejection always occurs in both breasts at the same time and lasts for an average of 2 minutes (Prime, Geddes, & Hartmann, 2007).

When a baby breastfeeds, his suckling sends nerve impulses to the mother's brain, where her hypothalamus signals her posterior pituitary to release oxytocin in bursts into her bloodstream (Rossoni et al., 2008). In addition to the physical sensations of the baby's suckling, his softness and warmth may also promote milk ejection. The mother's emotional state (relaxed or tense) can also affect milk ejection. During early breastfeeding, it may take a few minutes for milk ejection to occur as the mother's body becomes conditioned to this response. But with time and conditioning, milk ejection becomes faster and more automatic, sometimes occurring even without a baby at the breast.

• •

Most mothers have several milk ejections per breastfeeding, but most feel only one and some mothers feel none.

Number of milk ejections per breastfeeding. According to Australian research, the average number of milk ejections at each breastfeeding session is 3 to 4, with a range of 1 to 17 (Cobo, 1993; Kent et al., 2008; Ramsay, Mitoulas et al., 2005).

Mothers' perceptions of milk ejection. Australian researchers used ultrasound to observe milk ejection with 45 mothers during 166 breastfeeding sessions and found that 88% of study mothers could feel their first milk ejection, but none felt subsequent milk ejections (Ramsay et al., 2004). In another Australian study of 11 breastfeeding mothers, four reported feeling more than one milk ejection (Ramsay, Mitoulas et al., 2005). Breast pumping has been found to produce the same number of milk ejections as breastfeeding. In one Australian study, mothers had multiple milk ejections during 95% of their breast pumping sessions (Ramsay, Mitoulas et al., 2005).

Some mothers feel milk ejection as tingling, pressure, pins-and-needles, a feeling of "drawing" or "rushing down," increased thirst, milk leakage from the other breast, even pain, while others feel nothing (Ramsay et al., 2004; Ramsay, Mitoulas et al., 2005). During the first week or two after birth, it may also be felt as uterine cramping or as tension across the shoulder blades. Mothers feel milk ejection at varying levels of intensity. Some consider the feelings mild and others very intense. Feelings of nausea, intestinal pain, and vaginal bleeding have been associated with milk ejection (Prime et al., 2007). A small percentage of mothers report strong negative emotions—such as dread, anxiety, or anger—for 30 to 60 seconds just before milk ejection, with the intensity of these feelings increasing with breast fullness. This is known as D-MER, or depression associated with the milk-ejection reflex. For more details on this phenomenon, see the website www.d-mer.org.

When milk ejection occurs. When a baby breastfeeds, on average, it takes about a minute or so of suckling for a milk ejection to occur (Ramsay et al., 2004). The most reliable indicators of milk ejection are audible swallowing during breastfeeding and visibly faster milk flow during milk expression.

• •

A mother's perceptions and feelings can trigger milk ejection, and feelings of anxiety, anger, and tension can sometimes block it.

It is not unusual for milk ejections to occur in lactating mothers in response to stimuli other than breastfeeding, such as hearing another baby cry or having loving thoughts about their baby. This is because milk ejection is in part a conditioned response, so other familiar sights, smells, sounds, touch, and thoughts can sometimes trigger it. One Australian breastfeeding researcher told the story of one of his exclusively-pumping study mothers who covered her breast pump with a towel because otherwise whenever she looked at her pump it triggered milk ejection. One Canadian article described the experiences of three women with damaged nerve pathways between breast and brain. Because they were unable to feel the sensations of breastfeeding, they learned to trigger milk ejections with mental imagery while their babies were at the breast (Cowley, 2005).

Milk ejection occurs after about a minute of actively suckling.

Researchers from Colombia and the U.K. reported cases of "spontaneous milk ejection" (Cobo, 1993; McNeilly & McNeilly, 1978). Other physical responses that occur before breastfeeding have also been documented. U.K. researchers found that mothers often begin releasing oxytocin when their baby begins to fuss and as they get ready to breastfeed (McNeilly, Robinson, Houston, & Howie, 1983). Japanese research has also found that breast skin temperature begins to rise even before breastfeeding begins (Kimura & Matsuoka, 2007).

A mother's emotions can also trigger or inhibit milk ejection. For example, feeling upset, frustrated, stressed, or angry, releases the stress hormone epinephrine (adrenaline), which may dampen the body's response or delay milk ejection (Prime et al., 2007). It is not unusual for mothers of preterm babies to express less milk after receiving bad news about their baby's condition (Chatterton et al., 2000). Anticipating pain can also delay milk ejection.

There can also be physical causes of inhibited milk ejection. For example, the feeling of ice against a mother's skin, excessive alcohol intake, and some medications have been found to block milk ejection (Lawrence & Lawrence, 2005; Newton & Newton, 1948).

The normal stresses of motherhood, fatigue, and lack of sleep have not been found to affect milk volumes (Hill, Aldag, Chatterton, & Zinaman, 2005c). But if a mother's milk ejection seems inhibited or delayed for any reason, to encourage milk ejection, suggest she try relaxation techniques (such as childbirth breathing), warm compresses, or breast massage. Another strategy is to wait until she is feeling calmer and more relaxed to breastfeed or express milk. In a crisis, if her milk ejection is consistently delayed or inhibited, this may temporarily slow her milk production. If this happens, encourage her to continue breastfeeding and/or expressing. Assure her that with time and stimulation milk ejection and production will quickly return to normal.

MILK PRODUCTION

Basic Dynamics of Milk Production

There are four basic dynamics affecting milk production.

In the book, *The Breastfeeding Mother's Guide to Making More Milk* (West & Marasco, 2009), lactation consultants Diana West and Lisa Marasco describe what they call the "Milk Supply Equation" (below), which describes the basic forces affecting milk production. If any of the following are missing, milk production may be compromised:

Sufficient glandular tissue

+ Enough intact nerve pathways and milk ducts

+ Adequate hormones and functional hormone receptors

+ Frequent and effective milk removal and breast stimulation

= Ample milk production

• •

Each breast produces milk independently, and milk volume can vary greatly between left and right breast.

Milk ejection always occurs in both breasts simultaneously because it is triggered by hormones released into the mother's blood (see previous section). But after the first few days postpartum, milk production in each breast is regulated independently based on milk removal. In fact, a mother can establish or maintain milk production in just one breast, even after milk production in the unused breast ceases. (This is one alternative to complete weaning for the mother who has recurring mastitis or abscess in the same breast.) U.S. and Australian studies have measured milk production by breast and found that the left and right breasts rarely produce the same volume of milk and differences are often significant (Engstrom, Meier, Jegier, Motykowski, & Zuleger, 2007; Ramsay, Mitoulas et al., 2005).

If the mother who's baby is gaining weight normally is concerned because one of her breasts produces much more milk, explain that what matters to the baby is getting enough milk overall, not whether milk production in each breast is the same. In some cases, differences in production may be due to breast usage, especially if a mother or baby often favors one breast over the other. In most cases, though, differences in output are more likely because one breast is just a naturally larger milk producer. One U.S. study of 95 exclusively expressing mothers found that 70% produced more milk from their right breast and that milk output by breast was not associated with a mother's dominant hand, number of children, or previous breastfeeding experience (Hill, Aldag, Zinaman, & Chatterton, 2007). If the mother is concerned about obvious differences in breast size due to uneven but full milk production, reassure her that the breasts usually return to pre-pregnancy size after breastfeeding ends or even sooner (Kent, Mitoulas, Cox, Owens, & Hartmann, 1999).

Amount of Glandular Tissue

Some mothers lack the milk-producing glands needed to achieve full milk production.

Sometimes called breast hypoplasia or insufficient glandular tissue, mothers with this condition may have breasts with obvious areas of glandular tissue in a mostly soft breast because much of their glandular tissue is missing (Wilson-Clay & Hoover, 2008). Physical characteristics of this condition include widely spaced breasts (more than 1.5 inches or about 4 cm apart); large differences in breast size (asymmetry); tubular, irregular, or cone-shaped breasts rather than rounded, especially in the lower quadrants; and possibly bulbous-looking areolae (Huggins, Petok, & Mireles, 2000). Many of these mothers report no breast changes during pregnancy. For more details, see p. 703- "Underdeveloped Breasts."

There is great variability among mothers in breast size and shape, as well as how much of the breasts is glandular tissue (Geddes, 2007), and it is important never to assume from a mother's breast shape or lack of breast changes during pregnancy that she will not produce enough milk for her baby. However, whenever possible, mothers with these physical characteristics should be monitored closely without planting the seeds of doubt. One way to explain it to a mother is that "not all women with breasts of this shape have challenges with milk production, but some do, so let's plan to keep a careful eye on your baby's weight gain during the first few weeks."

If concerned about a mother's glandular tissue, moniter her closely without planting seeds of doubt.

Some mothers have too much glandular tissue in the breast.

In addition to the lack of glandular tissue described in the previous point, some women fall at the other end of the spectrum and have what's called "hyperplastic" or "hypertrophic" breasts, meaning overdevelopment of glandular tissue. This may occur in one breast or both (Lawrence & Lawrence, 2005). For details on one type of overdevelopment of the breast that occurs during pregnancy (called "gestational gigantomastia"), see p. 705- "Rapid Overdevelopment of the Breasts."

Condition of Nerves and Milk Ducts

Breast surgery or injury can sever nerves and may affect milk production.

If a mother has a history of breast surgery or injury (including nipple or areola scarring), this has the potential to affect milk ejection by damaging her nerve pathways between brain and breast. Intact nerve pathways allow nerve impulses to trigger the release of the hormone oxytocin, which is needed for milk ejection (see previous section, "Milk Ejection [Let-Down or Milk Release]"). The mother with a history of breast surgery or injury will know if these nerve pathways have been affected because she will lose some or all sensation in her nipple and areola. A mother who can feel both touch and temperature on her nipple and areola is unlikely to have problems with milk ejection during breastfeeding (West & Hirsch, 2008). For more details, see p. 706- "Breast Surgery or Injury."

When a mother's nerve pathways are damaged, until they grow back, or "reinnervate," she may achieve milk ejection only with the help of mental imagery (Cowley, 2005), touch in other areas of the breasts and body, acupressure, the use of a synthetic oxytocin nasal spray, or by applying pressure to the breasts during breastfeeding or pumping via breast compression or other types of hand pressure.

Severe engorgement and breast surgery or injury could damage or sever milk ducts, which may affect milk production.

Severe engorgement, if prolonged and extreme, can in rare cases cause enough damage to a mother's breast to affect long-term milk production. If a mother has had breast surgery or a breast injury, the following factors may affect the impact on her milk production.

Location of an implant and any incision or injury. Surgical incisions or injuries around the areola are more likely to cause nerve damage and severed milk ducts than incisions in the fold under the breast, in the armpit, or in the navel. For more details, see p. 706- "Breast Surgery or Injury."

Anatomical differences. The previous section "Breast Anatomy" described research that found there are between 4 and 17 lobes in the breast. When breast surgery or injury occurs, the number of working ducts and lobes a mother has may partly determine whether it has a major or minor effect on her milk production. For example, if two milk ducts are cut during surgery in a mother with four working milk ducts, this could significantly affect her milk production, but cutting two milk ducts in a mother with 15 working ducts may have little noticeable effect (Geddes, 2007). Milk ducts can eventually grow back or "recannalize," but this takes time. Neither the mother nor her healthcare provider will probably know how many working lobes and ducts she has, but this might be one reason a mother's milk production is affected after a surgery she was told should not affect her ability to breastfeed.

Breast injury can also affect milk supply.

Hormonal Levels and Receptors

For adequate milk production, a mother's hormones should be in balance, and her hormones and receptors should interact well.

Although hormones are not usually a major player in milk production (see next section), if a mother's hormonal levels are far enough out of the normal range, she may produce too much or too little milk (Edge & Segatore, 1993; Marasco, 2006). But there is more to a mother's hormonal dynamic. Her body's response to a hormone will be partly determined by how many receptors for this hormone she has and how many are activated. As described in more detail later, during the first few weeks after birth, milk removal is responsible for the activation of the prolactin receptors, and the more receptors that are activated, the more milk the mother will produce for that baby.

Another aspect of the hormonal influence on lactation is whether the hormone and its receptor work together normally. In their book *The Breastfeeding Mother's Guide to Making More Milk,* lactation consultants Diana West and Lisa Marasco liken the relationship between the hormone and its receptor to that of a lock and key, with both being necessary (West & Marasco, 2009). Even if hormonal levels are within the normal range, if there are too many locks and not enough keys or vice versa, the hormone will not have the expected effect. And if the hormone and its receptor do not work well together (i.e., the lock is rusty and the key can't open it), this can blunt the effect of that hormone. For example, the "insulin resistance" that occurs with Type 2 diabetes refers to the "resistance" the mother's insulin receptors have to binding with the insulin her body produces. She makes enough insulin; her body just can't use it efficiently.

Although we still don't understand completely all the hormonal intricacies affecting milk production, we know that the hormones described below play a role.

The hormones affecting lactation play different roles during pregnancy, birth, and breastfeeding.

Before birth. A pregnant mother has high blood levels of estrogen, placental lactogen, prolactin, and progesterone, which stimulate her breast tissue to develop and prepare for milk production. Although the mother begins producing colostrum, the first milk, mid-pregnancy, another role progesterone plays is to inhibit significant milk production until after birth (Czank, Henderson, Kent, Tat Lai, & Hartmann, 2007). This growth of breast tissue and the beginning of milk production is called "secretory differentiation" or "lactogenesis I." Hormones that regulate the mother's metabolism, such as growth hormone, glucocorticoids, thyroid hormone, and insulin also prepare the breast during pregnancy (Neville, McFadden, & Forsyth, 2002; Pang & Hartmann, 2007).

After birth. The delivery of the placenta triggers the hormonal chain of events that causes milk production to rapidly increase, called "secretory activation," "lactogenesis II," or the milk "coming in." Secretion of placental lactogen ends with the delivery of the placenta which produced it. Estrogen and progesterone blood levels fall quickly and stay low for the first months of breastfeeding, while prolactin (the "milk-producing hormone") levels decrease over the weeks but remain higher overall (Pang & Hartmann, 2007). Other hormones crucial to regulating the mother's metabolic changes, such as cortisol, thyroid-stimulating hormone, and insulin, are also important to milk production (Czank, Henderson et al., 2007).

Prolactin, cortisol, thyroid-stimulating hormone and insulin are all important in milk production.

A mother's prolactin blood levels rise and fall with each breastfeeding and milk expression (see next point). Prolactin milk levels, on the other hand, vary by breast fullness, with higher levels occurring with greater milk production and lower levels occurring with full breasts as milk production slows. Milk prolactin levels also vary by time of day, with the highest levels usually occurring between 2 am and 6 am (Cregan, De Mello, Kershaw, McDougall, & Hartmann, 2002). Australian researchers suggested this may be because the breast tends to be drained most fully in the late evening, leading to greater milk production in the early morning hours. Some studies have found that sleep itself can increase prolactin levels (Freeman, Kanyicska, Lerant, & Nagy, 2000). The release of prolactin and oxytocin together may contribute to the intense feeling of oneness with the baby that many mothers experience (Uvnas-Moberg, 2003).

Oxytocin is released during labor, causing the muscles of the uterus to contract. After birth, oxytocin release triggers delivery of the placenta. During breastfeeding, oxytocin release triggers milk ejection by causing contractions of the band-like cells surrounding the alveoli (see previous section "Milk Ejection (Let-Down or Milk Release)." Oxytocin release after birth also causes the uterus to contract and return quickly to its pre-pregnancy size, which is why many mothers experience uterine cramps during milk ejection in the first week after birth.

After the hormonal chain of events that occurs during the first days after birth, it appears hormones play only a minor role in establishing and maintaining milk production (Cox, Owens, & Hartmann, 1996; De Coopman, 1993). The hormonal influence on milk production is sometimes referred to as "endocrine control." After that, the most important aspect of establishing ample milk production is draining the breast often and well, which is sometimes referred to as "autocrine" or local control.

• •

The first 2 weeks after birth may be a critical period for activating enough prolactin receptors in the breast for ample long-term milk production.

Each time a baby breastfeeds or a mother expresses her milk, her blood prolactin levels increase. When a baby begins breastfeeding, the mother's blood prolactin levels start to rise. During the early months, they peak about 45 minutes after the baby starts breastfeeding and return to baseline levels within 3 hours or so.

During the first 10 days after birth, a mother's prolactin response to breast stimulation is at its peak (Cox et al., 1996). Within 45 minutes of starting breastfeeding, her blood prolactin levels may be double or triple her baseline levels, sometimes rising as much as 20 to 30 times higher (Noel, Suh, & Frantz, 1974). As the weeks and months pass, even with ample milk production, baseline prolactin blood levels and prolactin surges after breastfeeding gradually decrease. Months after birth, the prolactin levels of breastfeeding mothers are still higher than those of non-breastfeeding mothers, but the difference is not nearly as great (Table 10.1).

According to the "prolactin receptor theory," the higher and more consistently a mother's blood prolactin levels rise during this critical first 2 weeks after birth, the more prolactin receptors are activated in her breasts, increasing her milk production potential for that baby (de Carvalho, 1983). This activation of prolactin receptors starts anew with the birth of each baby. If for whatever reason a mother does not drain her breasts often and well during these first 2 weeks, fewer prolactin receptors may be activated and her milk production potential may be more limited without consistent effort to increase it. After the first 2 weeks, when her hormonal levels naturally decline, most mothers find it requires much more time and work to boost milk production. In rare cases, it may even be impossible. (For more details, see p. 603- "Relactation and Induced Lactation"). During these first 2 weeks, encourage the mother to use this hormonal advantage to "set" her milk production potential at "ample." Prolactin also works to keep the milk-making cells (alveoli) open and prevent involution.

Table 10.1. Prolactin Levels, Normal Range

Stage	Baseline (ng/mL)	After Suckling (ng/mL)
Woman in childbearing years (not lactating or pregnant)	2-20	n/a
Third trimester of pregnancy	150-250	n/a
Pregnant at term	200-500	n/a
First 10 days after birth	200	400
10 days-3 months	60-110	70-220
3-6 months	50	100
6-12 months	30-40	45-80

(Cox et al., 1996; West & Marasco, 2009)

Breast stimulation and milk removal are important to milk production (see next section), but so too are the "softer" aspects of breastfeeding: the mother's feelings and her baby's touch. The earlier section "Milk Ejection (Let-Down or Milk Release)" described the impact of the mother's emotions on milk ejection, which can affect milk removal and therefore production. Research has also found that a mother's hormonal response to milk-making is also affected by the presence or absence of her baby's touch.

The mother's emotions and her baby's touch have a hormonal effect on milk production.

Skin-to-skin contact after birth, for example, has been associated with increased oxytocin blood levels in the mother, which is important to milk production and has been associated with long-term effects on breastfeeding duration and the mother-baby relationship (Matthiesen, Ransjo-Arvidson, Nissen, & Uvnas-Moberg, 2001; Uvnas-Moberg, 2003). One Swedish study measured the hormonal levels of 63 mothers during the first 2 days postpartum and found that the more minutes mothers and babies spent in skin-to-skin contact before breastfeeding, the lower the mother's blood levels of the stress hormone cortisol, which is associated with greater relaxation (Handlin et al., 2009). Chapter 1 described the effects on breastfeeding dynamics when mother and baby enjoy an intimate, private environment after birth where they can relax together and cultivate a right-brained connection. This hormonally-enhancing right-brain connection supports a mother's hormonal response to breastfeeding and milk production.

Skin-to-skin contact after birth stimulates mothers' levels of oxytocin.

One reason many mothers who exclusively express their milk struggle with milk production is because they miss much of the "touch" and emotional aspects of breastfeeding, making them "hormonally challenged" (see p. 466- "Establishing Full Milk Production After Birth"). A U.S. study found that even 1 hour of skin-to-skin contact per day with preterm babies and their exclusively expressing mothers increased milk output (Hurst, Valentine, Renfro, Burns, & Ferlic, 1997).

Much is still unknown about how the interaction of a mother's hormones influences milk production. However, an association has been found between the following health conditions (which can cause or be caused by a hormonal imbalance or an abnormal response of hormones and their receptors) and milk production or infant weight gain (West & Marasco, 2009):

Some health conditions in the mother can affect her hormonal levels or her hormonal responses, which may affect milk production.

- **Obesity** (Mok et al., 2008), for details, see p. 526- "Obesity"
- **Diabetes** of any type (Hartmann & Cregan, 2001), for details see p. 759- "Diabetes Mellitus"
- **Hypertension**, or high blood pressure (Neifert et al., 1990)
- **Anemia** (Henly et al., 1995; Rioux, Savoie, & Allard, 2006)
- **Excess blood loss after birth**, more than 500 mL, which may reduce or inhibit pituitary function (Sert, Tetiker, Kirim, & Kocak, 2003; Willis & Livingstone, 1995)
- **Placental problems**, such as retained placenta (Neifert, McDonough, & Neville, 1981) or placental insufficiency during pregnancy, which may inhibit the growth of the baby or breast tissue or even cause the mother's milk to "come in" before birth

- **Thyroid imbalance or disease**, resulting in either too much or too little thyroid hormones (Marasco, 2006), for details see p. 767- "Thyroid Problems"
- **Polycystic Ovary Syndrome** (PCOS) (Glueck, Salehi, Aregawi, Sieve, & Wang, 2007; Marasco, Marmet, & Shell, 2000), for details see p. 764- "Polycystic Ovary Syndrome (PCOS)"
- **Luteal phase defect** (Bodley & Powers, 1999), which causes low progesterone levels during the second half of a woman's menstrual cycle and can cause infertility or lack of breast tissue growth during pregnancy
- **Gestational ovarian theca lutein cysts**, which can cause a jump in testosterone levels, inhibiting milk production for weeks after birth (Betzold, Hoover, & Snyder, 2004; Hoover, Barbalinardo, & Platia, 2002) For details, see p. 763.

Although some mothers with these conditions make ample milk, if a mother has one or more of the above, she should be considered at risk for low milk production and (like any mother) be encouraged to use optimal breastfeeding practices by breastfeeding early and often and making sure the baby takes the breast deeply (see chapters 1 and 2). Encourage close monitoring of the baby's weight gain after birth without planting the seeds of doubt.

How Well and Often Milk Is Removed

When all other aspects of the "milk supply equation" are in place, milk removal becomes the primary driver that determines rate of milk production.

The mother's physical characteristics described in the previous sections—how much glandular tissue she has, the condition of her nerves and milk ducts, and her hormonal levels and receptors—may significantly inhibit milk production when there are major deviations from the norm. But under some circumstances, milk removal can provide the stimulation needed to overcome other issues. Hormones, for example, prepare the breasts for milk production during pregnancy and cause the cascade of events that lead to milk increase after birth (the "endocrine control" of milk production mentioned earlier). But with breast stimulation and milk removal, even women who have never been pregnant can make milk (see p. 613- "Unique to Induced Lactation"). When the other aspects of the "milk supply equation" are functioning normally, this "autocrine" or local control is the primary driver of milk production and its basic dynamics are described in this section.

Milk removal is the primary driver of milk production.

Focusing on "rate of milk production" rather than "milk supply" may make it easier to understand how to use milk production's underlying dynamics.

Some people refer to a mother's "milk supply," a concept that implies a set volume of milk. But milk production is not static. It can vary from day to day and even over the course of a day. A more useful concept for understanding milk-making is "rate of milk production," which puts the focus on how fast or slow a mother makes milk.

Patterns of milk removal can vary greatly by culture, which influences milk production.

Breastfeeding rhythm—the heart of local control of milk production—varies tremendously from place to place. As U.S. researcher Kathleen Kennedy noted, a "breastfeeding" means something very different to mothers in different cultures (Kennedy, 2010). A Western mother, for example, may consider a "breastfeeding" a lengthy, ritualized activity that involves changing the baby's diaper, making herself a drink, turning off her phone, settling into a certain chair, and then putting her baby to breast for an extended time. In contrast, a mother in a developing country may keep her baby on her body, putting him to breast at the slightest cue for just a few minutes 15 to 20 times each day. These two babies may have about the same daily milk intake, but the immense cultural differences in their feeding rhythms may affect a mother's rate of milk production.

Many Western attitudes about feeding are based on bottle-feeding norms, such as the belief that babies should feed at set intervals, every few hours. Another is the belief that as babies get older they should take fewer and larger feedings. However, there are basic differences between breastfeeding and bottle-feeding and between mother's milk and infant formulas, so the same expectations cannot be applied to both. For example, U.S. research has found significant differences in the amount of milk taken by breastfed and formula-fed babies. On average, babies fed formula consume 15% more milk at 3 months, 23% more at 6 months, 20% more at 9 months, and 18% more at 12 months (Heinig, Nommsen, Peerson, Lonnerdal, & Dewey, 1993). And Australian research found that among breastfeeding babies the number of feedings per day does not change between 1 and 6 months of age (Kent et al., 2006). If a Western mother disregards her breastfed baby's feeding cues and manipulates his feeding pattern based on formula-feeding norms, this can sometimes lead to milk production issues.

Milk production is best regulated without "rules" by encouraging the mother to be responsive to her baby's feeding cues. If the mother allows her baby to drive the process without trying to manipulate it, they are more likely to avoid low milk production and overabundant milk production. Efforts to manipulate the process are more likely to create these challenges (Smillie, Campbell, & Iwinski, 2005).

Degree of Breast Fullness

One of the most influential dynamics affecting a mother's rate of milk production is how full her breasts are.

Our knowledge about milk production increased dramatically during the 1990s and 2000s, thanks in large part to the work of a Western Australian research team led by Peter Hartmann. With the help of local breastfeeding volunteers, this team used a high-tech approach to learn more about how the breast makes milk. In some studies, they used techniques from the field of topography, which measures mountain terrains, to chart physical changes in the breasts and determine how much milk the breasts hold (Cregan & Hartmann, 1999). They used sensitive scales (to 2g) to weigh babies before and after feedings to determine exactly how much milk a baby takes at each breast, at each feeding, and during a 24-hour period (Daly, Owens, & Hartmann, 1993). And they used ultrasound to learn more about milk ejection during feedings (Ramsay et al., 2004). Their findings indicate that one of the primary factors that affects how quickly or slowly milk is made is how full a mother's breasts are, or her degree of breast fullness.

Drained breasts make milk faster and full breasts make milk slower.

Full breasts make milk slower. As the breast becomes full of milk, two dynamics cause its rate of milk production to slow.

1. **FIL.** As the volume of milk in the breast increases so, too, does the amount of the peptide or whey protein known as "feedback inhibitor of lactation" (FIL for short), which slows milk production (Knight, Peaker, & Wilde, 1998; Prentice, 1989; Wilde, Addey, Boddy, & Peaker, 1995).
2. **Internal pressure from the milk** can slow milk production by reducing blood flow to the breast and compressing the milk-making cells, which can cause them to temporarily slow down or even stop production.

As the breasts fill with more and more milk, the combination of increasing FIL and increasing internal pressure causes milk production to become slower and slower.

Drained breasts make milk faster. The opposite is also true. Milk production speeds up when a mother's breasts are drained more fully. This is how a baby adjusts his mother's milk production as needed. If he wants more milk, he breastfeeds more often and he breastfeeds longer, taking a larger percentage of the available milk, causing the breasts to produce milk faster and faster.

Although many assume that babies take all of the available milk when they breastfeed, Australian research found that, on average, babies take 67% of the milk in the breasts (Kent, 2007). This means that after an average feeding, 33% (or a third of the milk) is left in the breast. One way a mother can increase her rate of milk production is to drain her breasts more fully, perhaps 90% to 95% instead of 67%. She might do this by breastfeeding the baby more than once from each breast, by expressing milk after breastfeeding, or by doing both. The more fully drained a mother's breasts are at the end of a feeding and the more times a day they are well drained, the faster her rate of milk production. If needed, she can also use this dynamic for the opposite effect. By feeding less often on one breast and allowing this breast to stay fuller, a mother with overabundant milk can slow her rate of milk production.

Drained breasts make milk faster than full breasts.

Within 1 day and even from feeding to feeding, rate of milk production can change dramatically. For example, after one study mother's breasts became full after 6 hours without milk removal, her rate of milk production per breast was measured at 22 mL (about 2/3 oz.) per hour (Daly, Kent, Owens, & Hartmann, 1996). By breastfeeding from that breast every 90 minutes and draining her breasts more completely, her rate of production per breast increased quickly to 56 mL (nearly 2 oz.) per hour—more than double the previous rate. As researchers wrote in one review article:

> ...[T]he breast can rapidly change its rate of milk synthesis from one interfeed interval to the next. This is a newly discovered property of the human mammary gland. In the past, it has been assumed that the rate of milk synthesis of a breast could change significantly only over a period of days (Daly & Hartmann, 1995, p. 30).

This review article also noted that the average rate of milk production over 24 hours in these mothers was only 64% of the fastest milk production measured, which meant these mothers had a much greater milk-making potential.

With frequent milk removal, three different physical processes act to speed milk production.

The short-term increase in milk-production when milk is removed from the breast described in the previous point is only part of the picture. More recently, scientists described several processes stimulated by frequent milk removal that work together over time to speed milk production even more (Czank, Henderson et al., 2007):

1. **Short-term**: Frequent milk removal minimizes FIL and pressure in the breast, leading to faster milk production.

2. **Medium-term**: Faster milk production speeds the metabolic activity of key enzymes used in milk-making, speeding milk production more.
3. **Long-term**: Over time frequent milk removal stimulates the growth and development of more glandular, milk-making tissue (why induced lactation works), also increasing the speed of milk production.

Breast Storage Capacity

A mother's breast storage capacity is the maximum volume of milk available to her baby when her breast is at its fullest and is unrelated to breast size.

In addition to "degree of breast fullness" described in the previous section, a mother's breast storage capacity also partly determines her rate of milk production. Breast storage capacity is defined as the maximum volume of milk available to the baby when the breast is at its fullest, and it can vary greatly from mother to mother. This individual difference helps explain why feeding rhythms can vary so greatly from one breastfeeding couple to another. One Australian study of 71 breastfeeding mothers and babies found a breast storage capacity range among its mothers of 74 to 382 g (2.6 to 12.9 oz.) per breast (Kent et al., 2006). Another Australian study found an even broader range among its mothers, from 81 to 606 mL (2.7 to 20.5 oz.) (Daly et al., 1993). The mother in this second study with the largest breast storage capacity accumulated up to 90% of her baby's daily milk intake in both breasts, while the one with the smallest storage capacity accumulated at most up to 20% of her baby's daily milk intake in both breasts.

Breast storage capacity is unrelated to breast size.

Breast storage capacity is not related to breast size, so a smaller-breasted mother may have a large capacity and a large-breasted mother may have a small capacity.

• •

Mothers with both large and small storage capacities can make ample milk for their babies, but their feeding rhythms often vary.

Depending on cultural practices, after about the first month postpartum, mothers with a large storage capacity often have far different feeding rhythms than those with a small storage capacity. Because by definition the breasts of a mother with a large storage capacity can hold more milk, her baby may be satisfied with one breast at most feedings, may feed fewer times per day overall, and may sleep longer at night. The breasts of a mother with a small storage capacity hold less milk, so to achieve the same daily milk intake, her baby may take both breasts at each feeding, feed more times per day, and feed more often at night. For more details on how storage capacity affects breastfeeding rhythm, see p. 79- "Rhythm and Storage Capacity."

Although storage capacity affects feeding rhythm, it does not affect a mother's ability to produce ample milk for her baby. In the study of 71 babies mentioned in the previous point, Australian researchers found that all of the study babies whose mothers had a small storage capacity had healthy weight gains (Kent et al., 2006). There were no issues with low milk supply or slow weight gain. These babies just fed more times each day than the babies whose mothers had a large capacity.

• •

Breast storage capacity determines how long it takes for a mother's breasts to become full enough for the rate of milk production to slow.

While "full breasts make milk slower," the time it takes to become full varies by both rate of milk production and breast storage capacity. A woman with a small breast storage capacity may feel full with 3 ounces (89 mL) of milk in each breast, and this fullness could cause her rate of milk production to slow. Whereas a woman with a larger storage capacity would not yet feel full with this same 3 ounces (89 mL) in her breasts, allowing her to go longer between feedings without her rate of milk production slowing.

The term "intercept time" has been used by researchers to describe the point at which breast fullness causes milk production to slow to a below-average rate (Daly et al., 1996). In this Australian study, rate of milk production was measured in four breastfeeding women with full milk production, and their "intercept time" ranged from 6 to 12 hours.

Some observations can provide clues to a mother's breast storage capacity.

Australian researchers use sophisticated technology to determine a mother's breast storage capacity (Cregan & Hartmann, 1999; Kent et al., 1999). But simple observations can provide clues in individual mothers. For example, in mothers who exclusively express their milk and do not get up at night to express, in general, women with larger storage capacities can express 300 mL (10 oz.) or more at their first morning expression. The mother with a small storage capacity, on the other hand, may awaken before morning with breast discomfort, yet be unable to express more than 150 mL (5 oz.) or so (Mohrbacher, 1996). When test-weighing is used during breastfeeding, a baby's maximum intake at one breastfeeding will also provide clues.

A mother's breast storage capacity can vary from baby to baby and change as her milk production increases or decreases.

Australian research found that there was a relationship between the peak volume of milk that could be stored in a mother's breast and her overall milk production (Kent et al., 1999). This means that if a mother breastfeeds twins, her breast storage capacity would probably be greater than when the same mother breastfeeds a single baby. U.S. pediatrician Christina Smillie noted that the stretching of a mother's milk-producing glands with greater milk production might be analogous to the stretching of a non-breastfeeding baby's stomach to eventually hold an unphysiologic 8 ounces (237 mL) of formula after gradually being fed larger and larger volumes by bottle (Smillie et al., 2005).

Misconceptions About Milk Production

Contrary to popular belief, drinking more fluids is not associated with greater milk production.

When a mother is concerned about her milk production, often the first advice she is given is to drink more fluids. But one U.S. study found that when mothers drank 25% more fluids than when they "drank to thirst," there was no statistically significant difference in milk production (Dusdieker, Booth, Stumbo, & Eichenberger, 1985). In fact, during the "more fluids" period, the mothers produced slightly less milk. A Canadian pilot study of 10 mothers found no statistically significant difference in milk production when mothers increased their fluid intake to 50% higher than usual or 50% lower than usual (Morse, Ewing, Gamble, & Donahue, 1992).

Drinking more does not increase a mother's milk supply.

A mother's diet is unlikely to affect her milk production unless it is extreme.

Even when food is scarce, mothers make ample milk for their babies. This is because a mother's diet is only one source of the energy and nutrients she needs to make milk. Energy and most nutrients can also be drawn from the body stores laid down during pregnancy (Hopkinson, 2007). Even mildly malnourished mothers in developing countries produce ample, good quality milk for their babies, and supplementing mothers' diets has not been found to boost milk production or improve the quality of the milk (Prentice et al., 1983).

Only when famine or near famine conditions last for weeks does a mother's milk production or milk quality suffer (Prentice, Goldberg, & Prentice, 1994). One Dutch study found that even in famine conditions, milk production may be only slightly affected among previously well-nourished mothers with good body stores (Smith, 1947). Among Western mothers, those whose diet may be extreme enough to affect milk production include women on severe, long-term diets, those with eating disorders, and those with a history of bariatric surgery. For more details, see the chapter "Nutrition, Exercise, and Lifestyle Issues."

Many mothers misinterpret their baby's behavior and other "false alarms" as indicators of low milk production.

Most newborns have some periods when they are irritable, wakeful at night, and want to breastfeed often or even constantly for part of the day, and these are not necessarily signs of low milk production. In many cases, mothers' crises of confidence over milk production (the most common reason mothers give for ending breastfeeding prematurely) are not due to actual low milk production (Hill & Humenick, 1989; Hillervik-Lindquist, 1991; Hillervik-Lindquist, Hofvander, & Sjolin, 1991). Especially during the first month, when milk production is increasing to meet a baby's growing needs, these baby behaviors should be understood as normal aspects of infancy. As long as a baby is gaining weight normally, they are not signs of low milk production.

Night waking and irritability do not mean that a mother's supply is low.

Other "false alarms" that sometimes concern mothers are their inability to express much milk (a learned skill that improves with practice), soft breasts (which after the first few weeks usually occurs after the hormones of childbirth settle down), no milk leakage (not all mothers leak), not feeling milk ejection (many mothers do not), milk looks thin (this is how human milk is supposed to look), and baby's willingness to take a bottle after breastfeeding (it flows so fast, babies may overfeed, even if full at the breast).

Milk Production Norms

Making Milk During the First Year and Beyond

Knowing average milk production can be useful in some situations, but the best gauge of adequate production is the baby's weight gain and growth.

This section includes the milk production averages and ranges for the mother exclusively breastfeeding her baby for the first 6 months. The ranges of milk production norms are large, but keep in mind it's not the number of ounces, milliliters, or grams a baby consumes per day that determines whether a mother's production is too low, too high, or just right. The best gauge of milk adequacy is the baby's weight gain and growth. In one Australian study of 71 healthy, thriving breastfed babies from 1 to 6 months of age, the difference in daily milk intake was nearly threefold (between 15.5 and 43 oz. [440 to 1220 g]) (Kent et al., 2006). For details on healthy growth in exclusively breastfed babies, see p. 203- "Growth from Birth to 12 Months."

In mid-pregnancy, mothers begin producing colostrum.

Production of colostrum begins about mid-pregnancy, but the mother's high blood levels of progesterone inhibit significant milk production until after birth (Czank, Henderson et al., 2007). Many pregnant mothers leak colostrum and can express small amounts. No association has yet been found between the amount of colostrum leaked or expressed during pregnancy and a mother's milk production later.

• •

On their first day of life, newborns take at the breast, on average, 37 to 56 mL (1.2-1.9 oz.) of colostrum, with milk intake doubling on the 2nd day.

The volume of colostrum a newborn receives at the breast during the first day varies greatly from one mother-baby pair to another. Some have also suggested that a newborn may receive a larger amount of colostrum if the first breastfeeding occurs within the first hour after birth than if the first feeding occurs later (West & Marasco, 2009). An Australian study of 9 babies found that 24-hour milk intake on the first day ranged from 7 to 123 mL (0.25 to 4.2 oz.), with an average daily intake of 37 mL (1.3 oz.) and average intake per feeding of 7 mL (0.25 oz.) (Saint, Smith, & Hartmann, 1984). A U.S. study of 13 mothers found 24-hour milk production on the first day of life averaged 56 mL (1.9 oz.), and on the 2nd day increased to 185 mL (6.2 oz.), with a range of 12-379 mL [0.4-12.8 oz.]) (Neville et al., 1988). By the 2nd day, a Dutch study of 18 mothers and babies estimated the average milk intake per feeding was 14 mL (0.5 oz.), with a range of daily intake from 44 to 335 mL (1.5 to 11.3 oz.) (Houston, Howie, & McNeilly, 1983). When breastfeeding is going well, the baby's milk intake increases as milk production increases and the baby's stomach expands in size (Zangen et al., 2001).

• •

Within 20 to 40 hours after birth, milk production begins to increase dramatically.

The delivery of the placenta triggers the hormonal chain of events that causes milk production to rapidly increase, referred to as "secretory activation," "lactogenesis II," or the milk "coming in" (Pang & Hartmann, 2007). With the placenta delivered, a mother's placental lactogen, progesterone, and estrogen levels fall quickly, while prolactin levels remain high, causing a dramatic upswing in milk production (Pang & Hartmann, 2007). Although this process begins about 20 to 40 hours after birth, mothers don't usually perceive their milk as "coming in" until a little later--50 to 60 hours after birth (Smith & Riordan, 2010).

One U.S. study documented the milk output of 13 mothers and included in its daily totals the milk the baby took at the breast (measured by test-weighing) plus milk spilled, spit up, or leaked (Neville et al., 1988). The following mean daily milk outputs illustrate the amazing increase in milk production in the first 4 days after birth:

- Day 1: 56 mL
- Day 2: 185 mL
- Day 3: 393 mL
- Day 4: 580 mL

How soon after birth a mother's milk increase occurs depends in part on whether she has breastfed a previous baby. Experienced breastfeeding mothers experience increased milk production earlier than first-time mothers (Dewey, Nommsen-Rivers, Heinig, & Cohen, 2003). One U.K. study estimated that women who breastfed a previous baby were about 1 day ahead of first-time mothers, who produced about 3 to 4 ounces (142 mL) less milk on Day 3 than the experienced breastfeeding mothers (Ingram, Woolridge, Greenwood, & McGrath, 1999). See the later section, "Delay in Milk Increase After Birth" for more details about circumstances and conditions that can cause a delay in this process.

When a mother's milk production rapidly increases after birth, this process goes from one driven primarily by a mother's hormonal changes to one driven primarily by breast stimulation and milk removal (Neville et al., 2002). U.S. research has found that the mother's perception of milk increase after birth (feelings of fullness and heaviness) is usually reliable (Nommsen-Rivers, Heinig, Cohen, & Dewey, 2008). These feelings of fullness usually last for a couple of weeks after birth (Humenick et al., 1994).

The number of times per day a mother breastfeeds or expresses milk during the first days after birth is associated with early milk volumes and milk volumes at 6 weeks postpartum. One U.S. study of mothers exclusively expressing milk found early frequency of breast stimulation was associated with milk output on Day 4, which was also associated with milk output at 6 weeks (Hill & Aldag, 2005). Other U.S. research comparing mothers exclusive expressing with breastfeeding mothers also found an association between early frequency of breast stimulation and milk production weeks later (Hill, Aldag, Chatterton, & Zinaman, 2005b; Hill et al., 2005c).

The number of times that mothers empty their breasts in the early days is associated with milk volume at 6 weeks.

• •

When breastfeeding is going well, by the end of the first week, a mother's milk production has increased from an average of 37 mL to 56 mL (1.2-1.9 oz.) on the first day to a mean of 610 mL (20.6 oz.) per day by Day 7 (Neville et al., 1988).

By the end of the first week postpartum, average milk production increases more than ten-fold over the first day.

• •

Although many think of colostrum, transitional milk, and mature milk as three separate and distinct types of milk, they actually reflect a continuum of changes that occur after birth as the mother's hormones shift and her breasts begin making more milk.

The milk changes gradually from colostrum to mature milk within 2 to 3 weeks.

Even before a mother notices an increase in her milk production, her milk has already started to change. A drop in progesterone with stable levels of prolactin cause the spaces between her milk-making cells (lactocytes) to close, so the milk and its components can no longer leak out of the alveoli. With these "tight junctions" in place, as milk production ramps up, the milk stays in the alveoli and its composition begins to change. As more of some components (fat, lactose, citrate, and potassium) remain in the milk-producing cells, their concentrations increase, causing other components (immunoprotective proteins, sodium, and chloride) to decrease in concentration. Increase in milk volume also changes the concentrations of some components. Scientists can tell when a mother's milk increase occurs by measuring the concentrations of specific milk components (Czank, Henderson et al., 2007).

Over the first 2 to 3 weeks, as a mother's milk undergoes these changes, she may notice her milk becoming whiter and thinner-looking. There is a wide range of colors and consistencies considered normal for colostrum, transitional milk, and mature milk. Colostrum, for example, may be clear, golden, white, and other colors. As many as 15% of mothers may have blood in their colostrum (known as "rusty-pipe syndrome"). For details, see p. 702. It may appear very thick or it may be thinner. Colostrum is a concentrated form of nourishment and immunities that provides the baby with protection from illness and infection and prepares his digestive system for the greater volumes of milk to come. For the normal range of colors for mature milk, see p. 464- "Handling and Preparing Milk."

Milk production continues to increase in most mothers from Weeks 1 through 5.

With frequent feedings, the mother's milk production continues to increase. Babies 2 to 3 weeks old usually take about 2 to 3 ounces (59 to 89 mL) at the breast, taking daily about 20 to 25 ounces (591 to 750 mL) of milk. To increase the mother's milk production to meet his growing needs, babies often have periods of longer, more frequent breastfeeding, which are sometimes referred to as "growth spurts."

During Weeks 4 and 5, many babies continue to take more milk per feeding as their stomachs grow in size. An average breastfeeding is about 3 to 5 ounces (89 to 118 mL), with daily milk intake increasing to an average of about 25 to 35 ounces (750 to 1034 mL) per day (Kent et al., 2006). In one U.S. study, 98 mothers of term breastfeeding babies did test-weights to measure milk intake at every feeding around the clock for the first 6 weeks of life, and researchers found that babies' milk intake increased rapidly during the first 3 weeks of life, increasing slightly during Weeks 4 and 5, and staying stable from Weeks 5 to 6 (Hill, Aldag, Chatterton, & Zinaman, 2005a).

When working with individual mothers and babies, however, keep in mind that not every breastfeeding couple is average. One study of 71 1- to 6-month-old exclusively breastfed babies found a large range of daily milk intake among healthy, thriving babies, from 15.5 to 43 ounces or 440 to 1220 grams (Kent et al., 2006).

After milk production reaches its peak at about 5 weeks, it stays relatively stable until it begins to decline when the baby starts other foods.

On average, at about 5 weeks postpartum, most mothers produce nearly as much milk per day as their breastfed baby will ever need (Allen, Keller, Archer, & Neville, 1991). After 5 weeks of age, a baby's daily milk intake reaches a plateau. When at about 6 months the baby starts solid foods, milk production starts to decline because solid foods take the place of mother's milk in baby's diet (Islam, Peerson, Ahmed, Dewey, & Brown, 2006). The reason breastfed babies don't need increasing amounts of milk between 1 and 6 months is because their rate of growth (along with their metabolism) during this period slows (Butte, 2005). So even though they get bigger and heavier, their slowing growth rate offsets the need for more milk. For more details, see p. 203- "Growth from Birth to 12 Months."

Milk composition changes over time.

One aspect of mother's milk that changes as baby grows is its ratio of whey protein to casein. Unlike most mammal milks, at birth human milk is higher in whey protein than casein. Whey proteins (which include lysozyme, lactoferrin, and secretory IgA) are easily and quickly digested by human babies and are responsible for the soft curds in babies' stools (Czank, Mitoulas, & Hartmann, 2007). Cow's milk (and most infant formulas) is about 80% casein protein, which is good for calves' multi-stomach digestive system, but difficult for human babies to digest. During the first month or so, when the baby's digestive system is most immature, the ratio of whey protein to casein protein in human milk is about 90:10 (Kunz & Lonnerdal, 1992). Over time, as the baby's digestive system matures, this ratio changes. By about 6 weeks, the ratio is 80:20. By about 6 months, this ratio is 60:40. In later lactation, it is 50:50.

Milk fat content can vary as much as ten-fold among mothers (Agostoni et al., 2001), but the average percentage of fat in mother's milk has also been found to change over time, with the milk of mothers with older babies significantly higher in fat than the milk of mothers with younger babies. One U.S. study compared the milk fat content of 34 mothers with breastfeeding babies older than a year (12 to 39 months) and 27 mothers with breastfeeding babies 2 to 4 months old (Mandel, Lubetzky, Dollberg, Barak, & Mimouni, 2005). The researchers found that the milk mothers made for the older babies was about 50% higher in fat than the milk made for the younger babies. Other U.S. research also found a similar increase of about 50% in fat content later in lactation (Dewey, Finley, & Lonnerdal, 1984). Fat content of milk has also been found to change over the course of a day, with milk expressed in the evening (when the breast is more drained) higher in fat than milk expressed in the morning (Lubetzky, Mimouni, Dollberg, Salomon, & Mandel, 2007).

After 1 year, milk production varies, depending on how much the baby breastfeeds, while the mother's breast tissue decreases.

By the time the breastfeeding baby is 15 months old and is eating many other foods, daily milk production has been measured at between 95 and 315 mL per day (Kent et al., 1999; Neville et al., 1991). But milk production at this stage is dependent upon how much breastfeeding the baby does, as research done in Zaire (where breastfeeding older babies is the norm) found mothers' producing, on average, 300 mL per day at 30 months postpartum (Hennart, Delogne-Desnoeck, Vis, & Robyn, 1981).

A mother's breast tissue is at its peak between 1 and 6 months postpartum. As her baby starts taking other foods, breast tissue usually decreases significantly between 6 and 9 months (Kent, 2007). By 15 months, most mothers' breasts have returned to their pre-pregnancy size, even when they are producing significant volumes of milk (Kent et al., 1999).

With weaning, the mother's glandular tissue involutes and milk production stops.

As a baby weans, the glandular tissue in the breast involutes, which means the milk-making glands shut down and the breast reverts to its pre-pregnancy state. First the milk-making cells (lactocytes) die, and then the fat cells in the breast differentiate to fill the space they occupied, changing the internal landscape of the breast (Watson, 2006). As milk production slows and stops, the milk increases in sodium, chloride, fat, and protein and decreases in lactose and potassium (Hartmann & Kulski, 1978).

After complete weaning, mothers can usually express milk for at least 6 weeks (Kent, 2007). Anecdotally, women have reported being able to express a little milk for years after lactation ended.

Making Milk for Twins, Triplets, and More

Most mothers can produce enough milk for twins, triplets, and even quadruplets.

The same milk-production dynamics described earlier in this chapter apply equally to mothers of multiples. The only real difference is the volume of milk needed. To exclusively breastfeed, the mother of twins, triplets, and quadruplets will need double, triple, or quadruple the milk needed by the mother of one baby.

If babies from a multiple pregnancy are born healthy and breastfeed effectively, all the average mother needs to know is that she can produce enough milk for all of her babies by breastfeeding on cue. One Australian study of eight mothers of twins and one mother of triplets found that all of the twin mothers except one produced double the milk of a mother of one baby (Saint, Maggiore, & Hartmann, 1986). The mother of triplets in this study produced 3.08 kg (109 oz.) of milk per day. In one amazing U.S. case report, a mother of quadruplets "exclusively" breastfed her babies for 6 months, starting solids at the appropriate age and continuing to breastfeed in addition to other foods for 12 months (Berlin, 2007). The word "exclusively" is in quotation marks because one of the quadruplets had the metabolic disorder PKU, and as a result, needed a small amount of phenylalanine-free formula each day. (For details on PKU, see p. 312- "PKU")

One U.S. mother of quadruplets born at 34 weeks by cesarean delivery reported that within the first month she produced so much milk that when her babies slept for 2 hour stretches she could express enough milk for their supplemental feedings, which were primarily mother's milk (Mead, Chuffo, Lawlor-Klean, & Meier, 1992). These babies breastfed until they were 12, 15, 15, and 18 months old.

But even when milk production is no problem, finding the time to breastfeed and manage the rest of life's demands can be. Tell the mother to expect each baby will need to breastfeed at least eight times every 24 hours. See the next point for strategies.

Having support and help is also vital. One Japanese study of 1,529 mothers of twins, 234 mothers of triplets, 20 mothers of quadruplets, and 4 mothers of quintuplets found that mothers of multiples had a significantly shorter duration of breastfeeding than mothers of single babies and that they were 1.83 times more likely to decide not to breastfeed when their husband did not help with child-rearing (Yokoyama & Ooki, 2004).

• •

There is no one right way to breastfeed multiples; encourage each mother to work out her own system.

Deciding which babies breastfeed when. Some mothers of multiples prefer as a time-saver to always breastfeed two babies at once. Most mothers prefer to breastfeed their babies separately at some feedings to enjoy some one-on-one time with each baby or because one baby needs extra help at the breast. Babies' breastfeeding patterns may vary, with one baby breastfeeding more often than the other. If one baby does not breastfeed as effectively as his sibling(s), suggest the mother try breastfeeding him at the same time as a more effective sibling. The more effective baby may better stimulate milk ejection, and the faster flow of milk may help the less effective baby get more milk more quickly. If that doesn't help, try to determine the cause of the baby's ineffective feeding. (Is he preterm? Does he have a tongue tie? Is he ill? Does he have a neurological impairment?) After finding the cause, provide suggestions addressing that issue.

Which baby gets which breast when. There are different ways to decide which baby gets which breast. Some mothers just breastfeed with no particular plan, offering whichever breast feels fullest to whichever baby seems hungriest at the moment. Other mothers keep each baby on the same breast for an entire day, alternating breasts every day. Allowing each baby to spend time at both breasts provides varied visual stimulation, which enhances eye development. Some mothers of twins assign each baby a particular breast that he receives at every feeding and never varies. If one baby breastfeeds less effectively, offering both breasts to each baby ensures both breasts are well stimulated to maintain milk production.

Keeping track of breastfeeding. Some mothers of multiples keep a daily written log of which baby breastfed when and on which breast along with diaper output. Other mothers don't keep track of either feedings or diapers. If both babies gain weight well, no record-keeping is needed. If a baby is not gaining weight well, suggest the mother record frequency and length of breastfeeding and diaper output for a few days. Life with multiples can be unbelievably hectic, and if a baby is placid or sleepy, he may not be breastfeeding often or long enough to meet his needs.

Night breastfeeding. Encourage the mother to find well-supported feeding positions that allow her to rest while she breastfeeds. For position ideas, see p. 47- "Breastfeeding Two Babies." Many multiples sleep in one crib or bed because they sleep better when they are touching. If a crib is used, it may make night feedings easier if it is in the room where mother sleeps, so she is near when the babies feed at night. One option is to fasten the crib to the side of the mother's bed, adjust the mattress level to hers, and remove the side rail closest to her bed for easy access to the babies at night. The mother can then pull into her bed whichever baby wants to breastfeed, feed him semi-reclined or lying on her side, and return him to the crib after he's finished or—if she falls asleep—when another baby awakens to feed.

Another alternative, which is common in Japan, is for the mother to sleep on a mattress or futon on the floor. The sleeping surface could be in the babies' room or the mother's room so that the mother can lie down with the babies and sleep during feedings. If the mother wants to bring the babies into her bed, be sure she knows about safe sleeping options (see p. 90- "Where Should Babies Sleep?").

• •

If due to health issues one or more babies aren't breastfeeding after birth, talk to the mother about expressing her milk.

When one or more babies are not yet breastfeeding, the mother can provide milk for him/them by expressing her milk. For details, see p. 466- "Establishing Full Milk Production After Birth."

• •

Breastfeeding multiples does not have to be "all or nothing"; partial breastfeeding is almost always a better option than no breastfeeding.

Either by choice or by circumstance, some mothers partially breastfed twins, triplets, and higher order multiples. One case report describes a mother who partially breastfed all four of her quadruplets until one weaned abruptly at 12 months (Auer & Gromada, 1998). The other three continued breastfeeding a couple times each day until 30 months of age.

If a mother is feeling overwhelmed or believes her life would be easier if she could share feedings with others, talk to her about the option of partial breastfeeding. In one U.S. study of 123 mothers of twins, after birth 110 (89%) initiated either breastfeeding or milk expression, and the mothers who persisted continued to provide a high percentage of mother's milk feedings through 28 weeks (Damato, Dowling, Madigan, & Thanattherakul, 2005). Another article based on this study data reported that of those mothers who had weaned by 9 weeks, the most common reason given (by 40% or 12 mothers) was their perceptions of inadequate milk production (Damato, Dowling, Standing, & Schuster, 2005). Of the mothers who weaned between 9 and 28 weeks, the most common reason given (by 32% or 12 mothers) was the extra time and/or burden involved in breastfeeding and/or milk expression. However, illness in the mother and/or babies was mentioned as one reason for weaning by 33% of the mothers at 9 weeks and 8% of the mothers at 28 weeks.

Low Milk Production

A baby's weight gain issues are not always due to low milk production.

Low milk production is not always the cause of excess weight loss after birth or slow weight gain later. Some health problems cause babies to gain weight slowly even with ample milk intake. (For details, see p. 224- "Slow Weight Gain with Good Milk Intake.") In other cases, mothers produce abundant milk, but their babies can't breastfeed effectively due to unusual anatomy, breathing problems, sensory integration issues, neurological impairment, preterm birth, or other issues. Before assuming low milk production is the cause of slow weight gain, be sure to rule out other factors. (See the chapter, "Weight Gain and Growth.") Before suggesting strategies, it is best to find the cause, in the meantime making sure the baby gets the milk he needs and that steps are taken to safeguard the mother's milk production.

Determining a Mother's Milk Production

When there is concern about a baby's weight after Day 3 or 4, test-weighing and milk expression can be used to help gauge milk production.

If a baby's weight loss after birth is in the normal range and he is gaining weight and growing well, ample milk production is assumed. If baby's weight loss within the first few days is greater than 10%, the first step is to help the baby take the breast deeper, use breast compression, and make sure baby takes the breast at least 10 to 12 times per day. If the baby's weight doesn't improve, supplements may be needed (see p. 234- "When and How to Supplement").

The following two strategies may be useful to determine a mother's milk production after milk increase on Day 3 or 4. They are not usually helpful before then because milk production and intake are relatively low.

Test-weighing. Watching for signs of milk intake as a baby breastfeeds is not a reliable gauge of milk production. One U.S. study found that neither mothers nor lactation consultants could accurately estimate preterm babies' milk intake at the breast by listening for swallowing and watching for wide jaw movements (Meier, Engstrom, Fleming, Streeter, & Lawrence, 1996). However, one reliable way to gauge milk intake at the breast is by using a very accurate (to 2 g) electronic baby scale for pre- and post-feed weights (Meier et al., 1994a). These scales are available in many hospitals and lactation clinics. In some areas they can be rented for home use from breast pump rental stations. For average intake at the breast per feeding by age, see Table 6.5 on p. 237- "When and How to Supplement", keeping in mind that feeding amounts will vary at different times of day. One test-weight does not provide enough information to gauge a baby's daily intake. So although it can rule out ineffective breastfeeding and low milk production, it does not reveal whether a baby is consistently effective at the breast or his daily milk intake. If the mother has the scale for home use, doing 24-hour test-weights provides much more information. For more details, see p. 841- "Scales for Test-Weighing."

Milk expression. Expressing milk can rule out low milk production as a cause of weight issues if a mother can express ample milk at several sessions. (The first session should not be used as a final gauge because milk may have accumulated in the breast.) However, milk expression is a less reliable way to confirm low milk production because all mothers cannot express milk effectively, especially right away. For example, one Australian study of 28 breastfeeding mothers with established and ample milk production found 11% were unable to express much milk using any of the seven pump cycling patterns tested (Kent, Ramsay, Doherty, Larsson, & Hartmann, 2003). For many women, milk expression is a learned skill that takes time and practice to master. Even when the most effective type of pump (usually a rental pump) is used, factors unrelated to milk production—such as fit and responsiveness—can affect a mother's yield. For details, see p. 825 in the "Tools and Products" appendix.

Milk expression is a less reliable way to determine milk supply than infant weight gain as not all mothers with full supply can express milk.

Delayed Milk Increase After Birth

A mother's milk production is considered delayed when she does not notice breast changes or fullness by about 72 hours postpartum.

When a mother's milk does not increase within the first 3 days after birth, U.S. researchers suggest three general categories of causes: 1) hormonal issues that prevent the breast from responding normally, such as retained placenta, ovarian tumor, or subnormal pituitary function, 2) causes related to the breast that could limit milk production, such as a history of breast surgery or underdeveloped breast tissue, and 3) ineffective or infrequent milk removal after birth (Neville & Morton, 2001). See Table 10.2 on the next page for a more detailed list of possible causes. Delays in milk increase are common in cultures where the medical model is used to manage birth and interventions and separation of mother and baby are the norm. For example, one U.S. study found that 22% of its 280 mothers had a delay in milk increase (Dewey et al., 2003). For this reason, its authors suggest that all mothers and babies be evaluated at 72 to 96 hours postpartum.

Table 10.2. Factors that May Delay Milk Increase after Birth

Mother Factors

- First-time mother
- Overweight, obese, or excessive weight gain during pregnancy
- Breast/nipple issues, such as underdeveloped breasts, a history of breast surgery or injury, or unusual breast or nipple anatomy
- Other health conditions that may affect mother's hormonal levels or her body's response to hormones, such as Type-I diabetes, polycystic ovary syndrome (PCOS), thyroid or pituitary issues, hypertension, luteal phase defect, prolactin resistance, gestational ovarian theca lutein cysts
- Medications

Baby Factors

- Any condition that reduces baby's breastfeeding effectiveness (unusual oral anatomy, birth injuries, breathing problems, health or neurological issues, etc.)

Birth-Related Factors

- Long labor or traumatic or unusually stressful birth, increasing cortisol levels
- Preterm birth, cutting short breast tissue development
- Retained placenta or other placental issues, affecting hormonal levels or breast tissue development
- Blood loss of more than 500 mL (more than a pint), affecting hormonal levels

Postpartum Factors

- Little or no breastfeeding or milk expression
- Separation of mother and baby, little or no skin-to-skin or body contact

A mother's hormonal levels and health issues may affect early milk increase.

First-time mothers. Mothers with older children previously experienced the breast tissue growth of pregnancy, which research has found results in milk increase, on average, about a day earlier than in first-time mothers (Ingram et al., 1999).

Overweight and obesity. Obesity, overweight, and excessive weight gain during pregnancy have been associated with delayed milk increase after birth (Chapman & Perez-Escamilla, 1999; Hilson, Rasmussen, & Kjolhede, 2004; Rasmussen, 2007). Obesity has also been associated with a decreased prolactin response to baby's suckling (Rasmussen & Kjolhede, 2004). However, these associations may not be entirely due to biological effects, as U.S. research has also found that overweight and obese women are less likely to put their newborns to the breast within the first 2 hours after birth, which has also been associated with a delay in milk increase (Bystrova, Matthiesen et al., 2007; Kugyelka, Rasmussen, & Frongillo, 2004). Until more information is available, obesity should be considered a red flag to closely monitor mother and baby after birth. For more details, see p. 526- "Obesity."

Other health conditions. Conditions that affect a mother's hormonal levels or her body's response to hormones include Type-I diabetes (Hartmann & Cregan, 2001), polycystic ovary syndrome (PCOS) (Marasco et al., 2000; Vanky, Isaksen, Moen, & Carlsen, 2008), thyroid or pituitary issues (Marasco, 2006; Schrager & Sabo, 2001), hypertension (Neifert et al., 1990), luteal phase defect (Bodley & Powers, 1999), prolactin resistance (Zargar et al., 2000), and gestational ovarian theca lutein cysts (Betzold et al., 2004; Hoover et al., 2002). For details on these conditions, see their sections in the chapter "Health Issues—Mother."

Medications. One drug that can potentially decrease milk production is the decongestant pseudoephedrine (Aljazaf et al., 2003). A small, preliminary U.S. study found an association between serotonin-reuptake inhibiting drugs often taken for depression and delay in milk production after birth (Marshall et al., 2010).

• •

Breast and nipple issues may be a factor in delayed milk increase.

Underdeveloped breasts. In some unusual cases, a mother's milk-producing glands may not have developed fully. Also known as "insufficient glandular tissue," or "hypoplastic breasts," many mothers with this condition have bulbous areolae or widely spaced breasts (more than 1.5 inches or about 4 cm apart), large differences in breast size, or tubular or cone-shaped breasts rather than rounded (Huggins et al., 2000). When the breasts are felt, there may be some obvious patches of glandular tissue in a mostly soft breast (Wilson-Clay, 2008). Mothers with this condition often notice no breast changes during pregnancy or breast fullness after birth. Although the change to mature milk happens on schedule, the volumes are too low to be felt as fullness. These symptoms should be considered a red flag to monitor mother and baby closely after birth. Depending on how much milk-making tissue she has and her breastfeeding dynamics, she may be able to continue to increase her milk production over time and eventually exclusively breastfeed later babies (Huggins et al., 2000; Wilson-Clay, 2008). For more details, see p. 703- "Underdeveloped Breasts."

Breast injury or surgery may increase the risk of low milk supply.

A history of breast surgery or injury. Some types of breast surgery or injury, such as breast reduction surgery, put a mother at increased risk of inadequate milk production. This may not actually be a delay in milk increase, but rather a symptom of overall low milk production. A surgical incision near the areola may also cause nerve damage, which may inhibit milk ejection and compromise milk transfer. For details, see p. 706- "Breast Surgery or Injury."

Unusual nipple anatomy or nipple piercing. Because unusual nipple anatomy may make it more challenging for a newborn to take the breast, it may affect milk transfer. Flat or inverted nipples were associated with delayed milk increase in one U.S. study (Dewey et al., 2003) and one Iranian study of first-time mothers (Vazirinejad, Darakhshan, Esmaeili, & Hadadian, 2009). The Iranian study included within its category of "maternal breast variations" abnormally large breasts and large, flat, and inverted nipples.

Nipple piercing can also affect milk transfer after birth. Although there are several case reports of mothers who successfully breastfed after a nipple piercing (Lee, 1995; Wilson-Clay & Hoover, 2008), there are also case reports of mothers whose complications from the piercing caused milk duct obstruction and reduced milk transfer during breastfeeding and milk expression (Garbin, Deacon, Rowan, Hartmann, & Geddes, 2009). For more details, see p. 665- "Nipple Piercing."

Some aspects of the labor and birth may delay milk increase after birth.

Long labor or traumatic birth. Stress can increase the level of cortisol in a mother's bloodstream, affecting her hormonal balance. One Guatemalan study found high levels of cortisol in mothers after a difficult birth and delayed lactogenesis II (Grajeda & Perez-Escamilla, 2002). Both U.S. and New Zealand research have found an association between an exhausting labor or physically or psychologically traumatic birth and a delay in milk increase (Beck & Watson, 2008; Chen, Nommsen-Rivers, Dewey, & Lonnerdal, 1998; Dewey, 2001). One U.S. study found that more than 1 hour spent pushing during stage II labor was associated with delayed milk increase (Dewey et al., 2003). For more details, see p. 55- "Birth Practices and Breastfeeding."

Cesarean birth. Some U.S. studies have found an association between caesarean delivery and delayed lactation, but it is unclear whether this is a result of the physical stress of a surgical delivery or the delay in the first breastfeeding and fewer feedings in the early days (Dewey et al., 2003; Evans, Evans, Royal, Esterman, & James, 2003). Other studies have not found this association (Kulski, Smith, & Hartmann, 1981; Patel, Liebling, & Murphy, 2003). In one small study, women who gave birth by caesarean and offered the breast sooner had an earlier increase in milk production than those who offered their infants the breast later (Sozmen, 1982). One U.S. randomized clinical trial of 60 breastfeeding mothers found that adding six breast pumping sessions between 24 and 72 hours after a caesarean birth did not stimulate a faster increase in milk production (Chapman, Young, Ferris, & Perez-Escamilla, 2001). The pumping was also associated with a shorter duration of breastfeeding among first-time mothers.

Preterm birth. A mother whose breast tissue grows and develops during 40 weeks of pregnancy may make more milk earlier than a mother whose breast tissue growth is cut short when her pregnancy ends at 30 weeks. One small Australian study of 22 mothers of preterm babies found that 82% expressed milk with significant variations in milk composition associated with low milk production (Cregan et al., 2002). U.S. research found when comparing mothers breastfeeding full-term babies with mothers expressing milk for preterm babies that frequency of breast stimulation accounted for 49% of the variance in milk production at Week 6, whereas the baby's gestational age at birth only accounted for about 11% (Hill et al., 2005b). Make sure a mother in this situation knows that during the first month postpartum with frequent breast stimulation breast tissue growth continues (Cox et al., 1999).

Retained placenta or other placental issues. U.S. lactation consultants Diana West and Lisa Marasco wrote "Anything that compromises placental function can also affect breast development during pregnancy" (West & Marasco, 2009, p. 127). This is because some of the hormones needed for breast development are released by the placenta. In some cases, an unusually low birthweight for gestational age (SGA) or a diagnosis of intrauterine growth retardation (IUGR) may be a red flag for placental issues. If placental fragments stay attached in a mother's uterus after birth, they can continue to release progesterone, preventing the hormonal chain of events needed for milk increase (Neifert et al., 1981). This is more likely if the placenta was slow to deliver or the birth attendant used tension to speed its delivery. Ask the mother if her placenta was delivered intact or if her birth attendant manually removed the placenta, as manual removal may increase the risk of retained fragments. One way to rule out retained placenta is for the mother's healthcare provider to do a blood test for beta human chorionic gonadotropin (β-hCG).

Blood loss of more than 500 mL (a pint). An association has been found between mild to moderate postpartum hemorrhage and low milk production (Willis & Livingstone, 1995). Some also note an association between postpartum hemorrhage and hypothyroidism, which can also affect milk production (D. West, personal communication, March 3, 2010). Extreme blood loss during delivery or at other times can cause a condition known as Sheehan's Syndrome, in which lack of blood flow to the pituitary renders it permanently nonfunctional, making both lactation and future pregnancy impossible (Schrager & Sabo, 2001; Sert et al., 2003). However, this is rare and usually mothers with excess postpartum bleeding get off to a slow start, but with careful attention to good breastfeeding dynamics and milk removal, they produce ample milk.

• •

Postpartum practices and early breastfeeding dynamics play a significant role in how quickly milk increases.

How soon after birth and how often a baby breastfeeds on the first day of life has been found to affect how quickly a mother's milk production increases. One Russian study found a positive association between the timing of the first feeding and milk intake on Day 4 (Bystrova, Widstrom et al., 2007). Newborns who breastfed for the first time within 2 hours of birth took, on average, 55% more milk on Day 4 (284 mL or 9.6 oz.) as compared with the babies whose first feeding occurred more than 2 hours after birth (184 mL or 6.2 oz.). One Japanese study of 140 mothers and babies found that the babies who had breastfed 7 to 11 times on their first day consumed 86% more milk on Day 3 than the babies who breastfed fewer than seven times (Yamauchi & Yamanouchi, 1990). The difference in milk intake between these two groups continued to be significant through the 5th day of life.

How often a baby breastfeeds on Day 1 affects how quickly her milk supply increases.

How much time a mother and baby spend touching or in skin-to-skin contact during the early days also affects a mother's hormonal levels, which can affect milk production. After a normal, unmedicated delivery, the movements of newborns in skin-to-skin contact with their mothers was found to increase their mothers' blood oxytocin levels (Matthiesen et al., 2001). Even an hour of mother-baby skin-to-skin contact was associated with increased milk output in mothers of preterm babies (Hurst et al., 1997).

Many factors can all contribute to low milk production after 1 week.

For details, see p. 220- in the section "Slow Weight Gain" in the chapter "Weight Gain and Growth."

Strategies for Making More Milk

The mother needing to boost milk production may first need help in processing her feelings.

A mother who is struggling with milk-production issues needs an empathetic ear. As author and lactation consultant Lisa Marasco wrote:

> Some mothers may initially be in denial that their breasts may not be doing their expected job and may need gentle help in facing the reality of their situation. For others, there may be feelings of guilt and self-condemnation, especially if the problem first becomes evident by the baby's inadequate growth. Tears of grief are common, and there is sometimes anger at the healthcare providers and educators who taught her how important breastfeeding was but did not warn her about such potential problems.

> So often the resources brought to the situation concentrate largely on the physical aspects of breastfeeding to the neglect of the emotions of the mother. Women experiencing any degree of lactation failure are facing a loss that is not generally appreciated in our culture, and we are in a key position as breastfeeding supporters to extend empathy and help assuage some of the grief. Sometimes, affected women need to hear that they are not at fault for what has happened and that they have indeed done their very best, whatever the outcome (Marasco, 2005, p. 28).

Listening and acknowledging the mother's feelings can help her feel ready to take the next step: sorting through her choices and deciding how she wants to proceed.

With low milk production, the first priority is to feed the baby and the second is to safeguard the mother's milk production.

No matter what the cause of low milk production, the first priority is to feed the baby. How this is done will depend on the situation. For example, some expressed milk in a cup and solid foods may be all a slow-gaining older baby needs while his mother is working to increase milk production. For the more vulnerable newborn, however, if breastfeeding is not meeting all of his needs for milk, the next best option is to feed him expressed mother's milk. If there is not enough to meet his needs, donor human milk is the next best choice. If there is not enough human milk of any kind available, feeding infant formula will be necessary.

Supplementing with extra milk can be critical to supporting breastfeeding. When a baby is stressed by hunger, he can become weakened and ineffective at the breast. The strategy of withholding milk until the baby "gets hungry enough" can put a small baby at risk for dehydration and electrolyte imbalance (hypernatremia), which may require hospitalization to balance electolytes before supplements are given.

When a baby breastfeeds ineffectively, milk expression may be necessary to safeguard the mother's milk production. The number of expressions per day will depend on the baby's age, the amount of milk needed, and how far the mother is from full milk production (see next section). In general, any mother needing to use milk expression to boost her production should choose the most effective method available to her, which in developed countries is a hospital-grade rental breast pump. For details on expression methods, see p. 453- "Milk Expression Methods."

Finding the cause(s) of low milk production will help determine the most effective strategies for making more milk.

The most common cause of low milk production is the baby spending too little time actively suckling at the breast, but when low production has another cause, increasing the time spent breastfeeding will not necessarily be an effective solution. In mothers with hormonal issues, such as thyroid imbalance, polycystic ovary syndrome, luteal phase defects, and other physical conditions, medical treatment may be the best milk-enhancing strategy. (See Table 10.3 for medical tests to determine possible hormonal causes.) If the mother's milk production is compromised by breast surgery or underdeveloped breast tissue, using the basic strategies described in the next section may not be enough to stimulate full milk production, but they may help her provide a greater percentage of her baby's daily milk intake.

Table 10.3. Tests for Hormonal Causes of Early Low Milk Production

Suggest the mother ask her healthcare provider about testing her blood levels of:
Testosterone—If elevated, an ultrasound can confirm the presence of gestational ovarian theca lutein cysts, which can delay milk increase for weeks postpartum.
TSH—If thyroid levels are high or low (normal range during pregnancy is 0.5-2.5 mIU/L), appropriate medication can be prescribed (Mandel, Spencer, & Hollowell, 2005).
Prolactin—Tests done before and 45 minutes after breastfeeding will show if there is a prolactin surge with breastfeeding (which may be double or more); if levels are low or there is no prolactin surge after breastfeeding, galactogogues may help improve milk production (see later section).
β-hCG—If levels are high, this may indicate retained placenta, which ultrasound can confirm.
Hemoglobin—If low, treat for anemia.

Adapted from (Amir, 2006; Betzold et al., 2004; West & Marasco, 2009)

If the baby's breastfeeding effectiveness is compromised due to tongue tie, other unusual oral anatomy, breathing problems, neurological impairment, prematurity, or other health conditions, treating or addressing the baby's health issue directly while using milk expression to boost the mother's production may the best option.

• •

Encourage any mother working to boost milk production to accept all offers of help and take good care of herself.

For most mothers, getting more rest, eating a more nutritious diet, and drinking more fluids will not boost milk production. But these can be important to a mother's morale and her ability to cope. Encourage the mother to accept all offers of assistance and offer to help her formulate a daily plan that will maximize her time spent boosting milk production while giving her the time needed to nurture her relationship with her baby, care for other children, and handle other responsibilities.

Using Basic Dynamics to Boost Milk Production

When a mother's milk production is low or faltering, first review the basics.

When considering strategies to boost production, start with these questions:

- **How many times per day does she breastfeed or express her milk?** Rather than discussing how many hours apart baby feeds are (i.e., "every 3 hours"), ask her to describe about what time she breastfeeds or expresses during a typical day and add them together for her daily total.
- **About how long does she breastfeed or express each breast at each session?** Has this changed recently? If using a pump, is she single or double pumping?
- **What is her longest stretch between breast drainings?** Stretches longer than about 8 hours cause some mothers' production to slow over time.
- **If expressing, what method or pump is she using?** If she's pumping,

ask her the brand and model she uses to decide whether it is effective enough for her situation. If she's using a breast pump also ask her when she last had her breast pump fit checked. Even if she had a good fit at first, fit can change with time and pumping (Meier, 2004; Wilson-Clay & Hoover, 2008). See p. 825- "Breast Pumps."

- **How much time does she spend each day holding her baby or in skin-to-skin contact?** Time spent touching can enhance milk-making (Hurst et al., 1997).
- **Discuss other factors that might affect her milk production**, such as any medications she is taking, a history of infertility, chest or breast surgery, and any health problems (see Table 3.3 on p. 112).

Table 10.4. Factors That May Contribute to Low Milk Production after 1 Week

Less-Than Optimal Breastfeeding Dynamics

- Shallow breastfeeding—Can decrease milk transfer; may be due to positioning issues or poor fit (large nipple, small mouth)
- Too little active suckling time at the breast—Scheduled, limited, or infrequent feedings, sleepy baby (overdressed?), overuse of swaddling or soothers (pacifier/dummy, swing), mother's mental health issues
- Delay in early milk production due to less-than-optimal breastfeeding start
- Feeding baby other liquids or solid foods (formula, water, juice, cereal, etc.)—Which delay or replace breastfeeding

Baby Factors

- Temperament—Placid/sleepy or difficult to settle for feedings
- Anatomy or health issues that can cause ineffective suckling—Unusual oral anatomy (tongue tie, cleft palate, etc.), illness, preterm birth, birth injury (hematoma, broken bone, torticollis), respiratory problems, sensory processing problems, neurological impairment (high/low tone)
- Health issues that can cause slow weight gain with healthy milk intake—Cardiac defect, cystic fibrosis (baby tastes salty), metabolic, respiratory, other disorders

Mother Factors

- Breast/Nipple Issues—Breast surgery or injury (severed milk ducts or nerve damage preventing milk ejection), inadequate glandular tissue (hypoplastic breasts), unusual nipple anatomy or nipple piercing (may decrease or prevent milk transfer)
- Health and Medication Issues—Serious illness, drugs/herbs that decrease milk production or are incompatible with breastfeeding, any conditions that may affect a mother's hormonal levels (obesity, thyroid, pituitary, ovarian cyst [many types]), hormonal contraceptives

To make milk faster, suggest breastfeeding strategies that drain the breasts more fully and more often.

As described in the earlier section "Degree of Breast Fullness," two different dynamics cause full breasts to make milk slower: 1) internal pressure from the milk, which reduces blood flow in the breasts and compresses milk-making cells, and 2) higher levels of the peptide or whey protein "feedback inhibitor of lactation," or FIL. As the breasts become fuller, the combination of increasing FIL and increasing internal pressure causes milk production to become slower and slower.

But the opposite is also true. A mother's rate of milk production speeds when her breasts are more fully drained. On average, babies take 67% of the milk in the breasts, which means after feeding, 33% (or a third of the milk) is left in the breast (Kent, 2007). One way to increase the rate of milk production is to drain 90% to 95% of the milk instead of 67%. Suggest the mother experiment with the following breastfeeding strategies and see which help her best use this dynamic.

Make sure the baby takes the breast deeply and transfers milk effectively. The following strategies can increase a mother's rate of milk production only if the baby removes milk effectively at the breast. Suggest the mother listen for sounds of the baby's swallows after every suckle or every other suckle for the first 10 minutes or so of breastfeeding, with occasional pauses. If needed, a very accurate baby scale (to 2 g) can be used to determine a baby's milk intake by weighing him before and after breastfeeding (Meier et al., 1994b). If the mother can express enough milk for a full feeding, but the baby does not transfer this much milk during a breastfeeding, milk production may not be the problem and more breastfeeding will not be the answer. Suggest the mother use the strategies described in chapter 1 to find an effective feeding position and to be sure the baby takes the breast deeply. Shallow breastfeeding can reduce the baby's milk intake and drain the breast unevenly, which can slow milk production (Mizuno et al., 2008). Also see the chapters "Challenges at the Breast" and "Health Issues—Baby" for conditions that can cause ineffective breastfeeding.

Offer each breast more than once at each feeding. Suggest the mother offer the other breast each time the baby comes off the breast. If at any point the baby does not stay active (just mouthing the breast rather than actively suckling and swallowing) or if he falls asleep quickly, suggest the mother use breast compression (see next paragraph) to keep him active at that breast longer. If possible and baby is able and willing, encourage the baby to take each breast at least twice.

Use breast compression or alternate breast massage. If the baby stops suckling actively, breast compression or alternate breast massage can increase milk flow, providing positive reinforcement to keep him interested in feeding actively longer. According to U.S. research, this increases the milk's fat content, one indicator of a more drained breast (Stutte, 1988). For a description of this technique, see p. 804 in the "Techniques" appendix.

Breastfeed more times each day. Breastfeeding more often gives the mother more time each day with "drained breasts" and less time each day with "full breasts," which can increase the rate of milk production between feedings (Daly et al., 1993). Over time frequent milk removal increases the rate of milk production via other mechanisms (Czank, Henderson et al., 2007). Over the medium term, more frequent milk removal speeds the metabolic activity of key enzymes used in milk-making, increasing the rate of milk production. Over the long-term, frequent milk removal stimulates the growth and development of more milk-making tissue in the breast, increasing the rate of milk production even more.

Guide the sleeping baby to the breast. To help increase the number of daily breastfeedings, the baby can be gently guided to the breast when drowsy or in a light sleep. U.K. research has found that laying sleeping babies tummy down on mothers' semi-reclined body triggers inborn feeding behaviors, which can lead to effective breastfeeding, even in late preterm babies (Colson, DeRooy, & Hawdon, 2003).

Avoid soothers and keep all suckling at the breast. Suggest the mother keep her baby on her body as much as possible to trigger feeding behaviors and provide all suckling at the breast. Swaddling and soothers, such as pacifiers/dummies and swings, can reduce time spent breastfeeding (Binns & Scott, 2002; Bystrova, Matthiesen et al., 2007). If supplements are needed and the baby can suckle effectively, encourage the mother to consider using an at-breast supplementer (see p. 815) to increase breast stimulation.

• •

Milk expression can drain the breasts more fully and speed the rate of milk production.

If the breastfeeding strategies described above are not enough to reach full milk production or the baby breastfeeds ineffectively, suggest the mother consider using milk expression to drain her breasts more fully. Be prepared to discuss expression choices. The first choice for any mother attempting to boost milk production is a rental-grade pump with a double-pump kit, which has been found to be more effective than hand expression (Slusher et al., 2007). If she chooses to pump, talk about pump models, pump fit, using sensory stimulation (including warmth) to trigger more milk ejections, and how to use her pump settings to get the most milk at each expression (see p. 449- "How to Express More Milk").

Also offer to help her formulate a daily plan that will not overwhelm her. Encourage her to respond to her baby if he cries while she's expressing, and if she begins to feel overwhelmed, to review and revise her daily plan to concentrate on those aspects that work best for her and eliminate the others. Tell her that for every Plan A, there is a Plan B, and mothers often need to change what they're doing as they see what works and what doesn't. If the baby is not breastfeeding effectively or will not breastfeed more often, the following milk-expression strategies may be key to boosting milk production. But the ultimate goal in most cases is to move away from milk expression to full breastfeeding as soon as possible.

Mik expression can boost milk production.

Express milk after feedings. Milk expression can be used as many times per day as practical to drain the mother's breasts more fully after breastfeeding to speed milk production. If the baby is very ineffective at the breast, to make her daily routine more manageable, the mother may need to limit the baby to a set period of breastfeeding (perhaps with an at-breast supplementer so he doesn't need to be fed again), with a higher priority given to the time spent expressing until the baby becomes more effective. Let the mother know that even if she doesn't express much milk at first, the main purpose of expressing is to stimulate faster milk production.

Express milk between feedings. Most mothers express more milk for supplementation by waiting to express an hour or more after breastfeeding. This stimulates milk production, too, and usually gives the mother of an effective feeder more milk for her efforts than expressing right after a breastfeeding. Let the mother decide if she would prefer to keep all feeding-related activities together by expressing right after feedings or if she would rather express at another time and get more milk.

Use breast massage during pumping and hand expression after. One U.S. study found that 86% of its 66 mothers of preterm babies expressed an average of 93% more milk when they used breast massage during pumping and hand expression after pumping to drain their breasts more completely (Morton et al., 2009). A U.K. study also found that breast massage during breast pumping increased milk output an average of 42% (88 mL vs. 125 mL) (Jones, Dimmock, & Spencer, 2001).

Express long enough so that the breast is well drained. Suggest the mother express up to 20 to 30 minutes per breast at each session, or at least 2 minutes after the last drop of milk. The more fully she can drain her breasts, the faster her rate of milk production.

From time to time "power pump." The purpose of this short-term strategy is to fit in more daily pumpings and give milk production a quick boost. One version of power pumping credited to U.S. lactation consultant Catherine Watson Genna involves putting the pump in an area the mother passes often and will be comfortable sitting or standing (West & Marasco, 2009). During a several-day period, every time she passes the pump, she uses it for 5 to 10 minutes, pumping into the same bottle and using the same pump pieces without cleaning them for 4 to 6 hours (the length of time milk is considered safe at most room temperatures). After this time, she combines and refrigerates the milk and cleans the pump parts. Because the milk is not refrigerated right away and the pump pieces are not cleaned after each use, this strategy is recommended only for mothers of full-term healthy babies.

Suggest the mother keep the longest stretch between breast drainings shorter than 8 hours.

Because full breasts make milk slower, long stretches between breastfeeding and/or milk expressions (usually at night) can slow a mother's milk production. Ask her the length of her current longest stretch. To avoid giving her body the message to slow milk production for part of the day, suggest she avoid going longer than 8 hours without either breastfeeding or milk expression. If her baby sleeps longer than 8 hours at night, she will need to decide whether to wake the baby to breastfeed or express her milk. For some small-capacity mothers, even 8 hours may be long enough to cause milk production to slow.

Galactogogues

A galactogogue is any substance—drug, herb, food, drink—that speeds milk production.

Galactogogues, or milk-enhancing substances, have been used worldwide through much of human history (Humphrey, 2003). Some have been passed down by word of mouth from generation to generation. And some—but not all—have been scientifically studied (see next point). They include prescription drugs, herbal preparations (powders, tablets, capsules, tinctures, and teas), and even some foods and drinks.

Galactogogues are most effective when combined with breast drainage.

For any mother considering using a galactogogue that is not a food, suggest she discuss it with her healthcare provider in light of her health history, as some are contraindicated in specific situations (i.e., metoclopramide in a mother with a history of depression). All galactogogues are most effective when used in combination with frequent and effective breast drainage and will have little to no effect without it. Also, galactogogues are most effective when they treat the underlying cause of a mother's low milk production.

• •

Domperidone and metoclopramide are prescribed drugs that raise prolactin levels, boosting milk production in some mothers with low production.

In the U.S., no drugs have been officially recognized by the Food and Drug Administration (FDA) as galactogogues. But some drugs used for other health problems have been found to boost milk production in some mothers as a side effect of increased blood prolactin levels. In the U.S., this makes prescribing these drugs to enhance milk-making an "off-label" use. One small Canadian study found that both domperidone and metoclopramide had a greater effect on prolactin levels in first-time mothers (Brown, Fernandes, Grant, Hutsul, & McCoshen, 2000).

Domperidone (Motilium™). This prescribed drug is widely used internationally to treat nausea and reflux disease, and to increase milk production. Like metroclopramide (see later in this point), taking domperidone prevents the release of dopamine which increases a mother's blood prolactin levels (Hofmeyr, Van Iddekinge, & Blott, 1985). But unlike metoclopramide, domperidone does not cross the blood-brain barrier, so central nervous system side effects are less likely (Hale, 2008). Also, because domperidone has a large molecular weight and high protein-binding, only low levels pass into mother's milk (Barone, 1999). For these reasons, domperidone is considered compatible with breastfeeding by the American Academy of Pediatrics (AAP, 2001) and is rated an L1 (safest) in *Medications and Mothers' Milk* (Hale, 2008). However, due to serious reactions in compromised chemotherapy patients who received high doses of domperidone by IV, in June 2004 the U.S. FDA advised it not be prescribed for breastfeeding mothers. Although readily available and frequently used to increase milk production in Canada and other parts of the world, domperidone is not available through most pharmacies in the U.S. However, it can be ordered with a prescription at U.S. compounding pharmacies and legally (for personal use) without a prescription directly from pharmacies outside the U.S. For current details on obtaining domperidone see the following link: http://www.lowmilksupply.org/domperidone-obtain.shtml.

Domperidone increases mik supply with low risk of central-nervous-system side effects.

Research has found that at its recommended dose of 10 to 40 mg three to four times per day (Gabay, 2002), domperidone increases milk production significantly in some mothers. One controlled, double-blind Canadian study of low-producing mothers of preterm babies found it increased milk production an average of 28% over the placebo group between 2 and 7 days after it was started (da Silva, Knoppert, Angelini, & Forret, 2001). However, not all mothers respond to domperidone this way. An Australian study of six low-producing mothers of preterm babies found that domperidone did not increase production in one-third (two) of its mothers (Wan et al., 2008). In the mothers whose milk production increased, this increase varied by dose, with three of the four mothers seeing a greater increase at 60 mg per day (367%) than at 30 mg per day (215%). Side effects were also dose-related, with the most common being dry mouth, headaches, and abdominal cramps. Both the mothers whose milk increased and those whose didn't had significantly higher blood prolactin levels. The underlying causes of the mothers' low milk production were not examined, so those whose milk didn't increase likely had issues unrelated to their prolactin levels, such as lack of sufficient glandular tissue, hormonal issues such as insulin resistance or high testosterone, or hypothyroidism.

In another Canadian study, 46 mothers of preterm babies born at less than 31 weeks gestation who experienced "lactation failure" were randomized into either the domperidone or placebo group and took it for 14 days (Campbell-Yeo et al., 2010). Mother's milk volumes in the domperidone group increased 267% during the 14 days and only 18.5% in the placebo group. Prolactin levels increased 97% in the domperidone group and 17% in the placebo group. Milk protein levels decreased 9.6% in the domperidone group and increased 3.6% in the placebo group, but both were considered within normal limits.

Some lactation professionals who work extensively with mothers with low milk production have found that some do not respond to domperidone at doses lower than 120 mg per day (West & Marasco, 2009). This dose has been found to be safe for as long as 12 years in those taking it for gastrointestinal problems (Reddymasu, Soykan, & McCallum, 2007; Soykan, Sarosiek, & McCallum, 1997).

Metoclopramide (Reglan™ or Maxeran™). Doses of 30 to 45 mg per day of this drug were found to be effective at increasing milk production within several days, while doses of 15 mg per day were not (Hale, 2008). When given within the first month postpartum at 10 mg doses three times per day for 7 to 14 days, this drug increased milk production an average of 110% in some mothers with low milk production (Ehrenkranz & Ackerman, 1986). Even among low-producing mothers of babies 8- to 12-months old, it was found to increase milk production by 72% (Kauppila et al., 1983). A study of 32 mothers in India who had low or no milk production during the first 3 weeks after birth found increased milk production in 67% of those who previously had no milk and in 100% of those who previously had low milk (Gupta & Gupta, 1985). A U.K. study of 37 women found that 5 mg doses had little effect on milk production, but 10 mg and 15 mg doses taken over 2 weeks increased milk output by 42 mL and 50 mL per feeding, respectively (Kauppila, Kivinen, & Ylikorkala, 1981).

When metoclopramide is started is important, as well as the mother-baby breastfeeding dynamics, as metroclopramide taken during the first few days after birth may not be an effective intervention. Studies done in the U.S. and Iran within the first few days of birth found that taking metoclopramide did not boost milk production 96 hours postpartum when mothers' blood prolactin levels are naturally high (Hansen, McAndrew, Harris, & Zimmerman, 2005) and that mothers who practiced "perfect" breastfeeding dynamics after birth produced just as much milk as those taking 30 mg of metroclopramide per day (Sakha & Behbahan, 2008).

Timing of metoclopramide is important. It may not be effective the first few days after birth.

When metoclopramide (or domperidone) is discontinued, a mother's milk production may slow, but not usually to the level it was before she started it. However, this may not be true if the mother's low milk production is due to inadequate glandular tissue or other types of primary lactation failure. To minimize this decrease in milk production, a mother can taper off this drug gradually by 10 mg per week (Hale, 2008). Because metoclopramide crosses the blood-brain barrier, one side effect is depression, so it is not recommended for women with a history of depression. The incidence of side effects from metoclopramide (headache, weakness, fatigue, depression) increase when it is taken for longer than a month, which is not recommended (Anfinson, 2002). This drug is rated an L2 (safer) in *Medications and Mothers' Milk* and the AAP considers it a drug whose effects on breastfeeding infants are unknown but may be of concern (AAP, 2001). Concerns about this drug are due in part to the side effect known as "tardive dyskinesia," which is a neurological problem that causes involuntary movements, which may become permanent in a small percentage of those who take this medication.

Other prescription drugs have also been found to boost milk production.

Other prescription drugs found to increase milk production include the antipsychotic medications sulpiride and chlorpromazine, recombinant human growth hormone (hGH), and thyrotropin-releasing hormone (TRH), which is given as a nasal spray. In some mothers with diabetes or polycystic ovary syndrome (PCOS), the drug metformin (Glucophase™), which sensitizes insulin receptors, has improved milk production (West & Marasco, 2009).

One review of the research on galactogogues concluded that due to concerns about serious side effects and little research on other drugs, metoclopramide and domperidone are better options as galactogogues (Gabay, 2002). Another review concluded that galactogogues do not enhance milk-making when good breastfeeding dynamics are practiced and mothers receive lactation support (Anderson & Valdes, 2007).

A variety of medicinal herbs have been used worldwide to enhance milk production.

Many herbal preparations have been used to enhance milk production for generations by breastfeeding mothers in traditional cultures (Humphrey, 2003).

Use with caution. However, some herbs contain active ingredients used in prescription medications, so they should be used with caution. Suggest any mother considering herbal galactogogues do so only under the guidance of someone well-versed in their use, such as a certified herbalist, so their quality and possible interactions with other herbs and medications can be evaluated. At this writing, in the U.S. no regulatory agency monitors herbal preparations for consistency, and their quality can vary widely. A U.S. study found that one in five Ayurvedic herbal products sold in Boston contained dangerous levels of heavy metals, such as mercury and lead (Saper et al., 2004). The website www.ConsumerLab.com provides subscribers with information on the quality of specific brands of herbal preparations.

Fenugreek, blessed thistle and other herbs have been used to boost milk production.

Different formulations and doses. Herbs are available in many forms, including powdered, tablet, capsule, tincture, and teas. A mother may respond better to one form than another, and different mothers may respond better to lower or higher doses. Teas can be especially tricky because the amount of active ingredient increases with longer steeping.

Fenugreek and blessed thistle. Fenugreek seed and blessed thistle are two herbal galactogogues that have been used for generations in Egypt and India and are recommended by popular authors of breastfeeding books (Huggins, 2005; Newman & Pitman, 2006). Fenugreek is used in cooking and in artificial maple syrup. When it is taken at doses high enough to boost milk production (usually three capsules three to four times per day), mothers often report their sweat and urine smell like maple syrup. One small non-placebo controlled U.S. study found that when 10 mothers of preterm babies took three fenugreek capsules three times daily within a week their milk output doubled from a mean of 207 mL to 464 mL with no adverse effects (Swafford & Berens, 2000). Fenugreek can be taken alone or with blessed thistle (three capsules three times per day), and mothers report that it usually takes 24 to 72 hours to notice an increase in milk production (Huggins, 2005). In the U.S., fenugreek is an herbal Generally

Recognized as Safe (GRAS). A reported adverse event was suspected GI bleeding in a 30-week preemie after his mother began taking fenugreek, but it was never confirmed as the cause (Hale, 2008). There have been two reports of allergic reactions (Patil, Niphadkar, & Bapat, 1997). Fenugreek decreases blood sugar, so caution is recommended with diabetic mothers (Hale, 2008).

Other herbal galactogogues. A wide variety of other herbs have been recommended for boosting milk production, including goat's rue, alfalfa, fennel, nettle, and shatavari. Not all herbs recommended as galactogogues are considered safe during pregnancy (West & Marasco, 2009). Although there are few published studies on herbal galactogogues, in one Peruvian study, 50 breastfeeding mothers took micronized Silymarin (a *Silybum marianum* extract), which increased their milk production 86% over 63 days compared with a 32% increase among those taking a placebo (Di Pierro, Callegari, Carotenuto, & Tapia, 2008).

For more details. An excellent resource about dosages and quality sources for the herbs mentioned above and many others is the book *The Breastfeeding Mother's Guide to Making More Milk*, by U.S. lactation consultants Diana West and Lisa Marasco. Some of this information is also available on these authors' website at the following link: http://www.lowmilksupply.org/herbalgalactagogues.shtml.

• •

Some foods and drinks are recommended in various cultures to enhance milk production.

Many traditional cultures consider food medicinal as well as nutritional, and specific foods are chosen and avoided by new mothers based on their properties. For example, in the Ayurvedic tradition of eastern India, foods believed to enhance milk-making include pumpkin, sunflower, and sesame seeds, as well as rice pudding with milk and sugar (Jacobson, 2007). In China, foods thought to regulate body warmth and fluids are recommended, such as chicken and seaweed soups, cooked papaya, millet, rice, anise, fennel, dill, cumin, caraway, and ginger.

Grains, such as oatmeal, have a reputation among North American mothers for speeding milk production, and grain-based drinks are recommended in many cultures. In Mexico, a drink commonly made for breastfeeding mothers contains oats or cornmeal simmered in milk. In Europe, coffee-substitutes made from roasted grains, especially barley, are recommended for speeding milk production. For more details, see www.mother-food.com.

Strategies for Supplementing That Enhance Milk-Making

The amount of supplement needed will depend on the baby's weight gain.

When a breastfed baby needs to be supplemented, his mother needs to strike a delicate balance between giving her baby the least amount of supplements needed, while actively breastfeeding as much as possible to stimulate faster milk production. Babies need to be well nourished to gain weight and thrive, and also to breastfeed effectively. If a baby with low milk intake becomes weak, this can compromise his ability to breastfeed. For details on choices of supplement and amount of milk needed by age, see p. 234- "When and How to Supplement."

Discuss the mother's feeding method options and the advantages of using an at-breast supplementer to increase breast stimulation.

An at-breast supplementer, also known as a tube-feeding device, can provide needed supplement while baby suckles at the breast, keeping the baby actively breastfeeding for longer to stimulate more milk production. It also avoids the need for the mother to spend more time feeding the baby again after breastfeeding. Not all mothers are comfortable using an at-breast supplementer (Borucki, 2005), so discuss the range of feeding options and support her in her choice. Her decision may depend in part on whether she is close to full milk production, making some milk, or making little or no milk, as well as the baby's ability to take milk from the breast effectively. For the pros and cons of each supplemental feeding method, see p. 814- Table B.1.

If a mother supplements by bottle, encourage her to use techniques and products that reinforce breastfeeding.

The mother supplementing her baby with feeding bottles and nipples/teats has options available to her that can work for or against continued breastfeeding. For details on how nipple flow, nipple shape, feeding technique, and other aspects of bottle-feeding can be tailored to encourage breastfeeding, see p. 819- "Feeding Bottles."

If a mother cannot produce enough milk to exclusively breastfeed, she needs empathy, support, and a chance to grieve her loss before making decisions.

When it becomes obvious that a mother is unable to fully nourish her baby at the breast, this can be emotionally devastating, and she may need some help in processing this loss. As author Lisa Marasco wrote:

> When a primary lactation failure is evident, great sensitivity is needed in guiding the mother through the process of deciding how she wants to proceed. Remember that she is facing a complex situation that does not offer a guarantee of full results, and that she may even have come to us hesitantly, afraid of 'fanaticism' that ignores the emotions and realities of her situation. As much as we want to see her do what it takes to breastfeed her baby, anything that feels like subtle pressure can heap more guilt upon her, resulting in anger and resentment toward us and anyone else who she feels does not appreciate the difficulty and hard work involved.
>
> An approach that may be helpful is to present information...[about] all of the possible tangible techniques to increase milk supply, but at the same time also emphasizing the relational and nurturing aspects of the nursing relationship so that the milk is not her only focus" (Marasco, 2005, p. 29).

When full breastfeeding is not an option, discuss the possibility of partially breastfeeding with supplements (Thorley, 2005). Depending on how much milk-making tissue she has and her breastfeeding dynamics, she may also find—like the mother inducing lactation—that with frequent breastfeeding her milk production may continue to increase over time (Huggins et al., 2000). Frequent breastfeeding causes more milk-making glandular tissue to grow, so even if she must continue to supplement with this baby, she may eventually be able to eliminate the supplement after solid foods are started or exclusively breastfeed later babies (Wilson-Clay & Hoover, 2008). One case report described a mother who exclusively breastfed a subsequent baby after receiving progesterone treatment during pregnancy to treat a luteal-phase defect (Bodley & Powers, 1999).

Overabundant Milk Production

Causes of overabundant milk production may be partly anatomical and partly cultural.

Milk production is best regulated by a baby's appetite. However, some mothers are just naturally large milk producers, and in many cultures, the "breastfeeding rules" mothers receive cause them to manipulate their baby's feeding rhythms, which can cause milk production to be too high (also known as "hyperlactation") or too low. As U.S pediatrician Christina Smillie wrote:

> ...[I]n the absence of a cultural history of easy and ubiquitous breastfeeding, and without an established understanding of the physiology of breastfeeding and lactation, health care providers now often pass on to mothers historical recommendations and rules about breastfeeding for which there are no clear physiological rationale. Many of these rules—at least so many minutes on a side, always feed on both sides, always offer the full side—probably date back to those days of 4-hour feeds, and are essentially strategies for maximizing milk production. Thus, as more and more women are breastfeeding in the United States, we are seeing more women who already have plenty of milk trying to breastfeed according to these culturally defined rules...
>
> Although normal variations in maternal anatomy and physiology and certain infant temperaments can certainly interact to create this clinical picture, more commonly, the initial cause of hyperlactation is cultural misinformation about optimal breastfeeding practices. Moreover, even when there are maternal or infant primary predispositions to rapid milk production, homeostatic mechanisms should normally lead to self-correction. However, cultural ideas about breastfeeding can interfere with these physiological mechanisms (Smillie et al., 2005).

When a mother is not pregnant or breastfeeding, milk production (or "galactorrhea") is usually caused by health problems or medications.

On occasion, a woman who is not pregnant or breastfeeding begins producing milk from both breasts. Called "galactorrhea," a mother with this condition should be referred to her healthcare provider for evaluation (Edge & Segatore, 1993). Because this mother is not breastfeeding, strictly speaking, this is an entirely different category than the overabundant milk production described in this section. But some mothers refer to this experience as "overproduction." This is a sign of elevated prolactin levels, which may be caused by a benign pituitary tumor (adenoma), an overactive thyroid (thyroxicosis), or other health problem (Lawrence & Lawrence, 2005). Galactorrhea can also be a side effect of some medications, such as tricyclic antidepressants, theophylline, amphetamines, and some contraceptives (Wichman & Cunningham, 2008).

Coping with Too Much Milk

Overabundant milk production can make breastfeeding challenging for the baby.

Many breastfeeding mothers think that making lots of milk is a plus not a minus. But when a mother overproduces, there can be real drawbacks to both her and her baby.

Difficulty coping with a fast milk flow. With overabundant milk production, milk flow is usually very fast, especially during the first milk ejection, which depending on the baby may lead to some of the following breastfeeding behaviors (Smillie et al., 2005):

- Pulling back, clamping down, or using biting or chewing mouth movements at the breast to slow milk flow
- Coming on and off the breast
- Keeping the breast loosely in his mouth while milk flows in

Some babies fuss during milk ejection, coughing, sputtering, or arching away. Many swallow lots of air when gulping milk, spit up regularly, and pass lots of gas. Although many believe excess gas is due to swallowed air, this is not the case, as air cannot pass from the stomach to the intestines. It is usually caused by high volumes of low-fat milk passing quickly through baby's intestines (see later point). Other common symptoms include refusal to breastfeed while falling asleep and general colicky or fussy behaviors. If the fussy behavior occurs during feedings, the cause is most likely difficulty coping with fast milk flow. If it occurs after feedings, it may be due to too much low-fat milk. Other possible symptoms include refusal to breastfeed even when obviously hungry, stopping breastfeeding when offered the other breast, and complete breast refusal (nursing strike).

Babies may have difficulties coping with too much milk.

Some of the above are also described as symptoms of an "overactive let-down reflex" (Andrusiak & Larose-Kuzenko, 1987), which research has not yet distinguished from overabundant milk production. Some of these symptoms may also occur in the baby with reflux disease and hypersensitivity, intolerance, or allergy.

Symptoms of taking high milk volume may include::

- Very fast weight gain, with some babies exceeding the average weight gain of 2 pounds (900 g) per month during the first 3 months by double or more
- Fussiness between feedings
- Continuous feeding cues even after taking ample milk
- Explosive green or watery stools

Constant feeding. Many of these babies always seem to be ravenous and unsatisfied despite large weight gains, which convinces many mothers that their problem is not too much milk but low milk production (Smillie et al., 2005). These behaviors can occur when a baby gets mostly high-sugar/low-fat milk at the breast. There may be so much milk in a full, overproducing breast, that the baby cannot drain it well enough to reach the fattier milk. Fat triggers the release in a baby's gut of a peptide called cholecystokinin (CCK), which aids in digestion and in regulation of intake, leaving a baby feeling satisfied and relaxed after a full meal. Breastfed babies may release more CCK than formula-fed babies (Marchini, Simoni, Bartolini, & Linden, 1993), but a breastfed baby taking mostly high-sugar/low-fat milk presumably releases less CCK, leaving him feeling unsatisfied, despite consuming large amounts (Smillie et al., 2005).

Stools that are green or watery or contain mucus or blood. The sugar in this high-sugar/low-fat milk is mostly lactose (milk sugar), and if the baby receives enough of it, it may overwhelm his gut, causing watery or green stools (Woolridge & Fisher, 1988). Green stools may also be a normal variation or a symptom of the baby's sensitivity to a food or medication he receives directly or indirectly through his mother's milk. For more details, see p. 517- "Is Baby Reacting to Something in Mother's Diet." Some clinicians have questioned whether the combination of colicky symptoms and mucus or blood in the stools—which are usually associated with allergy—might instead be symptoms of overabundant milk production alone (Smillie et al., 2005). If so, slowing mother's milk production (see next section) will resolve these symptoms.

To make milk flow more manageable for the baby, suggest laid-back breastfeeding positions and other strategies.

Before a mother's milk production has begun to slow (see next section), the following suggestions may help the baby cope with the fast milk flow.

- Try feeding positions that use gravity to give the baby more control over milk flow, such as the laid-back positions described and illustrated in chapter 1.
- Offer the breast more often, before it gets so full.
- Breastfeed when the baby is drowsy or sleepy, which can mean calmer feedings.
- Try frequent burping and breaks so that baby can pace himself during feeding.

Gravity can give baby more control during feeding sessions.

Rather than offering the baby a full breast, some recommend expressing the first milk ejection to decrease flow and make breastfeeding more manageable for the baby. The drawback to this strategy is that with the first milk ejection the mother expresses, on average, 45% of the available milk (Kent et al., 2008). So if she regularly expresses milk before breastfeeding, it can boost her milk production, making overproduction worse instead of better.

Overabundant milk production can make breastfeeding uncomfortable for the mother and increase her risk of mastitis.

Overproducing mothers may have any or all of the following common symptoms:

- **Profuse milk leakage** during and between feedings.
- **Painful nipples.** When an overwhelmed baby clamps down on the breast, chews, or clenches his jaw to slow milk flow, this may sometimes cause pinched, injured, or infected nipples (Smillie et al., 2005).
- **Painful breasts.** Many overproducing mothers experience milk ejections (especially the first) as painful or "knife-like" (Livingstone, 1996). With fast milk production, breast fullness and tenderness commonly cause discomfort, with some mothers feeling full even shortly after breastfeeding. Recurring mastitis of all types (plugged ducts, breast infections, abscess) are associated with overabundant milk production due to regularly occurring and prolonged periods of breast fullness.

Strategies for Making Less Milk

Before slowing milk production, be absolutely sure the behaviors and symptoms are not due to other causes.

The symptoms described in the previous section, such as gulping, coughing, and sputtering at the breast by the baby or the mother's nipple pain or recurring mastitis may have other causes, so before slowing milk production, be sure to rule them out. A baby with respiratory problems, sensory processing issues, a short frenulum, or a neurological impairment, for example, might find it difficult to cope with even an average milk flow. And recurring mastitis and painful breastfeeding can occur when a baby breastfeeds ineffectively for other reasons. Slowing a mother's milk production when overproduction is not the cause will not address the real issue and can lead to slow weight gain, failure to thrive, and low milk production.

Make special note of the baby's weight gain, as in most cases of overabundant milk production, a baby will be gaining weight at double or more of the expected weight gain of 2 pounds (900 g) per month. Although a small percentage of babies shut down or feed poorly with overabundant milk flow, if a baby is gaining in the normal range or below, overabundant milk production may not be the cause of baby's or mother's symptoms. No matter what the underlying cause, if a baby is not gaining more weight than average, slowing milk production is unlikely to help.

• •

It may be difficult to convince a mother to slow her milk production.

Even when a baby is gaining much more than the average 2 pounds (900 grams) per month and suffering from the symptoms previously described, it is often difficult to convince a mother to agree to slow her milk production because she may interpret her baby's behaviors as signs of hunger, leading her to believe that her milk production is low, not high. She may be worried that she doesn't have enough milk. Where breastfeeding is not yet the cultural norm, mothers may also be influenced by cultural messages about how easy it is to "lose her milk." In *The Breastfeeding Atlas,* U.S. lactation consultants Barbara Wilson-Clay and Kay Hoover suggest using pre- and post-feed test weights to show a mother exactly how much milk her baby takes at feedings to provide objective information that links her baby's unhappiness at the breast with too much, not too little milk (Wilson-Clay, 2008, p. 80).

Mothers may be convinced that their supplies are too low--not too high.

• •

When overabundant milk production is confirmed, suggest strategies to slow production using the dynamic "full breasts make milk slower."

As described earlier in this chapter, two different dynamics cause full breasts to make milk slower: 1) internal pressure from milk filling the breasts, which reduces blood flow and compresses milk-making cells, and 2) higher levels of the peptide or whey protein known as "feedback inhibitor of lactation," or FIL. As the breasts become fuller, the combination of increasing FIL and increasing internal pressure cause milk production to become slower and slower. These dynamics can be used to slow milk production in an overproducing mother without limiting her baby's time at the breast.

One breast per feeding or for 3-hour periods. In some cases of mild-to-moderate overproduction, limiting a baby to one breast per feeding (returning the baby to that breast more than once if needed) may be enough to bring milk production under control. In other cases, offering the same breast each time the baby shows feeding cues within a 3-hour window and alternating breasts every 3 hours can do the trick. During this time if the unused breast feels full or uncomfortable, the mother removes (by breastfeeding or expressing) the minimum amount of milk needed to keep her comfortable. However, in some cases, other measures are needed to resolve the symptoms.

Full drainage and block feeding. One Dutch article described a strategy the author called the "full drainage and block feeding" (FDBF) method and the experiences of four mothers who used it to slow milk production (van Veldhuizen-Staas, 2007). The first step was using an effective breast pump to drain both breasts as fully as possible (Berghuijs, 2000), then putting the baby immediately to the breast. Any time during the next 3 hours the baby showed feeding cues, the mothers offered the same breast. After 3 hours, the mothers began offering the other breast at all feedings for the next 3 hours. Depending on the severity of the mother's overproduction, the time blocks were increased to 4, 6, 8, or for one mother, 12 hours. For some mothers, no further use of the breast pump was needed; for others, draining the breast fully one or two more times helped.

A more right-brained approach. During her years in practice at her U.S. breastfeeding clinic, pediatrician Christina Smillie estimated seeing more than 1400 overproducing mothers and their babies. In response, she developed a variation of this strategy called "modified block feeding," which she considered less rule-oriented or "left-brained" and more supportive of a mother's intuition and her right-brained connection with her baby (Smillie et al., 2005). The underlying goal of this strategy is to help mothers avoid breastfeeding rules and learn to use their own and their baby's comfort as their guide.

She described her approach as alternately draining each breast well, and then leaving it full longer than before to slow milk production. Depending on the level of the mother's milk production, she recommended for a period of several days to a week the mother use a breast pump once each day to drain her breasts a fully as possible. The purpose of this drainage was to minimize the risk of mastitis in the mother and give the baby access to the high-fat milk that encouraged longer intervals between feedings. As in the previous strategy, the mother offered the same breast for periods of time, but rather than using the clock to determine when to switch breasts, she divided the day into unequal blocks of time based on the mother's lifestyle (Table 10.5) and alternated the breast used in the morning each day (C. Smillie, personal communication, January 30, 2010). The purpose of alternating the "morning breast" was to avoid uneven stimulation and slow milk production faster. Smillie defined "morning" as the time the mother considers herself up for the day until lunchtime, "afternoon" as lunchtime to dinnertime, "evening" as dinner time until bedtime, and "night" from bedtime until she's up for the day. These times can vary from day to day. The breast listed in each block of time (L=left, R=right) should be favored, with the breast in parentheses used whenever it feels right to mother or baby. During the mother's usual sleeping hours, Smillie encouraged her to do what felt right to her. She also encouraged mothers to use this strategy for 5 days only, as she found that when she didn't give a specific end date, some mothers continued it for weeks and even months. If used long-term, this strategy could become just another rule-based system that could artificially make milk production too high or too low. The goal is for the mother to learn to breastfeed by "feel" in a right-brained way by responding to her baby and to avoid external breastfeeding "rules," which were likely what caused her overproduction.

Table 10.5. A Right-Brained Strategy to Slow Milk Production

	Day 1	Day 2	Day 3	Day 4	Day 5:Done
Morning	L (R)	R (L)	L (R)	R (L)	L (R)
Afternoon	R (L)	L (R)	R (L)	L (R)	R (L)
Evening	L (R)	R (L)	L (R)	R (L)	L (R)
Night	Any	Any	Any	Any	Any

(C. Smillie, personal communication, January 30, 2010)

If needed, some drugs and/or medicinal herbs can be used to slow milk production.

If the methods in the previous point are not enough to resolve the mother's or baby's symptoms, the mother may want to consult with her healthcare provider about using drugs or medicinal herbs (sometimes referred to as "anti-galactogogues") to slow milk production.

Pseudoephedrine. One Australian study of eight lactating women found that when compared to a placebo a single 60-mg dose of this common decongestant (Sudafed™) reduced milk production by a mean of 24%. U.S. lactation consultant Barbara Wilson-Clay noted in *The Breastfeeding Atlas* that some mothers in her practice who took this medication under the guidance of their healthcare providers responded best when they took one 60 mg dose before bedtime and others got better results when this daily dose was spread evenly throughout the day (Wilson-Clay & Hoover, 2008). It's important that the original formula be used and not the "PE" version available in many U.S. pharmacies. Due to its effect on milk production, this drug is not usually recommended in breastfeeding mothers, but it passes into milk in very low levels (0.4-0.6% of the maternal dose), and no side effects have been reported in breastfeeding babies (Hale, 2008). Some have found its effect on milk production is greater after about 4 months postpartum (D. West, personal communication, March 3, 2010).

Combined oral contraceptives. For overabundant milk production after 3 weeks postpartum, some physicians prescribe a 4- to 7-day course of low-dose oral contraceptive pills with estrogen and progesterone once per day (Wilson-Clay & Hoover, 2008). Vaginal bleeding may occur after this treatment, and it may disrupt the effects of breastfeeding on the mother's fertility.

Sage. Before using a medicinal herb, suggest the mother consult with an herbalist, particularly when using sage, as its essential oil is toxic, and this form should be avoided. To use sage to slow milk production, steep 1 tablespoon of fresh whole leaf dried herb in 1 cup (0.25 L) of boiling water for 10 to 15 minutes. Drink 3 to 6 cups per day until milk production has slowed enough that the mother's and baby's symptoms have resolved, then discontinue (Humphrey, 2003).

RESOURCES FOR PARENTS

Websites

www.lowmilksupply.org –A resource for mothers created by the authors of *The Breastfeeding Mother's Guide to Making More Milk* (below).

www.MobiMotherhood.org –A website for mothers experiencing breastfeeding challenges. MOBI is an acronym for "mothers overcoming breastfeeding issues."

Books

Humphrey, S. (2003). *The nursing mother's herbal*. Minneapolis, MN: Fairview Press.

West, D., & Marasco, L. (2009). *The breastfeeding mother's guide to making more milk*. New York, NY: McGraw Hill.

REFERENCES

AAP. (2001). Transfer of drugs and other chemicals into human milk. *Pediatrics, 108*(3), 776-789.

Agostoni, C., Marangoni, F., Lammardo, A. M., Giovannini, M., Riva, E., & Galli, C. (2001). Breastfeeding duration, milk fat composition and developmental indices at 1 year of life among breastfed infants. *Prostaglandins Leukotrienes and Essential Fatty Acids, 64*(2), 105-109.

Aljazaf, K., Hale, T. W., Ilett, K. F., Hartmann, P. E., Mitoulas, L. R., Kristensen, J. H., et al. (2003). Pseudoephedrine: effects on milk production in women and estimation of infant exposure via breastmilk. *British Journal of Clinical Pharmacology, 56*(1), 18-24.

Allen, J. C., Keller, R. P., Archer, P., & Neville, M. C. (1991). Studies in human lactation: milk composition and daily secretion rates of macronutrients in the first year of lactation. *American Journal of Clinical Nutrition, 54*(1), 69-80.

Amir, L. H. (2006). Breastfeeding--managing 'supply' difficulties. *Australian Family Physician, 35*(9), 686-689.

Anderson, P. O., & Valdes, V. (2007). A critical review of pharmaceutical galactagogues. *Breastfeeding Medicine, 2*(4), 229-242.

Andrusiak, F., Larose-Kuzenko, M. (1987). *The effects of an overactive let-down reflex* (Vol. 13). Garden City Park, NY: Avery Publishing Group, Inc.

Anfinson, T. J. (2002). Akathisia, panic, agoraphobia, and major depression following brief exposure to metoclopramide. *Psychopharmacology Bulletin, 36*(1), 82-93.

Auer, C., & Gromada, K. K. (1998). A case report of breastfeeding quadruplets: factors perceived as affecting breastfeeding. *Journal of Human Lactation, 14*(2), 135-141.

BabyCenter.com. (2007). Breastfeeding your baby index. Retrieved June 4, 2007, from http:www.babycenter.com/baby/babybreastfeed/index

Barone, J. A. (1999). Domperidone: a peripherally acting dopamine2-receptor antagonist. *Annals of Pharmacotherapy, 33*(4), 429-440.

Beck, C. T., & Watson, S. (2008). Impact of birth trauma on breast-feeding: a tale of two pathways. *Nursing Research, 57*(4), 228-236.

Berghuijs, S. (2000). Casus. *Nederlandse Verniging van Lactatiekundigen Info*, 31-32.

Berlin, C. M. (2007). "Exclusive" breastfeeding of quadruplets. *Breastfeeding Medicine, 2*(2), 125-126.

Berry, C. A., Thomas, E. C., Piper, K. M., & Cregan, M. D. (2007). The histology and cytology of the human mammary gland and breastmilk. In T. W. Hale & P. E. Hartmann (Eds.), *Hale and Hartmann's Textbook of Human Lactation* (pp. 35-47). Amarillo, TX: Hale Publishing.

Betzold, C. M., Hoover, K. L., & Snyder, C. L. (2004). Delayed lactogenesis II: a comparison of four cases. *Journal of Midwifery & Women's Health, 49*(2), 132-137.

Binns, C. W., & Scott, J. A. (2002). Using pacifiers: what are breastfeeding mothers doing? *Breastfeeding Review, 10*(2), 21-25.

Bodley, V., & Powers, D. (1999). Patient with insufficient glandular tissue experiences milk supply increase attributed to progesterone treatment for luteal phase defect. *Journal of Human Lactation, 15*(4), 339-343.

Borucki, L. C. (2005). Breastfeeding mothers' experiences using a supplemental feeding tube device: finding an alternative. *Journal of Human Lactation, 21*(4), 429-438.

Brown, T. E., Fernandes, P. A., Grant, L. J., Hutsul, J. A., & McCoshen, J. A. (2000). Effect of parity on pituitary prolactin response to metoclopramide and domperidone: implications for the enhancement of lactation. *Journal of the Society for Gynecologic Investigation, 7*(1), 65-69.

Butte, N. F. (2005). Energy requirements of infants. *Public Health Nutr, 8*(7A), 953-967.

Bystrova, K., Matthiesen, A. S., Widstrom, A. M., Ransjo-Arvidson, A. B., Welles-Nystrom, B., Vorontsov, I., et al. (2007). The effect of Russian Maternity Home routines on breastfeeding and neonatal weight loss with special reference to swaddling. *Early Human Development, 83*(1), 29-39.

Bystrova, K., Widstrom, A. M., Matthiesen, A. S., Ransjo-Arvidson, A. B., Welles-Nystrom, B., Vorontsov, I., et al. (2007). Early lactation performance in primiparous and multiparous women in relation to different maternity home practices. A randomised trial in St. Petersburg. *International Breastfeeding Journal, 2*, 9.

Campbell-Yeo, M. L., Allen, A. C., Joseph, K. S., Ledwidge, J. M., Caddell, K., Allen, V. M., et al. (2010). Effect of domperidone on the composition of preterm human breast milk. *Pediatrics, 125*(1), e107-114.

Chapman, D. J., & Perez-Escamilla, R. (1999). Identification of risk factors for delayed onset of lactation. *Journal of the American Dietetic Association, 99*(4), 450-454; quiz 455-456.

Chapman, D. J., Young, S., Ferris, A. M., & Perez-Escamilla, R. (2001). Impact of breast pumping on lactogenesis stage II after cesarean delivery: a randomized clinical trial. *Pediatrics, 107*(6), E94.

Chatterton, R. T., Jr., Hill, P. D., Aldag, J. C., Hodges, K. R., Belknap, S. M., & Zinaman, M. J. (2000). Relation of plasma oxytocin and prolactin concentrations to milk production in mothers of preterm infants: influence of stress. *Journal of Clinical Endocrinology and Metabolism, 85*(10), 3661-3668.

Chen, D. C., Nommsen-Rivers, L., Dewey, K. G., & Lonnerdal, B. (1998). Stress during labor and delivery and early lactation performance. *American Journal of Clinical Nutrition, 68*(2), 335-344.

Cobo, E. (1993). Characteristics of the spontaneous milk ejecting activity occurring during human lactation. *Journal of Perinatal Medicine, 21*(1), 77-85.

Colson, S., DeRooy, L., & Hawdon, J. (2003). Biological Nurturing increases duration of breastfeeding for a vulnerable cohort. *MIDIRS Midwifery Digest, 13*(1), 92-97.

Cowley, K. C. (2005). Psychogenic and pharmacologic induction of the let-down reflex can facilitate breastfeeding by tetraplegic women: a report of 3 cases. *Archives of Physical Medicine and Rehabilitation, 86*(6), 1261-1264.

Cox, D. B., Kent, J. C., Casey, T. M., Owens, R. A., & Hartmann, P. E. (1999). Breast growth and the urinary excretion of lactose during human pregnancy and early lactation: endocrine relationships. *Experimental Physiology, 84*(2), 421-434.

Cox, D. B., Owens, R. A., & Hartmann, P. E. (1996). Blood and milk prolactin and the rate of milk synthesis in women. *Experimental Physiology, 81*(6), 1007-1020.

Cregan, M. D., De Mello, T. R., Kershaw, D., McDougall, K., & Hartmann, P. E. (2002). Initiation of lactation in women after preterm delivery. *Acta Obstet Gynecol Scand, 81*(9), 870-877.

Cregan, M. D., & Hartmann, P. E. (1999). Computerized breast measurement from conception to weaning: clinical implications. *Journal of Human Lactation, 15*(2), 89-96.

Czank, C., Henderson, J. J., Kent, J. C., Tat Lai, C., & Hartmann, P. E. (2007). Hormonal control of the lactation cycle. In T. W. Hale & P. E. Hartmann (Eds.), *Hale & Hartmann's Textbook of Human Lactation* (pp. 89-111). Amarillo, TX: Hale Publishing.

Czank, C., Mitoulas, L., & Hartmann, P. E. (2007). Human milk composition-nitrogen and energy content. In T. W. Hale & P. E. Hartmann (Eds.), *Hale & Hartmann's Textbook of Human Lactation* (pp. 75-88). Amarillo, TX: Hale Publishing.

da Silva, O. P., Knoppert, D. C., Angelini, M. M., & Forret, P. A. (2001). Effect of domperidone on milk production in mothers of premature newborns: a randomized, double-blind, placebo-controlled trial. *Canadian Medical Association Journal, 164*(1), 17-21.

Daly, S. E., & Hartmann, P. E. (1995). Infant demand and milk supply. Part 2: The short-term control of milk synthesis in lactating women. *Journal of Human Lactation, 11*(1), 27-37.

Daly, S. E., Kent, J. C., Owens, R. A., & Hartmann, P. E. (1996). Frequency and degree of milk removal and the short-term control of human milk synthesis. *Experimental Physiology, 81*(5), 861-875.

Daly, S. E., Owens, R. A., & Hartmann, P. E. (1993). The short-term synthesis and infant-regulated removal of milk in lactating women. *Experimental Physiology, 78*(2), 209-220.

Damato, E. G., Dowling, D. A., Madigan, E. A., & Thanattherakul, C. (2005). Duration of breastfeeding for mothers of twins. *Journal of Obstetric, Gynecologic, and Neonatal Nursing, 34*(2), 201-209.

Damato, E. G., Dowling, D. A., Standing, T. S., & Schuster, S. D. (2005). Explanation for cessation of breastfeeding in mothers of twins. *Journal of Human Lactation, 21*(3), 296-304.

de Carvalho, M., et al. (1983). Effect of frequent breast feeding on early milk production and infant weight gain. *Pediatrics, 72*, 307-311.

De Coopman, J. (1993). Breastfeeding after pituitary resection: support for a theory of autocrine control of milk supply? *Journal of Human Lactation, 9*(1), 35-40.

Dewey, K. G. (2001). Maternal and fetal stress are associated with impaired lactogenesis in humans. *Journal of Nutrition, 131*(11), 3012S-3015S.

Dewey, K. G., Finley, D. A., & Lonnerdal, B. (1984). Breast milk volume and composition during late lactation (7-20 months). *Journal of Pediatric Gastroenterology and Nutrition, 3*(5), 713-720.

Dewey, K. G., Nommsen-Rivers, L. A., Heinig, M. J., & Cohen, R. J. (2003). Risk factors for suboptimal infant breastfeeding behavior, delayed onset of lactation, and excess neonatal weight loss. *Pediatrics, 112*(3 Pt 1), 607-619.

Di Pierro, F., Callegari, A., Carotenuto, D., & Tapia, M. M. (2008). Clinical efficacy, safety and tolerability of BIO-C (micronized Silymarin) as a galactagogue. *Acta Biomed, 79*(3), 205-210.

Doucet, S., Soussignan, R., Sagot, P., & Schaal, B. (2009). The secretion of areolar (Montgomery's) glands from lactating women elicits selective, unconditional responses in neonates. *PLoS One, 4*(10), e7579.

Dusdieker, L. B., Booth, B. M., Stumbo, P. J., & Eichenberger, J. M. (1985). Effect of supplemental fluids on human milk production. *Journal of Pediatrics, 106*(2), 207-211.

Edge, D. S., & Segatore, M. (1993). Assessment and management of galactorrhea. *Nurse Practitioner, 18*(6), 35-36, 38, 43-34, passim.

Ehrenkranz, R. A., & Ackerman, B. A. (1986). Metoclopramide effect on faltering milk production by mothers of premature infants. *Pediatrics, 78*(4), 614-620.

Engstrom, J. L., Meier, P. P., Jegier, B., Motykowski, J. E., & Zuleger, J. L. (2007). Comparison of milk output from the right and left breasts during simultaneous pumping in mothers of very low birthweight infants. *Breastfeeding Medicine, 2*(2), 83-91.

Evans, K. C., Evans, R. G., Royal, R., Esterman, A. J., & James, S. L. (2003). Effect of caesarean section on breast milk transfer to the normal term newborn over the first week of life. *Archives of Disease in Childhood. Fetal and Neonatal Edition, 88*(5), F380-382.

Freeman, M. E., Kanyicska, B., Lerant, A., & Nagy, G. (2000). Prolactin: structure, function, and regulation of secretion. *Physiological Reviews, 80*(4), 1523-1631.

Gabay, M. P. (2002). Galactogogues: medications that induce lactation. *Journal of Human Lactation, 18*(3), 274-279.

Garbin, C. P., Deacon, J. P., Rowan, M. K., Hartmann, P. E., & Geddes, D. T. (2009). Association of nipple piercing with abnormal milk production and breastfeeding. *Journal of the American Medical Association, 301*(24), 2550-2551.

Geddes, D. T. (2007). Inside the lactating breast: the latest anatomy research. *Journal of Midwifery & Women's Health, 52*(6), 556-563.

Glueck, C. J., Salehi, M., Aregawi, D., Sieve, L., & Wang, P. (2007). Polycystic Ovary Syndrome: pathophysiology, endocrinopathy, treatment, and lactation. In T. W. Hale & P. E. Hartmann (Eds.), *Hale & Hartmann's Textbook of Lactation* (pp. 343-353). Amarillo, TX: Hale Publishing.

Going, J. J., & Moffat, D. F. (2004). Escaping from Flatland: clinical and biological aspects of human mammary duct anatomy in three dimensions. *Journal of Pathology, 203*(1), 538-544.

Grajeda, R., & Perez-Escamilla, R. (2002). Stress during labor and delivery is associated with delayed onset of lactation among urban Guatemalan women. *Journal of Nutrition, 132*(10), 3055-3060.

Gupta, A. P., & Gupta, P. K. (1985). Metoclopramide as a lactogogue. *Clinical Pediatrics, 24*(5), 269-272.

Hale, T. (2008). *Medications and Mothers' Milk* (13 ed.). Amarillo, TX: Hale Publishing.

Handlin, L., Jonas, W., Petersson, M., Ejdeback, M., Ransjo-Arvidson, A. B., Nissen, E., et al. (2009). Effects of sucking and skin-to-skin contact on maternal ACTH and cortisol levels during the second day postpartum-influence of epidural analgesia and oxytocin in the perinatal period. *Breastfeeding Medicine, 4*(4), 207-220.

Hansen, W. F., McAndrew, S., Harris, K., & Zimmerman, M. B. (2005). Metoclopramide effect on breastfeeding the preterm infant: a randomized trial. *Obstetrics and Gynecology, 105*(2), 383-389.

Hartmann, P., & Cregan, M. (2001). Lactogenesis and the effects of insulin-dependent diabetes mellitus and prematurity. *Journal of Nutrition, 131*(11), 3016S-3020S.

Hartmann, P. E., & Kulski, J. K. (1978). Changes in the composition of the mammary secretion of women after abrupt termination of breast feeding. *Journal of Physiology, 275*, 1-11.

Heinig, M. J., Nommsen, L. A., Peerson, J. M., Lonnerdal, B., & Dewey, K. G. (1993). Energy and protein intakes of breast-fed and formula-fed infants during the first year of life and their association with growth velocity: the DARLING Study. *American Journal of Clinical Nutrition, 58*(2), 152-161.

Henly, S. J., Anderson, C. M., Avery, M. D., Hills-Bonczyk, S. G., Potter, S., & Duckett, L. J. (1995). Anemia and insufficient milk in first-time mothers. *Birth, 22*(2), 86-92.

Hennart, P., Delogne-Desnoeck, J., Vis, H., & Robyn, C. (1981). Serum levels of prolactin and milk production in women during a lactation period of thirty months. *Clinical Endocrinology, 14*(4), 349-353.

Hill, P. D., & Aldag, J. C. (2005). Milk volume on day 4 and income predictive of lactation adequacy at 6 weeks of mothers of nonnursing preterm infants. *Journal of Perinatal and Neonatal Nursing, 19*(3), 273-282.

Hill, P. D., Aldag, J. C., Chatterton, R. T., & Zinaman, M. (2005a). Comparison of milk output between mothers of preterm and term infants: the first 6 weeks after birth. *Journal of Human Lactation, 21*(1), 22-30.

Hill, P. D., Aldag, J. C., Chatterton, R. T., & Zinaman, M. (2005b). Primary and secondary mediators' influence on milk output in lactating mothers of preterm and term infants. *Journal of Human Lactation, 21*(2), 138-150.

Hill, P. D., Aldag, J. C., Chatterton, R. T., & Zinaman, M. (2005c). Psychological distress and milk volume in lactating mothers. *Western Journal of Nursing Research, 27*(6), 676-693; discussion 694-700.

Hill, P. D., Aldag, J. C., Zinaman, M., & Chatterton, R. T., Jr. (2007). Comparison of milk output between breasts in pump-dependent mothers. *Journal of Human Lactation, 23*(4), 333-337.

Hill, P. D., & Humenick, S. S. (1989). Insufficient milk supply. *Image - the Journal of Nursing Scholarship, 21*(3), 145-148.

Hillervik-Lindquist, C. (1991). Studies on perceived breast milk insufficiency. A prospective study in a group of Swedish women. *Acta Paediatrica Scandinavica. Supplement, 376*, 1-27.

Hillervik-Lindquist, C., Hofvander, Y., & Sjolin, S. (1991). Studies on perceived breast milk insufficiency. III. Consequences for breast milk consumption and growth. *Acta Paediatrica Scandinavica, 80*(3), 297-303.

Hilson, J. A., Rasmussen, K. M., & Kjolhede, C. L. (2004). High prepregnant body mass index is associated with poor lactation outcomes among white, rural women independent of psychosocial and demographic correlates. *Journal of Human Lactation, 20*(1), 18-29.

Hofmeyr, G. J., Van Iddekinge, B., & Blott, J. A. (1985). Domperidone: secretion in breast milk and effect on puerperal prolactin levels. *British Journal of Obstetrics and Gynaecology, 92*(2), 141-144.

Hoover, K. L., Barbalinardo, L. H., & Platia, M. P. (2002). Delayed lactogenesis II secondary to gestational ovarian theca lutein cysts in two normal singleton pregnancies. *Journal of Human Lactation, 18*(3), 264-268.

Hopkinson, J. (2007). Nutrition in Lactation. In T. W. Hale & P. E. Hartmann (Eds.), *Hale & Hartmann's Textbook of Human Lactation* (pp. 371-386). Amarillo, TX: Hale Publishing.

Houston, M. J., Howie, P. W., & McNeilly, A. S. (1983). Factors affecting the duration of breast feeding: 1. Measurement of breast milk intake in the first week of life. *Early Human Development, 8*(1), 49-54.

Huggins, K. E. (2005). *The Nursing Mother's Companion* (20th Anniversary ed.). Boston, MA: Harvard Common Press.

Huggins, K. E., Petok, E. S., & Mireles, O. (2000). Markers of lactation insufficiency: A study of 34 mothers. In *Current Issues in Clinical Lactation*. Boston, MA: Jones and Bartlett.

Hull, V., Thapa, S., & Pratomo, H. (1990). Breast-feeding in the modern health sector in Indonesia: the mother's perspective. *Social Science and Medicine, 30*(5), 625-633.

Humenick, S. S., Hill, P. D., & Anderson, M. A. (1994). Breast engorgement: patterns and selected outcomes. *Journal of Human Lactation, 10*(2), 87-93.

Humphrey, S. (2003). *The Nursing Mother's Herbal*. Minneapolis, MN: Fairview Press.

Hurst, N. M., Valentine, C. J., Renfro, L., Burns, P., & Ferlic, L. (1997). Skin-to-skin holding in the neonatal intensive care unit influences maternal milk volume. *Journal of Perinatology, 17*(3), 213-217.

Ingram, J. C., Woolridge, M. W., Greenwood, R. J., & McGrath, L. (1999). Maternal predictors of early breast milk output. *Acta Paediatrica, 88*(5), 493-499.

Islam, M. M., Peerson, J. M., Ahmed, T., Dewey, K. G., & Brown, K. H. (2006). Effects of varied energy density of complementary foods on breast-milk intakes and total energy consumption by healthy, breastfed Bangladeshi children. *American Journal of Clinical Nutrition, 83*(4), 851-858.

Jacobson, H. (2007). *Mother Food: A Breastfeeding Diet Guide with Lactogenic Foods and Herbs - Build Milk Supply, Boost Immunity, Lift Depression, Detox, Lose Weight, Optimize a Baby's IQ, and Reduce Colic and Allergies*. Ashland, OR: Rosalind Press.

Jones, E., Dimmock, P. W., & Spencer, S. A. (2001). A randomised controlled trial to compare methods of milk expression after preterm delivery. *Archives of Disease in Childhood. Fetal and Neonatal Edition, 85*(2), F91-95.

Kauppila, A., Arvela, P., Koivisto, M., Kivinen, S., Ylikorkala, O., & Pelkonen, O. (1983). Metoclopramide and breast feeding: transfer into milk and the newborn. *European Journal of Clinical Pharmacology, 25*(6), 819-823.

Kauppila, A., Kivinen, S., & Ylikorkala, O. (1981). A dose response relation between improved lactation and metoclopramide. *Lancet, 1*(8231), 1175-1177.

Kennedy, K. I. (2010). Fertility, sexuality, and contraception during lactation. In J. Riordan & K. Wambach (Eds.), *Breastfeeding and Human Lactation* (4th ed., pp. 705-736). Boston, MA: Jones and Bartlett.

Kent, J. C. (2007). How breastfeeding works. *Journal of Midwifery & Women's Health, 52*(6), 564-570.

Kent, J. C., Mitoulas, L., Cox, D. B., Owens, R. A., & Hartmann, P. E. (1999). Breast volume and milk production during extended lactation in women. *Experimental Physiology, 84*(2), 435-447.

Kent, J. C., Mitoulas, L. R., Cregan, M. D., Geddes, D. T., Larsson, M., Doherty, D. A., et al. (2008). Importance of vacuum for breastmilk expression. *Breastfeeding Medicine, 3*(1), 11-19.

Kent, J. C., Mitoulas, L. R., Cregan, M. D., Ramsay, D. T., Doherty, D. A., & Hartmann, P. E. (2006). Volume and frequency of breastfeedings and fat content of breast milk throughout the day. *Pediatrics, 117*(3), e387-395.

Kent, J. C., Ramsay, D. T., Doherty, D., Larsson, M., & Hartmann, P. E. (2003). Response of breasts to different stimulation patterns of an electric breast pump. *Journal of Human Lactation, 19*(2), 179-186; quiz 187-178, 218.

Kimura, C., & Matsuoka, M. (2007). Changes in breast skin temperature during the course of breastfeeding. *Journal of Human Lactation, 23*(1), 60-69.

Knight, C. H., Peaker, M., & Wilde, C. J. (1998). Local control of mammary development and function. *Reviews of Reproduction, 3*(2), 104-112.

Kugyelka, J. G., Rasmussen, K. M., & Frongillo, E. A. (2004). Maternal obesity is negatively associated with breastfeeding success among Hispanic but not Black women. *Journal of Nutrition, 134*(7), 1746-1753.

Kulski, J. K., Smith, M., & Hartmann, P. E. (1981). Normal and caesarian section delivery and the initiation of lactation in women. *Australian Journal of Experimental Biology and Medical Science, 59*(4), 405-412.

Kunz, C., & Lonnerdal, B. (1992). Re-evaluation of the whey protein/casein ratio of human milk. *Acta Paediatrica, 81*(2), 107-112.

Lawrence, R. A., & Lawrence, R. M. (2005). *Breastfeeding: A Guide for the Medical Profession*. Philadelphia, PA: Elsevier Mosby.

Lee, N. (1995). More on pierced nipples. *Journal of Human Lactation, 11*(2), 89.

Livingstone, V. (1996). Too much of a good thing. Maternal and infant hyperlactation syndromes. *Canadian Family Physician, 42*, 89-99.

Love, S. M., & Barsky, S. H. (2004). Anatomy of the nipple and breast ducts revisited. *Cancer, 101*(9), 1947-1957.

Lubetzky, R., Mimouni, F. B., Dollberg, S., Salomon, M., & Mandel, D. (2007). Consistent circadian variations in creamatocrit over the first 7 weeks of lactation: a longitudinal study. *Breastfeeding Medicine, 2*(1), 15-18.

Mandel, D., Lubetzky, R., Dollberg, S., Barak, S., & Mimouni, F. B. (2005). Fat and energy contents of expressed human breast milk in prolonged lactation. *Pediatrics, 116*(3), e432-435.

Mandel, S. J., Spencer, C. A., & Hollowell, J. G. (2005). Are detection and treatment of thyroid insufficiency in pregnancy feasible? *Thyroid, 15*(1), 44-53.

Marasco, L. (2005). Polycystic Ovary Syndrome. *Leaven, 41*(2), 27-29.

Marasco, L. (2006). The impact of thyroid dysfunction on lactation. *Breastfeeding Abstracts, 25*(2), 11-12.

Marasco, L., Marmet, C., & Shell, E. (2000). Polycystic ovary syndrome: a connection to insufficient milk supply? *Journal of Human Lactation, 16*(2), 143-148.

Marchini, G., Simoni, M. R., Bartolini, F., & Linden, A. (1993). The relationship of plasma cholecystokinin levels to different feeding routines in newborn infants. *Early Human Development, 35*(1), 31-35.

Marshall, A. M., Nommsen-Rivers, L. A., Hernandez, L. L., Dewey, K. G., Chantry, C. J., Gregerson, K. A., et al. (2010). Serotonin transport and metabolism in the mammary gland modulates secretory activation and involution. *Journal of Clinical Endocrinology and Metabolism, 95*(2), 837-846.

Matthiesen, A. S., Ransjo-Arvidson, A. B., Nissen, E., & Uvnas-Moberg, K. (2001). Postpartum maternal oxytocin release by newborns: effects of infant hand massage and sucking. *Birth, 28*(1), 13-19.

McLennan, J. D. (2001). Early termination of breast-feeding in periurban Santo Domingo, Dominican Republic: mothers' community perceptions and personal practices. *Revista Panamericana de Salud Publica, 9*(6), 362-367.

McNeilly, A. S., & McNeilly, J. R. (1978). Spontaneous milk ejection during lactation and its possible relevance to success of breast-feeding. *British Medical Journal, 2*(6135), 466-468.

McNeilly, A. S., Robinson, I. C., Houston, M. J., & Howie, P. W. (1983). Release of oxytocin and prolactin in response to suckling. *British Medical Journal (Clinical Research Ed.), 286*(6361), 257-259.

Mead, L. J., Chuffo, R., Lawlor-Klean, P., & Meier, P. P. (1992). Breastfeeding success with preterm quadruplets. *Journal of Obstetric, Gynecologic, and Neonatal Nursing, 21*(3), 221-227.

Meier, P. (2004). Choosing a correctly fitted breastshield for milk expression. *Medela Messenger, 21*(1), 8-9.

Meier, P. P., Engstrom, J. L., Crichton, C. L., Clark, D. R., Williams, M. M., & Mangurten, H. H. (1994a). A new scale for in-home test-weighing for mothers of preterm and high risk infants. *Journal of Human Lactation, 10*(3), 163-168.

Meier, P. P., Engstrom, J. L., Crichton, C. L., Clark, D. R., Williams, M. M., & Mangurten, H. H. (1994b). A new scale for in-home test-weighing for mothers of preterm and high risk infants. *Journal of Human Lactation, 10*(3), 163-168.

Meier, P. P., Engstrom, J. L., Fleming, B. A., Streeter, P. L., & Lawrence, P. B. (1996). Estimating milk intake of hospitalized preterm infants who breastfeed. *Journal of Human Lactation, 12*(1), 21-26.

Mizuno, K., Nishida, Y., Mizuno, N., Taki, M., Murase, M., & Itabashi, K. (2008). The important role of deep attachment in the uniform drainage of breast milk from mammary lobe. *Acta Paediatrica, 97*(9), 1200-1204.

Mohrbacher, N. (1996). Mothers who forgo breastfeeding for pumping. *Ameda/Egnell Circle of Caring, 9*(2), 1-2.

Mok, E., Multon, C., Piguel, L., Barroso, E., Goua, V., Christin, P., et al. (2008). Decreased full breastfeeding, altered practices, perceptions, and infant weight change of prepregnant obese women: a need for extra support. *Pediatrics, 121*(5), e1319-1324.

Morse, J. M., Ewing, G., Gamble, D., & Donahue, P. (1992). The effect of maternal fluid intake on breast milk supply: a pilot study. *Canadian Journal of Public Health. Revue Canadienne de Sante Publique Public Health, 83*(3), 213-216.

Morton, J., Hall, J. Y., Wong, R. J., Thairu, L., Benitz, W. E., & Rhine, W. D. (2009). Combining hand techniques with electric pumping increases milk production in mothers of preterm infants. *Journal of Perinatology, 29*(11), 757-764.

Neifert, M., DeMarzo, S., Seacat, J., Young, D., Leff, M., & Orleans, M. (1990). The influence of breast surgery, breast appearance, and pregnancy-induced breast changes on lactation sufficiency as measured by infant weight gain. *Birth, 17*(1), 31-38.

Neifert, M. R., McDonough, S. L., & Neville, M. C. (1981). Failure of lactogenesis associated with placental retention. *American Journal of Obstetrics and Gynecology, 140*(4), 477-478.

Neville, M. C., Allen, J. C., Archer, P. C., Casey, C. E., Seacat, J., Keller, R. P., et al. (1991). Studies in human lactation: milk volume and nutrient composition during weaning and lactogenesis. *American Journal of Clinical Nutrition, 54*(1), 81-92.

Neville, M. C., Keller, R., Seacat, J., Lutes, V., Neifert, M., Casey, C., et al. (1988). Studies in human lactation: milk volumes in lactating women during the onset of lactation and full lactation. *American Journal of Clinical Nutrition, 48*(6), 1375-1386.

Neville, M. C., McFadden, T. B., & Forsyth, I. (2002). Hormonal regulation of mammary differentiation and milk secretion. *Journal of Mammary Gland Biology and Neoplasia, 7*(1), 49-66.

Neville, M. C., & Morton, J. (2001). Physiology and endocrine changes underlying human lactogenesis II. *Journal of Nutrition, 131*(11), 3005S-3008S.

Newman, J., & Pitman, T. (2006). *The Ultimate Breastfeeding Book of Answers*. New York, New York: Three Rivers Press.

Newton, M., & Newton, N. R. (1948). The let-down reflex in human lactation. *Journal of Pediatrics, 33*(6), 698-704.

Noel, G. L., Suh, H. K., & Frantz, A. G. (1974). Prolactin release during nursing and breast stimulation in postpartum and nonpostpartum subjects. *Journal of Clinical Endocrinology and Metabolism, 38*(3), 413-423.

Nommsen-Rivers, L. A., Heinig, M. J., Cohen, R. J., & Dewey, K. G. (2008). Newborn wet and soiled diaper counts and timing of onset of lactation as indicators of breastfeeding inadequacy. *Journal of Human Lactation, 24*(1), 27-33.

Pang, W. W., & Hartmann, P. E. (2007). Initiation of human lactation: secretory differentiation and secretory activation. *Journal of Mammary Gland Biology and Neoplasia, 12*(4), 211-221.

Patel, R. R., Liebling, R. E., & Murphy, D. J. (2003). Effect of operative delivery in the second stage of labor on breastfeeding success. *Birth, 30*(4), 255-260.

Patil, S. P., Niphadkar, P. V., & Bapat, M. M. (1997). Allergy to fenugreek (Trigonella foenum graecum). *Annals of Allergy, Asthma, and Immunology, 78*(3), 297-300.

Pisacane, A., & Continisio, P. (2004). Breastfeeding and perceived changes in the appearance of the breasts: a retrospective study. *Acta Paediatrica, 93*(10), 1346-1348.

Prentice, A. (1989). Evidence for local feedback control of human milk secretion. . *Biochemical Society Transactions, 17*, 489-492.

Prentice, A. M., Goldberg, G. R., & Prentice, A. (1994). Body mass index and lactation performance. *European Journal of Clinical Nutrition, 48 Suppl 3*, S78-86; discussion S86-79.

Prentice, A. M., Roberts, S. B., Prentice, A., Paul, A. A., Watkinson, M., Watkinson, A. A., et al. (1983). Dietary supplementation of lactating Gambian women. I. Effect on breast-milk volume and quality. *Human Nutrition. Clinical Nutrition, 37*(1), 53-64.

Prime, D. K., Geddes, D. T., & Hartmann, P. E. (2007). Oxytocin: Milk ejection and maternal-infant well-being. In T. W. Hale & P. E. Hartmann (Eds.), *Hale & Hartmann's Textbook of Human Lactation* (pp. 141-155). Amarillo, TX: Hale Publishing.

Ramsay, D. T., Kent, J. C., Hartmann, R. A., & Hartmann, P. E. (2005). Anatomy of the lactating human breast redefined with ultrasound imaging. *Journal of Anatomy, 206*(6), 525-534.

Ramsay, D. T., Kent, J. C., Owens, R. A., & Hartmann, P. E. (2004). Ultrasound imaging of milk ejection in the breast of lactating women. *Pediatrics, 113*(2), 361-367.

Ramsay, D. T., Mitoulas, L. R., Kent, J. C., Larsson, M., & Hartmann, P. E. (2005). The use of ultrasound to characterize milk ejection in women using an electric breast pump. *Journal of Human Lactation, 21*(4), 421-428.

Rasmussen, K. M. (2007). Association of maternal obesity before conception with poor lactation performance. *Annual Review of Nutrition, 27*, 103-121.

Rasmussen, K. M., & Kjolhede, C. L. (2004). Prepregnant overweight and obesity diminish the prolactin response to suckling in the first week postpartum. *Pediatrics, 113*(5), e465-471.

Reddymasu, S. C., Soykan, I., & McCallum, R. W. (2007). Domperidone: review of pharmacology and clinical applications in gastroenterology. *American Journal of Gastroenterology, 102*(9), 2036-2045.

Rinker, B., Veneracion, M., & Walsh, C. P. (2008). The effect of breastfeeding on breast aesthetics. *Aesthetic Surgery Journal, 28*(5), 534-537.

Rioux, F. M., Savoie, N., & Allard, J. (2006). Is there a link between postpartum anemia and discontinuation of breastfeeding? *Canadian Journal of Dietetic Practice and Research, 67*(2), 72-76.

Rossoni, E., Feng, J., Tirozzi, B., Brown, D., Leng, G., & Moos, F. (2008). Emergent synchronous bursting of oxytocin neuronal network. *PLoS Computational Biology, 4*(7), e1000123.

Saint, L., Maggiore, P., & Hartmann, P. E. (1986). Yield and nutrient content of milk in eight women breast-feeding twins and one woman breast-feeding triplets. *British Journal of Nutrition, 56*(1), 49-58.

Saint, L., Smith, M., & Hartmann, P. E. (1984). The yield and nutrient content of colostrum and milk of women from giving birth to 1 month post-partum. *British Journal of Nutrition, 52*(1), 87-95.

Sakha, K., & Behbahan, A. G. (2008). Training for perfect breastfeeding or metoclopramide: which one can promote lactation in nursing mothers? *Breastfeeding Medicine, 3*(2), 120-123.

Saper, R. B., Kales, S. N., Paquin, J., Burns, M. J., Eisenberg, D. M., Davis, R. B., et al. (2004). Heavy metal content of ayurvedic herbal medicine products. *Journal of the American Medical Association, 292*(23), 2868-2873.

Schaal, B., Doucet, S., Sagot, P., Hertling, E., & Soussignan, R. (2006). Human breast areolae as scent organs: morphological data and possible involvement in maternal-neonatal coadaptation. *Developmental Psychobiology, 48*(2), 100-110.

Schrager, S., & Sabo, L. (2001). Sheehan syndrome: a rare complication of postpartum hemorrhage. *Journal of the American Board of Family Practice, 14*(5), 389-391.

Sert, M., Tetiker, T., Kirim, S., & Kocak, M. (2003). Clinical report of 28 patients with Sheehan's syndrome. *Endocrine Journal, 50*(3), 297-301.

Slusher, T., Slusher, I. L., Biomdo, M., Bode-Thomas, F., Curtis, B. A., & Meier, P. (2007). Electric breast pump use increases maternal milk volume in African nurseries. *Journal of Tropical Pediatrics, 53*(2), 125-130.

Smillie, C. M., Campbell, S. H., & Iwinski, S. (2005). Hyperlactation: how left-brained 'rules' for breastfeeding can wreak havoc with a natural process. *Newborn and Infant Nursing Reviews, 5*(1), 49-58.

Smith, C. (1947). Effects of maternal undernutrition upon newborn infants in Holland (1944-1945). *Journal of Pediatrics, 30*, 229-243.

Smith, L., & Riordan, J. (2010). Postpartum care. In J. Riordan & K. Wambach (Eds.), *Breastfeeding and Human Lactation* (pp. 253-290). Boston, MA: Jones and Bartlett.

Soykan, I., Sarosiek, I., & McCallum, R. W. (1997). The effect of chronic oral domperidone therapy on gastrointestinal symptoms, gastric emptying, and quality of life in patients with gastroparesis. *American Journal of Gastroenterology, 92*(6), 976-980.

Sozmen, M. (1982). Effects of early suckling of cesarean-born babies on lactation. *Biology of the Neonate, 62*, 67-68.

Stutte, P. (1988). the effects of breast massage on volume and fat content of human milk. *Genesis, 10*(2), 22-25.

Swafford, S., & Berens, P. (2000). Effect of fenugreek on breast milk volume. *ABM News & Views, 6*(3), 21.

Thorley, V. (2005). Breast hypoplasia and breastfeeding: a case history. *Breastfeeding Review, 13*(2), 13-16.

Uvnas-Moberg, K. (2003). *The Oxytocin Factor: Tapping the Hormone of Calm, Love, and Healing*. Cambridge, MA: Da Capo Press.

van Veldhuizen-Staas, C. G. (2007). Overabundant milk supply: an alternative way to intervene by full drainage and block feeding. *International Breastfeeding Journal, 2*, 11.

Vanky, E., Isaksen, H., Moen, M. H., & Carlsen, S. M. (2008). Breastfeeding in polycystic ovary syndrome. *Acta Obstetricia et Gynecologica Scandinavica, 87*(5), 531-535.

Vazirinejad, R., Darakhshan, S., Esmaeili, A., & Hadadian, S. (2009). The effect of maternal breast variations on neonatal weight gain in the first seven days of life. *International Breastfeeding Journal, 4*, 13.

Wan, E. W., Davey, K., Page-Sharp, M., Hartmann, P. E., Simmer, K., & Ilett, K. F. (2008). Dose-effect study of domperidone as a galactagogue in preterm mothers with insufficient milk supply, and its transfer into milk. *British Journal of Clinical Pharmacology, 66*(2), 283-289.

Watson, C. J. (2006). Involution: apoptosis and tissue remodelling that convert the mammary gland from milk factory to a quiescent organ. *Breast Cancer Research, 8*(2), 203.

West, D., & Hirsch, E. (2008). *Breastfeeding after Breast and Nipple Procedures*. Amarillo, TX: Hale Publishing.

West, D., & Marasco, L. (2009). *The Breastfeeding Mother's Guide to Making More Milk*. New York, NY: McGraw Hill.

Wichman, C. L., & Cunningham, J. L. (2008). A case of venlafaxine-induced galactorrhea? *Journal of Clinical Psychopharmacology, 28*(5), 580-581.

Wilde, C. J., Addey, C. V., Boddy, L. M., & Peaker, M. (1995). Autocrine regulation of milk secretion by a protein in milk. *Biochemical Journal, 305 (Pt 1)*, 51-58.

Willis, C. E., & Livingstone, V. (1995). Infant insufficient milk syndrome associated with maternal postpartum hemorrhage. *Journal of Human Lactation, 11*(2), 123-126.

Wilson-Clay, B., & Hoover, K. (2008). *The Breastfeeding Atlas* (4th ed.). Manchaca, TX: LactNews Press.

Wilson-Clay, B., Hoover, K. (2008). *The Breastfeeding Atlas* (4th ed.). Manchaca, TX: LactNews Press.

Woolridge, M. W., & Fisher, C. (1988). Colic, "overfeeding", and symptoms of lactose malabsorption in the breast-fed baby: a possible artifact of feed management? *Lancet, 2*(8607), 382-384.

Yamauchi, Y., & Yamanouchi, I. (1990). Breast-feeding frequency during the first 24 hours after birth in full-term neonates. *Pediatrics, 86*(2), 171-175.

Yokoyama, Y., & Ooki, S. (2004). Breast-feeding and bottle-feeding of twins, triplets and higher order multiple births. *Nippon Koshu Eisei Zasshi, 51*(11), 969-974.

Zangen, S., Di Lorenzo, C., Zangen, T., Mertz, H., Schwankovsky, L., & Hyman, P. E. (2001). Rapid maturation of gastric relaxation in newborn infants. *Pediatric Research, 50*(5), 629-632.

Zargar, A. H., Salahuddin, M., Laway, B. A., Masoodi, S. R., Ganie, M. A., & Bhat, M. H. (2000). Puerperal alactogenesis with normal prolactin dynamics: is prolactin resistance the cause? *Fertility and Sterility, 74*(3), 598-600.

Milk Expression and Storage

Chapter 11

MILK EXPRESSION BASICS

Why Express Milk?

Milk expression is associated with longer breastfeeding duration.

Learning to express milk is one of the Baby Friendly Hospital Initiative's "Ten Steps to Successful Breastfeeding." Even when breastfeeding is going well, there are many reasons a mother may want or need to express her milk, which is why it is so common. One U.S. longitudinal mail survey of more than 3,600 mothers found that 85% of the mothers with babies 6 weeks to 4½ months old had expressed milk sometime since their baby's birth, 68% within the previous 2 weeks (Labiner-Wolfe, Fein, Shealy, & Wang, 2008). This survey found that milk expression was most common among first-time mothers and occurred less often as their babies got older.

Most mothers express milk at least sometime in the first 6 months postpartum.

A smaller U.S. retrospective study of 346 mothers found that during the first 6 months, 77% of the mothers whose babies received their milk used a breast pump to express (Geraghty, Khoury, & Kalkwarf, 2005). Just 10% of these mothers breastfed exclusively, giving no expressed milk or formula. Of the small number (5%) who exclusively pumped and bottle-fed their babies, all were mothers of preterm babies. The study found that mothers of full-term, healthy babies expressed as often as mothers of multiples and mothers of preterm babies.

One Australian study followed all mothers who gave birth in two urban Perth hospitals and found that between 1992 and 2002 the percentage of mothers expressing their milk doubled (Binns, Win, Zhao, & Scott, 2006). This increase may be due in part to an increasing public awareness of the importance of mother's milk to babies' health. This study and another Australian study of 587 mothers both found an association between milk expression and longer breastfeeding duration (Win, Binns, Zhao, Scott, & Oddy, 2006).

In the U.S., where more than half of mothers return to paid employment within their baby's first year, studies have also found that among low-income mothers, access to breast pumps increases breastfeeding incidence and duration. In an article describing a program in a Baby Friendly hospital in Boston that provided free double electric personal pumps to low-income families, its authors wrote that among African-American women, "the breastfeeding rate in this population increased by 54 percentage points primarily because all women received a breast pump" (Chamberlain, McMahon, Philipp, & Merewood, 2006, p. 97). A U.S. study of 208 low-income breastfeeding mothers who participated in a government food subsidy program found that providing rental electric breast pumps to mothers returning to work full-time increased the likelihood that they would not request formula by 5.5 times at 6 months and 3.0 times at 12 months (Meehan et al., 2008).

• •

Mothers express their milk for many reasons.

In an Australian study described previously, the most common reasons mothers gave for expressing milk (from most to least common) were: 1) so someone else could feed the baby, 2) to relieve engorgement, nipple pain, or mastitis, 3) to relieve discomfort from too much milk, and 4) to store extra milk. Other reasons included to increase milk production, to safeguard milk production while baby was having problems taking the breast or suckling well, to teach the baby to take a bottle, and to provide milk while mother was ill (Binns et al., 2006).

In the U.S. the reasons given were: 1) so someone else could feed the baby, 2) to store extra milk, 3) to relieve engorgement, and 4) to increase milk production. Other reasons included: to provide milk when the mother didn't want to breastfeed, to maintain milk production when baby couldn't breastfeed, to mix with cereal or food, and to provide milk when the mother had nipple pain (Labiner-Wolfe et al., 2008).

Prenatal hand-expression of colostrum may benefit some at-risk mothers and babies.

If a mother is at risk for low milk production after birth, one way to avoid the health risks associated with giving non-human milks in the early days is to express and store some colostrum during pregnancy. Examples of at-risk mothers include those with breast hypoplasia (inadequate glandular tissue), diabetes, polycystic ovary syndrome (PCOS), a history of breast surgery or injury, and multiple sclerosis.

Australian author, midwife, and lactation consultant Suzanne Cox created a protocol for prenatal expression of colostrum (Cox, 2006). She suggests the pregnant mother first discuss it with her healthcare provider and plan to begin learning manual expression at 34 weeks gestation, starting in the shower when her breasts are warm. Using a 1 or 3 mL syringe, the mother can draw up the drops as they are expressed and keep the syringe in the refrigerator between expressions. She suggests reusing the same syringe, freezing it either when it is full or after 2 days. If the mother expresses larger volumes of colostrum, she can collect it in a clean spoon or medicine cup, and then draw it up into the syringe. Although manual expression stimulates oxytocin release, Cox noted that this also occurs during eating, kissing, and cuddling, and research has found no association between nipple stimulation and miscarriage or preterm labor. For more details, see p. 559- "Effects on the Pregnancy."

How Much Milk to Expect

Most mothers need practice to express milk effectively.

On their first try, very few mothers express much milk; some only a few drops. Suggest the mother think of her first milk expressions as practice sessions and any milk as a bonus. Tell the mother that no matter what method she uses, milk expression is a learned skill and with practice she will get more milk. The key to effective milk expression is to condition her body to respond to the feel of her expression method with milk ejection. This can be as much psychological as it is physical (see next section). Even if a mother expresses just a few drops of milk, tell her she is doing well and encourage her to keep practicing and to expect more within a few days.

Mothers may need to practice milk expression before they are able to do it effectively.

When breastfeeding is going well, the milk available to express will increase over her baby's first 5 weeks or so.

On a baby's first day of life, mothers produce, on average, a little more than 1 ounce (about 37 mL) of colostrum, the first milk (Saint, Smith, & Hartmann, 1984). If breastfeeding goes well, by the time her baby is about 5 weeks old, the average mother will reach her peak milk production of 25 to 35 ounces (750 to 1035 mL) per day (Hill, Aldag, Chatterton, & Zinaman, 2005a). As milk production sharply increases during the first weeks, more milk is available for expression.

After about 5 weeks, daily milk production reaches its peak, and then stays relatively stable—within about 3 to 5 ounces (59 to 148 mL)—until the baby starts other foods at about 6 months, which causes production to gradually decrease (Cohen, Brown, Canahuati, Rivera, & Dewey, 1994). Table 11.1 illustrates how feeding amounts change as baby grows.

Table 11.1. Average Feeding Amount by Age

Baby's Age	Average Milk Per Feeding	Average Milk Intake Per Day
First week	1-2 oz. (30-59 mL)	10-20 oz. (300-600 mL) (after Day 4)
Weeks 2 and 3	2-3 oz. (59-89 mL)	15-25 oz. (450-750 mL)
Month 1-6	3-5 oz. (89-148 mL)	25-35 oz. (750-1035 mL)

(Mohrbacher & Kendall-Tackett, 2005)

Other factors affect how much milk a mother can express at a session.

Exclusively breastfeeding? If a baby also receives other foods or drinks, mothers produce less milk (Cohen et al., 1994; Islam, Peerson, Ahmed, Dewey, & Brown, 2006). Lower milk production means less milk available to express. If a mother is not exclusively breastfeeding, the volume of milk expressed will vary depending on how close she is to full milk production. For example, if a mother is supplying about half her baby's milk intake, she should expect to express about half of what a mother who is exclusively breastfeeding for a baby the same age would express.

Time elapsed since last breastfeeding or expression. The longer a mother waits to express, the more milk she is likely to express—to a point. If she waits 2 hours to express, she is likely to get more milk than if she expressed after 1 hour. But if a mother regularly waits so long to express that her breasts feel full, over time her milk production will slow, and she will express less milk. On average, a mother whose baby is exclusively breastfeeding should expect to express about half a feeding when she expresses between regular feedings and a full feeding if she expresses for a missed breastfeeding. See Table 11.1 for feeding amount by age when exclusively breastfeeding.

The mother's breast storage capacity. Her storage capacity is the maximum volume of milk available to the baby when the breast is at its fullest. Storage capacity varies among mothers and is not necessarily related to breast size. Mothers with a larger storage capacity may be able to express more milk at a session than mothers with a small storage capacity. For details, see p. 399-"Breast Storage Capacity."

Time of day. Most mothers express more milk in the morning than they do later in the day. This may be in part because babies older than a few weeks tend to feed less often during the night, leading to greater milk accumulation by morning (Kent et al., 2006).

Pump quality, fit, and practice time. When a mother expresses with a breast pump, other factors being equal, in general, pumps that cycle 40 to 60 times per minute tend to be more effective at expressing milk than pumps that cycle either more or fewer times per minute (Ramsay, Mitoulas, Kent, Larsson, & Hartmann, 2005).

Pump fit can also affect milk volume (Jones, Dimmock, & Spencer, 2001a; Meier, Motykowski, & Zuleger, 2004). A too-small nipple tunnel (the opening the nipple is drawn into during pumping) can compress milk ducts and slow milk flow. Also, fit can change with time and use, as mothers' nipples expand in size (Wilson-Clay & Hoover, 2008). A mother who had a good fit when she started pumping, may need a larger nipple tunnel as she pumps over time (Meier et al., 2004). For details, see p. 826- "Pump Fit."

Because milk ejection is, in part, a conditioned response, practice with a pump can help a mother's body learn to respond faster to its feel (Kent, Ramsay, Doherty, Larsson, & Hartmann, 2003). With practice, she can learn to trigger more milk ejections and express more milk.

Mothers who are stressed or upset may not be able to express milk effectively.

The mother's emotional state. If a mother feels upset, frustrated, stressed, or angry, this releases adrenaline, which blocks milk ejection (Prime, Geddes, & Hartmann, 2007). It is not unusual for mothers of preterm babies to pump less milk when they receive bad news about their baby's condition (Chatterton et al., 2000). If a mother is experiencing negative feelings and does not express as much milk as usual, suggest she take a break and express later when she is feeling calmer.

Typically, mothers express more milk from one breast than the other.

Studies that measure milk production have found the difference in milk output between breasts to be common and often significant (Engstrom, Meier, Jegier, Motykowski, & Zuleger, 2007; Ramsay et al., 2005). If a mother is concerned because one breast produces more milk, explain that what matters to the baby is getting enough milk overall, not whether each breast produces the same amount. Some differences in milk production may relate to breast usage, as some mothers favor one breast over the other. But one breast may simply be a naturally larger milk producer. One U.S. study of 95 exclusively expressing mothers found that milk output per breast was not associated with a mother's dominant hand, number of children, or previous breastfeeding experience (Hill, Aldag, Zinaman, & Chatterton, 2007). If the mother is concerned about differences in breast size, reassure her that her breasts will return to their pre-pregnancy size after she finishes breastfeeding.

If a baby takes more milk from a bottle than a mother can express, this does not necessarily mean her milk production is low.

Many babies take more milk from a bottle than during a breastfeeding because the bottle provides a more consistent milk flow, which can override a baby's appetite control mechanism and cause overfeeding (Li, Fein, & Grummer-Strawn, 2008; Taveras et al., 2004). At the breast, milk flow varies with milk ejection, so the baby feels full on less milk. Unless there are other signs of low milk production, taking more milk from the bottle does not necessarily indicate a problem with milk production.

The Role of Milk Ejection

During breastfeeding and milk expression, most milk leaves the breast only when a milk ejection occurs. Without a milk ejection, most milk stays in the breast. A milk ejection occurs when the hormone oxytocin is released into the mother's bloodstream, which causes muscles around the milk-producing glands to squeeze and milk ducts to widen, pushing milk out of the breast.

Triggering milk ejections—or let downs—is the key to effective milk expression.

Some mothers feel milk ejection as a tingling feeling, pressure, increased thirst, milk leakage, even pain, while others feel nothing (Ramsay, Kent, Owens, & Hartmann, 2004; Ramsay et al., 2005). When a baby breastfeeds, on average, it takes about a minute for a milk ejection to occur (Ramsay et al., 2004). The most reliable indicator of milk ejection is audible swallowing during breastfeeding and visibly faster milk flow during milk expression.

• •

Australian research found most women average three to four milk ejections during a breastfeeding, with a range of one to 17 (Cobo, 1993; Kent et al., 2008). One Australian study used ultrasound to observe milk ejection during 166 breastfeeding sessions with 45 mothers and found 88% of study mothers felt their first milk ejection, but none felt their subsequent milk ejections (Ramsay et al., 2004). In another Australian study of 11 breastfeeding mothers, four felt more than one milk ejection (Ramsay et al., 2005). Since so many mothers are unaware of more than one milk ejection, even among experienced breastfeeding mothers, many will not know to expect this during milk expression.

Most mothers have multiple milk ejections while breastfeeding and should expect this while expressing.

During breast pumping and breastfeeding, mothers experienced a comparable number of milk ejections (Ramsay & Hartmann, 2005). In this Australian study, multiple milk ejections occurred during 95% of its breast pumping sessions.

How to Express More Milk

More milk ejections during breastfeeding means more milk taken by the baby (Ramsay et al., 2004). This is also true during milk expression, but the law of diminishing returns also applies. Australian breast-pump research found that when the mother's set their breast pump at their highest comfortable vacuum setting, on average during the first milk ejection they expressed a little less than half of their available milk (Kent et al., 2008). "Available milk" is defined as a mother's breast fullness when she begins expressing multiplied by her breast storage capacity. If a mother expresses more milk than her baby takes at his largest breastfeeding, available milk during milk expression can exceed 100%.

With more milk ejections, more milk is expressed—to a point.

As the volume of milk in the breast decreases, milk flow slows. Less milk is expressed with each subsequent milk ejection. See Table 11.2 for the average results of 21 breastfeeding mothers using a hospital-grade double electric breast pump. In this Australian study, after two milk ejections, about 76% of the available milk was expressed (an average milk volume of 90 mL, or 3 ounces). This is 10% more than the 67% taken on average by a baby during a breastfeeding (Kent et al., 2006). With four milk ejections, on average, mothers express about 99% of the available milk. After four milk ejections, the amount of milk expressed continues to decrease. The fifth and sixth milk ejections yield only 7 mL, or about ¼ ounce each.

Table 11.2. Average Volume of Milk Expressed during Each Milk Ejection

Milk ejection	Average % of available milk expressed	Average volume of milk expressed
1st	45%	54 mL (1.8 oz.)
2nd	76%	37 mL (1.3 oz.)
3rd	88%	16 mL (0.5 oz.)
4th	99%	13 mL (0.4 oz.)
5th	104%	7 mL (0.2 oz.)
6th	109%	7 mL (0.2 oz.)
7th	111%	2 mL (0.1 oz.)

Adapted from Kent, 2008

Because these are averages, individual mothers may have different expression patterns, and some may express substantial amounts of milk as time goes on. Encourage each mother to notice as she practices milk expression her own milk output patterns and plan her expression sessions accordingly.

Triggering at least two milk ejections during a milk expression will drain the average mother's breasts as fully as the average breastfeeding baby. Triggering three to four milk ejections will drain her breasts more fully. This may be important if she is trying to stimulate faster milk production or if she needs to offset the effect of fewer milk expressions per day by draining her breasts more fully.

A mother's body can become conditioned to a specific feel and may need extra help when she starts expressing or changes method.

Milk ejection is in part a conditioned response (Kent et al., 2003). This means that when a mother's body becomes used to a particular feel, if this changes she may need extra help to trigger milk ejections. This can happen with an exclusively breastfeeding mother who starts expressing, with a mother who switches from one breast pump to another, or with a mother who switches from hand expression to a breast pump, or vice versa.

Milk ejection can become a conditional response.

An individual mother's responsiveness to different feels will also vary. In one Australian study, 28 mothers tested seven different breast pump cycling patterns (Kent et al., 2003). Half responded well to all seven patterns, while the other half responded well only to some patterns.

How comfortable a mother feels in her setting can also affect her milk flow.

A mother can sometimes get better results when she adjusts her environment.

She may do this in several ways.

Express milk in a familiar and comfortable place, perhaps always sitting in the same comfortable chair, with good arm and back support, so she can relax her entire body.

Minimize distractions. Some mothers start by turning off their phone, playing some relaxing music, and/or gathering what they need, such as a drink, a snack, or something to read. If the mother is at home and has older children, suggest she plan ahead for their needs. If the mother is away from home, suggest she find a comfortable, private place, where she can relax without worrying about interruptions.

Follow a pre-expression ritual. Preparing to express the same way each time can be a psychological trigger for relaxation and milk ejection. Possibilities include:

- Put a blanket or sweater around her shoulders for warmth.
- Use gentle breast massage, gently tap, rub, or roll her nipples for stimulation.
- Spend a minute or two relaxing by using childbirth breathing exercises or just sitting quietly, using mental imagery to picture a warm beach or other relaxing setting.

The mothers in one U.S. study expressed 121% more milk during the 2nd postpartum week while they listened to a 20-minute audiotape on relaxation and visual imagery than they did at other times (Feher, Berger, Johnson, & Wilde, 1989).

• •

If needed, a mother can use her senses and other cues to help trigger milk ejections.

Any of a mother's sensory pathways can trigger milk ejection, as well as her mind and emotions (Cobo, 1993). If at first a mother needs extra help triggering milk ejections, suggest she experiment with the strategies below to see which work best for her. Every mother is different, and she may find that one or two of these strategies work better for her than the others.

- **Sight:** Look at her baby or her baby's photo.
- **Smell:** Smell her baby's blanket or clothing.
- **Touch:** Apply warmth to her breasts using wet or dry heat. Interrupt expressing several times to massage her breasts again.
- **Taste:** Sip her favorite warm drink or have a snack to relax her.
- **Hearing:** Listen to a recording of her baby cooing or crying. If she's away from her baby, call and check on him, or call someone to chat to relax and distract her.
- **Mind/Feelings:** Close her eyes, relax, and imagine the feel of her baby's skin against hers or imagine her baby breastfeeding. Think about how much she loves her baby.

One Canadian article described three women whose nerve pathways between breast and brain were physically damaged and were able to trigger milk releases with mental imagery alone (Cowley, 2005).

• •

When using a breast pump, suggest the mother choose vacuum and cycle settings that produce faster milk flow for faster and greater milk yields.

Pump cycles. If the mother's pump has adjustable cycle speed and her body is conditioned to breastfeeding, suggest she start at a fast speed setting to trigger milk ejection more quickly. However, at milk ejection, suggest she set her pump's cycling speed to slow to drain her breasts faster. This mimics a baby's breastfeeding pattern. As her milk flow slows to a trickle, suggest she return to a fast cycle speed again to more quickly trigger the next milk ejection. Repeat until done, using her milk flow as her guide. She should use whichever pump settings produce faster milk flow.

Some breast pumps can cycle as fast as 120 cycles per minute (cpm), but Australian research found that 86% of mothers express no milk at all at this very fast cycle speed, so suggest the mother minimize any time spent at that setting (Ramsay et al., 2006). (In some pump models that cycle at 120 cpm, this is the first phase of what is referred to as "2-phase" pumping.) Before milk ejection, at a pump setting of 120 cpm mothers average only 1 to 2.7 mL of milk (Kent et al., 2008) compared with 10 mL (about 1/3 ounce) at 60 cpm (Ramsay et al., 2005).

Pump vacuum. Australian research has found that mothers get more milk faster when their pump vacuum is set at the highest comfortable setting during milk ejection (Kent et al., 2008). For more details, see p. 828- "Breast Pump Vacuum (Suction)" in the appendix "Tools and Products."

Pump cycles and vacuum can influence how much milk a mother can pump.

Encourage the mother to experiment with her pump controls, as individual mothers respond differently to the same stimuli. For example, one U.S. study found that when mothers began expressing with a pump set at a fixed cycle speed (50 cpm), time to milk ejection was delayed by a full minute when they switched to a pump that began at 120 cpm (Meier et al., 2008). As the mother experiments with her breast pump's settings, encourage her to use those settings that produce the fastest milk flow.

If milk ejection is an issue, suggest the mother express from one breast while the baby breastfeeds on the other.

In most cases, the baby will stimulate milk ejection quickly while the mother expresses from the other breast. Some mothers hand-express with their free hand, using pillows to help support the baby's weight at the other breast, or use a breast pump that can be operated with one hand. Expressing while the baby is at the breast can help condition a mother's body to the feel of her expression method, so that eventually she can have milk ejections when her baby is not at the breast.

If a mother's milk ejection is blocked or delayed because she is upset or stressed, suggest she try to relax or try expressing later.

A mother going through an emotional or physical crisis may find her milk ejection is temporarily affected. In extreme situations, this may temporarily affect her milk production. If this happens, encourage the mother to continue breastfeeding and/or expressing. Assure her that milk ejection and production will quickly return to normal.

MILK EXPRESSION METHODS

Choosing a Method

The most popular expression methods vary by locale.

In developing areas, hand expression is used more commonly than breast pumps because pumps are beyond many mothers' means and power sources are not always always available (Glynn & Goosen, 2005). In developed areas, mothers' preferences vary. One Australian study found that at 4 weeks postpartum, manual pumps were most popular (64%), followed by electric pumps (20%) and hand expression (16%) (Win et al., 2006). Another Australian study compared expression methods during the first 6 months postpartum in 1992 and 2002, and found in both years, 60% of mother used manual pumps, but over the course of this decade the use of electric pumps increased threefold (Binns et al., 2006).

Many U.S. mothers use more than one method and own more than one type of breast pump, which is why the following totals more than 100% (Labiner-Wolfe et al., 2008): electric breast pumps (60%), manual pumps (35%), combination pumps powered by battery and electricity (18%), hand expression (10%), and battery-powered pumps (3%).

A mother's expression needs will vary by preferences and frequency of expression.

If a mother asks for help in choosing an expression method, to better understand her situation, ask her the following questions:

- **How often will she express her milk?** The mother who is separated from her hospitalized baby will have very different milk-expression needs from the mother who wants to express milk for an occasional missed feeding.
- **Is she familiar with any methods and does she have a preference?** If so, discuss the pros and cons of her preferred method in her situation (see next point) and mention other methods that could also work well for her, so she can make an informed choice. If the mother has no preference, offer to describe the choices appropriate in her situation. For details on the suitability of different types of breast pumps for different situations, see Table 11.3 on p. 458.

Discuss the advantages and disadvantages of hand expression and breast pumps.

Some advantages of hand expression over a breast pump include:

- It's free of charge.
- The skin-to-skin contact more easily triggers milk ejection in some women compared to the feel of a plastic or glass pump flange.
- Some say it feels more "natural."
- It requires no electricity, batteries, or other external power sources.
- There are no "fit" issues.
- No special equipment is needed, and it is always available, even in emergencies.
- There is nothing to store or transport.
- Only the mother's hands need to be washed afterwards.

- It's the "green" way to express milk, with no use of power and no solid waste.

Some drawbacks of hand expression are:

- There is a learning curve.
- It requires physical effort and can become tiring.
- It may take more time if a mother expresses one breast at a time.
- It is not as effective as a hospital-grade breast pump at establishing milk production when a baby is not yet breastfeeding (Slusher et al., 2007).

Some advantages of breast pumps over hand expression include:

- Automatic pumps do the physical work of expressing for her.
- Double pumps usually express more milk in less time.
- Some mothers are more familiar with breast pumps.
- Some mothers don't know how to hand express or where to learn.
- Some mothers feel uncomfortable touching their breasts.
- Some mothers have limited hand movement or chronic wrist or hand pain.
- Some employers provide a breast pump at work.
- Double-pumping allows mothers to work while expressing.
- Hospital-grade breast pumps are more effective at establishing milk production when a baby is not yet breastfeeding (Slusher et al., 2007).

Disadvantages of breast pumps include:

- The most effective pumps are beyond some mothers' means and cheaper pumps may be ineffective or painful.
- Pump parts can break, get lost, or be left behind by mistake, rendering the pump nonfunctional.
- Power sources may not always be available.
- The pump's sound may draw unwelcome attention.
- A place to wash her pump parts may not always be available.

A combination of pumping and hand expression may yield more milk than either method alone.

Expressing milk does not have to be an "either/or" choice. Some U.S. research suggests that a mother may get significantly more milk by using hand expression after she pumps to drain her breasts more completely, especially while establishing her milk production after birth (Morton et al., 2009). U.K. research has also found that breast massage during breast pumping increases milk output significantly (Jones, Dimmock, & Spencer, 2001b). For details, see the later section "Establishing Milk Production."

If a mother can't express milk effectively with a pump, suggest she try hand expression.

While most mothers find breast pumps effective (Ortiz, McGilligan, & Kelly, 2004), a few mothers do not. If none of the suggestions for increasing pumping effectiveness has worked, suggest the mother try hand expression.

Hand Expression

Suggest the mother practice and experiment until hand expression works well for her.

Hand expression can relieve breast fullness, stimulate milk production, and provide milk for the baby. It is a useful skill that every breastfeeding mother should know.

If the expressed milk will be fed to her baby, suggest the mother first wash her hands well. The mother needs a clean collection container with a wide mouth, such as a cup. If she plans to feed her newborn after expressing, she could also use a clean spoon. To help her relax, encourage her to express in a private, comfortable place with good body support.

Hand expression is a useful skill every new mother should know.

Effective hand-expression techniques vary from mother to mother. What's most important is that each mother finds her own "sweet spot" on her breasts for best milk flow. Instructions that recommend finger placement using the areola as a guide can be misleading because of the large variation in areola size. Mothers with very large areolae may find their sweet spot within their areola and mothers with small areolae may find their sweet spot well away from it. When a mother is in the early learning stages, one U.S. video by Jane Morton, M.D. (see link below), suggests the mother apply small circle bandaids to these "sweet spots" to make them easier to find again the next time. Suggest the mother tailor any instructions to her own comfort and results.

Hand-expression instructions vary by instructor (Becker & Roberts, 2009). The following technique is a combination of several, including one from the World Health Organization (WHO, 2009):

1. Before expressing, spend some time gently massaging the breasts with hands and fingertips, a soft baby brush, or a warm towel.
2. Sit up, leaning slightly forward to allow gravity to help milk flow.
3. At the first expression, to find the "sweet spots" on the breast, start by putting thumb on top of the breast and fingers below the breast about 1.5 inches (4 cm) from the nipple. Apply steady pressure into the breast toward the chest wall a few times. If no milk comes, shift finger and thumb placement farther away or closer to the nipple and compress again a few times. Repeat, moving finger and thumb until slightly firmer breast tissue is felt and pressure yields milk. At future hand expressions, skip the "finding" phase and place fingers directly on this area.
4. Apply steady pressure into the breast toward the chest wall, not toward the nipple. The idea is to put pressure on areas of milk within the breast.
5. As this inward pressure is applied, compress the pads of the thumb and fingers together (pushing in, not pulling out toward the nipple), finding a good rhythm of press—compress—relax, like a baby's suckling pattern.
6. Alternate breasts every few minutes (5 or 6 times in total at each expression), rotating finger position, so that all areas of the breast are expressed and feel soft, which usually takes about 20 to 30 minutes.

Avoid sliding the fingers along the skin. See a video demonstration of one version of this technique at http://newborns.stanford.edu/Breastfeeding/HandExpression.html).

If the mother reports pain or discomfort, she may be compressing too hard, sliding her fingers along the skin, or squeezing the nipple itself, which can be both ineffective and painful. Ask her to describe what she is doing to determine what changes are needed.

With practice, a mother may be able to hand express while her baby breastfeeds or express both breasts simultaneously.

To hand-express milk while baby is at the breast, some mothers use pillows or cushions to support the baby's body, so they have both hands free. Some mothers learn to hand-express milk from both breasts simultaneously, with the right hand expressing the right breast and the left hand expressing the left breast, with collection containers on a stable surface at breast level.

The Warm Bottle Method

The Warm Bottle method is a low-tech way to provide relief to an engorged mother.

A kind of middle ground between hand expression and a breast pump, the Warm Bottle method can be ideal for an engorged mother without access to an effective breast pump who has not mastered hand expression or whose breasts are so taut that hand expression is difficult.

To use this method, a mother needs a glass bottle with a mouth about 2 inches (5 cm) wide and access to hot water.

Any clean glass bottle with a mouth diameter of at least 2 inches (5 cm) will work. A 1 liter or larger bottle is ideal. To use this method, suggest the mother:

- Slowly fill the bottle with hot water and let it stand for a few minutes.
- Wrap a cloth around the bottle and pour out the hot water.
- Allow the neck of the bottle to cool and then place the mouth over the mother's nipple and areola to form an airtight seal.
- As the bottle cools slowly, gentle suction is created, which draws the breast into the bottle's neck. The warmth of the bottle and the gentle suction usually triggers a milk ejection, expressing milk.
- When the milk flow slows, break the suction and remove the breast.
- If discomfort is felt break the suction. (Limit the time the bottle is on the breast.)
- Pour out the milk and repeat on the other breast.

If the glass bottle and the mother's hands are clean, this milk can be stored or fed. Avoid too-rapid cooling, as it causes more suction, which can lead to discomfort.

Breast Pumps

If a mother asks for help in choosing a breast pump, ask her about her situation, including how often she plans to pump.

For the mother who pumps daily for missed feedings, choosing the right type of pump can determine whether or not she meets her breastfeeding goals. Over the years, more effective pumps have become more generally available, but there are also painful and ineffective pumps on store shelves.

If a mother asks which pump is best for her, the answer will depend on her situation and her means. If a breast pump plays a major role in maintaining milk production, suggest the mother choose carefully. Examples include the mother who has a non-breastfeeding baby or the mother who is away from her young baby 30 or more hours per week and plans to provide only her milk for missed feedings.

The pump's type, cycles per minute (cpm), durability, and fit options determine whether it is suitable for specific situations.

One important factor to know when choosing an automatic or semi-automatic pump is its cycles per minute (cpm) - the number of times every minute the pump vacuum builds, peaks, and releases. This variable distinguishes, in part, more effective from less effective breast pumps. For a mother using her pump daily to replace missed feedings, in most cases the best choice would be an automatic double pump that generates at least 40 to 60 suction-and-release cycles per minute. A pump that can cycle in this range is generally considered most effective at establishing and maintaining milk production (Ramsay et al., 2005).

In addition to its cycling, another factor important for regular use is whether the pump offers different "fit options" or different diameter nipple tunnels (the area the mother's nipple is drawn into during pumping). Because one size does not fit all and because mother's fit can change with regular pumping (Meier et al., 2004; Wilson-Clay & Hoover, 2008), having access to multiple sizes is important. Durability also helps determine which pumps are designed for frequent use, so suggest the mother look for a pump with at least a 1-year warranty on the motor. Pump choices in this category include rental pumps and high-end, mother-owned double automatic pumps. See Table 11.3.

A mother who relies less on her breast pump for maintaining milk production will have more options, such as one who is away from her baby less than 30 hours per week or one who plans to provide other foods, such as formula or solids, for missed feedings.

When a mother misses feedings less often than once a day, this is generally considered "occasional use," and automatic pumps that generate 30 or fewer cycles per minute may be effective enough in this situation. Also an option for occasional use are semi-automatic pumps that require a mother to either generate or release pump suction by covering a hole or pushing a button or bar. Manual pumps—which are powered by squeezing a handle or some other physical action—also work well for some mothers in this situation, although some mothers tire of them quickly because they require muscle power to operate. They also require practice to find the rhythm that most quicly triggers milk ejection.

Individual mothers respond differently to different breast pumps, so there may be exceptions to the general guidelines in Table 11.3. There may also be situations that fall in between those listed, such as the mother who pumps for daily missed feedings 3 days per week rather than 5. This mother's best choice may depend on whether the 3 days she's away are in a row or if she has days at home with her baby in between.

Table 11.3. Types of Breast Pumps Best Suited for Different Situations

	Manual pump	**Semi-automatic pump**	**Automatic single/ double pump (<40 cpm)**	**Mother-owned automatic single/double pump (≥40 cpm, multiple fit options, 1-yr.warranty on motor)**	**Rental**
Pumping for <1 missed feedings/day	x	x	x	x	x
Pumping daily for missed feedings ≥5 days/week				x	x
Baby not breastfeeding: Establishing full milk production					x
Baby not breastfeeding: Maintaining full milk production				x	x

Adapted from (Jones & Tully, 2006) and (Mohrbacher & Stock, 2003)

Whatever breast pump a mother chooses, suggest she make sure she has a good fit.

The diameter of the nipple tunnel (the area the mother's breast is drawn into during pumping) varies among pumps. If the nipple tunnel is too large or small, this can result in less milk expressed, pain, or trauma. Some brands offer different nipple-tunnel sizes. For more details, see p. 826- "Pump Fit" in the appendix "Tools and Products."

Suggest a mother with less than 20 minutes to express consider a double breast pump; if single-pumping, suggest she frequently switch breasts.

Double pumps save time (Becker, McCormick, & Renfrew, 2008). If a mother uses a single pump, she must express one breast at a time, which usually takes about 20 to 30 minutes total. A double pump allows her to pump both breasts at the same time, which can cut her expression time in half.

Suggest the mother who is single-pumping switch breasts when the milk flow slows, usually every 5 to 7 minutes, and plan to express from each breast several times each pumping. Because both breasts should be well drained using this approach, the milk's fat content should be the same as if the mother double-pumped. Alternating breast stimulation may more effectively trigger milk ejection (Morton et al., 2009).

MILK STORAGE AND HANDLING

Milk Storage Guidelines

For Full-Term, Healthy Babies

The live cells in freshly expressed human milk kill bacteria, keeping milk fresh longer. Two Spanish studies found that when freshly expressed human milk is refrigerated its bacteria-killing properties stay active for the first few days, but begin to decline after 72 hours (Martinez-Costa et al., 2007; Silvestre, Lopez, March, Plaza, & Martinez-Costa, 2006).

Human milk takes longer to spoil than pasteurized cow's milk because its live cells kill bacteria.

• •

One U.S. study found no statistically significant differences between the bacterial levels of milk stored for 10 hours at room temperature and milk refrigerated for 10 hours, when a temperature range of 66°F to 72°F (19°C to 22°C) was maintained (Barger & Bull, 1987). But "room temperature" varies greatly by season and geography. While the temperature range used in this study is common in Chicago's temperate climate where this study took place, it is rare in tropical climates. Another U.S. study found that storing expressed milk at a slightly warmer temperature—77°F (25°C)—shortened safe storage time to 4 hours (Hamosh, Ellis, Pollock, Henderson, & Hamosh, 1996).

Storage guidelines for milk kept at room temperature vary by temperature.

Research done in Nigeria's tropical climate found that colostrum—which inhibits bacteria growth more effectively than mature milk—could be safely stored at 81°F to 90°F (27°C to 32°C) for up to 12 hours (Nwankwo, Offor, Okolo, & Omene, 1988).

• •

One U.S. study, which attempted to more closely replicate the conditions mothers face daily, found that milk stored at slightly below room temperature (60° F/15° C) stayed fresh for up to 24 hours (Hamosh et al., 1996).

Fresh milk can be safely stored in an insulated cooler bag with frozen ice packs for at least 24 hours.

• •

Suggest the mother store her milk in the back of the refrigerator and away from the door, where there is greater temperature fluctuation. Early research on refrigerated milk limited its study period to 24 hours (Pittard, Anderson, Cerutti, & Boxerbaum, 1985). Later research that extended the study period to 5 days found that bacterial counts continued to be low this entire time (Sosa & Barness, 1987). A Belgian study found that after 8 days of refrigeration some batches of milk actually had bacterial levels lower than when the milk was first expressed (Pardou, Serruys, Mascart-Lemone, Dramaix, & Vis, 1994). These researchers concluded that milk used within 8 days should be refrigerated, rather than frozen, because the antimicrobial qualities of human milk are better preserved by refrigeration.

Storage guidelines for milk kept in a refrigerator vary by criteria and the baby's health.

If bacterial count (one gauge of milk spoilage) is the only factor considered, the 8-day guideline for refrigerated milk makes sense. But when milk is refrigerated longer than 72 hours, other changes occur, such as a decrease in vitamin C levels and antioxidant properties (Buss, McGill, Darlow, & Winterbourn, 2001; Hanna et al., 2004). For this reason, some recommend mothers use refrigerated milk within a shorter time, such as 72 hours or 5 days (ABM, 2009; Meek, 2002). If a baby is ill or preterm, shorter guidelines may also be used (see later section "For the Hospitalized Baby").

Although it is always better to use expressed milk sooner rather than later, if a mother of a young baby finds an 8-day-old container of expressed milk in the back of her refrigerator, she should consider her situation. If she has more expressed milk available, she may decide to discard the older milk. But if her only other option is to give infant formula, using the stored milk would be the better choice. When in doubt, suggest the mother smell her milk. Spoiled milk usually smells sour.

Storage guidelines for frozen milk vary based on type of freezer.

Milk storage guidelines for frozen milk are based on the temperature fluctuation expected in each freezer type:

- Freezer compartment located inside a refrigerator—2 weeks
- Separate-door refrigerator/freezer—3 to 4 months
- Deep freeze—6 to 12 months

Suggest the mother store her milk in the back of the freezer away from the door and fluctuating temperatures. If stored in a refrigerator/freezer, suggest the mother put her milk on a rack or shelf above the freezer floor to avoid warming during the automatic defrost cycle (Walker, 2006). Before freezing, suggest the mother fill the container no more than about three-quarters full to allow for the normal expansion of the milk during freezing and to tighten bottle caps after the milk is completely frozen to allow displaced air to escape (Jones & Tully, 2006). For more details, see Table 11.4.

Before freezing too much milk, suggest the mother thaw some frozen milk to see if it smells soapy or rancid.

When a mother's cooled or frozen milk develops a soapy smell, this is probably due to high levels of lipase, the enzyme that breaks down fat. Depending on her milk lipase level, some mothers notice this change in smell and/or taste after a short time in the freezer, or later after the milk has been frozen longer. Freezing slows but does not stop the lipase from digesting the fat in the milk (Berkow et al., 1984; Bitman, Wood, Mehta, Hamosh, & Hamosh, 1983).

This milk is considered safe for the baby, and in most cases, the baby will accept it (Lawrence & Lawrence, 2005). But if the baby refuses the milk, the mother can prevent this change in smell and/or taste from occurring by scalding her milk before storing it, which will deactivate the lipase. This is done by heating the milk in a pan on the stove until it is bubbling around the edges, but not yet boiling, and then cooling the milk quickly (Jones & Tully, 2006). Although heating milk is not routinely recommended, if the baby will not accept expressed milk otherwise, this may be the only way the mother's milk can be used.

To avoid having to discard large amounts of frozen milk, suggest any mother planning to freeze her milk first freeze several test batches, thaw them after about a week, and smell the milk to see if its smell or taste has changed. If it has, suggest she check to see if her baby will take it. If the baby accepts it, the mother doesn't need to do anything else. If the baby rejects it, suggest she scald future batches before freezing.

Sour or rancid-smelling milk is probably unrelated to milk lipase levels. According to some milk storage experts, the most likely cause is chemical oxidation, rather than lipase-caused digestion of milk fat or bacterial contamination (Jones & Tully, 2006). Possible contributing factors are the mother's intake of polyunsaturated fats or free copper or iron ions in her water. In this case, heating the milk can actually speed oxidation, making the problem worse. While she is storing milk for her baby, suggest any mother whose expressed milk smells rancid or sour temporarily avoid her usual drinking water and any fish-oil or flaxseed supplements, as well as any foods like anchovies that contain rancid fats. While handling her milk, suggest she also avoid exposing it to her local water. It may also help to increase her antioxidant intake by taking beta carotene and vitamin E.

Table 11.4. Mature Milk Storage Times for Full-Term Healthy Babies at Home

Milk Storage/ Handling	**Deep Freeze** (0°F/ -18°C)	**Refrigerator/ Freezer** (variable 0°F/-18°C)	**Refrigerator** (39°F/4°C)	**Insulated Cooler with Ice Packs** (59°F/15°C)	**Room Temperature** (66°F-72°F/19°C-22°C)	(73°F-77°F/23°C-25°C)
Fresh	Ideal: 6 mos. Okay: 12 mos.	3-4 Months	Ideal: 72 Hours Okay: 8 days	24 Hours	6-10 Hours	4 Hours
Frozen, Thawed in Fridge	Do Not Refreeze	Do Not Refreeze	24 Hours	Do Not Store	4 Hours	4 Hours
Thawed, Warmed, Not Fed	Do Not Refreeze	Do Not Refreeze	4 Hours	Do Not Store	Until Feeding Ends	Until Feeding Ends
Warmed, Fed	Discard	Discard	Discard	Discard	Until Feeding Ends	Until Feeding Ends

(Jones & Tully, 2006; LLLI, 2008)

Milk that collects in breast shells, or "drip milk," should be discarded.

Milk that collects in breast shells tends to be lower in fat than actively expressed milk (Lucas, Gibbs, & Baum, 1978). It has also been found to contain higher levels of common skin bacteria (Gessler, Bischoff, Wiegand, Essers, & Bossart, 2004), probably due to prolonged skin contact. For these reasons, current guidelines recommend mothers discard this "drip milk" rather than storing it or feeding it to their babies (Jones & Tully, 2006).

Current guidelines recommend against refreezing thawed human milk.

The safety of refreezing thawed milk is most likely only going to be a major issue during a power outage for the mother with a large stash of frozen milk. One U.S. study researched the effects of refreezing milk using donor milk expressed by mothers who used no special sanitary precautions (Rechtman, Lee, & Berg, 2006). The frozen milk was thawed at refrigerator temperature (39° F /4°C) overnight, separated into different sample batches, and refrozen to -80°C (-110°F). These sample batches were later thawed to room temperature (73°F/23°C) and each batch exposed to one of the following conditions: 46°F (8°C) for 8 or 24 hours,

73°F (23°C) for 4 or 8 hours, multiple freeze-thaw cycles of varying lengths, and the control batch kept at a steady -4°F (-20°C). None of the batches developed unacceptable bacterial counts and vitamin content remained at adequate levels. As of this writing, guidelines to not refreeze milk have not yet been changed to reflect this research.

• •

Current guidelines recommend against saving any milk left in the container after a feeding.

Mothers are often told to discard any milk left after a feeding because the milk mixes with the baby's saliva. Although no published studies have examined the safety of keeping leftover milk, a college student researched this scenario for her unpublished senior thesis (Brusseau, 1998). In her study, she divided fresh milk donated from six women into two bottles, one of which was warmed and partially fed to their babies. The leftover milk and the milk in the bottle not fed (the control milk) were cultured immediately after feeding and 12, 24, 36, and 48 hours later. The only milk with increased total bacterial counts was one batch of the warmed and fed milk from a mother who had not followed instructions and had donated previously frozen instead of fresh milk. All other batches of milk showed no change in total bacterial counts within 48 hours after feeding.

Don't save milk left in a container after feeding.

• •

Each batch of milk should be labeled with the date, and in some cases, the baby's name and the time it was expressed.

Including the day, month, and year on the milk-storage container will allow the milk to be used in the order it was expressed. If the milk will be given in a group setting, such as a hospital or day-care facility, the baby's name should also be written on each container. If the mother is expressing milk for her preterm baby or to donate to a milk bank, she may also be asked to label it with the time of day it was expressed.

• •

To avoid waste, store milk in amounts no larger than the baby might take at a feeding.

For the baby older than about 1 month, suggest the mother start by freezing her milk in 2- to 4-ounce (60-118 mL) quantities, which is about how much babies on average take from the breast (Kent et al., 2006). Small amounts thaw and warm faster, and less milk will be discarded if the baby does not take it all. If the baby wants more milk, it can always be added. Before she learns how much milk is right for her baby, suggest she store some smaller 1- to 2-ounce (30-59 mL) amounts to provide a little extra if needed.

• •

On average, breastfed babies take much less milk per day than babies fed formula.

Although there is a large range of normal milk intakes among breastfeeding babies (Kent et al., 2006), the baby receiving only mother's milk usually takes less milk per day than the baby receiving formula. One U.S. study found that at 4 months of age breastfeeding babies consumed on average 25% fewer calories than formula-fed babies of the same age, even though their weight gains were comparable (Butte, Garza, Smith, & Nichols, 1984). Another U.S. study found that at 6 months breastfed babies, on average, consume 23% less milk than their formula-feeding counterparts (Heinig, Nommsen, Peerson, Lonnerdal, & Dewey, 1993). This could be important information for the mother who is gauging her baby's milk needs on her neighbor's formula-fed baby. (For more details on the reasons for this difference, see p. 207- "Growth from Birth to 12 Months."

When batches of expressed milk are combined, the milk should be dated according to the oldest milk. For example, if refrigerated milk from May 10 is combined with milk expressed on May 11, the combined batch should be dated May 10. Although some groups recommend restricting batches to milk expressed the same day (ABM, 2009), at this writing there is no evidence to support this restriction.

The mother can combine milk expressed at different times.

Fresh milk can be added directly to refrigerated milk without cooling it first. Fresh milk can be added to frozen milk, as long as there is less fresh milk than frozen milk, and it is first cooled for about an hour, so it does not thaw the top layer.

A Brazilian study found low levels of live yeast in human milk that was previously frozen and thawed (Rosa, Novak, de Almeida, Medonca-Hagler, & Hagler, 1990) and concluded that freezing milk may not kill yeast. However, the researchers acknowledge the possibility that the milk became contaminated with live yeast during its handling. There is currently no evidence to indicate that milk expressed and stored during a nipple infection or thrush in baby's mouth can cause a recurrence. If the mother is concerned, an alternative to discarding stored milk is to boil it before feeding, as boiling kills yeast.

It is unknown whether milk stored during a candida infection can cause a recurrence.

For Hospitalized Babies

Any mother of a preterm or sick baby needs to ask about milk-storage protocols at her hospital. In some institutions, sterile storage containers are provided and special labeling processes followed (Hurst & Meier, 2010). The hospital may also specify how much milk to put in each container and provide storage times for refrigerated and frozen milk that differ from those for home use. For sick or preterm babies, the Human Milk Banking Association of North America recommends expressed milk be refrigerated immediately, rather than allowing it to stay at room temperature. Milk storage guidelines will also differ if fortifier is added to the mother's milk (Jones & Tully, 2006). Human milk is not sterile, and bacteriologic screening is not usually recommended because there are currently no generally agreed upon acceptable levels of bacteria in the milk (Jones & Tully, 2006; Law, Urias, Lertzman, Robson, & Romance, 1989).

Suggest the mother of a hospitalized baby check with the staff for its milk storage guidelines, which vary by institution.

Preterm and sick babies are at higher risk for serious and even life-threatening health problems, so stricter hygiene precautions are needed. Simple steps like hand-washing before expressing milk can be critical in preventing contamination of the milk (Novak, Da Silva, Hagler, & Figueiredo, 2000). For more details, see p. 355- "Milk Handling and Safety."

Stricter hygiene precautions are needed when storing milk for ill or preterm babies.

In previous years, breast-washing and discarding the first drops of milk were routinely recommended to mothers of vulnerable babies to try to decrease milk contamination. However, research found no difference in milk contamination when these procedures were followed, so they are no longer recommended (Jones & Tully, 2006).

Washing the breast before expressing and discarding the first few drops of milk are no longer recommended.

Handling and Preparing Milk

Before storing milk, any reusable storage container should be washed in hot, soapy water, rinsed well, and air dried.

Washing, rinsing, and drying storage containers, along with good hand-washing by the mother, have been found sufficient to prevent milk contamination (Jones & Tully, 2006; Pittard, Geddes, Brown, Mintz, & Hulsey, 1991). Regular sterilization or sanitization of milk storage containers or pump parts is not currently recommended because no benefits to these extra procedures have been found.

Expressed milk separates into layers over time and its color may vary.

Layers. Because most mothers are familiar with the appearance of homogenized cow's milk, some worry when their expressed milk separates into milk and cream. Reassure the mother this separation is normal in any milk that is not homogenized. Before the milk is fed to the baby, suggest it first be swirled gently to mix the layers.

Colors. Usually human milk appears either bluish, yellowish, or even brownish in color. When a mother consumes some foods, food dyes, and medications, her milk may change color to pink or pink-orange (orange soda or gelatins), green (kelp or green drinks) , and even black (minocycline) (Lawrence & Lawrence, 2005). Frozen milk may take on a yellowish color, but it is not spoiled unless it smells or tastes sour.

Suggest the mother thaw frozen milk gently and gradually, keeping heat low.

Freezing and heating human milk destroys some of its immune properties that kill bacteria, making it more vulnerable to contamination. When thawing or warming milk, keep heat low, using one of the following methods:

- Thaw in the refrigerator overnight. Once thawed, milk can be refrigerated for up to 24 hours.
- Hold the container under cool running water for a few minutes.
- Hold the container in water that has been previously heated on the stove. If the water cools and the milk is not yet thawed, remove the container of milk and reheat the water. Do not heat the milk on the stove burner directly.

If using water to thaw or warm the milk, tilt or hold the container, so the water cannot seep under the lid. Thawed milk should not be kept at room temperature. It should be either fed immediately or refrigerated (Jones & Tully, 2006).

Before feeding, expressed milk can be warmed to between room and body temperature.

Older babies often willingly drink chilled milk directly from the refrigerator (Jones & Tully, 2006; LLLI, 2008). But for a small baby, cold milk may lower body temperature. To warm milk before feeding, hold the container under warm running water or hold it in a pan of water that has been previously heated on the stove.

A microwave should not be used to thaw or warm mother's milk.

Two U.S. studies found that heating human milk in a microwave oven destroys much of its anti-infective factors, such as IgA (Quan et al., 1992; Sigman, Burke, Swarner, & Shavlik, 1989). They also found that microwaves heat liquids unevenly, so even if the milk is swirled or shaken afterwards, "hot spots" remain that can burn the baby's throat.

In the U.S., according to the Centers for Disease Control and Prevention, the American Academy of Pediatrics, and the Occupational Safety and Health Administration (OSHA), human milk is not considered a biohazardous material, so rubber gloves are not needed when human milk is handled or fed, nor is a separate refrigerator required (CDC, 1994). At workplaces and at child care facilities, human milk can be stored along with other foods in a common refrigerator and no special precautions are needed.

Human milk is not a biohazardous substance, so no gloves or other special precautions are needed when handling it.

Storage Containers

Any food-grade container with a tight-fitting, solid lid (rather than one with a nipple/teat) can be used to store expressed milk. If the baby gets most of his nourishment from direct breastfeeding and only occasionally receives expressed milk, the type of storage container is not a major concern. But when a baby receives most of his nourishment from expressed milk, the storage container should be chosen carefully.

Glass and plastic containers with solid, tight-fitting lids are recommended for both hospital and home use.

Unfortunately, there are few studies on storage containers and their conclusions are conflicting, so current recommendations are based on very limited information. For example, one U.S. study found that more of the milk's leukocytes adhered to glass rather than plastic, which led to the recommendation that fresh milk be stored in plastic (Paxson & Cress, 1979). At that time, glass continued to be recommended for freezing because freezing kills most leukocytes anyway. A second U.S. study found that different types of leukocytes react differently to glass (Pittard & Bill, 1981). A third U.S. study convinced many to recommend glass again when it was found that over time many of the leukocytes were released from the glass, and after 24 hours milk stored in glass had more leukocytes than the milk stored in plastic (Goldblum, Garza, Johnson, Harrist, & Nichols, 1981).

Some recommend glass as a good first choice for freezing milk because it is the least porous, thus providing the best protection.

Some caution against storing milk in polycarbonate plastic containers, which contain the chemical bisphenol-A (BPA), due to concerns that under certain conditions this chemical could leach into the milk, which is associated with potential health risks (LLLI, 2008).

Many mothers find milk storage bags have practical advantages. They take up less storage space than hard-sided containers and can be attached directly to breast pump attachments in place of a bottle. Because they are not reused, there is less to wash.

Milk freezer bags can be used to store expressed milk for home use.

Types of milk bags. Some types of milk bags are sturdier than others. For example, some bags called "bottle liners" are made primarily for feeding rather than milk storage. These feeding bags tend to be thinner and more prone to splitting. If this type of bag is used to store milk, suggest the mother safeguard her milk by first inserting her bag of milk inside another bag before sealing and storing.

Why home use only? Milk freezer bags are not usually recommended for hospitalized babies because they are not airtight like hard-sided containers, and there is a greater risk of leaking (Jones & Tully, 2006; Walker, 2006). One U.S. study found a 60% decrease in some antibodies when milk was stored in bags, along with a partial loss of milk fat, which adhered to the sides of the bags (Goldblum et al., 1981). However, only the thin, "bottle liners" were studied, so these findings may not apply to the thicker freezer bags, and these results have not been duplicated. Some recommend milk freezer bags only for milk intended to be stored for less than 72 hours (ABM, 2009).

Sandwich bags. Storing expressed milk in plastic sandwich bags is not recommended because they are thin and tear easily (Jones & Tully, 2006).

Stainless steel storage containers are not recommended because fewer live cells survive.

Two studies from India compared the survival of live cells in freshly expressed milk when stored in glass or polypropylene plastic storage containers and in stainless steel containers. One study compared glass to stainless steel and found that more live cells survived and fewer stuck to the sides in glass, rather than stainless steel containers (Williamson & Murti, 1996). In the other study, significantly more live cells survived in the polypropylene plastic containers than the stainless steel containers (Manohar, Williamson, & Koppikar, 1997).

MILK EXPRESSION STRATEGIES

When Baby Isn't Breastfeeding

In some situations, effective milk expression is vital to longer breastfeeding duration.

Effective milk expression becomes critical when a baby cannot breastfeed after birth due to illness, prematurity, or other reasons, and expression must take the baby's place in establishing milk production. Effective expression is also vital when a mother needs to maintain her milk production temporarily, such as during a nursing strike and when a mother takes a medication that is incompatible with breastfeeding. This section describes expression strategies that can help mothers in different situations meet their breastfeeding goals.

Establishing Full Milk Production After Birth

Some mothers have negative feelings about exclusive milk expression, especially at first.

Mothers who are unexpectedly faced with milk expression instead of a breastfeeding baby may need to talk about their feelings and make some emotional adjustments. Some of these mothers feel odd or awkward. Some have mentioned feeling "like a cow." If the baby is ill or very preterm, a mother may need to grieve the normal birth and breastfeeding she was expecting before she can accept her situation. One Australian longitudinal study of 17 mothers and fathers of very-low-birthweight preterm babies found that the mothers had very mixed emotions about milk expression, considering it a symbol of both their connection to their baby and their disconnection from their baby while others provided primary care (Sweet, 2008).

When mothers are expressing milk for their babies, they may need to grieve normal breastfeeding before they can accept their situation.

Some mothers decide to exclusively express their milk and bottle-feed when their baby could be breastfeeding.

In some developed areas, increasing numbers of mothers are choosing to forgo breastfeeding for exclusive milk expression. This may be due to increased recognition of the importance of mother's milk to baby's health, along with greater access to effective expression methods.

Mothers give many reasons for this decision (Mohrbacher, 1996). Some become so comfortable expressing for their hospitalized preterm baby that it seems easier to continue this familiar routine after discharge (Geraghty et al., 2005). Some are faced with a breastfeeding problem they can't solve. Some erroneously think it will save them time, especially during the intense early weeks. Some are emotionally uncomfortable with the intimacy of breastfeeding.

If a mother could be breastfeeding, offer to help her meet her own goals before discussing transitioning baby to the breast.

The most important thing to say first to any mother wanting information about exclusive milk expression is: "I can help you. I have the information you need to make this work." When mothers are told first why they should transition to breastfeeding, they often tune this out and contact someone else.

When a mother knows exclusive expressing is possible and that she can learn how to do it, it is important for her to know that exclusive expressing takes much more time and work than direct breastfeeding—often double or triple the time due to the time it takes to express, feed, and clean equipment. Some mothers are unaware of this and may be motivated by this information to breastfeed instead.

The mother struggling with a breastfeeding problem needs to know that most problems are fixable and how to solve hers. However, in some cases, she may say that she and her baby are so stressed from working on breastfeeding that they need a break. If so, be sure she knows that even if she takes a break from breastfeeding, she can go back to it later when she and her baby are feeling more relaxed and ready. For details, see the later section on p. 476, "Transitioning to the Breast."

Stage 1: The First Few Days

If the mother's goal is to establish full milk production, encourage her to try to get there by around Day 10 postpartum.

Full milk production is about 750 to 1035 mL (25 to 35 ounces) per baby per day (Butte et al., 1984; Hurst & Meier, 2010). Make sure the mother knows that once she reaches this level, this is as much milk as her baby will ever need, no matter how big he gets (see p. 401- "Making Milk During the First Year and Beyond"). A mother's body is hormonally primed and ready to make milk during the first weeks after birth, and the research-based milk-expression strategies in this section and the next can be used to help her reach this goal.

Suggest the mother start expressing as soon as she can after birth and, if possible, use a multi-user (rental) automatic double breast pump.

Start expressing early. How soon after birth mothers start expressing milk can make a significant difference in their long-term milk production, especially among those with preterm babies. One U.S. study of 87 very-low-birthweight babies found that more mothers who began pumping within the first 6 hours after birth were successfully lactating at 40 weeks gestation than the mothers who started pumping later (Furman, Minich, & Hack, 2002). Other U.S. studies also found that the longer a mother delays milk expression after birth, the greater the risk of low milk production at 6 weeks (Hill, Aldag, Chatterton, & Zinaman, 2005c; Hopkinson, Schanler, & Garza, 1988).

Choose an effective expression method. In a Cochrane Review article that evaluated research on methods of milk expression (Becker et al., 2008), its authors noted that even in developing countries where hand expression is the norm, research has found that double electric rental pumps stimulate greater milk production during the first weeks (Slusher et al., 2007). The Human Milk Banking Association of North American, an independent organization whose research-based guidelines are used by many hospitals to establish milk expression protocols, recommends the use of a multi-user (rental) pump to establish milk production (Jones & Tully, 2006).

Double pumping saves time. This same Cochrane review article concluded that research is mixed on whether double (simultaneous) pumping increases milk production more effectively than single (sequential) pumping. However, it noted that double-pumping saves mothers time. This can help make exclusive expression a practical option for more women.

If pumping, be sure she has a good pump fit. When a breast pump's nipple tunnel is too large or too small, this can compromise effective milk expression and/or cause nipple pain and trauma. For details, see the p. 826- "Pump Fit" in appendix "Tools and Products."

A bad pump fit can cause pain and nipple trauma.

If a mother doesn't have access to an automatic double rental pump or the means to afford one, help her determine the most effective method available to her.

Using breast massage and hand expression with pumping drains the breasts more fully, which enhances short- and long-term milk production.

One U.S. study of 66 mothers of preterm babies found that 86% of its study mothers expressed an average of 93% more milk when they used breast massage during pumping and hand expression after pumping to drain their breasts more completely (Morton et al., 2009). This study also found that rather than milk production decreasing after 2 or 3 weeks of exclusive milk expression, as was reported in other studies (Bishara, Dunn, Merko, & Darling, 2009; Hill, Aldag, Chatterton, & Zinaman, 2005b), the massaging and hand-expressing mothers continued to increase their milk production up to 8 weeks after birth. For details see the online video at: http://newborns.stanford.edu/Breastfeeding/MaxProduction.html.

A U.K. study also found that breast massage during breast pumping increases milk output an average of 42% (88 mL vs. 125 mL) (Jones et al., 2001b). One preliminary Japanese study of 11 mothers with babies in the NICU found that during the first 48 hours after birth when midwives hand-expressed mothers' breasts this yielded three times more milk than the breast pump alone (Ohyama, 2007).

Massage, hand expression, and skin-to-skin contact may offset some of the hormonal challenges of exclusive expression.

Expressing milk often and long enough each day to establish full milk production can be difficult. The exclusively expressing mother may also be at a disadvantage because she lacks the hormonal stimulation breastfeeding provides, including body warmth, skin-to-skin contact, and the loving emotions often felt when baby is at the breast.

In addition to draining the breast more completely, adding breast massage and hand expression to breast pumping may help a mother reach full milk production more effectively because they provide physical/hormonal stimulation that is more like breastfeeding. This also may be why U.S. research on mothers of preterm babies in the NICU found that even an hour of skin-to-skin time with their babies each day was associated with more milk expressed (Hurst, Valentine, Renfro, Burns, & Ferlic, 1997).

During the first few days, suggest the mother express at least 8 to 10 times daily for 10 to 15 minutes and to expect very little milk.

Because most mothers produce very little milk in the early days, some suggest mothers think of these early milk expressions as "putting in their order" for more milk later. Some mothers express drops, others as much as a teaspoon (5 mL). Most do not express much more than this at first. However, each time a mother removes milk from her breasts it signals her body to increase milk production. Make sure the mother knows that the colostrum, or first milk, is concentrated nourishment and immunities, providing her baby with protection from illness and infection, and that no amount is too small to save and give to her baby.

Establishing full milk production via expression alone requires regular, frequent, and effective milk removal. In general, the more often and more fully the mother expresses, the more milk she will produce (Hill et al., 2005c; Morton et al., 2009). To stimulate full milk production, the exclusively expressing mother should plan to express her milk at least as often as a baby would be breastfeeding, no less than 8 to 10 times each day. As a visual reminder, some suggest each morning the mother place 10 candies or other snacks by her pump to help her meet this daily goal.

Intensive milk expression during the first few days and weeks appears to be key to adequate long-term milk production.

One U.S. study compared milk production of 95 mothers expressing for their preterm babies with 98 mothers of full-term, healthy breastfeeding babies and found that 49% of the difference in milk volumes at 6 weeks was due to frequency of early breast stimulation (Hill et al., 2005b). These researchers also found that milk volumes as early as Day 4 were associated with greater milk volumes at 6 weeks (Hill & Aldag, 2005).

Intense pumping during the first few days is key to establishing a long-term supply.

Mothers are sometimes told not to worry about expressing milk in the beginning because they can always increase their milk production later when the baby starts breastfeeding. But following this well-meaning advice can seriously undermine a mother's ability to meet her long-term breastfeeding goals. Later, after the hormones of childbirth have settled down, increasing milk production is usually more difficult and in rare cases may be impossible for some mothers.

Until the mother has reached full milk production, suggest she not go longer than 5 hours between expressions.

When a mother's breasts become full of milk and stay full, two dynamics signal her body to decrease her rate of milk production:

1. The accumulation in her breasts of a milk whey protein or peptide called "feedback inhibitor of lactation" (FIL for short) (Prentice, 1989).
2. Internal pressure from breast fullness.

Most newborns take, on average, one long 4- to 5-hour sleep stretch, which may or may not be at night. When a mother allows her breasts to stay full longer than an average newborn goes between feedings, the "full breasts make milk slower" dynamic may work against her desire to increase milk production (Daly, Owens, & Hartmann, 1993). By expressing her breasts more often, she can use the "drained breasts make milk faster" dynamic to get closer to her goal. For details, see p. 397- "Degree of Breast Fullness."

If the baby is in the special-care nursery, suggest the mother ask about expressing milk at her baby's bedside.

If mothers with ill or preterm babies are limited to expressing milk away from their babies, they often delay milk expression to talk to their baby's healthcare provider or because the expression room is unavailable. Making it easier to express more often is one good reason to make it possible for mothers to express at their baby's bedside (Hurst & Meier, 2010). Another good reason is the message it sends about the importance of milk expression. The sensory stimulation of looking at and touching her baby may also help her express more milk. If the option of expressing at the baby's bedside is not offered, suggest the mother request it.

Stage 2: From Milk Increase to Full Production

During the first 2 weeks postpartum, frequent expression is vital to reaching full milk production.

During the critical first 2 weeks postpartum, whenever a mother breastfeeds or expresses her milk, her blood prolactin levels (a milk-enhancing hormone) increase. Higher blood prolactin levels activate the prolactin receptors in her breasts that determine milk production. U.S. research indicates that the number of prolactin receptors activated during these early weeks may influence the peak milk production for that baby (de Carvalho, Robertson, Friedman, & Klaus, 1983). Most mothers find that trying to increase milk production after the first 2 weeks takes more time and work, and in some rare cases, it may even be impossible. For details, see p. 413- "Strategies for Making More Milk" in the chapter, "Making Milk."

In the U.S. study that compared milk production of 95 mothers expressing for their preterm babies with 98 mothers of breastfeeding babies, the mothers exclusively expressing pumped, on average, six times per day during the critical first 2 weeks. The breastfeeding mothers, on the other hand, averaged nine feedings per day, or 50% more breast drainings (Hill et al., 2005b). Nearly 52% of the expressing mothers produced inadequate milk volumes at Week 6, compared with only 17% of the breastfeeding mothers (some of whom gave unnecessary supplements). The researchers concluded that the difference in early breast stimulation accounted for 49% of the variance in milk output between these groups.

Beginning on Day 3 or 4, suggest the mother express longer, up to 20 to 30 minutes at each session, until she reaches full milk production.

Because "drained breasts make milk faster," longer and more complete milk expression stimulates full milk production faster (Morton et al., 2009). If the mother is pumping, encourage her to use breast massage during and hand expression after to express more milk and to increase her milk production faster (see previous section). When she reaches full milk production—at least 750 to 1035 mL (25 to 35 ounces) per day per baby—most mothers can decrease their expression time without slowing milk production.

Rather than trying to express her milk at regular time intervals, suggest she focus on the total number of expressions per day.

In some hospitals, mothers are told to express milk at specific intervals (i.e., "every 3 hours"). However, for many mothers, this makes expressing more challenging because life often interferes. Medical appointments, visitors, and other distractions can often postpone regular expressions, ultimately decreasing mothers' daily total.

Suggest instead that the mother focus on her daily goal of 8 to 10 expressions and that she express whenever it is most convenient for her, trying to avoid stretches longer than 5 hours or so until she reaches full milk production. Typically, breastfeeding babies do not feed at regular intervals, so there is nothing magical about expressing by the clock (Benson, 2001). Vastly more important to meeting her long-term milk production goals is her total number of breast drainings per day (Hill et al., 2005c). By keeping the focus there, many mothers find it easier to fit in the recommended number of daily expressions and reach full production more quickly. On some days, it might be easier for a mother to express her milk every hour for part of the day followed by a longer 4-hour stretch, and this is fine. This expression pattern is actually closer to how a baby breastfeeds.

If the mother is planning to provide her milk on a short-term basis, help her tailor her expression routine to her goals.

Some mothers who did not intend to breastfeed decide to provide their milk for their preterm or sick newborns on a short-term basis while they are especially vulnerable (Hurst & Meier, 2010). In this case, less intensive efforts to reach a lower level of milk production could be the focus, rather than stimulating full milk production.

Preterm birth affects milk production, but less than other factors.

Giving birth early affects a mother's ability to produce milk since the breast tissue growth she would normally experience during pregnancy is cut short. One small Australian study of 22 mothers expressing milk for preterm babies focused on some specific milk components associated with milk increase on Day 3 or 4 (citrate, lactose, sodium, and protein) and found that if one or more of these components was off by at least three standard deviations, there was an increased risk of low milk production (Cregan, De Mello, Kershaw, McDougall, & Hartmann, 2002).

However, the U.S. study previously described that compared 95 mothers expressing for preterm babies with 98 breastfeeding mothers concluded that length of gestation accounted for only 11% of the variation in milk volumes at 6 weeks and that frequency of breast stimulation had a more than fourfold greater effect (Hill et al., 2005c).

If the mother is expressing for more than one baby, it will probably take her longer to reach full milk production.

Mothers of twins, triplets, and higher-order multiples will obviously need much more milk than the mother of a single baby. To reach full milk production, suggest she continue with the longer and continued night-time expressions of Stage 2 until she is producing at least 750 mL (25 ounces) per baby per day. Then she can proceed to Stage 3.

If the mother has not reached full production by Day 10, consider other ways of boosting production.

See the later section on p. 475, "When Milk Production Needs a Boost."

Research on the use of oxytocin during milk expression is mixed.

Studies on oxytocin tablets and nasal spray and have not found more milk expressed (Prime et al., 2007). One U.K. study found no benefit to using oxytocin nasal spray 3 to 5 minutes before milk expression during the first 5 days of life. Although the mothers using the oxytocin spray expressed more milk at first, by the 5th day, there were no differences between the 21 mothers who used the oxytocin spray and the 21 mothers who used the placebo spray (Fewtrell, Loh, Blake, Ridout, & Hawdon, 2006).

Table 11.5. Milk Expression Strategies for Mothers Exclusively Expressing

	Stage 1: Birth to Day 3 or 4	Stage 2: Day 3 or 4 to Full Production	Stage 3: At Full Production
# daily expressions	8-10	8-10	5-7
Expression duration per breast	≥ 10-15 min.	≥ 20-30 min.	≥ 10-15 min.
Longest stretch	≤ 5 hours	≤ 5 hours	≤ 8 hours

Stage 3: At Full Milk Production

Once a mother has reached full milk production, suggest she decrease the number and length of expressions and monitor her daily milk yield.

When a mother reaches 750 mL (25 ounces) of milk per day, this means enough prolactin receptors have been activated to allow her to experiment with her expression routine without putting her milk production at long-term risk. In this situation, even if production dips, she should be able to quickly bring it back up again, as long as she doesn't allow her production to stay low longer than a week or two.

Decrease milk expressions to five to seven times per day. The number of times each day a mother needs to express her milk to maintain production will vary among mothers, depending on breast storage capacity (see next section). Encourage the mother to start by experimenting within the parameters in Table 11.5. In most cases, five to seven expressions per day are necessary to maintain long-term milk production. However, some mothers with a very small breast storage capacity may notice a decrease at seven daily expressions. If this happens, this means the mother will need to express milk more times per day to maintain her milk production.

Decrease expression time to 10 to 15 minutes. For most mothers, this is long enough. If milk production slows, the mother may need to express longer.

Suggest that mothers try sleeping 8 hours at night without expressing.

When a mother is ready to try sleeping at night without expressing milk, suggest she start by expressing as the last thing she does before going to sleep at night and the first thing she does when she awakens in the morning. Her experience will provide clues to her breast storage capacity. In general, women with larger storage capacities can do this without too much breast discomfort or painful fullness. For their first morning expression, they may express 300 mL (10 ounces) or more. The mother with a small storage capacity, on the other hand, may awaken before morning with breast discomfort, yet be unable to express more than 150 mL (5 ounces) or so (Mohrbacher, 1996).

Maintaining Full Milk Production

Sometimes breastfeeding mothers need to use exclusive expression to maintain an already established milk production.

Examples of those who need to maintain milk production with expression include mothers:

- Whose breastfeeding baby is on strike.
- Who must temporarily interrupt breastfeeding due to the need for an incompatible drug or a diagnostic test using radioactive compounds.
- Who are facing hospitalization (either of them or their baby), which involves separation.
- Who are away from baby on a business or personal trip.

Temporary interruptions of breastfeeding for any reason can be both emotionally and physically stressful for mother and baby. If it is abrupt, the stress is compounded. The mother may feel stressed about expressing and worry about how her baby will react to the change and/or her absence. She may also worry about mastitis and maintaining milk production. She may need emotional support during this time and a listening ear.

Her baby may find a change in feeding methods stressful (for options, see p. 811-"Alternative Feeding Methods" in the appendix "Tools and Products") and/or the introduction of new foods. If the baby and mother are not usually separated, this will add to their stress. If so, encourage the mother to ask the baby's caregiver to give him lots of cuddling and holding to help make up for her absence and the loss of breastfeeding.

The 'Magic Number' and Other Basics

In light of new information, giving all mothers the same guidelines for maintaining milk production no longer makes sense.

Some older studies drew conclusions about the average number of minutes and daily milk expressions needed to maintain milk production (de Carvalho, Anderson, Glangreco, & Pittard, 1985). One U.S. study of 32 mothers of preterm babies born at 28 to 30 weeks gestation concluded that to maintain milk production mothers needed to express at least five times per day for a total of more than 100 minutes (Hopkinson et al., 1988). However, this study was done before breast storage capacity (see next point) was understood. With our expanding understanding of the impact of individual differences, recommending that all mothers express for the same number of minutes and number of daily milk expressions no longer makes sense. An expression plan needs to be tailored to each mother, based on their breast storage capacity and other individual differences.

• •

The number of daily expressions needed to maintain production will vary by a mother's breast storage capacity and other factors.

Whether a mother is breastfeeding or expressing, the basic dynamics of milk production remain the same:

- **Drained breasts make milk faster.** When breasts are drained often and well, this sends the signal to the breasts to make milk faster.
- **Full breasts make milk slower.** The accumulation of the whey protein or peptide known as feedback inhibitor of lactation (FIL) and the internal pressure of breast fullness both send signals to the mother's body to slow down milk-making (Prentice, 1989). The more milk that fills the breast, the slower it is produced.

Breast storage capacity. How long it takes for a mother's breasts to become full depends on this variable, which refers to the maximum volume of milk available to the baby when the breast is at its fullest. Breast size is determined mostly by fatty tissue, so storage capacity is unrelated to breast size (Daly et al., 1993).

Large-capacity mothers can comfortably store more milk without feeling full and, therefore, need to express less often to maintain production. They also tend to express more milk each time. Small-capacity mothers feel full faster and need to express more often for the same daily milk yield. Both mothers can make ample milk, but the number of daily expressions needed to maintain production can vary greatly.

To use breast storage capacity as her guide, suggest the mother be aware of feelings of breast fullness, ideally never allowing herself to get too full or stay that way too long without expressing. When her breasts get and stay too full, this puts her at risk for both slowed milk production and mastitis (see p. 681- "Mastitis").

A mother's "magic number" is the number of daily expressions she needs to maintain her milk supply.

Her "magic number." Depending on her breast storage capacity, each mother has a specific number of daily expressions that will maintain her milk production over the long term. This is her "magic number." (For more, see p. 590.) If she is exclusively expressing, she can determine her magic number by reaching full production and then experimenting. For most, the magic number will be somewhere between five and seven expressions per day. If a mother has a very small capacity, it may be more; if very large, it may be less. However, some large-capacity mothers who cut back to fewer than five daily milk expressions report that production stays steady for a month or two, then declines precipitously. The mother will know she has found her magic number when her milk production stays steady without dropping.

The length of each expression. This factor can affect her magic number because increasing the length of her expressions ("drained breasts make milk faster") can sometimes offset fewer daily milk expressions (Mohrbacher, 1996).

The longest stretch between. Because full breasts make milk slower, very long stretches between expressions is another factor that may slow milk production. Mothers with a large storage capacity sometimes push the envelope and go as long as 10 to 12 hours as their longest daily stretch. Be sure to ask any mother with milk production issues about this variable. In some cases, a sagging milk production can be boosted simply by decreasing the longest stretch.

• •

When a mother using a breast pump reaches full production, she may be able to switch to a smaller, more portable pump.

With her prolactin receptors activated and a full milk production of at least 750 mL (25 ounces) per day per baby, many mothers can maintain milk production with breast pumps less effective than the multi-user, rental models. There are a wide range of automatic double pumps that provide at least 40 cycles per minute (see the previous "Breast Pumps" section) available for sale, some that include carry bags with insulated milk-cooling areas. When they change pumps, many mothers find that their milk ejection is temporarily affected due to the new feel. If so, see p. 449- "How to Express More Milk."

Automatic double pumps that provide fewer than 40 cpm are not recommended for mothers pumping exclusively (Jones & Tully, 2006). These, as well as semi-automatic and manual pumps, are recommended for occasional use.

Suggest that at least once a week the mother write down her 24-hour milk yield, so she can respond quickly if it decreases.

Keeping an eye on her milk yield is important, because the faster a mother responds to a drop in milk production, the sooner she'll rebound. If she works to increase her milk production within a week or two, it is usually fairly easy to recover from a drop, but if she waits 3 to 4 weeks or longer, it may be difficult to bring it up. For strategies, see the next section.

When Milk Production Needs a Boost

When a mother's milk production is low or faltering, first review the basics.

When considering strategies to boost production, start with these questions:

- **How many times per day does she express her milk?** If she tells you how many hours apart her expressions are, this is not enough information. Ask her to go through a typical day describing the times she expresses and then add them together for her daily total.
- **How long does she express per breast each time?** Has this changed recently? If using a pump, is she single or double pumping?
- **What is her longest stretch between expressions?** Stretches longer than about 8 hours will cause many mothers' production to decrease over time.
- **What expression method or pump is she using?** If she's pumping, ask her which brand and model she uses to determine whether it is effective enough for her situation.
- **When was the last time her pump fit was checked?** Even if she had a good fit at first, fit can change with time and pumping (Meier et al., 2004; Wilson-Clay & Hoover, 2008). See p. 826- "Pump Fit."
- **How much daily skin-to-skin contact with her baby does she have?** Skin-to-skin contact is associated with more milk expressed (Hurst et al., 1997).
- **What is her goal?** A mother planning to express short-term may not want to spend as much time on milk production as one who intends to express long term.

Other strategies can also help boost milk production.

Discuss other factors that might affect milk production, such as any medications she is taking, a history of breast surgery, and any health problems. See p. 390- "Milk Production" for a more complete list. Explore possible strategies.

- **Express more times per day.** More than eight expressions per day will increase milk production in most mothers. (For small-capacity mothers, this number may be higher.)
- **Express longer.** Suggest she keep expressing until 2 minutes after the last drop of milk or 20 to 30 minutes, whichever comes first.
- **Massage while expressing.** This has been found to yield more milk (Jones et al., 2001b; Morton et al., 2009).
- **Hand express after pumping.** By draining the breasts more fully each time and adding more skin-to-skin contact, this can also boost milk production (Morton et al., 2009).

- **Consider prescription and herbal medicines**. Some that have been found to boost milk production are metoclopramide (Reglan) and domperidone (Motilium). For details, see p. 419- "Galactogogues." Offer to provide information to the mother and her healthcare provider, so they evaluate them in light of her medical history.

Full Milk Production Achieved: What Next?

After achieving full milk production, be sure the mother knows her options.

When a mother achieves full milk production, she may wonder where to go from there. Expressing milk for a non-breastfeeding baby brings many rewards. Mothers say it feels great to see their baby grow and thrive on their milk, and it sets their mind at ease to know they're giving their baby the best (Mohrbacher, 1996). Mother's milk is recommended for at least a baby's first year (Gartner et al., 2005). But even motivated mothers find it difficult to make exclusive expression work long-term because it takes at least twice the time and effort (sometimes more) of direct breastfeeding.

Be sure the mother knows that transitioning her baby to the breast is an option—no matter how long she's been expressing. Make sure she knows, too, that if she decides instead to wean from expressing, there are ways to do it that are comfortable and safe.

Transitioning to the Breast

Babies of any age can be transitioned to the breast.

As described in the first chapter, babies are hardwired to breastfeed. Adoptive breastfeeding in Australia involves transitioning 6- to 12-month-old babies to the breast because adoptions are not allowed to take place there before this age (Gribble, 2005a). Breast-seeking behaviors have been observed in babies older than 1 year (Gribble, 2005b; Smillie, 2008).

Transitioning to the breast is possible no matter how long a mother has been expressing.

Think of this as a learning process that requires time and patience. The mother may sometimes feel awkward, anxious, or frustrated. Encourage her to consider their first attempts as "getting acquainted" sessions, enjoy the cuddling, and keep trying.

During this transition, make the breast a pleasant place to be.

Never let the breast become a battleground. While near the breast, give the baby lots of skin-to-skin and eye contact. Smile, talk, and enjoy each other. If the baby wants to move away, allow him to do so and come back to it at another time. If the baby fusses or cries at the breast, encourage the mother to stop and comfort him, so the baby does not associate the breast with frustration or unhappiness.

Start by making the breast available to the baby in laid-back breastfeeding positions.

These "biological nurturing" positions make the most of babies' innate feeding behaviors. For details, see Chapter 1.

If the baby doesn't take the breast at first, suggest the mother try while he's asleep or half-asleep.

In her DVD, *Biological Nurturing: Laid-Back Breastfeeding*, U.K. midwife and researcher Suzanne Colson illustrates how inborn feeding behaviors continue to be triggered when babies are asleep (Colson, 2008). Babies refusing the breast can be placed on their mothers' semi-reclined bodies while asleep, which can facilitate this process. Because sleep seems to "blunt" feeding reflexes, some babies take the breast more easily when drowsy or asleep.

Other strategies and tools may also help babies transition to the breast more easily.

See the chapter "Challenges at the Breast" for an overview of mother and baby issues that can affect breastfeeding and the section "Achieving Settled Breastfeeding" for specific strategies and tools. See also p. 614- "Transitioning Baby to the Breast" in the chapter, "Relacation, Induced Lactation, and Emergencies."

It may take time for the baby to take the breast easily and well.

The mother may feel discouraged if her baby does not take to breastfeeding quickly. Assure her that the early feedings are the most challenging, and that with time and practice, it will get easier.

If the mother is anxious about not knowing how much milk her baby takes from the breast, tell her how to gauge milk intake.

One emotional barrier that prevents many mothers from transitioning from exclusive expression to direct breastfeeding is their worries about their baby's milk intake at the breast. This may be an especially difficult barrier for mothers of babies born preterm or ill. Many of these mothers find it comforting to follow the routines that kept their babies alive in the hospital. They may consider breastfeeding risky for their vulnerable babies, even after the baby is no longer at risk and could breastfeed effectively and well. As described in the chapter, "The Preterm Baby," suggest the mother think of breastfeeding as a normal behavior (like walking and talking) that her baby is hardwired to do and that she can help facilitate.

Also share with the mother expected weight gains when breastfeeding and share less reliable signs she can use at home, such as diaper output and behavior after breastfeeding. Encourage her to notice her baby's diaper output and post-feeding behavior before transitioning to the breast, so that she'll be more aware of what to look for afterward.

If, in spite of this information, a mother is still very anxious about not knowing how much her baby takes at the breast, suggest for the first week she arrange for a daily weight check with her baby's healthcare provider. If she has the means and an accurate baby scale (to 2 g) is available for rent, suggest she consider a weekly rental, so she can do daily weight checks at home. This may help set her mind at ease during this transition. These scales are often available where mothers rent breast pumps.

Weaning from Exclusive Expression

Like any other weaning, it is more comfortable and less risky to wean from expression gradually.

If a mother decides to wean from expression, rather than transitioning her baby to the breast, there are several approaches she can use alone or in combination to make this more gradual.

If at any time during weaning her breasts feel very full, encourage her to express to comfort without expressing fully. Letting her breasts stay full increases the risk of pain and mastitis. With this in mind, possible approaches include:

- **Eliminate one daily pumping every 3 days or so**, leaving for last the first morning and last evening expressions. This gives her milk production time to adjust downward before dropping another expression. When an expression is dropped, adjust the timing so all expressions are about the same time interval apart. Repeat until fully weaned from expressing.

- **Gradually increase the intervals between expressions.** For example, if she had been expressing every 3 hours during the day, delay to 4 to 5 hours, and wait 3 days or so to increase the intervals again. Repeat until she no longer feels the need to express.
- **Keep the number of expressions the same, but stop sooner.** For example, if she was expressing 120 mL (4 ounces) at each expression, stop after 90 mL (3 ounces). Give her body 3 days or so to adjust and repeat until she no longer feels the need to express.

While the mother weans from milk expression, assure her that expressing to comfort as needed is in her best interest.

Whether a mother chooses one or combines several of the previous approaches, expressing to comfort as needed will not prolong the process. It will simply make it more comfortable and prevent painful fullness from developing into mastitis. The goal is a gradual weaning with a minimum of risk and discomfort.

Another milk-expression strategy sometimes recommended during weaning (especially for mothers with a hardened area in her breast [blocked duct] that won't go away) is to fully drain the breasts, and then go for longer and longer stretches without expressing (S. Burger, personal communication, November 18, 2009). Encourage the mother to use whichever of these milk-expression strategies works best for her.

When Missing Feedings Regularly

Whether a mother is regularly separated from her baby due to employment, school, or other commitments, she can continue to breastfeed and maintain her milk production. See p. 588- "Returning to Work" in the chapter, "Employment" for specific tips for planning daily routines and milk expression strategies to help maintain milk production over the long term.

Storing Milk While Exclusively Breastfeeding

Expressing both breasts about 30 to 60 minutes after a morning breastfeeding usually yields the most milk for storage without affecting breastfeeding.

Several approaches can be used to express and store milk while a mother is exclusively breastfeeding. Because babies take, on average, less than 70% of the milk in the breast at a feeding (Kent, 2007), there will usually be some milk left to express, even right after a breastfeeding. But if the mother waits a little while, there will be more. Most women get more milk in the morning than later in the day, and babies tend to have longer stretches between feedings then. (See p. 446 "How Much Milk to Expect.")

If the baby wants to breastfeed soon after expressing both breasts, encourage her to do so.

If an hour passes between a milk expression and the next breastfeeding, the baby's feeding pattern will not usually be affected. However, if the baby wants to feed sooner, encourage the mother to breastfeed anyway. Most babies will be patient with the slower milk flow. The baby may simply feed longer, take each breast more than once, or want to breastfeed again sooner than usual.

Some mothers feel more comfortable expressing from one breast and leaving the other fuller in case the baby wants to breastfeed. This can work especially well if the baby usually takes one breast at a feeding, but this way the mother will usually get less milk for storage than if she expresses from both breasts.

Another option is to express milk from one breast during or between breastfeedings.

RESOURCES FOR PARENTS

Pumping Instructions and Log

Hoover, K., & Wilson-Clay, B. Pumping milk for your preterm baby. Available from http://www.lactnews.com/products/pumpingforpreterm.

A 4-page booklet with full-color photos, a weekly pumping log, and low literacy text with instructions for the mother exclusively pumping from birth. Available in English and Spanish.

Websites

http://newborns.stanford.edu/Breastfeeding/HandExpression.html For a 7.5 minute video demonstrating manual expression technique.

http://newborns.stanford.edu/Breastfeeding/MaxProduction.html. For a 9.5 minute video demonstrating "hands-on pumping," which incorporates manual expression and massage.

www.ameda.com For pumping articles, low-literacy sheets for mothers, videos and podcasts.

DVDs

Frantz, K. Breastfeeding techniques that work, volume 6: Hand expression. Available from www.geddesproduction.com.

REFERENCES

ABM. (2009). Protocol #8: Human milk storage information for home use for healthy full-term infants. Retrieved January 27, 2010, from http://www.bfmed.org/Resources/Protocols.aspx.

Barger, J., & Bull, P. (1987). A comparison of the bacterial composition of breast milk stored at room temperature and stored in the refrigerator. *International Journal of Childbirth Education*, 29-30.

Becker, G. E., McCormick, F. M., & Renfrew, M. J. (2008). Methods of milk expression for lactating women. *Cochrane Database of Systematic Reviews*(4), CD006170.

Becker, G. E., & Roberts, T. (2009). Do we agree? Using a delphi technique to develop consensus on skills of hand expression. *Journal of Human Lactation, 25*(2), 220-225.

Benson, S. (2001). What is normal? A study of normal breastfeeding dyads during the first sixty hours of life. *Breastfeeding Review, 9*(1), 27-32.

Berkow, S. E., Freed, L. M., Hamosh, M., Bitman, J., Wood, D. L., Happ, B., et al. (1984). Lipases and lipids in human milk: effect of freeze-thawing and storage. *Pediatric Research, 18*(12), 1257-1262.

Binns, C. W., Win, N. N., Zhao, Y., & Scott, J. A. (2006). Trends in the expression of breastmilk 1993-2003. *Breastfeeding Review, 14*(3), 5-9.

Bishara, R., Dunn, M. S., Merko, S. E., & Darling, P. (2009). Volume of Foremilk, Hindmilk, and Total Milk Produced by Mothers of Very Preterm Infants Born at Less Than 28 Weeks of Gestation. *Journal of Human Lactation, 25*(3), 272-279.

Bitman, J., Wood, D. L., Mehta, N. R., Hamosh, P., & Hamosh, M. (1983). Lipolysis of triglycerides of human milk during storage at low temperatures: a note of caution. *Journal of Pediatric Gastroenterology and Nutrition, 2*(3), 521-524.

Brusseau, R. (1998). Bacterial analysis of refrigerated human milk following infant feeding. Unpublished senior thesis. Concordia University.

Buss, I. H., McGill, F., Darlow, B. A., & Winterbourn, C. C. (2001). Vitamin C is reduced in human milk after storage. *Acta Paediatrica, 90*(7), 813-815.

Butte, N. F., Garza, C., Smith, E. O., & Nichols, B. L. (1984). Human milk intake and growth in exclusively breast-fed infants. *Journal of Pediatrics, 104*(2), 187-195.

CDC. (1994). Guidelines for preventing transmission of human immunodeficiency virus through transplantation of human tissue and organs. Centers for Disease Control and Prevention. *MMWR Recommdations and Reports, 43*(RR-8), 1-17.

Chamberlain, L. B., McMahon, M., Philipp, B. L., & Merewood, A. (2006). Breast pump access in the inner city: a hospital-based initiative to provide breast pumps for low-income women. *Journal of Human Lactation, 22*(1), 94-98.

Chatterton, R. T., Jr., Hill, P. D., Aldag, J. C., Hodges, K. R., Belknap, S. M., & Zinaman, M. J. (2000). Relation of plasma oxytocin and prolactin concentrations to milk production in mothers of preterm infants: influence of stress. *Journal of Clinical Endocrinology and Metabolism, 85*(10), 3661-3668.

Cobo, E. (1993). Characteristics of the spontaneous milk ejecting activity occurring during human lactation. *Journal of Perinatal Medicine, 21*(1), 77-85.

Cohen, R. J., Brown, K. H., Canahuati, J., Rivera, L. L., & Dewey, K. G. (1994). Effects of age of introduction of complementary foods on infant breast milk intake, total energy intake, and growth: a randomised intervention study in Honduras. *Lancet, 344*(8918), 288-293.

Colson, S. (Writer) (2008). Biological Nurturing: Laid-Back Breastfeeding. Hythe, Kent, UK: The Nurturing Project.

Cowley, K. C. (2005). Psychogenic and pharmacologic induction of the let-down reflex can facilitate breastfeeding by tetraplegic women: a report of 3 cases. *Archives of Physical Medicine and Rehabilitationl, 86*(6), 1261-1264.

Cox, S. G. (2006). Expressing and storing colostrum antenatally for use in the newborn period. *Breastfeeding Review, 14*(3), 11-16.

Cregan, M. D., De Mello, T. R., Kershaw, D., McDougall, K., & Hartmann, P. E. (2002). Initiation of lactation in women after preterm delivery. *Acta Obstetricia et Gynecologica Scandinavica, 81*(9), 870-877.

Daly, S. E., Owens, R. A., & Hartmann, P. E. (1993). The short-term synthesis and infant-regulated removal of milk in lactating women. *Experimental Physiology, 78*(2), 209-220.

de Carvalho, M., Anderson, D. M., Glangreco, A., & Pittard, W. B., 3rd. (1985). Frequency of milk expression and milk production by mothers of nonnursing premature neonates. *American Journal of Diseases of Children, 139*, 483-485.

de Carvalho, M., Robertson, S., Friedman, A., & Klaus, M. (1983). Effect of frequent breast-feeding on early milk production and infant weight gain. *Pediatrics, 72*(3), 307-311.

Engstrom, J. L., Meier, P. P., Jegier, B., Motykowski, J. E., & Zuleger, J. L. (2007). Comparison of milk output from the right and left breasts during simultaneous pumping in mothers of very low birthweight infants. *Breastfeeding Medicine, 2*(2), 83-91.

Feher, S. D., Berger, L. R., Johnson, J. D., & Wilde, J. B. (1989). Increasing breast milk production for premature infants with a relaxation/imagery audiotape. *Pediatrics, 83*(1), 57-60.

Fewtrell, M. S., Loh, K. L., Blake, A., Ridout, D. A., & Hawdon, J. (2006). Randomised, double blind trial of oxytocin nasal spray in mothers expressing breast milk for preterm infants. *Archives of Disease in Childhood. Fetal and Neonatal Edition, 91*(3), F169-174.

Furman, L., Minich, N., & Hack, M. (2002). Correlates of lactation in mothers of very low birth weight infants. *Pediatrics, 109*(4), e57.

Gartner, L. M., Morton, J., Lawrence, R. A., Naylor, A. J., O'Hare, D., Schanler, R. J., et al. (2005). Breastfeeding and the use of human milk. *Pediatrics, 115*(2), 496-506.

Geraghty, S. R., Khoury, J. C., & Kalkwarf, H. J. (2005). Human milk pumping rates of mothers of singletons and mothers of multiples. *Journal of Human Lactation, 21*(4), 413-420.

Gessler, P., Bischoff, G. A., Wiegand, D., Essers, B., & Bossart, W. (2004). Cytomegalovirus-associated necrotizing enterocolitis in a preterm twin after breastfeeding. *Journal of Perinatology, 24*(2), 124-126.

Glynn, L., & Goosen, L. (2005). Manual expression of breast milk. *Journal of Human Lactation, 21*(2), 184-185.

Goldblum, R. M., Garza, C., Johnson, C. A., Harrist, R., & Nichols, B. L. (1981). Human milk banking I: Effects of container upon immunologic factors in mature milk. *Nutrition Research, 1*(449-459).

Gribble, K. D. (2005a). Adoptive breastfeeding. *Breastfeeding Review, 13*(3), 6.

Gribble, K. D. (2005b). Post-institutionalized adopted children who seek breastfeeding from their new mothers. *Journal of Prenatal & Perinatal Psychology & Health, 19*(3), 217-235.

Hamosh, M., Ellis, L. A., Pollock, D. R., Henderson, T. R., & Hamosh, P. (1996). Breastfeeding and the working mother: effect of time and temperature of short-term storage on proteolysis, lipolysis, and bacterial growth in milk. *Pediatrics, 97*(4), 492-498.

Hanna, N., Ahmed, K., Anwar, M., Petrova, A., Hiatt, M., & Hegyi, T. (2004). Effect of storage on breast milk antioxidant activity. *Archives of Disease in Childhood. Fetal and Neonatal Edition, 89*(6), F518-520.

Heinig, M. J., Nommsen, L. A., Peerson, J. M., Lonnerdal, B., & Dewey, K. G. (1993). Energy and protein intakes of breast-fed and formula-fed infants during the first year of life and their association with growth velocity: the DARLING Study. *American Journal of Clinical Nutrition, 58*(2), 152-161.

Hill, P. D., & Aldag, J. C. (2005). Milk volume on day 4 and income predictive of lactation adequacy at 6 weeks of mothers of nonnursing preterm infants. *Journal of Perinatal and Neonatal Nursing, 19*(3), 273-282.

Hill, P. D., Aldag, J. C., Chatterton, R. T., & Zinaman, M. (2005a). Comparison of milk output between mothers of preterm and term infants: the first 6 weeks after birth. *J Hum Lact, 21*(1), 22-30.

Hill, P. D., Aldag, J. C., Chatterton, R. T., & Zinaman, M. (2005b). Comparison of milk output between mothers of preterm and term infants: the first 6 weeks after birth. *Journal of Human Lactation, 21*(1), 22-30.

Hill, P. D., Aldag, J. C., Chatterton, R. T., & Zinaman, M. (2005c). Primary and secondary mediators' influence on milk output in lactating mothers of preterm and term infants. *Journal of Human Lactation, 21*(2), 138-150.

Hill, P. D., Aldag, J. C., Zinaman, M., & Chatterton, R. T., Jr. (2007). Comparison of milk output between breasts in pump-dependent mothers. *Journal of Human Lactation, 23*(4), 333-337.

Hopkinson, J. M., Schanler, R. J., & Garza, C. (1988). Milk production by mothers of premature infants. *Pediatrics, 81*(6), 815-820.

Hurst, N. M., & Meier, P. P. (2010). Breastfeeding the Preterm Infant. In J. Riordan (Ed.), *Breastfeeding and Human Lactation* (4th ed., pp. 425-470). Boston, MA: Jones and Bartlett.

Hurst, N. M., Valentine, C. J., Renfro, L., Burns, P., & Ferlic, L. (1997). Skin-to-skin holding in the neonatal intensive care unit influences maternal milk volume. *Journal of Perinatology, 17*(3), 213-217.

Islam, M. M., Peerson, J. M., Ahmed, T., Dewey, K. G., & Brown, K. H. (2006). Effects of varied energy density of complementary foods on breast-milk intakes and total energy consumption by healthy, breastfed Bangladeshi children. *American Journal of Clinical Nutrition, 83*(4), 851-858.

Jones, E., Dimmock, P. W., & Spencer, S. A. (2001a). A randomised controlled trial to compare methods of milk expression after preterm delivery. *Archives of Disease in Childhood. Fetal and Neonatal Edition, 85*(2), F91-95.

Jones, E., Dimmock, P. W., & Spencer, S. A. (2001b). A randomised controlled trial to compare methods of milk expression after preterm delivery. *Archives of Disease in Childhood. Fetal and Neonatal Edition, 85*(2), F91-95.

Jones, F., & Tully, M. R. (2006). *Best Practices for Expressing, Storing and Handling Human Milk* (2nd ed.). Raleigh, NC: Human Milk Banking Association of North America.

Kent, J. C. (2007). How breastfeeding works. *Journal of Midwifery & Women's Health, 52*(6), 564-570.

Kent, J. C., Mitoulas, L. R., Cregan, M. D., Geddes, D. T., Larsson, M., Doherty, D. A., et al. (2008). Importance of vacuum for breastmilk expression. *Breastfeeding Medicine, 3*(1), 11-19.

Kent, J. C., Mitoulas, L. R., Cregan, M. D., Ramsay, D. T., Doherty, D. A., & Hartmann, P. E. (2006). Volume and frequency of breastfeedings and fat content of breast milk throughout the day. *Pediatrics, 117*(3), e387-395.

Kent, J. C., Ramsay, D. T., Doherty, D., Larsson, M., & Hartmann, P. E. (2003). Response of breasts to different stimulation patterns of an electric breast pump. *Journal of Human Lactation, 19*(2), 179-186; quiz 187-178, 218.

Labiner-Wolfe, J., Fein, S. B., Shealy, K. R., & Wang, C. (2008). Prevalence of breast milk expression and associated factors. *Pediatrics, 122 Suppl 2*, S63-68.

Law, B. J., Urias, B. A., Lertzman, J., Robson, D., & Romance, L. (1989). Is ingestion of milk-associated bacteria by premature infants fed raw human milk controlled by routine bacteriologic screening? *Journal of Clinical Microbiology, 27*(7), 1560-1566.

Lawrence, R. A., & Lawrence, R. M. (2005). *Breastfeeding: A Guide for the Medical Profession*. Philadelphia, PA: Elsevier Mosby.

Li, R., Fein, S. B., & Grummer-Strawn, L. M. (2008). Association of breastfeeding intensity and bottle-emptying behaviors at early infancy with infants' risk for excess weight at late infancy. *Pediatrics, 122 Suppl 2*, S77-84.

LLLI. (2008). Storing human milk. Schaumburg, IL: La Leche League International.

Lucas, A., Gibbs, J. A., & Baum, J. D. (1978). The biology of human drip breast milk. *Early Human Development, 2*(4), 351-361.

Manohar, A. A., Williamson, M., & Koppikar, G. V. (1997). Effect of storage of colostrum in various containers. *Indian Pediatrics, 34*(4), 293-295.

Martinez-Costa, C., Silvestre, M. D., Lopez, M. C., Plaza, A., Miranda, M., & Guijarro, R. (2007). Effects of refrigeration on the bactericidal activity of human milk: a preliminary study. *Journal of Pediatric Gastroenterology and Nutrition, 45*(2), 275-277.

Meehan, K., Harrison, G. G., Afifi, A. A., Nickel, N., Jenks, E., & Ramirez, A. (2008). The association between an electric pump loan program and the timing of requests for formula by working mothers in WIC. *Journal of Human Lactation, 24*(2), 150-158.

Meek, J. Y. (2002). *American Academy of Pediatrics New Mother's Guide to Breastfeeding*. New York, New York: Bantam Books.

Meier, P., Motykowski, J. E., & Zuleger, J. L. (2004). Choosing a correctly-fitted breastshield for milk expression. *Medela Messenger, 21*, 8-9.

Meier, P. P., Engstrom, J. L., Hurst, N. M., Ackerman, B., Allen, M., Motykowski, J. E., et al. (2008). A comparison of the efficiency, efficacy, comfort, and convenience of two hospital-grade electric breast pumps for mothers of very low birthweight infants. *Breastfeeding Medicine, 3*(3), 141-150.

Mohrbacher, N. (1996). Mothers who forgo breastfeeding for pumping. *Ameda/Egnell Circle of Caring, 9*(2), 1-2.

Mohrbacher, N., & Kendall-Tackett, K. (2005). *Breastfeeding Made Simple: Seven Natural Laws for Nursing Mothers*. Oakland, CA: New Harbinger Publications.

Mohrbacher, N., & Stock, J. (2003). *The Breastfeeding Answer Book*. Schaumburg, IL: La Leche League International.

Morton, J., Hall, J. Y., Wong, R. J., Thairu, L., Benitz, W. E., & Rhine, W. D. (2009). Combining hand techniques with electric pumping increases milk production in mothers of preterm infants. *Journal of Perinatology, 29*(11), 757-764.

Novak, F. R., Da Silva, A. V., Hagler, A. N., & Figueiredo, A. M. (2000). Contamination of expressed human breast milk with an epidemic multiresistant Staphylococcus aureus clone. *Journal of Medical Microbiology, 49*(12), 1109-1117.

Nwankwo, M. U., Offor, E., Okolo, A. A., & Omene, J. A. (1988). Bacterial growth in expressed breast-milk. *Annals of Tropical Paediatrics, 8*(2), 92-95.

Ohyama, M. (2007). Which is more effective, manual- or electric-expression in the first 48 hours after delivery in a setting of mother-infant separation? Preliminary report. *Breastfeeding Medicine, 2*(3), 179.

Ortiz, J., McGilligan, K., & Kelly, P. (2004). Duration of breast milk expression among working mothers enrolled in an employer-sponsored lactation program. *Pediatr Nurs, 30*(2), 111-119.

Pardou, A., Serruys, E., Mascart-Lemone, F., Dramaix, M., & Vis, H. L. (1994). Human milk banking: influence of storage processes and of bacterial contamination on some milk constituents. *Biology of the Neonate, 65*(5), 302-309.

Paxson, C. L., Jr., & Cress, C. C. (1979). Survival of human milk leukocytes. *Journal of Pediatrics, 94*(1), 61-64.

Pittard, W. B., 3rd, Anderson, D. M., Cerutti, E. R., & Boxerbaum, B. (1985). Bacteriostatic qualities of human milk. *Journal of Pediatrics, 107*(2), 240-243.

Pittard, W. B., 3rd, & Bill, K. (1981). Human milk banking. Effect of refrigeration on cellular components. *Clinical Pediatrics (Philadelphia), 20*(1), 31-33.

Pittard, W. B., 3rd, Geddes, K. M., Brown, S., Mintz, S., & Hulsey, T. C. (1991). Bacterial contamination of human milk: container type and method of expression. *American Journal of Perinatology, 8*(1), 25-27.

Prentice, A. (1989). Evidence for local feedback control of human milk secretion. . *Biochemical Society Transactions, 17*, 489-492.

Prime, D. K., Geddes, D. T., & Hartmann, P. E. (2007). Oxytocin: Milk ejection and maternal-infant well-being. In T. W. Hale & P. E. Hartmann (Eds.), *Hale & Hartmann's Textbook of Human Lactation* (pp. 141-155). Amarillo, TX: Hale Publishing.

Quan, R., Yang, C., Rubinstein, S., Lewiston, N. J., Sunshine, P., Stevenson, D. K., et al. (1992). Effects of microwave radiation on anti-infective factors in human milk. *Pediatrics, 89*(4 Pt 1), 667-669.

Ramsay, D. T., & Hartmann, P. E. (2005). Milk removal from the breast. *Breastfeeding Review, 13*(1), 5-7.

Ramsay, D. T., Kent, J. C., Owens, R. A., & Hartmann, P. E. (2004). Ultrasound imaging of milk ejection in the breast of lactating women. *Pediatrics, 113*(2), 361-367.

Ramsay, D. T., Mitoulas, L. R., Kent, J. C., Cregan, M. D., Doherty, D. A., Larsson, M., et al. (2006). Milk flow rates can be used to identify and investigate milk ejection in women expressing breast milk using an electric breast pump. *Breastfeeding Medicine, 1*(1), 14-23.

Ramsay, D. T., Mitoulas, L. R., Kent, J. C., Larsson, M., & Hartmann, P. E. (2005). The use of ultrasound to characterize milk ejection in women using an electric breast pump. *Journal of Human Lactation, 21*(4), 421-428.

Rechtman, D. J., Lee, M. L., & Berg, H. (2006). Effect of environmental conditions on unpasteurized donor human milk. *Breastfeeding Medicine, 1*(1), 24-26.

Rosa, C. A., Novak, F. R., de Almeida, J. A., Medonca-Hagler, L. C., & Hagler, A. (1990). Yeasts from human milk collected in Rio de Janeiro, Brazil. *Revista de Microbiologia, 21*(4), 361-363.

Saint, L., Smith, M., & Hartmann, P. E. (1984). The yield and nutrient content of colostrum and milk of women from giving birth to 1 month post-partum. *British Journal of Nutrition, 52*(1), 87-95.

Sigman, M., Burke, K. I., Swarner, O. W., & Shavlik, G. W. (1989). Effects of microwaving human milk: changes in IgA content and bacterial count. *Journal of the American Dietetic Association, 89*(5), 690-692.

Silvestre, D., Lopez, M. C., March, L., Plaza, A., & Martinez-Costa, C. (2006). Bactericidal activity of human milk: stability during storage. *British Journal of Biomedical Science, 63*(2), 59-62.

Slusher, T., Slusher, I. L., Biomdo, M., Bode-Thomas, F., Curtis, B. A., & Meier, P. (2007). Electric breast pump use increases maternal milk volume in African nurseries. *Journal of Tropical Pediatrics, 53*(2), 125-130.

Smillie, C. (2008). How infants learn to feed: A neurbehavioral model. In C. W. Genna (Ed.), *Supporting Sucking Skills in Breastfeeding Infants* (pp. 79-95). Boston, MA: Jones and Bartlett.

Sosa, R., & Barness, L. (1987). Bacterial growth in refrigerated human milk. *American Journal of Diseases of Children, 141*(1), 111-112.

Sweet, L. (2008). Expressed breast milk as 'connection' and its influence on the construction of 'motherhood' for mothers of preterm infants: a qualitative study. *International Breastfeeding Journal, 3*, 30.

Taveras, E. M., Scanlon, K. S., Birch, L., Rifas-Shiman, S. L., Rich-Edwards, J. W., & Gillman, M. W. (2004). Association of Breastfeeding With Maternal Control of Infant Feeding at Age 1 Year. *Pediatrics, 114*(5), e577-583.

Walker, M. (2006). *Breastfeeding Management for the Clinician: Using the Evidence*. Boston, MA: Jones and Bartlett.

WHO. (2009). *Infant and young child feeding: Model Chapter for textbooks for medical students and allied health professionals*. Geneva, Switzerland: World Health Organization.

Williamson, M. T., & Murti, P. K. (1996). Effects of storage, time, temperature, and composition of containers on biologic components of human milk. *Journal of Human Lactation, 12*(1), 31-35.

Wilson-Clay, B., & Hoover, K. (2008). *The Breastfeeding Atlas* (4th ed.). Manchaca, TX: LactNews Press.

Win, N. N., Binns, C. W., Zhao, Y., Scott, J. A., & Oddy, W. H. (2006). Breastfeeding duration in mothers who express breast milk: a cohort study. *International Breastfeeding Journal, 1*, 28.

Sexuality, Fertility, Pregnancy, and Tandem Nursing

Chapter 12

BREASTFEEDING AND SEXUALITY

Changes in Sexual Desire and a Couple's Relationship

During the early postpartum, many breastfeeding mothers feel less sexual desire than they did before their pregnancy.

Whether a couple is married or living together, gay or straight, after a baby's birth, there are many dynamics that can decrease a mother's sexual desire and create tension in their relationship.

- The often-unexpected time and energy it takes to care for a newborn—nonstop days and sleepless nights—which can cause extreme fatigue and mood swings
- Much of a mother's emotional energy is focused on her intense love and feelings of oneness with her baby, often to the exclusion of others
- Changing feelings about their relationship, i.e., some have trouble seeing their partners both as parents and lovers
- Little uninterrupted "couple time"
- Feelings of being "touched out" after intense breastfeeding, making the mother less responsive to her partner's touch
- Birth-related physical or emotional issues, such as discomfort from episiotomy stitches or grief from a disappointing or traumatic birth
- Baby-related challenges, such as health problems or colic
- Hormonal shifts that can contribute to mood swings
- Fears of pregnancy or worries about contraception

Sexual desire and activity may decrease during the first 6 weeks postpartum.

One U.K. cross-sectional study of 484 mothers' sexual experiences during the first 6 months postpartum found that 67% had sex less often than before pregnancy, and only 5% had sex more often (Barrett et al., 2000). Comparing sex before and after birth, 38% described it as "less good," 47% "about the same," and 10% "improved."

If a mother feels less interested in sex, encourage her to talk about it with her partner.

When sex becomes a lower priority for long periods, the mother's partner may feel hurt and confused. The birth of a baby is one of the most stressful times for a couple, and during times of change, couples need to communicate openly. When vague feelings of unhappiness surface, it is time to talk. The mother's partner may need reassurance that her lack of sexual desire is not a personal rejection, but a common response to caring for a young baby. The mother may feel better knowing that her partner will not insist on something she is not comfortable giving and will work with her to find other ways acceptable to them both to strengthen and deepen their relationship.

Some breastfeeding mothers report heightened sexual responsiveness after birth.

For some, the deep feelings of inner peace that can come with breastfeeding spills over into their sexual relationship with their partner. The warmth and tenderness that caring for an infant stimulates sometimes enhance sexual desire and a deeper sexual bond between a mother and her partner. One mother said, "There's something about nursing a baby that gives you an all's-right-with-the-world feeling. I feel so loving toward my whole family, not just toward my baby. Sex just seems to be a natural expression of this good feeling" (Kenny, 1973, p. 220).

Some couples find the full breasts and rounded curves of pregnancy and lactation make a mother more attractive and womanly. Some have fewer worries about pregnancy at these times, allowing for freer sexual expression.

Research is mixed on the effects of breastfeeding on a mothers' postpartum sexuality.

Sex-research pioneers Masters and Johnson found that breastfeeding mothers were more comfortable with their sexuality and more anxious to resume sexual relations with their partners than formula-feeding mothers (Masters & Johnson, 1966). But many social, cultural, and psychological factors affect the expression of a woman's sexuality. So it is not surprising that research is mixed and conclusions vary by country and culture. Research from the Philippines and Bangladesh, for example, indicate that breastfeeding mothers are less interested in sex after childbirth than non-breastfeeding mothers (Islam & Khan, 1993; Udry & Deang, 1993). Research from the U.S. and U.K. found no differences (Grudzinskas & Atkinson, 1984; Robson, Brant, & Kumar, 1981). Research from Kuwait concluded that breastfeeding mothers were more sexually active than those who formula-fed (al Bustan, el Tomi, Faiwalla, & Manav, 1995). Some suggest breastfeeding may be a "swing factor," sometimes enhancing sexual desire and sometimes an obstacle to its expression (Kennedy, 2010).

Two fascinating U.S. studies found that exposure to breastfeeding mothers can affect other women's sexuality. In these studies non-pregnant, non-lactating women smelled a breastfeeding mother's scent (via pads worn on the breastfeeding mother's breast or armpit), which affected them hormonally by either increasing their sexual desire for their partner (or if they didn't have a partner increasing their sexual fantasies) or by regulating their menstrual cycles (Jacob et al., 2004; Spencer et al., 2004).

After the birth of a baby, it can be challenging to find a time and a place to make love and fit "couple time" into a routine.

There is an almost psychic link between many breastfeeding mothers and babies that makes them so closely attuned to each other that the baby wakes up whenever the mother feels strong emotions, including sexual arousal. Fortunately, this type of "radar" is usually short-lived, occurring only while the baby is small. As the baby matures and becomes less dependent upon the mother, the intensity of the mother-baby relationship diminishes.

Time spent together as a couple, whether or not it involves sex, is vital. After the birth of a baby, changes often happen quickly. Ideally, the mother and her partner should support each other as they adjust to their new life as a family. Especially while sex is at a premium, their relationship will more likely stay strong if they make it a priority to be intimate in other ways. If breastfeeding and baby care leave the mother feeling "touched out," for example, suggest she find other ways to be romantic with her partner, such as sharing a favorite meal served by candlelight.

In the early postpartum period, one way the mother's partner can show real caring and love is by pitching in and taking care of household chores—perhaps the best foreplay. Most mothers find it overwhelming to keep up with housework while caring for a tiny baby. If her partner does the housework, the mother may find it easier to relax and find time for sex. In many cases, a mother may need to point out what needs to be done, as her partner may be oblivious to unfinished tasks. Suggest the mother be openly appreciative of her partner's efforts to make their life easier—whether it's by doing household chores or by being patient when the baby consumes most of her time and energy.

Although some couples think they need to arrange for time away from the baby for "couple time," this is not a requirement. Many breastfeeding mothers are more comfortable and relaxed when their baby is near and schedule their couple time at home or take their baby along when they go out with their partner.

A good relationship may lead to better breastfeeding support.

One Brazilian study of 153 families found that the quality of a couple's relationship was not associated with breastfeeding duration, but that a good relationship between the couple was associated with good breastfeeding support from the mother's partner (Falceto, Giugliani, & Fernandes, 2004).

Breastfeeding and Sex: The Practical Details

Most couples resume sex by 5 to 7 weeks postpartum.

In the U.S., many mothers are advised by their healthcare providers to wait until their 6-week postpartum checkup before resuming sex. However, many women start earlier. Two U.K. studies found that 51% of mothers had resumed intercourse by Week 5 postpartum and 62% by Week 7 or 8 (Barrett et al., 2000; Grudzinskas & Atkinson, 1984). Two studies conducted in the Philippines found that 60% of women began having sex again by Week 7 or 8 (Ramos, Kennedy, & Visness, 1996; Udry & Deang, 1993).

Low estrogen levels may cause vaginal dryness, which is easily remedied with lubricants.

All women have low estrogen levels for the first month or two after birth. But breastfeeding extends this period of low estrogen for at least 6 months, and sometimes for the entire duration of lactation (Kennedy, 2010). Low estrogen levels may cause vaginal dryness, tightness, and tenderness. If the mother finds intercourse painful or uncomfortable, more foreplay may help. If that is not enough, suggest she try using a water-based lubricant, such as K-Y jelly. Another option is prescribed estrogen-based creams or suppositories, which research has found helpful with no apparent effect on lactation (Wisniewski & Wilkinson, 1991).

Some women leak milk while having sex.

The hormonal changes during lovemaking stimulate a milk ejection in some women. If either the mother or her partner finds this to be an issue, suggest she feed the baby or express milk before making love to reduce milk flow. She or her partner can stop the flow by applying pressure to the nipples. A towel on hand to catch leaked milk may also help.

Fondling and lovemaking do not need to be restricted during breastfeeding. A mother's breasts should not be considered "off limits," unless the mother wants them to be. Some enjoy the presence of mother's milk during lovemaking.

Some cultures prohibit sexual relations during breastfeeding or until the child reaches a certain age or developmental milestone.

In her classic book, *A Practical Guide to Breastfeeding*, Jan Riordan, EdD wrote: "Pressures and problems of sexual relations while lactating are as ancient as woman herself. Physicians during the 17th century recommended breastfeeding, but insisted that sexual relations during lactation would spoil the milk and endanger the life of the child" (Riordan, 1983, pp. 338-339). Because alternatives to breastfeeding led to higher rates of infant death, wet nurses became popular, allowing mothers to stop breastfeeding to meet their husbands' sexual needs without compromising their babies' health.

Due to the high value placed on child-spacing, some cultures insist on complete abstinence from sex for a specific period of time—from a few weeks to a year or even longer. In some places, resumption of sexual relations is determined by a developmental milestone, such as the eruption of the baby's teeth or the beginning of crawling or walking (Ford & Beach, 1950).

BREASTFEEDING, FERTILITY, AND CONTRACEPTION

The Effect of Breastfeeding on Fertility

Breastfeeding delays the return of a mother's fertility after birth.

The hormones released in the mother when her baby breastfeeds interact with many body processes to prolong the period of infertility after birth. One study from Argentina found that breastfeeding affects the development of the egg (ovum) within the ovary (Velasquez, Creus et al., 2006; Velasquez, Trigo, Creus, Campo, & Croxatto, 2006).

In cultures where exclusive breastfeeding is the norm, the effect of breastfeeding on fertility is greater.

However, the child-spacing effect of breastfeeding in a large population depends in part on the breastfeeding rhythm common in that culture, as well as duration of breastfeeding and the use of other contraceptives. In cultures where mothers breastfeed exclusively and intensely, the effect on fertility is greater. In cultures where mothers encourage longer intervals between feedings, follow feeding schedules, or mix breastfeeding with formula use, the effect on fertility is less. One study demonstrated the profound effect of cultural practices on fertility by analyzing the number of pregnancies prevented by breastfeeding in different countries (Becker, Rutstein, & Labbok, 2003). According to the researchers' calculations, no breastfeeding in Brazil would increase the number of births per year by only 1% to 4%, whereas no breastfeeding in Uganda would increase the number of births annually by 50%.

In some traditional societies, breastfeeding alone is responsible for a typical child-spacing of several years. For example, in the !Kung tribe of Botswana, Africa, despite the absence of sexual taboos during breastfeeding, births were spaced an average of 44 months apart (Konner & Worthman, 1980). The !Kung children are given free access to the breast and may feed briefly several times per hour around the clock for the first year of life. At this end of the spectrum, exclusive and intensive breastfeeding followed by a gradual introduction of solid foods and continued breastfeeding day and night has been reported to delay ovulation for up to 4 years (McNeilly, 2001).

This birth-spacing effect of breastfeeding is nature's way of making sure a mother can give her baby her full attention and her body has a chance to recover from pregnancy and childbirth. In both developing and industrialized nations, adequate spacing can be crucial to the survival of both mother and child. An analysis of research done in 17 countries concluded that a spacing of at least 36 to 59 months is optimal for both mother and child health outcomes in developing countries (Rutstein, 2005). In the U.S., studies have indicated that spacing of at least 28 months reduces maternity-related risks significantly (Klerman, Cliver, & Goldenberg, 1998; Zhu, Rolfs, Nangle, & Horan, 1999).

Before the Menses Resume

The time between birth and the first breastfeeding is one of the first aspects of breastfeeding rhythm associated with fertility, with a shorter time between birth and the first breastfeeding associated with a longer delay in the return of menses, (Kennedy, 2010; WHO, 1998b).

A baby's breastfeeding rhythm plays a major role in the timing of a mother's return to fertility.

The World Health Organization did a prospective study of more than 4,000 breastfeeding women in seven countries and found that 7 of the 10 factors significantly associated with the delay in menstruation after birth involved babies' breastfeeding rhythms (WHO, 1998a; WHO, 1998b). But there's more about breastfeeding that affects fertility than just the hormones released from active suckling. One Chilean study of 99 mother/baby pairs found that suckling activity and length were not associated with a delay in the return of menses, but time at the breast in non-suckling pauses was (Prieto, Cardenas, & Croxatto, 1999). So, sensory aspects of breastfeeding other than suckling may also affect a mother's return to fertility.

Breastfeeding rhythms have a profound effect on fertility and the return of menses.

Breastfeeding rhythm varies tremendously from place to place. As U.S. researcher Kathleen Kennedy noted, it is challenging to try to pinpoint exactly how many times and how long a mother needs to breastfeed each day to suppress fertility because a "breastfeeding" means something so different to different mothers (Kennedy, 2010). A Western mother, for example, may consider a "breastfeeding" a lengthy, ritualized activity, which may involve changing the baby's diaper, making herself a drink, turning off her phone, settling into a certain chair, and then putting her baby to breast for an extended time. A mother in a developing country, in contrast, may keep her baby on her body, putting him to breast at the slightest cue for just a few minutes 15 to 20 times each day. These two babies may get about the same amount of milk in 24 hours, but the immense differences in their rhythms make it difficult to quantify the "breastfeeding" needed to delay fertility.

Generally speaking, breastfeeding exclusively and often day and night—with no long stretches between feedings—produces a longer period of infertility after birth than scheduled or supplemented breastfeeding. This is because baby's time at the breast affects a mother's hormonal balance. One randomized 2-month intervention trial with 141 low-income mothers in Honduras found that when one group fed their babies a supplemental food provided at 4 months of age, 20% more of these mothers were menstruating at 6 months as compared with the mothers who exclusively breastfed between 4 and 6 months (Dewey, Cohen, Rivera, Canahuati, & Brown, 1997). When a mother begins to give her baby other foods, this decreases the amount of time at the breast and alters a mother's hormonal balance. A Chilean study found that ovulation before the first menstrual period occurred more often in women who supplemented their baby by bottle (Diaz et al., 1991).

Depending on her individual body chemistry (see next point), a mother will eventually reach a "tipping point" when her hormonal levels change enough to permit menstruation and ovulation (Labbok, Valdes, & Aravena, 2002). For details on how breastfeeding can be used reliably to space babies, see "Lactational Amenorrhea Method (LAM)" in the next section.

• •

A mother's body chemistry also plays a major role in when her fertility returns.

Population studies reveal how breastfeeding rhythms affect the return to fertility in large groups, but averages do not always apply to individual mothers and babies. Because we do not yet fully understand all of the hormonal interactions and body processes involved in how breastfeeding suppresses fertility, it is impossible to accurately predict when an individual mother will return to fertility (McNeilly, 2001).

Body chemistry explains in part why return to fertility can vary so widely among mothers whose babies have similar breastfeeding rhythms and suckling stimulation. It also explains in part why some mothers who exclusively breastfeed day and night resume their menses within 8 weeks of giving birth, while others resume their menses at 12 months, 24 months, or longer, even when their baby has long sleep stretches or receives regular supplements.

A mother's body chemistry does not usually change from one pregnancy to the next, which explains why research found that the single most significant predictor of when a mother will begin menstruating after birth is her experience after a previous pregnancy (WHO, 1998b). However, if the breastfeeding rhythm varies greatly from one baby to the next, this could cause a mother's return to fertility to also vary (Labbok et al., 2002; Labbok, 2007).

• •

A mother's nutritional status has been found to have little effect on the return of fertility.

Some studies led researchers to believe that breastfeeding mothers with more fat stores and better nutrition began menstruating earlier than breastfeeding mothers with less fat stores and poorer nutrition, but these studies did not control for breastfeeding frequency or supplementation of the baby (Frisch 1988; Prema, Naidu, Neelakumari, & Ramalakshmi, 1981). Research that controlled for these factors concluded that a mother's fat stores and nutritional status have little effect on the return of menses and fertility (Kurz, Habicht, Rasmussen, & Schwager, 1993; Wasalathanthri & Tennekoon, 2001).

• •

Most breastfeeding mothers of younger babies menstruate before ovulating.

Breastfeeding increases the likelihood that a mother's first menstruation will be anovulatory (not preceded by ovulation), especially if she begins menstruating during her baby's first 6 months of life. Because pregnancy is impossible without ovulation, some mothers refer to this as their "warning" period. Mothers who breastfeed exclusively and intensely may have up to three menstrual cycles before they are able to conceive (Labbok, 2007).

The longer a mother's menses are delayed by breastfeeding, the more likely she is to ovulate before her first menstruation. In one Australian study, mothers whose babies were older than 1 year were more than 2.5 times more likely to ovulate before their first menstrual period than mothers whose babies were younger than 3 months (Lewis, Brown, Renfree, & Short, 1991). According to one Indian study, the younger the baby when the mother's menses returned, the more anovulatory cycles the mother was likely to have (Singh, Suchindran, & Singh, 1993). In this study, after 9 months postpartum, though, no differences in fertility were associated with continuing to breastfeed. The effect of breastfeeding on fertility as children mature will depend in large part on the amount of time they spend at the breast, which is much more variable in older children.

A mother's body does not respond to milk expression in the same way it responds to breastfeeding.

A mother's hormonal response to milk expression may not be the same as breastfeeding, so a mother should not assume that expressing her milk will have the same effect on her fertility (Labbok, 2007). See the later section "Lactational Amenorrhea Method" for research on milk expression on fertility in employed mothers.

After solid foods are started, how the solids are given and the breastfeeding rhythm can affect when the mother's menses return.

When solid foods are started, the way they're given can affect whether a mother's menses returns quickly or whether her period of natural fertility is prolonged. To delay the return of her menses as long as possible, a mother can:

- Breastfeed before offering solid foods
- Introduce solid foods gradually
- Continue breastfeeding often day and night, going no longer than 4 hours without breastfeeding during the day and 6 hours at night (Labbok, 2007)

To speed the return of her menses, she can give solids before breastfeeding, introduce lots of solid foods quickly, and increase the intervals between breastfeeding.

As a baby breastfeeds less, the chances of ovulating before menstruating increase.

Some changes that can alter a mother's hormonal balance and increase her odds of ovulating before menstruating include:

- Starting solid foods or significant increasing other foods (fluids or solids)
- Sleeping longer at night
- Decreasing breastfeeding frequency
- Decreasing total time at the breast
- Weaning from the breast

Be sure the mother knows that any changes that decrease breastfeeding frequency increase the possibility of ovulation and pregnancy (Kauffman, 2007).

If a mother wants to become fertile before her menses have returned, one option is to cut back on breastfeeding.

The intensity of breastfeeding needed to suppress fertility will vary from mother to mother, depending on body chemistry. If a mother wants her fertility to return sooner than it would naturally, suggest she gradually increase the intervals between breastfeedings and/or give her baby more other foods. One expert suggests that because the hormonal response to breastfeeding is greater at night, the mother begin by limiting night feedings (Labbok, 2008). When a mother's breast stimulation has decreased enough to cross her own individual hormonal threshold, her fertility will return. Most mothers will become fertile without having to wean from the breast completely, but there are exceptions (see next point).

Hormonal medical treatments have been used to speed breastfeeding mothers' return to fertility, but the research on their safety and efficacy is still preliminary. At this writing, decreasing breastfeeding is the recommended approach (Kauffman, 2007).

Rarely, a mother may find it impossible to become pregnant until her baby is completely weaned from the breast.

For some unusually sensitive mothers who previously breastfed exclusively and intensely, even token breastfeeding can be enough to prevent pregnancy (Gray et al., 1990). In these rare cases, even after a mother has begun menstruating regularly, she may be unable to become pregnant. In this situation, the mother will need to weigh the risks to her current baby of weaning with the benefits of returning to fertility. Once a mother stops breastfeeding completely, fertility usually returns within about 30 days (Kauffman, 2007).

After the Menses Resume

After 8 weeks postpartum, if a mother has vaginal bleeding for 2 days or more or if she has a bleed that she considers to be like a menses, she should assume she's able to become pregnant.

In some women, light bleeding or spotting is the first indication of their return to fertility (Labbok, 2008). One U.S. study found that ovulation was nearly 10 times more likely to precede "regular" or "heavy" bleeding, as opposed to "spotting" or "light" bleeding (Campbell & Gray, 1993). If the mother does not want to conceive again soon, make sure she knows that bleeding increases her chances of getting pregnant.

Continuing to breastfeed after the menses resume reduces a mother's chances of conceiving and maintaining a pregnancy.

Even after a mother begins menstruating again, at first breastfeeding reduces her chances of conceiving. One Chilean study found that when mothers breastfed intensely day and night, each month of breastfeeding after menstruation resumed reduced a mother's chances of conceiving by more than 7% (Diaz et al., 1992). This is because, in many cases, the hormones of breastfeeding cause a deficient egg and follicle and a deficient luteal phase, and the hormonal levels in the second half of the menstrual cycle are too low to maintain a pregnancy.

After menstruation resumes, an increase in breastfeeding or milk expression may suppress it again, but the mother should consider herself fertile.

Sometimes a sudden increase in a baby's breastfeeding (such as during an illness) or a mother's milk expression can cause a mother who was menstruating to temporarily stop. The amount of extra stimulation needed to suppress menstruation will vary from mother to mother. If this happens, suggest the mother consider herself potentially fertile.

Breastfeeding and Contraception

Cultural and religious values will affect the family planning choices a mother finds acceptable, as well as other factors.

A method that is popular and effective in one culture may be unacceptable in another (Chertok & Zimmerman, 2007). Before discussing options, ask the mother what family planning options she is considering and which types of methods she would not find acceptable. Other information that might rule in or rule out some methods include (Labbok, Nichols-Johnson, & Valdes-Anderson, 2006):

- Her breastfeeding rhythm and her baby's age (LAM and hormonal methods)
- Her age (hormonal methods)

- Her partner's opinion
- Her childbearing goals (temporary or permanent methods)
- Her health (temporary or permanent methods, hormonal methods)
- Her financial resources, healthcare options and the availability of methods

Non-Hormonal Methods

Some of the non-hormonal methods support breastfeeding. At the very least, they have no effect on breastfeeding because there is nothing to pass into the milk, affect milk production, or alter milk composition. Be sure the mother who is fully breastfeeding a baby younger than 6 months is aware of the Lactational Amenorrhea Method, or LAM (see next section), as it is a reliable interim option while the mother considers other longer-term alternatives.

Non-hormonal methods of contraception are considered the first choice for breastfeeding mothers since they have no negative impact on breastfeeding.

Lactational Amenorrhea Method (LAM)

Lactational Amenorrhea Method, or LAM, is a temporary family planning method that does not require abstinence and has been found to be at least 98% reliable during the first 6 months postpartum in studies around the world (Kennedy, 2010; Labbok, 2007). This method consists of breastfeeding rhythms (see next point) that provide more than a prolonged period of natural infertility. Because LAM also promotes optimal breastfeeding, it leads to better health outcomes for mothers and babies, saves money that would otherwise be spent on supplements and contraceptives, and gives mothers control over their fertility. LAM is also acceptable to virtually all religious groups.

If the baby is less than 6 months old, the mother is fully breastfeeding and her menses has not resumed, her chance of becoming pregnant is about the same as if she were on the birth-control pill.

Lactational Amenorrhea method (LAM) is an important source of contraception worldwide.

Some reasons mothers give for choosing LAM over other methods is 1) they want a break from using a device or taking a prescribed medication, 2) they want more time before deciding on a long-term or permanent method of contraception, or 3) they prefer a natural method of child-spacing (Labbok, 2007). LAM's effectiveness is independent of a mother's education, religion, country of origin, and available breastfeeding support.

LAM has its roots in a meeting of two dozen researchers held in August 1988 in Bellagio, Italy, whose combined opinion is referred to as the Bellagio Consensus. After evaluating the research on breastfeeding and fertility from developed and developing countries, these researchers came to a better understanding of how an individual mother could use her natural delay in menses as a method of contraception. This led to the development in 1990 of the algorithm that became known as LAM 6 at the Institute for Reproductive Health in Georgetown University in Washington DC (*Guidelines: Breastfeeding, family planning, and the Lactational Amenorrhea Method--LAM*, 1994). For details about this algorithm, see the next point.

• •

Mothers are taught LAM by asking them these three questions:

For LAM to be effective, the answer to three specific questions must be "no."

1. Have your menses returned? (Defined as two consecutive days of bleeding after 8 weeks postpartum or a vaginal bleed the mother considers a menses.)

2. Are you supplementing regularly or allowing long periods without breastfeeding either day or night?
3. Is your baby more than 6 months old?

When a mother can answer "no" to all three questions, she has less than a 2% chance of pregnancy. She should then ask herself these questions regularly. When a mother's answer to any question is "yes," to avoid pregnancy, she should begin using another method of contraception.

To better research and understand LAM, breastfeeding patterns needed to be defined.

The key to suppression of fertility through breastfeeding is frequent breastfeeding day and night. To make it easier for mothers and healthcare providers to understand the impact of feeding on fertility, researchers defined breastfeeding patterns by dividing three main categories—full, partial, and token breastfeeding—into six subcategories:

Full breastfeeding

The key to suppressing fertility through breastfeeding is breastfeeding day and night.

- Exclusive breastfeeding—Baby receives only mother's milk and no other liquids or solids.
- Almost exclusive breastfeeding—Along with breastfeeding, baby receives no more than two mouthfuls daily of other foods, drinks, and/or vitamins/minerals.

Partial breastfeeding

- High partial breastfeeding—Breastfeeding is the vast majority of feedings.
- Medium partial breastfeeding—About half of all feedings are at the breast.
- Low partial breastfeeding—The vast majority of daily feedings are not at the breast.

Token breastfeeding

- The baby breastfeeds minimally, occasionally, or irregularly, not necessarily daily.

The mother can rely on LAM with confidence when she breastfeeds exclusively or almost exclusively (the patterns in "full breastfeeding" category), at least until her menses return, her breastfeeding pattern changes, or her baby turns 6 months old. Research indicates that high partial breastfeeding—with supplements comprising no more than 5% to 15% of a baby's feedings—can also effectively suppress a mother's fertility, especially if she breastfeeds first before giving the supplements. However, if the mother increases supplementation or her baby begins going longer without breastfeeding day or night, she is at increased risk of becoming fertile (Gray et al., 1990). Medium partial breastfeeding delays return of fertility for some mothers, but is not a reliable method to prevent pregnancy. Low partial and token breastfeeding have little effect on fertility.

Some studies have found LAM effective under certain conditions after the first 6 months.

LAM was originally limited to 6 months because this is when introduction of other foods is recommended. But several studies have found that if the mother's menses have not returned, solids are given after the baby breastfeeds, and the mother does not go without breastfeeding for longer than 4 hours during the day and 6 hours at night, very few pregnancies occur (Cooney, Nyirabukeye, Labbok, Hoser, & Ballard, 1996; Kazi, Kennedy, Visness, & Khan, 1995; Kennedy,

2002). One study done in Rwanda, where return of menses occurs on average 12 months postpartum, use of a modified LAM was extended from 6 to 9 months with no reported pregnancies (Cooney et al., 1996). In this extended version of LAM, mothers were also asked the question: "Are you fully or nearly fully breastfeeding your baby during the first 6 months?" and if the baby was between 7 and 9 months, "Are you breastfeeding before giving other foods, so that the baby's hunger is satisfied first with breastmilk, and then with other foods?"

• •

Studies have found that mothers using LAM breastfeed longer and return to fertility later, even where breastfeeding is the norm.

One report found that mothers who used LAM breastfed more often, and at 6 months, they were less likely to have menstruated than other exclusively breastfeeding women (Labbok, 2007).

• •

LAM appears to be slightly less effective in employed mothers expressing milk.

One Chilean study found LAM to be about 95% effective in preventing pregnancy for women who hand-expressed their milk at work (Valdes, Labbok, Pugin, & Perez, 2000), as with the 98% or more effectiveness found in other studies among mothers practicing LAM who were not separated from their babies. In the study of employed mothers, nearly half of the 170 mothers provided their milk exclusively for 6 months, despite their separation from their babies, and half of these women (28.2% of the total) were still not menstruating at 6 months.

Other Natural Methods

Other natural methods involve abstaining from sex during a woman's fertile times.

When a woman uses Natural Family Planning (NFP)—sometimes referred to as the Sympto-Thermal Method—she observes and interprets her body's signs of ovulation, such as changes in her temperature, the consistency of her cervical mucus, and her cervical opening. Because no drugs or products are involved, NFP is safe for mother and baby and does not affect breastfeeding. Training in NFP takes time and usually costs money, and to effectively prevent pregnancy, both the mother and her partner must agree to abstain from intercourse during fertile times.

For the mother who wants to prevent pregnancy without using artificial contraceptives, one option is to start by using LAM (see previous section) and begin NFP when LAM no longer applies. When used correctly, NFP has been found to be 91% to 99% effective (*Guidelines: Breastfeeding, family planning, and the Lactational Amenorrhea Method--LAM*, 1994). When NFP is used incorrectly, it is much less effective.

Another natural method is complete abstinence of sexual relations during breastfeeding, which is practiced in some cultures. Other natural methods involve different criteria for timing intercourse during a mother's infertile times, such as the Ovulation, Post-Ovulation, and Calendar Methods. When practiced perfectly, these methods vary in effectiveness from 91% to 98% (Labbok et al., 2006).

• •

It may be more difficult to recognize the signs of returning fertility when NFP is learned while the mother is breastfeeding.

These fertility signs can be more subtle during breastfeeding than during a woman's regular monthly cycles. Although some breastfeeding mothers notice an obvious change in their cervical mucus before their first postpartum ovulation, some women find their mucus pattern confusing. If a woman also takes her temperature upon awakening in the morning, the rise in her temperature can be used as another indication of ovulation. But if her sleep is disturbed during the night, temperature readings may be unreliable.

One U.S. multicenter study found that breastfeeding mothers using NFP, but not LAM, could nearly always determine when they were fertile, but misidentified many nonfertile days as fertile, resulting in unnecessary abstinence from intercourse (Kennedy et al., 1995). Using LAM during the first 6 months postpartum allowed mothers to avoid much of this unnecessary abstinence (Kennedy et al., 1991). If the mother has not previously learned NFP and she wants to begin while she is breastfeeding, suggest she contact an instructor from the Couple to Couple League (www.ccli.org/).

Barrier Methods and Spermicides

Condoms, diaphragms, and other barriers can be used alone or with other methods.

For the breastfeeding mother, barrier methods, such as condoms, diaphragms, contraceptive sponges, and cervical caps, have advantages over other contraceptive methods. They do not affect breastfeeding, they are easily available in most places, some provide protection from sexually transmitted diseases, they tend to be relatively inexpensive, and they can be used along with other methods. For example, if the mother is using NFP to determine her fertile times (see previous section), barrier methods can be used only when she is fertile, rather than abstaining from intercourse. When used correctly, condoms and diaphragms are generally considered to be very effective in preventing pregnancy (Kennedy, 2010).

Barrier methods of contraception have no impact on breastfeeding.

Barrier methods also have some disadvantages. Unless lubricated condoms are used, they can cause irritation due to vaginal dryness from low estrogen levels during early breastfeeding. Diaphragms require a physical exam for refitting after the mother gives birth and whenever her weight varies by more than 10 lbs. (4.5 kg).

Spermicides used alone or with a barrier method do not affect breastfeeding.

Spermicides can reduce the transmission of some infections and provide welcome lubrication during early breastfeeding (Labbok, 2008). However, some brands may cause irritation in sensitive people, and small amounts may be absorbed and pass into a mother's milk, but no effects on babies have been reported (Kennedy, 2010). Use of spermicides is considered compatible with breastfeeding.

Non-Hormonal IUDs

Non-hormonal IUDs reliably prevent pregnancy and are compatible with breastfeeding.

An intrauterine device (IUD) is a device inserted into a woman's uterus and left in place long-term. It works by altering a mother's hormonal state to prevent fertilization or implantation of a fertilized egg (Labbok, 2007). Highly effective at preventing pregnancy, a non-hormonal IUD does not affect milk production, milk composition, or the breastfeeding baby (Kennedy, 2010).

To reduce risk of expulsion or uterine perforation, IUDs should be inserted within 2 days of birth or after 6 weeks postpartum.

Breastfeeding mothers whose IUD was inserted more than 2 days after birth have reported excess vaginal bleeding or strong uterine contractions at milk ejection (Labbok, 2007). Spontaneous expulsion of an IUD has been associated with timing of insertion. To reduce the risk of expulsion, IUD insertion is recommended within the first 2 days after birth or after 4-to-6-weeks postpartum (Chi, Potts, Wilkens, & Champion, 1989; Labbok et al., 2006; Labbok, 2007).

Although one early U.S. study found an increased risk of uterine perforation among breastfeeding mothers with IUDs (Heartwell & Schlesselman, 1983), later, larger studies found no increased risk when the IUDs were inserted by experienced clinicians (Chi et al., 1989; Farr & Rivera, 1992). Breastfeeding mothers had less pain at IUD insertion and fewer removals for bleeding and pain than non-breastfeeding mothers, and these differences were attributed to the hormonal effects of lactation (Farr & Rivera, 1992).

Surgical Sterilization

Vasectomy and tubal ligation effectively prevent pregnancy, but surgery on the mother may cause an interruption of breastfeeding.

Both of these surgeries involve physically blocking the pathway between sperm and egg. Surgical sterilization should be considered permanent, as reversal cannot be guaranteed. Fewer risks are associated with a vasectomy, which may be done as an office procedure. Surgery on the mother's partner obviously has no effect on breastfeeding.

When a breastfeeding mother has a tubal ligation, however, she faces the risks associated with any surgery, and if performed after birth, there will be a temporary interruption of breastfeeding during the vulnerable early postpartum period (see chapter 2). Also, the pain from the surgery may make breastfeeding uncomfortable afterwards. Suggest the mother planning a tubal ligation after birth give herself enough time between birth and her surgery to express milk for any missed feedings.

Surgical methods of birth control will not impact breastfeeding but mother and baby will be apart and mothers should plan for this.

A full or partial hysterectomy will not affect breastfeeding, other than the challenges faced after any surgery.

The removal of a mother's uterus and/or ovaries will not affect her milk production, which is regulated by hormones secreted by her hypothalamus and pituitary glands. However, when a breastfeeding mother undergoes any surgery, she may need help in maintaining breastfeeding during her hospital stay. For details, see "Health Issues—Mother."

Hormonal Methods

Hormonal methods are not the first choices for a breastfeeding mother due to concerns about milk production and theoretical risks to the baby.

Progestin and estrogen, the hormones used in hormonal methods, are considered compatible with breastfeeding (AAP, 2001). But the World Health Organization, the Academy of Breastfeeding Medicine, and other health organizations consider these methods second and third choices for the breastfeeding mother because small amounts of these hormones pass into the milk, and during the early months of life, a baby is least able to metabolize and excrete both natural and synthetic steroids (Kennedy, 2010; WHO, 2004). There is also the possibility that estrogen and progestin may undermine optimal breastfeeding by decreasing milk production, although this has not been confirmed by research (Truitt, Fraser, Grimes, Gallo, & Schulz, 2003a; Truitt, Fraser, Grimes, Gallo, & Schulz, 2003b). Some experts recommend that hormonal methods be discouraged in some specific situations, such as when mother or baby has health issues, the baby is younger than 6 weeks old (progestin-only methods) or 6 months old (methods containing estrogen), the mother has confirmed low milk production or a history of breast surgery, other causes of milk production problems, multiple births, or her baby was born preterm (Labbok, 2007).

Progestin-Only Methods

Progestin-only hormonal methods, which may be compatible with breastfeeding, are considered the second choice for breastfeeding mothers.

Progestin-only methods prevent pregnancy by thickening cervical mucus, making sperm penetration more difficult, blocking ovulation, and thinning the uterine lining. However, since the onset of lactation occurs due to the rapid fall in natural progestins, the use of these methods in the early postpartum period may disrupt lactation. While studies have not identified any problems with later use of these methods, clinically, there are many anecdotal reports of decreased lactation when these methods are started. All of the following progestin-only methods are not available in all areas, and there are differences among them that may make one a better choice than another.

- **Progestin-only minipill** is most effective when taken at about the same time each day. It is slightly less effective (and less forgiving of missed pills) than the combined pill containing estrogen. Irregular bleeding, a commonly reported side effect of the minipill, is less likely while breastfeeding.
- **Progestin-releasing vaginal ring** is inserted in the vagina and removed for a week every 21 days (Massai et al., 2005).
- **Progestin-only IUD** works like a non-hormonal IUD with the addition of small amounts of progestin released into the mother's system over time. These provide the same degree of pregnancy prevention and breastfeeding outcomes as non-hormonal IUDs (Shaamash, Sayed, Hussien, & Shaaban, 2005). However, a recent study has identified a profound negative impact of this method on lactation (Chen, Creinin, Reeves, & Schwarz, 2009).
- **Progestin-only injectable** (i.e. Depo-Provera) is injected every 3 months. Since it is not reversible, care should be taken in its use during lactation.
- **Progestin-only implant** (i.e. Norplant or Implanon) is inserted under a woman's skin and prevents pregnancy for up to 5 years. Some implants, such as Nesterone or Elcometrine, deliver an orally inactive progesterone that baby cannot absorb, making it a better choice for breastfeeding mothers (Diaz, 2002).

Timed-released methods are used extensively in many U.S. public health departments because they provide highly effective and continuous protection from pregnancy over a long period of time independent of human error. One noteworthy difference among these methods is that the amount of hormone available to the baby through the milk is less with pills and implants and more with injectables, such as Depo-Provera, and the progestin-only IUD (Kennedy, 2010; King, 2007; Shikary et al., 1987).

Mothers should not start progestin-only methods before 6 weeks postpartum.

Most recommend breastfeeding mothers start progestin-only methods no earlier than 6 weeks postpartum.

Controversy exists about how soon after birth breastfeeding mothers should start using progestin-only methods. The World Health Organization and the International Planned Parenthood Federation recommend delaying these methods until breastfeeding has been well established for at least 6 weeks (IPPF, 2002; WHO, 2004). The American College of Obstetricians and Gynecologists recommends waiting at least 2 weeks postpartum to start the progestin-only pills and 6 weeks for implants, injectables, and progestin-only IUDs (ACOG, 2007). Despite these recommendations, many healthcare providers inject mothers they consider to be at high risk of pregnancy with Depo-Provera right after birth, due to worries they may become pregnant before their first postpartum checkup. However, if lactating, the risk of pregnancy in the first 6 to 12 weeks approaches zero, leading to overlap of protection and the possible risk of a negative impact on lactation.

Effects of the hormones on milk production. One concern about early use of these methods is their effect on the hormonal balance needed to establish milk production. In the first days after birth, the biological trigger for the rapid increase in milk production (called lactogenesis II or secretory activation) is the sharp drop in progesterone that occurs after the delivery of the placenta (Pang & Hartmann, 2007). If a mother receives an injection of progestin (a synthetic progesterone) right after delivery, this might alter her hormonal state enough to block milk production.

Hormonal contraceptives may negatively affect milk production.

Very few studies have been done on the use of progestin-only methods during the first 6 weeks, but a 1997 overview on the then-published research concluded that "the use of such contraceptive methods should be delayed for at least 3 days after birth" to allow the natural drop in progesterone to occur before mature milk production begins (Kennedy, Short, & Tully, 1997, p. 347).

In one U.S. study of 95 urban mothers, those who received a Depo-Provera injection at hospital discharge (likely 48 to 72 hours after birth) had a higher rate of exclusive breastfeeding at 1 week (70% vs. 64%) and 8 weeks (26% vs. 19%) than the mothers who used non-hormonal contraception. There were no statistically significant differences between the two groups in feeding frequency or introduction of formula supplements.

Another U.S. study of 319 mostly low-income Hispanic urban mothers examined the effects on breastfeeding of early initiation of progestin-only contraception (Halderman & Nelson, 2002). In this study, mothers were given a choice of non-hormonal methods and progestin-only implants, injectables, or pills. Mothers who chose the pills began taking them at home, while those who opted for implants and injectables received them between 6.25 and 132 hours (a mean of 52 hours) after birth. At 2, 4, and 6 weeks postpartum, the percentage of mothers exclusively breastfeeding in the hormonal contraception group were equal to or greater than those in the non-hormonal group. The same was true among those who received the Depo-Provera injection. At 2 weeks, 41% were exclusively breastfeeding, compared with 37% of the mothers in the non-hormonal group. At 4 weeks, the two groups breastfed comparably: 32% vs. 31%. And at 6 weeks, 37% of the mothers who received the Depo-Provera injection breastfed exclusively compared with 35% of the mothers using non-hormonal contraception. Because breastfeeding was not defined in these studies, the impact of these methods on milk production is not clear.

When considering the timing of starting progestin-only methods, suggest the mother and her healthcare provider factor in the period of natural infertility breastfeeding provides while her baby is primarily breastfeeding. (See the previous section on LAM.)

Effects of the hormones on the baby. In addition to concerns about milk production, there is a concern that the newborn may have difficulty metabolizing the hormones during the early postpartum period (Diaz, 2002; Kennedy, 2010). However, one expert writes, "The direct effect on the nursing infant is generally unknown, but it is believed to be minimal to none as natural progesterone is poorly bioavailable to the infant via milk" (Hale, 2008, p. 796). In other words, even if the baby receives progesterone in the milk, it will not be well absorbed from the gut (Shabaan 1991). And as of this writing, research has followed the breastfed children of mothers who used progestin-only methods for up to 17 years, with no long-term effects found on growth or development, including sexual development (Nilsson et al., 1986; Pardthaisong, Yenchit, & Gray, 1992).

One South African study found that when mothers were given appropriate information about the risks and benefits, they were able to make informed decisions about when to start progestin-only contraceptives based on their own situation and individual considerations (Hani, Moss, Cooper, Morroni, & Hoffman, 2003).

• •

There are anecdotal clinical reports of breastfeeding mothers having a drop in milk production after they start progestin-only methods.

These individual case reports are one reason these methods are considered the second choice for breastfeeding mothers, rather than the first. However, there is little research to confirm this effect. One three-center study done in Hungary and Thailand found a 12% decrease in milk volume among mothers taking the progestin-only minipill (the mothers using non-hormonal methods had a 6% decrease) (Tankeyoon et al., 1984). But few studies randomized or introduced the method in the first 2 days. Most research, with later introduction of these methods, found no statistically significant association between the use of progestin-only methods and decreased milk production, altered breastfeeding rhythms, or slowed infant growth or development, whether mothers used progestin-only minipills (McCann, Moggia, Higgins, Potts, & Becker, 1989; Moggia et al., 1991; Sinchai et al., 1995), injectables (Halderman & Nelson, 2002; Hannon et al., 1997), vaginal rings (Massai et al., 2005; Shaaban, 1991; Sivin et al., 1997), or implants (Reinprayoon et al., 2000; Schiappacasse, Diaz, Zepeda, Alvarado, & Herreros, 2002; Taneepanichskul et al., 2006).

In fact, some studies reported that mothers using progestin-only methods had slightly better milk volumes and longer duration of breastfeeding than mothers using non-hormonal methods (Halderman & Nelson, 2002; Koetsawang, 1987; Sinchai et al., 1995).

Methods Containing Estrogen

Contraceptive methods containing estrogen, the third choice for breastfeeding mothers, are not recommended until the baby is at least 6 months old.

Contraceptives containing estrogen are considered the third and last choice for breastfeeding mothers because estrogen has been found to decrease milk production and breastfeeding duration. The most common of these methods is the combined oral contraceptive pill, which is taken daily and contains both estrogen and progestin. Other combined methods include the contraceptive patch, the combined injectable, and the combined vaginal ring, all of which, like Depo-Provera (see previous section), give continuous highly effective protection from pregnancy and are immune to human error. These methods are not recommended for women over 35 who smoke and those with clotting problems, estrogen-dependent cancers, or severe migraines (Labbok, 2007). A disadvantage of the combined injectable is its inability to be discontinued if milk production problems develop.

If possible, mothers should avoid contraceptives containing estrogen for the first 6 months.

Concerns first arose about the use of combined oral contraceptives by breastfeeding mothers when higher-estrogen pills taken during the first weeks postpartum were found to decrease milk production between 20% and 40% (Koetsawang, 1987; WHO, 1988). When the newer combined oral contraceptives with lower-dose estrogen were started after full milk production is established, they appeared to have less effect on both breastfeeding duration and milk production, but due to the previously documented risks of these methods, both the World Health Organization and the International Planned Parenthood Federation recommend that breastfeeding mothers avoid them until their baby is at least 6 months old, when the introduction of solid foods can offset any decrease in milk production (IPPF, 2002; Kennedy, 2010; WHO, 2004).

The breastfed baby of a mother on combined oral contraceptives receives no more estrogen than he would receive from his mother during breastfeeding.

Both estrogen and progestin are considered compatible with breastfeeding by the American Academy of Pediatrics (AAP, 2001). One U.S. author wrote, "...the transfer of estradiol [estrogen] to human milk will be low and will not exceed the transfer during physiologic conditions when the mother has resumed ovulating" (Hale, 2008, p. 349). Hormonal contraceptives have been used by breastfeeding mothers for several decades and no short- or long-term effects of estrogen on breastfeeding babies have been reported.

Previous concerns about changes in milk composition with combined contraceptives appear to be unfounded.

Although some early studies noted slight changes in milk composition in mothers using hormonal contraception, later studies found no cause for concern (Dorea & Miazaki, 1999; Dorea & Myazaki, 1998; Fraser, 1991). The changes observed were within the normal variations in milk composition from feeding to feeding and day to day (Labbok, 2007).

If a breastfeeding mother uses a method containing estrogen, suggest she keep breastfeeding and monitor her baby's weight gain.

A breastfeeding mother using a contraceptive method containing estrogen should watch for any signs of decreased milk production. Suggest she schedule regular checkups with her baby's healthcare provider to monitor his weight gain, the most reliable gauge of adequate milk intake.

Emergency Contraception

An emergency contraceptive contains a high dose of progestin, but breastfeeding can continue uninterrupted.

One Chilean study measured breastfeeding mothers' blood and milk levels of levonorgesterol after receiving the single 1.5 mg dose used for emergency contraception (Gainer et al., 2007). The estimated infant exposure to this drug during the first 8 hours, when the levels were highest, was 1.0 µg, and during the first 24 hours was 1.6 µg. In light of the relative infant dose (RID) of this drug, Thomas Hale, author of *Medications and Mother's Milk,* considers this exposure "no risk at all for an infant" and recommends continued breastfeeding without interruption (T.W. Hale, personal communication, October 8, 2009).

RESOURCES FOR PARENTS

Websites

www.ccli.org -- Couple to Couple League, an organization that teaches Natural Family Planning (NFP)

Books

Bumgarner, N. (2000). *Mothering your nursing toddler*. Rev. ed. Schaumburg, Illinois: La Leche League International.

Couple to Couple League. (2007). *The art of natural family planning.* Cincinnati, OH: Couple to Couple League.

REFERENCES

AAP. (2001). Transfer of drugs and other chemicals into human milk. *Pediatrics, 108*(3), 776-789.

ACOG. (2007). ACOG Committee Opinion No. 361: Breastfeeding: maternal and infant aspects. *Obstetrics and Gynecology, 109*(2 Pt 1), 479-480.

al Bustan, M. A., el Tomi, N. F., Faiwalla, M. F., & Manav, V. (1995). Maternal sexuality during pregnancy and after childbirth in Muslim Kuwaiti women. *Archives of Sexual Behavior, 24*(2), 207-215.

Barrett, G., Pendry, E., Peacock, J., Victor, C., Thakar, R., & Manyonda, I. (2000). Women's sexual health after childbirth. *British Journal of Obstetrics and Gynaecology, 107*(2), 186-195.

Becker, S., Rutstein, S., & Labbok, M. H. (2003). Estimation of births averted due to breastfeeding and increases in levels of contraception needed to substitute for breastfeeding. *Journal of Biosocial Science, 35*(4), 559-574.

Campbell, O. M., & Gray, R. H. (1993). Characteristics and determinants of postpartum ovarian function in women in the United States. *American Journal of Obstetrics and Gynecology, 169*(1), 55-60.

Chen, B. A., Creinin, M. D., Reeves, M. F., & Schwarz, E. B. (2009). Breastfeeding continuation among women using the levonorgestrel-releasing intrauterine device after vaginal delivery. [abstract]. *Contraception, 80*, 204.

Chertok, I. R., & Zimmerman, D. R. (2007). Contraceptive considerations for breastfeeding women within Jewish law. *International Breastfeeding Journal, 2*, 1.

Chi, I. C., Potts, M., Wilkens, L. R., & Champion, C. B. (1989). Performance of the copper T-380A intrauterine device in breastfeeding women. *Contraception, 39*(6), 603-618.

Cooney, K. A., Nyirabukeye, T., Labbok, M. H., Hoser, P. H., & Ballard, E. (1996). An assessment of the nine-month lactational amenorrhea method (MAMA-9) in Rwanda. *Studies in Family Planning, 27*(3), 102-171.

Dewey, K. G., Cohen, R. J., Rivera, L. L., Canahuati, J., & Brown, K. H. (1997). Effects of age at introduction of complementary foods to breast-fed infants on duration of lactational amenorrhea in Honduran women. *American Journal of Clinical Nutrition, 65*(5), 1403-1409.

Diaz, S. (2002). Contraceptive implants and lactation. *Contraception, 65*(1), 39-46.

Diaz, S., Aravena, R., Cardenas, H., Casado, M. E., Miranda, P., Schiappacasse, V., et al. (1991). Contraceptive efficacy of lactational amenorrhea in urban Chilean women. *Contraception, 43*(4), 335-352.

Diaz, S., Cardenas, H., Brandeis, A., Miranda, P., Salvatierra, A. M., & Croxatto, H. B. (1992). Relative contributions of anovulation and luteal phase defect to the reduced pregnancy rate of breastfeeding women. *Fertility and Sterility, 58*(3), 498-503.

Dorea, J. G., & Miazaki, E. S. (1999). The effects of oral contraceptive use on iron and copper concentrations in breast milk. *Fertility and Sterility, 72*(2), 297-301.

Dorea, J. G., & Myazaki, E. (1998). Calcium and phosphorus in milk of Brazilian mothers using oral contraceptives. *Journal of the American College of Nutrition, 17*(6), 642-646.

Falceto, O. G., Giugliani, E. R., & Fernandes, C. L. (2004). Couples' relationships and breastfeeding: is there an association? *Journal of Human Lactation, 20*(1), 46-55.

Farr, G., & Rivera, R. (1992). Interactions between intrauterine contraceptive device use and breast-feeding status at time of intrauterine contraceptive device insertion: analysis of TCu-380A acceptors in developing countries. *American Journal of Obstetrics and Gynecology, 167*(1), 144-151.

Ford, C., & Beach, F. (1950). *Patterns of sexual behavior*. New York: Harper & Row.

Fraser, I. S. (1991). A review of the use of progestogen-only minipills for contraception during lactation. *Reproduction, Fertility, and Development, 3*(3), 245-254.

Frisch, R. E. (1988). Fatness and fertility. *Scientific American, 258*(3), 88-95.

Gainer, E., Massai, R., Lillo, S., Reyes, V., Forcelledo, M. L., Caviedes, R., et al. (2007). Levonorgestrel pharmacokinetics in plasma and milk of lactating women who take 1.5 mg for emergency contraception. *Human Reproduction, 22*(6), 1578-1584.

Gray, R. H., Campbell, O. M., Apelo, R., Eslami, S. S., Zacur, H., Ramos, R. M., et al. (1990). Risk of ovulation during lactation. *Lancet, 335*(8680), 25-29.

Grudzinskas, J. G., & Atkinson, L. (1984). Sexual function during the puerperium. *Archives of Sexual Behavior, 13*(1), 85-91.

Guidelines: Breastfeeding, family planning, and the Lactational Amenorrhea Method--LAM. (1994). Washington, DC: Institute for Reproductive Health, Georgetown University.

Halderman, L. D., & Nelson, A. L. (2002). Impact of early postpartum administration of progestin-only hormonal contraceptives compared with nonhormonal contraceptives on short-term breast-feeding patterns. *American Journal of Obstetrics and Gynecology, 186*(6), 1250-1256; discussion 1256-1258.

Hale, T. (2008). *Medications and Mothers' Milk* (13 ed.). Amarillo, TX: Hale Publishing.

Hani, A., Moss, M., Cooper, D., Morroni, C., & Hoffman, M. (2003). Informed choice--the timing of postpartum contraceptive initiation. *South African Medical Journal, 93*(11), 862-864.

Hannon, P. R., Duggan, A. K., Serwint, J. R., Vogelhut, J. W., Witter, F., & DeAngelis, C. (1997). The influence of medroxyprogesterone on the duration of breast-feeding in mothers in an urban community. *Archives of Pediatrics and Adolescent Medicine, 151*(5), 490-496.

Heartwell, S. F., & Schlesselman, S. (1983). Risk of uterine perforation among users of intrauterine devices. *Obstetrics and Gynecology, 61*(1), 31-36.

IPPF. (2002). IMAP statement on hormonal methods of contraception. *IPPF Medical Bulletin, 36*(5), 1-8.

Islam, M. M., & Khan, H. T. A. (1993). Pattern of coital frequency in rural Bangladesh. *Journal of Family Welfare, 39*, 38-43.

Jacob, S., Spencer, N. A., Bullivant, S. B., Sellergren, S. A., Mennella, J. A., & McClintock, M. K. (2004). Effects of breastfeeding chemosignals on the human menstrual cycle. *Human Reproduction, 19*(2), 422-429.

Kauffman, R. P. (2007). Reproductive bioenergetics, infertility, and ovulation induction in the lactating female. In T. W. Hale & P. F. Hartmann (Eds.), *Hale & Hartmann's Textbok of Human Lactation* (pp. 319-342). Amarillo, TX: Hale Publishing.

Kazi, A., Kennedy, K. I., Visness, C. M., & Khan, T. (1995). Effectiveness of the lactational amenorrhea method in Pakistan. *Fertility and Sterility, 64*(4), 717-723.

Kennedy, K. I. (2002). Efficacy and effectiveness of LAM. In M. K. Davis, C. Isaacs, L. A. Hanson & A. L. Wright (Eds.), *Advances in experimental medicine and biology: integrating population outcomes, biolgoical mechanims and research methods in the study of human milk and lactation* (2002/05/25 ed., pp. 207-216). New York: Kluwer Academic/Plenum Publishers.

Kennedy, K. I. (2010). Fertility, sexuality, and contraception during lactation. In J. Riordan & K. Wambach (Eds.), *Breastfeeding and human lactation* (4th ed., pp. 705-736). Boston, MA: Jones and Bartlett.

Kennedy, K. I., Gross, B. A., Parenteau-Carreau, S., Flynn, A. M., Brown, J. B., & Visness, C. M. (1995). Breastfeeding and the symptothermal method. *Studies in Family Planning, 26*(2), 107-115.

Kennedy, K. I., Parenteau-Carreau, S., Flynn, A., Gross, B., Brown, J. B., & Visness, C. (1991). The natural family planning--lactational amenorrhea method interface: observations from a prospective study of breastfeeding users of natural family planning. *American Journal of Obstetrics and Gynecology, 165*(6 Pt 2), 2020-2026.

Kennedy, K. I., Short, R. V., & Tully, M. R. (1997). Premature introduction of progestin-only contraceptive methods during lactation. *Contraception, 55*(6), 347-350.

Kenny, J. A. (1973). Sexuality of pregnant and breastfeeding women. *Archives of Sexual Behavior, 2*(3), 215-229.

King, J. (2007). Contraception and lactation. *Journal of Midwifery & Women's Health, 52*(6), 614-620.

Klerman, L. V., Cliver, S. P., & Goldenberg, R. L. (1998). The impact of short interpregnancy intervals on pregnancy outcomes in a low-income population. *American Journal of Public Health, 88*(8), 1182-1185.

Koetsawang, S. (1987). The effects of contraceptive methods on the quality and quantity of breastmilk. *International Journal of Gynaecology and Obstetrics, 25(suppl)*, 115-128.

Konner, M., & Worthman, C. (1980). Nursing frequency, gonadal function, and birth spacing among !Kung hunter-gatherers. *Science, 207*(4432), 788-791.

Kurz, K. M., Habicht, J. P., Rasmussen, K. M., & Schwager, S. J. (1993). Effects of maternal nutritional status and maternal energy supplementation on length of postpartum amenorrhea among Guatemalan women. *American Journal of Clinical Nutrition, 58*(5), 636-642.

Labbok, M., Nichols-Johnson, V., & Valdes-Anderson, V. (2006). ABM clinical protocol #13: contraception during breastfeeding. *Breastfeeding Medicine, 1*(1), 43-51.

Labbok, M., Valdes, V., & Aravena, R. (2002). Determinants of menses return in lactating women. In M. K. Davis, C. Isaacs, L. A. Hanson & A. L. Wright (Eds.), *Advances in experimental medicine and biology: integrating population outcomes, biological mechanisms and research methods in the study of human milk and lactation* (pp. 285-287). New York: Kluwer Academic Plenum Publishers.

Labbok, M. H. (2007). Breastfeeding, birth spacing, and family planning. In T. W. Hale & P. F. Hartmann (Eds.), *Hale & Hartmann's textbook of human lactation* (pp. 305-318). Amarillo, TX: Hale Publishing.

Labbok, M. H. (2008). *Breastfeeding, fertility, and family planning*. Accessed on March 11, 2010 from http://www.glowm.com/index.html?p=glowm.cml/section_view&articleid=396&recordset=&value=396

Lewis, P. R., Brown, J. B., Renfree, M. B., & Short, R. V. (1991). The resumption of ovulation and menstruation in a well-nourished population of women breastfeeding for an extended period of time. *Fertility and Sterility, 55*(3), 529-536.

Massai, R., Makarainen, L., Kuukankorpi, A., Klipping, C., Duijkers, I., & Dieben, T. (2005). The combined contraceptive vaginal ring and bone mineral density in healthy pre-menopausal women. *Human Reproduction, 20*(10), 2764-2768.

Masters, W., & Johnson, V. (1966). *Human sexual response*. Boston, MA: Little, Brown & Company.

McCann, M. F., Moggia, A. V., Higgins, J. E., Potts, M., & Becker, C. (1989). The effects of a progestin-only oral contraceptive (levonorgestrel 0.03 mg) on breast-feeding. *Contraception, 40*(6), 635-648.

McNeilly, A. S. (2001). Neuroendocrine changes and fertility in breast-feeding women. *Progress in Brain Research, 133*, 207-214.

Moggia, A. V., Harris, G. S., Dunson, T. R., Diaz, R., Moggia, M. S., Ferrer, M. A., et al. (1991). A comparative study of a progestin-only oral contraceptive versus non-hormonal methods in lactating women in Buenos Aires, Argentina. *Contraception, 44*(1), 31-43.

Nilsson, S., Mellbin, T., Hofvander, Y., Sundelin, C., Valentin, J., & Nygren, K. G. (1986). Long-term follow-up of children breast-fed by mothers using oral contraceptives. *Contraception, 34*(5), 443-457.

Pang, W. W., & Hartmann, P. E. (2007). Initiation of human lactation: secretory differentiation and secretory activation. *Journal of Mammary Gland Biology and Neoplasia, 12*(4), 211-221.

Pardthaisong, T., Yenchit, C., & Gray, R. (1992). The long-term growth and development of children exposed to Depo-Provera during pregnancy or lactation. *Contraception, 45*(4), 313-324.

Prema, K., Naidu, A. N., Neelakumari, S., & Ramalakshmi, B. A. (1981). Nutrition-fertility interaction in lactating women of low income groups. *British Journal of Nutrition, 45*(3), 461-467.

Prieto, C. R., Cardenas, H., & Croxatto, H. B. (1999). Variability of breast sucking, associated milk transfer and the duration of lactational amenorrhoea. *Journal of Reproduction and Fertility, 115*(2), 193-200.

Ramos, R., Kennedy, K. I., & Visness, C. M. (1996). Effectiveness of lactational amenorrhoea in prevention of pregnancy in Manila, the Philippines: non-comparative prospective trail. *British Medical Journal, 313*(7062), 909-912.

Reinprayoon, D., Taneepanichskul, S., Bunyavejchevin, S., Thaithumyanon, P., Punnahitananda, S., Tosukhowong, P., et al. (2000). Effects of the etonogestrel-releasing contraceptive implant (Implanon on parameters of breastfeeding compared to those of an intrauterine device. *Contraception, 62*(5), 239-246.

Riordan, J. (1983). *A practical guide to breastfeeding*. St. Louis, MO: The C.V. Mosby Company.

Robson, K. M., Brant, H. A., & Kumar, R. (1981). Maternal sexuality during first pregnancy and after childbirth. *British Journal of Obstetrics and Gynaecology, 88*(9), 882-889.

Rutstein, S. O. (2005). Effects of preceding birth intervals on neonatal, infant and under-five years mortality and nutritional status in developing countries: evidence from the demographic and health surveys. *International Journal of Gynaecology and Obstetrics, 89 Suppl 1*, S7-24.

Schiappacasse, V., Diaz, S., Zepeda, A., Alvarado, R., & Herreros, C. (2002). Health and growth of infants breastfed by Norplant contraceptive implants users: a six-year follow-up study. *Contraception, 66*(1), 57-65.

Shaaban, M. M. (1991). Contraception with progestogens and progesterone during lactation. *Journal of Steroid Biochemistry and Molecular Biology, 40*(4-6), 705-710.

Shaamash, A. H., Sayed, G. H., Hussien, M. M., & Shaaban, M. M. (2005). A comparative study of the levonorgestrel-releasing intrauterine system Mirena versus the Copper T380A intrauterine device during lactation: breast-feeding performance, infant growth and infant development. *Contraception, 72*(5), 346-351.

Shikary, Z. K., Betrabet, S. S., Patel, Z. M., Patel, S., Joshi, J. V., Toddywala, V. S., et al. (1987). ICMR task force study on hormonal contraception. Transfer of levonorgestrel (LNG) administered through different drug delivery systems from the maternal circulation into the newborn infant's circulation via breast milk. *Contraception, 35*(5), 477-486.

Sinchai, W., Sethavanich, S., Asavapiriyanont, S., Sittipiyasakul, V., Sirikanchanakul, R., Udomkiatsakul, P., et al. (1995). Effects of a progestogen-only pill (Exluton) and an intrauterine device (Multiload Cu250) on breastfeeding. *Advances in Contraception, 11*(2), 143-155.

Singh, K. K., Suchindran, C. M., & Singh, K. (1993). Effects of breast feeding after resumption of menstruation on waiting time to next conception. *Human Biology, 65*(1), 71-86.

Sivin, I., Diaz, S., Croxatto, H. B., Miranda, P., Shaaban, M., Sayed, E. H., et al. (1997). Contraceptives for lactating women: a comparative trial of a progesterone-releasing vaginal ring and the copper T 380A IUD. *Contraception, 55*(4), 225-232.

Spencer, N. A., McClintock, M. K., Sellergren, S. A., Bullivant, S., Jacob, S., & Mennella, J. A. (2004). Social chemosignals from breastfeeding women increase sexual motivation. *Hormones and Behavior, 46*(3), 362-370.

Taneepanichskul, S., Reinprayoon, D., Thaithumyanon, P., Praisuwanna, P., Tosukhowong, P., & Dieben, T. (2006). Effects of the etonogestrel-releasing implant Implanon and a nonmedicated intrauterine device on the growth of breast-fed infants. *Contraception, 73*(4), 368-371.

Tankeyoon, M., Dusitsin, N., Chalapati, S., Koetsawang, S., Saibiang, S., Sas, M., et al. (1984). Effects of hormonal contraceptives on milk volume and infant growth. WHO Special Programme of Research, Development and Research Training in Human Reproduction Task force on oral contraceptives. *Contraception, 30*(6), 505-522.

Truitt, S. T., Fraser, A. B., Grimes, D. A., Gallo, M. F., & Schulz, K. F. (2003a). Combined hormonal versus nonhormonal versus progestin-only contraception in lactation. *Cochrane Database of Systematic Reviews*(2), CD003988.

Truitt, S. T., Fraser, A. B., Grimes, D. A., Gallo, M. F., & Schulz, K. F. (2003b). Hormonal contraception during lactation. systematic review of randomized controlled trials. *Contraception, 68*(4), 233-238.

Udry, J. R., & Deang, L. (1993). Determinants of coitus after childbirth. *Journal of Biosocial Science, 25*(1), 117-125.

Valdes, V., Labbok, M. H., Pugin, E., & Perez, A. (2000). The efficacy of the lactational amenorrhea method (LAM) among working women. *Contraception, 62*(5), 217-219.

Velasquez, E. V., Creus, S., Trigo, R. V., Cigorraga, S. B., Pellizzari, E. H., Croxatto, H. B., et al. (2006). Pituitary-ovarian axis during lactational amenorrhoea. II. Longitudinal assessment of serum FSH polymorphism before and after recovery of menstrual cycles. *Human Reproduction, 21*(4), 916-923.

Velasquez, E. V., Trigo, R. V., Creus, S., Campo, S., & Croxatto, H. B. (2006). Pituitary-ovarian axis during lactational amenorrhoea. I. Longitudinal assessment of follicular growth, gonadotrophins, sex steroids and inhibin levels before and after recovery of menstrual cyclicity. *Human Reproduction, 21*(4), 909-915.

Wasalathanthri, S., & Tennekoon, K. H. (2001). Lactational amenorrhea/anovulation and some of their determinants: a comparison of well-nourished and undernourished women. *Fertility and Sterility, 76*(2), 317-325.

WHO. (1988). Effects of hormonal contraceptives on breast milk composition and infant growth. *Studies in Family Planning, 19*, 36-69.

WHO. (1998a). The World Health Organization Multinational Study of Breast-feeding and Lactational Amenorrhea. I. Description of infant feeding patterns and of the return of menses. World Health Organization Task Force on Methods for the Natural Regulation of Fertility. *Fertility and Sterility, 70*(3), 448-460.

WHO. (1998b). The World Health Organization Multinational Study of Breast-feeding and Lactational Amenorrhea. II. Factors associated with the length of amenorrhea. World Health Organization Task Force on Methods for the Natural Regulation of Fertility. *Fertility and Sterility, 70*(3), 461-471.

WHO. (2004). *Selected practice recommendations for contraceptive use* (2nd ed.). Geneva, Switzerland: WHO Reproductive Health Research Division.

Zhu, B. P., Rolfs, R. T., Nangle, B. E., & Horan, J. M. (1999). Effect of the interval between pregnancies on perinatal outcomes. *New England Journal of Medicine, 340*(8), 589-594.

Nutrition, Exercise, and Lifestyle Issues

Chapter 13

NUTRITION

Nutrition Basics

When talking to mothers, keep nutrition information simple and basic.

The same basic nutrition guidelines apply to the breastfeeding mother as apply to the rest of the family. To make her diet more nutrient-dense, suggest the mother choose fresh foods as close to their natural state as possible. Fresh fruits and vegetables, whole grain breads and cereals, and foods rich in calcium and protein are all good choices. The specific foods a mother chooses from these categories will vary according to her personal preferences, culture, climate, and family finances.

Nutrition-dense foods, such as fruits and vegetables and whole grains, are good choices for new mothers.

Keep diet information simple. Perceiving nutrition information as complicated may convince a mother not to breastfeed. According to one breastfeeding book written for doctors: "...[O]ne barrier to breastfeeding for some women is the 'diet rules' they see as being too hard to follow or too restrictive" (Lawrence & Lawrence, 2005, p. 317).

Suggest busy mothers keep nutritious foods on hand that don't require much preparation.

The biggest challenge for many breastfeeding mothers is finding the time for food shopping and cooking. But many foods are both nutritious and easy to eat as snacks or quick meals, such as cheese and crackers, yogurt, nuts, whole-grain bread, sprouts, sliced tomatoes, fresh fruits, whole or sliced raw vegetables, and hard-boiled eggs. Some mothers find smaller, more frequent meals easier to manage than three larger meals. Suggest the mother see if she feels better when she has a healthy snack and drink whenever she breastfeeds, rather than preparing larger meals. Some dietetic professionals recommend frozen and canned fruits and vegetables when fresh foods are not available to reduce preparation time and make it easier for the mother to eat more of these healthy foods (C. Lovelady, personal communication, February 15, 2010).

Other ways to simplify meal preparation include planning meals a week at a time to cut down on trips to buy food and washing and cutting vegetables in large batches for snacking or adding to a salad or main dish. Suggest when she cooks to make double batches of main dishes and freeze half for quick meals on hectic days. She (or a helper) can also use a slow cooker ("crock pot") to start dinner in the morning that will be ready during the hectic early evening hours. If others ask how they can help, suggest asking for meals. For some families, take-out meals may also be an option.

Even when food is scarce, breastfeeding mothers make ample milk.

A mother's diet is only one source of the energy and nutrients she needs to make milk. Energy and most nutrients can also be drawn from the body stores laid down during pregnancy (Hopkinson, 2007). Even mildly malnourished mothers in developing countries produce plenty of good quality milk for their babies. In one study from Gambia, a developing country where food supplies to mothers were limited, when mothers were given nutritional supplements, their babies did not gain more weight than the babies of women whose diets were not supplemented (Prentice et al., 1983). A meta-analysis examining research from around the globe found that only when famine or near famine conditions last weeks does a mother's milk production or milk quality suffer (Prentice, Goldberg, & Prentice, 1994). One Dutch study found that even in famine conditions, milk production may be only slightly affected among previously well-nourished mothers with good body stores (Smith, 1947).

Activity levels also affect mothers' nutritional needs. During the first 4 or 5 weeks after birth, most mothers are less physically active than they are at other times in their lives (Butte & King, 2005). This also reduces their need for calories.

Suggest the mother "eat to hunger," rather than counting calories.

Milk production has been estimated to use about 500 calories per day (IOM, 2005), with some of this energy coming from a mother's body stores. There is no need for an average-weight mother to keep careful track of her caloric intake. She can simply "eat to hunger," or use her appetite as her guide. Most mothers tend to feel hungrier while breastfeeding, so encourage her to trust her appetite and choose nutritious foods because they give her more energy and increase her resistance to illness. If a mother is overweight when she gives birth, limiting sweetened drinks and high-fat snack foods can help her bring her weight down during breastfeeding (see later section on weight loss).

The types of fatty acids in a mother's milk will vary with the fats she eats.

While the overall fat content of a mother's milk remains stable, the amounts of different types of fat vary by diet. For example, mothers who eat more unsaturated fats (mainly found in fish, nuts, seeds and oils from plants) tend to produce milk higher in unsaturated fats than mothers who eat more animal products (Hopkinson, 2007). Mothers who take fish oil or cod liver oil supplements produce milk richer in DHA (Olafsdottir, Thorsdottir, Wagner, & Elmadfa, 2006). These appear to be normal variations.

If a mother goes on a fast, be sure she knows that any changes in her baby's breastfeeding patterns or behavior are temporary.

Israeli research has looked at both milk composition and babies' behavior during the 24-hour fast of Yom Kippur in 48 breastfeeding women with babies between 1 and 6 months of age (Zimmerman et al., 2009). After mothers abstained from all food and drink for 24 hours, their milk was higher in sodium, calcium, and protein and lower in phosphorus and lactose. During the fast, some mothers indicated their babies wanted to breastfeed more often or seemed fussier than usual. The researchers suggest reassuring mothers in this situation that any changes in breastfeeding pattern or behavior is temporary and will return to normal after the fast, as long as the mother breastfeeds whenever the baby shows feeding cues.

Chronically undernourished mothers who do not get enough to eat may make milk lower in some vitamins.

A malnourished mother without good body stores and an inadequate diet is at risk of making milk lower than normal in some vitamins, including A, D, B_6, or B_{12} (Hopkinson, 2007). In this case, an improved diet or vitamin supplements would bring milk vitamin levels back to normal (see the section "Vitamin/Mineral Supplements").

Fluids

Suggest the breastfeeding mother "drink to thirst."

Following this guideline should provide all the fluids a breastfeeding mother needs (USDA, 2005). Most mothers feel thirstier more often while they are breastfeeding, so they may find themselves drinking more fluids than they were drinking before . Encourage the mother to take a drink at the first sign of thirst, rather than waiting until she is feeling parched. If a mother notices feeling thirsty while her baby breastfeeds, suggest she routinely have a drink handy when they get ready to feed.

While water is always a good choice, other fluids, such as fruit and vegetable juices, milk, and soups, can satisfy a mother's thirst and provide needed nutrients.

• •

Contrary to popular belief, drinking more fluids is not associated with greater milk production.

When a mother is concerned about her milk production, often the first advice she is given is to drink more fluids. But one U.S. study found that when mothers drank 25% more fluids than when they "drank to thirst," there was no statistically significant difference in milk production (Dusdieker, Booth, Stumbo, & Eichenberger, 1985). In fact, during the "more fluids" period, the mothers produced slightly less milk. A Canadian pilot study of 10 mothers found no statistically significant difference in milk production when mothers increased their fluid intake to 50% higher than usual or 50% lower than usual (Morse, Ewing, Gamble, & Donahue, 1992).

• •

A mother will know if she is drinking enough fluids by her stools and the color of her urine.

Pale yellow urine indicates a mother is probably drinking enough fluids. Constipation (hard, dry stools) and darker, more concentrated urine with a stronger smell are signs that a mother needs to drink more (Bronner, 2010). When a mother is constipated, she can avoid the need for commercial laxatives by drinking more liquids and eating more fresh and dried fruits (prunes and pears especially) and raw vegetables , as well as whole grains.

• •

A mother does not need to "drink milk to make milk."

Cow's milk is not consumed by older children and adults in many parts of the world because most nationalities are lactose intolerant later in life. After dairy farming became widespread among northern European peoples, these cultures developed a tolerance for cow's milk in adulthood.

Drinking cow's milk is not essential for breastfeeding mothers. Milk is one possible source of calcium, but if the mother does not like milk or if she or her baby is sensitive to milk, there are other calcium sources. Because yogurt and cheeses are processed, some mothers and babies who are sensitive to straight cow's milk can tolerate them. Other excellent sources of calcium are foods fortified with calcium like soy milk, rice milk, almond milk, tofu, and orange juice. Good sources of calcium that require eating larger amounts include bok choy, Chinese mustard greens, sesame seeds, kale, white beans, Brazil nuts, and broccoli (Hopkinson, 2007).

Vitamin/Mineral Supplements

Well-nourished breastfeeding mothers may not need vitamin/mineral supplements.

While supplements may benefit mothers who are malnourished or on a restricted diet (see next point), the best way for a well-nourished breastfeeding mother to get the nutrients she needs is through a balanced diet.

The undernourished or vitamin/mineral-deficient mother will benefit from supplements.

The woman who is chronically undernourished or is on a very restricted diet may eventually develop vitamin or mineral deficiencies that can lead to a decrease in the levels of some vitamins or minerals in her milk, such as iodine, A, D, B_6, or B_{12}, which may affect her baby's health. Mothers at risk include those on very restricted vegetarian diets, those with intestinal parasites, and those with a history of gastric bypass or other bariatric surgery (see later section on bariatric surgery). Other women at risk are those with Crohn's disease and other malabsorption disorders. In this case, vitamin-and-mineral supplements may be warranted, if the mother's diet is not rich in calcium-containing foods.

Some vitamin and mineral deficiencies may affect levels in mothers' milk.

Due to depletion of the ozone layer and warnings about sun exposure, the percentage of women and children suffering from vitamin D deficiency is on the rise, especially among those in northern latitudes (Hanley & Davison, 2005). Unlike other vitamins, vitamin D was never meant to come from our diet. Rather, it is made by the body when our skin is exposed to the sun. When a mother is vitamin D deficient, vitamin D supplements can both restore her own vitamin D levels and increase the amount in her milk, which can benefit her baby (see p. 242- "Vitamin Supplements" in the chapter "Weight Gain and Growth").

Caution the mother not to take much more than the recommended allowance for fat-soluble vitamins, which may be stored in fat.

Water-soluble vitamins, which include vitamins C and the B-complex vitamins (thiamin [B_1], riboflavin [B_2], niacin [B_3], pantothenic acid [B_5], pyridoxine [B_6], biotin [B_7], foci acid or folate [B_9], and cobalamin [B_{12}]) are flushed through a mother's system daily and do not accumulate. Fat-soluble vitamins, which are stored in fat and tissue, include vitamins A, D, E , and K,. Vitamins A, E, and K should not be taken in larger than the recommended doses unless the mother has a deficiency and is being treated to bring her levels up to normal. Vitamin A, for example, is secreted into human milk and is stored in the liver. Doses of more than 5,000 IUs per day are not recommended for adults (Hale, 2008).

Vitamin D is also considered a fat-soluble vitamin, but it behaves more like a hormone because it is made in our bodies during skin exposure to the sun. Due to the rise in vitamin D deficiencies in northern climes, larger-than-recommended doses may be beneficial to many mothers and babies. See p. 242- "Vitamin Supplements."

Foods to Eat or Avoid

There are no specific foods that should be consumed or avoided during breastfeeding.

A mother with healthy eating habits does not usually need to change her diet while she is breastfeeding. She doesn't have to drink cow's milk or eat any other specific foods, and no specific foods should be avoided. Although exceptions exist, most breastfeeding mothers can eat anything they like in moderation—including chocolate and spicy foods—without any effect on their baby.

During pregnancy and breastfeeding, all mammal young are exposed to the flavors of the foods their mothers eat through amniotic fluid and their mother's milk. This helps babies recognize safe foods when they are ready to expand their diet beyond milk (Forestell & Mennella, 2007; Mennella, 2007; Mennella, Jagnow, & Beauchamp, 2001). A Danish study found that some food flavor compounds appeared in mother's milk within 1 to 2 hours after ingestion (Hausner, Bredie, Molgaard, Petersen, & Moller, 2008). In one U.S. study, an hour or two after breastfeeding the mothers swallowed concentrated capsules of garlic extract and their milk acquired a distinct garlicky smell, but the babies who were fed this garlicky milk did not refuse it or act fussy. Instead, they drank more milk than usual (Mennella & Beauchamp, 1991a).

When a breastfeeding mother eats foods with different flavors, this gives her baby a preview of the tastes he'll experience later from solids.

Mothers do not need to eat or avoid any specific foods.

When mothers make a particular food a regular part of their diet during pregnancy and breastfeeding, their babies are more likely to accept it later as a solid food. In one U.S. study, pregnant mothers drank either carrot juice or water 4 days a week for 3 weeks (Mennella et al., 2001). When carrots were introduced to their babies later as a solid food, the babies' enjoyment of them was rated higher by the mothers who drank the carrot juice than by the mothers who drank the water. This variability in the flavor of the milk may be one reason why children who were breastfed as babies tend to have fewer feeding problems later (Lawrence & Lawrence, 2005, p. 349).

Is Baby Reacting to Something in Mother's Diet?

When a baby is fretful or gassy, many mothers wrongly assume something they ate is the cause.

Fussiness and gassiness are normal during the newborn period and are unlikely to be caused by something in the mother's diet. During the first year, only about 5% of breastfed babies react to a food their mother consumes, with cow's milk being the most common food babies react to (Kvenshagen, Halvorsen, & Jacobsen, 2008).

Most mothers can eat any food they like in moderation without any effect on their breastfeeding baby. Yet many breastfeeding mothers are told to avoid specific foods, which vary from culture to culture. For example, Chinese and Southeast Asian women are advised to avoid cold liquids because they are not good for the baby (Davis, 2001). Some Hispanic women are cautioned to avoid pork, chili, and tomatoes, while some African American mothers are warned to avoid onions (Taylor, 1985). In Australia, cabbage, chocolates, spicy foods, peas, onions, and cauliflower are thought to cause colic, gas, diarrhea, and rashes in the breastfeeding baby.

As described in the previous section, it is usually an advantage to a breastfeeding baby for his mother to eat a varied diet because the flavors from the foods she eats change the taste of her milk, providing her baby with a preview of the tastes he'll experience at the family table when he is older (Mennella, 2007).

Even when a baby *does* react to a food in the mother's diet, the specific food that causes a reaction will vary from baby to baby. So telling all breastfeeding mothers to avoid the same foods will do no good. Plus perceived "diet rules" dissuade some mothers from breastfeeding (Gabriel, Gabriel, & Lawrence, 1986).

Before assuming the baby is reacting to something in the mother's diet, ask if the baby has been given anything other than her milk.

When a baby fusses, some mothers assume it was due to something they ate, even if the baby is also receiving non-human milks or other foods. Because the percentage of breastfeeding babies who react to foods their mothers eat is small (see previous point), it is far more likely a baby will react to a food he is given directly, such as formula or solids, rather than to a food in his mother's diet.

Ask the mother if her baby is given teas or other remedies for colic or crying. Ask if other adults or children might be feeding the baby something other than her milk. Ask specifically if the baby is receiving supplemental feedings from the baby's father or a caregiver, as she may not think of this.

Ask if mother or baby is taking any medications, vitamins, or supplements, and whether the feeding problem started after they were introduced.

On average only about 1% of a mother's dose of medication passes into her milk, but a very sensitive baby may still have a reaction. If the baby's feeding problems started after the mother began taking the drug, vitamins, or other supplements, this will provide a clue. If a drug or supplement may be a cause, suggest the mother ask her healthcare provider for an alternative.

Ask how many caffeinated drinks the mother consumes daily, as too much caffeine can make a baby irritable and wakeful.

Very little caffeine (about 1.5% of the maternal dose) passes into a mother's milk (Berlin, Denson, Daniel, & Ward, 1984). But it takes much longer for caffeine to clear a young baby's system as compared with an older baby. For more details, see the next section.

A reaction to a food in the mother's diet is more likely if there is a family history of allergy and the baby has physical symptoms.

Although a baby affected by a food his mother eats is an exception to the rule, it can happen (Hill et al., 2005). Symptoms of food hypersensitivity, intolerance, or allergy include:

- Skin problems, such as eczema, dermatitis, hives, rash, dry skin (Martorell et al., 2006)
- Gastrointestinal problems, such as vomiting, diarrhea, blood or mucus in stools (Pumberger, Pomberger, & Geissler, 2001; Schach & Haight, 2002)
- Respiratory problems, such as congestion, runny nose, wheezing, coughing
- Crying during or after feedings (also a symptom of overabundant milk production and reflux disease)
- Difficulty going to sleep and staying asleep (Kahn, Mozin, Rebuffat, Sottiaux, & Muller, 1989; Kahn et al., 1987)

When a baby has a reaction like these, there is likely to be a family history of allergy. If one parent has allergies, the baby has a 20-40% risk of being allergic, and if both parents have allergies, the baby's risk increases to 50-80% (Ferreira & Seidman, 2007b).

If the baby has an acute reaction to a new food in mother's diet, symptoms may appear within an hour, but usually resolve within 24 hours.

If a baby seems to react acutely to something in the mother's diet, ask her if she has recently consumed a new food, especially one that is either strong or spicy, or if she has eaten a large amount of one food. If too much of one food is the issue, eating it in more moderate amounts may be enough to resolve the reaction.

Case reports document two Swiss breastfed babies who developed a rash within 1 hour after their mothers ate a dish with red pepper, with the rash disappearing within 12 to 48 hours (Cooper & Cooper, 1996). Based on many years of clinical experience, physicians Ruth and Robert Lawrence wrote that typically a baby's reaction to a food eaten by the mother resolves within 24 hours (Lawrence & Lawrence, 2005, p. 349).

The most common food to cause a reaction in babies through mother's milk is cow's milk, followed by other protein foods.

The overall incidence of reaction to cow's milk in the first year of life is estimated to be about 5%, with the most common reactions being pain behavior and gastrointestinal and respiratory symptoms (Kvenshagen et al., 2008). In one Danish study of 1749 newborns followed for their first year, only 0.5% (9) of the exclusively breastfed babies reacted to cow's milk in their mother's diet, and all of these babies were given infant formula in their first days of life while in the hospital, in some cases without the mother's knowledge (Host, Husby, & Osterballe, 1988). The younger the baby when cow's milk is introduced, the more likely it is to sensitize a baby to allergy.

Cow's milk is the most common allergen for babies.

After one group of study mothers consumed dairy, Finnish researchers isolated a cow's milk antibody (the protein beta-lactoglobulin) in the mothers' milk. The researchers detected this protein in the milk within 1 to 2 hours after consumption (Sorva, Makinen-Kiljunen, & Juntunen-Backman, 1994). A U.S. study reported that the level of another cow's milk protein (IgG) was higher in the milk of mothers of colicky babies as compared with other mothers (Clyne & Kulczycki, 1991). In this study, the level of this cow's milk protein was even higher in the milk of the mothers with colicky babies than in infant formula (up to 8.5 μg/mL vs. up to 6.4 μg/mL).

In another U.S. study, 35 of 66 mothers of colicky babies reported a decrease in their babies' colicky behavior when they eliminated milk and milk products from their diets (Jakobsson & Lindberg, 1983). The behaviors reappeared twice when the mothers ate dairy as a challenge. In an Australian study of 90 mothers with colicky babies, more foods were eliminated, including dairy, eggs, peanuts, tree nuts, wheat, soy, and fish (Hill et al., 2005). This change in diet decreased colic symptoms on average by only 21%.

When a mother eliminates a food she's been eating regularly, it may take weeks for the baby's reaction to subside.

Eliminating a food for a day or two will usually resolve a baby's acute reaction to a new food, but if the baby reacts to a food the mother eats often, it may take longer for it to clear her system and for the baby to feel better. Also, symptoms like congestion, eczema, wheezing, sleep disturbances, and crying often start gradually, so it may take time before the connection between the mother's diet and the baby's reaction becomes obvious.

When a mother goes on a dairy-free diet, for example, some babies respond within a few days, but it often takes 2 to 3 weeks for the cow's milk protein to clear from her system and the baby's reaction to subside (Vartabedian, 2007).

Some mothers worry that their bone health may be at risk when they reduce their calcium intake by eliminating dairy. A Finnish study examined the effect on bone mineral density of eliminating cow's milk from a breastfeeding mother's diet and concluded that elimination of dairy for a few months was not associated with loss of bone mineral density (Holmberg-Marttila et al., 2001). If the mother or her healthcare provider is concerned, the mother can take calcium supplements.

Other protein foods that may cause reactions in breastfed babies are soy, egg white (Casas, Bottcher, Duchen, & Bjorksten, 2000), peanuts (Vadas, Wai, Burks, & Perelman, 2001), fish, wheat, nuts, corn, and pork.

If a mother makes any major changes in her diet, suggest she eliminate no more than one or two foods at a time, so she can more easily pinpoint the cause. Also suggest that she get skilled help from a registered dietitian in evaluating her diet.

The mother can usually eat any offending foods again within 6 months or so.

Although children's allergic reactions to some foods may be permanent, a reaction to cow's milk is usually outgrown, often by 1 year (Ferreira & Seidman, 2007a). Although the offending food should not be given directly to the baby before 1 year, suggest the mother try adding it to her diet when her baby is 6 months old and see what happens.

If an elimination diet doesn't solve the problem, consider a new treatment along with it.

If more help is needed, suggest the mother talk to her healthcare provider about the possibility of prescribing a digestive enzyme, called Pancrease MT4, which is usually taken by those with cystic fibrosis to help break down their food more completely. The treatment involves taking two tablets with each meal and one with each snack (Schach & Haight, 2002). By breaking down the offending food more thoroughly, allergens are less likely to pass intact into the mother's milk and cause a reaction in her baby.

In one preliminary U.S. study on this treatment, 16 breastfeeding mothers whose babies had bloody stools eliminated dairy, soy, nuts, strawberries, and chocolate from their diet and began taking the Pancrease MT4 as directed (Repucci, 1999). In 13 of the babies, their bloody stools resolved and colic symptoms decreased while the mothers continued to breastfeed. More studies are needed with a control group as well as a treatment group to better evaluate its efficacy. But in the meantime, this could be suggested as an alternative to switching a breastfed baby to hydrolyzed or elemental cow's milk formula.

If a baby has bloody stools and eliminating dairy from the mother's diet does not resolve them, they will likely clear in time with continued breastfeeding.

Although in some studies, elimination of dairy from the mother's diet resolved babies' bloody stools (Pumberger et al., 2001), this symptom is not always caused by allergy or sensitivity. A Finnish study of 40 babies between 1 and 6 months old with bloody stools found, after elimination diets and dairy challenges, that only 18% had a cow's milk allergy (Arvola et al., 2006). Among these babies, 68% were exclusively breastfed, 12% were exclusively formula-fed, and 20% were fed both. In the babies receiving formula, a special amino acid-derived formula (Neocate) was used during the elimination diet. The researchers found that a viral particle aggregates in the intestinal mucosa of 20% of the babies, which indicates a virus may have triggered the bleeding in some. The mean duration of bloody stools was 10 days and a significant percentage of these babies also had other symptoms: mucous stools (73%), watery stools (38%), abdominal pain (58%), vomiting (18%), respiratory infection (22%), and fever (8%). During the first follow-up, 80% of the babies still had occasional bloody stools, and in nearly 58%, it lasted for more than 2 weeks. They found that when compared to a control group of babies without rectal bleeding, the intestinal levels of "good bacteria," such as *bifidobacterium* and *lactobacillus*, were 5 to 6 times lower among the babies with rectal bleeding, which the researchers suggested could be due to the diluting effect of diarrhea. They suggested probiotics as an intervention to bring gut flora back to more normal levels, and they concluded that "rectal bleeding in infants is generally a benign and self-limiting disorder" (Arvola et al., 2006, p. e761). They recommended elimination diets whenever a baby has bloody stools, since this resolved the symptoms of some babies, but they noted that in the vast majority of cases, this symptom was not an indicator of a serious health problem.

Elimination diets may be appropriate when babies have bloody stools.

If the baby's healthcare provider recommends suspending breastfeeding during a trial of hypoallergenic formula, suggest the mother discuss the possibility of continuing to breastfeed, as no negative outcomes have been associated with this (Sicherer, 2003).

Caffeine, Chocolate, and Herbal Teas

Moderate caffeine intake by the mother is not a problem for most breastfeeding babies.

Very little caffeine (about 1.5% of the maternal dose) passes into a mother's milk (Berlin et al., 1984). But it takes much longer for caffeine to clear a young baby's system as compared with an older baby. The half-life of caffeine is about 96 hours in a newborn, 14 hours in a 3- to 5-month-old baby, 2.6 hours in a baby older than 6 months, and 5 hours in an adult (Hale, 2008, p. 139). Two U.S. studies found that most mothers need to drink more than five cups of coffee before their breastfeeding baby is affected (Nehlig & Debry, 1994; Ryu, 1985a; Ryu, 1985b).

Breastfeeding mothers can drink up to five cups of coffee before their babies are affected.

If a mother is worried that her baby is reacting to caffeine, ask her how much caffeine she's getting from all sources.

Sources of caffeine include coffee, iced and hot teas, colas, other caffeine-containing soft drinks (be sure to ask about serving size), and any over-the-counter caffeine-containing drugs, such as some pain relievers, cold remedies, and diuretics.

If a mother consumes daily 750 mg of caffeine or more—the amount of caffeine in five 5-oz (150 mL) cups of coffee—and her baby seems irritable, fussy, and doesn't sleep long, suggest she substitute caffeine-free beverages for a week or two. Eliminating caffeine suddenly may cause headaches, but if caffeine is affecting her baby, within 3 to 7 days she should notice a difference.

Chocolate contains a substance similar to caffeine, but in much smaller amounts.

Chocolate contains theobromine, which is similar to caffeine and can produce the same effect if consumed in large amounts (Berlin & Daniel, 1981). Although the theobromine in chocolate is similar to caffeine, there is much less theobromine in chocolate than caffeine in coffee. A small cup of brewed drip coffee contains about 130 mg of caffeine, a cup of decaffeinated coffee contains about 3 mg of caffeine, and 1 ounce of milk chocolate contains about 6 mg of theobromine. Moderate consumption of chocolate does not usually cause problems in breastfeeding babies (Lawrence & Lawrence, 2005, p. 349).

Herbs can act like drugs, and some herbal teas may affect breastfeeding.

Many of today's modern medicines come from the herbs used in teas and home remedies. Like drugs, herbs can act as stimulants or tranquilizers and can also affect other body processes. Licorice, for example, can increase blood pressure, so it should be avoided by mothers with hypertension (Humphrey, 2003, p. 42; Lawrence & Lawrence, 2005, pp. 403-404). Before using an herb, it is important to learn about its use.

Some herbs can affect breastfeeding. For example, in significant amounts sage, peppermint, and parsley can reduce a mother's milk production (Humphrey, 2003). While major brands of herbal teas are safe for breastfeeding mothers, teas marketed as "private" brands or teas brewed from individual herbs should be used with caution.

Suggest the mother prepare herbal teas as directed and drink them in moderation.

If the mother is concerned about her herbal tea consumption, mention that the strength of a tea depends on its preparation. The longer the tea leaves are steeped, the stronger the tea. By decreasing her steeping time, the mother can decrease the tea's potency.

While breastfeeding, suggest the mother strive for moderation in all foods and drinks so that reactions are less likely to occur. A mother who drinks a few cups of herbal tea each day is unlikely to have a problem. But reactions are more likely if she drinks a quart (.946 liter) or more of tea each day, or if the tea is potent or contains active ingredients.

Bone Health

Breastfeeding appears to have a neutral or positive effect on a woman's bone health.

Although mothers lose bone mineral density while breastfeeding, they regain it after weaning (Carranza-Lira & Mera, 2002; Ensom, Liu, & Stephenson, 2002). One U.S. study that examined calcium absorption during breastfeeding found that a breastfeeding mother's intestinal calcium absorption increases after her menses resume and after weaning, which may help compensate for the calcium lost to human milk (Kalkwarf, Specker, Heubi, Vieira, & Yergey, 1996; Ritchie et al., 1998). This also appears to be true among adolescent mothers (Ward, Adams, & Mughal, 2005). This increased calcium absorption may coincide with rising estrogen levels. One Japanese study found that breastfeeding women had significantly higher bone metabolism than women who were mostly formula-feeding (Yamaga, Taga, Minaguchi, & Sato, 1996). One Italian study of 308 mothers found that bone mineral density appeared to be even higher after weaning than before pregnancy (Polatti, Capuzzo, Viazzo, Colleoni, & Klersy, 1999).

Several studies examined the effect of breastfeeding on long-term bone health. One Australian study of 174 women found that as duration of breastfeeding increased, risk of hip fracture after menopause decreased in a dose-response relationship (Cumming & Klineberg, 1993). Another U.S. study compared bone mineral density and osteoporosis or osteopenia in a group of women with at least six children who breastfed each for 6 months or more with a group of childless women (Henderson, Sowers, Kutzko, & Jannausch, 2000). Even with many pregnancies, extended lactation, and no recovery intervals, these mothers had comparable bone mineral densities and no increased incidence of osteoporosis or osteopenia.

The main predictor of bone loss later in life appears to be low calcium intake from childhood to early adulthood (Cross, Hillman, Allen, Krause, & Vieira, 1995).

• •

Calcium intake from food or supplements during breastfeeding does not seem to affect calcium levels in milk or bone mineral density.

The calcium needed for milk production does not appear to come from a mother's dietary calcium intake (Kent, Arthur, Mitoulas, & Hartmann, 2009). Instead, it appears to come from a combination of calcium drawn from the mother's bones (Holmberg-Marttila & Sievanen, 1999) and a decrease in the calcium excreted in her urine (King, 2001).

For a mother eating a varied and nutritious diet, there appears to be no benefit to taking extra calcium while breastfeeding. Research suggests that calcium supplementation during and after lactation has little to no effect on calcium absorption and bone mineral density (Allen, 1998; Kalkwarf, Specker, & Ho, 1999; Kolthoff, Eiken, Kristensen, & Nielsen, 1998). In fact, taking in too much calcium puts a mother at risk for kidney stones and urinary tract infections (Prentice, 1994). However, if a mother's diet is low in calcium, increasing calcium in her diet (see previous point on excellent and good sources of calcium) has been associated with less bone loss during pregnancy and breastfeeding (O'Brien et al., 2006).

A diet rich in calcium decreases women's bone loss during pregnancy and breastfeeding.

The Vegetarian Mother

Ask the vegetarian mother what specific foods she avoids.

Vegetarian diets cover a wide range. Some vegetarians avoid red meat, but eat poultry, seafood, milk products, and eggs. Ovo-lacto-vegetarians avoid all red meat, seafood, and poultry (flesh foods), but eat milk products and eggs. Lacto-vegetarians avoid flesh foods and eggs, but eat milk products. Ovo-vegetarians avoid flesh foods and milk products, but eat eggs. All of these diets include some form of animal protein.

Due to a risk of vitamin B_{12} deficiency, vitamin supplements are usually recommended for those whose vegetarian diets include no animal protein, such as vegan and macrobiotic diets, and those consuming very little animal protein (see next point).

Mothers on vegan or macrobiotic diets needs B_{12} supplements.

• •

When a mother consumes no animal products, taking vitamin B_{12} supplements prevents vitamin B_{12} deficiency in her and her breastfeeding baby.

Because the primary source of vitamin B_{12} is animal protein, vegan and macrobiotic diets—vegetarian diets including no animal products—put both mother and baby at risk of developing a vitamin B_{12} deficiency. If a vitamin B_{12} deficiency is caught early, any neurological problems may be reversed when treated with vitamin B_{12} supplements (Casella, Valente, de Navarro, & Kok, 2005); if not caught early, they may be irreversible.

Symptoms in the baby often develop first. They can appear within the first few months of life, but may go unrecognized until the 2nd year (CDC, 2003; Roschitz et al., 2005). The first symptoms are often irritability and disinterest in feeding, vomiting, drowsiness, weak cry, and motor development regression

(Weiss, Fogelman, & Bennett, 2004). Failure-to-thrive can follow, along with neurological symptoms, like low muscle tone and involuntary movements. The mother may have no symptoms, but blood or milk testing will detect her vitamin deficiency. Two studies document vitamin B_{12} deficiency in Dutch and U.S. mothers on macrobiotic diets (Dagnelie, van Staveren, Roos, Tuinstra, & Burema, 1992; Specker, 1994).

If the mother on a vegan or macrobiotic diet does not want to consume animal products, to safeguard her baby's long-term health and development, suggest she take vitamin B_{12} supplements or eat fortified soy products.

Mothers on macrobiotic diets tend to have lower levels of environmental contaminants in their milk than mothers who eat animal products.

A Dutch study found lower levels of PCBs (an environmental contaminant) in the milk of mothers on macrobiotic diets as compared to mothers who ate animal products (Dagnelie et al., 1992). Environmental contaminants are stored mostly in fat, and vegetarian diets tend to be lower in fat than those including animal products.

Weight and Weight Loss

Weight Loss

Many—but not all—breastfeeding mothers lose weight gradually during the first 6 months postpartum.

During the early weeks after birth, breastfeeding mothers tend to be less active than before giving birth and less active than non-breastfeeding mothers (Bronner, 2010). But because some of the fat reserves laid down during pregnancy are mobilized for milk production, they still tend to lose weight. The U.S. Institute of Medicine estimates that breastfeeding mothers who "eat to hunger" lose on average about 0.8 kg (1.6 pounds) per month during the first 6 months of lactation (IOM, 2005). These are averages, and some women gain weight while breastfeeding. A recent U.S. study of 24 mothers compared mothers exclusively breastfeeding with those doing mixed feeding and concluded that exclusive breastfeeding promotes greater weight loss than mixed feeding (Hatsu, McDougald, & Anderson, 2008).

Overall, however, the research on breastfeeding and weight loss is mixed. One U.S. systematic review of 28 studies could not draw conclusions, in part because the research did not use consistent definitions of breastfeeding.(Fraser & Grimes, 2003). A meta-analysis of the research from the Agency for Healthcare Research and Quality (AHRQ) concluded that when women were followed for 1 to 2 years after birth, the effect of breastfeeding on a mother's return to prepregnancy weight was negligible, in part due to the many other factors affecting her weight (Ip et al., 2007).

Breastfeeding mothers lose an average of 1.6 pounds per month in the first 6 months postpartum.

Some research indicates that weight loss during breastfeeding may specifically target a woman's hips and thighs. One small U.S. study of 24 women at 1 month postpartum found that mothers who breastfed either exclusively or partially had slimmer hips and weighed less than women whose babies received only formula (Kramer, Stunkard, Marshall, McKinney, & Liebschutz, 1993). Other later studies confirmed this finding (Butte & Hopkinson, 1998; Wosje & Kalkwarf, 2004).

On average, after 6 months, weight tends to become more stable unless the mother eats fewer calories and begins exercising regularly (Bronner, 2010).

There are good reasons for mothers to want to return to their prepregnancy weight other than concerns about attractiveness. Research has found an association between retaining weight more than 6 months after birth and obesity later in life (Rooney, Schauberger, & Mathiason, 2005).

If a breastfeeding mother wants to lose weight faster, suggest she eat less and exercise, but avoid extreme weight-loss programs.

If a mother chooses to eat less to lose weight, encourage her to eat nutrient-dense foods and consider a vitamin-and-mineral supplement. Although a minimum of 1800 calories per day is usually recommended during breastfeeding, one study found that eating as little as 1500 calories per day during the first 6 months of breastfeeding did not affect milk production or composition (Strode, Dewey, & Lonnerdal, 1986). But even if her milk production is not affected, eating poorly can compromise a mother's health and energy by depleting her reserves. Encourage the mother to eat a healthy diet for her own sake to increase her resistance to illness and maintain her energy.

One U.S. study found that when breastfeeding mothers lowered their calorie intake by 25 percent, they safely lost about 1 pound (0.45 kg) per week without affecting their baby's growth (Dusdieker, Hemingway, & Stumbo, 1994). Another U.S. study found that when 40 overweight women cut 500 calories from their daily diet and added a 45-minute exercise routine 4 days a week, the mothers in the diet-and-exercise group lost more weight than the mothers in the control group, while the average weight gain stayed the same among the babies in both groups (Lovelady, Garner, Moreno, & Williams, 2000).

To promote faster weight loss, suggest the mother begin by increasing her activity level and eliminating 100 calories per day from her diet. If she wants to do more, suggest she plan to eat at least 1800 calories per day in nutrient-dense foods.

Severe low-carbohydrate diets are not recommended for breastfeeding mothers.

Some experts have expressed concern about severe low-carbohydrate diets. Although at this writing, no research is available on the effects of the first phase of the low-carbohydrate diets popularized by Dr. Atkins on milk production or composition, experts have expressed concerns (Heinig & Doberne, 2004). At this writing, no evidence exists that low-carb diets are more effective for losing weight in the long run than low-calorie diets. A systematic review of the research found no weight-loss benefit to "low-carb" diets over low-calorie diets after 12 months (Bravata et al., 2003). If a mother wants to try a low-carb diet, suggest she consider a more moderate version, such as the maintenance phase of the South Beach diet, which includes a larger variety of nutritious foods. Suggest she also discuss her diet options with a nutrition professional, such as a registered dietitian, so that she can choose the diet most compatible with any other health issues.

A moderate low-carbohydrate diet can be appropriate for breastfeeding mothers.

Underweight/Eating Disorders

Mothers who are underweight, undernourished, or have eating disorders are at risk for vitamin deficiencies.

When a breastfeeding mother is undernourished, she runs the risk of using up her own nutritional stores to provide for her baby. Until her stores are depleted, her milk composition will remain normal. One Italian study of 1272 women found that being underweight before pregnancy was not associated with lower initiation or duration of breastfeeding (Giovannini, Radaelli, Banderali, & Riva, 2007).

However, even if she is not vitamin deficient, depleting her own reserves may leave a mother with less energy and a lower resistance to illness. If she becomes chronically malnourished and vitamin deficient, her milk levels of vitamin A, D, B_6, and B_{12} may fall below normal. With extreme malnutrition over a period of weeks, her milk production may eventually decrease (Smith, 1947). For details, see the previous sections "Nutrition Basics" and "Vitamin/Mineral Supplements." If a mother is malnourished, the most cost- and resource-effective strategy is to supplement the mother, rather than the baby.

• •

Women with a history of eating disorders have a greater incidence of preterm birth, but breastfeeding appears to be unaffected.

One Danish study examined the pregnancy and breastfeeding outcomes of 140 women 10 years after hospitalization for anorexia nervosa (Brinch, Isager, & Tolstrup, 1988). Fifty of these women had given birth, but they gave birth less often, delivering only about one-third the number of children as other women their age . There were twice as many preterm births as expected and six times more infant deaths. These women breastfed for about the same mean time as other women and did well from a mental-health perspective during pregnancy and postpartum.

• •

Some mothers with eating disorders embrace breastfeeding; others reject it.

Twice during pregnancy and twice during the first months postpartum, one U.K. study interviewed 16 women with eating disorders since adolescence (Stapleton, Fielder, & Kirkham, 2008). All but one had received treatment. Most (11 of 16) started breastfeeding after birth, and some of these mothers were "desperate" to breastfeed because it affirmed they were good mothers and because they felt they could eat foods they would not otherwise eat for fear of gaining weight. Feeling pride in their body's ability to nourish their infants helped to soften some mothers' negative body image.

Breastfeeding may be helpful for women with eating disorders.

Other mothers (5 of 16) rejected breastfeeding because they believed it was incompatible with their restrictive eating, bingeing/purging behaviors, and/or intense exercise regimens, and they felt that their emotional need to get back to these behaviors quickly after birth outweighed the importance of breastfeeding.

Nine of the 16 mothers did not share their eating disorder with their healthcare providers. Those who did worried that knowing about their eating disorder might make their healthcare provider more likely to criticize them or keep a closer eye on them. The researchers noted that pregnancy and the early postpartum period provides a window of opportunity for these women to change their self-image and adopt healthier behaviors .

Obesity

With few exceptions, mothers who are obese before pregnancy are less likely to breastfeed at birth, and if they do, they tend to wean earlier.

In a systematic review of 22 studies published before 2007, its Australian authors noted that obesity appears to be detrimental to breastfeeding, but they could not say for sure if the physical dynamics of obesity are responsible (Amir & Donath, 2007). There are many biological, psychological, behavioral, and cultural factors affecting breastfeeding outcomes, and it is unclear with obese women how much of a role each of these factors plays. Most of the studies reviewed used the World Health Organization's definitions: normal weight BMI (body mass index) <25, overweight BMI 25≥30, obese BMI >30.

When comparing breastfeeding initiation among obese and normal-weight women, this review noted that in areas where virtually all women breastfeed, obese women began breastfeeding at the same rate as normal-weight women. Some examples include a study conducted with 1078 women in northwest Russia, where only 1.3% of babies were never breastfed (Grjibovski, Yngve, Bygren, & Sjostrom, 2005), and two studies done in Western Australia, where breastfeeding initiation rates are estimated to be 96% (Oddy et al., 2006; Scott, Binns, Graham, & Oddy, 2006).

However, even in areas were virtually all women breastfeed at birth, overweight and obese women stop breastfeeding earlier. One Australian study of 1803 women found that overweight and obese women were more likely to have weaned their babies by 6 months than normal-weight women (Oddy et al., 2006). In Denmark, where 98% of women breastfeed, one study of 37,459 Danish women found that the greater the prepregnant BMI, the earlier breastfeeding stopped (Baker, Michaelsen, Sorensen, & Rasmussen, 2007).

One exception is overweight and obese U.S. black mothers. Two U.S. studies have found that U.S. black overweight and obese mothers breastfeed at the same rate and duration as normal-weight black mothers (Kugyelka, Rasmussen, & Frongillo, 2004; Liu, Smith, Dobre, & Ferguson, 2009). The reasons for this ethnic difference is not clear, but the authors suggest that it could be partly biological, noting a study that found fewer years of life lost among obese black women when compared with obese white women (Fontaine, Redden, Wang, Westfall, & Allison, 2003). Cultural values, such as attitudes about women's body weight, may also be a factor (see next page).

Obese women have increased risk for early breastfeeding cessation than women of normal weight.

• •

Excessive weight gain during pregnancy has also been linked to less breastfeeding.

In one U.S. study, if women gained much more weight during pregnancy than recommended by the U.S. Institute of Medicine (25 to 35 lbs. or 19.8 to 26 kg), they were more likely not to breastfeed at birth or to stop breastfeeding early (Hilson, Rasmussen, & Kjolhede, 2006; IOM, 1990). This held true whether at conception they were underweight, at normal weight, overweight, or obese, but the heavier at conception the women were, the greater the effect. For example, the duration of exclusive breastfeeding was 1 week shorter for women who were underweight or overweight at conception and 3 weeks shorter for women who were obese at conception.

• •

Some biological factors may affect breastfeeding in overweight and obese mothers.

The following factors are at least partly biological.

Delay in milk increase after birth. Several U.S. studies found an association between obesity and a delay in milk increase after birth (lactogenesis II) (Chapman & Perez-Escamilla, 1999; Chapman & Perez-Escamilla, 2000; Dewey, Nommsen-Rivers, Heinig, & Cohen, 2003; Hilson, Rasmussen, & Kjolhede, 2004). One U.S. study of 151 women found that those who were obese had a significantly greater chance of having a cesarean birth, which has also been associated with a delay in milk increase (Hilson et al., 2004). Animal studies have found a link between obesity and reduced milk production in rats and cows (Flint, Travers, Barber, Binart, & Kelly, 2005; Morrow, 1976; Rasmussen, 1998).

However, this may not be entirely related to the biological effects of obesity, as U.S. research has also found that overweight and obese women are less likely to put their newborns to the breast within the first 2 hours after birth, which has also been associated with a delay in milk increase (Bystrova et al., 2007; Kugyelka et al., 2004).

Decreased prolactin response to baby's suckling. One U.S. study measured mothers' blood prolactin and progesterone levels after birth and found that the prolactin response to baby's suckling was lower among overweight and obese mothers on Day 2, but not on Day 7 (Rasmussen & Kjolhede, 2004). The researchers measured blood progesterone levels because they thought that higher progesterone levels in obese mothers (progesterone is stored in fatty tissue) might explain the delay in milk production, but there was no difference in the blood progesterone levels between the groups.

Large breasts. Although not all overweight and obese women have large breasts, many do, and this can sometimes make finding a comfortable breastfeeding position more challenging. If a mother finds it difficult to get comfortable, she may postpone breastfeeding, which may also affect how early her milk increases. Her baby may also have a more difficult time taking the breast deeply, which can also affect timing of milk increase and overall milk production.

Related medical conditions. Overweight and obese mothers are more likely to suffer from medical conditions that can affect early breastfeeding, such as diabetes, which has been linked to later milk increase, and polycystic ovary syndrome (PCOS) (Arthur, Smith, & Hartmann, 1989; Neubauer et al., 1993). For details, see the chapter, "Health Issues—Mother." One French study found that the babies of obese women weighed less at 1 and 3 months when compared with babies of normal-weight women (Mok et al., 2008).

• •

Cultural beliefs and mothers' self-image may also affect breastfeeding behaviors in overweight and obese women.

How a culture views overweight and obesity can affect breastfeeding behaviors. In most Western cultures, for example, obesity is seen as a negative, so mothers may be reluctant to expose their bodies while breastfeeding (see next point). In one French study, the main reason given by obese women for deciding not to breastfeed was "decency" (Mok et al., 2008). This study also found that despite the greater number of breastfeeding problems obese women had in the first 3 months, they were less likely to seek help.

In these cultures, when compared to normal-weight women, obese women are more likely to have body-image dissatisfaction and low self-esteem, and to suffer from postpartum depression (Lacoursiere, Baksh, Bloebaum, & Varner, 2006; Matz, Foster, Faith, & Wadden, 2002; Sarwer, Wadden, & Foster, 1998). How a mother feels about her body can also affect her desire to breastfeed. Mothers who are unhappy with their body shape or weight have been found to be less likely to breastfeed (Barnes, Stein, Smith, & Pollock, 1997).

Culture can influence obese women's breastfeeding duration.

Yet in some cultures, there does not seem to be a link between mothers' weight and breastfeeding rates. One example is the Cree women in northern Quebec, Canada, where overweight and obesity are common (Vallianatos et al., 2006). One possible reason obese U.S. black mothers breastfeed at the same rates as normal-weight black mothers is because their culture has a more positive view of obesity (Kugyelka et al., 2004; Liu et al., 2009). If a culture does not consider obesity a negative, its mothers may be less likely to feel embarrassed or self-conscious about exposing their bodies around others.

Overweight and obesity are red flags for breastfeeding problems, but practical help can overcome them.

One survey of 31 U.S. healthcare providers who counsel breastfeeding mothers in New York state found that these clinicians were unaware that overweight and obese women are at higher risk for breastfeeding failure (Rasmussen, Lee, Ledkovsky, & Kjolhede, 2006). The authors suggest that breastfeeding supporters do more to provide these mothers with extra support, but first awareness of this risk factor needs to be raised.

During pregnancy, nutritional counseling can help an obese mother prepare for breastfeeding. One simple suggestion is that the mother choose nutrient-rich foods and avoid non-nutritious choices, such as soda and candy (Jevitt, Hernandez, & Groer, 2007). The obese mother can also reduce her chances of needing a cesarean birth by arranging for labor support and learning non-drug pain management techniques.

After birth, suggest the mother plan to keep her baby skin-to-skin on her chest and breastfeed as soon as possible, ideally within the first 2 hours after birth, as this may promote an earlier increase in milk production (see chapter 2). Encourage her to limit separation and plan for lots of body contact with her baby and frequent feedings.

U.S. lactation consultant Kay Hoover, M.Ed., IBCLC interviewed several obese breastfeeding mothers about the practical challenges they faced after the early postpartum period (Hoover, 2008). Their responses fell into four general areas:

Finding a comfortable breastfeeding position. Hoover described these mothers' fear of suffocating their baby with their large, heavy breasts. She also described four cases in her own practice of babies who would not take the breast when the heavy breast was resting on their chest. After repositioning the babies so this weight was not their chest, the babies took the breast and fed well. See the first chapter for laid-back breastfeeding positions that provide alternatives to more challenging upright positions.

Finding a well-fitting bra. Large bras are expensive and may be available only through mail-order. Some of the mothers Hoover interviewed described their efforts to make do with ill-fitting bras. She recommended mothers have at least three well-fitted bras.

Breastfeeding in public. Obese mothers often must expose more of their bodies during breastfeeding than normal-weight women. To provide more coverage, some wore a tank top or T-shirt with holes cut in the breast area under their shirt. One mother said, "It took a long time to feel comfortable enough with myself to be able to breastfeed in public. I finally decided that breastfeeding was best for my baby, so 'tough' if they have a problem seeing my fat rolls" (Hoover, 2008, p. 6).

Using a breast pump. Standard breast pump flanges were not large enough for some of these women, and larger flanges were not easily available. Double-pumping also presented logistical challenges.

Another common challenge faced by obese mothers is inflammation of the breast skin folds, sometimes caused by clothing friction, which can cause itching, burning, and pain. Also called "intertrigo," this can be prevented or treated with daily cleaning and drying of the skin folds. It may also help to wear a supportive bra, avoiding those that constrict breast tissue. If the mother develops a skin infection, suggest she ask her healthcare provider about a topical antifungal or antibiotic.

An overweight or obese mother may have an unrealistic view of her baby's weight.

One Japanese study of 1,496 women found that many mothers had unrealistic views of their baby's weight (Yakura, 1997). Many (23% to 58%) rated their normal-weight babies as obese, especially among those who dieted during adolescence. These mothers used both appropriate (frequent exercise) and inappropriate strategies to try to prevent future obesity in their children. Inappropriate strategies included reducing the frequency of breastfeeding, diluting formula, and not allowing snacking between meals.

Gastric Bypass and Other Bariatric Surgeries

Mothers with a history of bariatric surgery need to take vitamin and mineral supplements to avoid deficiencies.

Bariatric surgeries limit the amount of food the digestive system can hold by bypassing part of it or restricting its size with bands. Eighty-five percent of bariatric-surgery patients are women, and 80% of these women are in their childbearing years, so many may have questions about breastfeeding (Blankenship, 2008; Stefanski, 2006).

Dramatic weight loss is the purpose of bariatric surgery, and in some cases, it can be life-saving. It works by severely limiting the amount of food a person can consume. Weight loss averages 25% to 35% of original body weight by 18 months, and after the surgery, average calories per day decreases to 1,100 at 1 year and 1,300 at 18 months (Brolin, Robertson, Kenler, & Cody, 1994; Buchwald et al., 2004). Although one study done by Swedish researchers found no effect on milk production when breastfeeding mothers (who had not had bariatric surgery) consumed 1,500 calories per day for the first 6 months, as a rule, the caloric restriction among mothers with a history of bariatric surgery is even greater than this (Strode et al., 1986).

Women who have had gastric bypass surgery may have a B_{12} deficiency.

Along with concerns about low caloric intake, these surgeries also affect a mother's ability to absorb nutrients from her food. For example, 1 to 9 years after bariatric surgery 30% to 70% were found to have vitamin B_{12} deficiencies (Amaral, Thompson, Caldwell, Martin, & Randall, 1985). A vitamin B_{12} deficiency in a breastfeeding mother puts her baby at risk for neurological and other health issues (for more details, see the section "The Vegetarian Mother"). At least two cases of vitamin B_{12} deficiencies have been reported among breastfeeding babies whose mothers had a history of bariatric surgery (Grange & Finlay, 1994; Wardinsky et al., 1995). Bariatric surgery has also been associated with folate, calcium, and iron deficiencies (Amaral, Thompson, Caldwell, Martin, & Randall, 1984; Mason, Jalagani, & Vinik, 2005). For these reasons, after bariatric surgery, vitamin-and-mineral supplements are recommended.

Encourage the mother to learn about milk production, follow her nutritional guidelines carefully, and monitor her baby's weight.

Little is currently known about breastfeeding after bariatric surgery, so encourage the mother to share her history with her baby's healthcare provider, follow her own nutritional recommendations carefully (both diet and supplementation), and if exclusively breastfeeding, be sure her baby's weight is routinely monitored. In some cases, it also may be helpful for the mother's healthcare provider to do blood tests or other appropriate procedures to rule out vitamin-and-mineral deficiencies (Bronner, 2010).

As with all mothers, suggest she also educate herself about how to know her baby is getting enough milk and what she can do to maximize her milk production. Although cases have been reported of failure-to-thrive in breastfeeding babies after bariatric surgery, other possible causes were not ruled out (Martens, Martin, & Berlin, 1990).

EXERCISE

Moderate exercise has been found to improve a mother's cardiovascular fitness, blood lipid profiles, and insulin response (Lovelady, Fuller, Geigerman, Hunter, & Kinsella, 2004; Lovelady, Hunter, & Geigerman, 2003; Lovelady, Nommsen-Rivers, McCrory, & Dewey, 1995).

Moderate exercise benefits the breastfeeding mother in many ways.

Exercise also has emotional benefits. One U.S. prospective, randomized, controlled trial of 202 adults found that exercise can alleviate depression as effectively as anti-depressant medications (Blumenthal et al., 2007). An Australian qualitative study of six breastfeeding mothers enrolled in a formal exercise program reported some of the benefits the mothers enjoyed (Rich, Currie, & McMahon, 2004):

- A greater feeling of well-being
- Improved body image and easier weight control
- Enhanced relationships with others, including their baby

Exercise has a positive effect on women's physical and emotional well-being.

Some mothers considered exercise a great stress-reliever that made them less frazzled when their baby was unsettled. Some mothers expressed concern about decreased milk production when exercising began, but over time this did not seem to be an issue. A U.S. study of 156 adults found that exercise provided significant therapeutic benefit to those with major depression (Babyak et al., 2000).

• •

U.S. studies found no effect of exercise on milk production (Dewey, Lovelady, Nommsen-Rivers, McCrory, & Lonnerdal, 1994; Lovelady, Lonnerdal, & Dewey, 1990). Even when mothers both exercise and eat less to lose weight, milk production appears unaffected (Lovelady, 2004). Also, no significant differences in milk composition have been found after moderate exercise (Carey, Quinn, & Goodwin, 1997; Larson-Meyer, 2002; McCrory, 2000).

Milk production or composition is not affected by moderate exercise.

An Australian cohort study of 587 mothers interviewed them seven times from birth to 12 months postpartum and found that "exercise does not affect breastfeeding outcomes at the usual levels of activity undertaken by mothers" (Su, Zhao, Binns, Scott, & Oddy, 2007).

• •

In one U.S. study, researchers analyzed mothers' milk before and after extreme exercise and compared the babies' acceptance of the before-exercise milk with the milk expressed after exercise (Wallace, Inbar, & Ernsthausen, 1992). The mothers' milk was higher in lactic acid after extreme exercise, and the babies—who were fed the milk by medicine dropper—were judged by the authors to be

Exercising to exhaustion increases levels of lactic acid in a mother's milk, but there is no need to postpone breastfeeding.

less accepting of the after-exercise milk. Oddly, the researchers did not consider the impact of the medicine-dropper feeding method (which was new to the babies) on the babies' reactions. This study was widely publicized, along with its recommendations that mothers breastfeed their babies before exercising or provide expressed milk for feeding afterwards and avoid breastfeeding for as long as 90 minutes after exercise. In a later study that attempted to replicate this using familiar bottles to feed the babies the post-exercise, high-lactic-acid milk, researchers found that even after maximal exercise there was no difference in the babies' acceptance of the pre-and post-exercise milk (Wright, Quinn, & Carey, 2002). In a review of the literature, U.S researchers concluded that "altered acceptance of breastmilk due to higher lactic acid concentrations post-exercise is not likely to be a problem in most cases" (Dewey & McCrory, 1994, p. 450S).

When a mother starts exercising after birth, suggest she talk to her healthcare provider, and then start gradually.

In a review of the literature, one author suggests that if a mother wants to start exercising before 6 weeks postpartum to first discuss it with her healthcare provider, and then start slowly and gradually, being alert to her comfort (Larson-Meyer, 2002). If the exercise feels good, it's probably all right. But if the mother feels very tired, dehydrated, or if anything hurts, she needs to stop. She should see her healthcare provider if she notices more bright red vaginal bleeding than she would see during her menstrual cycle.

It may make it easier for a new mother to exercise more often if she includes her baby.

Lack of time can make exercising difficult to fit into daily routines. If so, suggest ways a mother can combine exercise with other activities she does with her baby. For example, walking with her baby in a stroller or a baby carrier provides both exercise and a change of scene. If the weather is bad, suggest the mother walk inside an enclosed shopping mall. There are also special strollers designed for running or jogging with a baby. Exercise videos and DVDs can be played at home. Some exercise books for new mothers feature routines that include the baby. In one Australian study, mothers reported that exercise became more fun when their baby was included (Rich et al., 2004).

GROOMING: HAIR CARE, TANNING, AND PIERCINGS

No evidence exists that a mother's use of hair-care products will affect her breastfeeding baby.

Some chemicals in hair-care products, such as hair dyes and permanents, may be absorbed through a mother's skin, but even so, there is no report of a breastfeeding baby being affected. If a mother's scalp is healthy and intact, less will be absorbed than if the skin on her scalp is scratched or abraded.

No evidence exists that a mother's use of a tanning bed will affect her breastfeeding baby.

Ultraviolet light is used in tanning beds to create a tan. Mothers are also exposed to ultraviolet light when outdoors and exposed to the sun.

Over the years, nipple piercing has become more common (Sadove & Clayman, 2008). One U.K. study of more than 10,000 people aged 16 and older found that 10% (1,934) had body piercings other than the earlobe. Of these, 9% (143) had nipple piercings, with twice as many men as women, most were 16-to-24 years old (Bone, Ncube, Nichols, & Noah, 2008).

Some mothers with pierced nipples have successfully breastfed, but some have had breastfeeding problems.

Several reported examples exist of mothers successfully breastfeeding with pierced nipples (Wilson-Clay & Hoover, 2008, pp. 68, 177). One report describes a mother who removed the ring from one of her nipples after birth and breastfed from one breast only (Lee, 1995). For a review of possible breastfeeding problems associated with nipple piercing and questions to ask a mother with pierced nipples, see p. 665 in the section "Nipple Piercing" in the chapter, "Nipple Issues."

ALCOHOL, NICOTINE, AND RECREATIONAL DRUGS

Alcohol

An occasional alcoholic drink is considered compatible with breastfeeding.

Specific recommendations on alcohol and breastfeeding vary. The American Academy of Pediatrics (AAP) Committee on Drugs categorizes alcohol when it is not taken in large amounts as a "maternal medication usually compatible with breastfeeding" (see later point) ("Transfer of drugs and other chemicals into human milk," 2001). In its 2005 policy statement on breastfeeding, the AAP Committee on Breastfeeding discouraged regular alcohol consumption and wrote: "An occasional celebratory single, small alcoholic drink is acceptable, but breastfeeding should be avoided for 2 hours after the drink" (Gartner et al., 2005, p. 497). In *Medications and Mother's Milk*, Hale wrote: "Significant amounts of alcohol are secreted into breastmilk, although it is not considered harmful to the infant if the amount and duration are limited" (Hale, 2008, p. 354).

A small amount of alcohol is acceptable for the breastfeeding mother.

An Australian systematic review of the literature concluded with the following recommendations for breastfeeding mothers: No alcohol in the first month. After the first month, limit alcohol intake to one to two standard drinks per day and drink them just after breastfeeding to limit the amount of alcohol the baby receives. If a mother wants to drink more than this, express milk before drinking and consider skipping one breastfeed (Giglia & Binns, 2006).

One U.S. study found that at 3 months postpartum, 36% of U.S. breastfeeding mothers consumed alcohol, with the majority drinking fewer than three alcoholic drinks per week (Breslow, Falk, Fein, & Grummer-Strawn, 2007). In an Australian study, more than 40% of breastfeeding women drank alcohol during the first year, with the majority having up to two drinks per week (Giglia & Binns, 2007). Mothers who drank more than two alcoholic drinks per day were nearly twice as likely to stop breastfeeding than mothers who drank less (Giglia, Binns, Alfonso, Scott, & Oddy, 2008).

Alcohol clears a mother's bloodstream quickly, so she can usually minimize her baby's exposure by drinking right after breastfeeding.

After an alcoholic drink without food, a mother's blood alcohol levels peak at about 30 to 60 minutes, 60 to 90 minutes with food (Lawton, 1985). Even if she doesn't express her milk, alcohol passes quickly out of her milk and bloodstream. It takes a 120-pound woman 2 to 3 hours to completely eliminate from her body the alcohol in one regular serving of beer or wine (Schulte, 1995).

However, the more alcohol a mother drinks, the longer it takes for it to clear her body. Canadian researchers (Ho, Collantes, Kapur, Moretti, & Koren, 2001) created a chart using average alcohol elimination time and factoring in mother's weight, time since drinking began, and number of drinks. To view this chart, go to : http://www.pubmedcentral.nih.gov/articlerender.fcgi?artid=2213923.

The Health Council of the Netherlands provides breastfeeding mothers with a simpler calculation: if the mother has had a standard drink (10g of alcohol), she should not breastfeed for 3 hours; if she's had more drinks, multiply the 3-hour period by the number of drinks (Health Council of the Netherlands, 2005).

The amount of alcohol that reaches the breastfeeding baby also depends upon whether she drinks with or without food, and whether or not she expresses her milk before drinking (see next point).

Both eating a meal and expressing milk before drinking decrease alcohol availability in a mother's system.

One U.S. study found that along with eating a meal before drinking, breastfeeding and expressing milk before drinking alcohol reduced alcohol availability in the mother's body (Pepino & Mennella, 2008). These effects were found to add to one another, so if a mother both ate a meal (reducing alcohol availability by 38%) and expressed her milk within the hour before drinking, this reduced the total availability of alcohol in her system by 58%.

The researchers suggested that the change in metabolism triggered by milk expression may exist to speed nutrient processing to more efficiently meet the increased energy demands of lactation. The researchers also noted that when this dynamic is better understood, it may be used to help maximize the effect of medications taken by breastfeeding women. Just as some medications should be taken with or between meals, so too medications may someday be timed with breastfeeding.

Alcohol disrupts a mother's hormonal balance and decreases the amount of milk the baby takes at the breast.

Some cultural folklore considers beer to have special properties to relax a breastfeeding mother and enhance her milk flow and production. When studies found that beer increased mothers' prolactin levels, this was thought to validate this belief (Carlson, Wasser, & Reidelberger, 1985; De Rosa, Corsello, Ruffilli, Della Casa, & Pasargiklian, 1981; Koletzko & Lehner, 2000). However, a body of research led by U.S. scientist Julie Mennella has found that far from enhancing milk flow, when mothers drank alcohol, their babies' breastfed more often, but consumed 20% to 27% less milk (Mennella, 1998; Mennella, 2001; Mennella & Beauchamp, 1993). Although babies took less milk for the first 4 hours after their mothers' drank alcohol, they compensated by feeding more often and by taking more milk 8 to 16 hours after this exposure (Mennella, 2001).

In one of these studies, a noticeable change in the odor of the mothers' milk paralleled the changes in alcohol concentration in the milk (Mennella & Beauchamp, 1991b). In an effort to determine if the change in the milk's flavor caused this decrease in milk intake, babies were fed bottles of expressed milk, one set of bottles with alcohol flavor added and another set without (Mennella, 1997). The babies took significantly more of the alcohol-flavored milk than the plain milk, so the researchers concluded that the babies did not take less from the breast because they rejected the milk's alcohol flavor.

One mechanism behind the babies' reduced milk intake at the breast was later found to be hormonal. The U.S. researchers found that while mothers' prolactin blood levels increased after drinking alcohol—mirroring the findings of earlier research—their oxytocin levels significantly decreased, which could inhibit milk ejection (Cobo, 1973; Mennella, Pepino, & Teff, 2005). The researchers concluded that while alcohol may relax a mother, it disrupts the hormonal balance needed for breastfeeding, reducing the availability of her milk to her baby.

Alcohol lowers oxytocin, which can impair milk ejection.

Later research by this same U.S. team found that a mother's prolactin response to alcohol varied depending on whether her blood alcohol levels were increasing or decreasing (Mennella & Pepino, 2008). If the mother pumped while blood alcohol increased, her prolactin levels increased, but if she pumped while her blood alcohol levels decreased, her prolactin response was delayed. A mother's body responses to suckling are complex and alcohol's effects on these dynamics are not yet fully understood.

• •

Exposure to alcohol in mother's milk causes babies to sleep less.

Although according to some folklore, babies sleep better after a breastfeeding mother drinks alcohol, one U.S. study found that alcohol produced the opposite effect (Mennella & Gerrish, 1998). Although the babies who were fed their mother's expressed milk with alcohol added fell asleep sooner, they slept for a significantly shorter time during the 3.5 hours after receiving the spiked expressed milk than they did when they were fed plain mother's milk. When non-alcoholic vanilla-flavored milk was tried instead of the alcohol-flavored milk, no difference in sleep patterns was found. The researchers concluded that the alcohol changed the babies' sleep-wake patterns, resulting in less sleep overall. When the time of the study was extended to 24 hours, the researchers found that the babies initially spent less time in active sleep, which they compensated for by spending more time in active sleep in the 20.5 hours after the initial alcohol exposure (Mennella & Garcia-Gomez, 2001).

• •

When a mother drinks large amounts of alcohol or drinks regularly over time, her breastfed baby may experience side effects.

Although the American Academy of Pediatrics Committee on Drugs considers alcohol compatible with breastfeeding if consumed occasionally and in small amounts, it lists possible side effects when a breastfeeding mother drinks large amounts, including drowsiness... deep sleep, weakness, decrease in linear growth, abnormal weight gain . It also notes that "maternal ingestion of 1 g/kg daily decreases milk-ejection reflex" ("Transfer of drugs and other chemicals into human milk," 2001, p. 779).

Research is mixed on whether long-term moderate to heavy drinking affects a breastfed baby's motor development. One U.S. study found that when mothers who breastfed for at least 3 months consumed two or more alcoholic drinks per day, their babies scored slightly below normal on motor development at 1 year (Little, Anderson, Ervin, Worthington-Roberts, & Clarren, 1989). Mental development was normal in both groups. However, babies in the "breastfed" group included those who received up to 16 ounces (480 ml) per day of cow's milk or formula. When researchers attempted to replicate this study and extend it to 18 months, no such association was found (Little, Northstone, & Golding, 2002).

• •

To determine if a mother is abusing alcohol, ask how many alcoholic drinks she has each day, week, and month.

A mother with a drinking problem is unlikely to volunteer this information. When asked how much she drinks, she may admit only to drinking occasionally. To better clarify her drinking habits, ask her for the specific number of drinks she has daily, weekly, and monthly. If alcohol abuse is suspected, discuss the risks of caring for an infant when intoxicated and the danger of bed-sharing if an adult has had too much to drink (see chapter 2). If alcohol abuse is suspected, contact her healthcare provider and refer her to a substance abuse counselor.

Nicotine

If a mother smokes, encourage her to breastfeed and to quit smoking or cut down as much as possible.

Although many smoking mothers consider formula-feeding "safer" than breastfeeding (see next point), the opposite is true. When a mother smokes and does not breastfeed, it increases her own health risks and her baby's risk of infection, respiratory illness, respiratory allergy, asthma, and sudden infant death syndrome (Guedes & Souza, 2009; Karmaus et al., 2008; Klonoff-Cohen et al., 1995; Ladomenou, Kafatos, & Galanakis, 2009; Yilmaz, Hizli et al., 2009). One U.S. case-control study examined the relationship between sudden infant death syndrome (SIDS) and smoking and found that while "overall breastfeeding was protective for SIDS...this effect was evident only among nonsmokers (Klonoff-Cohen et al., 1995)." In other words, smoking negated breastfeeding's protective effect and babies of smoking breastfeeding mothers had a rate of SIDS equal to nonsmoking bottle-feeding mothers.

It is generally safer for a smoking mother to breastfeed than to formula feed. But mothers should not expose their babies to second-hand smoke.

In addition to the obvious lack of antibodies in formula, there may be other reasons for these differences in health outcomes. One U.S. study found an association between not breastfeeding and reduced lung function at age 10 years (Ogbuanu, Karmaus, Arshad, Kurukulaaratchy, & Ewart, 2009). A Turkish study found that when mothers smoked, but did not breastfeed, their 6-month-old babies had lower blood levels of the antioxidant vitamins A, C, and E (Yilmaz, Isik Agras et al., 2009). The bloods levels of these vitamins were not lower, however, in the babies whose smoking mothers breastfed.

No matter how a baby is fed, exposure to environmental or passive smoking can be harmful (see last point in the section), but breastfeeding can offset some of the negative health outcomes associated with passive smoking (Nafstad, Jaakkola, Hagen, Botten, & Kongerud, 1996). One Greek study of 240 babies found an increased incidence of the lower respiratory infection bronchiolitis in families who smoked, except when babies were breastfed (Chatzimichael et al., 2007). Another Greek study also found an increased incidence of all types of infections during the first year of life in families where at least one parent smoked, except in those who breastfed (Ladomenou et al., 2009).

Smoking during pregnancy has been associated with lower birthweight, greater risk of preterm birth, and other health risks to mother and baby (Einarson & Riordan, 2009). This can be a strong motivator for many mothers to quit before birth (Giglia, Binns, & Alfonso, 2006; O'Campo, Faden, Brown, & Gielen, 1992). The more cigarettes smoked, the greater the chances the baby may be affected. One case of nicotine withdrawal symptoms was reported in the 48-hour-old breastfed baby of a mother who smoked heavily during pregnancy (Vagnarelli et al., 2006).

If the mother can't or doesn't want to stop smoking, see the later point on minimizing baby's exposure to nicotine.

• •

Mothers who smoke are less likely to breastfeed, and those who do breastfeed are more likely to wean earlier, but the causes may not be physical.

Although it is tempting to look for physical causes for these breastfeeding differences, a mother's intent to breastfeed and her decision to start breastfeeding at birth could not possibly be influenced by the physical effects of smoking . Yet research confirmed that smoking mothers are less likely to both plan to breastfeed and initiate breastfeeding (Liu, Rosenberg, & Sandoval, 2006; Ringel et al., 2001). Some research provides clues to the social and psychological factors at work For example, one study that examined the infant-feeding decisions of 4,000 women in the U.S. south in the 1960s found a trend that heavier smokers were more likely to breastfeed. This study was done at a time when women with more education and income were less likely to breastfeed and poorer, less educated women (who are also more likely to be smokers) were more likely to breastfeed (Underwood, Hester, Laffitte, & Gregg, 1965). In this study, 58% of those smoking more than one pack per day initiated breastfeeding compared with 46% of the nonsmokers.

However, when determining the reasons smoking mothers wean earlier than nonsmokers, the physical effects of smoking must be considered. For example, does nicotine affect a mother's hormonal levels, milk ejection, milk production, and/or milk composition? In two reviews of the literature, Australian physician Lisa Amir analyzed the merits of the studies often cited as proof of these physical effects of smoking on breastfeeding and concluded that the evidence is weak (Amir, 2001; Amir & Donath, 2003). According to Amir, it is unlikely that the physical effects of smoking are responsible for the differences consistently seen in breastfeeding duration.

For example, for every small study that found an association between smoking and decreased milk production, another had the opposite finding (Vio, Salazar, & Infante, 1991; Widstrom, Werner, Matthiesen, Svensson, & Uvnas-Moberg, 1991). Amir noted that when she used a stepwise regression to analyze the data from a U.S. study of mothers expressing milk for preterm babies, she found that smoking only accounted for 8% of the difference in milk production between the smoking and nonsmoking mothers, while day of initiation and frequency of expression accounted for 56% (Hopkinson, Schanler, Fraley, & Garza, 1992). When she examined the association between smoking and milk ejection and smoking and prolactin levels, she found the evidence weak and conflicting.

So what are the causes of these differences in breastfeeding duration? In a Canadian study, researchers surveyed 228 mothers and found that earlier weaning in smoking mothers had less to do with the physical effects of smoking and more to do with mothers' anxiety about how smoking affects their milk and their baby (Ratner, Johnson, & Bottorff, 1999). They concluded that most smoking women wean to formula earlier because they think it is "safer." In a Canadian longitudinal study of 80 breastfeeding mothers of 9- to 12-month-olds, 14% of the mothers listed the following reason for weaning from the breast:

"Breastfeeding did not allow me to drink alcohol or smoke as much as I want" (Rempel, 2004).

A more recent U.S. survey of 204 mothers confirmed that despite the recommendations that smoking mothers breastfeed for better health outcomes, 80% of its mothers believed that breastfeeding women should not smoke at all (Bogen, Davies, Barnhart, Lucero, & Moss, 2008). Only 25% of the study mothers who were current smokers considered it acceptable for a breastfeeding mother to smoke even one cigarette per day, and only 2% thought it was acceptable for breastfeeding mothers to use nicotine replacement therapies to help them quit smoking (see next point). Another qualitative U.S. study of 44 low-income women found these women thought smoking while breastfeeding could harm their baby and that smoking made their milk toxic and addictive (Goldade, Nichter, Adrian, Tesler, & Muramoto, 2008). They reported being unable to stop smoking and receiving little encouragement to breastfeed.

What about those who advise mothers about breastfeeding and smoking? The American Academy of Pediatrics' 2005 policy statement on breastfeeding tells pediatricians "Tobacco smoking by mothers is not a contraindication to breastfeeding…" (Gartner et al., 2005, p. 497). Yet a descriptive study of 209 U.S. pediatricians found that less than half told smoking mothers it was safe to breastfeed (Lucero et al., 2009). Most were likely to recommend formula feeding and were unsure about the safety of nicotine replacement therapies for breastfeeding mothers.

In light of these findings, it is not surprising that at both 10 weeks and 6 months more than twice as many nonsmoking mothers are breastfeeding (Haug et al., 1998; Jedrychowski et al., 2008; Liu et al., 2006). More education about smoking and breastfeeding is obviously needed among both mothers and healthcare providers.

• •

Nicotine-replacement products used to quit smoking are compatible with breastfeeding.

These products provide blood nicotine levels high enough to prevent or reduce withdrawal symptoms without the tars, carbon monoxide, and lung irritants that come with smoking and without the "buzz." According to a Cochrane Review article, use of these products increases the chances of successfully quitting smoking by 50% to 70% (Stead, Perea, Bullen, Mant, & Lancaster, 2008). They come in a variety of forms.

Nicotine gums, lozenges, tablets, inhalers, and nasal sprays are used intermittently over the course of the day, so blood and milk nicotine levels rise and fall. When using these products, suggest the same strategy recommended for the smoking mother (see next point): use them after breastfeeding and if possible wait a couple of hours before the next breastfeeding, when nicotine levels in blood and milk are lower (Hale, 2008). If a baby wants to breastfeed before that time, though, suggest the mother go ahead. Nicotine gums have been found to produce blood levels averaging only 30% to 60% of those produced by smoking (Schatz, 1998). Nicotine blood levels from inhalers are only about 12% (Hale, 2008). On average, one of these replacement products would provide about as much nicotine per day as less than one pack of cigarettes (Schatz, 1998).

Transdermal nicotine patches provide a steady level of nicotine in the mother's blood and milk, which if used correctly, should be lower than smoking. Suggest the mother remove the patch at bedtime for lower nicotine levels at night (Schatz,

1998). One Australian study of 15 breastfeeding mothers found that while on the patch their babies received 70% less nicotine and its metabolite cotinine than while smoking, while milk intake remained stable. The researchers wrote: "Undertaking maternal smoking cessation with the nicotine patch is, therefore, a safer option than continued smoking" (Ilett et al., 2003, p. 516).

• •

Some prescribed medications are used for smoking cessation.

One is the antidepressant bupropion (Zyban or Wellbutrin). The American Academy of Pediatrics considers this a drug "whose effect on nursing infants is unknown but may be of concern" ("Transfer of drugs and other chemicals into human milk," 2001). In *Medications and Mother's Milk,* Hale rates it an L3, and although plasma levels in breastfed babies are undetectable, he cites anecdotal reports of milk production issues (Hale, 2008).

• •

If a breastfeeding mother continues to smoke, suggest strategies to minimize her baby's exposure to nicotine and passive smoke.

Nicotine and cotinine (a byproduct of nicotine breakdown) are concentrated in mother's milk. U.K. research found that on average nicotine levels were three times higher in the mothers' milk than in her blood (Luck & Nau, 1984; Luck & Nau, 1985). One Canadian study comparing urine cotinine levels in smokers' breastfed and non-breastfed babies found five times more cotinine in the urine of smokers' breastfed babies than in those who did not breastfeed (Becker et al., 1999). Cotinine inhaled from passive smoke has been associated with increased incidence of respiratory problems, but cotinine in mother's milk has not. To reduce a breastfed baby's exposure to nicotine, suggest these strategies:

Nicotine and cotinine, a metabolite of nicotine, concentrate in mothers' milk.

Smoke fewer cigarettes per day. While quitting is ideal, if she won't or can't, suggest she cut back on the number of cigarettes she smokes per day to decrease her baby's exposure to nicotine. It may motivate the mother to cut back to know about several studies that have found a link between smoking and increased incidence of colic, even in non-breastfeeding mothers (Canivet, Ostergren, Jakobsson, Dejin-Karlsson, & Hagander, 2008; Reijneveld, Lanting, Crone, & Van Wouwe, 2005; Shenassa & Brown, 2004).

Smoke after breastfeeding. The half-life of nicotine—the amount of time it takes for half the nicotine to be eliminated from the body— is 95 minutes (Steldinger, Luck, & Nau, 1988). After smoking a cigarette, a breastfeeding mother's blood and milk nicotine levels first rise and then fall over time. One Swedish study found that smoking right before breastfeeding caused a ten-fold increase in the amount of nicotine the baby received (Dahlstrom, Lundell, Curvall, & Thapper, 1990). Smoking after breastfeeding and waiting a couple of hours before the next breastfeeding allows the milk nicotine levels to fall before the baby takes the breast again. However, if the baby wants to breastfeed sooner, breastfeeding is better than giving formula (Myr, 2004). Another incentive to smoke after breastfeeding comes from a U.S. study of 15 mothers and babies, which found that the babies spent significantly less time sleeping when the mothers smoked right before breastfeeding (Mennella, Yourshaw, & Morgan, 2007).

Smoke outside or in a separate room. No matter how a baby is fed, breathing cigarette smoke ("passive smoking") poses health risks for everyone in the family. One German study found that nicotine levels in the hair and in spinal and heart fluids in non-breastfed babies who died of SIDS were five times higher than in the babies who had been breastfed, leading the researchers to conclude that passive smoke may be more important to health than exposure to nicotine derivatives through breastfeeding (Bajanowski et al., 2008). Exposure to passive smoking has been found to increase the incidence of infections in non-breastfed babies, but breastfeeding provides some protection against infection (Ladomenou et al., 2009). Encourage the mother to make anywhere her baby spends a lot of time (home, car) smoke-free.

Recreational Drugs

Women at risk for drug abuse may have misconceptions about breastfeeding.

In low-income urban areas, drug abuse among mothers may be common and coexist with other contraindications to breastfeeding. But misconceptions also abound. One U.S. study of 393 mothers giving birth in three District of Columbia inner-city hospitals found that of the 51% who initiated breastfeeding 16% had documented contraindications to breastfeeding (England et al., 2003). The top two contraindications were cocaine use (75%) and HIV-positive status (28%), which accounted for 94% of those with contraindications, as well as tuberculosis (5%), PCP use (5%), and heroin use (3%).

The most common reason given for not breastfeeding was "I didn't want to," which was consistent with a lack of cultural support for breastfeeding in these populations. The second most common reason given (by 25% of the mothers) was concerns about "passing dangerous things to their babies." However, of these mothers, only 46% had a documented contraindication. Of those with a documented contraindication, only 42% reported this as their reason for not breastfeeding. The researchers wrote, "In our study, we could find no documentation of any breastfeeding contraindications in over half of the women who reported that they didn't want to breastfeed because they 'did not want to pass dangerous things'...[raising] the possibility that misperceptions regarding breastfeeding contraindications may have contributed to low breastfeeding initiation rates...." (England et al., 2003, p. 28). When working with populations at risk for drug abuse, it may be helpful to discuss breastfeeding contraindications with mothers.

• •

Not all women with a history of drug abuse should be encouraged to breastfeed.

The Academy of Breastfeeding Medicine's protocol on breastfeeding and the drug-dependent woman lists criteria that can be used to determine who should and who should not be supported and encouraged to breastfeed (Jansson, 2009). Those who *should* be supported in their desire to breastfeed are those who:

- Have not used illicit drugs for at least 90 days before birth and can maintain sobriety as an outpatient
- Are in substance-abuse treatment programs and give consent for their healthcare provider to have access to their treatment progress
- Plan to continue with their treatment program postpartum
- Received consistent prenatal care
- Had a urine test that was negative for illicit drugs at childbirth
- Are not taking psychiatric medication contraindicated during breastfeeding
- And are on stable methodone-replacement therapy, irrespective of the dose

Women who *should not* be encouraged to breastfeed include those who:

- Did not have prenatal care
- Took illicit drugs within 30 days of giving birth
- Refused treatment for substance abuse
- Had a positive urine test for illicit drugs at birth
- Are actively using drugs

Even if a mother does not breastfeed or withholds breastfeeding for the recommended length of time after drug use, she has a responsibility to keep her baby safe. While on drugs, recommend she arrange for her baby to be cared for by someone sober, as drug use at the very least puts the baby at risk for inadequate care.

When under the influence of illicit drugs, no matter how her baby is fed a mother's ability to provide adequate care is impaired.

One U.S. overview article on breastfeeding in mothers on methadone treatment for opiate addiction lists the following behaviors as common among their newborns (Jansson, Velez, & Harrow, 2004): irritability, rapid fluctuation between sleeping and waking, high muscle tone (causing jaw clenching and arching), uncoordinated sucking/swallowing, hypersensitivity to stimulation, nasal congestion, and vomiting. Some of these babies require medication for withdrawal symptoms before they can breastfeed well. One study found that rooming-in among methadone-treated mothers reduced both symptoms and the need for withdrawal medication (Abrahams et al., 2007). The babies who roomed-in with their mothers were also more likely to be discharged home with their mothers compared with babies who were separated from their mothers in the hospital. Abandonment of drug-exposed babies is a serious issue in some areas, and the researchers suggested that rooming-in may also promote better attachment and mothering.

Infant exposure to drugs during pregnancy or breastfeeding can cause symptoms that make breastfeeding challenging.

Mother's drug abuse during pregnancy may cause infant symptoms that make breastfeeding challenging.

Amphetamines

Amphetamines, such as dextroamphetamine, are powerful central nervous system stimulants. When prescribed for ADHD, this drug is considered compatible with breastfeeding (Hale, 2008; Ilett, Hackett, Kristensen, & Kohan, 2007). However, when taken in larger-than-prescribed amounts, amphetamines accumulate in the milk and can pose hazards to both the breastfeeding mother and her baby. Reported symptoms include irritability and sleeplessness ("Transfer of drugs and other chemicals into human milk," 2001). According to Hale's *Medications and Mother's Milk*, mothers "should be strongly advised to withhold breastfeeding for 24 hours following the non-clinical use of dextroamphetamine" (Hale, 2008, p. 274). In a 2009 Australian study of two mothers who injected methylamphetamines, its authors recommended breastfeeding be withheld for 48 hours (Bartu, Dusci, & Ilett, 2009).

If taken in prescribed doses, amphetamines are compatible with breastfeeding, but when abused, there are risks to mother and baby.

Cocaine

Cocaine is on the American Academy of Pediatrics Committee on Drugs list of "Drugs of Abuse Contraindicated during Breastfeeding" because it passes into the mother's milk in significant amounts and can cause cocaine intoxication

After taking cocaine, a mother should pump and dump for at least 24 hours.

in the breastfeeding baby ("Transfer of drugs and other chemicals into human milk," 2001; Winecker et al., 2001). Reported symptoms in the baby include irritability, vomiting, dilated pupils, tremors, and increased heart and respiratory rates. Although the effects on the mother can fade as quickly as 20 to 30 minutes, cocaine is metabolized slowly. Cocaine has been found in adults' urine for up to 7 days and even longer in babies' urine. Cocaine has been found in mother's milk for as long as 36 hours (Chasnoff, Lewis, & Squires, 1987). Because illicit drugs are rarely pure, cocaine may also contain other drugs that may be harmful to the breastfeeding baby.

Topical cocaine can also be hazardous to babies. In one case report, a mother applied cocaine to her nipples to relieve soreness. Three hours later she put the baby to the breast with a nipple shield, and the baby developed convulsions and breathing problems (Chaney, Franke, & Wadlington, 1988).

Hallucinogenic Drugs

Hallucinogenic drugs, such as Angel Dust, Ecstacy, and LSD, are contraindicated during breastfeeding.

Significant amounts of PCP (Angel Dust), gamma hyroxybutyric acid (Ecstasy), and LSD transfer into human milk, making them hazardous to the breastfeeding baby. Hale's *Medications and Mother's Milk* provides specific information on these drugs:

PCP (half-life of 24-51 hours)—Because it is stored in fatty tissue, PCP can be detected in mother's urine for 14-30 days. One mother who took PCP 41 days before she began lactating still had significant milk levels after her baby was born (Kaufman, Petrucha, Pitts, & Weekes, 1983).

Ecstacy (half-life of 20-60 minutes)—Depending on dose, recommend the mother pump and dump for at least 12-24 hours.

LSD (half-life of 3 hours)—This very potent drug crosses the blood-brain barrier and may cause hallucinations in the baby. LSD can be found in the mother's urine for 34-120 hours.

Heroin/Methadone

Heroin use by the mother is contraindicated during breastfeeding.

Heroin is on the American Academy of Pediatrics Committee on Drugs list of "Drugs of Abuse Contraindicated during Breastfeeding" ("Transfer of drugs and other chemicals into human milk," 2001). When abused, significant amounts of heroin pass into the mother's milk and can cause heroin addiction in the breastfeeding baby. Reported symptoms in the baby include tremors, restlessness, vomiting, and poor feeding.

• •

At all doses, methadone, an effective treatment for heroin addiction, is considered compatible with breastfeeding.

In its 1994 statement, the American Academy of Pediatrics Committee on Drugs considered methadone as compatible with breastfeeding up to a dose of 20 mg per day, but this maximum limit was removed in its 2001 publication ("Transfer of drugs and other chemicals into human milk," 2001). Milk levels of methadone in women on higher doses were found to remain within acceptable ranges (Begg, Malpas, Hackett, & Ilett, 2001; Jansson, Choo, Velez, Harrow et al., 2008; Jansson et al., 2007) . One U.S. study on long-term breastfeeding found methadone concentrations in blood and milk were low up to 6 months postpartum (Jansson, Choo, Velez, Lowe, & Huestis, 2008).

Although some research found breastfeeding may help to prevent withdrawal symptoms (known as "neonatal abstinence syndrome") in babies of mothers on methadone treatment (Abdel-Latif et al., 2006), other research has not (Jansson, Choo, Velez, Harrow et al., 2008). One Canadian study found that rooming-in after birth resulted in fewer cases of withdrawal in babies of mothers on heroin or methadone (Abrahams et al., 2007). Because milk levels of methadone are low, some suggest that the oxytocin released during skin-to-skin contact may be the reason some studies found breastfeeding decreased withdrawal symptoms (Phillips, Merewood, & O'Brien, 2003). Whatever the reason, some researchers advise women on higher-dose methadone maintenance to wean from breastfeeding gradually because in one New Zealand study, sudden weaning resulted in more withdrawal symptoms among its babies (Malpas & Darlow, 1999).

Breastfeeding may not prevent withdrawal symptoms in the baby of a mother on methadone treatment, but rooming-in may.

Methodone-maintained mothers can breastfeed.

Marijuana

Marijuana is on the American Academy of Pediatrics Committee on Drugs list of "Drugs of Abuse Contraindicated during Breastfeeding" ("Transfer of drugs and other chemicals into human milk," 2001). But many mothers have questions about it. Canada's Motherisk Program's Alcohol and Substance Use Helpline reportedly receives about three phone calls per week about the use of marijuana by breastfeeding mothers (Djulus, Moretti, & Koren, 2005).

Marijuana use is contraindicated during breastfeeding.

Marijuana, which comes from the leaves of the *Cannabis sativa* plant, is most commonly smoked, but can also be eaten. THC, the active ingredient in marijuana, accumulates in mother's milk. In heavy users, the level of THC in milk and blood may be as high as 8 to 1 (Perez-Reyes & Wall, 1982). Although its half-life is 25 to 57 hours (Hale, 2008), when a mother uses marijuana regularly, THC is stored in body fat, increasing its half-life up to 4 days (Djulus et al., 2005). After marijuana use by a breastfeeding mother, THC can be detected in her baby's urine for up to 3 weeks (Hale, 2008). Exposure to passive smoke would increase the amount of THC the baby receives. One study found an association between marijuana exposure via mother's milk during a baby's first month of life and decreased motor development at 1 year (Astley & Little, 1990). Because illicit drugs are rarely pure, marijuana may be laced with other drugs or substances that could be harmful to the breastfeeding baby.

RESOURCES FOR PARENTS

Handouts

Low-Carbohydrate Diets

Doberne, K. et al. (2004). Weight loss during lactation: are low-carbohydrate diets a good choice? ILCA Inside Track . This article can be accessed at www.feedyourbaby.com/ped/Dieting.pdf.

Gastric Bypass or Other Bariatric Surgeries

Kombol, P. (2008). Breastfeeding after weight loss surgery. ILCA Inside Track.

Books

Nutrition and Weight Loss

Behan, E. (2007). *Eat well, lose weight while breastfeeding.* New York: Ballantine Books.

Is Baby Reacting to Something in Mother's Diet?

Vartabedian, B. (2007). *Colic solved.* New York: Ballantine Books.

REFERENCES

Abdel-Latif, M. E., Pinner, J., Clews, S., Cooke, F., Lui, K., & Oei, J. (2006). Effects of breast milk on the severity and outcome of neonatal abstinence syndrome among infants of drug-dependent mothers. *Pediatrics, 117*(6), e1163-1169.

Abrahams, R. R., Kelly, S. A., Payne, S., Thiessen, P. N., Mackintosh, J., & Janssen, P. A. (2007). Rooming-in compared with standard care for newborns of mothers using methadone or heroin. *Canadian Family Physician, 53*(10), 1722-1730.

Allen, L. H. (1998). Women's dietary calcium requirements are not increased by pregnancy or lactation. *American Journal of Clinical Nutrition, 67*(4), 591-592.

Amaral, J. F., Thompson, W. R., Caldwell, M. D., Martin, H. F., & Randall, H. T. (1984). Prospective metabolic evaluation of 150 consecutive patients who underwent gastric exclusion. *American Journal of Surgery, 147*(4), 468-476.

Amaral, J. F., Thompson, W. R., Caldwell, M. D., Martin, H. F., & Randall, H. T. (1985). Prospective hematologic evaluation of gastric exclusion surgery for morbid obesity. *Annals of Surgery, 201*(2), 186-193.

Amir, L. H. (2001). Maternal smoking and reduced duration of breastfeeding: a review of possible mechanisms. *Early Human Development, 64*(1), 45-67.

Amir, L. H., & Donath, S. (2007). A systematic review of maternal obesity and breastfeeding intention, initiation and duration. *BMC Pregnancy Childbirth, 7*, 9.

Amir, L. H., & Donath, S. M. (2003). Does maternal smoking have a negative physiological effect on breastfeeding? The epidemiological evidence. *Breastfeeding Review, 11*(2), 19-29.

Arthur, P. G., Smith, M., & Hartmann, P. E. (1989). Milk lactose, citrate, and glucose as markers of lactogenesis in normal and diabetic women. *Journal of Pediatric Gastroenterology and Nutrition, 9*(4), 488-496.

Arvola, T., Ruuska, T., Keranen, J., Hyoty, H., Salminen, S., & Isolauri, E. (2006). Rectal bleeding in infancy: clinical, allergological, and microbiological examination. *Pediatrics, 117*(4), e760-768.

Astley, S. J., & Little, R. E. (1990). Maternal marijuana use during lactation and infant development at one year. *Neurotoxicology and Teratology, 12*(2), 161-168.

Babyak, M., Blumenthal, J. A., Herman, S., Khatri, P., Doraiswamy, M., Moore, K., et al. (2000). Exercise treatment for major depression: maintenance of therapeutic benefit at 10 months. *Psychosomatic Medicine, 62*(5), 633-638.

Bajanowski, T., Brinkmann, B., Mitchell, E. A., Vennemann, M. M., Leukel, H. W., Larsch, K. P., et al. (2008). Nicotine and cotinine in infants dying from sudden infant death syndrome. *International Journal of Legal Medicine, 122*(1), 23-28.

Baker, J. L., Michaelsen, K. F., Sorensen, T. I., & Rasmussen, K. M. (2007). High prepregnant body mass index is associated with early termination of full and any breastfeeding in Danish women. *American Journal of Clinical Nutrition, 86*(2), 404-411.

Barnes, J., Stein, A., Smith, T., & Pollock, J. I. (1997). Extreme attitudes to body shape, social and psychological factors and a reluctance to breast feed. ALSPAC Study Team. Avon Longitudinal Study of Pregnancy and Childhood. *Journal of the Royal Society of Medicine, 90*(10), 551-559.

Bartu, A., Dusci, L. J., & Ilett, K. F. (2009). Transfer of methylamphetamine and amphetamine into breast milk following recreational use of methylamphetamine. *British Journal of Clinical Pharmacology, 67*(4), 455-459.

Becker, A. B., Manfreda, J., Ferguson, A. C., Dimich-Ward, H., Watson, W. T., & Chan-Yeung, M. (1999). Breast-feeding and environmental tobacco smoke exposure. *Archives of Pediatrics and Adolescent Medicine, 153*(7), 689-691.

Begg, E. J., Malpas, T. J., Hackett, L. P., & Ilett, K. F. (2001). Distribution of R- and S-methadone into human milk during multiple, medium to high oral dosing. *British Journal of Clinical Pharmacology, 52*(6), 681-685.

Berlin, C. M., Jr., & Daniel, C. H. (1981). Excretion of theobromine in human milk and saliva. *Pediatric Research, 15*, 492.

Berlin, C. M., Jr., Denson, H. M., Daniel, C. H., & Ward, R. M. (1984). Disposition of dietary caffeine in milk, saliva, and plasma of lactating women. *Pediatrics, 73*(1), 59-63.

Blankenship, J. (2008). Bariatric surgery: Implications for women's health. *Women's Health Report*, pp. 1, 3, 4.

Blumenthal, J. A., Babyak, M. A., Doraiswamy, P. M., Watkins, L., Hoffman, B. M., Barbour, K. A., et al. (2007). Exercise and pharmacotherapy in the treatment of major depressive disorder. *Psychosomatic Medicine, 69*(7), 587-596.

Bogen, D. L., Davies, E. D., Barnhart, W. C., Lucero, C. A., & Moss, D. R. (2008). What do mothers think about concurrent breast-feeding and smoking? *Ambulatory Pediatrics, 8*(3), 200-204.

Bone, A., Ncube, F., Nichols, T., & Noah, N. D. (2008). Body piercing in England: a survey of piercing at sites other than earlobe. *BMJ, 336*(7658), 1426-1428.

Bravata, D. M., Sanders, L., Huang, J., Krumholz, H. M., Olkin, I., & Gardner, C. D. (2003). Efficacy and safety of low-carbohydrate diets: a systematic review. *Journal of the American Medical Association, 289*(14), 1837-1850.

Breslow, R. A., Falk, D. E., Fein, S. B., & Grummer-Strawn, L. M. (2007). Alcohol consumption among breastfeeding women. *Breastfeeding Medicine, 2*(3), 152-157.

Brinch, M., Isager, T., & Tolstrup, K. (1988). Anorexia nervosa and motherhood: reproduction pattern and mothering behavior of 50 women. *Acta Psychiatrica Scandinavica, 77*(5), 611-617.

Brolin, R. L., Robertson, L. B., Kenler, H. A., & Cody, R. P. (1994). Weight loss and dietary intake after vertical banded gastroplasty and Roux-en-Y gastric bypass. *Annals of Surgery, 220*(6), 782-790.

Bronner, Y. L. (2010). Maternal Nutrition During Lactation. In J. Riordan & K. Wambach (Eds.), *Breastfeeding and Human Lactation* (4th ed., pp. 497-518). Boston, MA: Jones and Bartlett.

Buchwald, H., Avidor, Y., Braunwald, E., Jensen, M. D., Pories, W., Fahrbach, K., et al. (2004). Bariatric surgery: a systematic review and meta-analysis. *Journal of the American Medical Association, 292*(14), 1724-1737.

Butte, N. F., & Hopkinson, J. M. (1998). Body composition changes during lactation are highly variable among women. *Journal of Nutrition, 128*(2 Suppl), 381S-385S.

Butte, N. F., & King, J. C. (2005). Energy requirements during pregnancy and lactation. *Public Health Nutrition, 8*(7A), 1010-1027.

Bystrova, K., Widstrom, A. M., Matthiesen, A. S., Ransjo-Arvidson, A. B., Welles-Nystrom, B., Vorontsov, I., et al. (2007). Early lactation performance in primiparous and multiparous women in relation to different maternity home practices. A randomised trial in St. Petersburg. *International Breastfeeding Journal, 2*, 9.

Canivet, C. A., Ostergren, P. O., Jakobsson, I. L., Dejin-Karlsson, E., & Hagander, B. M. (2008). Infantile colic, maternal smoking and infant feeding at 5 weeks of age. *Scandanavian Journal of Public Health, 36*(3), 284-291.

Carey, G. B., Quinn, T. J., & Goodwin, S. E. (1997). Breast milk composition after exercise of different intensities. *Journal of Human Lactation, 13*(2), 115-120.

Carlson, H. E., Wasser, H. L., & Reidelberger, R. D. (1985). Beer-induced prolactin secretion: a clinical and laboratory study of the role of salsolinol. *Journal of Clinical Endocrinology and Metabolism, 60*(4), 673-677.

Carranza-Lira, S., & Mera, J. P. (2002). Influence of number of pregnancies and total breast-feeding time on bone mineral density. *International Journal of Fertility and Women's Medicine, 47*(4), 169-171.

Casas, R., Bottcher, M. F., Duchen, K., & Bjorksten, B. (2000). Detection of IgA antibodies to cat, beta-lactoglobulin, and ovalbumin allergens in human milk. *Journal of Allergy and Clinical Immunology, 105*(6 Pt 1), 1236-1240.

Casella, E. B., Valente, M., de Navarro, J. M., & Kok, F. (2005). Vitamin B^{12} deficiency in infancy as a cause of developmental regression. *Brain and Development, 27*(8), 592-594.

CDC. (2003). Neurologic impairment in children associated with maternal dietary deficiency of cobalamin--Georgia, 2001. *Journal of the American Medical Association, 289*(8), 979-980.

Chaney, N. E., Franke, J., & Wadlington, W. B. (1988). Cocaine convulsions in a breast-feeding baby. *Journal of Pediatrics, 112*(1), 134-135.

Chapman, D. J., & Perez-Escamilla, R. (1999). Identification of risk factors for delayed onset of lactation. *Journal of the American Dietetic Association, 99*(4), 450-454; quiz 455-456.

Chapman, D. J., & Perez-Escamilla, R. (2000). Maternal perception of the onset of lactation is a valid, public health indicator of lactogenesis stage II. *Journal of Nutrition, 130*(12), 2972-2980.

Chasnoff, I. J., Lewis, D. E., & Squires, L. (1987). Cocaine intoxication in a breast-fed infant. *Pediatrics, 80*(6), 836-838.

Chatzimichael, A., Tsalkidis, A., Cassimos, D., Gardikis, S., Tripsianis, G., Deftereos, S., et al. (2007). The role of breastfeeding and passive smoking on the development of severe bronchiolitis in infants. *Minerva Pediatrica, 59*(3), 199-206.

Clyne, P. S., & Kulczycki, A., Jr. (1991). Human breast milk contains bovine IgG. Relationship to infant colic? *Pediatrics, 87*(4), 439-444.

Cobo, E. (1973). Effect of different doses of ethanol on the milk-ejecting reflex in lactating women. *American Journal of Obstetrics and Gynecology, 115*(6), 817-821.

Cooper, R. L., & Cooper, M. M. (1996). Red pepper-induced dermatitis in breast-fed infants. *Dermatology, 193*(1), 61-62.

Cross, N. A., Hillman, L. S., Allen, S. H., Krause, G. F., & Vieira, N. E. (1995). Calcium homeostasis and bone metabolism during pregnancy, lactation, and postweaning: a longitudinal study. *American Journal of Clinical Nutrition, 61*(3), 514-523.

Cumming, R. G., & Klineberg, R. J. (1993). Breastfeeding and other reproductive factors and the risk of hip fractures in elderly women. *International Journal of Epidemiology, 22*(4), 684-691.

Dagnelie, P. C., van Staveren, W. A., Roos, A. H., Tuinstra, L. G., & Burema, J. (1992). Nutrients and contaminants in human milk from mothers on macrobiotic and omnivorous diets. *European Journal of Clinical Nutrition, 46*(5), 355-366.

Dahlstrom, A., Lundell, B., Curvall, M., & Thapper, L. (1990). Nicotine and cotinine concentrations in the nursing mother and her infant. *Acta Paediatrica Scandanavica, 79*(2), 142-147.

Davis, R. E. (2001). The postpartum experience for southeast Asian women in the United States. *MCN; American Journal of Maternal Child Nursing, 26*(4), 208-213.

De Rosa, G., Corsello, S. M., Ruffilli, M. P., Della Casa, S., & Pasargiklian, E. (1981). Prolactin secretion after beer. *Lancet, 2*(8252), 934.

Dewey, K. G., Lovelady, C. A., Nommsen-Rivers, L. A., McCrory, M. A., & Lonnerdal, B. (1994). A randomized study of the effects of aerobic exercise by lactating women on breast-milk volume and composition. *New England Journal of Medicine, 330*(7), 449-453.

Dewey, K. G., & McCrory, M. A. (1994). Effects of dieting and physical activity on pregnancy and lactation. *American Journal of Clinical Nutrition, 59*(2 Suppl), 446S-452S; discussion 452S-453S.

Dewey, K. G., Nommsen-Rivers, L. A., Heinig, M. J., & Cohen, R. J. (2003). Risk factors for suboptimal infant breastfeeding behavior, delayed onset of lactation, and excess neonatal weight loss. *Pediatrics, 112*(3 Pt 1), 607-619.

Djulus, J., Moretti, M., & Koren, G. (2005). Marijuana use and breastfeeding. *Canadian Family Physician, 51*, 349-350.

Dusdieker, L. B., Booth, B. M., Stumbo, P. J., & Eichenberger, J. M. (1985). Effect of supplemental fluids on human milk production. *Journal of Pediatrics, 106*(2), 207-211.

Dusdieker, L. B., Hemingway, D. L., & Stumbo, P. J. (1994). Is milk production impaired by dieting during lactation? *American Journal of Clinical Nutrition, 59*(4), 833-840.

Einarson, A., & Riordan, S. (2009). Smoking in pregnancy and lactation: a review of risks and cessation strategies. *European Journal of Clinical Pharmacology, 65*(4), 325-330.

England, L., Brenner, R., Bhaskar, B., Simons-Morton, B., Das, A., Revenis, M., et al. (2003). Breastfeeding practices in a cohort of inner-city women: the role of contraindications. *BMC Public Health, 3*, 28.

Ensom, M. H., Liu, P. Y., & Stephenson, M. D. (2002). Effect of pregnancy on bone mineral density in healthy women. *Obstetrical and Gynecological Survey, 57*(2), 99-111.

Ferreira, C. T., & Seidman, E. (2007a). Food allergy: a practical update from the gastroenterological viewpoint. *J Pediatr (Rio J), 83*(1), 7-20.

Ferreira, C. T., & Seidman, E. (2007b). Food allergy: a practical update from the gastroenterological viewpoint. *Journal of Pediatric (Rio J), 83*(1), 7-20.

Flint, D. J., Travers, M. T., Barber, M. C., Binart, N., & Kelly, P. A. (2005). Diet-induced obesity impairs mammary development and lactogenesis in murine mammary gland. *American Journal of Physiology - Endocrinology & Metabolism, 288*(6), E1179-1187.

Fontaine, K. R., Redden, D. T., Wang, C., Westfall, A. O., & Allison, D. B. (2003). Years of life lost due to obesity. *Journal of the American Medical Association, 289*(2), 187-193.

Forestell, C. A., & Mennella, J. A. (2007). Early determinants of fruit and vegetable acceptance. *Pediatrics, 120*(6), 1247-1254.

Fraser, A. B., & Grimes, D. A. (2003). Effect of lactation on maternal body weight: a systematic review. *Obstetrical and Gynecological Survey, 58*(4), 265-269.

Gabriel, A., Gabriel, K. R., & Lawrence, R. A. (1986). Cultural values and biomedical knowledge: choices in infant feeding. Analysis of a survey. *Social Science and Medicine, 23*(5), 501-509.

Gartner, L. M., Morton, J., Lawrence, R. A., Naylor, A. J., O'Hare, D., Schanler, R. J., et al. (2005). Breastfeeding and the use of human milk. *Pediatrics, 115*(2), 496-506.

Giglia, R., & Binns, C. W. (2006). Alcohol and lactation: A systematic review. *Nutrition & Dietetics, 63*, 103-116.

Giglia, R. C., & Binns, C. W. (2007). Patterns of alcohol intake of pregnant and lactating women in Perth, Australia. *Drug and Alcohol Review, 26*(5), 493-500.

Giglia, R. C., Binns, C. W., & Alfonso, H. S. (2006). Which women stop smoking during pregnancy and the effect on breastfeeding duration. *BMC Public Health, 6*, 195.

Giglia, R. C., Binns, C. W., Alfonso, H. S., Scott, J. A., & Oddy, W. H. (2008). The effect of alcohol intake on breastfeeding duration in Australian women. *Acta Paediatrica, 97*(5), 624-629.

Giovannini, M., Radaelli, G., Banderali, G., & Riva, E. (2007). Low prepregnant body mass index and breastfeeding practices. *Journal of Human Lactation, 23*(1), 44-51.

Goldade, K., Nichter, M., Adrian, S., Tesler, L., & Muramoto, M. (2008). Breastfeeding and smoking among low-income women: results of a longitudinal qualitative study. *Birth, 35*(3), 230-240.

Grange, D. K., & Finlay, J. L. (1994). Nutritional vitamin B_{12} deficiency in a breastfed infant following maternal gastric bypass. *Pediatric Hematology and Oncology, 11*(3), 311-318.

Grjibovski, A. M., Yngve, A., Bygren, L. O., & Sjostrom, M. (2005). Socio-demographic determinants of initiation and duration of breastfeeding in northwest Russia. *Acta Paediatrica, 94*(5), 588-594.

Guedes, H. T., & Souza, L. S. (2009). Exposure to maternal smoking in the first year of life interferes in breast-feeding protective effect against the onset of respiratory allergy from birth to 5 yr. *Pediatric Allergy and Immunology, 20*(1), 30-34.

Hale, T. (2008). *Medications and Mothers' Milk* (13th ed.). Amarillo, TX: Hale Publishing.

Hanley, D. A., & Davison, K. S. (2005). Vitamin D insufficiency in North America. *Journal of Nutrition, 135*(2), 332-337.

Hatsu, I. E., McDougald, D. M., & Anderson, A. K. (2008). Effect of infant feeding on maternal body composition. *International Breastfeeding Journal, 3*, 18.

Haug, K., Irgens, L. M., Baste, V., Markestad, T., Skjaerven, R., & Schreuder, P. (1998). Secular trends in breastfeeding and parental smoking. *Acta Paediatrica, 87*(10), 1023-1027.

Hausner, H., Bredie, W. L., Molgaard, C., Petersen, M. A., & Moller, P. (2008). Differential transfer of dietary flavour compounds into human breast milk. *Physiology and Behavior, 95*(1-2), 118-124.

Health Council of the Netherlands. (2005). *Risks of Alcohol Consumption Related to Conception, Pregnancy and Breastfeeding*. Retrieved on March 11, 2010 from http://www.gezondheidsraad.nl/en/publications/risks-alcohol-consumption-related-conception-pregnancy-and-breastfeeding.

Heinig, M. J., & Doberne, K. (2004). Weighing the risks: the use of low-carbohydrate diets during lactation. *Journal of Human Lactation, 20*(3), 283-285.

Henderson, P. H., 3rd, Sowers, M., Kutzko, K. E., & Jannausch, M. L. (2000). Bone mineral density in grand multiparous women with extended lactation. *American Journal of Obstetrics and Gynecology, 182*(6), 1371-1377.

Hill, D. J., Roy, N., Heine, R. G., Hosking, C. S., Francis, D. E., Brown, J., et al. (2005). Effect of a low-allergen maternal diet on colic among breastfed infants: a randomized, controlled trial. *Pediatrics, 116*(5), e709-715.

Hilson, J. A., Rasmussen, K. M., & Kjolhede, C. L. (2004). High prepregnant body mass index is associated with poor lactation outcomes among white, rural women independent of psychosocial and demographic correlates. *Journal of Human Lactation, 20*(1), 18-29.

Hilson, J. A., Rasmussen, K. M., & Kjolhede, C. L. (2006). Excessive weight gain during pregnancy is associated with earlier termination of breast-feeding among White women. *Journal of Nutrition, 136*(1), 140-146.

Ho, E., Collantes, A., Kapur, B. M., Moretti, M., & Koren, G. (2001). Alcohol and breast feeding: calculation of time to zero level in milk. *Biology of the Neonate, 80*(3), 219-222.

Holmberg-Marttila, D., & Sievanen, H. (1999). Prevalence of bone mineral changes during postpartum amenorrhea and after resumption of menstruation. *American Journal of Obstetrics and Gynecology, 180*(3 Pt 1), 537-538.

Holmberg-Marttila, D., Sievanen, H., Sarkkinen, E., Erkkila, A., Salminen, S., & Isolauri, E. (2001). Do combined elimination diet and prolonged breastfeeding of an atopic infant jeopardise maternal bone health? *Clinical and Experimental Allergy, 31*(1), 88-94.

Hoover, K. L. (2008). Maternal obesity: Problems of breastfeeding with large breasts. *Women's Health Report*, pp. 6,10.

Hopkinson, J. (2007). Nutrition in lactation. In T. W. Hale & P. E. Hartmann (Eds.), *Hale & Hartmann's textbook of human lactation* (pp. 371-386). Amarillo, TX: Hale Publishing.

Hopkinson, J. M., Schanler, R. J., Fraley, J. K., & Garza, C. (1992). Milk production by mothers of premature infants: influence of cigarette smoking. *Pediatrics, 90*(6), 934-938.

Host, A., Husby, S., & Osterballe, O. (1988). A prospective study of cow's milk allergy in exclusively breast-fed infants. Incidence, pathogenetic role of early inadvertent exposure to cow's milk formula, and characterization of bovine milk protein in human milk. *Acta Paediatrica Scandanavica, 77*(5), 663-670.

Humphrey, S. (2003). The nursing mother's herbal. Minneapolis, MN: Fairview Press.

Ilett, K. F., Hackett, L. P., Kristensen, J. H., & Kohan, R. (2007). Transfer of dexamphetamine into breast milk during treatment for attention deficit hyperactivity disorder. *British Journal of Clinical Pharmacology, 63*(3), 371-375.

Ilett, K. F., Hale, T. W., Page-Sharp, M., Kristensen, J. H., Kohan, R., & Hackett, L. P. (2003). Use of nicotine patches in breast-feeding mothers: transfer of nicotine and cotinine into human milk. *Clinical Pharmacology and Therapeutics, 74*(6), 516-524.

IOM. (1990). *Nutrition during pregnancy. Part I, weight gain*. Washington, D.C.: National Academy Press.

IOM. (2005). *Dietary Reference Intakes for energy, carbohydrates, fiber, fat, fatty acids, cholesterol, protein, and amino acids.* Washington, DC: National Academy Press.

Ip, S., Chung, M., Raman, G., Chew, P., Magula, N., DeVine, D., et al. (2007). Breastfeeding and maternal and infant health outcomes in developed countries. *Evidence Report - Technology Assessment (Full Report)(153)*, 1-186.

Jakobsson, I., & Lindberg, T. (1983). Cow's milk proteins cause infantile colic in breast-fed infants: a double-blind crossover study. *Pediatrics, 71*(2), 268-271.

Jansson, L. M. (2009). ABM clinical protocol #21: Guidelines for breastfeeding and the drug-dependent woman. *Breastfeeding Medicine, 4*(4), 225-228.

Jansson, L.M., Choo, R.E., Harrow, C., Velez, M., Schroeder, J.R., Lowe, R., & Huestis, M.A. (2007). Concentrations of methadone in breast milk and plasma in the immediate perinatal period. *Journal of Human Lactation, 23*(2),184-190.

Jansson, L. M., Choo, R., Velez, M. L., Harrow, C., Schroeder, J. R., Shakleya, D. M., et al. (2008). Methadone maintenance and breastfeeding in the neonatal period. *Pediatrics, 121*(1), 106-114.

Jansson, L. M., Choo, R., Velez, M. L., Lowe, R., & Huestis, M. A. (2008). Methadone maintenance and long-term lactation. *Breastfeeding Medicine, 3*(1), 34-37.

Jansson, L. M., Choo, R. E., Harrow, C., Velez, M., Schroeder, J. R., Lowe, R., et al. (2007). Concentrations of methadone in breast milk and plasma in the immediate perinatal period. *Journal of Human Lactation, 23*(2), 184-190.

Jansson, L. M., Velez, M., & Harrow, C. (2004). Methadone maintenance and lactation: a review of the literature and current management guidelines. *Journal of Human Lactation, 20*(1), 62-71.

Jedrychowski, W., Perera, F., Mroz, E., Edwards, S., Flak, E., Rauh, V., et al. (2008). Prenatal exposure to passive smoking and duration of breastfeeding in nonsmoking women: Krakow inner city prospective cohort study. *Archives of Gynecology and Obstetrics, 278*(5), 411-417.

Jevitt, C., Hernandez, I., & Groer, M. (2007). Lactation complicated by overweight and obesity: supporting the mother and newborn. *Journal of Midwifery & Women's Health, 52*(6), 606-613.

Kahn, A., Mozin, M. J., Rebuffat, E., Sottiaux, M., & Muller, M. F. (1989). Milk intolerance in children with persistent sleeplessness: a prospective double-blind crossover evaluation. *Pediatrics, 84*(4), 595-603.

Kahn, A., Rebuffat, E., Blum, D., Casimir, G., Duchateau, J., Mozin, M. J., et al. (1987). Difficulty in initiating and maintaining sleep associated with cow's milk allergy in infants. *Sleep, 10*(2), 116-121.

Kalkwarf, H. J., Specker, B. L., Heubi, J. E., Vieira, N. E., & Yergey, A. L. (1996). Intestinal calcium absorption of women during lactation and after weaning. *American Journal of Clinical Nutrition, 63*(4), 526-531.

Kalkwarf, H. J., Specker, B. L., & Ho, M. (1999). Effects of calcium supplementation on calcium homeostasis and bone turnover in lactating women. *Journal of Clinical Endocrinology and Metabolism, 84*(2), 464-470.

Karmaus, W., Dobai, A. L., Ogbuanu, I., Arshard, S. H., Matthews, S., & Ewart, S. (2008). Long-term effects of breastfeeding, maternal smoking during pregnancy, and recurrent lower respiratory tract infections on asthma in children. *Journal of Asthma, 45*(8), 688-695.

Kaufman, K. R., Petrucha, R. A., Pitts, F. N., Jr., & Weekes, M. E. (1983). PCP in amniotic fluid and breast milk: case report. *Journal of Clinical Psychiatry, 44*(7), 269-270.

Kent, J. C., Arthur, P. G., Mitoulas, L. R., & Hartmann, P. E. (2009). Why calcium in breastmilk is independent of maternal dietary calcium and vitamin D. *Breastfeeding Review, 17*(2), 5-11.

King, J. C. (2001). Effect of reproduction on the bioavailability of calcium, zinc and selenium. *Journal of Nutrition, 131*(4 Suppl), 1355S-1358S.

Klonoff-Cohen, H. S., Edelstein, S. L., Lefkowitz, E. S., Srinivasan, I. P., Kaegi, D., Chang, J. C., et al. (1995). The effect of passive smoking and tobacco exposure through breast milk on sudden infant death syndrome. *Journal of the American Medical Association, 273*(10), 795-798.

Koletzko, B., & Lehner, F. (2000). Beer and breastfeeding. Advances in Experimental *Medicine and Biology, 478*, 23-28.

Kolthoff, N., Eiken, P., Kristensen, B., & Nielsen, S. P. (1998). Bone mineral changes during pregnancy and lactation: a longitudinal cohort study. *Clinical Science (London), 94*(4), 405-412.

Kramer, F. M., Stunkard, A. J., Marshall, K. A., McKinney, S., & Liebschutz, J. (1993). Breast-feeding reduces maternal lower-body fat. *Journal of the American Dietetic Association, 93*(4), 429-433.

Kugyelka, J. G., Rasmussen, K. M., & Frongillo, E. A. (2004). Maternal obesity is negatively associated with breastfeeding success among Hispanic but not Black women. *Journal of Nutrition, 134*(7), 1746-1753.

Kvenshagen, B., Halvorsen, R., & Jacobsen, M. (2008). Adverse reactions to milk in infants. *Acta Paediatrica, 97*(2), 196-200.

Lacoursiere, D. Y., Baksh, L., Bloebaum, L., & Varner, M. W. (2006). Maternal body mass index and self-reported postpartum depressive symptoms. *Maternal and Child Health Journal, 10*(4), 385-390.

Ladomenou, F., Kafatos, A., & Galanakis, E. (2009). Environmental tobacco smoke exposure as a risk factor for infections in infancy. *Acta Paediatrica, 98*(7), 1137-1141.

Larson-Meyer, D. E. (2002). Effect of postpartum exercise on mothers and their offspring: a review of the literature. *Obesity Research, 10*(8), 841-853.

Lawrence, R. A., & Lawrence, R. M. (2005). *Breastfeeding: A guide for the medical profession*. Philadelphia, PA: Elsevier Mosby.

Lawton, M. E. (1985). Alcohol in breast milk. *Australian and New Zealand Journal of Obstetrics and Gynaecology, 25*(1), 71-73.

Lee, N. (1995). More on pierced nipples. *Journal of Human Lactation, 11*(2), 89.

Little, R. E., Anderson, K. W., Ervin, C. H., Worthington-Roberts, B., & Clarren, S. K. (1989). Maternal alcohol use during breast-feeding and infant mental and motor development at one year. *New England Journal of Medicine, 321*(7), 425-430.

Little, R. E., Northstone, K., & Golding, J. (2002). Alcohol, breastfeeding, and development at 18 months. *Pediatrics, 109*(5), E72-72.

Liu, J., Rosenberg, K. D., & Sandoval, A. P. (2006). Breastfeeding duration and perinatal cigarette smoking in a population-based cohort. *American Journal of Public Health, 96*(2), 309-314.

Liu, J., Smith, M. G., Dobre, M. A., & Ferguson, J. E. (2009). Maternal obesity and breast-feeding practices among White and Black women. *Obesity (Silver Spring)*.

Lovelady, C. A. (2004). The impact of energy restriction and exercise in lactating women. *Advances in Experimental Medicine and Biology, 554*, 115-120.

Lovelady, C. A., Fuller, C. J., Geigerman, C. M., Hunter, C. P., & Kinsella, T. C. (2004). Immune status of physically active women during lactation. *Medicine and Science in Sports and Exercise, 36*(6), 1001-1007.

Lovelady, C. A., Garner, K. E., Moreno, K. L., & Williams, J. P. (2000). The effect of weight loss in overweight, lactating women on the growth of their infants. *New England Journal of Medicine, 342*(7), 449-453.

Lovelady, C. A., Hunter, C. P., & Geigerman, C. (2003). Effect of exercise on immunologic factors in breast milk. *Pediatrics, 111*(2), E148-152.

Lovelady, C. A., Lonnerdal, B., & Dewey, K. G. (1990). Lactation performance of exercising women. *American Journal of Clinical Nutrition, 52*(1), 103-109.

Lovelady, C. A., Nommsen-Rivers, L. A., McCrory, M. A., & Dewey, K. G. (1995). Effects of exercise on plasma lipids and metabolism of lactating women. *Medicine and Science in Sports and Exercise, 27*(1), 22-28.

Lucero, C. A., Moss, D. R., Davies, E. D., Colborn, K., Barnhart, W. C., & Bogen, D. L. (2009). An examination of attitudes, knowledge, and clinical practices among Pennsylvania pediatricians regarding breastfeeding and smoking. *Breastfeeding Medicine, 4*(2), 83-89.

Luck, W., & Nau, H. (1984). Nicotine and cotinine concentrations in serum and milk of nursing smokers. *British Journal of Clinical Pharmacology, 18*(1), 9-15.

Luck, W., & Nau, H. (1985). Nicotine and cotinine concentrations in serum and urine of infants exposed via passive smoking or milk from smoking mothers. *Journal of Pediatrics, 107*(5), 816-820.

Malpas, T. J., & Darlow, B. A. (1999). Neonatal abstinence syndrome following abrupt cessation of breastfeeding. *New Zealand Medical Journal, 112*(1080), 12-13.

Martens, W. S., 2nd, Martin, L. F., & Berlin, C. M., Jr. (1990). Failure of a nursing infant to thrive after the mother's gastric bypass for morbid obesity. *Pediatrics, 86*(5), 777-778.

Martorell, A., Plaza, A. M., Bone, J., Nevot, S., Garcia Ara, M. C., Echeverria, L., et al. (2006). Cow's milk protein allergy. A multi-centre study: clinical and epidemiological aspects. *Allergologia et Immunopathologia, 34*(2), 46-53.

Mason, M. E., Jalagani, H., & Vinik, A. I. (2005). Metabolic complications of bariatric surgery: diagnosis and management issues. *Gastroenterology Clinics of North America, 34*(1), 25-33.

Matz, P. E., Foster, G. D., Faith, M. S., & Wadden, T. A. (2002). Correlates of body image dissatisfaction among overweight women seeking weight loss. *Journal of Consulting and Clinical Psychology, 70*(4), 1040-1044.

McCrory, M. A. (2000). Aerobic exercise during lactation: safe, healthful, and compatible. *Journal of Human Lactation, 16*(2), 95-98.

Mennella, J. A. (1997). Infants' suckling responses to the flavor of alcohol in mothers' milk. *Alcoholism, Clinical and Experimental Research, 21*(4), 581-585.

Mennella, J. A. (1998). Short-term effects of maternal alcohol consumption on lactational performance. *Alcoholism, Clinical and Experimental Research, 22*(7), 1389-1392.

Mennella, J. A. (2001). Regulation of milk intake after exposure to alcohol in mothers' milk. *Alcoholism, Clinical and Experimental Research, 25*(4), 590-593.

Mennella, J. A. (2007). Chemical senses and the development of flavor preferences in humans. In T. W. Hale, P. E. Hartmann (Ed.), *Hale & Hartmann's Textbook of Human Lactation* (pp. 403-413). Amarillo, TX: Hale Publishing.

Mennella, J. A., & Beauchamp, G. K. (1991a). Maternal diet alters the sensory qualities of human milk and the nursling's behavior. *Pediatrics, 88*(4), 737-744.

Mennella, J. A., & Beauchamp, G. K. (1991b). The transfer of alcohol to human milk. Effects on flavor and the infant's behavior. *New England Journal of Medicine, 325*(14), 981-985.

Mennella, J. A., & Beauchamp, G. K. (1993). Beer, breast feeding and folklore. *Developmental Psychobiology, 26*, 459-466.

Mennella, J. A., & Garcia-Gomez, P. L. (2001). Sleep disturbances after acute exposure to alcohol in mothers' milk. *Alcohol, 25*(3), 153-158.

Mennella, J. A., & Gerrish, C. J. (1998). Effects of exposure to alcohol in mother's milk on infant sleep. *Pediatrics, 101*(5), E2.

Mennella, J. A., Jagnow, C. P., & Beauchamp, G. K. (2001). Prenatal and postnatal flavor learning by human infants. *Pediatrics, 107*(6), E88.

Mennella, J. A., & Pepino, M. Y. (2008). Biphasic effects of moderate drinking on prolactin during lactation. *Alcoholism, Clinical and Experimental Research, 32*(11), 1899-1908.

Mennella, J. A., Pepino, M. Y., & Teff, K. L. (2005). Acute alcohol consumption disrupts the hormonal milieu of lactating women. *Journal of Clinical Endocrinology and Metabolism, 90*(4), 1979-1985.

Mennella, J. A., Yourshaw, L. M., & Morgan, L. K. (2007). Breastfeeding and smoking: short-term effects on infant feeding and sleep. *Pediatrics, 120*(3), 497-502.

Mok, E., Multon, C., Piguel, L., Barroso, E., Goua, V., Christin, P., et al. (2008). Decreased full breastfeeding, altered practices, perceptions, and infant weight change of prepregnant obese women: a need for extra support. *Pediatrics, 121*(5), e1319-1324.

Morrow, D. A. (1976). Fat cow syndrome. *Journal of Dairy Science, 59*(9), 1625-1629.

Morse, J. M., Ewing, G., Gamble, D., & Donahue, P. (1992). The effect of maternal fluid intake on breast milk supply: a pilot study. *Canadian Journal of Public Health. Revue Canadienne de Sante Publique, 83*(3), 213-216.

Myr, R. (2004). Promoting, protecting, and supporting breastfeeding in a community with a high rate of tobacco use. *Journal of Human Lactation, 20*(4), 415-416.

Nafstad, P., Jaakkola, J. J., Hagen, J. A., Botten, G., & Kongerud, J. (1996). Breastfeeding, maternal smoking and lower respiratory tract infections. *European Respiratory Journal, 9*(12), 2623-2629.

Nehlig, A., & Debry, G. (1994). Consequences on the newborn of chronic maternal consumption of coffee during gestation and lactation: A review. *Journal of the American College of Nutrition, 13*(1), 6-21.

Neubauer, S. H., Ferris, A. M., Chase, C. G., Fanelli, J., Thompson, C. A., Lammi-Keefe, C. J., et al. (1993). Delayed lactogenesis in women with insulin-dependent diabetes mellitus. *American Journal of Clinical Nutrition, 58*(1), 54-60.

O'Brien, K. O., Donangelo, C. M., Zapata, C. L., Abrams, S. A., Spencer, E. M., & King, J. C. (2006). Bone calcium turnover during pregnancy and lactation in women with low calcium diets is associated with calcium intake and circulating insulin-like growth factor 1 concentrations. *American Journal of Clinical Nutrition, 83*(2), 317-323.

O'Campo, P., Faden, R. R., Brown, H., & Gielen, A. C. (1992). The impact of pregnancy on women's prenatal and postpartum smoking behavior. *American Journal of Preventive Medicine, 8*(1), 8-13.

Oddy, W. H., Li, J., Landsborough, L., Kendall, G. E., Henderson, S., & Downie, J. (2006). The association of maternal overweight and obesity with breastfeeding duration. *Journal of Pediatrics, 149*(2), 185-191.

Ogbuanu, I. U., Karmaus, W., Arshad, S. H., Kurukulaaratchy, R. J., & Ewart, S. (2009). Effect of breastfeeding duration on lung function at age 10 years: a prospective birth cohort study. *Thorax, 64*(1), 62-66.

Olafsdottir, A. S., Thorsdottir, I., Wagner, K. H., & Elmadfa, I. (2006). Polyunsaturated fatty acids in the diet and breast milk of lactating icelandic women with traditional fish and cod liver oil consumption. *Annals of Nutrition and Metabolism, 50*(3), 270-276.

Pepino, M. Y., & Mennella, J. A. (2008). Effects of breast pumping on the pharmacokinetics and pharmacodynamics of ethanol during lactation. *Clinical Pharmacology and Therapeutics, 84*(6), 710-714.

Perez-Reyes, M., & Wall, M. E. (1982). Presence of delta9-tetrahydrocannabinol in human milk. *New England Journal of Medicine, 307*(13), 819-820.

Phillips, B., Merewood, A., & O'Brien, S. (2003). Methadone and breastfeeding: New horizons. *Pediatrics, 111*(6), 1429-1430.

Polatti, F., Capuzzo, E., Viazzo, F., Colleoni, R., & Klersy, C. (1999). Bone mineral changes during and after lactation. *Obstetrics and Gynecology, 94*(1), 52-56.

Prentice, A. (1994). Maternal calcium requirements during pregnancy and lactation. *American Journal of Clinical Nutrition, 59*(2 Suppl), 477S-482S; discussion 482S-483S.

Prentice, A. M., Goldberg, G. R., & Prentice, A. (1994). Body mass index and lactation performance. *European Journal of Clinical Nutrition, 48 Suppl 3*, S78-86; discussion S86-79.

Prentice, A. M., Roberts, S. B., Prentice, A., Paul, A. A., Watkinson, M., Watkinson, A. A., et al. (1983). Dietary supplementation of lactating Gambian women. I. Effect on breast-milk volume and quality. *Human Nutrition. Clinical Nutrition, 37*(1), 53-64.

Pumberger, W., Pomberger, G., & Geissler, W. (2001). Proctocolitis in breast fed infants: a contribution to differential diagnosis of haematochezia in early childhood. *Postgraduate Medical Journal, 77*(906), 252-254.

Rasmussen, K. M. (1998). Effects of under- and overnutrition on lactation in laboratory rats. *Journal of Nutrition, 128*(2 Suppl), 390S-393S.

Rasmussen, K. M., & Kjolhede, C. L. (2004). Prepregnant overweight and obesity diminish the prolactin response to suckling in the first week postpartum. *Pediatrics, 113*(5), e465-471.

Rasmussen, K. M., Lee, V. E., Ledkovsky, T. B., & Kjolhede, C. L. (2006). A description of lactation counseling practices that are used with obese mothers. *Journal of Human Lactation, 22*(3), 322-327.

Ratner, P. A., Johnson, J. L., & Bottorff, J. L. (1999). Smoking relapse and early weaning among postpartum women: is there an association? *Birth, 26*(2), 76-82.

Reijneveld, S. A., Lanting, C. I., Crone, M. R., & Van Wouwe, J. P. (2005). Exposure to tobacco smoke and infant crying. *Acta Paediatrica, 94*(2), 217-221.

Rempel, L. A. (2004). Factors influencing the breastfeeding decisions of long-term breastfeeders. *Journal of Human Lactation, 20*(3), 306-318.

Repucci, A. (1999). Resolution of stool blood in breast-fed infants with maternal ingestion of pancreatic enzymes. *Journal of Pediatric Gastroenterology and Nutrition, 29*, 500A.

Rich, M., Currie, J., & McMahon, C. (2004). Physical exercise and the lactating woman: a qualitative pilot study of mothers' perceptions and experiences. *Breastfeeding Review, 12*(2), 11-17.

Ringel, S., Kahan, E., Greenberg, R., Arieli, S., Blay, A., & Berkovitch, M. (2001). Breastfeeding and smoking habits among Israeli women. *Israel Medical Association Journal, 3*(10), 739-742.

Ritchie, L. D., Fung, E. B., Halloran, B. P., Turnlund, J. R., Van Loan, M. D., Cann, C. E., et al. (1998). A longitudinal study of calcium homeostasis during human pregnancy and lactation and after resumption of menses. *American Journal of Clinical Nutrition, 67*(4), 693-701.

Rooney, B. L., Schauberger, C. W., & Mathiason, M. A. (2005). Impact of perinatal weight change on long-term obesity and obesity-related illnesses. *Obstetrics and Gynecology, 106*(6), 1349-1356.

Roschitz, B., Plecko, B., Huemer, M., Biebl, A., Foerster, H., & Sperl, W. (2005). Nutritional infantile vitamin B_{12} deficiency: pathobiochemical considerations in seven patients. *Archives of Disease in Childhood. Fetal and Neonatal Edition, 90*(3), F281-282.

Ryu, J. E. (1985a). Caffeine in human milk and in serum of breast-fed infants. *Developmental Pharmacology and Therapeutics, 8*(6), 329-337.

Ryu, J. E. (1985b). Effect of maternal caffeine consumption on heart rate and sleep time of breast-fed infants. *Developmental Pharmacology and Therapeutics, 8*(6), 355-363.

Sadove, R., & Clayman, M. A. (2008). Surgical procedure for reversal of nipple piercing. *Aesthetic Plastic Surgery, 32*(3), 563-565.

Sarwer, D. B., Wadden, T. A., & Foster, G. D. (1998). Assessment of body image dissatisfaction in obese women: specificity, severity, and clinical significance. *Journal of Consulting and Clinical Psychology, 66*(4), 651-654.

Schach, B., & Haight, M. (2002). Colic and food allergy in the breastfed infant: is it possible for an exclusively breastfed infant to suffer from food allergy? *Journal of Human Lactation, 18*(1), 50-52.

Schatz, B. S. (1998). Nicotine replacement products: implications for the breastfeeding mother. *Journal of Human Lactation, 14*(2), 161-163.

Schulte, P. (1995). Minimizing alcohol exposure of the breastfeeding infant. *Journal of Human Lactation, 11*(4), 317-319.

Scott, J. A., Binns, C. W., Graham, K. I., & Oddy, W. H. (2006). Temporal changes in the determinants of breastfeeding initiation. *Birth, 33*(1), 37-45.

Shenassa, E. D., & Brown, M. J. (2004). Maternal smoking and infantile gastrointestinal dysregulation: the case of colic. *Pediatrics, 114*(4), e497-505.

Sicherer, S. H. (2003). Clinical aspects of gastrointestinal food allergy in childhood. *Pediatrics, 111*(6 Pt 3), 1609-1616.

Smith, C. (1947). Effects of maternal undernutrition upon newborn infants in Holland (1944-1945). *Journal of Pediatrics, 30*, 229-243.

Sorva, R., Makinen-Kiljunen, S., & Juntunen-Backman, K. (1994). Beta-lactoglobulin secretion in human milk varies widely after cow's milk ingestion in mothers of infants with cow's milk allergy. *Journal of Allergy and Clinical Immunology, 93*(4), 787-792.

Specker, B. L. (1994). Nutritional concerns of lactating women consuming vegetarian diets. *American Journal of Clinical Nutrition, 59*(5 Suppl), 1182S-1186S.

Stapleton, H., Fielder, A., & Kirkham, M. (2008). Breast or bottle? Eating disordered childbearing women and infant-feeding decisions. *Maternal and Child Nutrition, 4*(2), 106-120.

Stead, L. F., Perea, R., Bullen, C., Mant, D., & Lancaster, T. (2008). Nicotine replacement therapy for smoking cessation (Publication no. 10.1002/14651858.CD00146.pub3). Retrieved 12 September 2009, from John Wiley & Sons, Ltd.:

Stefanski, J. (2006). Breast-feeding after bariatric surgery. *Today's Dietician, 8*(1), 47.

Steldinger, R., Luck, W., & Nau, H. (1988). Half lives of nicotine in milk of smoking mothers: implications for nursing. *Journal of Perinatal Medicine, 16*(3), 261-262.

Strode, M. A., Dewey, K. G., & Lonnerdal, B. (1986). Effects of short-term caloric restriction on lactational performance of well-nourished women. *Acta Paediatrica Scandanavica, 75*(2), 222-229.

Su, D., Zhao, Y., Binns, C., Scott, J., & Oddy, W. (2007). Breast-feeding mothers can exercise: results of a cohort study. *Public Health Nutrition, 10*(10), 1089-1093.

Taylor, M. M. (1985). *Transcultural aspects of breastfeeding--U.S.A.* (Vol. 2). Garden City Park, NY: Avery Publishing Group.

Transfer of drugs and other chemicals into human milk. (2001). *Pediatrics, 108*(3), 776-789.

Underwood, P., Hester, L. L., Laffitte, T., Jr., & Gregg, K. V. (1965). The relationship of smoking to the outcome of pregnancy. *American Journal of Obstetrics and Gynecology, 91*, 270-276.

USDA. (2005). *U.S. dietary guidelines for Americans*. Washington, DC: U.S. Department of Agriculture.

Vadas, P., Wai, Y., Burks, W., & Perelman, B. (2001). Detection of peanut allergens in breast milk of lactating women. *Journal of the American Medical Association, 285*(13), 1746-1748.

Vagnarelli, F., Amarri, S., Scaravelli, G., Pellegrini, M., Garcia-Algar, O., & Pichini, S. (2006). TDM grand rounds: neonatal nicotine withdrawal syndrome in an infant prenatally and postnatally exposed to heavy cigarette smoke. *Therapeutic Drug Monitoring, 28*(5), 585-588.

Vallianatos, H., Brennand, E. A., Raine, K., Stephen, Q., Petawabano, B., Dannenbaum, D., et al. (2006). Beliefs and practices of First Nation women about weight gain during pregnancy and lactation: implications for women's health. *Canadian Journal of Nursing Research, 38*(1), 102-119.

Vartabedian, B. (2007). *Colic solved: The essential guide to infant reflux and the care of your crying, difficult-to-soothe baby*. New York, NY: Ballantine Books.

Vio, F., Salazar, G., & Infante, C. (1991). Smoking during pregnancy and lactation and its effects on breast-milk volume. *American Journal of Clinical Nutrition, 54*(6), 1011-1016.

Wallace, J. P., Inbar, G., & Ernsthausen, K. (1992). Infant acceptance of postexercise breast milk. *Pediatrics, 89*(6 Pt 2), 1245-1247.

Ward, K. A., Adams, J. E., & Mughal, M. Z. (2005). Bone status during adolescence, pregnancy and lactation. *Current Opinion in Obstetrics and Gynecology, 17*(4), 435-439.

Wardinsky, T. D., Montes, R. G., Friederich, R. L., Broadhurst, R. B., Sinnhuber, V., & Bartholomew, D. (1995). Vitamin B_{12} deficiency associated with low breast-milk vitamin B_{12} concentration in an infant following maternal gastric bypass surgery. *Archives of Pediatrics and Adolescent Medicine, 149*(11), 1281-1284.

Weiss, R., Fogelman, Y., & Bennett, M. (2004). Severe vitamin B_{12} deficiency in an infant associated with a maternal deficiency and a strict vegetarian diet. *Journal of Pediatric Hematology/Oncology, 26*(4), 270-271.

Widstrom, A. M., Werner, S., Matthiesen, A. S., Svensson, K., & Uvnas-Moberg, K. (1991). Somatostatin levels in plasma in nonsmoking and smoking breast-feeding women. *Acta Paediatrica Scandanavica, 80*(1), 13-21.

Wilson-Clay, B., & Hoover, K. (2008). *The breastfeeding atlas* (4th ed.). Manchaca, TX: LactNews Press.

Winecker, R. E., Goldberger, B. A., Tebbett, I. R., Behnke, M., Eyler, F. D., Karlix, J. L., et al. (2001). Detection of cocaine and its metabolites in breast milk. *Journal of Forensic Sciences, 46*(5), 1221-1223.

Wosje, K. S., & Kalkwarf, H. J. (2004). Lactation, weaning, and calcium supplementation: effects on body composition in postpartum women. *American Journal of Clinical Nutrition, 80*(2), 423-429.

Wright, K. S., Quinn, T. J., & Carey, G. B. (2002). Infant acceptance of breast milk after maternal exercise. *Pediatrics, 109*(4), 585-589.

Yakura, N. (1997). Mothers' body perception biased to obesity and its effects on nursing behaviors. *Yonago Acta Medica, 40*, 127-145.

Yamaga, A., Taga, M., Minaguchi, H., & Sato, K. (1996). Changes in bone mass as determined by ultrasound and biochemical markers of bone turnover during pregnancy and puerperium: a longitudinal study. *Journal of Clinical Endocrinology and Metabolism, 81*(2), 752-756.

Yilmaz, G., Hizli, S., Karacan, C., Yurdakok, K., Coskun, T., & Dilmen, U. (2009). Effect of passive smoking on growth and infection rates of breast-fed and non-breast-fed infants. *Pediatrics International, 51*(3), 352-358.

Yilmaz, G., Isik Agras, P., Hizli, S., Karacan, C., Besler, H. T., Yurdakok, K., et al. (2009). The effect of passive smoking and breast feeding on serum antioxidant vitamin (A, C, E) levels in infants. *Acta Paediatrica, 98*(3), 531-536.

Zimmerman, D. R., Goldstein, L., Lahat, E., Braunstein, R., Stahi, D., Bar-Haim, A., et al. (2009). Effect of a 24+ hour fast on breast milk composition. *Journal of Human Lactation, 25*(2), 194-198.

Pregnancy and Tandem Nursing

Chapter
14

BREASTFEEDING DURING PREGNANCY

A pregnant mother may have mixed feelings about continuing to breastfeed.

Breastfeeding during a pregnancy and/or continuing to breastfeed both siblings after birth is not something most mothers plan. These practices are considered unusual or even unacceptable by many cultures. The mother may feel pressure to wean from the adults in her life, due to fears that breastfeeding will cause a miscarriage or be too stressful for the mother. But if her child is still avidly breastfeeding, she may also feel pressure to continue.

If helping a pregnant woman, start by helping her separate her own feelings from the feelings and opinions of others. Discuss her circumstances and her perception of her child's needs. Factors that may influence her decision include:

- Her child's age and his physical and emotional need to breastfeed
- Her breastfeeding-related discomforts, such as nipple pain
- Her previous breastfeeding experiences
- Pregnancy-related health issues, such as uterine pain or bleeding, a history of preterm birth, or weight loss during pregnancy
- Her partner's feelings about breastfeeding during pregnancy and tandem nursing

If the mother seems unsure about her feelings and there are no health issues affecting her situation, suggest she postpone a decision and take breastfeeding 1 day at a time.

• •

Due to changes in the milk and other factors, most children wean during pregnancy.

In two U.S. studies of women who became pregnant while breastfeeding, most children (57% and 69%) weaned before their sibling was born (Moscone & Moore, 1993; Newton & Theotokatos, 1979). Some reasons pregnancy often leads to weaning include:

- **Changes in the milk**. Most child-led weanings occurred during the 2nd trimester, when mature milk changes to low-volume, different-tasting colostrum.
- **Nipple pain**, a common side effect of the hormonal changes of pregnancy, which leads many mothers to breastfeed less often and to shorten feeding times.
- **The child's readiness to wean** independent of the pregnancy.

It is not possible to predict whether a child will wean during a pregnancy based on age alone, unless he is younger than 12 months. Although biologically babies need the milk before 12 months, some do wean at younger ages, which can sometimes be devastating to a mother.

Before 1 year, a child has a biological need for mother's milk, so he will not yet be developmentally ready to wean. But children mature at different rates, so after 1 year, age alone will not be an accurate predictor of weaning readiness. Also, some children wean during pregnancy, and then resume breastfeeding after the baby is born.

If a mother decides to wean or wants to determine if her child is ready to wean, suggest gentle weaning strategies.

Some specific strategies, such as "don't offer, don't refuse," substitution, and others, can help an unsure mother better gauge if her child is developmentally ready to wean. For a description of these strategies, see p. 188- "Gradual Weaning After 12 Months" in the chapter "Weaning from the Breast."

Give any mother who's decided to wean support and acceptance. Assure her that there are many ways, such as cuddling and focused attention, to meet her child's need for her. Also, be sure the mother knows that even if her child weans during pregnancy, this is no guarantee he won't want to breastfeed after the baby is born. If this happens and the mother does not want him to go to breast, suggest she offer him a taste of her milk in a spoon or cup. This mother may also appreciate receiving reassurance that she can meet her older child's needs in other ways.

Suggest the mother who plans to continue breastfeeding be flexible.

Although continued breastfeeding can help a mother meet her child's needs during a stressful and tiring time, encourage her to avoid assumptions about how breastfeeding will go. Emotions and physical comfort during pregnancy can be unpredictable. An open mind and flexibility to changing needs are keys to making breastfeeding during pregnancy a positive experience.

Concerns About the Unborn Baby

If the mother is well-nourished, breastfeeding during pregnancy should not deprive her unborn child.

To gain the recommended amount of weight during pregnancy, encourage the mother to get the rest she needs and eat nutrient-dense foods. She may also meet her nutrient and weight-gain goals more easily if she consumes more calories and takes a prenatal vitamin/mineral supplement.

In one U.S. study, the newborns of 57 mothers who breastfed during pregnancy were healthy at birth and born at the expected weights (Moscone & Moore, 1993). Another study of 253 rural Guatemalan women compared mothers who had weaned 6 months before conceiving with mothers who breastfed into the 2nd and 3rd trimester of pregnancy and found no significant difference in the babies' birthweights (Merchant, Martorell, & Haas, 1990). Although the growth of the baby in utero was not affected, this second study noted that the mothers who breastfed during pregnancy showed evidence of reduced maternal fat stores, despite consuming more of the nutritional supplements the researchers made available, compared to the other mothers. However, these were malnourished or undernourished mothers, and this issue would not apply to Western mothers on adequate diets.

Breastfeeding during pregnancy generally poses no risk to the fetus if the mother is healthy and well-nourished.

Mothers who are clinically malnourished may need nutritional supplements during pregnancy.

See the later section, "The Mother's Nutrition, Energy, and Health."

Effects on the Pregnancy

Uterine contractions occurring during breastfeeding are similar to those occurring during sexual relations.

As of this writing, no medical studies have determined the effect of breastfeeding on pregnancy outcomes. The uterine contractions experienced during breastfeeding are caused by the release of the hormone oxytocin from nipple stimulation and are a normal part of pregnancy. Uterine contractions also occur during sexual activity. Unless the couple has been asked to avoid sexual relations during a high-risk pregnancy, due to concerns about potential preterm labor, breastfeeding should not be contraindicated.

Some healthcare providers advise mothers to wean during pregnancy "just in case," but support for breastfeeding during pregnancy is increasing. In its 2008 breastfeeding position statement, the American Academy of Family Physicians wrote: "Breastfeeding during a subsequent pregnancy is not unusual. If the pregnancy is normal and the mother is healthy, breastfeeding during pregnancy is the mother's decision" (AAFP, 2008).

Some breastfeeding mothers feel stronger or more frequent contractions in later pregnancy. In one U.S. retrospective study, 53 of the 57 mothers who breastfed during pregnancy felt no breastfeeding-related contractions, and the four who did gave birth to healthy full-term babies (Moscone & Moore, 1993).

The mother with a high-risk or difficult pregnancy may be asked to wean.

There are no specific guidelines on which pregnancy complications are an indication for weaning, and prenatal caregivers vary widely in their recommendations. Mothers may be advised to wean when they are expecting twins, triplets, or more, have uterine pain or bleeding, have a history of or symptoms of preterm labor, or have less than appropriate weight gain during pregnancy. If a mother feels uncomfortable with the recommendations she is given, encourage her to get a second opinion from a breastfeeding-friendly caregiver.

Mother's Nutrition, Health, and Comfort

It is important for the pregnant, breastfeeding mother to stay well-nourished.

"Eat to hunger" and "drink to thirst" are the basic nutritional recommendations for breastfeeding mothers. Breastfeeding during pregnancy increases a mother's nutritional requirements (Bronner, 2010). Suggest the pregnant, breastfeeding mother expect to feel hungrier and thirstier than before her pregnancy and to increase her food and drink accordingly. Staying well-nourished will promote healthy weight gains for her and her children. See the chapter "Nutrition, Exercise, and Lifestyle Issues" for more specific suggestions for eating nutrient-dense foods.

A malnourished pregnant, breastfeeding mother and her children are at risk for lower-than-recommended weight gains.

A malnourished woman has few fat stores and may be vitamin deficient. Being malnourished may affect the mother's weight gain during pregnancy, the birthweight of her unborn baby, her newborn's weight gain while breastfeeding, and the weight gain of the breastfeeding older sibling. In this situation, providing nutritional supplements to the breastfeeding mother is the best strategy to counteract the malnourishment.

One study of 253 Guatemalan women found no significant difference in babies' birthweight when mothers who had weaned their older sibling more than 6 months before conception were compared with mothers who breastfed into the 2nd or 3rd trimester of pregnancy (Merchant et al., 1990). Even though these mothers were consuming nutritional supplements, the birthweights of the newborns tended to be lower the later in pregnancy they weaned the older sibling.

Another study found that malnourished Philippino women who breastfed during pregnancy had a poorer weight gain when compared with women who had weaned before pregnancy (Siega-Riz & Adair, 1993). A study of 113 children in Bhutan found that the children who weaned during their mothers' pregnancy had a reduced growth rate during the last months before weaning, when compared with children of the same age who had weaned or continued breastfeeding, but whose mothers were not pregnant (Bohler & Bergstrom, 1996). A Peruvian study of 133 pregnant women living in poverty found that an overlap between pregnancy and breastfeeding correlated with lower weight gains in the first month of the new baby's life (Marquis, Penny, Diaz, & Marin, 2002).

Breastfeeding may make it easier for a fatigued pregnant mother to rest with her child.

One advantage of continued breastfeeding during pregnancy is that it may make it easier for the mother to convince her baby or toddler to lie down and breastfeed when she wants to rest.

Nausea in early pregnancy may make breastfeeding more challenging.

Managing an active child can be difficult when a pregnant mother feels nauseated. For some pregnant mothers, breastfeeding does not increase feelings of nausea, but holding a squirming child does. Other mothers report increased feelings of nausea during breastfeeding, whether or not their child is active. This may be due in part to a mother's increased body awareness during breastfeeding. One strategy that may help is sharing frequent, small meals with her child to reduce both her nausea and her child's motivation to breastfeed, or limiting breastfeeding to a shorter time, such as the length of a favorite song.

As a mother's abdomen grows, breastfeeding may become more awkward.

In late pregnancy, as her lap disappears, a mother's large abdomen may make it difficult for her child to easily reach her nipple. If so, suggest she experiment by lying down and trying other positions. An older toddler can be incredibly creative and may breastfeed leaning over his reclining mother's side or over her shoulder when she's sitting. Most toddlers who are motivated to breastfeed will find a way.

For most breastfeeding mothers, the changing hormones of pregnancy cause sore or tender nipples and breasts.

Some women notice nipple and breast tenderness, even before missing their first menstrual period. Other women never experience this or notice it only late in pregnancy. The duration of nipple and breast soreness is also individual. Of the 39% of the women who reported nipple soreness in one U.S. study, most experienced it primarily during the first trimester (Moscone & Moore, 1993). In another U.S. study, 74% of the mothers reported their nipple soreness lasted for nearly the entire pregnancy, resolving only after their baby's birth (Newton & Theotokatos, 1979).

Nipple and breast pain convinces some mothers to wean during pregnancy. Mothers who continue breastfeeding learn to cope with the soreness in different ways. To make the soreness more manageable, suggest the mother try these strategies:

- Vary breastfeeding positions, making sure her child gets the nipple as far back in his mouth as possible.
- Use her childbirth breathing techniques while breastfeeding.
- Ask the child to try to be gentler or limit breastfeeding to a shorter time, assuring the child that the pain is not his fault.
- Hand-express until the milk ejection occurs, as milk flow can decrease pain.

During pregnancy, many mothers feel restless or irritable while breastfeeding.

Some pregnant mothers experience a feeling of restlessness or irritation with the older child while breastfeeding. Some refer to this as an "antsy" feeling. Two U.S. studies found that between 22% and 57% of their pregnant, breastfeeding mothers experienced this restlessness or irritation (Moscone & Moore, 1993; Newton & Theotokatos, 1979). If this occurs, suggest the mother try distracting herself with a book or with television.

The Child's Need for Milk

Most pregnant mothers notice a decrease in milk production as milk turns to colostrum.

The hormones that maintain a pregnancy also cause milk production to decrease. Most mothers (60% to 65%) report a significant decrease in milk during the 4th or 5th month of pregnancy (Moscone & Moore, 1993; Newton & Theotokatos, 1979). Some breastfeeding babies and toddlers respond to this decrease in milk by breastfeeding less or weaning. Some suddenly begin eating and drinking more other foods. The change in the milk's taste as it turns from mature milk to colostrum convinces some children to wean. The breastfeeding child old enough to talk will often comment on the change in flavor. Some who wean want to resume breastfeeding after the baby is born. Others continue to breastfeed during the pregnancy despite these changes.

If the breastfeeding baby is younger than 1 year, suggest the mother monitor his weight gain to make sure he continues to be well-nourished.

For the baby younger than one year, the natural pregnancy-related decrease in milk production could compromise his nutritional needs. Suggest the mother keep track of her baby's weight gain and, if needed, provide appropriate supplements.

The older breastfeeding child will not deprive the newborn of colostrum by breastfeeding during pregnancy.

As the milk changes to colostrum in preparation for the birth, reassure the mother that her breastfeeding child will not "use up" all the colostrum. No matter how often or long he breastfeeds, colostrum will still be available after birth for the newborn.

The increased hormones in the milk are compatible with breastfeeding the older child.

The hormones that maintain a pregnancy are found in mother's milk, but they are not harmful to the breastfeeding child. The small amount of these hormones the child receives will decrease as the mother's milk supply decreases. The baby in utero is exposed at a much higher level to the hormones produced by pregnancy than the breastfeeding child.

TANDEM NURSING

Tandem nursing may happen by design or by default and can be both joyful and stressful.

Mothers who decide not to actively wean during pregnancy may do so in happy anticipation of breastfeeding the older child and the newborn together, also known as tandem nursing. Others continue to breastfeed for their child's sake, without thinking much about tandem nursing. Others approach tandem nursing with concern or even dread. No matter what the mother's feelings during pregnancy, encourage her to avoid preconceived ideas about how she will feel and take tandem nursing 1 day at a time.

Planning During Pregnancy

If the older sibling is old enough to understand, suggest the mother prepare him for tandem nursing by discussing the newborn's needs.

If the older sibling is past 2 or 3, he can begin to learn to wait. One way for the mother to help prepare the older child is to talk to him about how she responded to his needs as a baby. She can also talk about how becoming a "big brother" or "big sister" means helping to take care of the newborn baby by talking to him, touching him gently, and letting him breastfeed first, since milk will be his only food.

Suggest the mother minimize her separation from the older sibling at birth, freeze meals, and arrange for household help.

Encourage the mother to plan a birth that takes into account the older sibling's need for her and minimizes separation. Unnecessary separation can make this stressful adjustment more difficult.

Preparing and freezing meals before the baby is born will help make mealtimes simpler during the baby's early weeks. Household help can also make this time easier. The mother's partner may take a major role, but if other family members or friends offer to help, be sure they understand their role is taking care of the house and helping with the older child, allowing the mother to focus on the newborn.

The Practical Details

During the first few days, suggest the newborn be given first priority at the breast.

The colostrum, or first milk, is a concentrated liquid with the nutrients and antibodies the newborn needs. There are small amounts of colostrum available until around the 3rd day after birth, when milk production increases. If the older child breastfeeds occasionally, the mother does not need to do anything special to make sure the newborn receives the colostrum he needs. But if the mother is concerned because the older child breastfeeds often, she can ask for help to make sure the newborn gets first priority at the breast. For example, the mother's partner or other helpers could give the older sibling focused attention or if appropriate, take him on special outings. This is a very short time, that may even be shorter when two children are breastfeeding, as more breastfeeding can stimulate the mother's milk production to increase sooner than usual. Encourage the mother to trust her own feelings on this.

The older sibling may ask to breastfeed more often in the early weeks, which may cause his stools to change.

When the older sibling sees the newborn breastfeeding, this may temporarily increase his interest in going to the breast. In addition to a source of nourishment, breastfeeding for the older sibling is also a source of comfort and closeness. When he feels anxious or threatened by the new baby, he may turn to the breast for reassurance that he is still loved. When he notices his mother's growing attachment to the baby, he may feel the need to reestablish his own relationship with her by breastfeeding and seeking her attention in other ways.

Colostrum and transitional milk can have a laxative effect on the older child, resulting in looser, more frequent stools. This should subside once the transitional milk is replaced by mature milk, which usually occurs about 2 weeks after birth.

Tandem nursing can help minimize engorgement and ensure abundant milk production.

If the mother is separated from the newborn and/or older sibling, engorgement can still occur. But if it does and the older sibling is willing to breastfeed, this can help reduce and relieve engorgement as the mother's milk increases. Some older siblings refuse the breast until it is softer, while others are thrilled by the new abundance of milk.

Normal breast hygiene is usually enough while tandem nursing, even in case of illness.

The tandem-nursing mother doesn't have to use special hygiene. Regular baths or showers, clean clothes, and reasonable cleanliness are enough. The Montgomery glands near the nipple secrete an anti-bacterial fluid, and babies are born with an immunity to most household (and sibling) bacteria, which is enhanced by the antibodies in the milk.

If one sibling has a cold or another common illness, the mother does not need to limit each child to one breast, because the children have already been exposed to the bacteria or virus that caused the illness by the time symptoms appear. When an illness becomes obvious, the siblings have already shared their mother's breasts for several days. One exception might be thrush, a fungal infection that is passed between mother and baby, or any other serious or highly contagious illness. In this case, the mother may want to consider limiting each child to one breast.

Suggest the mother be prepared to eat well, drink enough fluids, and get the rest she needs while tandem nursing.

Just like the mother of twins, the mother who is tandem nursing is likely to be hungrier and thirstier than when she was breastfeeding just one baby. See the chapter, "Nutrition, Exercise, and Lifestyle Issues" for ideas for nutritious snacks. Encourage her to have something easy on hand to eat every few hours and to drink to thirst. The concentration of her urine will tell her if she is drinking enough. If it is dark in color, or if she becomes constipated, she needs to drink more.

To get the rest she needs, encourage the mother to accept all offers of household help from family and friends, or if necessary hire household help. If this is not within her means, suggest she ask if a teenager in her neighborhood would be willing to come after school to play with older children and help with household chores.

The mother is the best one to decide how her children share the breast.

Each mother should feel free to manage the practicalities of tandem nursing in the way that works best within her own family dynamics. While the newborn has a greater physical need for the milk, tandem nursing is easier for some mothers if they can be flexible about who breastfeeds first, on what breast, and for how long (Gromada, 1992).

The newborn's needs. A mother may worry about whether the baby is getting the milk he needs when he and the older sibling share the breast. A mother may feel strongly about restricting the older sibling's breastfeeding to specific times or only after the baby has finished. If this arrangement works well for the older sibling, it is fine. But if not, reassure the mother that most women who tandem nurse find that because their milk is produced by supply and demand, they should have plenty of milk for both children, no matter when they breastfeed. While it may be best for the newborn to breastfeed first most of the time, switching from one breast to the other—rather than restricting each child to a side—is good for the baby as it promotes better eye development. If the mother is worried about her baby's milk intake, suggest that she monitor her baby's weight gain.

Encourage tandem-nursing mothers to find the arrangement that works well for them. She can balance her needs with the needs of her children.

The older sibling's needs. How the older sibling feels about sharing the breast and any breastfeeding restrictions will depend on his age and temperament. Some older children can handle restricting nursing to certain times and places; others find being asked to wait even for a few minutes is unbearable. Some regress after their sibling's birth and want to breastfeed like a newborn again. Also, the same child may react differently at different times. Encourage the mother to try different approaches—such as breastfeeding the children together, varying who breastfeeds when throughout the day, or giving her older child consistent breastfeeding times—until she finds what works best for them. When making these decisions, the mother's feelings are as important as the children's.

For her own comfort, the mother may want to encourage some consistency in the older sibling's breastfeeding, so that he doesn't breastfeed all day 1 day and not at all the next. Draining her breasts irregularly may increase her risk of mastitis.

The mother's needs. Discuss the mother's feelings about tandem nursing and ways to balance her own feelings with the needs of her children. For example, some mothers feel better about tandem nursing if they breastfeed both children together, which can cut down on time spent breastfeeding. Other mothers become restless or irritable when the children breastfeed together and enjoy tandem nursing more if they breastfeed separately. Some mothers feel most comfortable allowing the baby and older child to breastfeed on cue because there's less conflict. Others feel better about restricting the older sibling's breastfeeding to set times and places. Brainstorm with the mother to find practical ways to make tandem nursing subjectively better for her.

If a mother finds tandem nursing overwhelming or unpleasant, encourage her to find gradual and positive ways to wean her older child. (For specific suggestions, see p. 187- "Gradual Weaning After 12 Months" in the chapter "Weaning from the Breast")

Help from the mother's partner and use of a baby carrier can make it easier to meet both children's needs.

Using a baby sling or carrier can allow a mother to keep her baby close and still have a hand free for the older sibling. If the baby can breastfeed in the carrier, this allows the mother to give the older child her attention while the baby feeds.

The more active a role the mother's partner plays, the better. By spending a lot of time with the older sibling, entertaining him, and introducing him to fun activities, this decreases the pressure on the mother to provide for both children's needs.

Tandem nursing while away from home can sometimes be challenging.

One way to cut down on requests to breastfeed while out and about is to breastfeed both children before leaving home and offer snacks and drinks to the older sibling while away. For more suggestions on managing breastfeeding while away from home with an older child, see p. 190- "Gradual Weaning After 12 Months" in the chapter "Weaning from the Breast." If the mother knows she'll need to breastfeed both children while out, wearing clothing that permits discreet breastfeeding and using a shawl or blanket as a coverup can also make this easier.

Emotional Adjustments

Mothers react differently to tandem nursing.

Some mothers feel positively about tandem nursing; others do not. Because emotions can vary from mother to mother and day to day, do not assume that one mother's experience will be the same as another's or that a mother's feelings will remain the same over time.

Many mothers decide to tandem nurse because they are focused on the older sibling's needs. It is only natural for a mother to focus on the child she knows, rather than on the unborn baby, who is still a stranger to her. However, after birth, many mothers' feelings shift dramatically. The hormones of birth and breastfeeding—especially if the mother's experiences were positive—enhance her infatuation with the newborn in her arms. All of a sudden the older child looks so big, and the mother may feel resentful about taking time away from her newborn to breastfeed her older child.

Not every mother experiences such a dramatic shift in feelings. But if she does and if she made the decision to tandem nurse for the sake of the older sibling, she may feel guilty and alarmed. Assure her that these opposing feelings—first protective of the older child, then resentful of his demands—are common when a new baby joins the family.

Assure the mother that she might have these same negative feelings, even if the older sibling was not breastfeeding. But when breastfeeding is part of this dynamic, negative feelings often become focused there. Having these feelings does not mean she will never again enjoy breastfeeding her older child. If the mother is experiencing mood swings, tell her that feeling like she's on an emotional roller coaster after birth is common. In time, her strong feelings will diminish and she'll gain a clearer perspective.

If a mother finds the feelings associated with tandem nursing uncomfortable, suggest some possible adjustments.

While breastfeeding their newborn and older child together, some mothers become restless or irritable. Some describe their experience as a "creepy-crawly feeling" or have the urge to push their older child off the breast, which is sometimes referred to as "breastfeeding agitation" (Flower, 2003). Mothers who have this experience may worry that there's something wrong with them, so letting them know it is common enough to have earned a name may help them understand that this reaction is not a reflection of their true feelings about their older child. Some feel this way, even when the older sibling breastfeeds alone. An older child's teeth and gums may cause friction on the mother's nipple and areola, leading many to describe the "roughness" they feel when their older child suckles in comparison to the gentle suckle of their newborn. Some mothers don't notice these differences; others, however, find them disturbing. Some mothers experience the sensations from the older child's suckling as erotic.

Assure the mother that all of these feelings are common, and if she finds her feelings disturbing or uncomfortable, encourage her to make adjustments. For example, it may help reduce the sensations by varying her older child's breastfeeding position or breastfeeding her children separately rather than together. Some mothers find they can better handle these feelings by reducing their older child's time at the breast, keeping each breastfeeding short, but not eliminating or postponing them. Other mothers' breastfeed less often by distracting their older child with other activities, postponing breastfeeding, or before the older child asks to breastfeed, offering substitutions, such as snacks or drinks.

If the mother feels "touched out," suggest she arrange for a little time to herself each day.

"Touched out" is when a mother wants some physical space to herself because she has been cuddling, holding, and breastfeeding all day. Her children need her, her partner wants physical intimacy, and she may just want her body to herself.

Be sure the mother knows that these feelings are common. Although she may assume tandem nursing is the cause of her feelings, remind her that even if her older child was not breastfeeding, he would still seek her out for closeness and comfort. Suggest the mother arrange for a few minutes to herself each day, perhaps to take a bath or shower alone or go for a short walk. Even a little "alone time" can go a long way in improving a mother's mood.

It helps if the mother who's tandem nursing has a positive attitude and a sense of humor. When she can't muster these, encourage her to talk to someone who will listen sympathetically - her partner, a friend, other mothers who have tandem nursed, or others who are supportive of breastfeeding.

If the mother wants to wean the older child, discuss gradual, gentle weaning strategies.

A mother may begin tandem nursing with a positive attitude only to find that she feels very differently about it than she had imagined. A mother may decide to wean her older child if she has tried different ways of breastfeeding both children and still feels uncomfortable. Or she may make this decision suddenly and not want to try anything new. For gradual and gentle weaning strategies for the older child, see p. 187- "Gradual Weaning After 12 Months" in the chapter "Weaning from the Breast."

RESOURCES FOR PARENTS

Books

Bumgarner, N. (2000). *Mothering your nursing toddler* (Rev. ed.). Schaumburg, Illinois: La Leche League International.

Flower, H. (2003). *Adventures in tandem nursing.* Schaumburg, IL: La Leche League International.

REFERENCES

AAFP. (2008). American Academy of Family Physicians position paper: Family physicians supporting breastfeeding. Retrieved 10/11/09, 2009, from http://www.aafp.org/online/en/home/policy/policies/b/breastfeedingpositionpaper.printerview.html

Bohler, E., & Bergstrom, S. (1996). Child growth during weaning depends on whether mother is pregnant again. *Journal of Tropical Pediatrics, 42*(2), 104-109.

Bronner, Y. L. (2010). Maternal nutrition during lactation. In J. Riordan & K. Wambach (Eds.), *Breastfeeding and human lactation* (4th ed., pp. 497-518). Boston, MA: Jones and Bartlett.

Flower, H. D. (2003). *Adventures in tandem nursing*. Schaumburg, IL: La Leche League International.

Gromada, K. K. (1992). Breastfeeding more than one: Multiples and tandem breastfeeding. *NAACOGS Clinical Issues in Perinatal and Womens Health Nursing, 3*(4), 656-666.

Marquis, G. S., Penny, M. E., Diaz, J. M., & Marin, R. M. (2002). Postpartum consequences of an overlap of breastfeeding and pregnancy: Reduced breast milk intake and growth during early infancy. *Pediatrics, 109*(4), e56.

Merchant, K., Martorell, R., & Haas, J. (1990). Maternal and fetal responses to the stresses of lactation concurrent with pregnancy and of short recuperative intervals. *American Journal of Clinical Nutrition, 52*(2), 280-288.

Moscone, S. R., & Moore, M. J. (1993). Breastfeeding during pregnancy. *Journal of Human Lactation, 9*(2), 83-88.

Newton, N., & Theotokatos, M. (1979). Breastfeeding during pregnancy in 503 women: Does a psychobiological weaning mechanism exist in humans? *Emotion & Reproduction, 20B*, 845-849.

Siega-Riz, A. M., & Adair, L. S. (1993). Biological determinants of pregnancy weight gain in a Filipino population. *American Journal of Clinical Nutrition, 57*(3), 365-372.

Employment

Chapter 15

SETTING BREASTFEEDING GOALS

A mother's ideas about working and breastfeeding may be based on the experiences of women she knows, what she has read, what she has observed, or what she has seen portrayed in the media. Before discussing her goals, it may help to get a sense of what she knows and what her feelings are.

Before discussing the mother's goals, ask her what she has heard about working and breastfeeding and how she feels about it.

During a baby's first 6 months, exclusive breastfeeding is recommended. But if a baby will not be fully breastfed, the more mother's milk the baby receives, the better. Women have found many creative ways to fit full and partial breastfeeding into their lives, even with demanding jobs. Options include:

Make sure the mother knows that breastfeeding does not have to be "all or nothing."

There are many ways for mothers to combine employment and breastfeeding.

Exclusive breastfeeding by:

- Bringing the baby to work.
- Having the baby brought to work for feedings.
- Going to the baby for feedings.
- Reverse Cycle Breastfeeding - Baby takes most feedings while mother is at home and has his longest sleep stretch while mother is at work

Providing expressed mother's milk for all missed feedings by:

- Expressing milk at work during breaks.
- Expressing milk outside of work hours, such as before baby wakes in the morning, right after work, and after feedings at home.

Providing some expressed mother's milk and some other foods for missed feedings by:

- Expressing milk when together, but not when apart.
- Expressing milk when apart for some feedings.

Providing formula or other foods for all missed feedings and breastfeeding when together.

CONSIDERING EMPLOYMENT OPTIONS

Maternity Leave

Most countries offer partial or full pay to mothers for weeks or months after childbirth. The International Labour Organization (ILO) recommends a minimum paid maternity leave of 14 weeks. In the United States, however, there is no guaranteed paid maternity leave. At this writing, the Family Medical Leave Act (FMLA) guarantees up to 12 weeks of unpaid leave after childbirth, but only for women working for at least 1 year in companies with 50 or more

Most countries provide paid leave for women after childbirth; an exception is the United States.

employees. Some low-income U.S. mothers return to work as early as 1 to 2 weeks postpartum (Chamberlain, McMahon, Philipp, & Merewood, 2006; Roe, Whittington, Fein, & Teisl, 1999).

Suggest the mother take as long a maternity leave as possible to help get breastfeeding well established.

When mothers take at least 6 weeks of maternity leave, employed and stay-at-home mothers start breastfeeding at about the same rates (Calnen, 2007; Gielen, Faden, O'Campo, Brown, & Paige, 1991; Kurinij, Shiono, Ezrine, & Rhoads, 1989; Ong, Yap, Li, & Choo, 2005; Scott, Binns, Oddy, & Graham, 2006). Not so when maternity leave is less than 6 weeks. In the U.K., two large studies found an association between maternity leaves shorter than 6 weeks and lower breastfeeding initiation rates (Hawkins, Griffiths, Dezateux, & Law, 2007b; Noble, 2001). A U.S. study had similar findings (Fein & Roe, 1998). Low-income mothers tend to return to work earlier than higher-income mothers and tend to have jobs less likely to accommodate breastfeeding (Lindberg, 1996).

Longer maternity leaves are associated with longer breastfeeding duration (Authur, Saenz, & Replogle, 2003; Hills-Bonczyk, 1993; Kearney & Cronenwett, 1991; Roe et al., 1999; Ryan, Zhou, & Arensberg, 2006; Visness & Kennedy, 1997). One study of 1550 U.S. women concluded that each week of maternity leave increased breastfeeding duration by nearly half a week (Roe et al., 1999).

Work Schedules and Settings

Suggest the mother look into flexible work-schedule options.

Although some women have little flexibility in their jobs, some may discover more options than they expect. The following are some possible flexible work arrangements to consider:

- Part-time—Working fewer hours per week
- Job-sharing—Sharing one position with another person (another mother?)
- Phase back—Gradually increasing work hours from part-time to full-time
- Flex-time—Adjusting work hours to baby's routine
- Compressed work week—Working the same hours in fewer days
- Telecommuting—Working from home
- On-site day care—Going to baby for feedings as needed

On average, mothers working part-time breastfeed longer than mothers working full-time.

According to the research described below, in general, women working part-time breastfeed for about the same length of time as women staying at home. But in one U.S. study, by 6 months after birth, 26% of mothers working full time were breastfeeding, as compared with nearly 37% of mothers working part-time and 35% of mothers not working (Ryan et al., 2006).

- In the U.K., mothers employed part-time or self-employed were more likely to breastfeed for at least 4 months as compared with those employed full-time (Hawkins, Griffiths, Dezateux, & Law, 2007a).
- In Australia, mothers returning to full-time work before 12 months were less likely to be fully breastfeeding at 6 months or breastfeeding at all at 12 months (Scott et al., 2006).

- In Taiwan, only about 11% of the women who returned to work for 8 to 12 hour days were breastfeeding at 3 months as compared with the national breastfeeding average of 17% at 3 months (Chen, Wu, & Chie, 2006). Longer work days and less flexible break times were associated with earlier weaning.
- In New Zealand, at 4 months, 39% of the mothers who returned to work full-time were breastfeeding as compared with 57% of the women who stayed home (McLeod, Pullon, & Cookson, 2002).
- In Singapore, at 6 months, only 20% of the mothers working full-time were breastfeeding as compared with 31% of the mothers at home (Ong et al., 2005).

One U.S. study noted—not surprisingly—that as daily work hours increase, number of breastfeedings decrease (Roe et al., 1999).

Ask the mother to describe her work setting.

Some work settings are more conducive to breastfeeding than others. One U.S. study found that mothers in administrative and manual jobs stopped breastfeeding earlier than average, while women in service jobs breastfed as long as mothers at home and those in professional jobs (Kimbro, 2006). Other jobs found to be especially challenging include military (Stevens & Janke, 2003), security guard (Dunn, Zavela, Cline, & Cost, 2004), jobs with 12-hour rotating shifts (Witters-Green, 2003), and physicians during residency (Authur et al., 2003; Miller, Miller, & Chism, 1996).

Type of job the mother has influences breastfeeding duration.

If a mother has an inflexible work schedule or setting, explore the possibility of "reverse cycle breastfeeding."

"Reverse cycle breastfeeding" is when most feedings take place while the mother is home and the baby takes his longest sleep stretch while mother is at work. The mother may schedule her work hours during her baby's naturally occurring longest sleep period. Or the baby may choose to change his feeding rhythm so that he is awake and feeding more often when mother is home. Some mothers have been able to make breastfeeding work with challenging work schedules or settings by using this approach. If the baby falls into this pattern naturally, or the mother schedules her work around her baby, it can take much of the pressure off the mother to express her milk. However, it may not be easy to change a baby's sleep patterns to achieve this.

Worksite Lactation Support

Worksite lactation support increases breastfeeding duration.

In its *Guide to Breastfeeding Interventions*, the U.S. Centers for Disease Control and Prevention lists worksite lactation support as one of the interventions proven effective at increasing breastfeeding duration (Shealy, 2005). In one U.S. study of 462 U.S. women who took part in a worksite lactation support program, 97.5% began breastfeeding after birth. At 6 months, 58% were breastfeeding at a time when the U.S. breastfeeding rate at 6 months was only 32% (Ortiz, McGilligan, & Kelly, 2004).

The basic elements of a worksite lactation program—support, time, education, and place—can be tailored to different workplaces in different ways.

Worksite lactation support includes a variety of possible options that can be basic or extensive, depending on a workplace's size, preferences, and resources. The U.S. government's toolkit, *The Business Case for Breastfeeding* (HRSA, 2008), describes the basic elements using the acronym STEP:

- **Support**—Company-wide awareness of the program's benefits and a positive attitude.
- **Time**—A maternity-leave policy and paid or unpaid breaks for breastfeeding or milk expression during the workday.
- **Education**—Information on breastfeeding and balancing breastfeeding with work demands.
- **Place**—A comfortable, private area to breastfeed or express milk.

The U.S. Breastfeeding Committee offers examples of various levels of worksite lactation support on its web site (www.usbreastfeeding.org). One article suggests offering employers a "menu" of options (Click, 2006).

When talking to her boss, encourage the mother to focus on the benefits to her employer of providing worksite lactation support.

Many mothers are reluctant to discuss lactation support at work. Some women worry that asking for a time and place to breastfeed or express their milk will be seen as requesting special favors. Some feel awkward because breastfeeding feels so personal, and they are concerned that it may be perceived as unprofessional to discuss it. Both the mother and her employer stand to gain, but most employers are unaware of the benefits to them (Dunn et al., 2004; Libbus & Bullock, 2002). If a mother has information about how breastfeeding will benefit her employer financially, she may feel more comfortable about discussing her needs.

When a mother breastfeeds, her employer benefits too.

The impact of breastfeeding on family health has a significant positive impact on an employer's bottom line. The U.S. government's toolkit, *The Business Case for Breastfeeding*, focuses on three main areas that result in significant cost savings for businesses (HRSA, 2008):

1. Breastfeeding employees miss less work.
2. Breastfeeding lowers healthcare costs.
3. Supporting breastfeeding in the workplace results in lower employee turnover rates and greater productivity and loyalty.

One U.S. study indicated that the more mother's milk babies received, the less likely they were to become ill and be excluded from child care (Jones & Matheny, 1993). Another U.S. study found that in the first year of life, the extra medical costs of formula-feeding average between $331 and $475 per never-breastfed baby (Ball & Wright, 1999).

Employee retention also saves businesses money. A New Zealand study estimated that for each employee who returned to work after maternity leave, the company saved $75,000 (EEOTrust, 2001). At this writing, the national U.S. average for employee retention after birth is 59%. In comparison, Mutual of Omaha's lactation program led to an 83% retention rate after birth. A U.S. study of several companies with lactation programs found an average retention rate of 94% (Ortiz et al., 2004).

In some areas, employers may be required by law to provide a time and place for breastfeeding or milk expression.

Before the mother talks to her boss, suggest she check her national and state or provincial laws. In the U.S., some state laws require giving breastfeeding employees a time and place to pump. See http://www.llli.org/Law/LawMain.html for listings of breastfeeding laws by state.

When discussing breastfeeding laws, however, encourage the mother to bring up this subject carefully, so her employer does not see it as a veiled threat. Most U.S. worksite breastfeeding laws carry no penalty if not followed. Suggest the mother keep the main focus on how her company will benefit. In some areas, "Breastfeeding Friendly Employer" awards are offered through local health departments, which may provide positive incentives for local employers.

In the U.S., more worksite lactation support programs are available in large companies, in healthcare workplaces, and to office workers.

According to a 2007 survey, 26% of U.S. businesses provide lactation support for at least some employees (SHRM, 2007). This survey found that mothers were more likely to find lactation support in large companies with 500 employees or more (42%), as compared with medium companies with 99 to 499 employees (26%) and small companies with 1-99 employees (9%). Mothers working in healthcare settings were more likely to have a worksite lactation program, as compared with mothers in retail, government, or in other settings.

Common barriers to worksite lactation support can often be overcome with creative thinking and an open mind.

Barriers to worksite lactation support, such as the following, can usually be overcome:

Time away from work duties. If there is a concern about the time spent expressing milk at work, explain that many women can express their milk during regular break and meal times. If this is not enough time, the mother can ask to make up for time needed by coming in early or leaving later. She can also emphasize that the need to express at work is temporary, as most mothers stop expressing by the time their babies are 12 months old (Slusser, Lange, Dickson, Hawkes, & Cohen, 2004).

Discomfort with breastfeeding. It may help to choose words carefully. For example, use the word "lactation" instead of "breastfeeding." Avoid promotional materials with photos of breasts or breastfeeding. Get permission from other women in the workplace to share their stories, so the employer can more clearly see the need.

Resistance from other employees. This can be avoided by including other employees in the planning process or by providing staff training. To create a greater sense of fairness, some companies offer breastfeeding education and equipment to the fathers working for the company, as well as the mothers (Cohen, Lange, & Slusser, 2002). Share the financial benefits to the company as a whole and any specifics that might be appropriate, such as that the lactation breaks will be no longer than employees' usual breaks and mealtimes.

Lack of available space. If a mother doesn't have a private office, the space needed to breastfeed or express milk can be as small as 4 feet by 5 feet (1.5 by 2 meters), such as a modified storage room. Suggest the mother brainstorm with her employer about existing areas that could be used. For example, rather than a separate room, a screen could be used in the manager's office to create a private area for breastfeeding or milk expression.

Even without an official worksite lactation program, companies can still offer benefits and services that support breastfeeding.

In one survey of 157 U.S. businesses, only 28% of businesses provided specific lactation support services, yet many offered benefits that promote breastfeeding, such as (Dunn et al., 2004):

- Maternity leave of 3 months or more (85%)
- Flex-time, job sharing, or part-time employment options (72%)
- Refrigerator for storage of mother's milk (71%)
- Breaks for expressing milk or breastfeeding (62%)

Togetherness and Separation

Some mothers bring their baby to work or go to their baby for feedings during their workday.

Some companies either allow the mother to keep the baby in her work area or provide on-site child care. In a survey of U.S. businesses, 43% of small companies allowed mothers to bring their babies to work in emergencies (SHRM, 2007). Another survey of 157 U.S. companies in Colorado reported that 9% of the companies provided on-site child care (Dunn et al., 2004). See the website http://www.partingatwork.org/ for sample schedules, policy templates, and affidavits from parents and employers.

Breastfeeding even once during the work day reduces the number of times women need to pump.

Even if her baby is not at her workplace, a mother may be able to go to her baby for some or all feedings by choosing a caregiver near work rather than home. Breastfeeding even once during her workday reduces the time spent expressing milk or the amount of other foods her baby needs. Choosing a caregiver near work rather than home also reduces a mother's travel time away from the baby, thereby reducing her need to express milk.

When a mother misses feedings at work, she needs to decide if she will provide her milk for some or all of the missed feedings.

If the mother decides against expressing when she misses feedings, her baby is younger than 12 months, and she is unable to express enough milk outside her work hours to meet her baby's need, suggest she check with her baby's healthcare provider about what other foods to provide while at work. For more details, see the next section.

CONSIDERING MILK EXPRESSION OPTIONS

To Express or Not

If mother and baby are separated during the workday, milk expression offers several advantages.

When the employed mother has a baby younger than 1 year, she may want to consider expressing milk during her workday to:

- Stay more comfortable and avoid leaking
- Decrease her risk of mastitis
- Maintain her milk production
- Avoid the cost and health risks of mother's milk substitutes

When a mother planning to work full-time away from her young baby will not be expressing milk at work, discuss other options.

Although it is rare, some mothers with a very large breast storage capacity (for details, see p. 399- "Breast Storage Capacity") may be able to comfortably go for an 8-hour workday without expressing milk. In other unusual cases, large-capacity mothers have been able to express enough milk at home to meet their baby's need for milk during their work hours (Berggren, 2006). Mothers of older babies on solid foods may also be able to get through a workday without expressing because their milk production is already reduced. But most exclusively breastfeeding mothers will find that before the workday is over, they may have painful breast fullness, which increases the risk of mastitis. Most mothers who regularly go 8 hours or more without expressing also experience a rapid reduction in milk production. Expressing milk even once during the workday significantly increases comfort and helps maintain milk production overall.

Most mothers will need to express at least once during an 8-hour workday.

Before discussing options, ask first if the mother's workday will be longer than her baby's longest stretch between feedings at home. If she is already going this length of time without a problem, she does not need to make any changes. But if her time at work will be much longer than her current longest stretch at home and she will not be either breastfeeding or expressing milk during her workday, she may want to consider a "partial weaning." This is a way to reduce her milk production gradually so that she can be away from her baby for long stretches without breast fullness or pain, yet still have some milk for breastfeeding when she returns home.

There are different approaches to a partial weaning. One involves first noting the usual breastfeeding times. Then about a week or two before returning to work suggest the mother pick one feeding during the hours she'll be working, avoiding the first morning feeding when she would likely feel full already. If she is exclusively breastfeeding, her baby is likely younger than 6 months, so suggest she talk to her baby's healthcare provider about what to feed the baby instead and feed this at the missed breastfeeding. Continue to feed this food at about the same time every day. After dropping a breastfeeding, suggest she give her body at least 2 to 3 days before dropping another feeding. If her breasts become full, suggest she express just enough milk to feel comfortable and no more. This will cause her milk production to slow gradually without pain or risk of mastitis. When her breasts do not feel full for the entire time she'll be at work, she is ready.

Another approach to a partial weaning is to continue offering the breast first at all feedings while she is with her baby and offer the supplements in between. When the baby regularly takes as much supplement as he would take during her workday, she is ready.

Expression Methods

Hand expression and breast pumps each have advantages and disadvantages.

For details, see the chapter, "Milk Expression and Storage."

If a mother asks for help in choosing a breast pump, ask her how many hours per week she and her baby will be apart.

For the mother who does a lot of pumping, choosing the right breast pump can make the difference between meeting or not meeting her breastfeeding goals. Although over the years, more effective pumps have become more available, there are still painful and ineffective pumps on store shelves, so mothers need to choose carefully. The best choice for a mother will depend on her means and her situation.

For a mother in the following situation, her breast pump may play a major role in maintaining milk production, so suggest she choose carefully:

It's important that mothers choose a pump that will help them meet their breastfeeding goals.

- Away from her baby 30 or more hours per week
- Baby younger than 6 months old
- Wants to provide only mother's milk for missed feedings

In this situation one important feature is how many cycles per minute (cpm) the pump can generate. In most cases the recommendation is an automatic double pump that generates 40 to 60 suction-and-release cycles per minute. A pump that can cycle in this range is generally considered to be most effective at keeping up milk production. Pump choices in this category include rental pumps and mother-owned automatic double pumps that offer a 1-year warranty on the motor. For more details, see p. 456-"Breast Pumps" in the chapter "Milk Expression and Storage" and p. 825 "Breast Pumps." A mother in the following situations may rely less on her breast pump for maintaining milk production:

- Away from her baby part-time, less than 30 hours per week
- Plans to provide other foods for missed feedings in addition to her milk, such as mother's milk substitutes and/or solid foods

In these situations, a less effective pump recommended for "occasional use" might suffice, such as an automatic pump that generates 30 to 35 cycles per minute or less. Some mothers also use semi-automatic pumps that require a mother to either generate or release pump suction by covering a hole or pushing a button or bar. For some mothers away from their babies part-time, manual pumps also work well. But many mothers tire of them quickly because they require muscle power to use. They also require practice to find the rhythm that triggers her milk ejection.

Most mothers find it takes 10 to 15 minutes per breast to express their milk. With a single pump, a mother can only express one breast at a time, which means it takes about 20 to 30 minutes to express both breasts. A double pump allows her to pump both breasts at the same time, which can cut her expression time in half. Some mothers have also learned to hand express their milk from both breasts simultaneously in the same amount of time it takes to double-pump.

Any mother with less than 20 minutes to express her milk should consider a double breast pump.

If the pump opening—or "nipple tunnel"—the breast is drawn into during pumping is too large or too small, this can result in pain, trauma, and less milk expressed. For details, see p. 826 in the appendix "Tools and Products."

Suggest any mother using a breast pump make sure she has a good pump fit.

Planning Ahead for Work

Before returning to work, suggest the mother ask if her workplace provides a lactation room and/or breast pumps for employees. If there is no specific area for expressing milk, suggest she ask about a private office, empty conference room, storage room, or lounge. Where space is tight, a privacy screen can create a private area. The mother's car or a restroom can be used as a last resort. Although many mothers have resorted to using a restroom, it is far from ideal (Brown, Poag, & Kasprzycki, 2001; Miller et al., 1996; Rojjanasrirat, 2004; Stevens & Janke, 2003; Thompson & Bell, 1997; Witters-Green, 2003).

The mother expressing milk at work will need a private place, and if using a pump, she may need an electrical outlet.

For the mother hand-expressing, privacy, a comfortable chair, and a milk collection container are all that's needed. If she is using a breast pump, suggest she ask if there's an electrical outlet available. If not, some quality breast pumps can be powered by rechargeable batteries.

Some workplaces—usually large companies—provide either multi-user rental pumps or mother-owned breast pumps either at a discount or free of charge (Ortiz et al., 2004). Most workplaces expect employees to provide their own pumps.

When calculating the time needed to express milk at work, the total time will depend in part on the expression method the mother is using.

The time a mother needs for milk expression at work will depend in part on her method.

- **One breast at a time.** Plan for each expression to take between 20 and 30 minutes, plus clean-up and travel to and from her private area.
- **Both breasts at once.** Plan for each expression to take at least 10 to 15 minutes, plus clean-up and travel to and from her private area.

To reduce clean-up time, one option is for the mother to buy enough extra pump parts for all her pumpings at work, which she can wash at home after work.

The number of times a mother needs to express during her workday to maintain her milk production depends upon several factors:

Many mothers can fit milk expression into their usual breaks and mealtimes.

- Whether or not her baby is exclusively breastfed
- The number of hours they are apart, including travel time
- Her breast storage capacity

As a starting point, to calculate how many times a mother of a fully mother's-milk-fed baby younger than 6 months should plan to express her milk at work, suggest she divide the number of hours by three that she and her baby will be apart, including travel time. For example:

- Apart 12 hours, 4 expressions (12 ÷ 3 = 4)
- Apart 9 hours, 3 expressions (9 ÷ 3 = 3)

After following this routine at work for a while, she can adjust as needed. For more details, see the following section, "Daily Routines and Milk Production."

Most mothers with young babies working full-time express milk two to three times per day and spend less than an hour total expressing milk.

A U.S. study of 283 mothers working full-time tracked how many times each day they expressed milk at work and the time they spent doing it (Slusser et al., 2004). When their babies were between 3 and 6 months old, the mothers expressed milk at work on average 2.2 times per day and 85% spent an hour or less on milk expression. By 6 months, the mothers expressed milk, on average, 1.9 times per day, with 95% spending an hour or less on expression at work.

Most mothers stop expressing milk by their baby's first birthday.

As a baby eats more solid foods, he needs less milk (Cohen, Brown, Canahuati, Rivera, & Dewey, 1994; Islam, Peerson, Ahmed, Dewey, & Brown, 2006). As a baby's need for milk decreases, so does the mother's need to express milk. Most babies 1 year or older can drink other milks from a cup. By that time, most mothers have stopped expressing milk at work, even though they may continue to breastfeed at home. In one U.S. study of 332 women working for five companies that participated in a corporate lactation plan, mothers stopped expressing milk at work when their babies were a mean age of 9 months (Ortiz et al., 2004). The age at which the largest number of mothers stopped expressing milk was 12 months.

Suggest the mother consider where to store her milk at work.

Depending on the room temperature at her worksite and the length of her workday, a mother may or may not need to cool her expressed milk. See p. 459-"Milk Storage Guidelines" in the chapter "Milk Expression and Storage" for milk storage times for different room temperature ranges. The season and her local climate will affect whether or not her milk needs to be cooled while she travels from work to home.

As long as the mother follows the milk storage guidelines, any milk she stores at room temperature can be refrigerated and/or frozen later.

If the mother needs to cool her milk, she has several options:

- Pump bag cooler compartment cooled with reusable freezer packs
- Separate cooler bag cooled with freezer packs
- A private or shared refrigerator

To avoid the risk of milk loss or contamination, many women prefer to store their milk in a private rather than shared space.

According to the U.S. Centers for Disease Control and Prevention (CDC, 1988) and the U.S. Occupational Safety and Health Administration (OSHA) (Clark, 1992), no special precautions, such as rubber gloves or separate storage, are required for handling mother's milk, either in the workplace or at child care facilities. Contact with mother's milk is not considered an occupational exposure. This means that simple hand washing and cleaning up of spills is all that's needed (Nommsen-Rivers, 1997).

Mother's milk is not a biohazardous material and no special precautions are needed at work or at child care facilities.

Stored breastmilk is not a biohazard.

PRIORITIES DURING MATERNITY LEAVE

Baby Time

Suggest the mother think of her weeks or months at home after birth as a time of closeness and togetherness. It is also a time to think about her breastfeeding goals and plan for the future. Many of the choices she makes during this time will lay the foundation for her time back at work.

During the early weeks at home, suggest the mother focus on breastfeeding long and often to ensure ample milk production later.

One of the most important things she can do while on leave is to breastfeed long and often. This will help set her milk production at the level she will need long-term. Every time a mother breastfeeds, the hormone prolactin is released. With every breastfeeding, the level of prolactin in her blood rises. More prolactin in the blood—especially during the first 2 weeks after birth—activates the prolactin receptors in the breast, and the more prolactin receptors activated during this critical period, the greater the potential milk production for that baby (De Carvalho, 1983). For more details, see p. 392- "Hormonal Levels and Receptors."

Some mothers think ahead to their time back at work and wonder if their baby would adapt to their work routine more easily if they mimicked their work schedule at home. If breastfeeding is going well, milk production is best set by the baby, so during maternity leave suggest the mother not limit breastfeeding to certain times or feed at predetermined intervals, as this can ultimately undermine her long-term breastfeeding goals.

Suggest the mother wait until she returns to work to adopt her work schedule.

Let her know that a baby's ability to adapt increases with age. Before birth, a baby receives constant nourishment through the umbilical cord. During the early weeks, the baby learns to adjust to intermittent feedings, and this period is less stressful for the baby (and the whole family) if he is fed on cue, which is recommended to set healthy milk production (Gartner et al., 2005).

Mothers differ in their storage capacity, the amount of milk their breasts can comfortably hold before feeling full (for details, see p. 399- "Breast Storage Capacity"). This individual difference affects the number of times per day a

In the week or two before going back to work, suggest the mother make note of how many times each day her baby breastfeeds.

mother needs to drain her breasts well to keep her milk production stable after she goes back to work. To get a sense of her storage capacity, within a week or so of going back to work, suggest she make note of how many times each 24-hour day her baby breastfeeds. This will give her a general idea of how many times she will need to express milk while back at work to keep her milk production steady. See the later section, "Keeping Milk Production Stable: The 'Magic Number'."

Milk Expression Logistics

When to Express

If possible, before returning to work, suggest the mother allow 3 or 4 weeks to practice milk expression and store some milk.

Expressing milk is a learned skill. Most mothers find—no matter what method they use—that with practice they can express more milk more easily. A breastfeeding mother's body is conditioned to release her milk to the feel of her baby at the breast. Expressing milk feels different than breastfeeding, so it can take some time for her body to respond to this new feel in the same way (Kent, Ramsay, Doherty, Larsson, & Hartmann, 2003). Giving herself a few weeks to get comfortable with her expression method will allow her to go through this "conditioning phase" at home rather than at work, where she will have a more intense need to express quickly and effectively.

Mothers should give themselves a few weeks to get used to milk expression.

Another advantage of starting to express about a month before returning to work is that it gives the mother time to store a reserve of milk. If a mother begins expressing after her milk production reaches its peak, around 5 weeks after birth (Hill, Aldag, Chatterton, & Zinaman, 2005), and she expresses milk every morning about an hour after a breastfeeding, after some practice she should expect to get about half a feeding at each expression. During her first few expressions, suggest she expect to get very little milk while her body adjusts to the new feel of her expression method. After expressing for 4 weeks, she should have about 14 full feedings frozen as a back-up by the time she goes back to work.

A reserve of frozen milk is an especially good idea for the mother employed full-time who plans to provide her milk exclusively for her young baby. The mother can plan to express enough milk each day at work to feed the baby the next day, but it is always good to have some extra milk as a hedge against the unexpected.

Different mothers have different comfort levels with the volume of milk they want to have stored before returning to work. Some mothers feel anxious if they have less than a full week's worth of feedings. Others are happy to go back with just enough milk to cover their first day.

• •

During maternity leave, there are several ways a mother can express and store milk without interfering with breastfeeding.

One way is to store whatever milk the mother expresses to keep herself comfortable during the early weeks. Many mothers feel the need to "express to comfort" when their breasts feel full and their baby is unwilling to breastfeed. "Expressing to comfort" means expressing just enough milk to relieve breast fullness without stimulating more milk production. Any milk expressed can be frozen and combined with other batches expressed later.

Another way to store milk during this time is to plan a daily milk expression.

To avoid upsetting or shortchanging the baby, suggest the mother try to allow at least an hour between an expression and the next breastfeeding. On average, babies only take about 67% of the milk in the breast, so there is usually milk left to express after a feeding (Kent, 2007). To get the most milk for her efforts, suggest the mother:

- Try expressing in the morning, as most women get more milk then.
- Pump 30 to 60 minutes after a breastfeeding and at least an hour before the next breastfeeding.

To build a supply of stored breastmilk, mother can plan a daily milk expression before they return to work.

If the baby wants to breastfeed right after an expression, suggest the mother go ahead. Most babies are patient and do not mind feeding longer to get the milk they need. The mother can encourage the baby to go back and forth from breast to breast several times until done. Remind the mother that milk production is continuous, so even if only a few minutes have passed since she finished expressing, there will be some milk there for the baby. As Kerstin Berggren, author of *Working Without Weaning,* tells mothers: "The breasts are never empty. They are constantly replenishing" (K. Berggren, personal communication, January 19, 2010).

Another option is to express milk from one breast while the baby breastfeeds on the other breast. This works especially well for babies who prefer to take just one breast at a feeding.

• •

For a mother returning to work within the first few weeks after birth, more intense milk expression may make it possible for her to breastfeed longer.

The recommendation to delay regular milk expression after birth is geared to mothers who take at least a 6-week maternity leave. Mothers who return to work within 5 weeks of giving birth, however, will not have time to establish full milk production by breastfeeding alone (Hill et al., 2005). In the U.S., some low-income women go back to work as early as 2 weeks after birth (Chamberlain et al, 2006).

Encourage any mother in this situation to either make arrangements to express milk intensively when back at work (so that she is draining her breasts well at least 8 to 10 times total each day, including the times she breastfeeds the baby) or while on maternity leave use frequent milk expression in addition to breastfeeding to try to achieve full milk production before she returns to work. Mothers who express milk for their preterm babies are encouraged to reach full milk production (at least 25 oz. or 750 mL per day) by Day 10 to 14 postpartum at the latest. A mother who will be separated from her baby full time before about 5 weeks postpartum (the time it takes, on average, for a baby to establish full milk production by breastfeeding alone) may benefit from boosting her milk production with regular milk expression during her maternity leave before returning to work.

Storing Milk

How much milk a mother expresses each time during her baby's first month will depend in part on her baby's age and other factors.

On a baby's first day of life, on average, a mother produces about 1 ounce (30 mL) of colostrum, the first milk. When breastfeeding goes well, by the time her baby is about 40 days old, she will reach her peak production of, on average, 25 to 35 ounces (739 to 1030 mL) of milk (Hill et al., 2005). Milk production increases dramatically during the first weeks, making more milk available for expression over time. Once it reaches its peak at about 5 weeks, milk production stays relatively stable until about 6 months. Table 1 illustrates the increase in milk intake at feedings during baby's first month.

Table 15.1. Average Milk Intake by Age

Baby's Age	Ave. Milk Per/Feeding	Ave. Milk Per Day
First week	1-2 oz. (30-590 mL)	10-20 oz. (296-591 mL) (after Day 4)
Weeks 2 and 3	2-3 oz. (59-89 mL)	15-25 oz. (443-739 mL)
Months 1 to 6	3-5 oz. (89-147 mL)	25-35 oz. (739-1030 mL)

(Kent et al., 2006)

How much milk is expressed will also depend on whether the baby is exclusively breastfed (or if not, how much other milk or solids he receives each day), how much time has passed since the last breast draining, the time of day, the mother's emotional state, and other factors.

Pump quality, flange fit, and practice with a pump can affect how much milk is expressed. See the previous section "Expression Options" for details on pump choices and p. 825 in the appendix "Tools and Products." As described, the amount of practice a mother has expressing milk also affects her milk yield. Because milk ejection, or let-down, is partly a conditioned response, practice with a pump can help a mother's body learn to respond to its feel with more milk ejections, which results in more milk (Kent et al., 2008; Kent et al., 2003). For more details, see p. 446- "How Much Milk to Expect."

Mothers can combine milk expressed at different times, as long as the milk storage guidelines are followed.

At first a mother may express only a little milk, which she can add to other stored milk. If she combines milk from different days, suggest she label the container with the date of the oldest milk. She can add fresh milk to cooled milk. She can add fresh milk to frozen milk if it is cooled first and the amount added is less than that frozen. For more complete details, see p. 464- "Handling and Preparing Milk."

To avoid waste, suggest the mother store no more milk in a container than her baby will take at one feeding.

At this writing, milk storage recommendations say that after milk has been warmed and fed, any milk left should be discarded (Jones & Tully, 2006; Tully, 2005). Average milk intake at a breastfeeding is 3 to 4 ounces (88 to 118 mL), but every baby is different. One Australian study found the amount of milk 1- to 6-month-old babies took at a breastfeeding ranged from very little to about 8 ounces (236 mL) (Kent et al., 2006). Before she knows how much expressed milk her baby will take, suggest she also store some 1- to 2-ounce (30 to 59 mL) containers in case the baby wants a little more. More milk can always be added to the feeding, but leftover milk should not be saved. Smaller volumes also have the advantage of warming faster.

How Much Milk Baby Will Need

The mother can calculate how much milk her baby should need while she's at work based on how many hours they're apart.

One of the many plans a mother returning to work needs to make is how much milk to leave for her baby each day. On average, breastfeeding babies take about 25 ounces (750 mL) of milk each day (24-hour period), but babies differ. Among babies growing normally, there is a large range of daily milk intake, from 15 to 41 ounces (440 to 1220 mL) per day (Kent, 2007; Kent et al., 2006).

To help a mother calculate the amount of milk her baby will need while she's at work, add a little extra milk to account for big eaters and use 30 ounces (887 mL) per 24 hours as a benchmark. Then divide this amount by the portion of the day she and her baby are apart. For example:

Most babies of mothers working full time will need 10 to 15 ounces a day.

- **6 hours apart** (one-quarter of a 24-hour day) one-quarter of 30 ounces (887 mL) is 7.5 ounces (252 mL)
- **8 hours apart** (one-third of a 24-hour day) one-third of 30 ounces (887 mL) is 10 ounces (296 mL)
- **12 hours apart** (half of a 24-hour day) half of 30 ounces (887 mL) is 15 ounces (444 mL)

Most mothers working full-time are away from their babies for 8 to 12 hours per day, so most of these babies will need between 10 and 15 ounces (296 to 739 mL) of milk. This assumes that the mother breastfeeds often during the hours she and her baby are together. If the mother breastfeeds very little while at home or if her baby sleeps for very long stretches at night without breastfeeding, her baby will need more milk while she's at work.

• •

It may set a mother's mind at ease to know that her baby will need about the same amount of milk per day at 5 weeks as he will at 6 months.

Mothers often worry that as their babies grow bigger and heavier they will need more and more milk per day to meet their growing needs, which may feel like an impossible dilemma. Reassure the mother that while babies fed formula do take more and more milk over the months, this is not true for breastfeeding babies (Kent et al., 2006).

When breastfeeding is going well, baby's daily milk intake reaches its peak at about 5 weeks postpartum (Hill et al., 2005) and stays fairly stable until the baby starts taking other foods, ideally at about 6 months (Butte, Garza, Smith, & Nichols, 1984; Kent et al., 2006; Neville et al., 1988). So when a mother with full milk production returns to work, all she needs to do is keep it stable because as a baby gets older his rate of growth slows. Research has found that at 6 months, breastfeeding babies take, on average, 22% less milk per day than babies who are fed only formula (Heinig, Nommsen, Peerson, Lonnerdal, & Dewey, 1993). So if her baby is thriving at 5 weeks, about this level of milk production should meet her baby's needs for the duration. Knowing this can be immensely reassuring.

Sometimes as babies begin sleeping longer at night, it will appear that they need more milk, but it is only because they are taking more milk during their waking hours to make up for the missed night feedings. If an employed mother keeps her baby close at night, this will encourage night feeding, which reduces the amount of milk she needs to express during her workday.

Introducing a Bottle

If a mother is planning for her baby to feed by bottle while she's at work, suggest she wait until her baby is at least 3 to 4 weeks old to try bottle feeding.

It is not necessary for a mother to introduce the bottle while she is on maternity leave. She can delay bottles until she returns to work and have the caregiver introduce them then. But many mothers find that it sets their mind at ease to introduce the bottle earlier. If so, suggest she plan to wait to start bottles until her baby has been breastfeeding well for at least 3 to 4 weeks, to reduce the chance that giving the bottle may negatively impact breastfeeding.

Many parents are told to start the bottle as early as possible to "get the baby used to it." Some are warned not to wait too long or the baby won't take it. Research does not support these points of view. One U.S. study of 120 mothers and babies (Kearney & Cronenwett, 1991) found that most babies take the bottle easily whether started at 1 month, 2 months, or 3 to 6 months (Table 15.2).

Table 15.2. Infant Age and Acceptance of First Bottle

Age at first bottle-feeding	N	Refused Bottle (%)	Resisted (%)	Took Easily (%)
1 month	57	4	26	70
2 months	16	12	25	63
3-6 months	47	13	15	72

(Kearney & Cronenwett, 1991)

Suggest the mother try different types of bottle nipples/teats and choose a slow-flow nipple her baby accepts.

Adults are encouraged to eat slowly to activate our "appetite control mechanism," so that we feel full with less food. The same dynamic is true for babies. A baby is more likely to take more milk with a fast-flow bottle, which can lead to overfeeding (Li, Fein, & Grummer-Strawn, 2008; Taveras et al., 2006). A baby using a slow-flow nipple/teat is more likely to feel full on less milk, minimizing the milk the mother needs to provide while she's away.

Because babies have mouths with different shapes, one type of bottle and nipple will not be the best choice for all babies. Suggest the mother buy several types and styles and see which her baby prefers. For more details, see p. 819- "Feeding Bottles."

Suggest the mother plan for someone else, such as the caregiver, to introduce the bottle.

In many cases, the best person to introduce the bottle is the person who will be caring for the baby while the mother is at work, since the bottle will be a part of their relationship. This may go more smoothly if the caregiver has the chance to have a few visits and get to know the baby first.

If a baby is reluctant to take a bottle, there are many strategies to try and, if needed, other ways to feed the baby.

The following strategies may help a reluctant baby accept a bottle. Suggest the mother have the caregiver experiment to see what works best.

- **Have someone other than mother offer the bottle.** Most babies will not accept a bottle from mother or from someone else if mother is within earshot or even in the building because they know they could be breastfeeding.

- **Offer the bottle before baby is too hungry.** Babies tend to accept something new more easily if they are feeling calm rather than ravenous.
- **Offer short trials with the bottle at first**. If the baby resists, don't keep at it until baby is screaming. Let the baby play with it and put it away if the baby begins to seem unhappy.
- **Try different feeding positions**. Many babies like to be snuggled close when given a bottle, but some babies will not take a bottle when held in their usual breastfeeding position. Try instead to hold baby facing forward, with his back against the caregiver's chest or propped on raised legs, or try the bottle when baby is sitting in an infant seat.
- **Wrap the baby in mother's nightgown** or other clothing with the mother's smell on it while offering the bottle.
- **Warm the bottle nipple/teat to body temperature** by running warm water over it before offering it, or try dipping it in warm mother's milk. If baby is teething, try a nipple that has been chilled in the refrigerator.
- **Tap baby's lips with the bottle nipple**, wait until baby opens, and allow baby to draw the nipple into his mouth rather than pushing it in.
- **Move rhythmically when offering the bottle** to calm baby by walking, rocking, or swaying.
- **Experiment with different types of bottles and nipples**: Bottle nipples come in different materials and different shapes. Try different kinds until the baby finds one with which he is comfortable.
- **Try offering the bottle while baby is half-asleep.**
- **If baby is older, give him a bottle to play with** for a few days before attempting feeding.
- **Give some milk by spoon first** and then offer the bottle, or let baby suck on a finger and slip in the bottle along the side as he sucks.

There are a number of strategies mothers can try to help babies take a bottle when they need to be apart.

If none of these suggestions work, babies can be fed other ways, with a cup, spoon, or eyedropper.

• •

To help prevent the baby from preferring the bottle, limit bottles given by the baby's mother.

Babies can understand that their mother feeds them from the breast, while others feed them in other ways. One way to help keep a baby interested in breastfeeding is for the mother to restrict bottle-feeding to others and only breastfeed when she is with the baby.

• •

If a baby takes more from a bottle than a mother expressed for a missed breastfeeding, this does not necessarily mean the mother's milk production is low.

If a mother is concerned because her baby takes more from the bottle than she can express at one sitting, explain that this is likely due to the different flow rates of breast and bottle. The bottle flows consistently, but during breastfeeding there is an ebb and flow of milk as milk ejections occur. Due to this natural ebb and flow, a breastfeeding baby may feel full on less milk, whereas the faster, more consistent flow of the bottle may override a baby's "appetite control mechanism" and cause overfeeding (Li et al., 2008; Taveras et al., 2006). Taking more milk from the bottle than the mother expresses is not a reliable indicator of low milk production. Rather, it is more likely a reflection of these differences in feeding methods.

RETURNING TO WORK

Easing the Transition

It may make the transition back to work easier if the mother plans to work fewer days and/or fewer hours, even if only for a short time.

To make her first week back at work easier and less stressful, suggest the mother consider starting back to work near the end of her work week, such as on a Thursday or Friday, working shorter hours, or starting back to work part-time. These gradual ways to return to her work schedule may make the transition easier for both her and her baby.

Suggest the mother plan her work wardrobe with her need to breastfeed or express milk in mind.

The following wardrobe suggestions may make it easier to breastfeed or express milk at work:

- Have breast pads on hand and an extra top available in case of milk leakage.
- Wear two-piece outfits, so she can express or breastfeed without having to fully undress.
- Wear patterned tops rather than solid colors to better camouflage leaks or spilled milk.
- Have a jacket or sweater handy for use as a cover-up if needed.

It may help motivate the mother to accept help if she knows that breastfeeding is at greatest risk during the first 2 months back at work.

According to one U.S. study, during the first 2 months back at work, mothers are 2.2 times more likely to stop breastfeeding than mothers not yet back at work (Kimbro, 2006). If after returning to work she continues breastfeeding for 2 more months, her odds of continuing are about the same as a mother at home. Knowing this may motivate a mother to proactively take steps to reduce her stress during the first months at work.

Returning to work is a major adjustment for many mothers.

In one U.S. study, some of the many adjustments are described by mothers who returned to work on average 11 weeks after giving birth (Nichols & Roux, 2004). These mothers:

- Found it difficult to leave their babies.
- Had conflicting demands on their time and energy.
- Felt overloaded with work-family strains.
- Had challenges with child care and financial demands.
- Were sleep deprived and experienced mood changes.

Although the negatives outweighed the positives, the positives the mothers reported included learning to ask for and receive help, their enjoyment of motherhood, the realignment of their priorities and lifestyle to better reflect their new family dynamics, and the satisfaction they derived from their work.

There is no substitute for being in contact with other mothers who have been there. Mothers report that breastfeeding is easier with support and information. Some mothers find coworkers an important source of ongoing support (Rojjanasrirat, 2004).

Encourage the mother to seek support from other experienced working-and-breastfeeding mothers.

If there are no experienced breastfeeding mothers at work, suggest she get in touch with her local breastfeeding support groups. One U.S. study found that employed mothers who attended a breastfeeding support meeting within the first 6 weeks postpartum were three times more likely to breastfeed longer than 6 months and meet their own breastfeeding goals, as compared with mothers who didn't attend a meeting (Chezem & Friesen, 1999). Another U.S. study found that attending a worksite breastfeeding support group at a U.S. public health clinic was one of four significant predictors of breastfeeding duration for a group of mostly Latina mothers (Whaley, Meehan, Lange, Slusser, & Jenks, 2002).

Strategies to Minimize Milk Needed and Avoid Waste

How a mother plans her daily routine can affect how much milk she needs to express at work.

The following strategies can help keep expression to a minimum:

- **Plan to breastfeed at least twice before leaving the baby with the caregiver**: once when she awakens and again at the caregiver's when she drops her baby off before work.
- **Breastfeed as soon as she arrives at the caregiver's after work**. If her baby seems hungry just before she arrives, suggest the caregiver feed as little milk as possible, so the baby will want to breastfeed when she gets there.
- **Breastfeed often at home and continue breastfeeding at night**. As mentioned earlier, the baby needs a set amount of milk per 24-hour day. The less milk the baby takes at the breast while they're at home, the more milk he will need while the mother is at work.
- **Choose a caregiver close to work rather than home to cut down on travel time** and therefore time apart.

Depending on the length of a mother's workday, the first three strategies can cut the volume of milk needed significantly.

The amount of milk stored and the nipple/teat flow can affect how much milk is discarded and how much her baby needs to feel full.

To minimize the volume of milk the mother needs to express at work, suggest she:

- **Store her milk in the smallest amounts her baby will take**. The average breastfeeding is 3 to 4 ounces (88 to 118 mL), but every baby is different. Once she's back at work and knows how much her baby usually takes at a feeding, she will know how much milk to store. Suggest she also store some 1- to 2-ounce (30 to 59 mL) batches to avoid waste in case the baby wants just a little more.
- **Choose a slow-flow nipple** if her baby is fed by bottle. This allows the baby's "appetite control mechanism" to be triggered earlier, so the baby feels full on less milk. Nipple/teat package information is not always an accurate indicator of flow. Suggest the mother experiment with several brands by turning the bottle upside down and observing the rate of milk flow.

Keeping Milk Production Stable: The 'Magic Number'

One way to keep milk production stable over time is to maintain the same number of breast drainings per day (the "magic number").

To keep her milk production stable over the long term, suggest the mother continue to drain her breasts the same number of times per day after she goes back to work as she did while she was at home. Tell her to think of this as her "magic number." A mother's breast storage capacity will affect how many breast drainings per day she needs to keep milk production steady. Drained breasts make milk faster and full breasts make milk slower, and it takes more milk for large-capacity women to feel full. Many large-capacity women maintain their milk production on fewer breast drainings per day and express more milk at each session than other mothers. Small-capacity women feel full faster and must drain their breasts more times to get the same amount of milk. Both types of women can make plenty of milk for their babies overall, but their "magic number" can vary greatly.

Over time and as baby grows, many mothers in Western cultures gradually breastfeed fewer and fewer times each day. When the total number of daily breast drainings (breastfeedings plus milk expressions) drops below an individual mother's threshold (determined in large part by her breast storage capacity), her body will send the signal to reduce milk production (Daly, Kent, Owens, & Hartmann, 1996; Kent, 2007). For more details, see p. 399- "Breast Storage Capacity."

A woman's magic number is the number of times she needs to drain her breasts in order to maintain her milk production.

Once back at work, suggest that at least once per week the mother make note of how many times each day she drains her breasts. As babies begin sleeping longer at night, this "magic number" can decrease. Also Western mothers are often encouraged to follow bottle-feeding norms and encourage their babies to take larger and less frequent feedings. However, this is counter to breastfeeding norms (Kent et al., 2006).

It is not unusual for a mother to keep her number of milk expressions at work steady, but over time breastfeed fewer and fewer times per day at home. When a mother reports a decrease in milk production, be sure to ask her about her 24-hour total, breastfeedings at home, as well as milk expressions at work. Ask her how her "magic number" now compares to what it was when she was on maternity leave and breastfeeding. Increasing her number of daily breast drainings is often all that's needed to boost decreasing milk production.

To keep her milk production stable over the long term, suggest the mother limit her longest stretch without draining her breasts to 8 hours or less.

Because drained breasts make milk faster and full breasts make milk slower, long stretches between breastfeedings at night can slow a mother's milk production. When a mother is having milk production issues, ask her the length of her longest stretch. To avoid giving her body the message to slow milk production, suggest she try to avoid going more than 8 hours without either breastfeeding or expressing her milk. For example, if her baby sleeps 10 to 12 hours at night, to keep her milk production stable, she may need to either wake the baby to breastfeed or express her milk. For some small-capacity mothers, even 8 hours may be long enough to cause a decrease in milk production. For more details, see p. 399- "Breast Storage Capacity."

If a mother travels without her baby, suggest she use her "magic number" to determine the daily number of milk expressions needed. While on the road, she can either freeze her milk or discard it. If she's using a breast pump, suggest she make sure she has extra pump parts with her and, if needed, extra batteries. Mothers have come up with many creative solutions for storing their milk while traveling. Some find ways to freeze the milk and ship it back home on dry ice. If the trip is less than week, she can keep the milk refrigerated and carry it back in a cooler pack. For air travel in the U.S., the Transportation Security Administration (TSA) allows mothers to carry an unlimited volume of mother's milk, even if she is traveling without her baby.

If a mother's job requires travel, she can keep her milk production steady by using her "magic number" as her guide.

Mothers can maintain their milk production even while traveling on business.

Because solid foods take the place of mother's milk in a baby's diet (Cohen et al., 1994; Islam et al., 2006), as baby takes more solids, he takes less mother's milk. This is a normal part of breastfeeding, and a mother's production naturally adjusts downward as her baby takes more other foods and less milk. This is important to keep in mind when mothers report that they are expressing less milk at work than they did before. If the baby has started solid foods, this may be a normal change, and it may not be necessary for the mother to increase her milk production.

When a breastfed baby starts eating solid foods, milk production usually decreases.

Problem-Solving

When a mother says, "My baby is taking more milk than I express at work" or "I used to express more milk at work, but now I'm expressing less," don't assume that her milk production is the problem. First rule out other possibilities. To get to the root of the issue, ask her:

If a mother expresses less milk than her baby takes when they are apart or she expresses less milk than she used to, get more information before offering suggestions.

- The baby's age and how long she has been back at work.
- Is the baby fully mother's milk fed? If not, how much and what other foods does baby take?
- What is their total time apart, including travel time?
- How much milk (and any other foods) does baby take while mother is at work?
- What is the daily routine, including all breastfeedings, expressions, and other feedings?
- What was her "magic number" while on maternity leave and now?
- What is the longest stretch between breast drainings (usually at night)?

Example 1: Mother is expressing less milk at work than her baby takes.

Baby girl - 10 weeks old. Mother returned to work 2 weeks ago. Mother and baby are apart 8 hours per day 5 days a week. Baby is fully mother's milk fed and is taking 20 ounces (591 mL) per day from caregiver. "Magic number" during maternity leave: 8; now: 5. Daily routine:

- One breastfeeding at home in the morning
- Two milk expressions at work (expressing 12 ounces [355 mL] total)

- Two breastfeedings at home in the evening
- Baby sleeps 8 hours at night, the longest stretch

Baby is fed four 5-ounce (147 mL) bottles by the caregiver

- One bottle fed at arrival
- Two more bottles fed over the course of the day
- One more bottle fed just before mother arrives to take baby home

Conclusions: The mother is expressing the expected amount of milk. Eight hours apart is one-third of a 24-hour day. Using 30 ounces (887 mL) per day as a benchmark, she should expect to express about one-third of this or about 10 ounces (296 mL). She is expressing 12 ounces (355 mL).

She has two issues: her daily routine and her "magic number." Two simple changes in daily routine could reduce the amount of expressed milk she needs each day by half, from 20 ounces (592 mL) to 10 ounces (296 mL):

1. Instead of feeding the baby a bottle of expressed milk upon arrival at the caregiver's, she could breastfeed before leaving baby.
2. Before picking up the baby at the end of the day, she could ask the caregiver to hold off her baby with very little milk, and then breastfeed when she arrives.

Although her rate of milk production has not yet decreased, she has only been back at work for 2 weeks. She is at risk of slowed milk production, since her "magic number" has recently fallen from eight to five. Depending on her storage capacity, this may or may not be an issue for her. Make the mother aware of this so that she knows what adjustments to make to increase her rate of milk production if needed.

Example 2—Mother is expressing less milk at work than she did 2 months ago.

Baby boy - 8 months old. Mother returned to work 5 months ago. Mother and baby are apart 9 hours per day 5 days a week. Baby was fully mother's milk fed until 2 months ago, now is taking solid foods and 9 ounces (266 mL) of mother's milk per day from the caregiver. Mother used to express 12 ounces (355 mL) per day at work and now is able to express only 9 ounces (266 mL). "Magic number" during maternity leave was 8 and is now: 8. Her daily routine is:

- Two breastfeedings in the morning, one at home and one before mother leaves the caregiver's
- Three milk expressions at work (expressing 9 ounces (266 mL) total, which used to be 12 ounces (355 mL)
- Three breastfeedings at home in the evening
- Baby sleeps 8 hours at night, the longest stretch

Baby is fed two 4.5 ounce (134 mL) bottles by the caregiver.

- Mother breastfeeds when she leaves baby with caregiver
- Baby receives two bottles fed over the course of the day
- Mother feeds baby as soon as she arrives

Conclusions: Most likely the drop in milk expression from 12 ounces (355 mL) to 9 ounces (266 mL) is due to the baby's increasing intake of solid foods, which is replacing three ounces of milk each day. A gradually decreasing milk production as baby takes more and more solid foods is normal and expected. Reassure the mother that since she is keeping up with her baby's need for milk, there is no reason for her to try to increase her milk production.

• •

There are several reasons why a baby may take more milk than expected from the caregiver.

When a baby takes much more milk from the caregiver than expected, it can add tremendous stress to a mother's life. To determine the reason, do some detective work to see if changes can be made. When mothers are away from their babies between 8 and 12 hours, babies usually take, on average, 10 to 15 ounces (296 to 444 mL). Even so, every baby is different and the range of normal milk intake in healthy, thriving babies is large, from 15 to 41 ounces (440 to 1220 mL) per day (Kent, 2007; Kent, Mitoulas, Cox, Owens, & Hartmann, 1999; Kent et al., 2006).

Ask the mother what type of bottle nipple the caregiver uses to feed her baby. A fast-flow nipple can contribute to overfeeding. Some brands of nipples flow faster than others, so suggest the mother try a different brand.

Some caregivers use food as a way to keep babies content. No matter what the reason, one symptom of overfeeding is disinterest in breastfeeding later at home (Berggren, 2006). If a baby is growing and gaining well, but is breastfeeding very little at home, this may be one reason.

Another question to ask is how much milk the caregiver is discarding during the mother's workday. If there is much more milk in the bottle than the baby takes, this can be another contributing factor. Storing milk in smaller quantities may make a big difference.

• •

If a mother's milk production is low, try to find out why so that strategies to boost milk production address the root cause.

Be sure to consider:

- Her peak milk production—Has she ever fully breastfed? If not, she may not yet have reached full milk production.
- Her "magic number"—Has it dropped?
- Her longest stretch between breast drainings—Is it longer than 8 hours?
- Her method of milk expression—Has she ever been able to express the expected amount of milk? If so, consider pump fit and other strategies for improving the effectiveness of her method. (For details, see the chapter, "Milk Expression and Storage" and the appendix "Tools and Products.") If not, would she consider trying another method?

Example: Mother is expressing half of what her baby needs while they're apart.

Baby boy - 6 months old. Mother returned to work 4 months ago. Mother and baby are apart 8 hours per day 5 days a week. Baby is mostly mother's milk fed. Some formula supplements have been needed off and on. Mother expresses 6 ounces (180 mL) at work total. Baby needs 12 ounces (355 mL) per day. Mother has used galactogogues (milk-enhancing substances) to bring up rate of milk production, but every time she stops taking them, her milk production slows again. Mother wants her baby to be exclusively mother's milk fed. "Magic number" during maternity leave: 8 to 10; now: 5. Her daily routine:

- One breastfeeding at home before work
- Two milk expressions at work (expressing 6 ounces [177 ml] total)
- Two breastfeedings at home in the evening
- Baby began sleeping 10 to 12 hours at night—the longest stretch—at about 2 months of age.

Baby's is fed three 4-oz. (147 mL) bottles while with the caregiver.

Conclusions: The combination of the 10- to 12-hour sleep stretch at night and the drop in the "magic number" from 9 to 5 most likely explain this mother's difficulty in maintaining her milk production. She said that when her baby started sleeping so long at night, at first she got up to express her milk once during the night and that helped her store enough milk for her workday. She started dropping daily breastfeedings when her friends told her that a baby that age did not need so many feedings each day. After a better understanding of the dynamics working against her, this mother decided to breastfeed more at home and to get up once during the night to express her milk.

When a mother needs to increase her rate of milk production, be prepared to offer several approaches for her to consider and encourage her to act quickly.

Because mothers are different, one approach to increasing milk production will not appeal to all mothers. See p. 413 in the chapter, "Making Milk" for a range of strategies to suggest. Also, when a mother's milk production slows, the sooner she works to increase it, the more quickly she is likely to see results. The longer a mother waits, the more difficult it can be to boost milk production.

RESOURCES FOR PARENTS

Books

Berggren, K. (2006). *Working without weaning.* Amarillo TX: Hale Publishing.

Hicks, J. (2006). *Hirkani's daughters.* Schaumburg, IL: La Leche League International.

Pryor, G. & Huggins, K. (2007). *Nursing mother, working mother.* Boston: Harvard Commons Press.

Websites

http://www.usbreastfeeding.org/Publications.html

http://www.llli.org/NB/NBworking.html

http://www.workandpump.com/

http://www.kellymom.com/bf/pumping/bf-links-pumping.html

www.breastfeedingmadesimple.com

http://www.breastfeeding.asn.au/bfinfo/index.html

Maternity leaves and protection by country:

http://www.waba.org.my/whatwedo/womenandwork/pdf/
MaternityProtectionChart21May2006.pdf

U.S. worksite lactation laws:

http://www.llli.org/Law/LawBills.html

REFERENCES

Authur, C. R., Saenz, R.B., & Replogle, W.H. (2003). The employment-related breastfeeding decisions of physiican mothers. *Journal of the Mississippi State Medical Association, 44*, 383-387.

Ball, T. M., & Wright, A. L. (1999). Health care costs of formula-feeding in the first year of life. *Pediatrics, 103*(4 Pt 2), 870-876.

Berggren, K. (2006). *Working without weaning: A working mother's guide to breastfeeding*. Amarillo TX: Hale Publishing.

Brown, C. A., Poag, S., & Kasprzycki, C. (2001). Exploring large employers' and small employers' knowledge, attitudes, and practices on breastfeeding support in the workplace. *Journal of Human Lactation, 17*(1), 39-46.

Butte, N. F., Garza, C., Smith, E. O., & Nichols, B. L. (1984). Human milk intake and growth in exclusively breast-fed infants. *Journal of Pediatrics, 104*(2), 187-195.

Calnen, G. (2007). Paid maternity leave and its impact on breastfeeding in the United States: an historic, economic, political, and social perspective. *Breastfeeding Medicine, 2*(1), 34-44.

CDC. (1988). Perspectives in disease prevention and health promotion update: universal precautions for prevention of transmission of human immunodeficiency virus, hepatitis B virus, and other bloodborne pathogens in health-care settings. *MMWR, 37*(24), 377-388.

Chamberlain, L. B., McMahon, M., Philipp, B. L., & Merewood, A. (2006). Breast pump access in the inner city: a hospital-based initiative to provide breast pumps for low-income women. *Journal of Human Lactation, 22*(1), 94-98.

Chen, Y. C., Wu, Y. C., & Chie, W. C. (2006). Effects of work-related factors on the breastfeeding behavior of working mothers in a Taiwanese semiconductor manufacturer: a cross-sectional survey. *BMC Public Health, 6*, 160.

Chezem, J., & Friesen, C. (1999). Attendance at breast-feeding support meetings: relationship to demographic characteristics and duration of lactation in women planning postpartum employment. *Journal of the American Dietetic Association, 99*(1), 83-85.

Clark, R. A. (1992). Breast milk does not constitute occupational exposure as defined by standard. Washington, DC: Occupational Safety and Health Administration.

Click, E. R. (2006). Developing a worksite lactation program. *MCN; American Journal of Maternal Child Nursing, 31*(5), 313-317.

Cohen, R., Lange, L., & Slusser, W. (2002). A description of a male-focused breastfeeding promotion corporate lactation program. *Journal of Human Lactation, 18*(1), 61-65.

Cohen, R. J., Brown, K. H., Canahuati, J., Rivera, L. L., & Dewey, K. G. (1994). Effects of age of introduction of complementary foods on infant breast milk intake, total energy intake, and growth: a randomised intervention study in Honduras. *Lancet, 344*(8918), 288-293.

Daly, S. E., Kent, J. C., Owens, R. A., & Hartmann, P. E. (1996). Frequency and degree of milk removal and the short-term control of human milk synthesis. *Experimental Physiology, 81*(5), 861-875.

De Carvalho, M. (1983). Effect of frequent breast feeding on early milk production and infant weight gain. *Pediatrics, 72*, 307-311.

Dunn, B. F., Zavela, K. J., Cline, A. D., & Cost, P. A. (2004). Breastfeeding practices in Colorado businesses. *Journal of Human Lactation, 20*(2), 170-177.

EEOTrust. (2001). *New Zealand's best employers in work and life*. Retrieved February 19, 2010, from http://www.eeotrust.org.nz/content/docs/breastfeeding_sheets.pdf.

Fein, S. B., & Roe, B. (1998). The effect of work status on initiation and duration of breast-feeding. *American Journal of Public Health, 88*(7), 1042-1046.

Gartner, L. M., Morton, J., Lawrence, R. A., Naylor, A. J., O'Hare, D., Schanler, R. J., et al. (2005). Breastfeeding and the use of human milk. *Pediatrics, 115*(2), 496-506.

Gielen, A. C., Faden, R. R., O'Campo, P., Brown, C. H., & Paige, D. M. (1991). Maternal employment during the early postpartum period: effects on initiation and continuation of breast-feeding. *Pediatrics, 87*(3), 298-305.

Hawkins, S. S., Griffiths, L. J., Dezateux, C., & Law, C. (2007a). The impact of maternal employment on breast-feeding duration in the UK Millennium Cohort Study. *Public Health and Nutrition, 10*(9), 891-896.

Hawkins, S. S., Griffiths, L. J., Dezateux, C., & Law, C. (2007b). Maternal employment and breast-feeding initiation: findings from the Millennium Cohort Study. *Paediatric and Perinatal Epidemiology, 21*(3), 242-247.

Heinig, M. J., Nommsen, L. A., Peerson, J. M., Lonnerdal, B., & Dewey, K. G. (1993). Energy and protein intakes of breast-fed and formula-fed infants during the first year of life and their association with growth velocity: the DARLING Study. *American Journal of Clinical Nutrition, 58*(2), 152-161.

Hill, P. D., Aldag, J. C., Chatterton, R. T., & Zinaman, M. (2005). Comparison of milk output between mothers of preterm and term infants: the first 6 weeks after birth. *Journal of Human Lactation, 21*(1), 22-30.

Hills-Bonczyk, S. (1993). Women's experiences with combining breast-feeding and employment. *Journal of Nurse-Midwifery, 38*(5), 257-266.

HRSA. (2008). *The business case for breastfeeding*. Retrieved February 19, 2010, from http://www.womenshealth.gov/breastfeeding/programs/business-case/.

Islam, M. M., Peerson, J. M., Ahmed, T., Dewey, K. G., & Brown, K. H. (2006). Effects of varied energy density of complementary foods on breast-milk intakes and total energy consumption by healthy, breastfed Bangladeshi children. *American Journal of Clinical Nutrition, 83*(4), 851-858.

Jones, E. G., & Matheny, R. J. (1993). Relationship between infant feeding and exclusion rate from child care because of illness. *Journal of the American Dietetic Association, 93*(7), 809-811.

Jones, F., & Tully, M.R. (2006). *Best practice for expressing, storing and handling human milk in hospitals, homes and child care settings* (Second ed.). Raleigh, NC: Human Milk Banking Association of North America.

Kearney, M. H., & Cronenwett, L. (1991). Breastfeeding and employment. *Journal of Obstetric, Gynecologic, and Neonatal Nursing, 20*(6), 471-480.

Kent, J. C. (2007). How breastfeeding works. *Journal of Midwifery & Women's Health, 52*(6), 564-570.

Kent, J. C., Mitoulas, L., Cox, D. B., Owens, R. A., & Hartmann, P. E. (1999). Breast volume and milk production during extended lactation in women. *Experimental Physiology, 84*(2), 435-447.

Kent, J. C., Mitoulas, L. R., Cregan, M. D., Geddes, D. T., Larsson, M., Doherty, D. A., et al. (2008). Importance of vacuum for breastmilk expression. *Breastfeeding Medicine, 3*(1), 11-19.

Kent, J. C., Mitoulas, L. R., Cregan, M. D., Ramsay, D. T., Doherty, D. A., & Hartmann, P. E. (2006). Volume and frequency of breastfeedings and fat content of breast milk throughout the day. *Pediatrics, 117*(3), e387-395.

Kent, J. C., Ramsay, D. T., Doherty, D., Larsson, M., & Hartmann, P. E. (2003). Response of breasts to different stimulation patterns of an electric breast pump. *Journal of Human Lactation, 19*(2), 179-186; quiz 187-178, 218.

Kimbro, R. T. (2006). On-the-job moms: work and breastfeeding initiation and duration for a sample of low-income women. *Maternal and Child Health Journal, 10*(1), 19-26.

Kurinij, N., Shiono, P. H., Ezrine, S. F., & Rhoads, G. G. (1989). Does maternal employment affect breast-feeding? *American Journal of Public Health, 79*(9), 1247-1250.

Li, R., Fein, S. B., & Grummer-Strawn, L. M. (2008). Association of breastfeeding intensity and bottle-emptying behaviors at early infancy with infants' risk for excess weight at late infancy. *Pediatrics, 122 Suppl 2*, S77-84.

Libbus, M. K., & Bullock, L. F. (2002). Breastfeeding and employment: an assessment of employer attitudes. *Journal of Human Lactation, 18*(3), 247-251.

Lindberg, L. D. (1996). Trends in the relationship between breastfeeding and postpartum employment in the United States. *Social Biology, 43*, 191-202.

McLeod, D., Pullon, S., & Cookson, T. (2002). Factors influencing continuation of breastfeeding in a cohort of women. *Journal of Human Lactation, 18*(4), 335-343.

Miller, N. H., Miller, D. J., & Chism, M. (1996). Breastfeeding practices among resident physicians. *Pediatrics, 98*(3 Pt 1), 434-437.

Neville, M. C., Keller, R., Seacat, J., Lutes, V., Neifert, M., Casey, C., et al. (1988). Studies in human lactation: milk volumes in lactating women during the onset of lactation and full lactation. *American Journal of Clinical Nutrition, 48*(6), 1375-1386.

Nichols, M. R., & Roux, G. M. (2004). Maternal perspectives on postpartum return to the workplace. *Journal of Obstetric, Gynecologic, and Neonatal Nursing, 33*(4), 463-471.

Noble, S. (2001). Maternal employment and the initiation of breastfeeding. *Acta Paediatrica, 90*(4), 423-428.

Nommsen-Rivers, L. (1997). Universal precautions are not needed for health care workers handling breast milk. *Journal of Human Lactation, 13*(4), 267-268.

Ong, G., Yap, M., Li, F. L., & Choo, T. B. (2005). Impact of working status on breastfeeding in Singapore: evidence from the National Breastfeeding Survey 2001. *European Journal of Public Health, 15*(4), 424-430.

Ortiz, J., McGilligan, K., & Kelly, P. (2004). Duration of breast milk expression among working mothers enrolled in an employer-sponsored lactation program. *Pediatric Nursing, 30*(2), 111-119.

Roe, B., Whittington, L. A., Fein, S. B., & Teisl, M. F. (1999). Is there competition between breast-feeding and maternal employment? *Demography, 36*(2), 157-171.

Rojjanasrirat, W. (2004). Working women's breastfeeding experiences. *MCN; American Journal of Maternal Child Nursing, 29*(4), 222-227; quiz 228-229.

Ryan, A. S., Zhou, W., & Arensberg, M. B. (2006). The effect of employment status on breastfeeding in the United States. *Women's Health Issues, 16*(5), 243-251.

Scott, J. A., Binns, C. W., Oddy, W. H., & Graham, K. I. (2006). Predictors of breastfeeding duration: evidence from a cohort study. *Pediatrics, 117*(4), e646-655.

Shealy, K. (2005). *The CDC guide to breastfeeding interventions*. Retrieved February 19, 2010, from http://www.cdc.gov/breastfeeding/pdf/breastfeeding_interventions.pdf.

SHRM. (2007). *2007 benefits: A survey report by the Society for Human Resource Managers*. Alexandria, VA: Society for Human Resource Managers.

Slusser, W. M., Lange, L., Dickson, V., Hawkes, C., & Cohen, R. (2004). Breast milk expression in the workplace: a look at frequency and time. *Journal of Human Lactation, 20*(2), 164-169.

Stevens, K. V., & Janke, J. (2003). Breastfeeding experiences of active duty military women. *Military Medicine, 168*(5), 380-384.

Taveras, E. M., Rifas-Shiman, S. L., Scanlon, K. S., Grummer-Strawn, L. M., Sherry, B., & Gillman, M. W. (2006). To what extent is the protective effect of breastfeeding on future overweight explained by decreased maternal feeding restriction? *Pediatrics, 118*(6), 2341-2348.

Thompson, P. E., & Bell, P. (1997). Breast-feeding in the workplace: how to succeed. *Issues in Comprehensive Pediatric Nursing, 20*(1), 1-9.

Tully, M. R. (2005). Working and breastfeeding. *AWHONN Lifelines, 9*(3), 198-203.

Visness, C. M., & Kennedy, K. I. (1997). Maternal employment and breast-feeding: findings from the 1988 National Maternal and Infant Health Survey. *American Journal of Public Health, 87*(6), 945-950.

Whaley, S. E., Meehan, K., Lange, L., Slusser, W., & Jenks, E. (2002). Predictors of breastfeeding duration for employees of the Special Supplemental Nutrition Program for Women, Infants, and Children (WIC). *Journal of the American Dietetic Association, 102*(9), 1290-1293.

Witters-Green, R. (2003). Increasing brestfeeding rates in working mothers. *Families, Sytems & Health, 21*, 415-434.

Relactation, Induced Lactation, and Emergencies

Chapter 16

RELACTATION AND INDUCED LACTATION

Relactation is the process of increasing milk production in a woman who has been pregnant.

A mother may decide to relactate when she is still producing some milk or many years after her last pregnancy. The difference between relactation and increasing low milk production is one of degree. Most commonly, relactation occurs after the mother has spent weeks or months breastfeeding very little or not at all. She may or may not have begun breastfeeding after birth. Unlike the mother inducing lactation (see next point), this mother has experienced the breast tissue development that occurs during pregnancy. If she can transition the baby to the breast, breastfeed 10 to 12 times each day, spend lots of time each day touching and holding her baby, and there are no physical obstacles to making milk, over several weeks her odds of substantial milk production are good.

For mothers with prior breastfeeding experience, the odds of relactation are good.

Induced lactation is the process of stimulating milk production in a woman who has never been pregnant.

Although induced lactation was once referred to as "adoptive breastfeeding," with the availability of modern reproductive technologies, this term does not always apply. A mother may be adopting a baby or surrogacy may be involved (Biervliet, Maguiness, Hay, Killick, & Atkin, 2001, p. 5). A mother's ability to produce milk by inducing lactation is partly influenced by cultural beliefs. In cultures where breastfeeding is the norm, there are many documented cases of full milk production in mothers inducing lactation. In cultures where breastfeeding is not the norm, many believe full milk production is unlikely.

Success of induced lactation varies widely by cultural norm.

Gathering Information

Ask the mother her reasons for wanting to breastfeed and her goals and expectations.

Her reasons for breastfeeding. See the later section "Unique to Induced Lactation" for emotional benefits of inducing lactation for an adopted child. Mothers decide to relactate for a variety of reasons. The baby may not be thriving on formula due to intolerance or allergy. The baby may have a medical condition for which mother's milk is recommended. The mother may be unhappy at the loss of breastfeeding and want to reclaim it for herself and her baby. The mother may be breastfeeding an older baby or toddler and decide to relactate for a newly adopted child. Some mothers relactate and induce lactation to help a sick friend or relative. Discussing the mother's reasons for wanting to produce milk can help her clarify her feelings and goals.

If she is relactating for her youngest child, ask what happened with breastfeeding. In this case, the dynamics that caused her milk production to decrease may still exist and need to be addressed. If the mother had breastfeeding problems, ask about them. The cause may be simple misinformation, such as being told to breastfeed on a schedule, which led to slow weight gain and supplements, which decreased milk production. If so, provide the mother with information about milk production dynamics (see Chapter 11, "Making Milk"). If a mother had nipple pain and trauma, she may need to learn about helping her baby take the breast deeply or other causes may need to be explored, such as tongue tie. If the mother began formula-feeding after birth, ask her why and if these reasons are still important to her.

Her goals. When the mother shares her goals, ask what aspect of breastfeeding is most important to her. In one U.S. survey of 366 women who relactated, most were not as concerned about the amount of milk they produced as their ability nurture their baby at the breast (Auerbach & Avery, 1980). Some survey mothers decided to relactate for health reasons (baby's formula intolerance or health problems), but most relactated because they hoped breastfeeding would bring them emotionally closer to their babies. In hindsight, 75% of the women surveyed considered relactation a positive experience and their milk production was unrelated to their feelings of success.

It may take a month or more for mothers to reach full milk production.

Relactation expectations. Let the mother know that depending on how low her milk production is when she starts, it may take a month or more to reach full milk production. In a study done in India with 1,000 healthy mothers relactating for healthy babies less than 6 weeks old, those who had a "lactation gap" (time since last breastfeeding) of less than 15 days were able to stimulate full milk production within 3 to 5 days (Banapurmath, Banapurmath, & Kesaree, 2003). Those whose lactation gap was more than 15 days took longer than the 10-day study to reach full lactation. More than half of the 366 U.S. survey mothers who relactated established full production within 1 month (Auerbach & Avery, 1980). It took more than 1 month for full relactation in another 25%. The remaining mothers breastfed with supplements until their babies weaned. If the mother is concerned that she might not reach full relactation, assure her that even partial relactation is a huge boon to her and her baby, and if this is her end result, she will know she did everything possible.

Induced lactation expectations. Different mothers approach induced lactation with different goals. To clarify a mother's goals, a good starting point is to ask her how important milk production is to her. Some mothers consider substantial milk production their top priority. Others consider the closeness of breastfeeding and the amount of milk produced as equally important. Still others consider induced lactation primarily a way to increase their emotional closeness to their baby and care little about how much milk they produce. When a mother says closeness is her top priority, suggest she focus on the emotional aspects of breastfeeding and think of any milk she produces as an added bonus. In this case, her success is best gauged by her baby's willingness to take the breast and enjoy the comfort and security he receives there. If inducing full milk production is one of the mother's top priorities, offer to discuss her options in light of her specific situation.

Also let her know that all mothers inducing lactation who breastfeed long term eventually reach a stage where their baby's need for milk and their milk production match. Some mothers can discontinue formula supplements after 6 months, when solid foods take their place in the baby's diet. For some, it may be closer to 12 months, when their child is eating more solids. But all mothers and babies eventually reach the point when extra milk becomes unnecessary.

• •

Ask the mother her baby's age and their breastfeeding history, as well as any anatomy or health issues.

The baby's age, breastfeeding history, and current response to the breast. The baby's age and willingness to breastfeed may affect the process. In the survey of 366 U.S. mothers who relactated described in the previous point, the mothers who started relactating within 2 months of birth reported greater milk production than those who relactated more than 2 months after birth. If the mother is inducing lactation, ask if either she or her child have breastfed before. It was once thought the younger the baby, the more smoothly induced lactation was likely to go, but adopted toddlers often take to breastfeeding easily and enthusiastically (Gribble, 2005a). In Australia, adoptions are not allowed until at the earliest 6 to 12 months after birth, and many mothers have successfully transitioned their children to the breast at this age, and even much older.

Health or anatomy issues in mother or baby. Do mother and baby have any known medical conditions? Are they on any medications (be sure to ask about hormonal contraception)? Is there anything unusual about the mother's breasts or nipples (very large breasts, flat or inverted nipples)? Breastfeeding may go more smoothly with a healthy mother and baby with average anatomy. If mother or baby has unusual anatomy, such as inverted nipples, tongue-tie, etc., it may or may not affect breastfeeding. See the sections about their anatomy issues in other chapters.

• •

Ask about the mother's availability to her baby, her support network, and if appropriate, about any infertility issues.

Her daily responsibilities. If the mother has other children, ask how many and their ages. If she is employed, how many hours per week is she away from her baby? If she is employed and inducing lactation, is she planning to take maternity leave when her child arrives? If so, for how long? What other daily obligations does the mother have? Is she or her family under any unusual stress? If the mother has many commitments, ask her if she can take some time off and get help with her older children while she focuses on increasing her milk. Provide all mothers with full information on their options, as a mother's circumstances are not a reliable way to predict which mother will follow through and which will not (K. Gribble, personal communication, February 6, 2010).

Her available support. Ask the mother if she has a partner, and if so how her partner feels about her plans. Does she have household help or can she get it? Is she in contact other breastfeeding mothers? If not, refer her to a mother-to-mother support group and to the websites at the end of this chapter for online support. Make sure she knows the value of support and ask if she has family or friends who can give her day-to-day help and encouragement.

A mother's ability to relactate may depend, in part, on her other responsibilities and level of social support.

Infertility issues. Some causes of infertility in the mother may affect milk production. For example, if the mother is adopting a baby due to infertility, ask if the issue was with her, her partner, or both. Some physical conditions that prevent conception or sustaining a pregnancy may affect milk production. For example, Sheehan's syndrome, caused by extreme blood loss (after birth or at any time) that is severe enough to render the pituitary non-functional prevents both pregnancy and lactation (Schrager & Sabo, 2001; Sert, Tetiker, Kirim, & Kocak, 2003). Some types of hormonal imbalances may affect fertility, breast development, and milk production (see p. 395- "Hormonal Levels and Receptors"). In most cases, a mother with infertility issues will not know for sure if her milk production will be affected until she tries.

Strategies for Increasing Milk Production

One key to both relactation and induced lactation is persuading the baby to take the breast.

Because the process involved in relactating and inducing lactation are essentially the same, they share the same basic strategies. One critical aspect of both is persuading the baby to take the breast. Although some studies have found younger babies accept the breast more readily than older babies, children older than 12 months have also willingly taken to breastfeeding (Phillips, 1993). Research conducted internationally has documented breast-seeking behaviors in adopted children between 8 months and 12 years of age (Gribble, 2005d). Recognizing and triggering babies' breast-seeking behaviors (see Chapter 1) can make the transition to the breast easier. But every baby is different, and there is no way to know until the mother offers the breast how the baby will accept it. For specific strategies, see the later section "Helping Baby Accept the Breast" on p. 614.

Creating a Plan and Cultural Influences

Offer to help the mother create a plan based on her priorities and her situation.

The most important strategy for both relactation and induced lactation is frequent breast stimulation by breastfeeding and/or milk expression. Galactogogues, or milk-enhancing substances, are another option. For a mother considering using a galactogogue, this choice should be discussed with her healthcare provider in light of her health history, but her preferences also play a role. Some women may not have the time or money to express their milk with an automatic double pump, while others prefer milk expression over breastfeeding. However, if the mother seems uncomfortable with breastfeeding, explore this with her, as this may affect her willingness to transition her baby to the breast.

Offer to help the mother formulate a plan that incorporates the strategies with which she feels most at ease. If her plan incorporates strategies she feels uncomfortable with, she is unlikely to follow through.

Induced lactation. If the mother's goal is to breastfeed primarily for greater intimacy with her child, she may want to wait until the baby arrives and use only breastfeeding and body contact to induce lactation. However, if she feels strongly about stimulating substantial milk production before her baby arrives and she knows her baby's arrival date at least several months in advance, she may want to consider the induced lactation protocols described on p. 613-"Unique to Induced Lactation."

If her situation includes adoption, the type of adoption may make a difference. How far in advance will she know for certain of the baby's arrival? Is it a traditional U.S. adoption? In this case, sometimes things change right before the baby is scheduled to arrive, which may affect the mother's desire to produce milk in advance. In Australia, the baby will be older (6 to 12 months), so the mother is unlikely to be as focused on her milk production as a mother adopting a newborn. Is a surrogate carrying her baby? If so, she may have much more time and greater certainty about when the baby will be in her arms.

Discuss the following strategies with her in light of her priorities and situation and help her create a plan with which she feels comfortable.

In developing countries where breastfeeding is the norm, there is a long history of successful relactation and induced lactation. Researchers have documented full induced lactation in Africa, Indonesia, South America, India, Polynesia, and among Native Americans (Wieschhoff, 1940). In South Africa, researchers reported grandmothers inducing full or partial lactation for their grandchildren after their mothers left for an extended absence or returned to work (Slome, 1956). In a more recent study in Nigeria, by simply breastfeeding 8 to 10 times per day, six women induced full lactation within 3 to 4 weeks for babies whose mothers had died (Abejide et al., 1997). Where breastfeeding is the norm, mothers expect to produce enough milk for their babies and those around them support them in their efforts.

Cultural beliefs about breastfeeding and parenting practices may affect milk production.

But in countries where breastfeeding is not the yet the norm, even birth mothers doubt their ability to make enough milk, and mothers relactating and inducing lactation are less likely to reach full milk production. In one survey of 65 Western adoptive mothers who induced lactation, the mothers calculated their babies received 25% to 75% of their daily milk intake from the breast (Hormann, 1977). The mothers calculated these percentages by subtracting the amount of formula the baby took per day from the amount needed by an exclusively formula-fed baby. But these estimates were likely low because formula-fed babies, on average, consume 15% more milk at 3 months and 23% more at 6 months than exclusively breastfed babies (Heinig, Nommsen, Peerson, Lonnerdal, & Dewey, 1993). Only two of these survey mothers induced full lactation, and two mothers with pituitary disorders produced no milk.

After comparing the differences in outcomes among adoptive mothers inducing lactating in developed and developing countries, Australian researcher Karleen Gribble wrote:

In cultures where breastfeeding is the norm, mothers who relactate or induce lactation produce more milk.

> Adoptive mothers in developing countries may have greater milk production than mothers in the West because they are more knowledgeable about breastfeeding, practice frequent breastfeeding, remain in close physical contact with their children and live in cultures that are supportive of breastfeeding. They also have reproductive and breastfeeding histories that may make breastfeeding easier, though they are less likely to have pharmaceutical galactagogues available. Adoptive mothers in the West should be encouraged to maximize their milk supply by emulating the mothering styles of women in developing countries and developing a strong support network for breastfeeding. It may be that most adoptive mothers are physically capable of producing sufficient breastmilk for the child but that in the West, sociocultural factors act as preventatives (Gribble, 2004, p. 5).

Knowledge about breastfeeding. In developing countries, women learn about breastfeeding during their childhood by watching mothers around them breastfeed. But in Western cultures, most mothers either breastfeed behind closed doors or cover themselves, leaving new mothers ignorant and uncertain about how breastfeeding works.

Breastfeeding and parenting practices. Among birth mothers, differences in breastfeeding and parenting practices affect both milk production and return to fertility (see Chapter 13). As U.S. researcher Kathleen Kennedy noted, a Western mother may think of a "breastfeeding" as a lengthy, ritualized activity involving changing the baby's diaper, making herself a drink, turning off her phone, settling into a certain chair, and then putting her baby to breast for an extended time (Kennedy, 2010). However, a mother in a developing country may keep her baby on her body, putting him to breast at the slightest cue for just a few minutes 15 to 20 times each day (Lozoff & Brittenham, 1979). In developing countries, this greater body contact may enhance a mother's hormonal response to milk production. Western mothers, on the other hand, are encouraged to feed their babies at regular intervals, sleep separately, and avoid holding their babies "too much" for fear of "spoiling." As a result, Western babies spend much of their days in infant seats, strollers/prams, and cribs. For the mother relactating or inducing lactation in a developed country, attending breastfeeding mother-support groups (such as La Leche League and the Australian Breastfeeding Association), where mothers practice more responsive breastfeeding, can provide her with exposure to parenting practices that enhance milk production.

Bottles, because of their faster flow, may impair full relactation.

Attitudes about breastfeeding. In developing countries, birth and adoptive mothers are strongly encouraged and supported in their efforts to breastfeed because breastfeeding is a matter of life or death. One study of 1,000 relactating mothers in India estimated that babies partially breastfed were more than four times more likely to die during the first 6 weeks of life compared with those exclusively breastfed (Banapurmath et al., 2003). Babies not breastfed at all were more than 14 times more likely to die. When the timeframe was extended to 2 months, babies not breastfed were more than 23 times more likely to die. For this reason, in India, mothers relactating may be hospitalized to increase their odds of success (De, Pandit, Mishra, Pappu, & Chaudhuri, 2002). Breasts are considered primarily for feeding and comforting babies, and their exposure in public for breastfeeding is widely accepted (Dettwyler, 1995). Mothers also have confidence in their ability to breastfeed because they are surrounded by mothers producing ample milk. In Western countries, the breast has been sexualized and birth mothers doubt their milk-making abilities. Western mothers relactating or inducing lactation may be met with amazement, doubt, or criticism.

Supplemental feeding methods. In developing countries, most mothers relactating or inducing lactation supplement their babies with easy-to-clean, temporary methods, such as spoons and cups (Banapurmath et al., 2003). Feeding bottles—a long-term feeding method—are rarely used due to contamination risks. In developed countries, however, feeding bottles are common, and due to their fast flow, the baby is more likely to take more supplement than needed. In one study of relactation in 15 mothers in India, full relactation was achieved only when feeding bottles were stopped (Banapurmath, Banapurmath, & Kesaree, 1993). In a Nigerian study in which six mothers achieved full induced lactation, babies were supplemented only by cup or spoon (Abejide et al., 1997). Also, healthcare providers and the mother's family strongly urged them to induce lactation to ensure their baby's survival and provided practical help to accomplish this.

• •

Suggest the mother learn the basics of breastfeeding and the physical changes she can expect as she begins to produce more milk.

To understand the reasons behind the "how-tos" of relactation and induced lactation, it is helpful for the mother to understand the basic dynamics of milk production (see Chapter 11, "Making Milk"). She also needs to be able to gauge when her baby is getting enough milk at the breast and when he needs more supplement. Knowing how to help her baby take the breast deeply will help avoid nipple pain and increase her baby's breastfeeding effectiveness. The more she knows, the easier it is for her to adapt recommendations to her baby and her situation.

It can also be reassuring for the mother to know that she may experience some physical and emotional changes as her milk production increases:

- **Menstrual changes.** With increased breast stimulation, the mother may menstruate irregularly or stop menstruating altogether.
- **Breast changes.** Her areolae may darken and her breasts may become tender, feel fuller, hotter, or heavier, and increase in size.
- **Mood changes.** With lactation-related hormonal changes, some mothers find that with more oxytocin, prolactin, and other breastfeeding hormones in their system their mood improves. Others begin to feel warm, anxious, or nervous or become depressed, fatigued, tearful, or angry. Mood changes may make the mother feel overwhelmed or like giving up. Be sure the mother knows that mood changes are usually a sign she's about to notice increased milk production and to tap into her support network if she's feeling down.

Encourage any mother relactating or inducing lactation to accept all offers of help and to take good care of herself.

For most mothers, getting more rest, eating a more nutritious diet, and drinking more fluids will not boost milk production. But these can be important to a mother's morale and her ability to cope. Encourage the mother to accept all offers of assistance, and offer to help her formulate a daily plan that will maximize her time spent boosting milk production, while allowing her the time she needs to care for other children and to meet other responsibilities.

Breast Stimulation and Mother-Baby Body Contact

The most effective strategy for relactation and induced lactation is frequent, effective breastfeeding around the clock.

Breastfeed at least 10 to 12 times per day. Before a mother has milk to remove, nipple stimulation increases the release of prolactin, which contributes to growth of breast tissue. Regular breastfeeding stimulates milk production in a number of ways. In mothers producing some milk, it takes advantage of the "drained breasts make milk faster" dynamic (explained in the chapter "Making Milk"), which causes an increase in the rate of milk production between feedings by keeping pressure within the breast low and not allowing a build-up in the breast of the peptide or whey protein "feedback inhibitor of lactation" (Daly, Owens, & Hartmann, 1993). Over time frequent milk removal also increases milk production by speeding the metabolic activity of key enzymes used in milk-making and stimulating the growth and development of more milk-making tissue in the breast (Czank, Henderson, Kent, Tat Lai, & Hartmann, 2007).

Frequent milk removal increases production for relactating mothers.

Be sure the baby takes the breast deeply. Frequent breastfeeding can increase a mother's rate of milk production only if the baby stimulates the breast well and removes the milk effectively. Suggest the mother use the strategies described in Chapter 1 to find an effective feeding position and to be sure the baby takes the breast deeply. Shallow breastfeeding can reduce the baby's milk intake and drain the breast unevenly, which can slow milk production (Mizuno et al., 2008).

Offer each breast more than once at each feeding. Suggest that each time the baby comes off the breast the mother offer the other breast. If the baby does not stay active (just mouthing the breast rather than actively suckling and swallowing) or if he falls asleep quickly, suggest the mother use breast compression (see next paragraph) to keep him active at that breast longer. If possible, encourage the baby to take each breast at least twice.

Use breast compression or alternate breast massage. If the baby stops suckling actively, breast compression or alternate breast massage can increase milk flow, which helps to keep him feeding actively longer. For a description of this technique, see p. 804- "Breast Compression" in the "Techniques" appendix.

Guide the sleeping baby to the breast. To help increase the number of daily breastfeedings, the baby can be gently guided to the breast when drowsy or in a light sleep. U.K. research found that laying a sleeping baby tummy down on mother's semi-reclined body triggers inborn feeding behaviors, which can lead to effective breastfeeding during sleep, even in late preterm babies (Colson, DeRooy, & Hawdon, 2003).

Avoid soothers and keep all suckling at the breast. One way to increase the time spent at the breast is for the mother to keep all suckling at the breast. Swaddling and soothers, such as pacifiers/dummies and swings, can reduce time spent breastfeeding (Binns & Scott, 2002; Bystrova et al., 2007). Giving supplements with an at-breast supplementer can also increase breast stimulation by keeping the baby actively breastfeeding for longer.

Suggest the mother plan to keep her baby on her body as much as possible to trigger feeding behaviors and to enhance milk-making.

Research done in the U.S. and Sweden has found associations between mother-baby touch, enhanced hormonal responses in the mother, and increased milk production. After birth, newborns' touch increased mothers' blood oxytocin levels (Matthiesen, Ransjo-Arvidson, Nissen, & Uvnas-Moberg, 2001). In mothers of preterm babies, daily mother-baby skin-to-skin contact was associated with greater milk volumes expressed (Hurst, Valentine, Renfro, Burns, & Ferlic, 1997). Skin-to-skin contact before breastfeeding was associated with lower levels of stress hormones in the mother and a greater hormonal response to breastfeeding (Handlin et al., 2009).

To keep her baby against her body, encourage the mother to use a sling or baby carrier during the day (preferably one that allows her to breastfeed) and to spend as much of her time as practical with her breast accessible to her baby in laid-back breastfeeding positions, such as leaning back comfortably on her sofa (see Chapter 1). At night, encourage the mother to keep the baby close and to breastfeed often.

Milk expression can also be used to speed the rate of milk production.

If the baby is breastfeeding effectively, suggest the mother make breastfeeding a higher priority than milk expression. But if the mother is away from her baby regularly or the baby is not yet breastfeeding effectively, milk expression can be a useful tool. The first choice for any relactating mother is a hospital-grade rental pump with a double-pump kit, which has been found to be more effective at establishing milk production than hand expression (Slusher et al., 2007). Suggest the mother relactating or inducing lactation who is using a breast pump, double-pump at least once during the wee hours of the morning, when prolactin levels are naturally higher (Czank et al., 2007).

Where breast pumps are not available or are outside the mother's means, hand expression can be used (Banapurmath et al., 2003). One case study from Brazil describes a mother with low milk production who relactated at 8 weeks by deeper and more frequent breastfeeding, hand-expressing her milk after each breastfeeding, and feeding it to her baby (de Melo & Murta, 2009). Her milk volume quickly increased, which led to better weight gain and full milk production. After a previous average weight gain of 11 g per week, her baby gained, on average, 15 g per day the first week, and by the 2nd week, his weight gain averaged 25 g per day. In cases like this, donor human milk or infant formula could be used as a supplement to boost weight gain initially while the mother's milk production increased.

If the mother chooses to pump, discuss available pump models and pump fit, how to use sensory stimulation (including warmth) to trigger more milk ejections, and how to use her pump settings to get the most milk at each expression (see p. 449- "How to Express More Milk" in the chapter "Milk Expression and Storage"). Double-pumping is a huge time saver (Becker, McCormick, & Renfrew, 2008). Many mothers can double pump "hands-free" by cutting holes in a bra or using a tight top to hold the pump parts in place. Also suggest the following strategies.

Use breast massage during pumping and hand expression after pumping. One U.S. study found that 86% of its 66 mothers of preterm babies expressed an average of 93% more milk when they used breast massage during pumping and hand expression after pumping to drain their breasts more completely (Morton et al., 2009). A U.K. study also found that breast massage during breast pumping increased milk output an average of 42% (88 mL vs. 125 mL) (Jones, Dimmock, & Spencer, 2001).

Express long enough to drain the breast well. Suggest the mother express up to 20 to 30 minutes per breast at each session, or at least 2 minutes after the last drop of milk. The more fully she can drain her breasts, the faster her rate of milk production increases. As mentioned above, hand-expressing milk after pumping to more fully drain the breast increases milk production faster (Morton et al., 2009).

Express milk after or between breastfeedings. If the mother is highly motivated and does not find adding milk expression to her routine too overwhelming, she can express as many times per day as practical after or between breastfeedings. Let the mother know that even if she doesn't express much milk at first, its main purpose is to stimulate faster milk production. Because most mothers express more milk by waiting an hour or more after breastfeeding to express, let the mother decide if she would prefer to keep all feeding-related activities together by expressing right after breastfeeding or if she would rather express at another time and get more milk for supplementation.

Mothers can increase their milk production if they also express milk in between feedings.

From time to time "power pump." The purpose of this short-term strategy is to fit in more daily pumpings and give milk production a quick boost. One version of power pumping credited to U.S. lactation consultant Catherine Watson Genna involves putting the pump in an area the mother passes often where she will be comfortable sitting or standing (West & Marasco, 2009). During a several-day period, every time she passes the pump, she uses it for 5 to 10 minutes, pumping into the same bottle and using the same pump pieces without cleaning them for a period of 4 to 6 hours (the length of time milk is considered safe at most room temperatures). After this time, she combines and refrigerates the milk and cleans the pump parts. Because the milk is not refrigerated right away and the pump parts are not cleaned after each use, this strategy is only suitable for mothers of full-term healthy babies.

Suggest the mother keep her longest stretch between breast drainings shorter than 8 hours.

Because full breasts make milk slower, long stretches between breastfeedings and/or milk expressions (usually at night) can slow a mother's milk production. Ask her the length of her current longest stretch. To avoid giving her body the message to slow milk production for part of the day, suggest she avoid going longer than 8 hours without either breastfeeding or expressing milk. If her baby sleeps longer than 8 hours at night, she will need to decide whether to wake the baby to breastfeed or express her milk. For some mothers with small breast-storage capacities (see the chapter "Making Milk"), even an 8-hour stretch may be long enough to cause milk production to slow.

Galactogogues

Prescribed and/or herbal galactogogues may help some mothers boost milk production.

For specific drugs and medicinal herbs and doses, see p. 419- "Galactogogues." For a mother considering using a galactogogue, this choice should be discussed with her healthcare provider in light of her health history, but her preferences also play a role. For example, one woman may prefer not to take prescription medicines, but be enthusiastic about taking medicinal herbs. Another woman may be uncomfortable taking medicinal herbs, but want to take prescribed medications. Others may want to do both.

In most cases, galactogogues are not necessary for full milk production.

Although galactogogues may be helpful in some cases, relactation and induced lactation can be accomplished without them.

Relactation. One study conducted in India randomly assigned relactating women into two groups (Seema, Patwari, & Satyanarayana, 1997). Group I breastfed frequently and received ongoing information and support from a health worker. Group II received this along with metoclopramide, a prescribed galactogogue. Time to full relactation, pattern of weight gain, rate of reduction of supplement, and total weight gain were all comparable between the two groups, with 92% of the mothers achieving full relactation and 6% partial relactatation. The researchers concluded that most mothers can fully relactate without using galactogogues.

Galactogogues can help mothers relactate or induce lactation. But they are not always necessary.

In a large study done in India in which no galactogogues were used, 83% of its 1,000 mothers with babies younger than 6 weeks reached full milk production within 10 days (Banapurmath et al., 2003). These mothers were instructed to breastfed at least every 2 hours, offer the breast whenever the baby showed interest, use hand expression to stimulate milk production, provide lots of skin-to-skin contact, and sleep with their babies at night. In another study on relactation from India, when breastfeeding 10 to 12 times per day for about 10 minutes per breast, 61% of the 139 relactating mothers achieved full milk production (including one mother relactating for twins) and 23% achieved partial milk production (De et al., 2002). These mothers were encouraged to supplement as needed by cup and spoon, sleep with the babies, and provide lots of skin-to-skin contact.

Induced lactation. Galactogogues may be helpful to some, but like relactation, induced lactation can be accomplished without them. When used, they can be given either before or after the baby arrives (Bryant, 2006). In one study of 27 mothers inducing lactation in Papua, New Guinea, 11 mothers who had never breastfed received a single injection of 100 mg of medroxyprogesterone (Depo-Provera) a week before beginning their efforts to induce lactation, then took 10 mg of metoclopramide (Reglan) or 25 mg of chlorpromazine (Thorazine) four times daily until they had enough milk to sustain their babies. The 16 mothers who had previously breastfed received the oral medication without the injection until adequate lactation was established (Nemba, 1994). In this study, 24 out of the 27 mothers induced full lactation.

Unique to Induced Lactation

Breastfeeding can help an adopted or foster child form healthy attachments and increase the mother's sensitivity to her child.

The importance of human milk to the normal health and development of any baby (and mother) are well known (Ip, Chung, Raman, Trikalinos, & Lau, 2009). But breastfeeding is much more than milk. The profound effects of breastfeeding on the mother-child relationship are especially valuable to adoptive families. In one Australian review article, researcher Karleen Gribble described the role breastfeeding played in helping adopted children, especially those with a history of abuse or neglect, form a close and healthy relationship with their new mothers (Gribble, 2006). The regular, intimate touch and the calming, relaxing, analgesic effect of breastfeeding can be key to an easier transition from the birth mother or an institution to the new family. For the adoptive breastfeeding mother, the relaxing hormones released during breastfeeding provide stress relief and enhance her sensitivity to her child (Uvnas-Moberg, 2003). In another article, Gribble reports that when children spend time in institutions before adoption, adoptive mothers believed that the primal experience of breastfeeding helped their children express grief over the loss of their birth mother and comforted them as they adjusted to their new family (Gribble, 2005d).

Breastfeeding can help adopted children form a close and healthy bond with their new mothers.

Breastfeeding can provide the same emotionally healing experiences to foster children. One case report about a medically fragile foster child described the improvements in physical and emotional health that occurred with breastfeeding (Gribble, 2005b). Its author suggested that mothers consider this option when the child is likely to be with the foster mother long term, especially for children who were previously breastfed or whose birth mother expressed a desire for their child to be breastfed. To allay any concerns about transmission of illness, such as HIV and HTLV-1 (see the chapter "Health Issues—Mother"), she suggests having foster mothers take blood tests (such as are used for milk donors). She noted that the biggest barriers to providing breastfeeding and human milk to foster children is social, as many social services personnel consider breastfeeding "an extra" or "a luxury," rather than a basic human need and right.

• •

A mother inducing lactation, with at least several months advance notice, can use prenatal induced lactation protocols before her baby arrives.

If milk production is high on a mother's priority list and she knows her baby's arrival date at least several months in advance, suggest she review with her healthcare provider the protocols developed by Canadian pediatrician Jack Newman and one of the first mothers to use them, Lenore Goldfarb (Goldfarb & Newman, 2000). The Web site www.asklenore.info describes these protocols in detail.

Three induced lactation protocols. At this writing, three protocols have been developed: the Regular Protocol, for women with at least 6 months before their baby's arrival, the Accelerated Protocol, for women with less than 6 months, and the Menopause Protocol, for women who have had surgical removal of their reproductive organs or naturally occurring menopause. To enhance breast tissue development, all three protocols involve taking one active oral contraceptive pill (containing 1 to 2 mg of progesterone and no more than 0.035 mg of estrogen) without interruption each day. To speed milk production, mothers also take daily domperidone, a prescribed medication. Before the baby arrives, the oral contraceptive is stopped (the timing varies among the protocol), which causes a drop in the mother's progesterone level, while the domperidone the mother continues to take stimulates an increase in her blood prolactin levels, causing her milk to "come in." This mimics (at much lower levels) the hormonal changes that naturally occur after birth. After the oral contraceptive is stopped, to further stimulate milk production, medicinal herbs are started and the mother begins pumping every 3 hours with an automatic double pump. Possible side effects of these protocols include prolonged breakthrough bleeding, increased blood pressure, and weight gain.

According to Goldfarb, even before the baby's arrival, mothers using the Regular Protocol produce 60% to 100% of their baby's milk needs, and mothers using the Accelerated Protocol produce 25% to 50%. However, at this writing, these results have not been published in peer-reviewed journals.

Suggest any mother considering using one of these protocols consult with her healthcare provider about the drugs and herbal medicines in light of her health history. Also be sure she knows that use of the oral contraceptives as recommended may not prevent pregnancy and that if hormonal contraceptives are contraindicated for her due to thrombosis, cardiac problems, or severe hypertension, she should not use these protocols.

Transitioning Baby to the Breast

Helping Baby Accept the Breast

If the baby balks at breastfeeding, it may help to first trigger her baby's inborn feeding behaviors and be patient.

Some babies take the breast easily and enthusiastically. Other babies accept it only with patience and encouragement. In one U.S. survey of 366 women who relactated, 39% reported their baby breastfed well at the first try, 32% were ambivalent about breastfeeding, and 28% refused to breastfeed (Auerbach & Avery, 1980). Within 1 week, 54% had taken the breast well, and by 10 days, it rose to 74%. On average, babies younger than 3 months and those who had previously breastfed went to the breast more easily.

Because breastfeeding is hardwired, most babies will eventually take the breast.

Babies fed for long periods with feeding bottles may at first be more reluctant to breastfeed than babies fed in other ways (Abejide et al., 1997). But because babies are hardwired to breastfeed, most will eventually take the breast. Breast-seeking behaviors have been reported from all over the world in adopted children aged 8 months to 12 years (Gribble, 2005d). One Australian article described six children between 12 and 48 months old who stimulated partial relactation in their mothers from suckling alone after being weaned for at least 6 months (Phillips, 1993). Suggest the mother start by spending some time each day holding her baby tummy down on her semi-reclined body, as this triggers inborn feeding behaviors (Colson, Meek, & Hawdon, 2008). (For more details, see Chapter 1.)

Suggest the adoptive mother focus first on her relationship with her child.

For an adoptive mother, before planning to put her child to the breast, suggest she first focus on their developing relationship. Because breastfeeding is an intimate act, children are more likely to take the breast when they trust and feel close to their new mother. When the adoptive mother welcomes her child to the family, at first she is a stranger to him. Before offering the breast, suggest she focus on ways to become emotionally closer, such as holding, carrying, co-sleeping, co-bathing, and being responsive to his needs. For the first few weeks, it may help to make their relationship exclusive if others are not allowed to hold the baby (Macrae & Gribble, 2006). The child's personality and past experiences with feeding will also affect his response to the breast. For example, if the child is used to being fed quickly with a fast-flow bottle, transitioning gradually by first shifting to a medium-flow bottle and then a slow-flow bottle can be gradual steps that allow him to experience feeding as something that is less overwhelming and more pleasurable before offering the breast.

For the older baby or toddler, it may help to first spend time around breastfeeding mothers and babies, so he can see this interaction, or read books with breastfeeding pictures. No matter what the child's age, patience and persistence are key.

If the baby continues to balk at the breast, suggest the mother try some basic strategies.

If a baby has never breastfed or hasn't breastfed for some time, it may take patience before he accepts the breast. When a mother begins offering the breast, suggest the following strategies.

- **Keep the breast a pleasant place to be**, not a battleground. If breastfeeding feels stressful, feed another way and instead give baby lots of cuddle time at the breast, especially while asleep (Smillie, 2008).
- **Spend time touching and skin-to-skin.** When not feeding, hold the baby and—if baby likes it—give skin-to-skin contact, perhaps by taking warm baths together.
- **Offer the breast while baby is in a light sleep or drowsy.** Some babies take the breast more easily when in a relaxed, sleepy state (Colson et al., 2003).
- **Use feeding positions baby likes best** and experiment, starting first with a semi-reclining position with baby tummy down and supported on mother's body.
- **Try breastfeeding in a private place without distractions.** This could be a quiet, darkened room or an area with dim lighting.
- **Trigger a milk ejection before baby goes to breast** to give an instant reward or try expressing milk first onto baby's lips.
- **Try breast shaping and/or support**. Using the breast sandwich, nipple tilting, and other techniques may help the baby take the breast deeper and better trigger active suckling. For details, see p. 802- "Breast Shaping" in the "Techniques" appendix.
- **Try breastfeeding in motion, while walking or rocking.**

- **Spend lots of time breastfeeding** whenever the baby breastfeeds well.
- **Supplement as needed** to make sure the baby gets the milk he needs to feel strong, calm, and open to breastfeeding.

Suggest the mother use the breast for comfort as well as for feeding.

In areas where breastfeeding is not yet the norm, some mothers are cautioned not to let the baby use their breast "like a pacifier," but offering the breast for comfort both enhances the mother's relationship with her baby and stimulates milk production. Suggest she take advantage of any and all ways to use her breast for comfort.

- Offer the breast whenever the baby wants to suckle, rather than a pacifier/dummy.
- Offer the breast when the baby is not too hungry or too full.
- When baby is at the breast, give lots of cuddling and skin-to-skin contact.
- Approach breastfeeding as a time the baby gets special attention and closeness, without concerns about the baby's response.

In some situations, tools and other strategies can help the baby accept the breast.

Drip expressed milk at the breast. If the baby goes to the breast, but won't stay there, ask a helper use a spoon or eyedropper to drip expressed milk on the breast or in the corner of his mouth. Swallowing triggers suckling, which can get baby started breastfeeding. Give more milk if baby comes off. In some studies, this is called the "drop and drip" method and has been used effectively to help relactating babies accept the breast (Banapurmath et al., 2003; Kesaree, 1993).

Feed a little milk first. Some babies are more willing to try breastfeeding if they are not very hungry. Suggest a mother give one-third to half a feeding and then offer the breast.

Try a thin, silicone nipple shield. In some situations, nipple shields can be a useful tool to transition a baby to the breast, especially if he has been fed by bottle, regularly received a pacifier, or the mother has inverted nipples. For details on use, fit, and application, see p. 834- "Nipple Shields."

Try an at-breast supplementer. If slow milk flow is an issue, a feeding-tube device will provide flow at the breast and may help the baby accept the breast or keep breastfeeding. If slow flow is not the cause, this may not be a good choice. For details, see p. 815- "At-Breast Supplementers" in the "Tools and Products" appendix.

Use the bottle as a transitional tool. If the bottle-fed baby will not yet take the breast or the mother chooses to supplement with the bottle, suggest the following strategies to encourage the transition to the breast or continued acceptance of the breast:

- When bottle-feeding, hold the bottle against the breast, so the baby gets used to feeding there.
- Wrap the bottle in a cloth and feed it against the exposed breast, so the baby cannot touch the bottle while feeding, but can feel the mother's skin.

- Try "bait and switch," where the mother begins by bottle-feeding the baby in a breastfeeding position, and while her baby is actively sucking and swallowing, pulls out the bottle teat and inserts her breast. (This can also be used with a pacifier/dummy.)

U.S. lactation consultant Dee Kassing describes other bottle-feeding strategies that may ease the transition to the breast by using the bottle to mimic breastfeeding (Kassing, 2002):

- Use a slow-flow nipple.
- Rather than inserting the bottle nipple/teat into the baby's mouth, brush it lightly against the baby's lips and wait for him to open wide before allowing him to draw it into his mouth.
- Use a wide based nipple that requires a wider gape as the baby feeds.

Ensuring Adequate Milk Intake

Discuss feeding methods for supplementing and their potential impact on milk production.

In the developing world where relactation and induced lactation are practiced successfully, mothers often use temporary feeding methods, such as a cup or a spoon, to give supplements between breastfeedings. Some studies have noted that babies supplemented by bottle have a more difficult time making the transition to full breastfeeding. Researchers who studied 15 relactating mothers in India wrote: "It was interesting to note that babies refused to suck at the breast once they were used to bottle feeding...In all these mothers, relactation was successful when bottle feeding was stopped" (Banapurmath et al., 1993, pp. 1330-1331). One reason for this may be the bottle's fast flow can cause babies to take more milk than they need, meaning less active suckling time at the breast. Because feeding bottles are a long-term feeding method (and in some parts of the world more socially acceptable than breastfeeding), mothers may be less motivated to discontinue them (Gribble, 2004).

An alternative to cups, spoons, and feeding bottles is an at-breast supplementer, also known as a tube-feeding device, which can provide the needed supplement while baby suckles at the breast. This feeding method may keep the baby actively breastfeeding longer to stimulate more milk production, and it may avoid the need for the mother to feed the baby again after breastfeeding. But it can also be "addictive" to both mother and baby and weaning from it may be difficult. Not all mothers are comfortable using an at-breast supplementer (Borucki, 2005), so discuss the range of feeding options and support her in her choice. Her decision may depend in part on whether she is close to full milk production, making some milk, or making little or no milk. For the pros and cons of each supplemental feeding method, see p. 814.

• •

As the young baby takes more milk from the breast, suggest his weight be checked regularly to be sure he gets enough—but not too much—supplement.

As the mother notices her young baby swallowing more milk and breastfeeding longer, she can start the process of gradually decreasing the amount of supplement given. Before doing so, however, suggest she have her baby weighed by his healthcare provider and schedule weight checks at least weekly on the same scale. If the baby is younger than 3 months and his weight gain slips below about 20 g (about two-thirds of an ounce) per day or about 140 g (5 oz.) per week, this is a sign the baby needs more supplement. (For weight gains appropriate for older children, see p. 205- Table 6.1.

The mother needs to strike the delicate balance of feeding the young baby the least amount of supplement needed, while actively breastfeeding as much as possible to stimulate faster milk production. Babies need to stay well nourished. If the mother cuts back on the supplement too quickly and the baby becomes weak from low milk intake, this can compromise his ability to breastfeed. On the other hand, if the mother gives too much supplement, the baby will be too full to breastfeed often or long enough to stimulate faster milk production. Regular weight checks will help the mother keep the baby's milk intake in the right range.

If babies 0-3 months skip below a weight gain of 20g per day or 140 g per week, more supplement is needed.

Sometimes milk production increases all at once rather than gradually. In one U.S. case report, a mother induced lactation for her adopted baby by breastfeeding with an at-breast supplementer, breast pumping every 3 to 4 hours, and taking metoclopramide, a prescribed galactogogue (Cheales-Siebenaler, 1999). The mother saw no milk for the first 3 months, then she started using oxytocin nasal spray, and she began to see sprays of milk each time she pumped. By the next week, she began pumping 4 ounces (118 mL) at each pumping. After that she was able to stop pumping and supplementing and fully breastfeed.

• •

If needed, test-weighing and milk expression can help a mother gauge her milk production.

The baby's weight gain is the best indicator of how close the mother's milk production is to meeting his needs. But if the mother wants more information, the following two strategies can tell her more about the baby's milk intake and her milk production.

Test-weighing. If the mother wants to know her baby's milk intake at the breast, one reliable way is by using a very accurate (to 2 g) electronic baby scale for pre- and post-feed weights (Meier et al., 1994). These scales are available in many hospitals and lactation clinics. In some areas, they can be rented for home use from breast pump rental stations. See Table 6.3 on p. 222 in the chapter "Weight Gain and Growth" for average milk intake at the breast per feeding by age. But make sure the mother knows that the amount of milk her baby consumes at one feeding will vary by his hunger (just like in adults) and by time of day. Although knowing averages can be helpful, be sure she is also aware that daily milk intake among healthy, thriving breastfed babies can vary by as much as three-fold (Kent et al., 2006). Also, one test-weight is not enough information to gauge a baby's 24-hour milk intake. If the mother has the scale for home use, doing test-weights around the clock provides much more information.

Milk expression. Expressing milk can provide clues to a mother's milk production, but it is less reliable than test-weighing because not all mothers can express milk effectively, especially in the beginning. One Australian study of 28 breastfeeding mothers with established and ample milk production found 11% were unable to express much milk using any of the seven pump cycling patterns tested (Kent, Ramsay, Doherty, Larsson, & Hartmann, 2003). Milk expression is a learned skill that takes many mothers time and practice to master. Even when the most effective pump (usually a rental pump) is used, factors unrelated to milk production—such as pump fit and a mother's responsiveness—can affect her yield. For details, see p. 825- "Breast Pumps" in the "Tools and Products" appendix.

Other signs of milk intake, such as audible swallowing and diaper output, are not completely reliable, but can provide clues on a daily basis.

Audible swallowing. When babies swallow milk at the breast, some describe the sound as "kah," "kah," "kah." After milk ejection, most babies swallow after every suckle or two, with occasional pauses. As breastfeeding continues, milk flow slows, and as a baby's hunger is satisfied, he swallows less often. If the mother can't hear her baby swallow at all, he may just be a quiet feeder. But if the baby's audible swallowing stops early in the feeding or he falls asleep quickly, suggest the mother help keep him actively breastfeeding longer by first helping him take the breast deeper and then using breast compression (see p. 804- "Breast Compression" in the "Techniques" appendix) for a faster milk flow.

Diaper output. Although two U.S. studies found that diaper output was not a completely reliable gauge of milk intake during the first 14 days of life (Nommsen-Rivers, Heinig, Cohen, & Dewey, 2008; Shrago, Reifsnider, & Insel, 2006), during the first 6 weeks, the number of stools per day can provide a general idea of whether a baby is getting enough milk. The mean number of stools per day among exclusively breastfeeding newborns was four, but some passed as many as eight per day. Because formula can be constipating, formula supplements can affect the number and consistency of a baby's stools, making diaper output an even less reliable indicator. When ultra-absorbent disposable diapers/nappies are used, wet diapers can be difficult to count. However, a baby's urine should always be light colored and not strong-smelling. One Indian study suggested its 1,000 relactating mothers expect their babies to have at least six urinations during the day and two at night, with the urine staying clear and colorless (Banapurmath et al., 2003).

During the first 6 weeks, number of stools per day can provide a general idea of whether babies are getting enough.

Keep track of stools and feedings. Although it is only a rough sign of milk intake, suggest that as the mother decreases the supplement, between regular weight checks, she make note every day of:

- The number of her baby's stools at least the size of a U.S. quarter (2.5 cm) or larger.
- How many feedings he takes at the breast and his response to them (active suckling? accepts the breast well?).
- Amount of supplement given, when given, and total given over 24 hours.

It can be reassuring for a mother to see her baby's stooling stay steady as she decreases the supplement. Although four stools per day the size of a U.S. quarter (2.5 cm) or larger are average at first, after 6 weeks of age stooling frequency often decreases, sometimes dramatically. Exclusively breastfed babies older than 6 weeks may go as a long as a week between stools, which is not a cause for concern as long as the baby is gaining weight well.

Whenever low milk intake is a possibility in a younger baby, the mother should know the signs of dehydration.

Knowing the signs of dehydration can be reassuring when the baby is thriving and can act as a warning if he's not. The following are signs the baby needs more supplement:

- Two or fewer wet diapers in 24 hours
- When skin is pinched, it stays pinched looking

- Extreme sleepiness or lethargy
- Dry mouth and eyes

Signs the baby's milk intake at the breast is increasing include less supplement taken, changes in stool consistency, and others.

Less supplement taken. As the baby takes more milk during breastfeeding, he will become more interested in the breast and less interested in finishing the supplement. When the mother notices this, suggest she reduce the amount of supplement. If she's using an at-breast supplementer, she might start the feeding without it and end the feeding with it.

Other signs of increasing mother's milk intake. When the baby is supplemented with formula, another sign of increasing mother's milk intake is looser and milder-smelling stools. If the baby was ill, his health and temperament may improve. A diaper rash or other skin condition may improve. The baby may become more alert and active, or if he was tense before, he may seem more relaxed.

Follow baby's lead. When the baby continues to gain at least 5 oz. (140 g) per week while the amount of supplement decreases, it means the mother's milk production is filling the gap. If, at any time, the baby starts spending more time at the breast (or suddenly seems finished faster), lets milk dribble out while suckling, or otherwise seems full, decrease the supplement at that feeding. If there is supplement left after several feedings in a row, cut back a little on the amount in the container. Unless it is obvious the supplement needs to be decreased faster, cutting back by a half-ounce (15 mL) per feeding works well for many mothers and babies, with a day or two in between cut-backs.

Less supplement in the morning, more in the afternoon. An alternative to cutting back the same amount at every feeding is to handle feedings differently at different times of day. Most mothers have the most milk available in the morning and less as the day goes on. Reducing supplements may work best by offering less at the first morning feeding and more in the evening. As the mother's milk production continues to increase, the first morning breastfeeding is usually the best time to eliminate the supplement completely. If the baby seems comfortable after receiving less supplement than usual, continue to gradually reduce the amount offered without leaving the baby hungry. Avoid giving him more supplement than he actually wants.

The mother may notice a dip in milk production around the time of menstruation.

Even if, due to the hormonal changes involved in menstruation, the mother's milk production decreases slightly at the beginning of menstrual bleeding, with a few days of increased breastfeeding, milk production usually rebounds.

BREASTFEEDING IN EMERGENCIES

During emergencies, breastfeeding is key to infant health and survival.

Even in developed countries during times of peace and plenty, babies fed non-human milks are at greater risk of illness and death (Chen & Rogan, 2004). However, during war, famine, drought, earthquake, hurricane, or other natural disasters, the risks of formula-feeding increase exponentially as conditions deteriorate and challenges, such as the following occur:

- Poor hygiene
- Limited or contaminated water supplies
- Less availability of food of all types, including infant formula
- Limited access to refrigeration and heat to warm formula and sterilize containers
- Increased exposure to illness from crowds
- Decreased availability of medical treatment

Breastfeeding during emergencies can mean the difference between life and death.

A baby fed non-human milks during an emergency is more likely to become ill from exposure to organisms in contaminated water and food and is at risk for underfeeding when formula becomes scarce. The non-breastfeeding baby is also more likely to become ill because he is lacking the antibodies and other immunities in mother's milk. In some emergencies, infant mortality related to formula-feeding has increased by as much as 25-fold (UNICEF, 2008).

Breastfeeding becomes vital during emergencies because it provides babies with unlimited safe food and water during their first 6 months, a safe partial food and water source afterward, and protection from illness. Along with all this, breastfeeding also enhances the close, loving bond between mother and baby, delays the mother's return to fertility, and enables her to nourish her baby with the more limited resources she has available.

While appropriate breastfeeding practices are important to all mothers and babies, during an emergency, they may make the difference between life and death. Suggest any mother in an emergency:

- Start breastfeeding within an hour or so of birth.
- Maintain as much mother-baby skin-to-skin contact as possible after birth for increased infant stability.
- Breastfeed often and well day and night.
- Breastfeed exclusively for the first 6 months.
- Offer appropriate solid foods to the baby at around 6 months of age.
- Continue breastfeeding for at least the first 2 years (WHO, 2001).

Malnourished and stressed mothers can produce ample milk for their babies.

Babies sometimes die unnecessarily due to common misconceptions about breastfeeding in emergencies. For example, in Iraq during the Gulf War, the misconception that women could not produce adequate milk when malnourished and under great stress led some officials, journalists, and relief workers to discourage breastfeeding (Burleigh, 1991). Although psychological stress can delay a mother's milk ejection, breastfeeding is most definitely possible and milk will continue to be produced if the mother keeps breastfeeding. One U.S. study found that perceived stress, sleep difficulty, and fatigue were not related to milk volume (Hill, Aldag, Chatterton, & Zinaman, 2005). In 1978 after a devastating earthquake in Guatemala, continued breastfeeding by local mothers played a key role in infant survival (Solomons & Butte, 1978).

Mothers' milk quality only suffers under famine conditions.

As described in Chapter 14, "Nutrition, Exercise, and Lifestyle Issues," women can produce ample milk even on very inadequate diets. A meta-analysis examining research from around the globe found that only when famine or near famine conditions continue for weeks does a mother's milk production or milk quality suffer (Prentice, Goldberg, & Prentice, 1994). One Dutch study found that even in famine conditions, milk production may be only slightly affected among previously well-nourished mothers with good body stores (Smith, 1947). If famine occurs, providing breastfeeding mothers with food is less costly and results in better health outcomes than providing formula for babies.

No association has yet been found between a mother's fluid intake and her milk production. One U.S. study found that increasing breastfeeding mother's fluid intake by 25% did not affect their milk production (Dusdieker, Booth, Stumbo, & Eichenberger, 1985).

In her article "Infant Feeding in Emergencies," UK author Marion Kelly wrote: "Since the ability to breastfeed is remarkably resistant to the effects of maternal undernutrition and psychological stress, the notion that many mothers who were breastfeeding pre-crisis will need to use breast-milk substitutes once disaster has struck should be rejected by those with responsibility for relief programmes" (Kelly, 1993, p. 111).

• •

Trained relief workers and experienced breastfeeding mothers can provide mothers with breastfeeding support.

In all cultures, breastfeeding support during emergencies is important. But in cultures where formula use is common, many women need help in gauging when their milk production is adequate and how to increase production if necessary. Even in countries like Sweden, where breastfeeding is the norm, women often worry about not making enough milk, even when their milk production is ample (Hillervik-Lindquist, 1991). "Perceived insufficient milk" does not necessarily mean the mother's milk production is low. It may be the result of a mother's misinterpretation of normal infant behaviors or unrealistic expectations of how often a newborn breastfeeds. For this reason, health workers in emergencies need to understand breastfeeding norms, so they can help mothers learn to gauge adequate milk production and encourage mothers to feed more often if they need to increase milk production.

Part of any relief effort should be the establishment of policies that make breastfeeding information and support a priority. Some have found an effective way to support breastfeeding is to find mothers who are currently breastfeeding in the affected areas or those who have previously breastfed with the knowledge and skills to help other mothers (Kelly, 1993). These women can counsel mothers on overcoming common challenges, such as nipple pain, low milk production, and mastitis; provide information on increasing milk production for those mostly breastfeeding; and provide information on relactation or induced lactation for those who had never breastfed or who had weaned prior to the emergency.

• •

Exclusive breastfeeding, wet nursing, induced lactation, and relactation should be encouraged in emergencies, as even partial milk production can save babies' lives.

To prevent infant deaths in an emergency, birth mothers who had previously weaned or never breastfed can be encouraged to relactate (Jelliffe & Jelliffe, 1977; WHO, 1998) and adoptive mothers can be encouraged to induce lactation. Even partial milk production provides a source of safe, uncontaminated food and protection from illness. See the previous sections for the strategies used for relactation and induced lactation.

In an emergency, the main focus should be on basic approaches, such as putting the baby to breast for feedings and for comfort and using hand expression for breast stimulation when the baby is not at the breast. Frequent mother-baby skin-to-skin contact day and night should also be encouraged. If available, galactogogues can be used to enhance milk production.

During emergencies, infant formula should only be given to those caring for babies who cannot fully breastfeed, along with intensive support to improve survival rates.

When a war or natural disaster occurs in a developing country, the first impulse among many in developed nations is to offer aid in the form of infant formula (Gribble, 2005c). But this can cause more problems than it solves. Because exclusive breastfeeding is not common anywhere in the world, even where breastfeeding is the norm, making formula available puts breastfeeding babies at risk. Providing formula to the affected areas can increase formula-related deaths, undermine mothers' confidence in breastfeeding, and create an unnecessary dependence on commercial products. Breastfeeding mothers may decide to start giving their babies formula because they think anything from developed countries is "better." In 1991, for example, during relief efforts in Iraq, although Kurdish mothers were told by British health personnel about the health risks of infant formula, many mothers "expressed skepticism on the grounds that the practice had originated in the West" (Kelly, 1993, p. 116). Relief workers need to know that when breastfeeding babies are fed formula it will decrease the mother's milk production and increase the baby's risk for formula-related illness and death. Use of infant formula actively and passively harms babies' immune systems, making them vulnerable to infection and death from diarrhea and pneumonia.

Providing infant formula during emergencies can undermine breastfeeding, increasing the risk of infant death.

When an emergency occurs in areas where breastfeeding is not yet the norm, health risks to babies increase when formula is no longer easily available and hygiene deteriorates. In these areas, relief workers wanting to support breastfeeding may encounter the extra challenge of dealing with traditional practices that undermine breastfeeding. During the war in Bosnia, for example, many formula-fed babies died when formula became scarce and safe preparation became a challenge. However, traditional practices, such as scheduled breastfeeding and early and regular use of formula, undermined mothers' milk production (Ademovic, 1998). Lack of access to infant formula can kill within a few days. After Hurricane Katrina in New Orleans, formula-fed infants died because they did not have access to formula or human milk.

If formula is provided in a crisis area, this should be done only under existing international guidelines (IFE, 2007), which include:

- Limiting formula distribution to specifically defined situations (WHA, 1994)
- Guaranteeing its availability as long as the baby requires it (until at least 6 months of age)
- Providing formula only in unbranded, generic packaging so sales are not promoted
- Distributing the formula only to babies younger than 12 months of age who are partially weaned along with clean water, fuel and containers for heating and sterilization, instructions and measuring tools, and extra medical support for formula-related illness, such as treatments for diarrhea, and specific plans for breastfeeding promotion to offset the availability of formula

Easily cleaned feeding cups may also need to be provided in areas where hygiene is poor to avoid the use of feeding bottles and nipples/teats, which are not recommended because they are easily contaminated. Extra food allowances may also be offered to breastfeeding mothers as an incentive for continued breastfeeding.

Promoting the survival of babies in emergencies must involve promotion of exclusive breastfeeding and measures that help women achieve this. This includes:

- Giving mothers priority access to food and other resources
- Providing "safe spaces" where mothers can care for their babies and receive breastfeeding help
- Preventing the uncontrolled distribution of infant formula or other milk products

RESOURCES FOR PARENTS

Relactation

Websites

http://www.who.int/child_adolescent_health/documents/who_chs_cah_98_14/en/ --World Health Organization's 1998 booklet, "Relactation: Review of Experience and Recommendations for Practice" is free and downloadable.

Induced Lactation

Websites

www.fourfriends.com/abrw/ --The Adoptive Breastfeeding Resource Website was established in 1997 and reflects a variety of viewpoints and perspectives from a worldwide pool of experts on induced lactation and an opportunity for adoptive mothers to interact.

www.asklenore.info –Location of the Protocols for Induced Lactation created by Lenore Goldfarb and Canadian pediatrician Jack Newman.

Breastfeeding in Emergencies

Websites

http://whqlibdoc.who.int/hq/2004/9241546069.pdf --World Health Organization's 2004 brochure "Guiding Principles for Feeding Infants and Young Children During Emergencies" is free and downloadable.

http://www.ennonline.net/ --U.K.'s Emergency Nutrition Network, whose Infant and Young Child Feeding in Emergencies (IFE) Core Group offers downloadable information for the public and relief workers on protecting breastfeeding during emergencies.

REFERENCES

Abejide, O. R., Tadese, M. A., Babajide, D. E., Torimiro, S. E., Davies-Adetugbo, A. A., & Makanjuola, R. O. (1997). Non-puerperal induced lactation in a Nigerian community: case reports. *Annals of Tropical Paediatrics, 17*(2), 109-114.

Ademovic, M. (1998). Breastfeeding during wartime means safe, available food for baby. *BFHI News, 8*, 2-3.

Auerbach, K. G., & Avery, J. L. (1980). Relactation: a study of 366 cases. *Pediatrics, 65*(2), 236-242.

Banapurmath, C. R., Banapurmath, S. C., & Kesaree, N. (1993). Initiation of relactation. *Indian Pediatrics, 30*(11), 1329-1332.

Banapurmath, S., Banapurmath, C. R., & Kesaree, N. (2003). Initiation of lactation and establishing relactation in outpatients. *Indian Pediatrics, 40*(4), 343-347.

Becker, G. E., McCormick, F. M., & Renfrew, M. J. (2008). Methods of milk expression for lactating women. *Cochrane Database of Systematic Reviews*(4), CD006170.

Biervliet, F. P., Maguiness, S. D., Hay, D. M., Killick, S. R., & Atkin, S. L. (2001). Induction of lactation in the intended mother of a surrogate pregnancy: case report. *Human Reproduction, 16*(3), 581-583.

Binns, C. W., & Scott, J. A. (2002). Using pacifiers: what are breastfeeding mothers doing? *Breastfeeding Review, 10*(2), 21-25.

Borucki, L. C. (2005). Breastfeeding mothers' experiences using a supplemental feeding tube device: finding an alternative. *Journal of Human Lactation, 21*(4), 429-438.

Bryant, C. A. (2006). Nursing the adopted infant. *Journal of the American Board of Family Medicine, 19*(4), 374-379.

Burleigh, P. (1991, June 10). Watching children starve to death: an exclusive look inside Iraq's devastated hospitals. *Time*, 36-37.

Bystrova, K., Matthiesen, A. S., Widstrom, A. M., Ransjo-Arvidson, A. B., Welles-Nystrom, B., Vorontsov, I., et al. (2007). The effect of Russian Maternity Home routines on breastfeeding and neonatal weight loss with special reference to swaddling. *Early Human Development, 83*(1), 29-39.

Cheales-Siebenaler, N. J. (1999). Induced lactation in an adoptive mother. *Journal of Human Lactation, 15*(1), 41-43.

Chen, A., & Rogan, W. J. (2004). Breastfeeding and the risk of postneonatal death in the United States. *Pediatrics, 113*(5), e435-439.

Colson, S., DeRooy, L., & Hawdon, J. (2003). Biological Nurturing increases duration of breastfeeding for a vulnerable cohort. *MIDIRS Midwifery Digest, 13*(1), 92-97.

Colson, S. D., Meek, J. H., & Hawdon, J. M. (2008). Optimal positions for the release of primitive neonatal reflexes stimulating breastfeeding. *Early Human Development, 84*(7), 441-449.

Czank, C., Henderson, J. J., Kent, J. C., Tat Lai, C., & Hartmann, P. E. (2007). Hormonal control of the lactation cycle. In T. W. Hale & P. E. Hartmann (Eds.), *Hale & Hartmann's Textbook of Lactation* (pp. 89-111). Amarillo, TX: Hale Publishing.

Daly, S. E., Owens, R. A., & Hartmann, P. E. (1993). The short-term synthesis and infant-regulated removal of milk in lactating women. *Experimental Physiology, 78*(2), 209-220.

de Melo, S. L., & Murta, E. F. (2009). Hypogalactia treated with hand expression and translactation without the use of galactagogues. *Journal of Human Lactation, 25*(4), 444-447.

De, N. C., Pandit, B., Mishra, S. K., Pappu, K., & Chaudhuri, S. K. (2002). Initiating the process of relactation: an Institute based study. *Indian Pediatrics, 39*(2), 173-178.

Dettwyler, K. A. (1995). Beauty and the breast. In P. Stuart-Macadam & K. A. Dettwyler (Eds.), *Breastfeeding: Biocultural Perspectives* (pp. 39-73). New York, NY: Aldine de Gruyter.

Dusdieker, L. B., Booth, B. M., Stumbo, P. J., & Eichenberger, J. M. (1985). Effect of supplemental fluids on human milk production. *Journal of Pediatrics, 106*(2), 207-211.

Goldfarb, L., & Newman, J. (2000). The protocols for induced lactation. Retrieved January 1, 2010, from http://www.asklenore.info/breastfeeding/induced_lactation/protocols_intro.html

Gribble, K. D. (2004). The influence of context on the success of adoptive breastfeeding: developing countries and the west. *Breastfeeding Review, 12*(1), 5-13.

Gribble, K. D. (2005a). Adoptive breastfeeding. *Breastfeeding Review, 13*(3), 6.

Gribble, K. D. (2005b). Breastfeeding of a medically fragile foster child. *Journal of Human Lactation, 21*(1), 42-46.

Gribble, K. D. (2005c). Infant feeding in the post-Indian Ocean Tsunami context: reports, theory and action. *Birth Issues, 14*(4), 121-127.

Gribble, K. D. (2005d). Post-institutionalized adopted children who seek breastfeeding from their new mothers. *Journal of Prenatal & Perinatal Psychology & Health, 19*(3), 217-235.

Gribble, K. D. (2006). Mental health, attachment and breastfeeding: implications for adopted children and their mothers. *International Breastfeeding Journal, 1*(1), 5.

Handlin, L., Jonas, W., Petersson, M., Ejdeback, M., Ransjo-Arvidson, A. B., Nissen, E., et al. (2009). Effects of sucking and skin-to-skin contact on maternal ACTH and cortisol levels during the second day postpartum-influence of epidural analgesia and oxytocin in the perinatal period. *Breastfeeding Medicine, 4*(4), 207-220.

Heinig, M. J., Nommsen, L. A., Peerson, J. M., Lonnerdal, B., & Dewey, K. G. (1993). Energy and protein intakes of breast-fed and formula-fed infants during the first year of life and their association with growth velocity: the DARLING Study. *American Journal of Clinical Nutrition, 58*(2), 152-161.

Hill, P. D., Aldag, J. C., Chatterton, R. T., & Zinaman, M. (2005). Psychological distress and milk volume in lactating mothers. *Western Journal of Nursing Research, 27*(6), 676-693; discussion 694-700.

Hillervik-Lindquist, C. (1991). Studies on perceived breast milk insufficiency. A prospective study in a group of Swedish women. *Acta Paediatrica Scandinavica. Supplement, 376*, 1-27.

Hormann, E. (1977). Breastfeeding the adopted baby. *Birth and the Family Journal, 4*, 165.

Hurst, N. M., Valentine, C. J., Renfro, L., Burns, P., & Ferlic, L. (1997). Skin-to-skin holding in the neonatal intensive care unit influences maternal milk volume. *Journal of Perinatology, 17*(3), 213-217.

IFE. (2007). *Infant and young child feeding in emergencies: operational guidance for emergency relief staff and programme managers*. Oxford, U.K.: Emergency Nutrition Network (ENN).

Ip, S., Chung, M., Raman, G., Trikalinos, T. A., & Lau, J. (2009). A summary of the Agency for Healthcare Research and Quality's evidence report on breastfeeding in developed countries. *Breastfeeding Medicine, 4 Suppl 1*, S17-30.

Jelliffe, D. B., & Jelliffe, E. F. P. (1977). Breast feeding: a key measure in large-scale disaster relief. *Disasters, 1*(3), 199-203.

Jones, E., Dimmock, P. W., & Spencer, S. A. (2001). A randomised controlled trial to compare methods of milk expression after preterm delivery. *Archives of Disease in Childhood. Fetal and Neonatal Edition, 85*(2), F91-95.

Kassing, D. (2002). Bottle-feeding as a tool to reinforce breastfeeding. *Journal of Human Lactation, 18*(1), 56-60.

Kelly, M. (1993). Infant feeding in emergencies. *Disasters, 17*(2), 110-121.

Kennedy, K. I. (2010). Fertility, sexuality, and contraception during lactation. In J. Riordan & K. Wambach (Eds.), *Breastfeeding and Human Lactation* (4th ed., pp. 705-736). Boston, MA: Jones and Bartlett.

Kent, J. C., Mitoulas, L. R., Cregan, M. D., Ramsay, D. T., Doherty, D. A., & Hartmann, P. E. (2006). Volume and frequency of breastfeedings and fat content of breast milk throughout the day. *Pediatrics, 117*(3), e387-395.

Kent, J. C., Ramsay, D. T., Doherty, D., Larsson, M., & Hartmann, P. E. (2003). Response of breasts to different stimulation patterns of an electric breast pump. *Journal of Human Lactation, 19*(2), 179-186; quiz 187-178, 218.

Kesaree, N. (1993). Drop and drip method. *Indian Pediatrics, 30*(2), 277-278.

Lozoff, B., & Brittenham, G. (1979). Infant care: cache or carry. *Journal of Pediatrics, 95*(3), 478-483.

Macrae, S., & Gribble, K. D. (2006). Why grandma can't pick up the baby. In S. Macrae & J. MacLeod (Eds.), *Adoption parenting: building a toolbox, creating connections*. Warren, NJ: EMK Press.

Matthiesen, A. S., Ransjo-Arvidson, A. B., Nissen, E., & Uvnas-Moberg, K. (2001). Postpartum maternal oxytocin release by newborns: effects of infant hand massage and sucking. *Birth, 28*(1), 13-19.

Meier, P. P., Engstrom, J. L., Crichton, C. L., Clark, D. R., Williams, M. M., & Mangurten, H. H. (1994). A new scale for in-home test-weighing for mothers of preterm and high risk infants. *Journal of Human Lactation, 10*(3), 163-168.

Mizuno, K., Nishida, Y., Mizuno, N., Taki, M., Murase, M., & Itabashi, K. (2008). The important role of deep attachment in the uniform drainage of breast milk from mammary lobe. *Acta Paediatrica, 97*(9), 1200-1204.

Morton, J., Hall, J. Y., Wong, R. J., Thairu, L., Benitz, W. E., & Rhine, W. D. (2009). Combining hand techniques with electric pumping increases milk production in mothers of preterm infants. *Journal of Perinatology, 29*(11), 757-764.

Nemba, K. (1994). Induced lactation: a study of 37 non-puerperal mothers. *Journal of Tropical Pediatrics, 40*(4), 240-242.

Nommsen-Rivers, L. A., Heinig, M. J., Cohen, R. J., & Dewey, K. G. (2008). Newborn wet and soiled diaper counts and timing of onset of lactation as indicators of breastfeeding inadequacy. *Journal of Human Lactation, 24*(1), 27-33.

Phillips, V. (1993). Relactation in mothers of children over 12 months. *Journal of Tropical Pediatrics, 39*(1), 45-48.

Prentice, A. M., Goldberg, G. R., & Prentice, A. (1994). Body mass index and lactation performance. *European Journal of Clinical Nutrition, 48 Suppl 3*, S78-86; discussion S86-79.

Schrager, S., & Sabo, L. (2001). Sheehan syndrome: a rare complication of postpartum hemorrhage. *Journal of the American Board of Family Practice, 14*(5), 389-391.

Seema, Patwari, A. K., & Satyanarayana, L. (1997). Relactation: an effective intervention to promote exclusive breastfeeding. *Journal of Tropical Pediatrics, 43*(4), 213-216.

Sert, M., Tetiker, T., Kirim, S., & Kocak, M. (2003). Clinical report of 28 patients with Sheehan's syndrome. *Endocrine Journal, 50*(3), 297-301.

Shrago, L. C., Reifsnider, E., & Insel, K. (2006). The Neonatal Bowel Output Study: indicators of adequate breast milk intake in neonates. *Pediatric Nursing, 32*(3), 195-201.

Slome, C. (1956). Nonpuerperal lactation in grandmothers. *Journal of Pediatrics, 49*(5), 550-552.

Slusher, T., Slusher, I. L., Biomdo, M., Bode-Thomas, F., Curtis, B. A., & Meier, P. (2007). Electric breast pump use increases maternal milk volume in African nurseries. *Journal of Tropical Pediatrics, 53*(2), 125-130.

Smillie, C. (2008). How infants learn to feed: A neurbehavioral model. In C. W. Genna (Ed.), *Supporting Sucking Skills in Breastfeeding Infants* (pp. 79-95). Boston, MA: Jones and Bartlett.

Smith, C. (1947). Effects of maternal undernutrition upon newborn infants in Holland (1944-1945). *Journal of Pediatrics, 30*, 229-243.

Solomons, N. W., & Butte, N. (1978). A view of the medical and nutritional consequences of the earthquake in Guatemala. *Public Health Reports, 93*(2), 161-169.

UNICEF. (2008). *The State of the World's Children: Maternal and Infant Health*. New York, NY: United Nations Children's Fund.

Uvnas-Moberg, K. (2003). *The Oxytocin Factor: Tapping the Hormone of Calm, Love, and Healing*. Cambridge, MA: Da Capo Press.

West, D., & Marasco, L. (2009). *The Breastfeeding Mother's Guide to Making More Milk*. New York, NY: McGraw Hill.

WHA. (1994). Resolution WHA 47.5. 47th World Health Assembly, May 9, 1994.

WHO. (1998). *Relacation: review of experience and recommendations for practice*. Geneva, Switzerland: World Health Organization.

WHO. (2001). *Optimal Duration of Exclusive Breastfeeding: Report of an Expert Consultation*. Retrieved 3/21/08. from http://www.who.int/nutrition/publications/optimal_duration_of_exc_bfeeding_report_eng.pdf.

Wieschhoff, H. (1940). Artificial stimulation of lactation in primitive cultures. *Bulletin of the History of Medicine, VIII*(10), 1403-1415.

Nipple Pain and Other Issues

Chapter 17

NIPPLE PAIN

In most cases, nipple pain is a solvable problem.

It is not unusual during the first 2 weeks of breastfeeding for a mother to have mild nipple pain that resolves as soon as her milk lets down (see next section). But moderate-to-severe pain and skin trauma are signs that either damage is being done or that the mother has a condition in need of treatment, such as mastitis or a bacterial or yeast infection. Unfortunately, many mothers who suffer from moderate-to-severe nipple pain do not seek help because they mistakenly believe or have been told that nipple pain is a normal part of breastfeeding.

Severe nipple pain is not normal.

Nipple pain increases a mother's risk of depression.

When breastfeeding is painful, a mother may begin to dread feedings, and this anxiety can lead to depression. Many studies (Li, Fein, & Grummer-Strawn, 2008; Sheehan, Krueger, Watt, Sword, & Bridle, 2001; Taveras et al., 2003; Woolridge, 1986) have found nipple pain among the most common reasons mothers give for premature weaning.

The effect of nipple pain on mood was described in an Australian study of 65 breastfeeding mothers who were asked to complete the Profile of Mood States (Amir, Dennerstein, Garland, Fisher, & Farish, 1996; Amir, Dennerstein, Garland, Fisher, & Farish, 1997). More than twice as many mothers with nipple pain rated as depressed as compared with the mothers without nipple pain (38% vs. 14%). After the nipple pain was resolved, about the same percentage of women in both groups rated as depressed. So when a mother is in pain and seems depressed, in some cases resolving her pain may also resolve her depression.

The intensity of a mother's pain may be affected by the severity of her nipple trauma and by her desire to breastfeed.

An Australian study of 69 mothers (Heads & Higgins, 1995) found that, not surprisingly, mothers whose nipples were more damaged felt more pain. But they also found an association between a mother's desire to breastfeed and her perception of nipple pain. Mothers with a strong desire to breastfeed perceived their pain as less than mothers who were not as motivated to breastfeed.

What's Normal at First?

Some mild nipple pain in the first 2 weeks is normal if it resolves with milk ejection and there is no skin trauma.

Most research (Centuori et al., 1999; Heads & Higgins, 1995; Hill & Humenick, 1993; Ziemer & Pigeon, 1993) indicates that 70% to 96% of Western women experience some nipple pain in the early weeks of breastfeeding. Called "transient soreness" by some (Smith & Riordan, 2010, p. 259), several U.S. and Australian studies (Henderson, Stamp, & Pincombe, 2001; Ziemer, Paone, Schupay, & Cole, 1990; Ziemer & Pigeon, 1993) found this nipple pain usually peaks on or around the 3rd day.

One possible reason this early nipple pain is so common is mothers' increased breast sensitivity after birth. Some theorize that mothers' heightened sensitivity to touch may promote the establishment of early milk production (Prime, Geddes, & Hartmann, 2007).

To reassure mothers experiencing this initial pain, lactation consultants Barbara Wilson-Clay and Kay Hoover share with mothers what they call the "30 second rule" (Wilson-Clay & Hoover, 2008, p. 47)—a mother can safely ignore nipple pain if she thinks her baby has taken the breast deeply and the pain resolves within 30 seconds. But if skin trauma develops or the pain lasts longer than 30 seconds, the mother should seek help.

Suggest the mother seek help if her nipple pain is intense or skin trauma develops.

If a mother experiences any of the following, suggest she seek help as soon as possible:

- Intense, toe-curling pain
- Pain lasting throughout the feeding
- Pain or a burning sensation between feedings
- Continuing pain with no improvement after a day or two of consistently trying to correct the cause

Continuing pain may also indicate the baby is not taking milk well from the breast.

Nipple Pain in the First Week

Ask the mother what day the pain started, when during the feeding she feels the pain, its intensity, and if there is trauma, where it is and what it looks like.

When the pain started may provide clues to possible causes (see Table 17.1).

- **After a couple days of comfortable breastfeeding.** Explore the possibility that breast fullness from an increase in milk production may be contributing to shallow breastfeeding. Suggest the mother breastfeed more often and use Reverse Pressure Softening (see p. 795 in the "Techniques" appendix) or express a little milk to soften the nipple and areola before putting the baby to breast.
- **At the beginning of the feeding.** If the baby is younger than 2 weeks old and the discomfort resolves after her milk starts to flow, this may be "transient soreness" or a sign of a shallow latch (also called shallow breastfeeding). If it lasts longer than about 30 seconds, suggest the mother try some of the positioning suggestions in the next section.
- **During the entire breastfeeding.** This mother needs help now. Possible causes include shallow breastfeeding, unusual infant oral anatomy (tongue tie, unusual palate, receding chin, etc.), strong suckling, or unusual nipple anatomy.
- **After feedings or in between.** If the mother is comfortable during breastfeeding and the pain starts afterwards, ask the mother to look at her nipple for any color changes when the pain begins. If there are color changes, consider vasospasm (white) or Raynaud's phenomenon (white, blue, and/or red).

The intensity and timing of the mother's pain will provide more clues. Again, transient nipple soreness typically peaks on or around the 3rd day.

There can also be visual clues to the cause of nipple pain and trauma:

- **Misshapen nipple after breastfeeding**. The nipple may look like the tip of a new tube of lipstick, flattened and pointed. If this happens consistently, this can lead to the damage described in the next point.
- **Cracks, bleeding, or a compression stripe** (a white line across the nipple face)—usually a sign of shallow breastfeeding (see the positioning

section in this chapter). Other possible causes include unusual oral anatomy in the baby, unusual nipple anatomy in the mother, or fast milk flow (baby squeezes the nipple in his mouth to slow the flow).

- **Starburst-shaped lesions in the center of the nipple** have been reported in engorged mothers, when milk flow is slowed by breast swelling (Wilson-Clay & Hoover, 2008, p. 49).

Ask the mother to describe her pain.

Her choice of words can provide clues. For example, she may describe the pain as dull or sharp, throbbing, stabbing, burning, or itchy.

Table 17.1. Nipple/Pain Trauma

Factors Contributing to Nipple Pain/Trauma in the First Week

More than one factor may be contributing to nipple pain. Consider:

Mother-Baby Factors

- Positioning/shallow breastfeeding—Nipple may look pinched or misshapen after feeding or areola may be bruised.
- Lips—Baby's lips sucked in.
- Suction—Baby removed from breast without first breaking suction.
- Fit—Nipple too large for baby's mouth.

Baby Factors

- Oral anatomy—Check for tongue-tie, short tongue, unusual palate, receding chin, tight labial frenulum.
- Strong or unusual suckling, clamping, biting, or clenching.

Mother Factors

- Engorgement—A taut breast can cause shallow breastfeeding.
- Vasospasm or Raynaud's phenomenon—Nipple changes color after feeding.
- Nipple anatomy—Nipple appears inverted, dimpled, etc.
- Use or misuse of pumps or products—(see next section) for pumps: check flange fit, level of suction, and cycling (not too slow in semi-automatic pumps); use of bottles or pacifiers/dummies; poorly fitting bras; wet breast pads, irritating creams/ointments

Mother-Baby Factors

Positioning and Shallow Latch

In the early weeks, shallow latch is one of the most common causes of nipple pain and trauma.

When the baby takes the breast deeply in his mouth, typically the mother's nipple extends to within about 5 mm of where baby's hard and soft palates join (Geddes, Kent, Mitoulas, & Hartmann, 2008; Jacobs, Dickinson, Hart, Doherty, & Faulkner, 2007). If the nipple reaches this depth, there is usually little friction or pressure, and breastfeeding is comfortable. Some call this area in the baby's mouth the "comfort zone" (Mohrbacher & Kendall-Tackett, 2005). Most cases of nipple pain and trauma can be resolved when the mother's nipple consistently reaches the comfort zone. When this happens, traumatized nipples can heal, even with continued breastfeeding.

• •

Ask the mother how she and her baby are positioned during breastfeeding and whether she supports her breast.

Dynamics that can contribute to shallow breastfeeding include:

Upright or side-lying feeding position, especially in the early weeks. See next point and the section "Gravity Can Help or Hinder" on p. 43 in the chapter, "Basic Breastfeeding Dynamics."

Unstable position. If a baby is held in a precarious position, the baby may shift during feedings, which can pull the nipple out of the comfort zone. If a baby feels unstable, he may also pull at the breast or clamp down.

Mothers should be comfortably seated when they breastfeed.

Supporting the breast at an unnatural level. When a mother supports her breast at a height different from its usual resting place, this can become tiring. If she releases it after her baby takes the breast, its weight may pull the nipple out of the comfort zone, leading to shallow breastfeeding. If this happens, suggest the mother either support her breast throughout the feeding or—even easier—use a feeding position that allows the baby to take the breast in its usual resting place. See p. 133 in the chapter "Challenges at the Breast" for positioning strategies for large-breasted mothers.

• •

At first, laid-back, semi-reclining feeding positions may make breastfeeding easier and more comfortable.

While the mother and baby are learning to breastfeed, suggest she start by leaning back into "biological nurturing" positions (see Chapter 1). U.K. research indicates that babies take the breast more easily on their tummies, supported by their mothers' semi-reclined body (Colson, Meek, & Hawdon, 2008). These positions simplify breastfeeding by making it unnecessary to teach "latch-on techniques" to every mother in order to achieve deep breastfeeding. In these positions, the effects of gravity on the mother's and baby's inborn feeding behaviors usually accomplish this automatically. In a study of 40 English and French mothers during the first month postpartum, when mothers used these laid-back positions:

> …there was no need to line up nose to nipple and wait for mouth gape or to assess tongue position as suggested by those teaching [positioning and attachment] skills. Gravity pulled the baby's chin and tongue forward. Together the anti-gravity reflexes often triggered the degree of mouth opening needed to achieve pain-free, neonatal self-attachment even when the baby appeared to be in light sleep (Colson et al., 2008, p. 448).

In upright or side-lying feeding positions, gravity pulls baby's body away and deep breastfeeding is more difficult to achieve. For details, see Chapter 1, "Basic Breastfeeding Dynamics."

• •

Breastfeeding while the baby sleeps can also increase a mother's breastfeeding comfort.

In laid-back feeding positions, U.K. research found that babies can breastfeed effectively even when asleep (Colson, DeRooy, & Howdon, 2003). The DVD "Biological Nurturing: Laid-Back Breastfeeding" illustrates how putting babies to breast while asleep "blunts" their feeding reflexes, making comfortable breastfeeding easier to achieve (Colson, 2008).

In laid-back, semi-reclining positions, many mothers have one or both hands free to help their baby. U.K. research provided some insights into mothers' inborn feeding behaviors, such as foot stroking, which triggers toe grasping, which releases lip and tongue reflexes, which helps the baby take the breast and feed. The researchers noted that mothers "appeared to trigger instinctively the right reflex at the right time" (Colson et al., 2008, p. 446).

Mothers' inborn feeding behaviors may also contribute to more comfortable breastfeeding.

Despite good feeding dynamics, nipple pain and trauma can occur when mothers and babies have fit issues or if they have the anatomical variations described in later sections—such as tongue tie, unusual palates, and unusual nipples.

If nipple pain is an issue when using laid-back feeding positions, the mother may need to give her baby more help or there may be other issues.

When a mother finds breastfeeding painful, ask "What if breastfeeding didn't hurt?" and try simple strategies, such as pulling down on babies' lips or chin after the baby has taken the breast in laid-back positions (Colson, 2009). See "Techniques" appendix for a description of breast shaping and asymmetrical latch, other approaches which may help.

Baby's Lips Sucked In

Ask the mother if her baby's top and bottom lips are flanged out when at the breast.

If either lip is sucked in, suggest she gently pull it out.

Removing Baby from Breast

Taking the baby off the breast without breaking suction first can cause nipple pain.

Whenever possible, encourage the mother to let the baby stay at the breast until he comes off on his own. But at those times when the mother needs to take the baby off the breast before he is finished, suggest first breaking the suction. The mother can do this by gently inserting a finger in the corner of the baby's mouth, pulling down on the baby's chin, or pressing down gently on the breast.

Fit

Both the mother's and baby's physical characteristics affect their breastfeeding "fit." For example, a tongue-tied baby might breastfeed well from a soft, flexible breast, but if the same baby tried to breastfeed from a taut breast, this could lead to problems, such as ineffective feeding and nipple trauma.

If a mother's nipples are too wide or long for her baby's mouth, this may cause nipple pain.

When breastfeeding is going well, a baby usually takes the nipple and some of the areola into his mouth. But if the mother's nipple is too wide or long for the baby to accommodate more than just the nipple itself, this can cause pain and trauma, as well as feeding aversion and ineffective milk removal (Wilson-Clay & Hoover, 2008).

If a too-large-nipple for a too-small-mouth causes pain and trauma, first every effort should be made to make breastfeeding work (optimizing how baby takes the breast, use of a nipple shield, or any other strategy that works). If nothing helps, reassure the mother that babies grow very quickly and that she can establish her milk production by expressing her milk until her baby's mouth grows enough to comfortably breastfeed, which will usually be within the first few weeks. See p. 466 in the chapter, "Milk Expression and Storage" for strategies on how to establish full milk production through milk expression.

Baby Factors

Oral Anatomy

Tongue tie

Ask the mother if anyone in their family is tongue tied, if she hears a clicking sound during breastfeeding, and if her baby can stick his tongue past his lower gum.

The frenulum is the string-like membrane that attaches the tongue to the floor of the mouth. A short frenulum, sometimes called tongue tie or ankyloglossia, may run in families (Ballard, Auer, & Khoury, 2002).

If tongue tie is the cause of nipple pain and trauma, this will likely be obvious within the first few days of breastfeeding (Ballard et al., 2002). One U.S. study found that 25% of tongue-tied babies had trouble breastfeeding (Messner, Lalakea, Aby, Macmahon, & Bair, 2000). In a U.K. study of 215 tongue-tied babies with breastfeeding problems, 77% of their mothers had nipple pain or trauma (Griffiths, 2004).

A baby's oral anatomy can cause nipple pain.

Different types of tongue tie affect breastfeeding dynamics differently. When a baby cannot extend his tongue past his lower gum, this is a sign of one of the four types of tongue tie (for more details see the section "Tongue Tie" on p. 118 in the chapter "Challenges at the Breast"). An Australian study of 24 tongue-tied babies having feeding problems used ultrasound during breastfeeding and found one group of babies (37%) had difficulty staying on the breast and took the breast shallowly, compressing the tip of the mother's nipple (Geddes, Langton, et al., 2008). The other group (46%) could stay on the breast and take the breast deeper, but compressed the base of the nipple. The mothers in both of these groups had nipple pain and reduced milk flow.

Difficulty staying on the breast and a clicking sound during breastfeeding are both signs that the baby cannot maintain suction at the breast and may not be taking milk effectively. When breastfeeding is painful, a baby with these issues should be checked for a short frenulum and other unusual oral anatomy.

• •

When breastfeeding a tongue-tied baby is painful, several strategies may help.

A good first step is to try to achieve deeper breastfeeding. But even with optimal breastfeeding dynamics, if feedings are still painful or ineffective, discuss clipping the frenulum and other options. For details, see p. 123 in the chapter, "Challenges at the Breast." In one U.K. study (Hogan, Westcott, & Griffiths, 2005), breastfeeding improved in 95% of the babies who had frenotomies.

Short tongue and receding chin

If a receding chin or short tongue is contributing to painful breastfeeding, suggest the mother position the baby tummy down for feedings.

When the baby breastfeeds on his tummy, gravity helps bring the tongue forward (Marmet & Shell, 2008). Research suggests that breastfeeding in these positions may make feedings go more smoothly for both mothers and babies (Colson et al., 2008).

Palate

Unusual palates—high, bubble, grooved—sometimes contribute to painful breastfeeding.

Unusual palates do not always cause painful breastfeeding. Types of palates reported to contribute to pain during breastfeeding include: bubble palate, grooved or channel palate, and high palate (Snyder, 1997). Babies who are intubated for long periods may develop grooves in their palates or high, narrow arches (Wilson-Clay & Hoover, 2008; Wolf & Glass, 1992)

An average (or "reference") infant palate is smooth and sloping. If a baby with an average palate is given a finger to suck pad side up, he will comfortably draw it back into his mouth about 1.5 inches (3.75 cm)—near where the soft and hard palates join—and the entire length of the finger will stay in contact with the palate. If a baby has a bubble palate, a gap will be felt above the finger, which may be shallow or deep, round or oval. Some babies with bubble palates are most comfortable with the nipple drawn up into the bubble, which can cause discomfort during breastfeeding.

The baby with a grooved or channel palate has a thin groove along the length of the palate, which may affect the baby's ability to maintain suction at the breast or, like a bubble, the groove may affect how deeply the baby draws the breast into his mouth. An average palate slopes up about a quarter inch (0.5 cm). A baby with a higher-than-average palate may have difficulty drawing the breast far enough back in his mouth for comfortable breastfeeding. A high palate may make it difficult for him to maintain suction, resulting in a clicking sound during breastfeeding.

As with a tongue tie, the infant's anatomy is only part of the story. Comfortable breastfeeding is also partly determined by the mother's breast and their breastfeeding position. If a mother has an inelastic nipple and taut breast tissue, for example, the "fit" between her breast and her baby's high palate may be less than ideal. However, if the mother's breast and nipple are more pliable, she might breastfeed comfortably. If a mother's breast is taut from engorgement or tissue swelling after birth, her comfort may improve quickly as the tautness subsides. Breastfeeding position can also be a factor. If gravity works against mother and baby, this can make a challenging fit even more challenging.

Suggest any baby with an unusual palate also be checked for tongue tie.

Experienced clinicians have noticed an association between unusual palates and tongue tie (Genna, 2008, p. 183). This may be because, as it develops, the baby's palate is shaped by its surroundings and can be molded by tongue movements (Palmer, 1998).

Tight labial frenulum

Ask the mother if her baby's lips flange out during breastfeeding.

The labial frenulum is the membrane that connects the lip with the gumline. A tight labial frenulum may contribute to ineffective breastfeeding or nipple pain and trauma (Wiessinger & Miller, 1995).

Torticollis

If baby keeps his head turned to one side, consider torticollis as a possible cause of nipple pain.

Ten percent of babies under 8 weeks old prefer to hold their heads to one side which can be a sign of torticollis, from the Latin words meaning "twisted neck." Torticollis is caused by a confined position in the womb (Boere-Boonekamp & van der Linden-Kuiper, 2001). When a baby's neck muscles are pulled to one side, this pulls his lower jaw, which can give a baby an asymmetrical look and possibly cause the baby pain (Mojab, 2007).

One U.S. article described 11 babies with asymmetrical lower jaws (Wall & Glass, 2006). All of the mothers had breastfeeding problems, including nipple pain, which may be the first symptom of undiagnosed torticollis. For strategies, see the chapter, "Challenges at the Breast."

Strong or Unusual Suckling

Some babies generate unusually high suction levels at the breast, which may contribute to painful feedings.

Most mothers are able to resolve painful breastfeeding by adjusting their positioning for deeper breastfeeding, by decreasing their engorgement, or with practice over time. But there are some mothers who continue to suffer painful feedings for weeks and even months.

One Australian study of 60 breastfeeding mothers compared the suction levels in babies' mouths during breastfeeding in 30 mothers who were comfortable breastfeeding with 30 who had continuing pain after other causes— candida, bacterial infection, vasospasm, dermatitis, infant tongue-tie, and torticollis— were ruled out (McClellan et al., 2008).

The babies in both groups spent about the same amount of time at the breast and about the same amount of time actively suckling. In the pain group, half of the mothers felt pain throughout the feeding, while the other half felt pain either at the beginning of the feeding or after a few minutes.

The study found that the babies of mothers in continuing pain generated significantly higher mean suction levels, both while actively suckling (152 mmHg vs. 97 mmHg) and when the suction was lowest (91 mmHg vs. 55 mmHg), as compared with the mothers who felt comfortable. The babies whose mothers were in pain also took less milk during breastfeeding despite the higher suction levels, which the researchers suggest is probably due to the pain disrupting the mothers' milk let-down.

Although the cause of the high suction levels isn't known, the researchers suggest that this may be one reason some women continue to find breastfeeding painful even after seeking help.

• •

Painful feedings can also occur when babies bunch or hump their tongues, clamp or clench at the breast, or do other kinds of unusual suckling.

Some babies are born with a tendency to clench or clamp down whenever something touches the inside of their mouth. This response (also known as "gum biting" among speech pathologists) is common among preterm babies, especially those born between 32 and 36 weeks gestation. But sometimes it occurs in a full-term baby. This may be due to a temporary immaturity in the baby that will be outgrown quickly (within days) or it may persist for some time.

Using laid-back feeding positions and having the baby take an active role in going to the breast can help cut down or eliminate clenching. When the baby goes to the breast, he will naturally extend his tongue before taking it, which will eliminate the touch of the breast to the lower gum ridge that can sometimes trigger this behavior.

If a baby bunches, humps, or sucks his tongue, suggest he be evaluated for tongue tie. Also consider the tongue exercises described in the "Techniques" appendix.

Mother Factors

Taut Breast Tissue

Taut breast tissue can make it difficult for the baby to draw the breast back to the comfort zone, leading to nipple pain and trauma.

When a mother's breast tissue is taut (either naturally occurring, due to engorgement, or from excess IV fluids during labor), the baby may be able to draw only the nipple into his mouth, leading to shallow breastfeeding, pain during feedings, and lower milk intake, which can aggravate engorgement.

Strategies to try include:

- Reverse pressure softening—a simple technique the mother can do herself (described on p. 795 in the "Technique" appendix) to push the swelling back into the breast, softening the nipple and areola.
- Expressing a little milk to soften nipple and areola.
- Breast shaping—see the "Techniques" appendix for descriptions.

When the baby is able to take the breast deeply, suggest the mother breastfeed more often to more quickly relieve her engorgement. See "Engorgement" in the chapter, "Breast Issues," for more strategies.

Some characteristics of the mother's breast or nipple may also lead to soreness.

Nipple Anatomy

Ask if one or both of the mother's nipples is flat or inverted or if there is anything unusual about her nipples.

Protruding (everted) nipples are not necessary for comfortable and effective breastfeeding, as many mothers can testify. But some studies have found that breastfeeding problems are more common among women with flat or inverted nipples and that these mothers may benefit from extra breastfeeding support and help in the early days (Dewey, Nommsen-Rivers, Heinig, & Cohen, 2003; Moore & Anderson, 2007). For details, see the later section "Flat and Inverted Nipples."

Vasospasm and Raynaud's Phenomenon

If the mother's nipple turns white after feedings and she describes her pain as "burning" or "shooting," consider vasospasm or Raynaud's phenomenon.

Vasospasm is a constriction of the blood vessels in the nipple that causes the nipple to blanch, or turn white. Compression of the nipple is a common cause, either due to shallow breastfeeding or the baby compressing the nipple to slow fast milk flow. When the nipple is compressed, it may look misshapen after feedings —pointed or creased, like the tip of a new tube of lipstick (Wilson-Clay & Hoover, 2008, p. 49). The blood flowing back to the nipple may cause a burning sensation, intense throbbing, or shooting pain.

Vasospasm strategies:

- **Try laid-back breastfeeding positions** if shallow breastfeeding is the cause. Also try breast shaping and other strategies to achieve deeper breastfeeding.
- **Apply warmth after feedings** via warm compresses, a heating pad, taking a warm shower, immersing the breasts in warm water (Walker, 2006), or using a hair dryer on warm. Warmth can prevent or relieve pain by increasing blood flow to the nipple Dressing warmly and avoiding exposing the nipple to air may help.
- **Avoid exposure to triggers such as cold, caffeine, alcohol, and nicotine**, which can cause vasoconstriction, as can some prescription drugs.
- **Take pain medication,** such as ibuprofen or whichever analgesia her healthcare provider recommends, to relieve the pain.
- **Consider prescription treatments for Raynaud's phenomenon** (below).

In one Canadian study, many mothers with diagnosed staphylococcus aureus infection of the nipple also suffered from vasospasms (Livingstone & Stringer, 1999). The interventions that resolved the vasospasms were instruction in improved breastfeeding technique, prescribed oral antibiotics, and avoiding nipple exposure to cold.

Raynaud's phenomenon, another possible cause of nipple vasospasm, is a vascular disorder that affects up to 20% of women of childbearing age (Anderson, Held, & Wright, 2004). Its triggers include exposure to cold and emotional stress, which cause narrowing of the arteries in fingers (and sometimes toes) that turns them white, blue, and/or red and causes painful tingling, burning, or numbness (Walker, 2006). Other triggers are caffeine, alcohol, nicotine, and some prescription drugs, such as beta blockers (Morino & Winn, 2007). A mother with Raynaud's phenomenon will probably have a history of these symptoms prior to delivery and many also have a history of migraine headaches or autoimmune disorders (Anderson et al., 2004).

For some mothers with Raynaud's, staying warm and avoiding cold is enough to prevent vasospasm and pain after feeding. For others, over-the-counter analgesics will keep them comfortable. If the pain is emotionally stressful for the mother, knowing the cause may provide needed reassurance (Morino & Winn, 2007). But if the pain is severe and this knowledge does not ease it, treatment may also be needed for breastfeeding to continue.

Raynaud's strategies:

Previously described strategies for vasospasms.

Prescribed treatments: Nifedipine, a calcium channel blocker that increases blood flow, is considered the most effective treatment. Recommended dose of 30 to 60 mg/day of sustained-release formulation is considered compatible with breastfeeding (Hale, 2008, p. 692). A 2-week course may be long enough to relieve the pain for most mothers without recurrence, but some may need to take it longer (Garrison, 2002).

Nitroglycerin ointment or spray (2%) is another possible treatment, although it may only be effective in 50% of the cases (Garrison, 2002). It is applied sparingly after feedings for 24 hours, and after that only when blanching occurs.

The effectiveness of nonprescription treatments, such as taking vitamin B_6 supplements, has not yet been determined.

Timing of nipple pain can help you narrow down its cause.

Nipple Pain at Any Time

Ask the mother her baby's age, when the pain started, if she's ever had nipple trauma, and if she has noticed any skin changes.

The baby's age can provide a clue. If the baby is older than about 4 months old, for example, teething may be a factor.

When the pain started. If nipple pain starts after weeks or months of comfortable breastfeeding, something has changed and the key is to find out what (see Figure 17.2). In an article for doctors, Australian physician and lactation consultant Lisa Amir asks the question: "What are the likely causes of the sudden onset of nipple pain in a breastfeeding woman?" and answers: Candida infection, eczema/dermatitis, vasospasm, pregnancy, trauma (such as a bite), and herpes infection (Amir, 2004).

Prior nipple trauma. Broken skin on the nipple increases a mother's risk of developing mastitis, as well as fungal and bacterial infections. One Canadian study of 227 mothers found that 64% of the mothers with moderate to severe nipple pain before 1 month after birth had bacterial infections (Livingstone, Willis, & Berkowitz, 1996).

Visible skin changes. The type of skin changes provides clues to possible causes. For example, an areola that looks inflamed , shiny, or appears to have white plaque may indicate candida or thrush (Francis-Morrill, Heinig, Pappagianis, & Dewey, 2004), pus in a traumatized nipple indicates a bacterial infection, a sore or lesions could be a herpes infection (Amir, 2004) or an infected Montgomery gland (Wilson-Clay & Hoover, 2008), and tiny pin-sized vesicles have been associated with impetigo (Thorley, 2000).

Ask the mother to describe the pain and what she thinks is the cause.

Type of pain may provide a clue. For example, if the pain is extreme and there is no broken skin or visible skin changes, consider candida or mastitis.

Mother's idea of the cause. The mother will know if there was an incident that caused skin damage, such as biting or pulling off the breast without breaking the suction.

Ask the mother if before the pain began she started using a breast pump or other product.

Table 17.2. Nipple Pain after 1 Month

Causes of Nipple Pain Starting after 1 Month

There may be more than one cause. Consider first:

Mother-Baby Interaction

- Positioning/shallow breastfeeding—older babies/toddlers may breastfeed acrobatically
- Candida/thrush—diagnosis/treatment needed

Baby Factors

- Teething and biting
- Pulling off the breast without breaking suction
- Unusual breastfeeding positions—usually an older baby or toddler

Mother Factors

- Overabundant milk production—can lead to unusual suckling to slow flow
- Blebs, blisters
- Dermatological problems—dermatitis, eczema, poison ivy/oak
- Sores—herpes, infected Montgomery glands
- Pregnancy—hormonal changes can cause nipple discomfort
- Referred pain—from mastitis, fibromyalgia, pulled muscle, pinched nerve, etc.
- Use or misuse of pumps or products—pumps: check flange fit, suction, and cycling; use of bottles or pacifiers/dummies; poorly fitting bras; wet breast pads, creams/ointments; contact with chlorine or other substances

Complications of Prior Broken Skin on the Nipple

- Mastitis
- Bacterial or fungal infection

Mother-Baby Factors

Candida/Thrush

Candidiasis is a fungal infection that can cause excruciating pain.

The pain associated with this fungal infection may be described as itching, burning, or stabbing. For details, see the later section, "Candida/Thrush."

Baby Factors

Teething and Biting

When a teething baby's gums feel sore, he may bear down on the breast, causing pain.

See the later section, "Teething and Biting."

Distractability and Acrobatic Breastfeeding Positions

If a distractible baby's pulling at the breast is causing nipple pain, suggest the mother have a finger ready to break suction.

As babies grow and become more aware of their surroundings, they may turn their heads to look at distractions without first breaking suction. If so, encourage the mother to be ready to break the suction. Over time, consistent removal from the breast discourages this behavior.

• •

If an older baby's acrobatic breastfeeding causes nipple pain, the mother can set limits.

Babies old enough to crawl and walk may want to take the breast in unusual positions that pull on the nipple, causing discomfort. Reassure the mother that breastfeeding needs to be good for them both and that it is fine for her to let her baby know that they will breastfeed only in positions that are comfortable for her, too.

Mother Factors

Overabundant Milk Production or Fast Milk Flow

Nipple pain may be due to a baby's attempt to make a fast milk flow more manageable.

When a mother has overabundant milk production or her milk flows very quickly, her baby may use his mouth or tongue to avoid being overwhelmed by milk. Lactation consultants Barbara Wilson-Clay and Kay Hoover note that some babies "...compress or crimp the nipple" to slow milk flow (Wilson-Clay & Hoover, 2008, p. 49). Suggest laid-back breastfeeding positions, as gravity may help baby better control milk flow without the need to compress the nipple.

Mastitis

A mother may perceive mastitis as nipple pain.

Depending on the location of her plugged duct, breast infection, or breast abscess, a mother's nipple pain may be a type of "referred pain" (see later section) that actually originates elsewhere, but that she perceives is in her nipple. In this case, the nipple pain will resolve when her mastitis resolves.

Blisters, Sores, Blebs, and Other Skin Problems

Blisters, sores, blebs, and any other skin problem can cause nipple pain.

For details, see the later sections.

Pregnancy

Due to hormonal changes, nipple pain during pregnancy is common.

Nipple tenderness may be one of the first symptoms of pregnancy, but this varies among women. Some feel nipple tenderness before missing their first menstrual period, while others experience it later. For strategies to make this type of nipple pain more manageable, see the section "Breastfeeding during Pregnancy" on p. 560 in the chapter "Sexuality, Fertility, Pregnancy, and Tandem Nursing."

Breast Pumps and Products

Breast pumps

Using a breast pump should not hurt, but if the flange doesn't fit or the vacuum is too high, pain and trauma can result.

Many mothers think "more is better" when it comes to pump vacuum. They mistakenly think that milk expression with a pump is like sucking a drink through a straw—the stronger the vacuum, the more milk they'll get. But that's not the way it works. Australian researchers found that setting the pump vacuum too high expressed less milk, because mothers became tense, inhibiting their milk let-down. The most effective vacuum setting is the highest that is comfortable (Kent et al., 2008; Ramsay et al., 2006).

So if a mother is experiences pain during or after pumping, the first suggestion is to try pumping at a lower vacuum setting.

The flange is the pump part a mother holds to her breast. Good flange fit is necessary for comfort and good milk flow. Flange fit is determined by the size of the opening (called the "nipple tunnel") the mother's nipple is drawn into while pumping. If the nipple tunnel is too small, her nipple may rub along its sides or get wedged. If the nipple tunnel is too large, too much areola may rub along the sides, causing pain and trauma. Both major pump companies, Ameda and Medela, offer a variety of flange sizes. For more details, see p. 826 in the "Tools and Products" appendix.

• •

Some breast pumps can generate unsafe vacuum levels or maintain vacuum too long.

One example is the old-style "bicycle-horn" hand pump. Some models have no vacuum control, which can result in too-high vacuum levels. Other types of hand pumps can be pulled or squeezed too vigorously. Some semi-automatic pumps, which require mothers press a button or plug a hole to start or release vacuum, cause nipple damage by maintaining vacuum for too long—some for up to 15 seconds—because they generate vacuum so slowly that it takes a long time to reach desired vacuum levels. Some mothers don't read their pump's instructions and neglect to release the vacuum when they should.

In some women, excessive pump vacuum has caused hemorrhages under the skin, called petechiae, which look like tiny, flat, round purple-red spots.

In contrast, what makes quality breast pumps safe and comfortable is their vacuum levels—high enough to express milk, but not so high as to cause tissue damage—and their quick and automatic release of vacuum, at least every 1 to 2 seconds.

Bottles and pacifiers/dummies

Some research suggests that the use of bottles and pacifiers may change the way some babies suckle, causing nipple pain.

One Italian study of 219 mothers found the use of a pacifier or feeding bottles in the hospital was associated with nipple pain at discharge (Centuori et al., 1999). Two Swedish studies found an association between bottle and pacifier use and the development of an "incorrect" sucking pattern during breastfeeding the researchers called "superficial nipple sucking," which could lead to nipple pain (Righard, 1998; Righard & Alade, 1997). A U.S. study of 328 mothers and newborns also found a link to bottle pacifier use in the first 48 hours and "sub-optimal breastfeeding behaviors" on Days 3 and 7 (Dewey et al., 2003).

If the baby has been receiving bottles, suggest to the mother that it might help the baby learn to suckle without causing pain if she used another feeding method to supplement. Discuss her options, which are described on p. 811 in the "Tools and Products" appendix.

Other products

Other products may also contribute to nipple pain and trauma.

These include:

- Bras that are so tight they compress the nipple, or bras with a rough seam that rubs and irritates the nipple.
- Topical creams or ointments (prescribed or over-the-counter), which can cause skin reactions (Cooper & Shaw, 1999; Huggins & Billon, 1993).
- Breast pads, when left wet for too long against the breast, can cause skin breakdown known as maceration (why our skin turns white and wrinkly after we've stayed in a bath too long).
- Any product that requires washing the nipple after using it, which can cause further irritation.

If any of these could be the cause of a mother's nipple pain, suggest she make a change, such as wearing a different bra, either discontinuing the nipple cream or ointment or asking her healthcare provider for a substitute, or trying a different product.

Referred Pain

An injury or condition elsewhere in a mother's body may be perceived as nipple pain.

When an injury or condition occurs along the same nerve pathway as the nipple, it may be perceived as nipple pain. Called "referred pain," this could be due to mastitis or an injury elsewhere. Ask the mother if she has a pulled muscle in her back, neck, or shoulder, if she has pain elsewhere in her body, or if she has been diagnosed with fibromyalgia.

Strategies for Nipple Pain and Trauma

When a mother has nipple pain, the first step should be to try to find the cause and, if possible, correct it. After that, comfort measures and treatments can be helpful, whether the cause is immediately correctable or not.

Comfort Measures

Comfort measures can provide pain relief during and after breastfeeding.

Commonly recommended comfort measures include:

- Take an analgesia that her healthcare provider recommends and is compatible with breastfeeding.
- Stimulate a milk ejection by expressing some milk before putting baby to breast.
- Breastfeed first on the least sore breast until the milk releases, then move the baby gently to the more painful breast.

- Apply a nipple-care product between feedings that decreases pain, such as USP-modified anhydrous lanolin or hydrogel pads (see next section).
- Wear breast shells between feedings to reduce clothing friction or pressure.

If breast shells are used, suggest the mother choose the shell backings with the large nipple openings (not the smaller openings designed for inverted nipples). To use breast shells safely, her bra cup must be large enough to accommodate the shells without putting undue pressure on her breasts. Consistent pressure on the breasts can cause mastitis in a mother already at increased risk for mastitis. Red circles on her breasts when she removes the shells indicate she needs a larger bra cup.

When the cause of painful breastfeeding cannot be corrected quickly, it may help to vary positions at each feeding.

Although varying positions at each feeding is not recommended when breastfeeding is going well, if the cause of the nipple pain cannot immediately be corrected, such as a short frenulum or an unusual palate, the mother may be more comfortable if she varies feeding positions, as spreading the pain and damage more evenly may make breastfeeding more tolerable. If the mother uses laid-back breastfeeding positions, she can adjust her baby's lie, so he approaches the breast from different angles at each feeding - vertically, horizontally, and diagonally. If she is upright, she can hold her baby at various angles in front of her body and along her side.

If the pain is severe enough that the mother does not want to breastfeed, suggest she express her milk while her nipples heal.

If the nipple pain is too intense for the mother to continue breastfeeding or she feels as though the pain is interfering with her relationship with her baby, she can express her milk and feed the milk to her baby for a short time using one of the alternative feeding methods described in the appendix "Tools and Products." For expression strategies to maintain her milk production, see p. 473 in the chapter, "Milk Expression and Storage."

Treatments for Nipple Trauma

Depending on the severity of the pain and trauma, different mothers will benefit from different approaches. In some cases, all a mother may need is to adjust her positioning and help her baby achieve deeper breastfeeding. If her pain and trauma are more severe, sharing comfort measures and strategies to speed healing may be important.

Moist Wound Healing

Mothers were once told to keep traumatized nipples dry, but wounds heal faster and pain is reduced with moist-wound healing treatments.

In the past, mothers with nipple damage were told to use drying techniques, such as a hair dryer set on low to dry the nipples, keeping bra flaps open, and using a sun lamp. However, researchers in the wound care field discovered decades ago that wounds actually heal 50% faster when the internal moisture of the skin is maintained and scabbing and crusting are avoided (Hinman & Maibach, 1963).

Internal moisture is not the same as surface wetness. Keeping a milk-soaked breast pad against the skin provides surface wetness, which can lead to chapping, skin breakdown, and slower healing. To maintain internal moisture, a moisture barrier must cover the nipple to prevent evaporation, drying, and scab formation.

Scabbing slows healing because it reduces the flow of nutrients to the wound and acts as a barrier to new cells, which must burrow under the scab. One drawback of scabbing unique to the breastfeeding mother is that nipple scabs pull off when baby breastfeeds, requiring the healing process to begin all over again.

To maintain a moisture barrier, the mother can use a product that maintains the usual amount of moisture on her nipples that is present in the skin, such as USP-modified anhydrous lanolin or hydrogel pads. If the moisture barrier is removed and she allows the skin to dry, healing will slow.

Maintaining a normal moisture balance has also been found to decrease pain, because the nerve endings are kept in a more normal environment and protected from outside stimuli (Mann Mertz, 1990).

Treatments by Stage of Nipple Trauma

Before considering using any of the following treatment options, the first step should always be to find and correct the cause of the trauma.

Appropriate treatment will vary by stage of trauma and by individual preferences.

The following four-stage system for rating nipple trauma was developed by this author to help standardize reporting of nipple trauma among healthcare providers and researchers (Lauwers & Swisher, 2005; Wilson-Clay & Hoover, 2008).

- **Stage I—Superficial Intact**, pain or irritation with no skin breakdown. May include redness, bruising, red spots, swelling.
- **Stage II—Superficial with Tissue Breakdown.** May include pain with possible abrasion, shallow crack or fissure, compression stripe, hematoma, and shallow ulceration.
- **Stage III—Partial Thickness Erosion**, skin breakdown involving the destruction of the epidermis to the lower layers of the dermis. May include deep fissure, blister, deep ulceration with more advanced erosion.
- **Stage IV—Full Thickness Erosion**, deeper damage through the dermis. May include full erosion of some parts of the dermis.

When choosing among the treatment options described in the following points, be sure to take into account the mother's preferences.

• •

Expressed milk is a treatment option appropriate for Stage I nipple trauma.

Using the mother's own expressed milk is sometimes recommended as an alternative to commercial products, because it is free, easily available, and has antibacterial properties. But when there is broken skin on the nipple, it dries quickly, so it does not provide moist wound healing. If the mother wants to use expressed milk as a treatment, suggest she first wash her hands, then express a few drops of her milk after breastfeeding and rub it gently into the skin, allowing her nipples to air dry afterward. In some cultures, skin irritations are commonly treated with human milk. The following studies examined its effects.

One Turkish study divided 90 mothers into three treatment groups on Day 1: 1) applied warm, wet compresses after breastfeeding 4 times per day, 2) applied expressed milk after all feedings and let it dry for a few minutes, and 3) kept nipples dry (Akkuzu & Taskin, 2000). The researchers found that the groups using warm, wet compresses and expressed milk developed the most cracks, which peaked on Day 3. Among these three groups, the mothers with cracked nipples who used expressed milk had a shorter duration of cracked nipples than the mothers who dried their nipples.

A U.S. study of 177 first-time mothers found no difference in pain intensity or breastfeeding duration in its four groups, all of whom received breastfeeding education: 1) expressed milk with air drying, 2) warm water compresses, 3) USP-modified lanolin, and 4) education only. The lanolin group, however, applied it only 4 times per day after feedings, rather than after every feeding as is recommended, losing the benefit of moist wound healing (Pugh et al., 1996).

An Iranian study compared expressed milk to peppermint water (a local treatment for nipple pain (Melli et al., 2007). In this study, 196 first-time mothers were randomized to one of two treatment groups: peppermint water or expressed milk. Only 9% of those who used peppermint water had nipple cracks compared with 27% who used expressed milk. Nipple pain was also lower in the peppermint water group.

USP-modified anhydrous lanolin is an option for Stage I and II nipple trauma.

Some studies indicate that if a mother applies enough USP-modified anhydrous lanolin after every breastfeeding to keep the nipples moist, this can reduce nipple pain and speed healing (Spangler & Hildebrandt, 1993). Some studies have found that when lanolin is not applied after every breastfeeding, it does not speed healing (Mohammadzadeh, Farhat, & Esmaeily, 2005; Pugh et al., 1996). For best results, suggest a mother apply just enough to keep the nipple moist between feeding, so it doesn't dry out. The baby's reaction needs to be a factor, too. In one study, mothers reported that after applying the lanolin ointment their babies had more difficulty taking the breast (Dodd & Chalmers, 2003, p. 492).

What makes USP modified anhydrous lanolin different from the lanolins used in the past is the removal of impurities that caused the skin reactions previously thought to be due to "wool allergy." Some brands contain higher levels of these impurities, which include pesticides, free lanolin alcohols, and detergents. The lower the levels of these impurities, the less likely a product is to elicit a reaction (Clark, Blondeel, Cronin, Oleffe, & Wilkinson, 1981).

Applying other topical creams and ointments (as well as oils and tea bags) to the nipple has drawbacks.

Depending on the ingredients in the nipple cream or ointment, drawbacks may include:

- An unfamiliar taste on the nipple, which can cause fussiness or breast refusal.
- The need to wash the nipple before breastfeeding, because it is unsafe for baby to ingest, which may involve rubbing the nipple and causing more damage.
- Clogged nipple pores, which can reduce oxygen to the wound and slow healing.
- Dry skin, if alcohol is one of the ingredients.
- Numbing baby's mouth or delaying mother's milk release, if numbing or anesthetic agents are included, such as in teething gels.

Applying vitamin E to the nipple—once a commonly recommended treatment—may cause:

- Skin reactions in mother. Although vitamin E rarely causes allergic reactions when ingested, it can when applied topically (Aeling, Panagotacos, & Andreozzi, 1973; Fisher, 1986, p. 151).
- Elevated vitamin levels in baby. Elevated vitamin E levels were found in babies after vitamin E was applied to damaged nipples (Marx, Izquierdo, Driscoll, Murray, & Epstein, 1985).

Some clinicians recommend applying olive oil to the nipple due to its anti-inflammatory properties, but this does not provide the advantages of moist wound healing, and there is the possibility of a reaction in mother or baby.

Although warm-water compresses are available to all mothers, they do not appear to be an effective treatment for nipple pain. In one Canadian study of 65 first-time mothers with nipple pain, warm water and tea-bag compresses were compared with no treatment. No difference was found between the effectiveness of the two types of compresses, and nearly 45% of the mothers dropped out of the study (Lavergne, 1997).

• •

Some types of hydrogel pads can be used with any stage of nipple trauma.

The U.S. Food and Drug Administration considers the use of hydrogels appropriate for all stages of skin damage (Dodd & Chalmers, 2003). Water-based and glycerin gel pads have been used for decades to speed wound healing in other parts of the body. But they were not commonly recommended for breastfeeding mothers until the publication of a 1997 journal article referring to them as "a new approach to an old problem" (Cable, Stewart, & Davis, 1997). However, within the next year, doubts were raised when a U.S. study found an association between their use and an increased incidence of infection.

Glycerin pads. In this U.S. study, 42 women with sore nipples were divided into two groups, both of whom received education about breastfeeding technique (Brent, Rudy, Redd, Rudy, & Roth, 1998). After feedings, one group used breast shells and USP-modified anhydrous lanolin; the other group used a glycerin-based hydrogel pad. Pain decreased significantly in both groups. This study was stopped early because significantly more women in the glycerin pad group developed infections (seven in the glycerin group compared with two in the breast shells/lanolin group). This was unexpected because the wound-healing literature indicated that these pads tended to decrease the rate of infection when used on other parts of the body.

In another study conducted by U.S. researchers and done in Latvia, 90 Latvian women with nipple pain were divided into three groups (Cadwell, Turner-Maffei, Blair, Brimdyr, & Maja McInerney, 2004). All mothers received instruction on breastfeeding technique. Thirty mothers wore glycerin gel pads between feedings, 30 applied USP-modified anhydrous lanolin and wore breast shells between feedings, and 30 received no products. None of the mothers developed an infection, and researchers found no difference in healing time or perception of pain among the three groups. The only difference was mothers' satisfaction with their treatment. All in the glycerin gel group were satisfied, whereas 9% (three) of the mothers in the other two groups were not.

Water-based pads. In a U.S. multicentered, prospective, randomized controlled clinical trial, researchers randomly assigned 106 mothers who had never breastfed to two groups within 24 hours after birth (Dodd & Chalmers, 2003). One group used USP-modified anhydrous lanolin. The other used water-based hydrogel pads. Both groups received instruction in breastfeeding technique and the use of their product. Before this study, both of these products were being routinely given to new mothers. The clinicians conducted this study to gain more information on which product gave better results. Although a "no products" group was part of the original study design, the research review board concluded it would be unethical to withhold products to mothers in pain. Because the last published study done on hydrogels in breastfeeding mothers found a high rate of infection, the researchers instructed each mother to wash her hands before handling the pad, to rinse the pads before breastfeeding, and rinse their breast before replacing the hydrogel on their breast to remove the baby's saliva (Brent et al., 1998). There were no infections in the hydrogel group and eight infections in the lanolin group, which was considered to be within normal limits. The researchers found a statistically significant difference in pain reduction between the two groups, with the mothers using the hydrogel pads reporting less pain. The mothers in the hydrogel group also used this product for fewer days than those in the lanolin group, a mean of 33 days versus 44 days.

• •

When choosing a hydrogel pad for a breastfeeding mother, ask some basic questions.

The answers to these questions may help choose a hydrogel pad.

Is this pad recommended for breastfeeding mothers? If not and the mother has a skin reaction to the product, the person or institution recommending it may be at legal risk. Also, some pads are not recommended for breastfeeding mothers because the residue they leave on the breast should not be ingested by babies (Davis, 2001).

How long does the pad last? The longer the wear time, the lower the long-term cost for the mother. At this writing, some pads can be used for only 4 hours, while others can be reused for up to 6 days.

Does the pad have a cloth backing? If so, rinsing the pad will wet the cloth and leave wet stains on mothers' clothing. Also, the need for a cloth backing indicates the product falls apart easily on its own and likely has a shorter wear time.

Does the pad have an adhesive border? The frequent removal of these pads for feeding or milk expression causes skin damage at the site of the adhesive (Ziemer, Cooper, & Pigeon, 1995).

• •

All-purpose nipple ointment (APNO) is a commonly recommended (but not yet researched) treatment that may be an option for Stage I, II, and III trauma.

Developed by Canadian pediatrician Jack Newman, this ointment requires a prescription and is created by a pharmacist, who mixes antibiotic, anti-fungal, and anti-inflammatory medications in the following proportions:

- Mupirocin 2% ointment (15 grams)
- Betamethasone 0.1% ointment (15 grams)
- Miconazole powder added so final concentration is 2% miconazole

According to Newman, APNO should be applied to the affected nipples sparingly after feedings, and when the pain is gone, the mother weans from it gradually over a week (Newman & Pitman, 2006, p. 110). Because the ingredients are absorbed into the mother's skin, the mother does not need to remove it before the next breastfeeding.

Topical ointments have not been found to effectively treat an active bacterial infection of the nipple (Livingstone & Stringer, 1999; Livingstone et al., 1996). If a mother's nipples show signs of an infection, such as visible pus, consider other treatments (see later section "Bacterial Infections").

In some unusual cases, a nipple shield may help reduce pain during breastfeeding.

Although a nipple shield may provide some pain relief, its use is not the best first choice. If pain and trauma are caused by shallow breastfeeding, using a nipple shield without first striving for deeper breastfeeding may not help. If the baby takes just the tip of the shield into his mouth, rather than the soft brim behind the tip, this would compress the nipple through the shield and cause continued pain.

But if the cause of the pain and trauma cannot be quickly corrected, a nipple shield may decrease the pain just enough to make breastfeeding tolerable for the mother until her baby either outgrows the problem or until it is corrected later, for example, a tongue-tied baby whose scheduled frenotomy has not yet taken place.

Blood swallowed from traumatized nipples is not harmful to the baby.

Assure the mother that any blood her baby swallows from damaged nipples will not be harmful to him. Emphasize that finding the cause of her nipple damage will allow her to correct it, so that her damaged nipples can heal and the bleeding will no longer be a concern.

Preventing Infections

Broken skin on the nipple increases a breastfeeding mother's risk of nipple infections and mastitis.

A mother's skin acts as a protective layer so that organisms cannot enter her body. Cracks or bleeding nipples create a point of entry for bacteria, fungi, and viruses on the nipple and within the breast. Many studies around the world have found an association between broken nipple skin and an increased incidence of mastitis (Amir, Forster, Lumley, & McLachlan, 2007; Fetherston, 1998; Foxman, D'Arcy, Gillespie, Bobo, & Schwartz, 2002; Kinlay, O'Connell, & Kinlay, 2001).

To prevent infection, some suggest mothers wash damaged nipples daily with mild soap, and after feedings, rinse the nipples and apply an antibiotic ointment.

If a mother had broken skin anywhere other than her nipple, the first recommendation would be to wash it with soap and water to prevent infection. In years past, breastfeeding mothers were told to avoid soap on their nipples, because it could be drying. But when there is nipple trauma, daily washing with warm soapy water and a warm water rinse in the bath or shower only makes sense.

When bacteria enter a wound, they create a sticky goo called a biofilm, which protects the bacteria and can prevent topical treatments from reaching the wound. A baby's saliva stimulates biofilm production. But gentle washing (known as "wound debridement") dislodges this biofilm to help prevent infection and promote healing (Ryan, 2007).

Cracked or bleeding nipples increase mother's risk of infection.

In their book, *The Breastfeeding Atlas*, Barbara Wilson-Clay and Kay Hoover recommend (based on a Cochrane review article) that mothers with nipple trauma use tap or saline water to rinse their nipples after every feeding (Fernandez, Griffiths, & Ussia, 2002; Wilson-Clay & Hoover, 2008). The purpose of this practice is to prevent the organisms in the baby's mouth from colonizing the wound. They also suggest that after rinsing, mothers apply a thin layer of mupirocin (Bactroban®) ointment to help prevent infection, which does not have to be removed and is compatible with continued breastfeeding (Hale, 2008, p. 666).

BACTERIAL, FUNGAL AND VIRAL NIPPLE INFECTIONS

Bacterial Infections

When a mother's nipples are not healing quickly or her pain continues despite correcting the cause, she may have a bacterial infection.

Although antibiotic ointments can sometimes prevent infection, once a bacterial infection is confirmed, the mother may need another type of treatment to resolve it.

In one Canadian study of 227 mothers with babies younger than 1 month, 64% of these mothers with moderate to severe pain along with nipple cracks, fissures, ulcers, and/or visible pus had *staphylococcus aureus* bacterial infections in their nipples (Livingstone & Stringer, 1999; Livingstone et al., 1996). An Australian study also found an association between nipple pain, fissures, and *staphylococcus aureus* (Amir, Garland, Dennerstein, & Farish, 1996).

To determine the most effective treatment for these infections, a Canadian study divided 84 mothers whose nipples cultured positive for *staphylococcus aureus* into four groups, each with a different treatment plan, and checked their progress 5 to 7 days later (Livingstone & Stringer, 1999). All of the treatment groups received instruction on breastfeeding technique. The percentage of mothers who improved varied by group:

- 9% in the instruction-only group.
- 16% in the group who applied the antibiotic ointment mupirocin after every feeding.
- 36% in the group who applied topical fusidic acid after every feeding.
- 79% in the group who received a 10-day course of oral antibiotics (dicloxacillin, cephalosporins, or erythromycin).

The researchers also found that within 7 days, 25% of the mothers not taking oral antibiotics developed mastitis, compared with 5% of the mothers taking oral antibiotics, so they stopped the study early due to ethical concerns, which may have affected the reliability of the results. The researchers concluded that oral antibiotics are an effective treatment in mothers with extremely sore, cracked nipples.

Impetigo, another type of bacterial infection, looks like watery, pinhead-sized blisters, and can be treated without interrupting breastfeeding.

Although impetigo rarely occurs on the breast or nipple, it is possible. In one Australian case, a mother reported unbroken, watery, pinhead-sized blisters in a line on her areola and nipple, and waves of pain in her breast (Thorley, 2000). When asked if her 15-month-old breastfeeding toddler had any blisters like this, she said she had seen some on his face, but thought they were chickenpox. The sores eventually scabbed over. The mother was diagnosed with impetigo and treated by her healthcare provider without interrupting breastfeeding.

Candida/Thrush

A yeast infection, also known as thrush or candidiasis, is an overgrowth of a fungus (yeast) that normally lives in our bodies.

Candida albicans, a one-celled organism, is a fungus that can cause thrush and vaginal yeast infections. It thrives in moist, dark environments, such as on the nipples, in the vagina, in the mouth, and in the baby's diaper area. This fungus normally lives in our bodies in balance with other organisms, but illness, pregnancy, antibiotic use, or other factors that throw the body out of balance can cause an unhealthy overgrowth. One U.S. study found that the use of bottles during the early weeks of breastfeeding increases the risk of candidiasis (Morrill, Heinig, Pappagianis, & Dewey, 2005).

If a mother's nipple pain starts within the first week after birth, a fungal infection is probably not the primary cause.

Typically, thrush takes some time to develop. During the first week of breastfeeding, nipple pain is much more likely to be caused by trauma from shallow breastfeeding or from a bacterial infection.

In some areas, thrush is common and the pain convinces many mothers to wean.

One U.S. study attempted to determine the incidence of thrush by comparing a control group of 40 non-pregnant, non-breastfeeding women with a study group of 100 low-income new mothers being seen at a Nevada clinic (Morrill et al., 2005). None of the mothers in the control group tested positive for candida. In the study group, however, after culturing the babies' mouths and the mothers' nipples/areola, breast folds, and milk 2 weeks after birth, the researchers found that 23% of the study group tested positive for candida, and 8% of these mothers already had thrush symptoms, such as burning nipples, painful breasts, stabbing pain in the breast, and shiny or flaky skin on the nipples/areola. By 9 weeks, 20% of these mothers had symptoms of a candida infection and 18% of their babies had obvious white patches in their mouths. Of the mothers and babies who cultured positive, 43% were still breastfeeding at 9 weeks, compared with 69% who were not. Of those who cultured positive at 2 weeks, 65% had weaned by 9 weeks, all reportedly due to pain. Of those who cultured negative at 2 weeks, 31% had weaned by 9 weeks, 38% due to pain and the other 62% for other reasons. The researchers acknowledged that this incidence of candida may not apply to other populations, because it could be related to hospital practices or the inadvertent spreading of candida by clinic personnel.

Few of the mothers with symptoms received treatment from their healthcare providers. Of the 20 women with symptoms, only five were treated for candida. Two of the five mothers who received treatment weaned before 9 weeks due to continuing pain. This may be in part because the candida infection was treated with nystatin, which in most cases is ineffective. One U.S. study found nystatin effective in babies in only 32% of cases, while oral fluconazole suspension was effective in 100% (Goins, Ascher, Waecker, Arnold, & Moorefield, 2002).

One symptom is not enough to determine whether thrush is causing a mother's nipple pain; a combination of symptoms is more reliable.

When a mother has nipple pain, it can be difficult to determine whether or not yeast is involved. Many mothers have been mistakenly treated for thrush only to discover their pain was from another cause, such as Raynaud's Phenomenon (Anderson et al., 2004) or a bacterial infection (Thomassen, Johansson, Wassberg, & Petrini, 1998). One U.S. survey found that 93% of U.S. physicians diagnose thrush based on symptoms only and do not use diagnostic tests (Brent, 2001).

In an effort to clarify which symptoms are reliable indicators of thrush, U.S. researchers studied 100 mothers and found that thrush is the likely cause of painful breastfeeding if a mother has the following symptoms together (Francis-Morrill et al., 2004):

- Shiny nipple/areola skin with stabbing pain
- Flaky nipple/areola skin and breast pain

If these symptoms appear alone, they are much less likely to indicate thrush.

In the baby, possible symptoms include:

- White patches on the baby's gums, cheeks, palate, tonsils, and/or tongue (if wiped off, they may look red or bleed)
- Diaper rash (may be simply red or red with raised dots)

Most babies have a white, milky coating on their tongue. This is not a sign of thrush unless white patches spread to the baby's cheeks and gums (Wilson-Clay & Hoover, 2008, p. 53). Some babies can have a yeast rash on their bottom, but not in their mouth.

Before a mother is treated for candida —especially if her baby has no symptoms— other possible causes of nipple pain should be ruled out, such as shallow breastfeeding, bacterial infection, mastitis, vasospasm/Raynaud's Phenomenon, and skin problems, such as eczema, psoriasis, and dermatitis (see later sections).

Shooting pains in the breast are unlikely to be due to candida in the milk ducts if that is the mother's only symptom.

Once it was thought that the most likely cause of shooting or burning pain in the breasts was a secondary yeast infection in or around the milk ducts, but research has found otherwise. One Swedish study found that three times more women with deep breast pain had bacterial infections rather than yeast infections (Thomassen et al., 1998). A U.S. study reported that 8 of 12 women with deep breast pain were treated with repeated courses of diflucon, a powerful anti-fungal drug before their histories revealed Raynaud's Phenomenon as the cause of their pain (Anderson et al., 2004). Another U.S. study compared expressed milk from 18 breastfeeding mothers without breast pain with the milk of 16 mothers with nipple and breast pain and detected no candida in the milk of either group (Hale, Bateman, Finkelman, & Berens, 2009). For more details, see the section "Deep Breast Pain" on p. 696 in the chapter, "Breast Issues."

Mothers with nipple damage may develop both bacterial and fungal infections and need treatment for both.

The all-purpose nipple ointment (see p. 649 in the "Treatments" section) is one treatment designed to help prevent both bacterial and fungal infections, although if a bacterial infection is confirmed, oral antibiotics may also be needed (see the section "Bacterial Infections").

Treatment options for thrush vary by practice and availability.

If thrush is diagnosed by a healthcare provider, to prevent recurrence, both mother and baby should be treated at the same time, even if one of them has no visible symptoms (Chetwynd, Ives, Payne, & Edens-Bartholomew, 2002).

Thrush treatment options for baby:

Over-the-counter treatments

- **Gentian violet**. To use: dip cotton swab in a 0.5% or 1% solution and swab inside baby's mouth on cheeks, gums, and tongue once or twice daily for 3 to 7 days. (Avoid stronger concentrations, which can cause sores in baby's mouth.) Stop after 4 days if symptoms are gone. Gentian violet can be used with other antifungals. Rat studies indicate gentian violet is only carcinogenic when ingested daily in large amounts (Newman & Pitman, 2006, p. 118). It stains clothing purple.

Treatments requiring a prescription

- **Nystatin suspension.** Apply 1 dropperful in each cheek 4 to 8 times daily for at least 2 weeks. It is most effective if used after every feeding. One U.S. study found nystatin effective in only 32% of its cases, while oral fluconazole suspension was effective in 100% (Goins et al., 2002).
- **Miconazole gel.** Apply the 25 mg gel (not available in the U.S.) 4 times daily. One German study found it faster and more effective than nystatin (Hoppe, 1997).
- **Clotrimazole gel**. Pharmacists make this oral gel by crushing a 10 mg clotrimazole lozenge and mixing it with 5 mL of glycerin or 3 mL of methylcellulose. Apply to baby's mouth every 3 hours for five applications (Amir & Hoover, 2002).
- **Fluconazole.** Give 6 mg/kg oral suspension via dropper as a first dose followed by 3 mg/kg/day once daily for 2 weeks (Amir & Hoover, 2002).

Treatment options for mother:

Over-the-counter treatments

- **Gentian violet.** Dip cotton swab in 0.5% or 1% solution and swab nipple/areola once or twice a day for 3 to 7 days. Stop after 4 days if pain is gone. It stains clothing purple. It can be used in combination with other antifungals.
- **Miconazole.** Cream or lotion (2%). Apply to nipples/areola 2 to 4 times daily for 7 days (Amir & Hoover, 2002).
- **Ketoconazole.** Cream (2%). Apply to nipples/areola 2 to 4 times daily at least 2 days after symptoms disappear (Amir & Hoover, 2002).

Treatments requiring a prescription

- **Clotrimazole**. Both over-the-counter and prescription versions are available. For OTC versions: Apply to nipples/areola after feedings 2 to 4 times daily for at least 2 days after symptoms disappear. Prescribed version: Pharmacists make a gel by crushing a 10 mg clotrimazole lozenge and mixing it with 5 mL of glycerin or 3 mL of methylcellulose. Apply to nipples/areola every 3 hours for five applications (Amir & Hoover, 2002).
- **Nystatin cream or ointment.** Apply 4 times per day for 14 days. Note: Nystatin is much less effective than other treatment options (see "baby" above).

- **Nystatin with triamcinolone (corticosteroid).** Use cream or ointment. Apply to nipples/areola 4 times daily until at least 2 days after symptoms disappear.
- **All-Purpose Nipple Ointment.** See p. 649 in "Treatment" section for components and use.
- **Oral fluconazole.** Used when topical treatments are ineffective. Take 400 mg loading dose, then 100 mg 2 times daily for at least 2 weeks. Continue for 1 week after pain is gone (Newman & Pitman, 2006, p. 120). The single-dose treatment for vaginal yeast infections will not usually be effective.

Breastfeeding can continue during thrush treatment; the mother may first feel worse before she feels better.

In mild cases of thrush, once treatment has begun, a mother may begin to feel relief in 1 to 2 days. In more severe cases, it can take 3 to 5 days or longer. When a mother is taking oral fluconazole, it may take a week or longer for the pain to disappear, because rather than killing the yeast, fluconazole prevents it from reproducing. Encourage the mother to take her medication for the full course, since the thrush may recur if she stops the medication when the symptoms disappear.

During treatment, the mother's symptoms may seem worse for a day or two before they improve. Suggest she rinse her nipples with clear water and air dry them after each breastfeeding, as thrush thrives on milk and moisture. Before the pain has gone, encourage her to use the comfort measures described earlier in this chapter.

After treatment, if there is a recurrence of thrush, encourage the mother to take precautions to prevent it from recurring again.

Thrush can be harbored in many places, and it can spread to other members of the family. If it recurs, suggest the mother:

- Ask for treatment for her partner and, if breastfeeding more than one, the other sibling.
- Wash her hands often, especially after changing diapers and using the toilet.
- Wash baby's hands often if he sucks thumb or fingers.
- If used, boil pacifiers, bottle nipples, or teethers once a day for 20 minutes to kill the thrush. After 1 week of treatment, discard them and buy new ones.
- If used, boil daily for 20 minutes all breast pump parts that touch the milk.
- If breast pads are used, use disposable pads and discard after each feeding.
- Wash toys that have been in the baby's mouth in hot, soapy water and rinse well.
- Use paper towels for hand drying. Discard after use.

Research indicates that freezing does not kill yeast (Rosa, Novak, de Almeida, Mendoca-Hagler, & Hagler, 1990), but no one is sure if expressed milk can cause a recurrence. Suggest the mother give the baby any milk that was expressed and stored during a thrush outbreak while they are being treated. If that is not possible or practical, suggest she boil the milk to kill any yeast before giving it to the baby.

Viral Herpes Infections

Herpes sores can occur on the nipple, are spread by contact, and can be dangerous to the newborn.

Herpes simplex 1 (cold sores) and 2 (genital herpes) are two different herpes viruses spread by contact with the sores. They are small, painful, fluid-filled, red-rimmed blisters that dry after a few days and form a scab. Genital herpes sores can be spread to the breast.

Herpes has proved fatal to newborn babies up to 3 weeks of age (Sullivan-Bolyai, Hull, Wilson, & Corey, 1983). If a pregnant woman or her partner has recurrent herpes, she should talk to a healthcare provider knowledgeable about herpes and breastfeeding to decide what precautions to take. If a sore on the nipple or breast is suspected of being herpes, a culture should be done and the results should be available within a few days.

If a mother is waiting for the results of her culture or herpes on the breast has been confirmed, she can continue to breastfeed if the sores can be covered, so the baby does not touch them. But if the sores are on the nipple, areola, or anywhere else the baby might touch while breastfeeding, the mother should express milk from that breast until the sores heal. She can continue to breastfeed on the unaffected breast. If the mother's hand or breast-pump parts touch the sores while expressing milk, they may contaminate her milk with the virus, and the milk should be discarded. If the mother's hand or breast-pump parts do not come touch the sores, the baby may be fed the milk.

• •

Serious complications from herpes are much less likely in babies older than 1 month.

Although herpes can be dangerous to a baby younger than 1 month, there are case reports of older babies touching their mother's herpes sores while breastfeeding without developing complications. There is also a documented case of a breastfeeding 15-month-old with a cold sore in his mouth who passed herpes to his mother's breast (Sealander & Kerr, 1989). Although an older baby is not likely to develop life-threatening complications from herpes, suggest the mother take steps to avoid spreading it to her child, as the sores can be very painful for a week or more and may make eating and drinking difficult (Newman & Pitman, 2006, p. 215).

OTHER SKIN PROBLEMS

Skin problems that occur anywhere else on the body can also occur on the breast and nipples and may be unrelated to breastfeeding.

Ask the mother to describe the skin problem and gather other information to help determine the cause.

Some questions to ask a mother with skin problems include:

Has the mother recently used any cream, ointment, pads, or other product on or near her nipples? Eczema and other types of dermatitis can develop on the nipples when irritating nipple products are used. Nipple inflammation can occur as a reaction to ingredients in some nystatin creams, a prescribed candida treatment (Cooper & Shaw, 1999; Huggins & Billon, 1993).

Has she used a new laundry product or toiletry product, like cologne, deodorant, hair spray, or powder near her breasts? In some mothers, these can cause irritation.

Has she used any devices on her nipples, like a breast pump, breast shells, nipple shields, or nipple suction devices? Too-high suction levels can sometimes cause skin damage, and exposure to the plastics of breast shells or pump flanges may cause a reaction in some sensitive mothers (Wilson-Clay & Hoover, 2008, p. 54).

Does she have a health problem and/or is she taking any medication? Skin problems can indicate an allergic reaction to some medications. Certain health problems increase the risk of skin reactions. For example, one mother with celiac disease, which increases the risk of dermatitis, developed painful eczema on her nipples while breastfeeding. With her second child, medical treatment resolved the eczema (Amir, 1993). When eczema is the cause, mothers may notice vesicles that erupt and become crusted (Wiener, 2006).

Is her baby eating solid foods, teething, or taking medication? Mothers can react to medication and/or teething gels in a baby's mouth. If the mother is sensitive to certain foods, eczema can develop on the mother's nipples when the baby breastfeeds with particles of these foods still in his mouth. Rinsing the baby's mouth with water before breastfeeding or eliminating the irritating food from the baby's diet for a while may help.

Does she or her child have a similar skin problem anywhere else on their bodies or a history of allergic skin reactions? Skin problems unrelated to breastfeeding can spread to the nipple. In that case, the mother may be familiar with the problem, such as psoriasis, and the treatments that work for her and just want to know the effect, if any, of these treatments on breastfeeding. A mother with poison ivy on the nipple probably has the rash in other areas, too. With poison ivy, as long as the mother's breasts and nipples have been washed and the oil from the plant removed, it is safe for the baby to breastfeed (Wilson-Clay & Hoover, 2008, p. 55). See also the example in the previous section of the mother and child with impetigo (Thorley, 2000). A history of allergic rashes or other skin reactions raises the strong possibility that the problem is dermatological rather than lactation-related (Porter & Schach, 2004).

• •

Continued pain, other symptoms, and slow or no healing are signs the mother should see her healthcare provider.

In a U.S. report of 20 mothers who saw a lactation consultant for unusual skin problems on or near the nipple and who were later referred to a dermatologist, the authors concluded that with appropriate treatment mothers with these unusual skin conditions were able to resume breastfeeding without pain within a few days (Huggins & Billon, 1993). They suggest that a mother with skin problems consider seeing a healthcare provider (specifically a dermatologist, if possible) when:

If a mother continues to have pain even after intervention, she should see her healthcare provider.

- She continues to feel significant pain during breastfeeding (especially burning or stinging pain), even when baby is taking the breast deeply.
- Nipple trauma heals unusually slowly or has stopped completely.
- Blisters, rash, scaling, crusting, or oozing sores appear on her nipples, are healing slowly, or healing has stopped.
- Nipples show no sign of improvement, even after treatment.

If a mother with eczema on her nipples does not improve with treatment, she should be seen by her healthcare provider to rule out Paget's disease.

Paget's disease is an uncommon form of breast cancer. It accounts for 1% to 3% of breast cancers and is sometimes mistaken for eczema (Chen, Sun, & Anderson, 2006). It usually appears on one nipple, comes on gradually, has an irregular but distinct edge, and the nipple is almost always affected, sometimes seeming to disappear. A mother whose eczema does not clear up within 3 weeks of treatment should see her healthcare provider right away to rule out this possibility (Barankin & Gross, 2004). Because its symptoms appear minor, many mothers postpone seeing their healthcare provider for as long as 30 weeks (Duff, 1998). If the mother waits this long, her odds of survival are much lower. Early detection is vital.

NIPPLE BLISTERS AND BLEBS

Blisters

A clear blister is usually caused by friction and/or high vacuum.

A blister may form on the tip of the nipple if the baby is breastfeeding shallowly and putting undue pressure on the end of the nipple. Discuss the basics of achieving deep breastfeeding (see the first chapter). A laid-back breastfeeding position may help, and achieving deeper breastfeeding may be all that's needed to reduce the pain and prevent the blister from recurring.

To open a blister, suggest the mother first apply warm, wet compresses before breastfeeding.

The moisture will soften and the heat will thin the skin, which may cause the blister to open. If not, see the later point on opening a bleb for more suggestions.

'Blebs' or Milk Blisters

A milk blister, or "bleb," may or may not be painful and appears to be associated with plugged milk ducts.

One type of white spot on the nipple is called a "bleb" or "milk blister." Its cause is still not fully understood. Some think a bleb could be a plug— perhaps caused by a granule of thickened milk—blocking the milk from flowing at the nipple. Some think blebs may be caused by a thin layer of skin blocking the opening of a milk duct from the outside. One medical textbook suggests they may be small pressure cysts that form at the end of the milk duct (Lawrence & Lawrence, 2005, p. 300).

Many have observed that these white spots sometimes coincide with bouts of mastitis, but the cause and effect is unclear (Newman & Pitman, 2006; Noble, 1991; Riordan & Wambach, 2010). Does the bleb cause the mastitis by blocking the flow of milk from the duct? Or does the bleb form as a result of the mastitis, which caused the milk to thicken in a duct? At this writing, no one knows for sure.

If the bleb is not painful, no treatment is needed. It may resolve on its own over time.

A white spot on the nipple may be due to other causes.

White nipple spots due to other causes may or may not be painful. These could be caused by a build-up of dead skin, like cradle cap, which can be removed by rubbing it with a lubricating oil like lecithin (Lawrence & Lawrence, 2005, p. 301; Wilson-Clay & Hoover, 2008, p. 56). In *The Breastfeeding Atlas*, lactation consultants Barbara Wilson-Clay and Kay Hoover note that some mothers report a white spot after the baby has bitten the nipple, which is caused by an accumulation of saliva and milk moisture under skin edges (p. 56). They recommend the mother clean it like she would any bite wound and apply topical antibiotic ointment to prevent infection (for details, see the "Preventing Infections" section on p. 650 earlier in this chapter).

Another possible cause of a white spot on the nipple is candida or thrush. When a mother has thrush, she may develop a small blister-like sore on her nipple. Before assuming a mother has a bleb, first rule out these other possibilities.

If a bleb is painful, there are several ways the mother can try to resolve it on her own.

First, suggest the mother apply wet heat to the bleb, either with warm compresses or by soaking the nipple in warm water (lying on her side in a bathtub or leaning forward into a sink or basin of warm water). Then suggest she rub the nipple with a damp cloth to remove any excess skin (Riordan & Wambach, 2010). Some also suggest lubricating the nipple with olive oil (Wilson-Clay & Hoover, 2008, p. 56). After this, suggest she try to express milk from that duct by compressing the areola behind the plug. In some cases, mothers can express a thickened string of milk, which may help open the duct and keep it open.

If the bleb is painful and persists despite these treatments, suggest the mother see her healthcare provider to open it.

The blister can be opened with a sterile needle. In some cases, when the duct is opened, milk from behind the plug will flow and bring relief. In other cases, it will be dry.

After the bleb has been opened, suggest the mother wash it with a mild soap and rinse well with water once a day to prevent infection. Another way to help prevent infection is to apply a thin layer of a topical antibiotic ointment, such as mupirocin, to her nipples after feedings. For more details, see the "Preventing Infections" section on p. 650 in this chapter.

To prevent recurring blebs, some dietary changes and lecithin supplements may help.

If a mother continues to experience recurring blebs and/or plugged ducts, some suggest reducing saturated fats in her diet and taking a lecithin supplement (Eglash, 1998). Suggested dosages of lecithin range from 1 tablespoon per day (Lawrence & Lawrence, 2005, p. 299) to 1 tablespoon 3 to 4 times a day or one to two 1,200 mg capsules 3 or 4 times per day (Newman & Pitman, 2006, p. 126).

FLAT AND INVERTED NIPPLES

Protruding (everted) nipples are not necessary for effective breastfeeding, as many mothers with flat and inverted nipples can testify. Most babies are happy to suck on anything they can get into their mouths, including adult arms, shoulders, and necks, none of which have protruding nipples.

Types of Nipples

Flat nipples do not protrude or become erect when stimulated or cold.

See **Figure 17.1.**

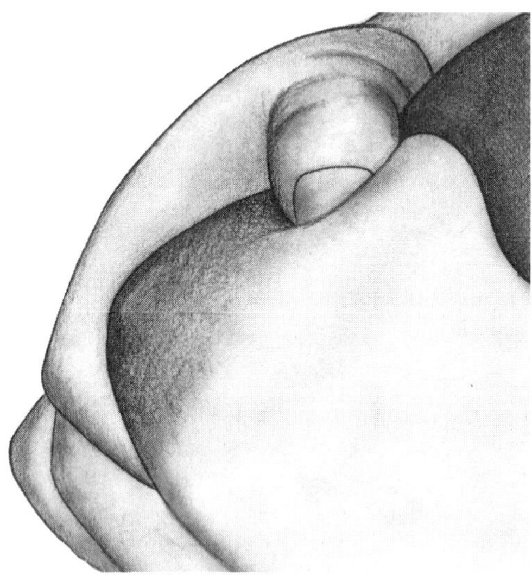

Figure 17.1. Flat nipple *©2010 Christian Bressler, used with permission*

Inverted nipples pull in rather than protrude when the mother's areola is compressed.

The mother can determine whether one or both of her nipples are inverted nipples by doing what some call the "pinch test," gently compressing the areola about an inch (2.5 cm) behind the base of the nipple. If her nipple protrudes, it is not inverted (even if it appears inverted at rest). If the nipple pulls in or becomes concave (**Figure 17.2**), it is a true inverted nipple.

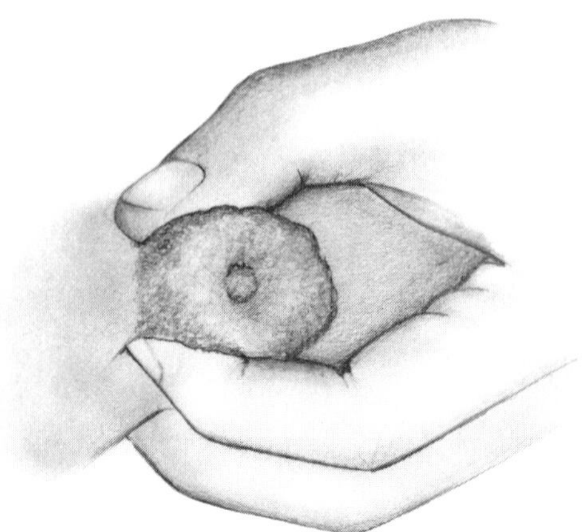

Figure 17.2. Inverted nipple *©2010 Christian Bressler, used with permission*

There are different types and terms for inverted nipples and explanations for their cause.

Nipple inversion has been described by many as being caused by tiny bands of connective tissue, called adhesions, that attach the nipple to the inner breast tissue and pull in the nipple. Some attribute nipple inversion to very short milk ducts that draw the nipple in (Chandler & Hill, 1990). Others assert that nipples invert because they contain less dense connective tissue beneath the nipple (Terrill & Stapleton, 1991). Some plastic surgeons have proposed a grading system for inverted nipples based on the amount of connective tissue (like scar tissue) they contain and how easily they can be made to protrude manually (Han & Hong, 1999).

There are different degrees of nipple inversion. Some invert only slightly, and a baby who suckles normally will draw them out with no difficulty. However, at first a preterm or sick baby may find the same nipples challenging. Other nipples invert moderately or severely, which means that when compressed they retract deeply and can make taking the breast difficult and in some extreme cases impossible.

A dimpled or folder nipple is a type of inverted nipple in which only a part of the nipple is inverted. It will not protrude or harden when stimulated, but the mother can pull it out with her fingers (Figure 17.3). It does not, however, stay out afterwards. Some types of dimpled and inverted nipples can cause nipple pain, especially in the early weeks. Barbara Wilson-Clay and Kay Hoover describe the experience of one mother with dimpled nipples whose nipple tissue inside the fold was adhered and breastfeeding and pumping left this inner tissue moist, causing skin breakdown from too much moisture (maceration) and bleeding (Wilson-Clay & Hoover, 2008, p. 43). In this case, the mother was able to resolve her problem by holding the nipple open until it dried and by keeping this area very clean.

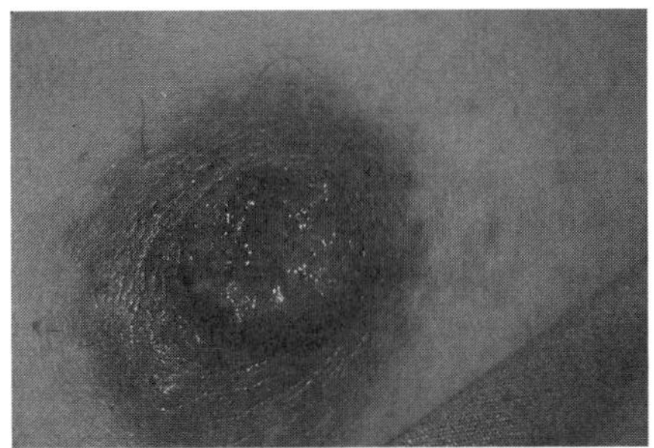
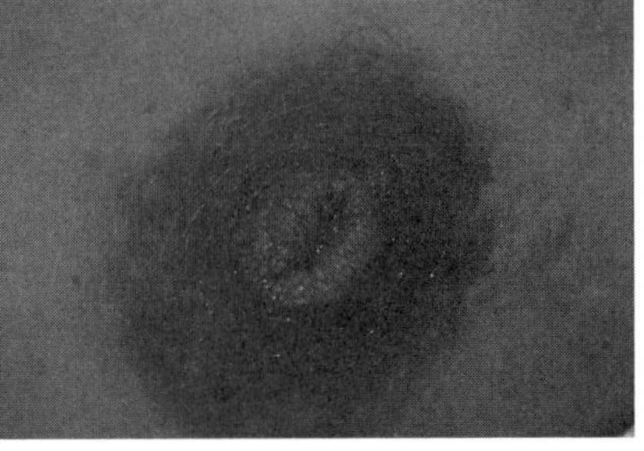

Figure 17.3. Dimpled nipple open after pumping (left) then closed (right).

B. Wilson-Clay and K. Hoover, The Breastfeeding Atlas, 4th ed. 2008

A mother may have one flat or inverted nipple and one nipple that protrudes.

It is also not unusual for a woman's nipples to vary. For example, although both of her nipples may be flat, one may protrude more than the other. In this case, her baby may show a preference for the more-protruding nipple..

Treatments for Flat or Inverted Nipples

During pregnancy, treatments to draw out flat and inverted nipples may cause more breastfeeding problems than they solve.

Treatments to draw out flat and inverted nipples during pregnancy—such as the Hoffman technique (the fingers are used to draw out inverted nipples) or wearing breast shells—have been commonly recommended for decades. But two U.K. studies found that identifying flat or inverted nipples during pregnancy and "treating" them with either of these approaches appeared to cause more breastfeeding problems than they solved (Alexander, Grant, & Campbell, 1992; MAIN, 1994). The first of these two studies, which followed 96 first-time mothers with flat or inverted nipples, found that more of those in the treatment group either decided not to breastfeed or stopped breastfeeding earlier than those whose nipples were not treated. The researchers expressed concern that telling a pregnant woman her nipples could be problematic may "act as a disincentive" to successful breastfeeding because it calls into question her ability to breastfeed. They concluded that during pregnancy recommending "breast shells may reduce the chances of successful breastfeeding" (Alexander et al., 1992, p. 1030). The second study, which followed 463 mothers with flat or inverted nipples, found that babies whose mothers did ***not*** receive treatment during pregnancy had fewer problems taking the breast than those whose mothers received treatments. They therefore recommended that healthcare professionals stop screening mothers during pregnancy for flat or inverted nipples. Due to these research findings, the U.K. Royal College of Midwives warns against focusing on "inadequate nipples," encouraging a focus instead on positioning after birth.

"Treating" flat or inverted nipples during pregnancy may cause more problems than it solves.

After birth, if a mother has flat nipples, ask if they were flat before birth to help determine if this is a short-term issue.

Consider the possibility that her nipples may have flattened due to engorgement or areola swelling from excess IV fluids given during labor. If so, see p. 795 in the "Techniques" appendix for a description of reverse pressure softening and manual expression of milk to soften the areola for easier breastfeeding.

Nipples drawn out by previous breastfeeding may flatten or invert again after weaning.

If a pregnant woman expresses concern that her nipples are inverted again after being drawn out by breastfeeding a previous baby, focus on her success and reassure her that her next baby should be able to draw them out again.

Early Breastfeeding

Flat and inverted nipples sometimes make breastfeeding challenging.

Some U.S. studies have found an association between flat and inverted nipples and early breastfeeding problems, such as ineffective breastfeeding and difficulty taking the breast (Dewey et al., 2003; Moore & Anderson, 2007). Because unusual nipple or breast anatomy may make it more challenging for a newborn to take the breast and achieve deep breastfeeding, it may also affect milk transfer and weight gain. Flat or inverted nipples were associated with delayed milk increase in one U.S. study (Dewey et al., 2003). An Iranian study of first-time mothers examined the effect of "maternal breast variations" (including flat and inverted nipples and "abnormally large breasts") on weight gain during the first 7 days (Vazirinejad, Darakhshan, Esmaeili, & Hadadian, 2009). At 7 days of life, the mean weight of the babies whose mothers had one or more of these "breast variations" was below birthweight, whereas the mean weight among the babies whose mothers did not was above birthweight.

Preventing Breastfeeding Difficulties

To prevent problems, suggest the mother try laid-back feeding positions.

These positions use gravity to help rather than hinder breastfeeding and may make the early learning period easier (Colson, 2008; Colson et al., 2008). For details, see the first chapter "Basic Breastfeeding Dynamics."

Suggest frequent breastfeeding after birth to prevent engorgement.

Engorgement can make breastfeeding challenging for mothers with protruding nipples and create even greater challenges for mothers with flat or inverted nipples. To keep the mother's breasts as soft and pliable as possible while her baby learns to breastfeed, encourage frequent feedings using the strategies described in the second chapter, "Breastfeeding Rhythms."

If possible, avoid artificial nipples in the first weeks.

In *The Breastfeeding Atlas* authors Wilson-Clay and Hoover suggest that after the "supernormal stimulus" of bottles and pacifiers/dummies, babies whose mothers have flat or inverted nipples may be more prone to breastfeeding problems than the average baby (Wilson-Clay & Hoover, 2008, p. 41). If possible, suggest the mother avoid artificial nipples during the early weeks of breastfeeding while baby is learning.

Difficulties Associated with Flat or Inverted Nipples

Baby Not Taking the Breast

If the baby takes one breast, suggest feeding often from that breast and try the following suggestions with the other breast.

Most mothers have one nipple that is easier for the baby to take. If the baby takes one breast well, suggest she feed often from that breast and express milk from the refused breast, while she tries the following strategies with it.

Suggest the mother express some milk on the nipple or in baby's mouth to entice him.

If the mother has a helper, suggest the helper drip some of the mother's milk onto the breast near the nipple with a spoon or eyedropper, while the mother leans back and helps baby to the breast. (Honey should not be used on the nipple, as it has been associated with infant botulism.)

Suggest the mother try to draw out her nipple.

Strategies and products for drawing out the nipple include:

Try pulling back slightly on the breast to help the nipple protrude (**Figure 17.4**). Rarely, a mother may need to pull back on the breast throughout the feeding.

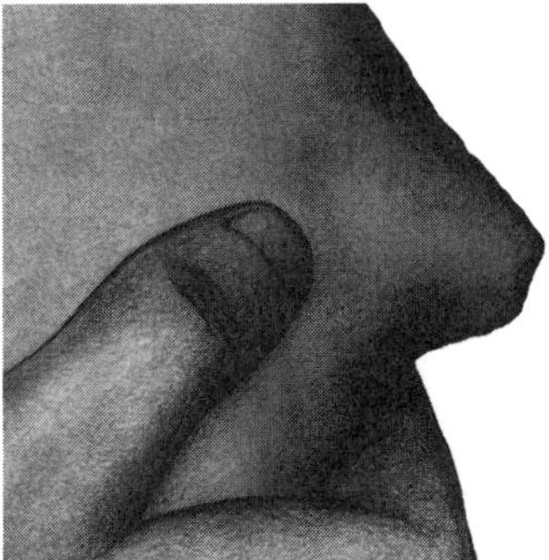

Figure 17.4. Inverted nipple protruding while mother pulls back breast tissue
©2010 Christian Bressler, used with permission

Nipple rolling. If the mother's nipples can be grasped, suggest she roll the nipple between thumb and index finger for a minute or two, and then quickly touch it with a moist, cold cloth or ice wrapped in a cloth. (Avoid prolonged ice on the nipple, as it can numb the breast and inhibit the milk ejection.)

Breast shaping or support. Breast sandwich, nipple tilting, and other techniques may help the baby take the breast deeper to trigger active suckling. For details, see p. 802 in the "Techniques" appendix.

Breast shells. These plastic devices—worn in the mother's bra before feedings—include a dome and a snap-on backing with a small opening designed to apply pressure to the areola and draw out the nipple. If used, suggest the mother restrict her wear time to no longer than 30 minutes before a breastfeeding, as consistent pressure on the breasts increases the risk of mastitis. Also suggest she use shells only if her bra cup is large enough to comfortably accommodate them. If the shells leave obvious red rings on her breast, her bra cup may be too small for safe use. For more details see p. 831- "Breast Shells."

Breast pump. Using a breast pump before feeding can soften the areola and help draw out the nipple. The suction generated by the breast pump pulls out the nipple uniformly from the center, which may make it easier for baby to take the breast.

Modified syringe. An alternative to a commercial product is a modified disposable syringe, which is available worldwide. In one Indian study (Kesaree, Banapurmath, Banapurmath, & Shamanur, 1993), the researchers describe how to transform a 10 or 20 mL syringe (depending on nipple size) into a small suction device that can be used to draw out an inverted nipple before feedings. (For details, see "Nipple Everters" on p. 832 in the "Tools and Products" appendix.) These researchers followed eight mothers with inverted nipples whose babies were unable to take their breast and who had been bottle-feeding for 28 to 103 days. After receiving positioning help and using the modified syringe for 30 to 60 seconds several times a day, seven of eight babies took the breast. Within 4 to 6 weeks, six of the eight women were exclusively breastfeeding.

Commercial suction devices. Along with the makeshift device described above, there are also available for sale in some areas manufactured products specifically designed to draw out inverted nipples.

Using a nipple shield may help the baby take the breast.

If the previous strategies do not work, suggest the mother try a nipple shield, a flexible silicone nipple worn over her nipple during feedings. A nipple shield provides a protruding nipple and has holes in the tip, so the baby receives milk at the breast. For details on fit, applying the shield, taking the breast with the shield, and weaning from the shield, see p. 835 in the "Tools and Products" appendix.

If none of these strategies work, suggest the mother express her milk, which may also help draw out her nipple, and feed it to her baby.

In some cases, depending on the type and degree of nipple inversion, manual expression may not be effective. In this case, a breast pump may not only express milk more effectively, it may also help draw out the nipple when the usual strategies fail. With some types of deeply inverted nipples, when the baby tries to take the breast, rather than compressing the mother's breast tissue under her areola, he may compress the buried nipple instead. In this case, the baby may not receive much milk and breastfeeding may be painful for the mother. A breast pump does not compress the mother's areola. It provides uniform suction on the nipple, drawing the nipple out and, in some cases, stretching the adhesions that hold it in.

How long a mother will need to pump will depend on the type of inverted nipple and the degree of inversion. For some mothers, one pumping is enough for the nipple to stay out. If so, the mother can start breastfeeding on that breast immediately. But if the nipple inverts again, the mother may need to continue pumping. Rarely, a mother may need to pump for days or weeks before her nipple is drawn out.

In some cases, after a mother's nipple has been drawn out by the pump, it may invert again when the baby pauses during breastfeeding. If this happens, the mother may need to pump for a short time to draw out the nipple and use a tube-feeding device at the breast to encourage more continuous suckling as a temporary transition to exclusive breastfeeding.

If the mother needs to pump exclusively for a time and feed her baby in other ways, discuss pumping and feeding methods with her. For details on how to establish full milk production with a pump, see the chapter "Milk Expression and Storage," and for feeding methods, see the "Tools and Products" appendix.

Nipple Pain

Depending on the type and degree of nipple inversion, some mothers experience persistent nipple pain.

A true inverted nipple or dimpled nipple may make the mother prone to nipple soreness, depending on its type and severity. Normal breastfeeding may even cause trauma in some types of inverted nipples. If the nipple retracts between feedings, the skin may stay moist, contributing to chapping. See "Treatment" section on p. 645 for suggestions.

Some mothers experience nipple pain for about 2 weeks, as their baby's sucking gradually draws out their nipples. Other mothers have persistent sore nipples for a longer time. Sometimes, instead of stretching, the adhesions remain tight, creating a point of stress that can cause cracks or blisters. When the mother's nipple can be drawn into the back of the baby's mouth and the baby begins breastfeeding effectively, many mothers will be able to breastfeed without discomfort. On rare occasions, a mother will continue to feel some discomfort even after the baby has begun breastfeeding well, because her nipple has undergone a radical change. In this case, see p. 644- "Comfort Measures" for ideas.

NIPPLE PIERCING

Mothers with pierced nipples have successfully breastfed.

Over the years, nipple piercing has become more common (Sadove & Clayman, 2008). One U.K. study of more than 10,000 women, aged 16 and older, found that 10% (1,934) had body piercings other than the earlobe. Of these, 9% (143) had nipple piercings, with twice as many men as women and most in the 16-to-24 age group (Bone, Ncube, Nichols, & Noah, 2008).

The literature includes several examples of mothers successfully breastfeeding with pierced nipples (Wilson-Clay & Hoover, 2008, pp. 68, 177). One case report describes a mother who removed the ring from one of her nipples after birth and breastfed from one breast only (Lee, 1995).

Possible breastfeeding complications from nipple piercing include altered nipple sensation, mastitis, and reduced milk production.

After a nipple piercing, healing usually takes 6 to 12 months, and there is a 10% to 20% increased risk of mastitis unrelated to lactation (Jacobs, Golombeck, Jonat, & Kiechle, 2003). In a review of 12 cases of infection and one case of abscess, the authors noted that all infections occurred between 3 and 9 months after the piercing (Bengualid, Singh, Singh, & Berger, 2008). In the U.K. study described in the previous point, 38% had some complications after a nipple piercing, with swelling, infection, and bleeding the most common. About 25% saw a healthcare provider as a result of the complications, with 1 in 100 hospitalized.

Although women have breastfed without problems after nipple piercing, in some cases, nipple scar tissue from the piercing may complicate a baby's attachment to the breast and block milk ducts (Armstrong, Caliendo, & Roberts, 2006). One Australian article described three mothers whose complications from their nipple piercing caused milk duct obstruction, which resulted in minimal milk transfer during breastfeeding and milk expression, despite frequent pumping (Garbin, Deacon, Rowan, Hartmann, & Geddes, 2009). One of these mothers chose to breastfed exclusively on the unpierced breast, so if a mother develops this problem, let her know that one-sided (unilateral) breastfeeding is an option.

Questions to ask a mother with pierced nipples include:

- Has she had any complications from her nipple piercing?
- Does she remove her nipple jewelry before breastfeeding?
- Are her nipples either numb or hypersensitive?
- Is there any obvious scarring on her nipples? If so, where?
- How much weight has her baby gained?
- Has she seen any nipple discharge other than milk?

Numbness of the nipples may affect milk ejection during breastfeeding. A healthy weight gain rules out these potential problems. Hypersensitivity could make breastfeeding painful. Scarring could affect milk flow. Encourage all mothers to remove their nipple jewelry before breastfeeding to prevent choking. If a mother is concerned about her nipple piercing closing before her baby weans, suggest she use temporary jewelry to keep it open (Martin, 2004).

TEETHING AND BITING

When a baby is teething, his gums may feel swollen and sore. As a result, he may breastfeed differently or chew on the nipple, as applying pressure on his gums can ease his discomfort.

Let the mother know that nipple pain from teething is temporary.

Nipple pain from teething will pass as the baby's teeth erupt. In the meantime, suggest the mother give the baby something cold to chew on before breastfeeding, like a cold, wet washcloth or a cold teething toy. For the baby on solids, a frozen bagel or frozen peas may help soothe baby's gums and make breastfeeding more comfortable.

Suggest the mother consult her baby's healthcare provider before giving her baby a pain-relieving drug or an over-the-counter preparation to numb his gums. These products may numb the baby's tongue (or the mother's breast), making breastfeeding difficult.

It is not necessary to wean from the breast after baby's teeth erupt.

Many mothers are told to stop breastfeeding at signs of their baby's first tooth, but many babies never bite, and those who try once usually never bite again.

If a baby is actively breastfeeding, he can't bite.

During breastfeeding, the nipple goes far back in baby's mouth, with the baby's lips and gums on the areola and the baby's tongue covering his lower gum (Jacobs et al., 2007). So even with teeth, a baby cannot bite while he is actively breastfeeding.

If a baby bites, suggest the mother try to stay calm and pull him in close.

Most mothers' first reaction to biting is to startle and pull the baby off the breast. After this reaction, most babies never bite again. But if a baby does bite again, suggest the mother try to stay calm. Pulling the baby off the breast with his teeth clamped down can cause more damage than the bite itself. If the mother yells, many babies will be startled. This can backfire in sensitive babies, who may respond by refusing the breast. (For details, see the section on "Nursing Strike" in the chapter "Challenges at the Breast.") Because bringing a baby "on strike" back to the breast can take much coaxing, suggest the mother try to stay calm if her baby bites again.

Rather than pulling the baby off the breast when he bites, suggest that she slip a finger between the baby's gums or teeth, which will release the nipple.

If a mother is worried, discuss ways to prevent biting.

If the baby has been biting persistently, suggest the following strategies:

- **Give the baby her complete attention during breastfeeding.** Eye contact, stroking, and talking decrease the odds the baby will bite to get her attention.
- **Learn to recognize the end of a breastfeeding.** Most biting occurs when the baby loses interest in breastfeeding. If a mother is alert, she may notice, for example, that tension develops in baby's jaw before he bites down. If she sees this sign, she can break the suction and take him off before he bites. Some babies chew or bite down near the end of a breastfeeding as a sign they are done.
- **Don't pressure a disinterested baby to breastfeed.** If the baby pushes mother away, suggest she offer again later.
- **Make sure the baby breastfeeds deeply.** Being well onto the breast will trigger active suckling and lessen the odds of biting.
- **Remove a sleeping baby who is not actively suckling from the breast.** To do this, suggest the mother gently insert her finger between baby's gums to release the nipple. If baby bites, he'll bite the finger instead of the breast.
- **Keep her milk production abundant.** Some babies bite when they are frustrated at the breast from too little milk. Unnecessary supplements

of formula, water, or juice or too early introduction of solid foods can decrease milk production.

- **Note behaviors that lead to biting.** Some babies bite when teased, pressured to breastfeed, or when the mother yells at older siblings. Suggest the mother notice what happened before her baby bit. Knowing the cause can prevent future biting.
- **Keep breastfeeding relaxed and positive.** Some babies bite when their mothers are tense. If the mother is frazzled, suggest she try deep breathing, relaxing music, or breastfeeding lying down or in a darkened room.
- **Give praise when baby doesn't bite.** Suggest the mother say, "Thank you" and "good baby" when he is gentle at the breast. Smiles, hugs, and kisses can help gently teach baby to breastfeed comfortably.

If biting becomes persistent, other strategies may help.

The following strategies may also discourage biting:

- **Stop the feeding.** Remove the temptation for baby to make mother jump again.
- **Offer a teether, such as a teething ring, a toy, or anything acceptable to bite.**
- **Set baby quickly on the floor.** After a few seconds of distress, comfort the baby to give the message that biting brings negative consequences.
- **Keep a finger near the baby's mouth ready to break the suction, if needed.** Some distractible babies try to turn and look with the nipple still in their mouths. If the mother responds consistently by breaking suction, baby will learn quickly that turning away means losing the nipple.

A baby needs to learn what to do with new teeth while breastfeeding. Babies don't understand that biting causes pain. They don't bite because of "meanness." Breastfeeding babies learn to associate their mother with feelings of security and comfort, as well as relief from hunger. These positive associations should help baby learn quickly.

REFERENCES

Aeling, J. L., Panagotacos, P. J., & Andreozzi, R. J. (1973). Letter: Allergic contact dermatitis to vitamin E aerosol deodorant. *Archives of Dermatology, 108*(4), 579-580

Akkuzu, G., & Taskin, L. (2000). Impacts of breast-care techniques on prevention of possible postpartum nipple problems. *Professional Care of Mother and Child, 10*(2), 38-41.

Alexander, J. M., Grant, A. M., & Campbell, M. J. (1992). Randomised controlled trial of breast shells and Hoffman's exercises for inverted and non-protractile nipples. *BMJ, 304*(6833), 1030-1032.

Amir, L. (1993). Eczema of the nipple and breast: a case report. *Journal of Human Lactation, 9*(3), 173-175.

Amir, L. (2004). Test your knowledge. Nipple pain in breastfeeding. *Australian Family Physician, 33*(1-2), 44-45.

Amir, L., & Hoover, K. (2002). Candidiasis and breastfeeding (Vol. 6). Schaumburg, IL: La Leche League International.

Amir, L. H., Dennerstein, L., Garland, S. M., Fisher, J., & Farish, S. J. (1996). Psychological aspects of nipple pain in lactating women. *Journal of Psychosomatic Obstetrics and Gynaecology, 17*(1), 53-58.

Amir, L. H., Dennerstein, L., Garland, S. M., Fisher, J., & Farish, S. J. (1997). Psychological aspects of nipple pain in lactating women. *Breastfeeding Review, 5*, 29-32.

Amir, L. H., Forster, D. A., Lumley, J., & McLachlan, H. (2007). A descriptive study of mastitis in Australian breastfeeding women: incidence and determinants. *BMC Public Health*, 7, 62.

Amir, L. H., Garland, S. M., Dennerstein, L., & Farish, S. J. (1996). Candida albicans: is it associated with nipple pain in lactating women? *Gynecologic and Obstetric Investigation, 41*(1), 30-34.

Anderson, J. E., Held, N., & Wright, K. (2004). Raynaud's phenomenon of the nipple: a treatable cause of painful breastfeeding. *Pediatrics, 113*(4), e360-364.

Ballard, J. L., Auer, C. E., & Khoury, J. C. (2002). Ankyloglossia: assessment, incidence, and effect of frenuloplasty on the breastfeeding dyad. *Pediatrics, 110*(5), e63.

Barankin, B., & Gross, M. S. (2004). Nipple and areolar eczema in the breastfeeding woman. *Journal of Cutaneous Medicine and Surgery, 8*(2), 126-130.

Bengualid, V., Singh, V., Singh, H., & Berger, J. (2008). Mycobacterium fortuitum and anaerobic breast abscess following nipple piercing: case presentation and review of the literature. *Journal of Adolescent Health, 42(*5), 530-532.

Boere-Boonekamp, M. M., & van der Linden-Kuiper, L. L. (2001). Positional preference: prevalence in infants and follow-up after two years. *Pediatrics, 107*(2), 339-343.

Bone, A., Ncube, F., Nichols, T., & Noah, N. D. (2008). Body piercing in England: a survey of piercing at sites other than earlobe. *BMJ, 336*(7658), 1426-1428.

Brent, N., Rudy, S. J., Redd, B., Rudy, T. E., & Roth, L. A. (1998). Sore nipples in breast-feeding women: a clinical trial of wound dressings vs conventional care. *Archives of Pediatrics and Adolescent Medicine, 152*(11), 1077-1082.

Brent, N. B. (2001). Thrush in the breastfeeding dyad: results of a survey on diagnosis and treatment. *Clinical Pediatrics, 40*(9), 503-506.

Cable, B., Stewart, M., & Davis, J. (1997). Nipple wound care: a new approach to an old problem. *Journal of Human Lactation, 13*(4), 313-318.

Cadwell, K., Turner-Maffei, C., Blair, A., Brimdyr, K., & Maja McInerney, Z. (2004). Pain reduction and treatment of sore nipples in nursing mothers. *Journal of Perinatal Education, 13*(1), 29-35.

Centuori, S., Burmaz, T., Ronfani, L., Fragiacomo, M., Quintero, S., Pavan, C., et al. (1999). Nipple care, sore nipples, and breastfeeding: a randomized trial. *Journal of Human Lactation*, 15(2), 125-130.

Chandler, P. J., Jr., & Hill, S. D. (1990). A direct surgical approach to correct the inverted nipple. *Plastic and Reconstructive Surgery, 86*(2), 352-354.

Chen, C. Y., Sun, L. M., & Anderson, B. O. (2006). Paget disease of the breast: changing patterns of incidence, clinical presentation, and treatment in the U.S. *Cancer, 107*(7), 1448-1458.

Chetwynd, E. M., Ives, T. J., Payne, P. M., & Edens-Bartholomew, N. (2002). Fluconazole for postpartum candidal mastitis and infant thrush. *Journal of Human Lactation, 18*(2), 168-171.

Clark, E. W., Blondeel, A., Cronin, E., Oleffe, J. A., & Wilkinson, D. S. (1981). Lanolin of reduced sensitizing potential. *Contact Dermatitis, 7*(2), 80-83.

Colson, S. (2008). *Biological Nurturing: Laid-Back Breastfeeding*. Hythe, Kent, UK: The Nurturing Project.

Colson, S. (2009). In N. Mohrbacher (Ed.). Hythe, Kent, UK.

Colson, S., DeRooy, L., Hawdon, J. (2003). Biological Nurturing increases duration of breastfeeding for a vulnerable cohort. *MIDIRS Midwifery Digest, 13*(1), 92-97.

Colson, S. D., Meek, J. H., & Hawdon, J. M. (2008). Optimal positions for the release of primitive neonatal reflexes stimulating breastfeeding. *Early Human Development, 84*(7), 441-449.

Cooper, S. M., & Shaw, S. (1999). Contact allergy to nystatin: an unusual allergen. *Contact Dermatitis, 41*(2), 120.

Davis, G. (2001). Safety of hydrogel dressings. *Journal of Human Lactation, 17*(2), 117.

Dewey, K. G., Nommsen-Rivers, L. A., Heinig, M. J., & Cohen, R. J. (2003). Risk factors for suboptimal infant breastfeeding behavior, delayed onset of lactation, and excess neonatal weight loss. *Pediatrics, 112*(3 Pt 1), 607-619.

Dodd, V., & Chalmers, C. (2003). Comparing the use of hydrogel dressings to lanolin ointment with lactating mothers. *Journal of Obstetric, Gynecologic, and Neonatal Nursing, 32*(4), 486-494.

Duff, M. (1998). Paget's disease of the nipple: A 14 year experience. *Irish Medical Journal, 91*(4), 1-5.

Eglash, A. (1998). Delayed milk ejection reflex and plugged ducts: Lecithin therapy. *ABM News and Views, 3*(1), 4.

Fernandez, R., Griffiths, R., & Ussia, C. (2002). Water for wound cleansing. *Cochrane Database Syst Rev*(4), CD003861.

Fetherston, C. (1998). Risk factors for lactation mastitis. *Journal of Human Lactation, 14*(2), 101-109.

Fisher, A. (1986). *Contact Dermatitis*. Philadelphia, PA: Lea & Febiger.

Foxman, B., D'Arcy, H., Gillespie, B., Bobo, J. K., & Schwartz, K. (2002). Lactation mastitis: occurrence and medical management among 946 breastfeeding women in the United States. *American Journal of Epidemiology, 155*(2), 103-114.

Francis-Morrill, J., Heinig, M. J., Pappagianis, D., & Dewey, K. G. (2004). Diagnostic value of signs and symptoms of mammary candidosis among lactating women. *Journal of Human Lactation, 20*(3), 288-295; quiz 296-289.

Garbin, C. P., Deacon, J. P., Rowan, M. K., Hartmann, P. E., & Geddes, D. T. (2009). Association of nipple piercing with abnormal milk production and breastfeeding. *Journal of the American Medical Association, 301*(24), 2550-2551.

Garrison, C. P. (2002). Nipple vasospasms, Raynaud's syndrome, and nifedipine. *Journal of Human Lactation, 18*(4), 382-385.

Geddes, D. T., Kent, J. C., Mitoulas, L. R., & Hartmann, P. E. (2008). Tongue movement and intra-oral vacuum in breastfeeding infants. *Early Human Development, 84*(7), 471-477.

Geddes, D. T., Langton, D. B., Gollow, I., Jacobs, L. A., Hartmann, P. E., & Simmer, K. (2008). Frenulotomy for breastfeeding infants with ankyloglossia: effect on milk removal and sucking mechanism as imaged by ultrasound. *Pediatrics, 122*(1), e188-194.

Genna, C. W. (2008). The influence of anatomic and strucural issues on sucking skills. In C. W. Genna (Ed.), *Supporting Sucking Skills in Breastfeeding Infants.* Boston, MA: Jones and Bartlett.

Goins, R. A., Ascher, D., Waecker, N., Arnold, J., & Moorefield, E. (2002). Comparison of fluconazole and nystatin oral suspensions for treatment of oral candidiasis in infants. *Pediatric Infectious Disease Journal, 21*(12), 1165-1167.

Griffiths, D. M. (2004). Do tongue ties affect breastfeeding? *Journal of Human Lactation, 20*(4), 409-414.

Hale, T. (2008). *Medications and Mothers' Milk* (13 ed.). Amarillo, TX: Hale Publishing.

Hale, T. W., Bateman, T. L., Finkelman, M. A., & Berens, P. D. (2009). The absence of Candida albicans in milk samples of women with clinical symptoms of ductal candidiasis. *Breastfeeding Medicine, 4*(2), 57-61.

Han, S., & Hong, Y. G. (1999). The inverted nipple: its grading and surgical correction. *Plastic and Reconstructive Surgery, 104*(2), 389-395; discussion 396-387.

Heads, J., & Higgins, L. C. (1995). Perceptions and correlates of nipple pain. *Breastfeeding Review, 3*(2), 59-64.

Henderson, A., Stamp, G., & Pincombe, J. (2001). Postpartum positioning and attachment education for increasing breastfeeding: a randomized trial. *Birth, 28*(4), 236-242.

Hill, P. D., & Humenick, S. S. (1993). Nipple pain during breastfeeding: The first two weeks and beyond. *Journal of Perinatal Education, 2*(2), 21-35.

Hinman, C. D., & Maibach, H. (1963). Effect of Air Exposure and Occlusion on Experimental Human Skin Wounds. *Nature, 200*, 377-378.

Hogan, M., Westcott, C., & Griffiths, M. (2005). Randomized, controlled trial of division of tongue-tie in infants with feeding problems. *Journal of Paediatrics and Child Health, 41*(5-6), 246-250.

Hoppe, J. E. (1997). Treatment of oropharyngeal candidiasis and candidal diaper dermatitis in neonates and infants: review and reappraisal. *Pediatric Infectious Disease Journal, 16*(9), 885-894.

Huggins, K. E., & Billon, S. F. (1993). Twenty cases of persistent sore nipples: collaboration between lactation consultant and dermatologist. *Journal of Human Lactation, 9*(3), 155-160.

Jacobs, L. A., Dickinson, J. E., Hart, P. D., Doherty, D. A., & Faulkner, S. J. (2007). Normal nipple position in term infants measured on breastfeeding ultrasound. *Journal of Human Lactation, 23*(1), 52-59.

Jacobs, V. R., Golombeck, K., Jonat, W., & Kiechle, M. (2003). Mastitis nonpuerperalis after nipple piercing: time to act. *International Journal of Fertility and Womens Medicine, 48*(5), 226-231.

Kent, J. C., Mitoulas, L. R., Cregan, M. D., Geddes, D. T., Larsson, M., Doherty, D. A., et al. (2008). Importance of vacuum for breastmilk expression. *Breastfeeding Medicine, 3*(1), 11-19.

Kesaree, N., Banapurmath, C. R., Banapurmath, S., & Shamanur, K. (1993). Treatment of inverted nipples using a disposable syringe. *Journal of Human Lactation, 9*(1), 27-29.

Kinlay, J. R., O'Connell, D. L., & Kinlay, S. (2001). Risk factors for mastitis in breastfeeding women: results of a prospective cohort study. *Australian and New Zealand Journal of Public Health, 25*(2), 115-120.

Lauwers, J., & Swisher, A. (2005). *Counseling the Nursing Mother* (4th ed.). Boston, MA: Jones and Bartlett.

Lavergne, N. A. (1997). Does application of tea bags to sore nipples while breastfeeding provide effective relief? *Journal of Obstetric, Gynecologic, and Neonatal Nursing, 26*(1), 53-58.

Lawrence, R. A., & Lawrence, R. M. (2005). *Breastfeeding: A Guide for the Medical Profession* (6th ed.). Philadelphia, PA: Elsevier Mosby.

Lee, N. (1995). More on pierced nipples. *Journal of Human Lactation, 11*(2), 89.

Li, R., Fein, S. B., & Grummer-Strawn, L. M. (2008). Association of breastfeeding intensity and bottle-emptying behaviors at early infancy with infants' risk for excess weight at late infancy. *Pediatrics, 122 Suppl 2*, S77-84.

Livingstone, V., & Stringer, L. J. (1999). The treatment of Staphyloccocus aureus infected sore nipples: a randomized comparative study. *Journal of Human Lactation, 15*(3), 241-246.

Livingstone, V. H., Willis, C. E., & Berkowitz, J. (1996). Staphylococcus aureus and sore nipples. *Canadian Family Physician, 42*, 654-659.

MAIN. (1994). Preparing for breast feeding: treatment of inverted and non-protractile nipples in pregnancy. The MAIN Trial Collaborative Group. *Midwifery, 10*(4), 200-214.

Mertz, P. M. (1990). Intervention: Dressing effects on wound healing. In: W. H. Eaglstein (Ed.), Wound care manual: New directions in wound healing (pp. 83-96). Princeton, NJ: Convatec.

Marmet, C., & Shell, E. (2008). Therapeutic positioning for Breastfeeding. In C. W. Genna (Ed.), *Supporting Sucking Skills in Breastfeeding Infants* (pp. 305-325). Boston, MA: Jones and Bartlett.

Martin, J. (2004). Is nipple piercing compatible with breastfeeding? *Journal of Human Lactation, 20*(3), 319-321.

Marx, C. M., Izquierdo, A., Driscoll, J. W., Murray, M. A., & Epstein, M. F. (1985). Vitamin E concentrations in serum of newborn infants after topical use of vitamin E by nursing mothers. *American Journal of Obstetrics and Gynecology, 152*(6 Pt 1), 668-670.

McClellan, H., Geddes, D., Kent, J., Garbin, C., Mitoulas, L., & Hartmann, P. (2008). Infants of mothers with persistent nipple pain exert strong sucking vacuums. *Acta Paediatrica, 97*(9), 1205-1209.

Melli, M. S., Rashidi, M. R., Nokhoodchi, A., Tagavi, S., Farzadi, L., Sadaghat, K., et al. (2007). A randomized trial of peppermint gel, lanolin ointment, and placebo gel to prevent nipple crack in primiparous breastfeeding women. *Medical Science Monitor, 13*(9), CR406-411.

Meltzer, D. I. (2005). Complications of body piercing. American Family Physician, 72(10), 2029-2034.

Messner, A. H., Lalakea, M. L., Aby, J., Macmahon, J., & Bair, E. (2000). Ankyloglossia: incidence and associated feeding difficulties. *Archives of Otolaryngology--Head & Neck Surgery, 126*(1), 36-39.

Mohammadzadeh, A., Farhat, A., & Esmaeily, H. (2005). The effect of breast milk and lanolin on sore nipples. *Saudi Medical Journal, 26*(8), 1231-1234.

Mohrbacher, N., & Kendall-Tackett, K. (2005). *Breastfeeding Made Simple: Seven Natural Laws for Nursing Mothers*. Oakland, CA: New Harbinger Publications.

Mojab, C. G. (2007). Congenital torticollis in the nursling. *Journal of Human Lactation, 23*(1), 12.

Moore, E. R., & Anderson, G. C. (2007). Randomized controlled trial of very early mother-infant skin-to-skin contact and breastfeeding status. *Journal of Midwifery and Women's Health, 52*(2), 116-125.

Morino, C., & Winn, S. M. (2007). Raynaud's phenomenon of the nipples: an elusive diagnosis. *Journal of Human Lactation, 23*(2), 191-193.

Morrill, J. F., Heinig, M. J., Pappagianis, D., & Dewey, K. G. (2005). Risk factors for mammary candidosis among lactating women. *Journal of Obstetric, Gynecologic, and Neonatal Nursing, 34*(1), 37-45.

Newman, J., & Pitman, T. (2006). *The Ultimate Breastfeeding Book of Answers*. New York, New York: Three Rivers Press.

Noble, R. (1991). Milk under the skin (milk blister)--A simple problem causing other breast conditions. *Breastfeeding Review, 2*(3), 118-119.

Palmer, B. (1998). The influence of breastfeeding on the development of the oral cavity: a commentary. *Journal of Human Lactation, 14*(2), 93-98.

Porter, J., & Schach, B. (2004). Treating sore, possibly infected nipples. *Journal of Human Lactation, 20*(2), 221-222.

Prime, D. K., Geddes, D. T., & Hartmann, P. E. (2007). Oxytocin: Milk ejection and maternal-infant well-being. In T. W. Hale, & P.E. Hartmann (Ed.), *Hale & Hartmann's Textbook of Human Lactation*. Amarillo, TX: Hale Publishing.

Pugh, L. C., Buchko, B. L., Bishop, B. A., Cochran, J. F., Smith, L. R., & Lerew, D. J. (1996). A comparison of topical agents to relieve nipple pain and enhance breastfeeding. *Birth, 23*(2), 88-93.

Ramsay, D. T., Mitoulas, L. R., Kent, J. C., Cregan, M. D., Doherty, D. A., Larsson, M., et al. (2006). Milk flow rates can be used to identify and investigate milk ejection in women expressing breast milk using an electric breast pump. *Breastfeeding Medicine, 1*(1), 14-23.

Righard, L. (1998). Are breastfeeding problems related to incorrect breastfeeding technique and the use of pacifiers and bottles? *Birth, 25*(1), 40-44.

Righard, L., & Alade, M. O. (1997). Breastfeeding and the use of pacifiers. *Birth, 24*(2), 116-120.

Riordan, J., & Wambach, K. (2010). Breast-related issues. In J. Riordan & K. Wambach (Eds.), *Breastfeeding and Human Lactation* (4th ed., pp. 291-324). Boston, MA: Jones and Bartlett.

Rosa, C. A., Novak, F. R., de Almeida, J. A. G., Mendoca-Hagler, L. C., & Hagler, A. N. (1990). Yeasts from human milk collected in Rio de Janeiro, Brazil. *Review of Microbiology, 21*(4), 261-363.

Ryan, T. J. (2007). Infection following soft tissue injury: its role in wound healing. *Current Opinion in Infectious Disease, 20*(2), 124-128.

Sadove, R., & Clayman, M. A. (2008). Surgical procedure for reversal of nipple piercing. *Aesthetic Plastic Surgery, 32*(3), 563-565.

Sealander, J. Y., & Kerr, C. P. (1989). Herpes simplex of the nipple: infant-to-mother transmission. *American Family Physician, 39*(3), 111-113.

Sheehan, D., Krueger, P., Watt, S., Sword, W., & Bridle, B. (2001). The Ontario Mother and Infant Survey: breastfeeding outcomes. *Journal of Human Lactation, 17*(3), 211-219.

Smith, L., & Riordan, J. (2010). Postpartum care. In J. Riordan & K. Wambach (Eds.), *Breastfeeding and Human Lactation* (4th ed., pp. 253-290). Boston: Jones and Bartlett.

Snyder, J. (1997). *Variation in infant palatal structure and breastfeeding.* Encino, CA: Lactation Institute.

Spangler, A., & Hildebrandt, E. (1993). The effect of modified lanolin on nipple pain/damage during the first 10 days of breastfeeding. *International Journal of Childbirth Education, 8*(3), 15-19.

Sullivan-Bolyai, J.Z., Fife, K.H., Jacobs, R.F., Miller, Z. & Corey, L. (1983). Disseminated neonatal herpes simplex virus type 1 from a maternal breast lesion. *Pediatrics,* 71: 455-57.

Taveras, E. M., Capra, A. M., Braveman, P. A., Jensvold, N. G., Escobar, G. J., & Lieu, T. A. (2003). Clinician support and psychosocial risk factors associated with breastfeeding discontinuation. *Pediatrics, 112*(1 Pt 1), 108-115.

Terrill, P. J., & Stapleton, M. J. (1991). The inverted nipple: to cut the ducts or not? *British Journal of Plastic Surgery*, 44(5), 372-377.

Thomassen, P., Johansson, V. A., Wassberg, C., & Petrini, B. (1998). Breast-feeding, pain and infection. *Gynecologic and Obstetric Investigation, 46*(2), 73-74.

Thorley, V. (2000). Impetigo on the areola and nipple. *Breastfeeding Review, 8*(2), 25-26.

Vazirinejad, R., Darakhshan, S., Esmaeili, A., & Hadadian, S. (2009). The effect of maternal breast variations on neonatal weight gain in the first seven days of life. *International Breastfeeding Journal, 4,* 13.

Walker, M. (2006). *Breastfeeding Management for the Clinician: Using the Evidence.* Boston, MA: Jones and Bartlett.

Wall, V., & Glass, R. (2006). Mandibular asymmetry and breastfeeding problems: experience from 11 cases. *Journal of Human Lactation, 22*(3), 328-334.

Wiener, S. (2006). Diagnosis and management of Candida of the nipple and breast. *Journal of Midwifery and Women's Health, 51*(2), 125-128.

Wiessinger, D., & Miller, M. (1995). Breastfeeding difficulties as a result of tight lingual and labial frena: a case report. *Journal of Human Lactation, 11*(4), 313-316.

Wilson-Clay, B., & Hoover, K. (2008). *The Breastfeeding Atlas* (4th ed.). Manchaca, TX:

LactNews Press.

Wolf, L., & Glass, R. (1992). *Feeding and Swallowing Disorders in Infancy.* Tucson, AZ: Therapy Skill Builders.

Woolridge, M. W. (1986). Aetiology of sore nipples. *Midwifery, 2*(4), 172-176.

Ziemer, M. M., Cooper, D. M., & Pigeon, J. G. (1995). Evaluation of a dressing to reduce nipple pain and improve nipple skin condition in breast-feeding women. *Nursing Research, 44*(6), 347-351.

Ziemer, M. M., Paone, J. P., Schupay, J., & Cole, E. (1990). Methods to prevent and manage nipple pain in breastfeeding women. *Western Journal of Nursing Research, 12*(6), 732-743; discussion 743-734.

Ziemer, M. M., & Pigeon, J. G. (1993). Skin changes and pain in the nipple during the 1st week of lactation. *Journal of Obstetric, Gynecologic, and Neonatal Nursing, 22*(3), 247-256.

Breast Issues

Chapter 18

ENGORGEMENT

Between the 2nd and 6th day after birth, a mother's breasts usually begin to feel tender, larger, and heavier. These sensations are caused by an increasing volume of milk, as well as an increased flow of blood and lymph to the breasts, which aids in milk production. If the baby takes the breast well and removes the milk often and effectively, these extra fluids will drain easily from the breasts. Within the next few weeks as milk production is established and the hormones of childbirth decrease, the mother's breasts begin to feel softer most of the time, even with increased milk production.

As milk production increases after birth, most mothers feel some breast fullness or engorgement, which usually subsides within a few weeks.

After birth, some breast fullness or engorgement is considered "physiologic," or normal. But if a baby breastfeeds infrequently or ineffectively and the breasts stay full of milk (sometimes called "milk stasis"), blood circulation slows. As pressure builds, proteins from the blood and milk seep into the breast tissues, causing swelling (Fetherston, 2001). This swelling can cause breast discomfort, warmth, and throbbing, which may extend into a mother's armpit area, where some milk-producing glands are located (called the "tail of Spence"). The skin on the mother's breasts may appear taut and shiny.

Infrequent or ineffective breastfeeding can lead to engorgement.

Engorgement may occur only in the areola ("areolar engorgement"), only in other areas in the breast ("peripheral engorgement"), or in both. It may also occur in one or both breasts, depending on the breastfeeding pattern. Engorgement may also cause a fever of up to 101°F/38.3°C (Riordan & Hoover, 2010), which is sometimes confused with a postpartum infection, resulting in unnecessary separation of mother and baby.

• •

If a mother's breasts (and ankles) begin to swell within the first day or two after birth—even before her milk increases—excess IV fluids given during labor may be the cause, rather than engorgement.

IV fluids given during labor can aggravate and prolong engorgement.

Some laboring mothers receive more IV fluids than ordered by their doctor (Gonik & Cotton, 1984). Also, one type of commonly used IV fluid (crystalloid) both adds to the body's fluid load and reduces the ability to process excess fluid, extending the amount of time it takes for swelling to resolve. If a mother in this situation also becomes engorged, this dynamic can delay the resolution of engorgement for up to 10 to 14 days (Cotterman, 2004; Gonik & Cotton, 1984; Park, Hauch, Curlin, Datta, & Bader, 1996).

• •

Frequent breastfeeding removes colostrum and the increasing volume of milk, which allows the extra blood and lymph to drain more easily, making breast fullness less likely to become painful engorgement.

To help minimize engorgement, keep mother and baby together after birth and encourage frequent and long breastfeeding.

With unrestricted access to the breast, a newborn may breastfeed often for short periods, such as a few minutes every hour, or for long stretches, even hours at a time, until the mother's milk becomes more abundant, or "comes in" (Benson, 2001). When a baby's inborn feeding reflexes are triggered, he can even feed effectively while asleep (Colson, 2008; Colson, DeRooy, & Hawdon, 2003). If the baby sleeps for long stretches, encourage the mother to guide her baby to the breast often to help relieve breast fullness, while providing the milk he needs.

One Australian study of 152 mothers and babies found that when babies breastfed from one breast for as long as they wanted before being offered the second breast, their mothers experienced significantly less engorgement than the mothers who were told to be sure their babies took both breasts at each feeding (Evans, Evans, & Simmer, 1995).

Another U.S. study of 54 women found that more mothers became engorged when they followed hospital instructions to restrict their baby's early feeding times (Moon & Humenick, 1989). In other words, the more minutes spent at each breast during early breastfeeding, the less engorgement later.

Engorgement can manifest differently among different mothers and in the same mother with different babies.

One U.S. study found that mothers who had breastfed previously became engorged sooner and more severely than first-time breastfeeding mothers (Hill & Humenick, 1994). A more recent study done in Russia by Swedish, Canadian, and Russian researchers also found that engorgement was significantly more pronounced earlier among mothers with older children (Bystrova et al., 2007).

Another U.S. study of 114 mothers evaluated breast fullness for the first 14 days and identified four different patterns of engorgement (Humenick, Hill, & Anderson, 1994):

- **Pattern 1**: Increasing engorgement, peaking between Day 3 and 6, then decreasing
- **Pattern 2**: Minimal, non-varying engorgement
- **Pattern 3:** Engorgement with more than one peak and less engorgement between
- **Pattern 4:** Intense engorgement during the entire first 2 weeks

The intervals between breastfeeds and the frequency and duration of breastfeeding were similar across these four patterns. Whichever pattern of engorgement a mother has, she should be encouraged to treat it as soon as possible.

If a mother says she feels engorged, ask for more information.

Some information to gather from the mother includes:

- **The age of the baby.** Engorgement usually starts 3 to 6 days after birth. If the baby is older than about 2 weeks, the mother may have breast fullness from missed or delayed feedings.
- **How often and long they breastfeed.** If the baby has not been breastfeeding often or falls asleep quickly, this may intensify engorgement.
- **How her breasts feel.** Is the skin on her breasts soft and elastic or stretched tight? Does her areola feel soft and elastic like her earlobe or hard like the tip of her nose? If her areola is soft and elastic, she may not need to use the techniques described below to soften the areola before putting her baby to the breast. If her areola is hard, these techniques may help her baby get farther onto the breast.

Engorgement should be treated as soon as possible to prevent complications.

If a mother treats engorgement promptly, its most extreme symptoms usually resolve within 12 to 48 hours. However, if engorgement is not treated promptly, it can take up to 7 to 14 days or longer for her symptoms to resolve (Humenick et al., 1994).

Possible complications of engorgement include:

- Feeding problems and weight gain issues
- Nipple pain and trauma
- Mastitis
- In extreme cases, unrelieved pressure can damage the milk-making tissue, which may compromise long-term milk production (Wilson-Clay & Hoover, 2008, p. 79).

If a mother has a history of breast surgery or injury, she may have sections of the breast that do not drain. If so, reassure her that milk ducts that do not connect to the nipple do not increase her risk for mastitis. Like the mother who does not breastfeed, those areas will quickly stop producing milk and revert to their pre-pregnancy state. Because these ducts are not exposed to outside organisms via the ductal system, they are unlikely to become infected. See also p. 709-"Initiating Breastfeeding."

Effective treatments for engorgement reduce swelling and pain and/or drain the milk often and well.

Treatments for engorgement have not been well studied, but strategies that drain milk from the breasts and reduce swelling will help it resolve faster. A mother doesn't have to do all of the following. Encourage her to use the strategies that work well and feel soothing.

Take anti-inflammatory and/or pain medications. A Cochrane review of the research on engorgement treatments (Snowden, Renfrew, & Woolridge, 2001) found that the only treatment proven effective was taking anti-inflammatory medication. Suggest the mother consult with her healthcare provider about the best medication for her.

Apply cold compresses between feedings to reduce swelling and relieve pain. Suggest the mother protect her skin by wrapping ice packs, gel packs, or a bag of frozen vegetables in a cloth and apply them to her breasts for about 20 minutes or so (Walker, 2006, pp. 385-386). Applying cold constricts the breast tissue and allows blood and lymph to drain from the breast more easily. Many mothers find this soothing.

Breastfeed often and long, allowing baby to "finish the first breast first" to better drain each breast. Suggest the mother plan to feed as often as the baby is willing, at least every couple of hours, allowing the baby to stay on one breast until he comes off on his own, rather than trying to drain both breasts equally (Evans et al., 1995).

If still feeling full, express milk. If the baby doesn't soften both breasts after breastfeeding, suggest the mother hand-express her milk or "pump to comfort" with an effective breast pump just long enough to make her breast(s) feel more comfortable. Another choice is the Warm Bottle Method described on p. 456 in the chapter "Milk Expression and Storage" that simply requires a wide-mouthed glass bottle. If a pump is used, suggest the mother use reverse pressure softening first (Cotterman, 2004), described on p. 795 in the "Techniques" appendix.

Research indicates that draining the engorged breasts is more effective at relieving discomfort than applying cabbage leaf extract or cold (Nikodem, Danziger, Gebka, Gulmezoglu, & Hofmeyr, 1993; Roberts, Reiter, & Schuster, 1998). For details, see next point.

Expressing milk can lessen engorgement.

Some mothers are told that they should not express their milk because it will increase their milk production and worsen the engorgement, but the opposite is true. Draining milk from the breast helps reduce congestion and, therefore, the engorgement faster.

Another milk expression strategy involves draining the breasts as fully as possible once or twice with an effective breast pump. A breast pump can sometimes remove more milk than a newborn, which also helps reduce breast congestion, allowing extra blood and lymph to drain more easily.

Help her relax and stimulate milk flow for better breast drainage by suggesting that she:

- Apply heat briefly before breastfeeding or milk expression by taking a warm shower or applying warm, moist heat for a minute or two. Prolonged heat is not recommended because it may increase swelling, making the engorgement worse (Walker, 2006, p. 385).
- Use gentle breast massage (Jones, Dimmock, & Spencer, 2001) to stimulate milk flow, massaging from the chest wall toward the areola and concentrating on the most engorged areas. If she can do it comfortably, suggest the mother use her fingertips to gently knead the breast in this direction. Massaging when the baby's suckling slows down has been found to increase milk intake and breast drainage (Stutte, Bowles, & Morman, 1988). Some combine warmth and massage by massaging in the shower or while leaning over a basin of warm water.

• •

Other treatments for engorgement have not been proven effective, but some mothers find them soothing or prefer them over others.

Cabbage leaves have long been recommended as a home remedy for engorgement. Although they do not prevent engorgement (Nikodem et al., 1993) or treat engorgement more effectively than chilled gelpaks (Roberts, 1995), most mothers preferred them to gelpaks. One Australian double-blind study compared the use of a cream containing cabbage leaf extract with a placebo cream in 21 engorged women and found no differences in outcome (Roberts et al., 1998).

To use cabbage leaves as a treatment for engorgement, rinse either refrigerated or room temperature cabbage leaves, strip the large vein, and cut a hole for the nipple (Roberts, Reiter, & Schuster, 1995). Suggest the mother apply the cabbage leaves directly to her breasts, wearing them inside her bra. When they wilt, usually within 2 to 4 hours, suggest she remove them and reapply fresh leaves. Any relief reported from the use of cabbage leaves occurred within 8 hours of application (Roberts, 1995).

Ultrasound as a possible treatment for engorgement was studied in Australia on 197 engorged breasts, with one thermal continuous ultrasound machine working normally and a sham machine that generated only heat in the control group. The engorgement resolved equally quickly in both groups (McLachlan, Milne, Lumley, & Walker, 1993).

Manual lymphatic drainage therapy. In *The Breastfeeding Atlas,* Barbara Wilson-Clay and Kay Hoover describe this technique, which involves gentle massage by trained massage therapists along the lymph drainage pathways to improve lymph flow. When nothing else helped, several mothers they referred for this treatment reported afterwards reduced discomfort and better milk yields while pumping (Wilson-Clay & Hoover, 2008, p. 78).

If taut, engorged breasts prevent the baby from breastfeeding well, suggest the mother use techniques to soften the areola.

If the engorged mother's nipple and areola become so flat and taut that the baby can take only the nipple, breastfeeding may become both painful and ineffective, aggravating the engorgement. If this happens, the following strategies may help:

- **Reverse Pressure Softening** is the best first strategy. It involves applying gentle consistent pressure with the fingers to move the swelling back into the body of the breast, softening the areola. (For details, see p. 795 in the "Techniques" appendix.)
- **Laid-back breastfeeding positions**, laying baby tummy down on mother's semi-reclined body and experimenting with different angles to find optimal breastfeeding dynamics. These positions allow gravity to draw breast swelling back into the body of the breast.
- **Express just enough milk to soften the areola**, either with manual expression, the Warm Bottle Method (see p. 456- "The Warm Bottle Method"), or an effective breast pump, using Reverse Pressure Softening first. Assure the mother that expressing milk will help to resolve her engorgement faster.
- **Breast shells.** Worn for about a half hour before feeding in a bra large enough to hold them comfortably, they can soften the areola and draw out the nipple.
- **Nipple shield.** Short-term use may help the baby take the breast and drain it well. As the engorgement resolves, suggest the mother wean from the shield. (For details on fit, application, and weaning from the shield, see p. 835 in the "Tools and Products" appendix.)

If, despite all of the above, the baby still cannot breastfeed, suggest the mother express her milk and feed it to her baby.

See p. 453- "Choosing a Method" for details on choosing an effective breast pump, and see p. 811- "Alternative Feeding Methods" for choosing an alternative feeding method.

If engorgement continues in one breast despite consistent treatment, suggest the mother see her healthcare provider to rule out other causes.

In rare cases, this may be a warning sign of another type of breast problem, such as a cyst or even breast cancer. If there is no other obvious cause, suggest the mother see her healthcare provider as soon as possible.

MASTITIS

Mastitis means inflammation of the breast and covers a range of symptoms from mild to severe.

"Itis" means inflammation, so "mastitis" refers to inflammation of the breast, whether or not the mother has a bacterial infection (Betzold, 2007). At the least severe end of the mastitis spectrum is subclinical mastitis, which we are only beginning to understand. It appears to make the milk saltier and causes milk production to decrease, but has no other obvious symptoms (Filteau et al., 1999). Next along the spectrum is a blocked duct that a mother can clear with one good breastfeeding. Further along this spectrum is a hardened area in the breast with a fever, which may or may not involve a bacterial infection. At the most severe end is a breast abscess, a pus-filled cyst, which may require hospitalization and drainage.

Blocked Ducts and Breast Infections

Mastitis is a common problem that occurs most often during the early weeks of breastfeeding.

The incidence of mastitis varies from study to study and depends in part on whether the study included only those mothers whose mastitis was diagnosed and treated by their healthcare providers or whether it included all mothers with symptoms of mastitis. Research indicates that only about half the mothers with mastitis symptoms contact their healthcare providers (Riordan & Nichols, 1990; Scott, Robertson, Fitzpatrick, Knight, & Mulholland, 2008).

Several prospective studies on mastitis have been done with large groups of breastfeeding mothers and have shed some light on the factors that put mothers at risk. In one case-control group of 306 mothers nested in a prospective study in Western Australia, the incidence of mastitis was 27% during the first 3 months postpartum, with a recurrence rate of 6.5% (Fetherston, 1998). The mothers in this study were referred from a local breastfeeding support program and had not necessarily reported their mastitis to their healthcare provider. The major predictors for mastitis were: stress, blocked ducts, a tight bra, nipple pain or the nipple looking misshapen after a feeding, a history of mastitis, milk appearing "thicker" than normal, and difficulty taking the breast.

In an Australian prospective cohort study of 1,075 breastfeeding women, the overall incidence of mastitis during the first 6 months postpartum was 20% (Kinlay, O'Connell, & Kinlay, 2001). These mothers were followed from birth and included all mothers who gave birth in two hospitals, not just those who contacted their healthcare providers with symptoms. The major risk factor for developing mastitis was cracked nipples.

A U.S. prospective study followed 946 breastfeeding mothers and found for the first 12 weeks after birth the incidence of mastitis was about half of the Australian studies—9.5%, but this study reported only "healthcare provider-diagnosed mastitis," which did not include the mothers who treated mastitis on their own (Foxman, D'Arcy, Gillespie, Bobo, & Schwartz, 2002). The main risk factors for mastitis in this group were: history of mastitis with a previous child and cracks and nipple sores during the same week as the mastitis.

An Australian study that combined a randomized controlled trial with a survey followed 1,193 breastfeeding women for 6 months. About 17% of the mothers experienced at least one bout of self-reported mastitis, with 53% occurring during the first 4 weeks and about 75% occurring during the first 8 weeks. The authors wrote that this study "...found no association between breastfeeding duration and mastitis" (Amir, Forster, Lumley, & McLachlan, 2007, p. 9), as most cases of mastitis occurred during the early postpartum period, so longer breastfeeding was not associated with more mastitis. Risk factors included longer duration of nipple pain and cracked nipples. The researchers cited prevention of nipple pain and trauma in the early weeks as one way to reduce the incidence of mastitis.

A Scottish longitudinal study followed 420 breastfeeding mothers for the first 6 months postpartum and found that 18% of its mothers had at least one episode of self-reported mastitis, with 53% of the episodes occurring in the first 4 weeks (Scott et al., 2008). About 10% of its mothers were told incorrectly that they needed to wean from the affected breast or to stop breastfeeding altogether.

Approximately 15%-20% of mothers experience mastitis.

Mastitis is not unknown in developing countries. One large, prospective study of 1,678 consecutive patients at a Ghana breast care clinic diagnosed 13% of the women with mastitis or abscess (Ohene-Yeboah & Amaning, 2008). This study included women and girls of all ages, so many of them were not breastfeeding or of childbearing age.

When a mother has mastitis, she may feel down, discouraged about breastfeeding, and worried about both herself and her baby.

U.S. research has found an association between inflammation and depression (Kendall-Tackett, 2007). The same substances that contribute to breast inflammation (see next section) also release the stress hormone cortisol. So, a mother with mastitis may also be at higher risk for depression.

If the mother is worried about continuing to breastfeed, reassure her that breastfeeding during mastitis is a vital part of her treatment (see later section) and that some immunological components in her milk are elevated during mastitis to protect her baby's health (Buescher & Hair, 2001). Keeping her milk flowing will prevent her mastitis from getting worse and will help her recover faster. Discuss possible causes to help the mother determine why it has happened and how to prevent it from recurring.

If the mother is in pain, encourage her to talk to her healthcare provider about pain medication compatible with breastfeeding, such as ibuprofen (Hale, 2008, pp. 488-489), an anti-inflammatory that may also help reduce her breast swelling more quickly. For details, see later section "Treatments" on p. 685. If the mother wants to wean, see this section for specific strategies.

Symptoms of Mastitis

Redness and tender areas or lumps in the breast are symptoms of a blocked duct.

This occurs when a milk duct or lobe is not draining well and has become inflamed. Pressure builds behind the plug and milk components leak into surrounding breast tissue, which causes inflammation. Sometimes referred to as "caking," this usually occurs in only one breast.

In some cases, expressed milk from a blocked duct may look thick or stringy, or this may be a sign of an impending blocked duct.

A blocked duct causes pressure within the breast to build (sometimes called "milk stasis"), which causes some of the milk to seep through the walls of the ducts into the breast tissue, leaving behind thickened or stringy milk that the mother may see when she expresses. Some mothers also report expressing what looks like a crystal, a grain of sand, or a long, thin strand of spaghetti, which may be accompanied by mucus. None of these are harmful to the baby. One Australian researcher suggested that thickened expressed milk may be a predictor of future mastitis (Fetherston, 1998).

A mother with mastitis may run a fever, even if she does not have a bacterial infection, and cultures cannot reliably tell the difference.

It is not always possible to know if breast inflammation is from infection or a blocked duct. The components of the milk, such as cytokines, that leak into surrounding tissues cause inflammation, which can cause a fever, even without bacterial infection (Fetherston, 2001; Kvist, Hall-Lord, & Larsson, 2007; Michie, Lockie, & Lynn, 2005). For this reason, blocked ducts can also cause flu-like symptoms, such as feeling achy and run-down, and very warm breasts.

Some experts suggest that symptoms can be used to determine whether a mother has a blocked duct or her inflammation is bacterial (Lawrence & Lawrence, 2005, p. 563). However, research does not support this approach and no currently available tests can distinguish a blocked duct from a bacterial infection. In one U.S. study, by counting bacteria and leukocyte colonies in milk, researchers were able to differentiate among full breasts (or "milk stasis"), a blocked duct, and a bacterial infection, but this test is not available to most clinicians (Thomsen, Espersen, & Maigaard, 1984).

Research indicates that the test routinely used to culture milk does not reliably distinguish a bacterial infection from a blocked duct, because a mother's skin and milk are not sterile and bacteria will always be present in both (Kvist, Larsson, Hall-Lord, Steen, & Schalen, 2008; Matheson, Aursnes, Horgen, Aabo, & Melby, 1988). In dairy cows, cultures are used successfully, in part because all the lobes drain into one udder. But in human mothers, breast lobes are anatomically separate, so during milk expression, milk from the healthy lobes mix with milk from the infected lobe, diluting bacterial counts (Wilson-Clay & Hoover, 2008, p. 85). Thankfully, the basic treatments for a blocked duct and breast infection are the same, so except in extreme cases, it is not necessary to tell the difference.

A Swedish study of 210 episodes of mastitis found that having a fever made no difference in how long a mother's mastitis lasted (Kvist, Hall-Lord, & Larsson, 2007). Mastitis symptoms resolved in about the same length of time whether a mother had a fever or not. The mothers with nipple damage, however, took longer to feel better than those without broken skin on the nipple.

Some symptoms are specific to a bacterial infection.

If the mother's symptoms become severe, no matter what the cause, suggest she contact her healthcare provider. Symptoms that indicate a bacterial infection and may require medical treatment include:

- Visible pus in a nipple crack or fissure
- Pus or blood in her milk
- Red streaks in her breast
- Any other sudden symptoms with no obvious cause, such as nausea and vomiting

If the mother has symptoms of a bacterial infection, encourage her to contact her healthcare provider to evaluate whether medication is needed. Whether or not a mother needs antibiotics, breastfeeding can and should continue. Sudden weaning puts a mother at risk of her mastitis worsening into a breast abscess, a much more serious condition.

If a mother has severe mastitis in both breasts and her baby is less than 2 weeks old, it may be a hospital-acquired infection.

Usually mastitis occurs in only one breast. Hospital-acquired (or "nosocomial") infections are often more severe than other types, because they tend to be drug-resistant strains. In this case, a mother's mastitis may result from exposure to virulent bacteria after a hospital birth or after a hospital stay for other reasons. This was once a major problem for all mothers, when hospital stays after birth were longer.

However, now infections that once existed only in the hospital, such as MRSA (methicillin-resistant Staphylococcus aureus), have spread to some communities as well (Salgado, Farr, & Calfee, 2003; Stafford et al., 2008). **If a mother develops an MRSA infection, the baby has already been exposed to it before her symptoms became obvious, so there is no reason to stop breastfeeding unless the baby is compromised (ill or born preterm).** If the baby's health is fragile, the mother's milk could be pasteurized before feeding it to him (Gastelum, Dassey, Mascola, & Yasuda, 2005; Kim et al., 2007), or if that is not an option, her milk may need to be discarded until it is clear of infection. Hand-washing and other routine hygiene practices should be recommended to help stop the spread of infection.

If the baby balks at breastfeeding from the affected breast, suggest the mother express her milk and keep breastfeeding on the other breast.

During mastitis, sodium and chloride levels rise in mother's milk, making the milk taste saltier. Some babies react to this change in taste by showing a strong preference for the unaffected breast, sometimes refusing the affected breast altogether. If the baby balks at taking the affected breast, see p. 146- "Strategies to Achieve Settled Breastfeeding." The mother can continue breastfeeding on the unaffected breast, expressing her milk often from the affected breast to help clear the mastitis and prevent that breast from becoming painfully full. Within a week after the mother's symptoms have cleared, her milk should lose its salty taste (Fetherston, Lai, & Hartmann, 2006) and the baby should go back to that breast as usual.

A mother's milk production may be slowed in the affected breast for about a week, but she can bring it back to normal quickly.

Because the inflammation of mastitis slows milk flow, this signals the mother's body to decrease milk production in the affected breast (Wambach, 2003). However, one Australian study found that within 7 days after the mastitis symptoms were gone, the mother's milk composition was back to normal (Fetherston et al., 2006). Suggest the mother bring her production back by breastfeeding and/or expressing often on the affected breast.

Mastitis Treatments

Mastitis treatment basics include analgesia, heat and/or cold, frequent breast drainage, and rest.

Analgesia. Any mother in pain should be encouraged to talk to her healthcare provider about appropriate analgesia that is compatible with breastfeeding. Ibuprofen, for example, is also an anti-inflammatory, which can help decrease her symptoms, as well as reduce pain, and is considered compatible with breastfeeding (Hale, 2008, pp. 488-489).

Apply heat and/or cold. Because heat can increase swelling, suggest limiting its use to short periods. Wet or dry heat can be applied to the affected area for 10 minutes or so before feedings, at least 3 times each day. Warm showers, warm compresses, a heating pad, or a water bottle can be used. Some mothers find it soothing to soak their breast by leaning over a basin of warm water or lying on their side in a warm bathtub. Suggest the mother remove any dried milk from the nipple with water before breastfeeding or expressing, and gently massage the area while it is warm. Between feedings, mothers can apply cold to reduce swelling, making sure to wrap any cold packs or packages of frozen vegetables in a cloth to protect her skin. Encourage the mother to choose heat and/or cold based on what she finds most effective and soothing.

Drain the breasts often and well, loosening any tight clothing, including her bra, for better milk flow (Osterman & Rahm, 2000). If she can comfortably go without a bra for a couple of days, this may help.

- **Breastfeed after applying heat** to aid milk flow and help unplug the affected duct, making sure the baby is taking the breast deeply to more evenly drain the breast (Mizuno et al., 2008). If the mother is not breastfeeding, encourage her to express her milk after applying heat.
- **Drain the affected breast at least every couple of hours day and night** to reduce fullness and keep the milk flowing. Breastfeed on the affected side first for as long as the breast feels tender or warm.
- **Use gentle breast massage** while the breast is warm, concentrating on any lumps or sore areas by using fingertips or the palm of her hand, moving from the armpit toward the nipple. Massage has been found to increase milk flow during breastfeeding and expressing (Jones et al., 2001; Stutte et al., 1988).
- **Vary feeding positions**, which may help unplug a duct as long as the baby takes the breast deeply in all the positions used. At least once during each feeding suggest the mother position the baby so his nose or chin points toward the plug (Riordan & Wambach, 2010). Laid-back breastfeeding positions allow a mother to do this comfortably by varying the angle of the baby's "lie" on her body. Some mothers with mastitis may benefit from occasionally breastfeeding on her hands and knees over her baby (Marmet & Shell, 2008). Suggest the mother use only positions that work well and are comfortable for her. If a mother is not breastfeeding, suggest she try the tips for increasing milk flow during milk expression on p. 449 in "How to Express More Milk."

Rest. Mastitis may be one sign a mother is fatigued or stressed. When her resistance to illness decreases, risk factors are more likely to lead to mastitis. If possible, suggest the mother take her baby to bed with her and stay there until she feels better. If it's not possible, suggest she postpone extra activities and plan to spend an hour or two each day relaxing with her baby with her feet up. Be sure she knows that rest is the key to recovery.

In a Swedish study, acupuncture was tested as a therapy for mastitis, but it was not found to improve outcomes (Kvist, Hall-Lord, Rydhstroem, & Larsson, 2007).

• •

The use of antibiotics to treat mastitis varies widely by country and may be over-used in some parts of the world.

The home treatments described in the previous point are the best first approach for any mother with symptoms of mastitis. Antibiotics will not address the underlying cause of the mastitis, but may be appropriate in severe cases and when an infection is obvious. The research on antibiotic use is mixed. The Academy of Breastfeeding Medicine's mastitis protocol recommends that "If symptoms are not improving within 12 to 24 hours or if the woman is acutely ill, antibiotics should be started" (ABM, 2008, p. 178).

However, Swedish research calls this recommendation into question. Researchers cultured the milk of 192 women with mastitis and 466 milk donors without mastitis in an attempt to learn more about the role various organisms play in this condition (Kvist et al., 2008). They found Staphylococcus aureus and Group B streptococci in the milk of mothers both with and without mastitis, and they found no correlation between the severity of the mothers' symptoms and the bacteria levels in their milk. They also found that bacterial counts did not differ between mothers treated with antibiotics and those using only home treatment. They concluded that milk cultures may not be an accurate gauge for determining whether or not a mother with mastitis has a bacterial infection and questioned the use of antibiotics to treat mastitis, especially high rates of use.

Some studies have found antibiotic treatment for mastitis to be as high as 77% to 97% of healthcare provider treated cases in the U.S. (Foxman et al., 2002; Wambach, 2003) and Australia (Fetherston, 1997; Kinlay, O'Connell, & Kinlay, 1998). A Finnish study that followed 664 women with mastitis reported that 38% were treated with antibiotics (Jonsson & Pulkkinen, 1994). In comparison, 15% of the mothers in another Swedish study were prescribed antibiotics, 3.3% (seven mothers) due to the severity of their symptoms and 11.4% (24 mothers) due to the results of their milk cultures (Kvist, Hall-Lord, & Larsson, 2007). After the study, 12% (21 mothers) contacted their healthcare providers with recurring symptoms, and 8 of these then received antibiotics. But of these eight mothers, five had previously received antibiotics while in the study, so only three of the study mothers (1.6%) who didn't receive antibiotics during the study appeared to need them later.

One U.S. study found that frequent removal of milk from the breasts decreased the duration of symptoms by 50%, as compared with the use of antibiotics alone (Osterman & Rahm, 2000).

• •

In some cases, treatment with antibiotics may be appropriate.

When a mother has a sore breast, fever, and flu-like symptoms, suggest she begin home treatment right away. Suggest she contact her healthcare provider if:

- After 24 hours of home treatment, her symptoms are the same or worse.
- She has been running a fever for some time.
- She has obvious signs of a bacterial infection, such as visible pus.
- Her temperature suddenly spikes higher.

If she has any of these signs, her healthcare provider may prescribe an antibiotic compatible with breastfeeding. The drugs usually given for a 10 to 14 day course are a penicillinase-resistant penicillin (such as cloxacillin or dicloxacillin) or a cephalosporin, such as cephalexin (250 mg to 500 mg per day). Mothers taking a shorter course of antibiotics may be at greater risk of recurrence (Lawrence & Lawrence, 2005, p. 566). Encourage the mother to take the full course of antibiotics even after she feels better. Antibiotics may help resolve a mother's symptoms, even if she doesn't have an infection, because they are also effective anti-inflammatory drugs (Walker, 2006, p. 392).

If there is no improvement within 2 days of antibiotic treatment, rule out cellulitis and other breast diseases and consider the need for a different drug.

If a mother does not respond to antibiotics within 2 days, the World Health Organization and the Academy of Breastfeeding Medicine recommend that her milk be cultured so another drug can be chosen that targets the specific organism involved (ABM, 2008; WHO, 2000).

Cellulitis may look like mastitis, but has a different cause and treatment.

Cellulitis is a condition that is sometimes mistaken for mastitis. It is an inflammation of the skin and underlying tissues, and a different organism is usually involved. The organism usually enters the body through broken skin, such as nipple trauma. It affects the connective tissue of the breast, rather than the milk-making tissues (Riordan & Wambach, 2010). The areas affected may look red and swollen and appear raised. If a mother has cellulitis, heat and massage can aggravate it, rather than help, and she will need different antibiotics. When the usual treatments are not working, suggest the mother have her healthcare provider evaluate her for cellulitis.

Other breast disease. If the mother's red and swollen breast does not improve within at least 72 hours of treatment with antibiotics, suggest she see her healthcare provider to rule other causes, some of which could be life-threatening. For example, the early stages of inflammatory breast cancer accounts for 1% to 5% of all breast cancers in the U.S. and can mimic mastitis (NCI, 2006). Its symptoms include redness, swelling and warmth in the breast without an obvious lump. This is caused by cancer cells blocking the mother's lymph nodes. As the disease progresses, the mother's skin may change color, appearing pink, purple, or bruised. Areas of the breast may also form ridges or look pitted, like the skin of an orange (called 'eau d'organge). The mother's nipple may become flattened, red, and crusty. Inflammatory breast cancer can be diagnosed by exam and confirmed with biopsy, mammogram, or ultrasound.

A possible alternative to antibiotics is swabbing the nipple and areola after feedings with a nisin solution.

Frequent use of antibiotics has produced many resistant strains of bacteria, which is one reason to use them sparingly. A Spanish pilot study examined an alternative mastitis treatment: the topical application of nisin, a food-grade microbial produced by the lactic acid bacterium Lactococcus lactis (Fernandez, Delgado, Herrero, Maldonado, & Rodriguez, 2008). Nisin is a bacteriocin, a substance produced by bacteria that kills other bacteria. In this study, eight mothers with mastitis in both breasts were divided into two groups. One group of four mothers applied a small amount of nisin solution (~0.1 mL) to the nipple and areola after every breastfeeding for 2 weeks, and the other group of four applied a solution without nisin. After 2 weeks, the symptoms completely resolved in the nisin group, whereas symptoms continued in the other group.

Staphylococcus aureus (even methicillin-resistant strains such as MRSA) responded to the nisin, and the level of Staph aureus in the milk of the nisin group declined throughout the 2 weeks of the study. In the non-nisin group, though, the level of Staph aureus in the milk increased slightly. A larger study is underway at this writing.

Most breast lumps are not caused by cancer, but this possibility and others, such as galactoceles and cysts, need to be ruled out if the mother's lump does not decrease in size after treatment (Dahlbeck, Donnelly, & Theriault, 1995; Marchant, 2002).

If a breast lump doesn't shrink within a few days of treatment, suggest the mother contact her healthcare provider to rule out other causes.

Causes of Mastitis

The most common risk factors for mastitis are periods of breast fullness, nipple pain or trauma, and sustained pressure on the breast.

Periods of breast fullness can sometimes occur even when breastfeeding is going well, but discuss possible causes with the mother.

- **Ineffective breastfeeding, leaving the breast full after feedings**. This may be from shallow breastfeeding, engorgement, or anatomical issues, such as inverted nipples, tongue-tie, or unusual palate. In one Australian study, all five mothers of babies with tongue tie developed mastitis (Fetherston, 1998). For details, see p. 118- "Tongue Issues."
- **Overabundant milk production.** Even when a baby breastfeeds effectively, if a mother produces much more milk than her baby takes, her breasts may feel full much of the time. If her baby's weight gain is well above average, this may be a possibility. For details, see p. 425- "Overabundant Milk Production."
- **Restricted breastfeeding**. This may occur when a mother schedules feedings or limits feeding length. Ask the mother to describe how she breastfeeds.
- **Missed feedings, supplements, or irregular feeding patterns**. Is her baby receiving bottles or a pacifier/dummy? Supplements and pacifiers can delay breastfeeding. Some babies are just naturally irregular feeders. Suggest the mother breastfeed or express her milk before her breasts feel full.
- **Baby sleeping for longer stretches day or night.** This may be due to normal growth and development. Ask whether her baby's breastfeeding pattern changed before she developed mastitis. Babies can breastfeed effectively, even while asleep (Colson, 2008; Colson et al., 2003).
- **Ineffective milk expression.** This may result from the use of an ineffective breast pump during extended times away from the baby.
- **Outside distractions that prevent or delay breastfeeding**. Ask if the mother has been unusually busy. A prime time for mastitis is around the holidays, when mothers are busy, distracted, and fatigued.
- **Too-rapid weaning.** This may cause too much breast fullness for too long.
- **Uneven breast drainage**. This is usually caused by shallow breastfeeding, during which the baby may drain some areas of the breast more than others.

One Japanese study of 37 mothers and babies found that when babies take the breast shallowly, the breast does not drain evenly, leaving some areas more drained and other areas less drained (Mizuno et al., 2008). Researchers determined the degree of drainage of different breast lobes by drawing milk from their corresponding nipple pores and measuring their milk fat content. High fat content indicated that the lobe was well drained during breastfeeding. Low fat content indicated not as much milk was taken from that lobe. The researchers found that the study babies who achieved deep breastfeeding drained the breast more evenly than those who breastfed shallowly.

Nipple trauma. Broken skin on the nipple provides a point of entry for bacteria. Ultrasound breast research has shown that after milk ejection, milk flows back into the ducts, making it possible for bacteria to be carried back with the milk (Ramsay, Kent, Owens, & Hartmann, 2004). Many studies have found an increased risk of mastitis after nipple trauma (Amir et al., 2007; Amir, Garland, & Lumley, 2006; Foxman et al., 2002; Kinlay et al., 2001).

One Canadian study (Livingstone, Willis, & Berkowitz, 1996) found that during the first month postpartum, 64% of its 227 mothers with moderate to severe nipple pain and nipple fissures tested positive for Staphylococcal aureus, the organism most commonly linked with infectious mastitis (Osterman & Rahm, 2000; Scott et al., 2008). Of the mothers not started on oral antibiotics, 25% subsequently developed mastitis. One Australian study concluded, "The prevention and improved management of nipple damage could potentially reduce the risk of ... developing mastitis" (Amir et al., 2007, p. 62). For strategies to prevent bacterial infection of the traumatized nipple, see p. 650- "Preventing Infections."

Consistent pressure on the breast. Firm pressure sustained on the breast can restrict milk flow, which can cause milk components to leak into the surrounding breast tissue and trigger inflammation. Examples include:

- **An ill-fitting bra** that binds part of the breast or one that provides little support, allowing the weight of heavy breasts to constrict milk ducts (Fetherston, 1998).
- **Breast shells** worn for hours in a bra with too-small cups, leaving indentations on the breast when removed (Fetherston, 1998).
- **Stomach-sleeping**, which can cause long-term breast tissue compression.
- **A tote or baby carrier** with straps that press into the breast for long periods.

Fatigue often precedes mastitis (Fetherston, 1998; Riordan & Nichols, 1990). For other, more unusual factors that can increase the risk of mastitis, see the next section.

If a mother with mastitis decides to wean, help her do it slowly and safely.

If a mother with mastitis weans too quickly, this could cause her mastitis to worsen or to develop into a breast abscess (see later section). To avoid a more serious health problem, suggest she wait until her mastitis clears, and then wean very slowly to avoid a recurrence.

Lactation consultants Barbara Wilson-Clay and Kay Hoover describe a slow-weaning plan after the surgical drainage of a breast abscess in *The Breastfeeding Atlas* (Wilson-Clay & Hoover, 2008, pp. 88-89). The mother exclusively expressed her milk with a breast pump and alternated between dropping a daily pumping, waiting several days, then gradually decreasing each pumping by a couple of minutes, and then waiting several days. Using this strategy, the mother was able to stop her milk production safely and comfortably over a period of several weeks. Any time during the weaning the mother felt any breast fullness, she pumped just enough milk to soften her breasts. That way she was able to cease milk production without causing more health problems.

Recurring Mastitis

Recurring mastitis can be demoralizing, even to a motivated mother.

Chronic mastitis can cause even the most dedicated mother to question her commitment to breastfeeding. It's important to listen carefully and acknowledge the mother's feelings, no matter how negative. Offer to help her try to determine the cause of the recurrences, and assure her that in most cases the cause can be found and eliminated, or treatment can be started that can break the cycle. If she decides to wean, emphasize the importance of weaning slowly and carefully (see previous point).

• •

To determine the cause, first ask her to describe her previous treatments.

Failure to fully recover from a previous mastitis is a common cause of recurring mastitis. It is especially likely if the last episode of mastitis was within the previous few weeks, although previous mastitis anytime puts a mother at greater risk of recurrence. Encourage the mother to be vigilant with home treatment until her mastitis is completely gone.

If the mother's mastitis recurs even after treatment with antibiotics, it is still possible that the original mastitis did not completely resolve. Repeated mastitis can happen—especially if the same risk factors are present—but it is usually a recurrence of the original mastitis, rather than a new case. Other possibilities include:

- A too-short course of antibiotics (less than 10 to 14 days), either due to her doctor's order or because she stopped taking them too soon.
- Prescription of an inappropriate antibiotic.
- Reinfection after finishing the medication by an organism carried in the baby's throat or nose (Wust, Rutsch, & Stocker, 1995).

If her mastitis recurs after she has taken an antibiotic for at least 10 days, suggest the mother ask her doctor to culture her milk and her baby's throat and nose to determine if another antibiotic might be more effective. If her baby's throat or nose cultures are positive, the baby may need treatment, too. One Australian study of 100 mothers with mastitis and 99 controls found an association between positive culture of the baby's nose and the mothers' mastitis (Amir et al., 2006). Because Staphylococcus aureus is the most common organism involved with mastitis, it is typically treated with the antibiotics effective against it. But sometimes other bacteria are involved, such as Streptococcus pneumoniae (Wust et al., 1995), Group B Streptococcus, or even tuberculosis (Gupta, Gupta, & Duggal, 1982), and another drug would be more effective. With the wider spread of MRSA, it is also possible that she has a drug-resistant strain of Staphylococcus aureus and a different drug would be more effective (Fortunov, Hulten, Hammerman, Mason, & Kaplan, 2006; Salgado et al., 2003; Stafford et al., 2008).

Talk to her about her usual breastfeeding patterns to see if any of the common causes of mastitis may be responsible for her recurrences.

Most often, recurring mastitis is triggered by one of its common causes:

- Periods of breast fullness
- Entry of bacteria in the breast due to nipple trauma
- Sustained pressure on the breast

See the previous section for more specific areas to explore, such as overabundant milk production, a change in feeding pattern, starting a new job, a recent nipple bite, trauma from using too-tight breast pump flanges, constrictive clothing, sleeping on her stomach, a new baby carrier that presses into her breast, etc. One of these may be the underlying cause responsible for her recurring mastitis.

Other, more unusual risk factors, along with fatigue and stress, may also contribute to recurring mastitis.

Fatigue or feeling "run down" often precedes mastitis (Fetherston, 1998; Riordan & Nichols, 1990), especially in mothers with more than one child (Fetherston, 2001). Anything that decreases a mother's resistance to illness or infection may make her more prone to mastitis, especially if she has other risk factors. In one survey of 91 breastfeeding mothers, those who had mastitis (about one-third) ranked fatigue first and stress second as major contributing factors (Riordan & Nichols, 1990). Several described family travel, hectic holidays, christenings, parties, and household moves as triggers. In a German review of 16 studies, its authors suggested that stress contributes to breast inflammation by releasing substances such as cytokines that trigger inflammation (Wockel, Abou-Dakn, Beggel, & Arck, 2008).

Other, more unusual factors that can contribute to recurring mastitis include:

- **Nipple bleb,** or "milk blister," blocking milk flow from one or more nipple pores. For details, see p. 658- "'Blebs' or Milk Blisters."

Any breast surgery increases the risk of mastitis.

- **Exclusive pumping**, which can lead to longer stretches between milk expressions than would usually occur with breastfeeding, causing periods of breast fullness.
- **Health issues** that increase a mother's susceptibility to infection, such as diabetes, IgA deficiency (Fetherston, Lai, & Hartmann, 2008), or anemia (Fetherston, 1998).
- **Nipple shield use** (did the mother begin using it due to ineffective breastfeeding?) or poor hygiene of the shield (Fetherston, 1998; Noble & Bovey, 1997).
- **Breast injury** from intense exercise or trauma, which may cause breast swelling and block milk flow (Fetherston, 1998).
- **Nipple piercing**, which allows bacteria to enter the breast (Jacobs, Golombeck, Jonat, & Kiechle, 2003; Trupiano et al., 2001).
- **Internal breast abnormalities**, scar tissue from previous breast surgery, abscess, cyst, or cancer that causes internal pressure on ducts and blocks milk flow (Dahlbeck et al., 1995; Marchant, 2002; Meguid, Oler, Numann, & Khan, 1995; Olsen & Gordon, 1990).

If the mastitis always recurs in the same area, there may be an internal cause. Any breast surgery—biopsy, breast reduction, breast augmentation, tumor, or cyst removal—increases the risk of mastitis due to internal scarring, which can cause pressure on the milk ducts. Unusual anatomy in a duct is another possible cause. Due to pressure on milk ducts, an existing breast lump from any cause may put a mother at increased risk. Since these causes cannot be easily corrected, a mother may choose to breastfeed only on the unaffected breast, gradually allowing milk production to stop on the affected side.

Recurring mastitis in the same location is also a warning sign of possible breast cancer. If the mastitis always occurs in the same breast and at the same spot, suggest the mother see her doctor to rule out this cause.

• •

Possible treatments for recurring mastitis are low-dose, long-term antibiotics, dietary changes, and lecithin supplements.

Some mothers have been able to break the cycle of chronic recurring mastitis with preventive, low-dose, long-term antibiotic treatment. Following a 10- to 14-day course of antibiotics to treat their current mastitis, these women were then prescribed low doses of antibiotics (i.e., 500 mg. erythromycin) taken daily for 2 to 3 months to prevent recurrence (Lawrence & Lawrence, 2005, p. 567).

If a mother continues to experience recurring mastitis, some suggest dietary changes, such as reducing saturated fat intake and taking a lecithin supplement (Eglash, 1998). Suggested dosages of lecithin range from 1 tablespoon (15 mL) per day (Lawrence & Lawrence, 2005, p. 299) to 1 tablespoon (15 mL) 3 to 4 times a day, or one to two 1,200 mg capsules 3 or 4 times per day (Newman & Pitman, 2006, p. 126).

Breast Abscess

Breast abscesses are uncommon and usually occur when mastitis is not treated well or doesn't respond to treatment.

A breast abscess is a walled-off area of pus in the breast with no opening for drainage, so it must be either aspirated or surgically drained. It is a serious and often painful condition that needs immediate medical attention.

Abscesses are categorized by location. Subareolar abscesses are just under the areola. Intramamamary abscesses are deeper within the breast. Abscesses may also have one pocket (unilocular) or multiple pockets, called multiocular abscesses. Thankfully, breast abscesses are relatively uncommon. When both self-reported and healthcare provider-treated mastitis are considered, research indicates they occur in about 3% of breastfeeding mothers who've had mastitis (Amir, Forster, McLachlan, & Lumley, 2004; Amir et al., 2007). One Swedish study found that among the more than 1.4 million women who gave birth in Sweden between 1987 and 2000 (not just those who had mastitis), the rate of abscess was 0.1% (Kvist & Rydhstroem, 2005). When an abscess occurs in a breastfeeding woman, it is usually the result of untreated mastitis, a delay in treatment, or incorrect treatment.

• •

In some areas, most abscesses culture positive for MRSA, an organism resistant to common antibiotics.

As resistant strains of bacteria spread into communities, incorrect treatment of abscesses may become more of an issue. One U.S. study reported that cases of community-acquired methicillin-resistant Staphylococcus aureus (MRSA) increased nine-fold in the Dallas, Texas area between 2003 and 2008, and that 63% of the breastfeeding study mothers diagnosed with breast abscesses cultured positive for MRSA (Stafford et al., 2008). Another U.S. study in Houston, Texas, found similar percentages of MRSA (63% to 64%) among its 33 study mothers with breast abscesses (Peterson, 2007).

Where community-acquired MRSA is becoming prevalent, suggest mothers wash their hands often. Healthcare providers need to be especially vigilant about using gloves and routinely disinfecting the everyday objects they touch, such as clipboards, pens, and computer keyboards, and the surfaces mothers and babies come in contact with, such as baby scales and breast pumps (Wilson-Clay, 2008).

• •

An ultrasound is preferred over a mammogram to identify an abscess and can also be used during treatment.

In many cases, the mother's healthcare provider may not be able to confirm an abscess by examination alone. A mammogram cannot distinguish an abscess from other masses, such as a tumor, and the breast squeezing involved in this procedure can be very painful for a mother with inflamed breasts. Ultrasound, on the other hand, can distinguish a breast abscess from solid masses, especially when performed by a technician familiar with the lactating breast. Confirming the existence, size, and location of the abscess allows the healthcare provider to determine whether or not surgical drainage is necessary or whether a less-invasive treatment is an option.

• •

For most abscesses, fine-needle aspiration and catheter drainage are effective treatments that are less invasive than surgery and make continued breastfeeding easier.

Until recent years, breast abscesses were usually treated by surgical drainage, which required hospitalization. But research indicates that a combination of ultrasonic imaging to locate the abscess and aspiration and flushing with a needle or catheter can eliminate the need for surgery 97% of the time (Christensen et al., 2005; Ulitzsch, Nyman, & Carlson, 2004). These procedures are much less invasive and can typically be done as an outpatient, which minimizes separation of mother and baby. Culturing the aspirated pus for organisms and treating the mother with appropriate antibiotics for at least 10 days is also a vital part of this treatment.

One Swedish study followed 43 breastfeeding women diagnosed with 56 abscesses (some women had more than one) (Ulitzsch et al., 2004). The ultrasound revealed the size and location of the abscess. For abscesses 3 cm or smaller, the researchers used fine-needle aspiration guided by ultrasound to aspirate and flush them with saline solution. For abscesses larger than 3 cm, they inserted catheters to drain and flush them. Some mothers (48%) needed the aspiration and flushing done only once for their abscesses to resolve; other mothers needed multiple aspirations and flushings (2 to 5) before their abscesses resolved. Catheters were left in the breast an average of 6 days (range: 1 to 25 days) before removal. Only one (2%) of the 43 mothers had surgical drainage.

A Danish study followed 151 women with abscesses, including 89 who were breastfeeding and 62 who developed abscesses while they were not lactating. The women were treated using fine-needle aspiration or a catheter as described in the previous study. After the first round of drainage, 97% of the breastfeeding study mothers recovered, with 1% having a recurrence and 2% needing surgery later. The researchers concluded that because these procedures do not require hospitalization or affect breastfeeding, they "should replace surgery as the first line of treatment in uncomplicated...breast abscess" (Christensen et al., 2005, p. 188).

Aspiration should not affect breastfeeding. If the catheter (or the incision if surgical drainage is used) is near her nipple or areola, the mother can continue breastfeeding on the unaffected breast. If the catheter or incision is far enough from the nipple so that the baby's mouth does not touch it when he breastfeeds, the mother may also be able to breastfeed on the affected breast. An abscess that is surgically drained is not usually closed, but remains open and is allowed to drain and heal from the inside out. As with any mother with mastitis, rest is a key part of the treatment.

When breastfeeding continues during abscess treatment, the mother may need to make some adjustments.

If the mother does not breastfeed on the affected side, encourage her to express her milk from that breast while her incision is healing to prevent engorgement. (For details, see the chapter "Milk Expression and Storage.")

Breastfeeding can continue on the affected breast after surgical drainage (ABM, 2008) and will not prevent healing, even though milk may seep out of the incision. The incision may heal more slowly, but continuing to breastfeed prevents the affected breast from becoming painfully full, prevents the mastitis from recurring, and decreases the odds that the baby will prefer the unaffected breast after healing.

Subclinical Mastitis

Subclinical mastitis in human mothers is controversial.

"Subclinical" means having no obvious symptoms. In the dairy industry, subclinical mastitis is well known and linked to decreased milk production in cows, but it is still unclear whether the same is true for human mothers.

Some African studies have defined subclinical mastitis as an increase in a mother's milk sodium and potassium content in the absence of weaning (Aryeetey, Marquis, Timms, Lartey, & Brakohiapa, 2008; Filteau et al., 1999; Kasonka et al., 2006). More recent studies have also found it may include an increase in some milk enzymes (Rasmussen et al., 2008). This is an area of interest and concern, because some research indicates that when an HIV-positive mother's milk undergoes these changes, her baby is at greater risk of becoming infected. Research from the U.K. on Bangladeshi women indicates that basic breastfeeding counseling, promoting early and exclusive breastfeeding, feeding on cue, and good breastfeeding technique reduces the percentage of women whose milk undergoes the changes in composition associated with subclinical mastitis (Flores & Filteau, 2002). Other research on breastfeeding mothers of 3- to 6-month-olds has found no significant decrease in milk production among mothers whose milk shows signs of subclinical mastitis (Aryeetey, Marquis, Brakohiapa, Timms, & Lartey, 2009).

At least one Australian researcher questions the current interpretations, because as she pointed out, these changes in mother's milk occur for reasons other than mastitis and weaning (Fetherston, 2001). Higher sodium and potassium levels are also normal during pregnancy and when milk production increases rapidly after birth. Australian research has also identified other situations in which a mother's milk increases in sodium and potassium, even when her breasts are healthy, such as preterm birth, nipple trauma, overabundant milk production, low milk production, and when a mother develops a systemic infection (Fetherston et al., 2006). More research is needed before firm conclusions about subclinical mastitis in human mothers can be drawn.

DEEP BREAST PAIN

A mother with breast pain may feel worried and upset.

When a mother has deep breast pain, in addition to the discomfort she is suffering, in the back of her mind, the mother may be worried that her pain indicates a serious physical problem, such as breast cancer. Recurring pain may also give her second thoughts about breastfeeding. Listen and acknowledge her feelings. Offer to help her determine the cause of her pain. Assure her that in most cases the cause of deep breast pain can be found and the pain relieved. Also encourage her to contact her healthcare provider for appropriate pain medication.

• •

Ask the age of her baby, where and when she feels the pain, and if she's had nipple pain or trauma or any other breastfeeding problems.

Some causes of deep breast pain can occur at any stage of breastfeeding, but some are more likely during the first weeks, while breastfeeding is getting established. For example, nipple pain and trauma, mastitis, vasospasm, Raynaud's Phenomenon, and strong let-down are more common during early breastfeeding. Referred pain from an injury can happen at any time.

The mother may feel the pain in one or both breasts. It may be localized in one area or radiate throughout the breasts. If the mother has (or had) nipple pain, nipple trauma, or mastitis, this may be a clue to its cause. The following are the most common causes of deep breast pain, along with how the symptoms of each are perceived.

If the pain is in one breast during or between feedings, consider:

- **Nipple pain and/or trauma**. The pain may be localized, but it is usually radiating. The pain resolves when breastfeeding no longer hurts and nipples have healed. Ask the mother if her nipples look misshapen after feedings. For more, see the chapter "Nipple Issues."
- **Mastitis**. The pain is usually localized, but it could be radiating. In severe cases, it could occur in both breasts. Most cases occur during the early weeks of breastfeeding (Amir et al., 2007). Ask the mother if there is a hard area in her breast or if she feels pain when she puts pressure on her breast. If breast pain continues after treatment for mastitis, suggest the mother see her healthcare provider to rule out abscess and other breast issues (Amir, 2003). See earlier section, "Mastitis." A Spanish study found that culturing the mother's milk for bacteria could distinguish mastitis from Raynaud's Phenomenon, as bacterial counts were significantly higher with mastitis than with Raynaud's (Delgado, Collado, Fernandez, & Rodriguez, 2009).
- **Nipple infection**. The pain may be localized or radiating. It occurs after nipple damage, and pus may be seen. If both nipples are infected, it could occur in both breasts. It is most likely due to bacterial infection (Thomassen, Johansson, Wassberg, & Petrini, 1998), but fungal infection (or both) is also possible. For details, see p. 651- "Bacterial Infections."

If the pain is in both breasts *during* feedings, consider:

- **Engorgement**. The pain is usually radiating and will resolve with engorgement. It occurs in the first 2 weeks of breastfeeding, and the breast tissue feels taut. It can occur later after missed feedings or long sleep stretches. See earlier section, "Engorgement."

- **Strong milk ejection**. The pain is usually radiating. One German study of 335 non-lactating women found a strong association between milk duct dilation and breast pain unrelated to their menstrual cycles (Peters, Diemer, Mecks, & Behnken, 2003). The wider the mothers' milk ducts while dilating, the greater their pain. Ultrasound research on breastfeeding women has indicated a large variation in duct size and a significant increase in ductal diameter during milk ejection (Ramsay et al., 2004), which may contribute to breast pain during feedings in some women (Walker, 2006, p. 397). Ask the mother if the pain starts shortly after feedings begin, when she hears her baby gulping. Overabundant milk production may increase the pain. This pain usually decreases over time, disappearing within a month of breastfeeding (Riordan & Wambach, 2010).

If the pain is in both breasts *between* feedings, consider:

- **Vasospasm or Raynaud's Phenomenon**. The pain is usually radiating. The nipple may turn white (blanch) after the baby releases the breast. If Raynaud's is involved, the nipple may then turn red and/or blue, and the mother may have a history of fingers blanching when cold. It usually begins during the early weeks of breastfeeding. For details and treatment options, see p. 639 in the chapter "Nipple Issues."
- **Referred pain from nipple pain and/or trauma.** The pain may be localized or radiating and will resolve when nipple pain and/or trauma resolves. It usually occurs during the early weeks of breastfeeding, but may occur later if nipple damage happens when baby is teething.

• •

If the common causes don't seem to fit, explore less common causes of deep breast pain.

If the pain is in one breast during or between feedings, consider:

- **Internal scarring from a previous breast surgery or injury**. The pain is usually localized. Ask the mother if she has had any breast enhancement or surgery. Ask her if she has ever sustained a breast injury. See last section in this chapter.
- **Ruptured breast implant**. The pain is usually localized. You may see changes in breast shape or skin changes (Walker, 2006).
- **Galactocele**. The pain is usually localized. You can usually feel an obvious lump within the breast. For details, see p. 699- "Breast Lumps."
- **Ductal ectasia**. The pain is usually localized and may also include burning, itching, and swelling of the nipple. For details, see p. 703- "Blood in the Milk or Nipple Discharge."
- **Referred pain from muscle strain or injury**. The pain may be localized or radiating and resolves when injury heals. An injury elsewhere in the body may be felt as breast pain if it is along the same nerve pathways. In the early weeks, this could be due to a birth injury, such as a pulled back or neck muscle. Later, it could be due to any injury, joint pain, or muscle strain, such as leaning over to breastfeed in uncomfortable positions. It may be felt in both breasts. Ask the mother if she has a pulled muscle, muscle strain, or any other injury. If so, suggest she use

laid-back breastfeeding positions, so she doesn't have to support her baby's weight.

- **Breast cancer**. The pain may be localized or radiating. If a mother's breast pain does not resolve after a couple of weeks, suggest she see her healthcare provider to rule this out. Between 8% and 15% of mothers later diagnosed with breast cancer report breast pain as one of their symptoms (Ohene-Yeboah & Amaning, 2008).

If the pain is in both breasts during feedings, consider:

- **Premenstrual pain**. The pain is usually radiating and peaks before a menstrual period when breasts swell with extra blood and lymph fluids. It can be felt during or between feedings and includes feeling of heaviness, fullness, and tenderness. Symptoms usually resolve soon after menstruation starts. If fibrocystic breast changes are a contributing factor, eliminating caffeine may help.

If the pain is in both breasts between feedings, consider:

- **Very large breasts** are heavy and can pull on the connective tissues above the breast. Ask the mother if she feels tenderness where the breasts join the chest wall and near the third rib when she applies gentle pressure above the breasts. A different style or better fitting bra may help relieve the pain.

Shooting pains in the breast between feedings are unlikely to be due to candida if that is the only symptom.

Once it was thought that the most likely cause of shooting or burning pain in the breasts between feedings was a secondary yeast infection in or around the milk ducts, but research has found otherwise. One Swedish study found that 3 times more women with deep breast pain had bacteria infections, rather than yeast infections (Thomassen et al., 1998). In one Canadian study, mothers with diagnosed Staphylococcus aureus infection of the nipple also suffered from vasospasms, which can cause deep breast pain (Livingstone & Stringer, 1999). The interventions that resolved the vasospasms were instruction in improved breastfeeding technique, prescribing oral antibiotics, and avoiding nipple exposure to cold. A U.S. study reported that 8 of 12 women with deep breast pain were treated with repeated courses of a powerful anti-fungal drug before their health history revealed that Raynaud's Phenomenon was the cause of their pain (Anderson, Held, & Wright, 2004). After treatment with prescription nifedipine, their pain resolved.

Another U.S. study compared the expressed milk from 18 breastfeeding mothers without breast pain or other symptoms with the milk of 16 mothers with stabbing or burning breast pain between feedings, as well as nipple pain or trauma (Hale, Bateman, Finkelman, & Berens, 2009). Accurate assay methods were unable to detect candida in the milk of either group. To further confuse the issue, some common yeast treatments, such as gentian violet and fluconazole, also act as an anti-inflammatory, so they may relieve some of a mother's symptoms, even if yeast is not the cause of her pain.

In an effort to clarify which symptoms are reliable indicators of candida infections, U.S. researchers studied 100 mothers and found that yeast is the likely cause of painful breastfeeding if a mother has the following symptoms together (Francis-Morrill, Heinig, Pappagianis, & Dewey, 2004):

- Shiny nipple/areola skin with stabbing pain
- Flaky nipple/areola skin and breast pain

If any of these symptoms appear alone, they are much less likely to predict thrush.

For more details, see p. 652- "Candida/Thrush."

BREAST LUMPS

When lactating, a woman's breasts typically feel lumpier than when she is not lactating.

Breast texture changes during lactation because more blood and lymph flow to the breasts and because the milk ducts fill and empty many times each day. Suggest the mother become familiar with the way her breasts feel during lactation by examining them regularly. With practice, she can learn to distinguish normal breast lumpiness from a lump that might need medical attention by noticing if it decreases in size after breastfeeding. If a lump's size stays constant or increases, suggest it be checked by a healthcare provider.

If a mother notices a lump that does not decrease in size after careful home treatment for mastitis, suggest she see her healthcare provider.

During breastfeeding, most lumps are either milk-filled glands or inflammation, such as mastitis. Some are benign tumors (fibromas) or milk-retention cysts (galactoceles). Only rarely are they cancerous.

If the mother's healthcare provider is not familiar with the lactating breast, suggest he or she consult with a knowledgeable colleague or that the mother find another healthcare provider experienced with breastfeeding mothers.

Suggest the mother plan to breastfeed right before her breasts are examined or a procedure is performed.

Breastfeeding right before an exam or procedure reduces the amount of milk in her breasts, making it easier to feel a lump and to perform procedures. If the mother brings the baby with her, she can breastfeed while she is waiting, keeping the amount of milk in her breasts at a minimum when she is seen.

Breastfeeding is compatible with most diagnostic tests.

Some of the diagnostic tests that might be used to diagnose a breast lump include:

X-rays. Mother's milk is not affected and a mother may breastfeed right after an x-ray.

Imaging scans (PET, MIBI, and EIT scans, and ultrasound). These imaging techniques do not interfere with breastfeeding or affect mother's milk (West & Hirsch, 2008). Unlike mammograms, ultrasound can effectively distinguish solid breast lumps from cysts, galactoceles, and abscesses.

A CAT scan or magnetic resonance imaging (MRI) does not interfere with breastfeeding or affect mother's milk, but as part of these procedures a mother may be injected with a radiopaque or radiocontrast agent, which allows blood vessels to be seen more clearly. The agents typically used with CAT scans are iodinated radiocontrast agents, but unlike other iodine agents, the iodine in these products stays bound to the molecule, which prevents the iodine from going into the milk. Agents used with an MRI typically contain gadolinium, which has been found to "penetrate milk poorly and would be virtually unabsorbed orally. Therefore, they are of little risk to a breastfeeding infant" (Hale, 2008, p. 1065). Some package inserts for these products suggest mothers interrupt breastfeeding for 24 hours after use, but this is usually not necessary. These preparations are also used in children for diagnostic purposes.

Mammograms use low-level x-rays and can be done on a lactating breast. Like other x-rays, mammograms do not affect the milk, so the mother can breastfeed afterward. But they are usually more difficult to read in younger women and during lactation because breast tissue is denser at those times. As women age, their breast tissue loses density, making mammography a more effective diagnostic tool. A mammogram can help determine the size and location of a known lump, but may not show early lumps or soft-tissue changes in the lactating breast.

The level of a mother's milk production will affect the quality of a mammogram. Greater milk production causes greater breast tissue density, making a mammogram harder to read. Conversely, lower milk production makes a mammogram easier to read. But breast tissue changes take time. It would take about a month after weaning before a difference would be noticeable in the quality of a mother's mammogram.

If a breastfeeding mother needs a mammogram, encourage her to look for a radiologist with experience reading mammograms of lactating women, bring her baby with her to the testing site, and breastfeed before the mammogram.

Fine-needle aspiration cytologic study. This quick, nearly painless procedure can determine the nature of a breast lump (sometimes avoiding the need for biopsy) and can often be done in an office or clinic, using local anesthesia, without interrupting breastfeeding.

A biopsy can usually be done without interrupting breastfeeding.

Suggest the mother make sure her healthcare provider knows she's breastfeeding before her breast biopsy, so compatible medications can be chosen. Also, suggest she request her surgeon avoid cutting milk ducts whenever possible. Because the location of the milk ducts is not obvious before surgery, suggest the mother request incisions be made in vertical lines like the spokes of a wheel to avoid the ducts (D. West, personal communication, November 6, 2009).

Fibrocystic changes in the breast are common, and pregnancy and breastfeeding may reduce the severity of symptoms.

As women age, the hormones of menstruation contribute to the development of benign cysts in the breasts. Sometimes these feel like dense, fibrous areas. At other times, they may feel like a smooth, round lump that can be easily moved around. Some women feel pain and tenderness as well, often intensified during menstruation. Because pregnancy and breastfeeding prevent or delay menstruation, many feel relief from their symptoms then. Reducing caffeine may reduce symptoms (Lawrence & Lawrence, 2005).

Any breast lump should be checked if it hasn't disappeared within a couple of weeks. Fine-needle aspiration will determine whether or not a lump is a benign cyst.

In *Breastfeeding: A Guide for the Medical Profession,* Drs. Ruth and Robert Lawrence describe the cause and treatment of galactoceles:

Galactoceles, or milk-filled cysts, are uncommon and harmless.

> Milk-retention cysts are uncommon and, when found, are almost exclusively a problem in lactating women. The contents at first are pure milk. Because of fluid absorption, they later contain thick, creamy, cheesy, or oily material. The swelling is smooth and rounded, and compression of it may cause milky fluid to exude from the nipple. Galactoceles are believed to be caused by blockage of a milk duct. The cyst may be aspirated to avoid surgery, but will fill up again. It can be removed surgically under local anesthesia without stopping the breastfeeding. Its presence does not require cessation of lactation. Firm diagnosis can be made by ultrasound; a cyst and milk will appear the same, whereas a tumor will be distinguishable (Lawrence & Lawrence, 2005, p. 299).

To avoid surgery, fine-needle aspiration, using a local anesthetic, can usually be done in a healthcare provider's office or clinic, which allows the contents of the cyst to be removed and its contents checked. Once a galactocele is confirmed, if it is not painful or growing, nothing need be done.

Preliminary Thai research on 16 women with galactoceles indicates that using a nylon probe to remove the obstruction in the milk duct causing the galactocele can reduce the incidence of recurrence (Auvichayapat et al., 2003). In this study, none of the 11 women whose galactocele was treated with the nylon probe had a recurrence, whereas 2 of the 5 who were treated with fine-needle aspiration had a recurrence.

Calcifications in the breast occur more commonly as women age.

During the aging process, calcium leaves the bones and travels to other areas of the body, landing in the arteries, joints, and breasts. Calcifications or microcalcifications in the breast are tiny deposits of calcium that can be detected only with a mammogram and occur in about 4% of women (Sickles & Abele, 1981). They appear to be more common in women who have breastfed. If a mammogram shows calcifications that are evenly distributed in both breasts, this is usually not a cause for concern. However, when they appear in clusters, this is considered a risk factor for cancer, so another mammogram is recommended within a few months (Uematsu, Kasami, & Yuen, 2009).

BLOOD IN THE MILK OR NIPPLE DISCHARGE

Assure the mother that blood in the milk usually disappears quickly and will not harm her baby.

When a mother sees blood in her milk, she may worry she has a serious health problem and that the blood will harm her baby. Suggest the mother contact her healthcare provider to discuss the blood, but assure her that bleeding from the breast in late pregnancy and the first few weeks postpartum is usually due to more harmless causes (see next point). Also assure her that it is fine to continue breastfeeding and that the bleeding will not harm her baby.

Blood in the milk is not uncommon; there are several likely causes.

Blood in the milk is probably much more common than we realize. When U.S. researchers examined the early milk of 72 women under a microscope, they detected red blood cells in 17, or 15%, of the asymptomatic breastfeeding women (Kline & Lash, 1964).

"Rusty-pipe syndrome," also known as "vascular engorgement," is one common cause of blood in the milk during pregnancy and early breastfeeding. It is caused by slight internal bleeding due to a combination of increased blood flow to the breasts and rapid development of the milk-producing glands (Kline & Lash, 1964). Most common in first-time mothers, this usually occurs in both breasts, although it may occur in one breast at first. When this is the cause, usually there is little or no discomfort. One Australian survey followed 32 Australian women who reported blood in the milk during pregnancy and lactation that could not be explained by other causes (O'Callaghan, 1981). Most reported that the blood cleared within 3 to 7 days after birth, with a few mothers reporting a brief reappearance a few weeks later.

Intraductal papillomas and fibrocystic changes are two other common causes of blood in the milk (Lawrence & Lawrence, 2005, p. 605). An intraductal papilloma is a benign wart-like growth in a milk duct that causes bleeding as it erodes. It usually occurs in only one breast, cannot be felt as a lump, and may or may not be accompanied by discomfort. The bleeding often stops spontaneously within a couple weeks of birth without treatment.

Breast or nipple trauma can cause blood in the milk when broken capillaries in the breast occur from rough handling, too-high breast pump vacuum levels, or use of a poor quality breast pump. Sometimes a mother cannot distinguish whether blood is coming from the nipple or inside the breast.

To rule out other, more serious causes, suggest the mother see her healthcare provider.

With the previously described causes, blood in the milk usually clears up without treatment within a couple of weeks after birth. However, if the mother continues to see blood in her milk after that, more serious causes, such as Paget's disease and other types of breast cancer, should be ruled out. Although breast cancer is unlikely, suggest the mother see her healthcare provider as soon as possible (Lang & Kuerer, 2007). Non-invasive tests, such as mammograms and MRIs, can be used to help determine the cause of the blood in her milk (Tokuda et al., 2009).

Milk expression during pregnancy and breastfeeding can produce secretions of different colors. Normal milk and colostrum can come in a variety of colors, including blue, green, brownish, yellow, gold, and clear.

A nipple discharge other than blood can be due to a variety of causes.

Pus, stringy-looking milk, or granules can sometimes be expressed during mastitis. See the previous section for more details.

Ductal ectasia is caused by the formation of an irritating lipid fluid in a dilated duct that causes inflammation and a sticky discharge, which can also be in different colors (Lawrence & Lawrence, 2005, p. 604). The mother may have no discomfort, or she may have burning pain, itching, and nipple swelling. Treatment includes warm compresses and antibiotics. If the mother is in discomfort, surgical removal of the duct is an option.

UNUSUAL BREAST DEVELOPMENT

Extra Nipples and Breast Tissue

Some mothers develop extra nipples, areolae, and/or breast tissue, usually along the milk line, which runs from the armpit to the groin.

About 1% to 2% of mothers have extra breasts and/or nipples, which are remnants from the embryonic development of the mammary ridge (Riordan & Wambach, 2010). Some extra breasts are breast tissue and no nipples; some are nipples, but no breast tissue. Some mothers have ducts that leak milk through the skin without breast or nipple (Wilson-Clay & Hoover, 2008). Some mothers develop multiple breasts.

Normal breast tissue extends into the armpit (known as the "tail of Spence"), which may become engorged as milk production increases (see the section "Engorgment"). But when a mother has extra breasts in the armpit or elsewhere, they may become engorged, but not drain into the main ductal system. If the extra breasts have a nipple (which may look like a mole), milk may leak from the nipple, and the mother may be able to express milk to relieve feelings of fullness. If the extra breasts do not have a nipple, suggest she apply cold compresses to reduce swelling faster. Without the release of milk, production will quickly stop, and the tissue will soften, just like the breasts of a mother who does not breastfeed.

Although most extra breasts and nipples occur along the milk line, some have developed elsewhere, such as on the buttocks or the back (Lawrence & Lawrence, 2005). The existence of extra breasts, nipples, or ducts should not affect breastfeeding, although these areas become engorged and even develop mastitis. A mother with extra nipples may have leakage when she breastfeeds. If so, suggest she use pads or cloths to absorb the leaked milk.

Underdeveloped Breasts

If a mother's milk-producing glands did not fully develop, she may be unable to produce enough milk for her baby.

One author estimates about 1 in 1,000 mothers have breast hypoplasia (Powers, 1999). Others refer to underdeveloped breasts as primary lactation failure or insufficient glandular tissue (Neifert, Seacat, & Jobe, 1985). Some mothers with this condition have unusually shaped breasts or areolae (see next point), because some of the normal glandular tissue is missing. These breasts usually feel like obvious patches of glandular tissue in a mostly soft breast (Wilson-Clay & Hoover, 2008).

Breast development is influenced by heredity, but it can also be affected during puberty by hypothyroidism (Pringle, Stanhope, Hindmarsh, & Brook, 1988) and ovarian cysts (Sharma, Bajpai, Mittal, Kabra, & Menon, 2006). In some parts of the world, a greater incidence of altered breast development has been found in girls exposed environmentally to agricultural chemicals (Guillette et al., 2006).

Although a mother in this situation may not be able to fully nourish her baby at the breast, the baby can partially breastfeed with supplements, either given at the breast with an at-breast supplementer or with another feeding method (Thorley, 2005). Depending on how much milk-making tissue she has and her breastfeeding dynamics, she may also be able to continue to increase her milk production over time (Huggins, Petok, & Mireles, 2000) and eventually exclusively breastfeed later babies (Wilson-Clay & Hoover, 2008). One case report describes a mother who exclusively breastfed a subsequent baby after receiving progesterone treatment during pregnancy to treat a luteal-phase defect (Bodley & Powers, 1999).

• •

Breast appearance, spacing, and lack of breast changes are red flags, but are not reliable indicators that a mother will have low milk production.

Among mothers there is great variability in breast size and shape, as well as how much of the breasts is glandular tissue (Geddes, 2007). One U.S. prospective study of 34 mothers found the following visual indicators among the mothers unable to produce enough milk (Huggins et al., 2000):

- Widely spaced breasts (more than 1.5 inches or about 4 cm apart)
- Large differences in breast size
- Tubular or cone-shaped (hypoplastic) breasts, rather than rounded

Some of these mothers also had bulbous-looking areolae. Many of the study mothers with low milk production noticed no breast changes during pregnancy or breast fullness after birth. The researchers adapted a rating system from another study to describe four categories of breast shapes: 1) round, normal breasts, 2) breasts lacking tissue underneath, 3) breasts lacking tissue underneath and along the sides, and 4) breasts with little tissue anywhere (von Heimburg, Exner, Kruft, & Lemperle, 1996).

It is important, however, never to assume from a mother's breast shape or lack of breast changes during pregnancy that she will not produce enough milk for her baby. One Australian study found that breast tissue growth continues during breastfeeding throughout the first month postpartum (Cox, Kent, Casey, Owens, & Hartmann, 1999). One of its study mothers had no noticeable breast tissue growth before birth, but produced plenty of milk for her baby and experienced significant breast tissue growth during the month after birth.

Whenever possible, mothers with these red flags should be monitored closely, without planting the seeds of doubt. *The Breastfeeding Atlas* features photos of women with these physical characteristics who made ample milk. Its authors write:

> Good counseling skills are critical when a woman presents with these markers, because they may not always predict difficulty with

breastfeeding. The LC must avoid creating anxiety or creating a loss of confidence. However, because the calibration of lactation occurs early in the process, women with unusual breasts deserve extra attention and extended follow-up to make sure they reach their full lactation potential (Wilson-Clay & Hoover, 2008, p. 62).

Rapid Overdevelopment of the Breasts

With pregnancy and early breastfeeding, most women experience some breast growth. However, gestational gigantomastia is an unusual condition that falls far outside the norm. During pregnancy, the mother's breast tissue become hypersensitive to pregnancy hormones and grow to double or triple their previous size (8 to 20 bra cup sizes or more), often completely incapacitating her (Lawrence & Lawrence, 2005). Although it can occur during a first pregnancy, it usually happens first during a second or third pregnancy and occurs equally in small-breasted and large-breasted women. Once considered extremely rare, it appears to be becoming more common (Craig, 2008).

Some breast growth is normal, but one type of rapid breast growth, called "gigantomastia," can be disabling.

The three types of gestational gigantomastia, which have different hormonal triggers, can be distinguished by when the excessive breast growth starts. In the first type, which is most common and responds well to antiprolactin hormone therapy, breast growth occurs when a mother becomes pregnant and continues through all three trimesters of pregnancy. In the second type, the next most common, rapid breast growth begins in the second trimester, lasts for 3 to 6 weeks, then slows. This second type is usually accompanied by high insulin blood levels. In the third type, the rarest, rapid breast growth occurs right before or right after birth and, at this writing, a hormone sensitivity has not yet been identified.

• •

In more than 80% of the cases, the breasts return to normal size after the baby is born, but gigantomastia recurs with each subsequent pregnancy, even if breast reduction surgery is done. In cases of extreme incapacitation, mastectomies have been performed during pregnancy.

Medical therapies other than surgery are available to treat gestational gigantomastia, which typically recurs with each pregnancy.

Recently developed medical therapies to treat and control this condition provide alternatives to breast surgery. To receive current information on effective treatments, suggest any mother with gestational gigantomastia ask her healthcare provider to contact Randall Craig, MD (hrcraigmd@yahoo.com), an Arizona doctor who specializes in this and other disorders.

BREAST SURGERY OR INJURY

Basic Considerations

If a mother with a history of breast surgery or injury is concerned about how much milk she'll produce, discuss her goals and options.

Some mothers have not given much thought to their breastfeeding goals, so it may help first to get a sense of what is important to her. Be sure the mother understands that breastfeeding does not have to be "all or nothing." From a health standpoint, some breastfeeding is almost always better than none. In terms of health outcomes, those who were partially breastfed as babies usually fall between those exclusively breastfed and those who have never breastfed (Horta, Bahl, Martines, & Victora, 2007; Ip et al., 2007). Ask the mother how she would feel about partial breastfeeding and let her know that any amount of her milk is a boon to her and her baby. Some mothers may embrace this idea, and others may reject it.

Also discuss the emotional aspects of breastfeeding, so she is aware that there is more involved than milk. Breastfeeding calms and comforts a baby, and the hormones of breastfeeding enhance mother-baby intimacy. Understanding her values, goals, and what aspects of breastfeeding are most important to her can help her in making decisions that are right for her.

Factors That Affect Breastfeeding

Ask the mother for the date and the details of her surgery or injury and if she's had any complications.

In the book, *The Breastfeeding Mother's Guide to Making More Milk* (West & Marasco, 2009), authors Diana West and Lisa Marasco describe the "Milk Supply Equation" (below). Breast surgery and injury primarily affect the first two of the physical dynamics needed for milk production:

Sufficient glandular tissue

+ Intact nerve pathways and milk ducts

+ Adequate hormones and hormone receptors

+ Frequent, effective milk removal and breast stimulation

= Good milk production

Incisions around the areola are more likely to cause nerve damage and severe milkducts than other types of incisions.

Surgery or injury details. If her breast surgery involved removing some of her milk-making glands (such as most types of breast reduction surgery), this will likely affect the volume of milk she can produce. The amount of breast tissue removed does not appear to affect breastfeeding outcomes (Cherchel, Azzam, & De Mey, 2007; Cruz-Korchin & Korchin, 2006; Hefter, Lindholm, & Elvenes, 2003). If the mother is unsure about how her surgery was done, suggest she contact her surgeon. If she's unclear on injury details, suggest she contact her healthcare provider.

Where her incisions or injuries are located. For good milk flow during breastfeeding, intact nerve pathways allow nerve impulses to travel from breast to brain and trigger the release of hormones needed for milk ejection. If critical nerve pathways are disrupted, achieving normal milk flow can be more challenging (Halbert, 1998). When facing the breasts, the primary nerve—the fourth intercostal—enters the areola between 1 o'clock and 4 o'clock on the right breast and 8 o'clock and 11 o'clock on the left breast (Schlenz, Kuzbari, Gruber, & Holle, 2000). So incisions around the areola (periareolar) are more likely to cause nerve damage and severed milk ducts than incisions in the fold under the breast (subglandular), in the armpit (axillary), or the navel (transumbilical);(Hurst, 1996; Neifert et al., 1990)

When her surgery was done or injury occurred. Nerves can regenerate (or grow back) over time. This "reinnervation" happens at a set rate (about 1 mm per month) and is not influenced by pregnancy or breastfeeding. So the more time that has passed since the surgery or injury, the more sensitive a mother's breasts and nipples are likely to become and the less nerve damage is likely to affect breastfeeding (West & Hirsch, 2008).

Milk ducts. In addition to nerve function, the number of intact milk ducts is also important to milk production. How much cutting milk ducts affects milk production depends in part on how many milk ducts a mother has to begin with. Nine milk ducts are average, but some mothers have as few as 4 and as many as 14 (Ramsay, Kent, Hartmann, & Hartmann, 2005). Unlike nerves, the regrowth of milk ducts occurs faster during pregnancy and breastfeeding. So if a mother had milk production issues with one child, she will likely produce more milk with each child afterward.

Milk ducts are more likely to be cut when surgical incisions are made around the areola or into the body of the breast, rather than incisions made in the fold under the breast, in the armpit, or through the navel.

Complications can occur with any surgery. Ask about changes in nipple sensation and any noticeable scarring, infection, or any subsequent surgery. Complications and additional surgeries may mean lower milk production (Hurst, 2003).

If she had breast surgery, ask her why it was done and if she has any other health issues.

If the mother decided to have surgery because her breasts did not develop normally, milk production problems may be due to a lack of milk-making tissue and be unrelated to her surgery. (For details, see the previous section "Underdeveloped Breasts.") A mother who had breast reduction surgery may also have other health conditions that can affect milk production, such as obesity, diabetes, hypothyroidism, or polycystic ovary syndrome (West & Hirsch, 2008).

If only one breast was affected by surgery or injury, full milk production is more likely.

If the mother has had surgery or sustained an injury on one breast only, breastfeeding may not be affected, as most mothers are capable of exclusively breastfeeding twins, triplets, and more. And even women who have had one breast removed via mastectomy have produced enough milk for their babies by breastfeeding often on the remaining breast.

The exception to this would be the mother with very asymmetrical breasts (which may have motivated her to have surgery on one breast), who may also have insufficient glandular tissue.

Ask the mother if she has either reduced or heightened nipple or breast sensitivity

Whenever surgery is performed on the breast, loss of sensation is common (see previous point). The more extensive the surgery or the larger the breast implant, typically the less breast sensation the mother feels. Some women experience unusual sensations or greater sensitivity after breast surgery.

After breast injury, women sometimes experience a loss of sensation, too. If there is no sensation at all, this means vital nerves have likely been damaged.

If a woman is considering breast surgery, suggest she talk to her surgeon about preserving breast functionality.

No matter what type of surgery a mother is considering—breast biopsy, tumor or cyst removal, breast augmentation or reduction, or breast lift—encourage her to talk to her surgeon about her desire to breastfeed and ask him or her to try to avoid as much as possible cutting milk ducts and nerves during the surgery. See the impact of specific procedures and recommended techniques in the later sections.

Preparing During Pregnancy

Discuss with the mother her breastfeeding goals and options

For details, see the first point in the last section.

During pregnancy, encourage the mother to learn all she can about normal breastfeeding.

Women with a history of breast surgery or injury are often overly focused on their special situation and assume that breastfeeding information geared toward the average mother does not apply to them. But these mothers have an even greater need than most to understand breastfeeding norms. With her doubts about her body, if she doesn't have realistic expectations, she may assume that even normal behaviors and feeding patterns mean that breastfeeding is not working.

Worries about insufficient milk are common, even among mothers without a history of breast surgery or injury. In fact, these worries are the most common reason mothers give for early weaning and are often unrelated to actual milk production (Hillervik-Lindquist, Hofvander, & Sjolin, 1991). After breast surgery or injury, a mother is even more likely to doubt breastfeeding. So encourage her to read books and visit websites with accurate, up-to-date breastfeeding information (see recommendations at the end of this chapter) and attend mother-support groups to learn from other mothers' experiences.

Suggest the mother use knowledgeable and supportive healthcare providers and breastfeeding friendly birthing facilities.

During and after birth, the mother needs people around her who can help her evaluate how breastfeeding is going based on reliable indicators. To help breastfeeding get off to the best possible start, encourage her to:

- Give birth at a Baby Friendly birthing facility in her area.
- Learn how to minimize interventions during labor and birth.
- Find skilled breastfeeding help, meet them during pregnancy, and keep their contact information on hand.
- Plan to see the baby's healthcare provider at least weekly for weight checks during the first month.

- Learn when supplements are needed and discuss feeding options (see next section).

Ask the mother if her nipple and breast sensitivity decreased after her surgery or injury.

Loss of all feeling in her breasts indicates nerve damage and puts her at risk for difficulty with milk ejection. It may help to know this in advance, so that she can plan ahead. For details, see previous and next sections.

Initiating Breastfeeding

To avoid early problems, encourage the mother to focus on achieving deep breastfeeding and minimizing engorgement.

By breastfeeding deeply (see chapter 1) and often (see chapter 2), a mother with a history of breast surgery or injury may be able to avoid some early breastfeeding problems. Mothers with any active breast tissue will probably have some breast fullness or engorgement, perhaps in areas where the milk is unable to drain due to severed ducts. However, reassure the mother in this situation that milk ducts that do not connect to the nipple do not put her at greater risk for mastitis. Like the mother who does not breastfeed, those areas of the breast will quickly stop producing milk and revert to their pre-pregnancy state. Because these ducts are not exposed to outside organisms via the ductal system, they are unlikely to become infected. Suggest she view breast swelling and engorgement as positive signs that her breasts are making milk and use the comfort measures described in the previous "Engorgement" section to ease any discomfort.

Discuss strategies if a mother's nerve damage prevents milk ejection.

A mother who can feel both touch and temperature on her areola and nipple is likely to experience normal milk ejection during breastfeeding (West & Hirsch, 2008). But a mother who has lost all sensation is at risk of impaired or inhibited milk ejection, at least until her nerves grow back or "reinnervate."

A mother whose nerve pathways are impaired may be able to achieve milk ejection only with the help of mental imagery, the use of a synthetic oxytocin nasal spray, or by applying pressure to the breasts during breastfeeding via breast compression (see "Techniques" appendix) or other types of hand pressure. Discuss these options with her to help her determine which might be feasible for her.

In some cases, nipple pain, blanching, and/or feeding problems may be related to nerve damage or scarring.

Although the pulling of scar tissue during breastfeeding can cause sharp nipple pain—especially with the first child a mother breastfeeds after her surgery—other causes are more likely. Suggest a mother in pain first rule out more common and treatable causes, such as shallow breastfeeding, bacterial nipple infection, vasospasm, and Raynaud's Phenomenon. For details, see the chapter "Nipple Issues."

Those who work extensively with breastfeeding mothers after breast surgery report that nipple blanching is common, perhaps due to disruption of nerves and/or blood supply (West, 2001; West & Hirsch, 2008). No matter what the cause, the treatments for vasospasm and Raynaud's Phenomenon may be helpful (see p. 639- "Vasospasm or Raynaud's Phenomenon").

Another commonly reported issue is difficulty taking the breast because the nipple and areola feel less "full." Special care to use good breastfeeding technique can help overcome this challenge (see chapter 1).

If a mother's milk production is likely to be low, suggest postpartum strategies that can help maximize it.

If a mother is likely to have less-than-full milk production, discuss ways to maximize her milk-making potential that will activate as many prolactin receptors as possible during the critical first few weeks. Not all mothers will want to try all the possibilities, but some options include using breast compression or massage during breastfeeding to increase milk removal, increasing feeding frequency, taking herbal or prescribed galactagogues, and expressing milk after and/or between breastfeedings. For details, see p. 413 in the chapter, "Making Milk."

The Need for Supplementation

Suggest the mother keep close tabs on her baby's weight and diaper output to gauge whether supplements are needed.

The most accurate way to determine whether a baby is getting enough milk is by monitoring his weight. Loss of up to 7% to 10% of birthweight within the first 3 to 4 days postpartum is considered in the normal range. After that, when breastfeeding is going well, babies tend to gain on average about an ounce (28 g) per day or about 6 ounces (170 g) per week. The need for supplements will depend on the baby's weight. If the baby is losing weight quickly, supplements are needed right away. However, if the baby's weight gain is slightly below average, there is time to try milk-enhancing strategies first. Diaper output, while not as reliable, can also be used as a rough gauge (Nommsen-Rivers, Heinig, Cohen, & Dewey, 2008). For details, see the chapters, "Weight Gain and Growth" and "Making Milk."

Ask the mother if she'd like to know about common breastfeeding outcomes after birth.

After breast surgery or injury, breastfeeding outcomes include:

- Full milk production with no need for supplements.
- Milk production sufficient for the first few weeks, but as the hormones of childbirth settle down and milk production becomes more dependent on the stimulation of milk removal, supplements become necessary (West & Hirsch, 2008).
- Little to no milk production, with supplements needed soon after birth.

Even a mother producing little milk may be able to exclusively breastfeed during the first few days. Some mothers with nerve damage find that even with frequent breastfeeding, reduced nerve stimulation results in decreased milk production over time.

If a baby is not receiving adequate milk at the breast, it is vital to rule out other causes—such as shallow breastfeeding, tongue tie, and others—before assuming it is due to previous breast surgery or injury. See p. 210 for the section "Slow Weight Gain" in the chapter "Weight Gain and Growth" for other possibilities.

If a baby doesn't need supplements within the first 5 or 6 weeks, chances are they won't be needed. Babies' milk intake typically increases during the first 5 weeks or so (Hill, Aldag, Chatterton, & Zinaman, 2005), then plateaus until solid foods are started (Neville et al., 1988). So unless other changes that affect milk production occur, such as decreasing feeding frequency, if a baby is still growing and thriving without supplements by 5 to 6 weeks of age, the baby will probably not need them.

When supplements are needed, encourage the mother to give enough—but not too much—and to consider her feeding options.

To stimulate her breasts to make as much milk as possible, the mother needs to strike a delicate balance between giving her baby the least amount of supplements needed, while actively breastfeeding as much as possible. Babies need to be well nourished to gain weight and thrive, and also to breastfeed effectively. If a baby does not get enough milk, he can become weak, which can compromise his ability to breastfeed. For more details, see p. 423- "Strategies for Supplementing That Enhance Milk-Making."

If supplements are needed, suggest the mother consider using an at-breast supplementer, also known as a tube-feeding device, which can keep her baby actively breastfeeding for longer, thereby stimulating more milk production. It also provides extra milk during breastfeeding, so the mother doesn't have to spend more time feeding her baby again later. Not all mothers are comfortable using an at-breast supplementer, so discuss feeding options and support her in her choice. Her decision may depend in part on whether she is close to full milk production, making some milk, or making little to no milk. For details on different feeding options, see the appendix "Tools and Products."

Breast Augmentation Surgery

Breast augmentation is one of the most common types of plastic surgery.

Also known as augmentation mammaplasty, it has been performed on many millions of women worldwide. During this surgical procedure, silicone- or saline-filled sacs are inserted into a pocket that is formed either between the chest muscles and the glandular tissue or under the muscles. The incision may be in the fold under the breast, near the armpit, around the edge of the areola, or rarely, through the navel. Another technique gaining in popularity is "biocompartmental breast lipostructuring." This involves injecting the mother's own fat from other parts of her body into her breasts for an increase of up to two cup sizes (Zocchi & Zuliani, 2008). This is likely to have less impact on breastfeeding than techniques involving incisions.

The location of the mother's incisions and the size of her implant may affect her breastfeeding outcome.

Two U.S. studies found that women who had breast surgery with incisions around the areola were at least 5 times more likely to have insufficient milk, as women who did not have breast surgery. However, the first of these studies did not differentiate between women who had breast augmentation and breast reduction surgery, which has a much greater potential affect on milk production (Neifert et al., 1990). The second study focused on 42 women with breast implants and 42 control women (Hurst, 1996). However, it did not control for factors that might have affected milk production, such as time elapsed since the surgery, implant size, implant location, and angle of insertion. It found that 64% of the mothers who underwent breast augmentation had insufficient milk production (defined as gaining less than 20 g/day while exclusively breastfeeding), as compared with 7% of the control mothers.

Research is mixed on the effect of incision location on nipple sensitivity. A U.S. study of 20 women with implants (Mofid, Klatsky, Singh, & Nahabedian, 2006) found no difference in nipple sensitivity among women who had breast implants inserted around the areola or in the fold under the breast, but this and a Brazilian study (Pitanguy, Vaena, Radwanski, Nunes, & Vargas, 2007) did find an association between larger implants (in previously small-breasted women) and reduced nipple sensitivity. Until there is more research, suggest any woman considering breast implant surgery avoid incisions around the areola and larger implants (West & Hirsch, 2008).

The placement of the implants above or below a mother's chest muscles may also affect lactation.

Placing the implant directly under the breast tissue (submammary), rather than either partially covered by the chest muscle (subpectoral) or almost completely covered by the chest muscle (transrectus), may put pressure on the milk-producing glands and reduce milk production (Hurst, 1996; Michalopoulos, 2007). In most breast augmentations today, the implants are placed below the muscles. If the mother is unsure about how the surgery was done, suggest she contact her surgeon.

After breast implant surgery, significant scarring and any subsequent surgery can cause discomfort and reduce milk production.

Scarring is the body's natural reaction to surgery. Severe scarring, known as capsular contracture, can cause discomfort during breastfeeding or put enough pressure on the milk-producing glands to cause a reduction in milk production (Strom, Baldwin, Sigurdson, & Schusterman, 1997). When scarring is severe, it may require more surgery to remove it, which can cause damage to nerves and milk ducts (Henriksen et al., 2003; Michalopoulos, 2007).

Concerns about silicone in the milk of mothers with implants have proved to be unfounded.

In the mid-1990s, concerns were raised about potential health risks to breastfed children of mothers with silicone breast implants, because several cases of unusual gastrointestinal disorders and autoimmune symptoms were found in small samples of these children (Levine & Ilowite, 1994; Teuber & Gershwin, 1994). A Danish cohort study compared health outcomes of children of 1,135 women with breast implants with 7,071 children of mothers who'd had breast reduction surgery (Kjoller et al., 1998) and found no significant increases in gastrointestinal problems, connective tissue diseases, or congenital malformations in either group.

In 2001, after reviewing the research, the American Academy of Pediatrics' Committee on Drugs wrote that when milk from mothers with silicone implants was compared with milk from mothers without implants, there was no difference found in the levels of silicon (silicone is elemental silicon bonded to oxygen) (AAP, 2001). The chair of this committee wrote: "It is unlikely that elemental silicon causes difficulty, because silicon is present in higher concentrations in cow's milk and formula than in the milk of humans with implants" (Berlin, 1994).

If the mother is concerned about silicone in her milk, let her know that research indicates that formula and cow's milk contain levels of silicon more than 10 times higher than the milk of mothers with implants (Semple, Lugowski, Baines, Smith, & McHugh, 1998). Silicone is also given directly to babies in some colic remedies, such as Mylicon® drops. It is a "ubiquitous substance found in all food, liquids, etc." (Hale, 2008, p. 872) and absorption by the babies' digestive tract is considered unlikely.

Like silicone implants, saline implants are made with a silicone envelope. They are filled with saline or salt water, a natural body fluid, so if a mother's saline implants leak or rupture, there should be no health risk to mother or baby.

In most types of breast surgery, there is more than one way for the surgery to be performed. An incision around or across the areola (periareolar or transareolar) would cut milk ducts and possibly major nerves. An incision in the fold under the breast is less likely to affect breastfeeding than an incision near the areola, as the milk ducts and vital nerves would not be involved. An incision near the armpit is also less likely to affect breastfeeding. See the earlier point for suggestions on the placement of the implant.

Suggest any woman planning future breast augmentation surgery request her surgeon use techniques least likely to damage nerves and milk ducts.

Surgeries involving removal of the nipple are most likely to negatively affect breastfeeding.

Be sure the mother knows, however, that even if the surgery is done following all the recommended procedures, it does not guarantee she will achieve full milk production. In a previously mentioned U.S. study of 42 women who had breast augmentation surgery, 48% of the mothers who had one of the recommended types of incisions and implant placement did not achieve full milk production (Hurst, 1996). Even under ideal conditions, it is possible for there to be complications that can impair lactation. As one researcher wrote: "With good surgical technique and proper postoperative management, most of the complications associated with surgery that may result in insufficient milk production can be minimized, but not always avoided" (Michalopoulos, 2007, p. 62).

Breast Reduction Surgery

Some breast reduction techniques affect breastfeeding outcomes more than others.

Also known as reduction mammaplasty, breast reduction surgery decreases breast size by removing either the fat within the breast via liposuction or by surgically removing breast tissue.

Liposuction is the breast reduction technique least likely to affect milk production, because only fatty tissue is removed and there is minimal scarring and nerve damage However, liposuction does not usually reduce breast size by more than two cup sizes (Spear, 2006), and it is not considered the best option for younger women, because their breasts tend to contain less fatty tissue (Nahai & Nahai, 2008).

Free nipple grafts put milk production most at risk, because this type of breast reduction surgery involves surgically removing the nipples from the breasts and reattaching them elsewhere to make the breasts look more symmetrical (Marshall, Callan, & Nicholson, 1994). This procedure, which is not as common as other techniques, severs all milk ducts, nerves, and blood vessels. Even so, due to regrowth of nerves and milk ducts, some mothers produce milk and a few produce ample milk (West & Hirsch, 2008).

Pedicle techniques and others. In addition to concerns about milk ducts and nerves, there are also concerns about maintaining a good blood supply to the nipple and areola after surgery, as too little blood flow can cause tissue death, a very serious complication that can greatly reduce lactation potential. To protect these vital arteries, while some parts of the breast are being removed during surgery, a section of the breast that includes these arteries, milk ducts, and nerves can be kept intact. These intact sections are called "pedicles," and the names of these surgical techniques ("inferior," "superior," and "medial" pedicle techniques) refer to the specific section of the breast used to create the pedicle. Different techniques can be used with different types and shapes of incisions, which make it impossible to tell from a mother's scar what type of surgery she had.

One Australian study of 30 women who had undergone breast reduction surgery and later breastfed found that the women who had the pedicle techniques produced more milk than the women who had free nipple grafts (nipples completely detached and then reattached) (Marshall et al., 1994).

Research on pedicle techniques. One Brazilian study of 49 women who had breast reduction surgery using an inferior pedicle technique (called transposition) were compared with 96 control mothers (Souto, Giugliani, Giugliani, & Schneider, 2003). This study distinguished between exclusive and partial breastfeeding and followed its mothers for an entire year. In the surgery group, the duration of exclusive breastfeeding was only 5 days as compared with 3 months in the control group. Duration of any breastfeeding in the surgery group was 58% at 1 month, 16% at 6 months, and 10% at 12 months, compared with the control group with rates of 94% at 1 month, 58% at 6 months, and 35% at 12 months.

Comparing different pedicle techniques. Although many studies have examined the effects of different types of breast reduction surgeries on lactation outcomes, unfortunately, consistent definitions of breastfeeding success have not been used, making it impossible to draw firm conclusions about the differences in techniques. An Italian study compared different breast reduction techniques and defined success as no supplementation needed during the first 3 weeks (Chiummariello et al., 2007; Chiummariello et al., 2008). Of its 368 women, the following percentages met this definition of success (with breast reduction surgery used): 60.7% (superior pedicle), 55.1% (lateral pedicle), 48% (medial pedicle), and 43.5% (inferior pedicle). One Puerto Rican study compared the breastfeeding outcomes of 164 women who underwent breast reduction surgery using different pedicle techniques with 151 women with large breasts who did not have breast reduction surgery and found almost no differences in outcomes between the two groups (Cruz & Korchin, 2007). Using a definition of success as 2 weeks of breastfeeding with or without supplements, the researchers found that all of the breast reduction techniques (superior, medial, and inferior pedicle) produced a success rate of about 62% and that the controls (no breast reduction surgery) also had a success rate of 62%. About 34% of both groups supplemented with formula during the first 2 weeks. This study reveals little about lactation potential after surgery, but indicates clearly the prevalence of early, unnecessary supplementation.

Research has not found an association between amount of tissue removed and breastfeeding outcomes.

Studies from Norway (Hefter et al., 2003), Puerto Rico (Cruz-Korchin & Korchin, 2006), and Belgium (Cherchel et al., 2007) found that the amount of breast tissue removed during breast reduction surgery was not associated with breastfeeding success.

Some mothers are discouraged from breastfeeding after surgery by their healthcare providers.

One Canadian study found that 9 of the 41 mothers who chose not to breastfeed were discouraged from initiating breastfeeding by their healthcare provider (Brzozowski, Niessen, Evans, & Hurst, 2000).

Breast Lift

In most cases, a breast lift will not affect breastfeeding.

Also known as mastopexy, a breast lift is used to reshape and reposition sagging breasts. It involves removing excess skin, but the nerves and milk-making glands are not usually affected and no breast tissue is removed. If a breast lift is done along with a breast augmentation, the risks would be the same as the two procedures combined (West & Hirsch, 2008).

Breast Injury

Ask the woman to describe her injury and her age when it occurred.

A woman who has had a breast injury may be worried about her milk production. The same basic considerations apply to her as to women with a history of breast surgery. Milk production should not be affected if her milk ducts and nerves were not damaged.

A loss of sensation in one or both breasts may indicate nerve damage. If so, her milk ejection may be affected in that breast. However, if only one breast is affected, in most cases, she'll be able to establish full milk production in the other breast. If both breasts are affected, see the previous section "Initiating Breastfeeding."

If the mother's nipples were burned, scarring may affect milk flow and skin elasticity, and may cause pain during breastfeeding.

Even second- and third-degree burns do not usually extend deeply enough into the breast to affect the milk-making glands. If the mother's nipples were burned and scarred, her ability to breastfeed would depend on how many nipple pores are blocked by scar tissue. The overall effect on breastfeeding will depend on how many milk ducts and corresponding nipple pores the mother has. Nine nipple pores and corresponding ducts are average, but some mothers have as few as 4 and as many as 14 (Ramsay et al., 2005). Scar tissue may also make the breast tissue less pliable, which may make taking the breast more challenging.

Some mothers with scarred nipples report that early breastfeeding is painful, although in some cases the pain resolves early. In one case report, the pain resolved within days of the birth (Faridi & Dewan, 2008).

Expressing colostrum during pregnancy indicates that at least some of the nipple pores are not blocked.

Expressing colostrum during pregnancy is not a reliable gauge of how much milk a mother will produce after birth. Many mothers who are unable to express colostrum go on to produce abundant milk. If during pregnancy the mother can express colostrum, however, it indicates that some of her nipples pores are not blocked.

RESOURCES FOR PARENTS

Websites

www.BFAR.org –An informational website for mothers who are breastfeeding after breast reduction surgery.

www.fda.gov/cdrh/breastimplants/index.html –A U.S. Food and Drug Administration (FDA) informational website on breast implants.

www.lowmilksupply.org –For mothers having milk production issues.

www.mobimotherhood.org –For mothers overcoming breastfeeding issues (MOBI).

Books on Normal Breastfeeding

Mohrbacher, N. S. & Kendall-Tackett, K. (2010). *Breastfeeding made simple: seven natural laws for nursing mothers, 2nd Edition.* Oakland, CA: New Harbinger Publications.

Books that Cover Breastfeeding after Breast Surgery or Injury

West, D. & Marasco, L. (2009). *The breastfeeding mother's guide to making more milk.* New York: McGraw Hill.

West, D. (2001). *Defining your own success: Breastfeeding after breast reduction surgery*. Schaumburg, IL: La Leche League International, 2001.

Resources for Professionals

West, D. & Hirsch, E. (2008). Breastfeeding after breast and nipple procedures: A guide for healthcare professionals. *Clinics in Human Lactation.* Amarillo: Hale Publishing.

REFERENCES

AAP. (2001). Transfer of drugs and other chemicals into human milk. *Pediatrics, 108*(3), 776-789.

ABM. (2008). ABM clinical protocol #4: mastitis. Revision, May 2008. *Breastfeeding Medicine, 3*(3), 177-180.

Amir, L. H. (2003). Breast pain in lactating women--mastitis or something else? *Australian Family Physician, 32*(3), 141-145.

Amir, L. H., Forster, D., McLachlan, H., & Lumley, J. (2004). Incidence of breast abscess in lactating women: report from an Australian cohort. *BJOG, 111*(12), 1378-1381.

Amir, L. H., Forster, D. A., Lumley, J., & McLachlan, H. (2007). A descriptive study of mastitis in Australian breastfeeding women: incidence and determinants. *BMC Public Health, 7*, 62.

Amir, L. H., Garland, S. M., & Lumley, J. (2006). A case-control study of mastitis: nasal carriage of Staphylococcus aureus. *BMC Fam Pract, 7*, 57.

Anderson, J. E., Held, N., & Wright, K. (2004). Raynaud's phenomenon of the nipple: a treatable cause of painful breastfeeding. *Pediatrics, 113*(4), e360-364.

Aryeetey, R. N., Marquis, G. S., Brakohiapa, L., Timms, L., & Lartey, A. (2009). Subclinical Mastitis May Not Reduce Breastmilk Intake During Established Lactation. *Breastfeeding Medicine*.

Aryeetey, R. N., Marquis, G. S., Timms, L., Lartey, A., & Brakohiapa, L. (2008). Subclinical mastitis is common among Ghanaian women lactating 3 to 4 months postpartum. *Journal of Human Lactation, 24*(3), 263-267.

Auvichayapat, P., Auvichayapat, N., Tong-un, T., Thinkhamrop, B., Vachirodom, D., & Uttravichien, T. (2003). A controlled trial of a new treatment for galactocele. *Journal of the Medical Association of Thailand, 86*(3), 257-261.

Benson, S. (2001). What is normal? A study of normal breastfeeding dyads during the first sixty hours of life. *Breastfeeding Review, 9*(1), 27-32.

Berlin, C. M., Jr. (1994). Silicone breast implants and breast-feeding. *Pediatrics, 94*(4 Pt 1), 547-549.

Betzold, C. M. (2007). An update on the recognition and management of lactational breast inflammation. *J Midwifery Womens Health, 52*(6), 595-605.

Bodley, V., & Powers, D. (1999). Patient with insufficient glandular tissue experiences milk supply increase attributed to progesterone treatment for luteal phase defect. *Journal of Human Lactation, 15*(4), 339-343.

Brzozowski, D., Niessen, M., Evans, H. B., & Hurst, L. N. (2000). Breast-feeding after inferior pedicle reduction mammaplasty. *Plastic and Reconstructive Surgery, 105*(2), 530-534.

Buescher, E. S., & Hair, P. S. (2001). Human milk anti-inflammatory component contents during acute mastitis. *Cellular Immunology, 210*(2), 87-95.

Bystrova, K., Widstrom, A. M., Matthiesen, A. S., Ransjo-Arvidson, A. B., Welles-Nystrom, B., Vorontsov, I., et al. (2007). Early lactation performance in primiparous and multiparous women in relation to different maternity home practices. A randomised trial in St. Petersburg. *Int Breastfeed J, 2*, 9.

Cherchel, A., Azzam, C., & De Mey, A. (2007). Breastfeeding after vertical reduction mammaplasty using a superior pedicle. *J Plast Reconstr Aesthet Surg, 60*(5), 465-470.

Chiummariello, S., Cigna, E., Buccheri, E. M., Dessy, L. A., Alfano, C., & Scuderi, N. (2007). Breastfeeding After Reduction Mammaplasty Using Different Techniques. *Aesthetic Plastic Surgery*.

Chiummariello, S., Cigna, E., Buccheri, E. M., Dessy, L. A., Alfano, C., & Scuderi, N. (2008). Breastfeeding after reduction mammaplasty using different techniques. *Aesthetic Plastic Surgery, 32*(2), 294-297.

Christensen, A. F., Al-Suliman, N., Nielsen, K. R., Vejborg, I., Severinsen, N., Christensen, H., et al. (2005). Ultrasound-guided drainage of breast abscesses: results in 151 patients. *British Journal of Radiology, 78*(927), 186-188.

Colson, S. (Writer) (2008). Biological Nurturing: Laid-Back Breastfeeding. Hythe, Kent, UK: The Nurturing Project.

Colson, S., DeRooy, L., & Hawdon, J. (2003). Biological Nurturing increases duration of breastfeeding for a vulnerable cohort. *MIDIRS Midwifery Digest, 13*(1), 92-97.

Cotterman, K. J. (2004). Reverse pressure softening: a simple tool to prepare areola for easier latching during engorgement. *Journal of Human Lactation, 20*(2), 227-237.

Cox, D. B., Kent, J. C., Casey, T. M., Owens, R. A., & Hartmann, P. E. (1999). Breast growth and the urinary excretion of lactose during human pregnancy and early lactation: endocrine relationships. *Experimental Physiology, 84*(2), 421-434.

Craig, H. R. (2008). *Gestational gigantomastia: Clinical and lactation management.* Paper presented at the International Lactation Consultant Association (ILCA) Conference, Las Vegas, NV.

Cruz-Korchin, N., & Korchin, L. (2006). Effect of pregnancy and breast-feeding on vertical mammaplasty. *Plastic and Reconstructive Surgery, 117*(1), 25-29.

Cruz, N. I., & Korchin, L. (2007). Lactational performance after breast reduction with different pedicles. *Plastic and Reconstructive Surgery, 120*(1), 35-40.

Dahlbeck, S. W., Donnelly, J. F., & Theriault, R. L. (1995). Differentiating inflammatory breast cancer from acute mastitis. *American Family Physician, 52*(3), 929-934.

Delgado, S., Collado, M. C., Fernandez, L., & Rodriguez, J. M. (2009). Bacterial analysis of breast milk: a tool to differentiate Raynaud's phenomenon from infectious mastitis during lactation. *Current Microbiology, 59*(1), 59-64.

Eglash, A. (1998). Delayed milk ejection reflex and plugged ducts: Lecithin therapy. *ABM News and Views, 3*(1), 4.

Evans, K., Evans, R., & Simmer, K. (1995). Effect of the method of breast feeding on breast engorgement, mastitis and infantile colic. *Acta Paediatrica, 84*(8), 849-852.

Faridi, M. M., & Dewan, P. (2008). Successful breastfeeding with breast malformations. *Journal of Human Lactation, 24*(4), 446-450.

Fernandez, L., Delgado, S., Herrero, H., Maldonado, A., & Rodriguez, J. M. (2008). The bacteriocin nisin, an effective agent for the treatment of staphylococcal mastitis during lactation. *Journal of Human Lactation, 24*(3), 311-316.

Fetherston, C. (1997). Management of lactation mastitis in a Western Australian cohort. *Breastfeeding Review, 5*(2), 13-19.

Fetherston, C. (1998). Risk factors for lactation mastitis. *Journal of Human Lactation, 14*(2), 101-109.

Fetherston, C. (2001). Mastitis in lactating women: physiology or pathology? *Breastfeeding Review, 9*(1), 5-12.

Fetherston, C. M., Lai, C. T., & Hartmann, P. E. (2006). Relationships between symptoms and changes in breast physiology during lactation mastitis. *Breastfeeding Medicine, 1*(3), 136-145.

Fetherston, C. M., Lai, C. T., & Hartmann, P. E. (2008). Recurrent blocked duct(s) in a mother with immunoglobulin A deficiency. *Breastfeeding Medicine, 3*(4), 261-265.

Filteau, S. M., Rice, A. L., Ball, J. J., Chakraborty, J., Stoltzfus, R., de Francisco, A., et al. (1999). Breast milk immune factors in Bangladeshi women supplemented postpartum with retinol or beta-carotene. *American Journal of Clinical Nutrition, 69*(5), 953-958.

Flores, M., & Filteau, S. (2002). Effect of lactation counselling on subclinical mastitis among Bangladeshi women. *Annals of Tropical Paediatrics, 22*(1), 85-88.

Fortunov, R. M., Hulten, K. G., Hammerman, W. A., Mason, E. O., Jr., & Kaplan, S. L. (2006). Community-acquired Staphylococcus aureus infections in term and near-term previously healthy neonates. *Pediatrics, 118*(3), 874-881.

Foxman, B., D'Arcy, H., Gillespie, B., Bobo, J. K., & Schwartz, K. (2002). Lactation mastitis: occurrence and medical management among 946 breastfeeding women in the United States. *American Journal of Epidemiology, 155*(2), 103-114.

Francis-Morrill, J., Heinig, M. J., Pappagianis, D., & Dewey, K. G. (2004). Diagnostic value of signs and symptoms of mammary candidosis among lactating women. *J Hum Lact, 20*(3), 288-295; quiz 296-289.

Gastelum, D. T., Dassey, D., Mascola, L., & Yasuda, L. M. (2005). Transmission of community-associated methicillin-resistant Staphylococcus aureus from breast milk in the neonatal intensive care unit. *Pediatric Infectious Disease Journal, 24*(12), 1122-1124.

Geddes, D. T. (2007). Inside the lactating breast: the latest anatomy research. *J Midwifery Womens Health, 52*(6), 556-563.

Gonik, G., & Cotton, D.B. (1984). Peripartum colloid osmotic pressure changes influence of intravenous hydration. *Am J Obstet Gynecol, 150,* 174-177.

Guillette, E. A., Conard, C., Lares, F., Aguilar, M. G., McLachlan, J., & Guillette, L. J., Jr. (2006). Altered breast development in young girls from an agricultural environment. *Environmental Health Perspectives, 114*(3), 471-475.

Gupta, R., Gupta, A. S., & Duggal, N. (1982). Tubercular mastitis. *International Surgery, 67*(4 Suppl), 422-424.

Halbert, L. A. (1998). Breastfeeding in the woman with a compromised nervous system. *Journal of Human Lactation, 14*(4), 327-331.

Hale, T. (2008). *Medications and Mothers' Milk* (13 ed.). Amarillo, TX: Hale Publishing.

Hale, T. W., Bateman, T. L., Finkelman, M. A., & Berens, P. D. (2009). The absence of Candida albicans in milk samples of women with clinical symptoms of ductal candidiasis. *Breastfeeding Medicine, 4*(2), 57-61.

Hefter, W., Lindholm, P., & Elvenes, O. P. (2003). Lactation and breast-feeding ability following lateral pedicle mammaplasty. *British Journal of Plastic Surgery, 56*(8), 746-751.

Henriksen, T. F., Holmich, L. R., Fryzek, J. P., Friis, S., McLaughlin, J. K., Hoyer, A. P., et al. (2003). Incidence and severity of short-term complications after breast augmentation: results from a nationwide breast implant registry. *Annals of Plastic Surgery, 51*(6), 531-539.

Hill, P. D., Aldag, J. C., Chatterton, R. T., & Zinaman, M. (2005). Comparison of milk output between mothers of preterm and term infants: the first 6 weeks after birth. *Journal of Human Lactation, 21*(1), 22-30.

Hill, P. D., & Humenick, S. S. (1994). The occurrence of breast engorgement. *Journal of Human Lactation, 10*(2), 79-86.

Hillervik-Lindquist, C., Hofvander, Y., & Sjolin, S. (1991). Studies on perceived breast milk insufficiency. III. Consequences for breast milk consumption and growth. *Acta Paediatrica Scandinavica, 80*(3), 297-303.

Horta, B., Bahl, R., Martines, J. C., & Victora, C. G. (2007). *Evidence on the long-term effects of breastfeeding: Systematic reviews and meta-analyses*. Retrieved. from.

Huggins, K. E., Petok, E. S., & Mireles, O. (2000). Markers of lactation insufficiency: A study of 34 mothers. In *Current Issues in Clinical Lactation*. Boston, MA: Jones and Bartlett.

Humenick, S. S., Hill, P. D., & Anderson, M. A. (1994). Breast engorgement: patterns and selected outcomes. *Journal of Human Lactation, 10*(2), 87-93.

Hurst, N. (2003). Breastfeeding after breast augmentation. *Journal of Human Lactation, 19*(1), 70-71.

Hurst, N. M. (1996). Lactation after augmentation mammoplasty. *Obstetrics and Gynecology, 87*(1), 30-34.

Ip, S., Chung, M., Raman, G., Chew, P., Magula, N., DeVine, D., et al. (2007). Breastfeeding and maternal and infant health outcomes in developed countries. *Evid Rep Technol Assess (Full Rep)*(153), 1-186.

Jacobs, V. R., Golombeck, K., Jonat, W., & Kiechle, M. (2003). Mastitis nonpuerperalis after nipple piercing: time to act. *International Journal of Fertility and Womens Medicine, 48*(5), 226-231.

Jones, E., Dimmock, P. W., & Spencer, S. A. (2001). A randomised controlled trial to compare methods of milk expression after preterm delivery. *Archives of Disease in Childhood. Fetal and Neonatal Edition, 85*(2), F91-95.

Jonsson, S., & Pulkkinen, M. O. (1994). Mastitis today: incidence, prevention and treatment. *Annales Chirurgiae et Gynaecologiae. Supplementum, 208*, 84-87.

Kasonka, L., Makasa, M., Marshall, T., Chisenga, M., Sinkala, M., Chintu, C., et al. (2006). Risk factors for subclinical mastitis among HIV-infected and uninfected women in Lusaka, Zambia. *Paediatric and Perinatal Epidemiology, 20*(5), 379-391.

Kendall-Tackett, K. (2007). A new paradigm for depression in new mothers: the central role of inflammation and how breastfeeding and anti-inflammatory treatments protect maternal mental health. *Int Breastfeed J, 2*, 6.

Kim, Y. H., Chang, S. S., Kim, Y. S., Kim, E. A., Yun, S. C., Kim, K. S., et al. (2007). Clinical outcomes in methicillin-resistant Staphylococcus aureus-colonized neonates in the neonatal intensive care unit. *Neonatology, 91*(4), 241-247.

Kinlay, J. R., O'Connell, D. L., & Kinlay, S. (1998). Incidence of mastitis in breastfeeding women during the six months after delivery: a prospective cohort study. *Medical Journal of Australia, 169*(6), 310-312.

Kinlay, J. R., O'Connell, D. L., & Kinlay, S. (2001). Risk factors for mastitis in breastfeeding women: results of a prospective cohort study. *Australian and New Zealand Journal of Public Health, 25*(2), 115-120.

Kjoller, K., McLaughlin, J. K., Friis, S., Blot, W. J., Mellemkjaer, L., Hogsted, C., et al. (1998). Health outcomes in offspring of mothers with breast implants. *Pediatrics, 102*(5), 1112-1115.

Kline, T. S., & Lash, S. R. (1964). The Bleeding Nipple of Pregnancy and Postpartum Period; a Cytologic and Histologic Study. *Acta Cytologica, 8*, 336-340.

Kvist, L. J., Hall-Lord, M. L., & Larsson, B. W. (2007). A descriptive study of Swedish women with symptoms of breast inflammation during lactation and their perceptions of the quality of care given at a breastfeeding clinic. *Int Breastfeed J, 2*, 2.

Kvist, L. J., Hall-Lord, M. L., Rydhstroem, H., & Larsson, B. W. (2007). A randomised-controlled trial in Sweden of acupuncture and care interventions for the relief of inflammatory symptoms of the breast during lactation. *Midwifery, 23*(2), 184-195.

Kvist, L. J., Larsson, B. W., Hall-Lord, M. L., Steen, A., & Schalen, C. (2008). The role of bacteria in lactational mastitis and some considerations of the use of antibiotic treatment. *Int Breastfeed J, 3*, 6.

Kvist, L. J., & Rydhstroem, H. (2005). Factors related to breast abscess after delivery: a population-based study. *BJOG, 112*(8), 1070-1074.

Lang, J. E., & Kuerer, H. M. (2007). Breast ductal secretions: clinical features, potential uses, and possible applications. *Cancer Control, 14*(4), 350-359.

Lawrence, R. A., & Lawrence, R. M. (2005). *Breastfeeding: A Guide for the Medical Profession*. Philadelphia, PA: Elsevier Mosby.

Levine, J. J., & Ilowite, N. T. (1994). Sclerodermalike esophageal disease in children breast-fed by mothers with silicone breast implants. *JAMA, 271*(3), 213-216.

Livingstone, V., & Stringer, L. J. (1999). The treatment of Staphyloccocus aureus infected sore nipples: a randomized comparative study. *J Hum Lact, 15*(3), 241-246.

Livingstone, V. H., Willis, C. E., & Berkowitz, J. (1996). Staphylococcus aureus and sore nipples. *Can Fam Physician, 42*, 654-659.

Marchant, D. J. (2002). Inflammation of the breast. *Obstetrics and Gynecology Clinics of North America, 29*(1), 89-102.

Marmet, C., & Shell, E. (2008). Therapeutic positioning for Breastfeeding. In C. W. Genna (Ed.), *Supporting Sucking Skills in Breastfeeding Infants* (pp. 305-325). Boston, MA: Jones and Bartlett.

Marshall, D. R., Callan, P. P., & Nicholson, W. (1994). Breastfeeding after reduction mammaplasty. *British Journal of Plastic Surgery, 47*(3), 167-169.

Matheson, I., Aursnes, I., Horgen, M., Aabo, O., & Melby, K. (1988). Bacteriological findings and clinical symptoms in relation to clinical outcome in puerperal mastitis. *Acta Obstetricia et Gynecologica Scandinavica, 67*(8), 723-726.

McLachlan, Z., Milne, E. J., Lumley, J., & Walker, B. L. (1993). Ultrasound treatment for breast engorgement: A randomised double blind trial. *Breastfeeding Review, 2*(7), 316-320.

Meguid, M. M., Oler, A., Numann, P. J., & Khan, S. (1995). Pathogenesis-based treatment of recurring subareolar breast abscesses. *Surgery, 118*(4), 775-782.

Michalopoulos, K. (2007). The effects of breast augmentation surgery on future ability to lactate. *Breast J, 13*(1), 62-67.

Michie, C., Lockie, F., & Lynn, W. (2005). The challenge of mastitis. *Breastfeeding Review, 13*(1), 13-16.

Mizuno, K., Nishida, Y., Mizuno, N., Taki, M., Murase, M., & Itabashi, K. (2008). The important role of deep attachment in the uniform drainage of breast milk from mammary lobe. *Acta Paediatrica, 97*(9), 1200-1204.

Mofid, M. M., Klatsky, S. A., Singh, N. K., & Nahabedian, M. Y. (2006). Nipple-areola complex sensitivity after primary breast augmentation: a comparison of periareolar and inframammary incision approaches. *Plastic and Reconstructive Surgery, 117*(6), 1694-1698.

Moon, J. L., & Humenick, S. S. (1989). Breast engorgement: contributing variables and variables amenable to nursing intervention. *Journal of Obstetric, Gynecologic, and Neonatal Nursing, 18*(4), 309-315.

Nahai, F. R., & Nahai, F. (2008). MOC-PSSM CME article: Breast reduction. *Plastic and Reconstructive Surgery, 121*(1 Suppl), 1-13.

National Cancer Institute. (2006). Inflammatory breast cancer: questions and answers. Retrieved February 12, 2010, from http://www.cancer.gov/cancertopics/factsheet/Sites-Types/IBC.

Neifert, M., DeMarzo, S., Seacat, J., Young, D., Leff, M., & Orleans, M. (1990). The influence of breast surgery, breast appearance, and pregnancy-induced breast changes on lactation sufficiency as measured by infant weight gain. *Birth, 17*(1), 31-38.

Neifert, M. R., Seacat, J. M., & Jobe, W. E. (1985). Lactation failure due to insufficient glandular development of the breast. *Pediatrics, 76*(5), 823-828.

Neville, M. C., Keller, R., Seacat, J., Lutes, V., Neifert, M., Casey, C., et al. (1988). Studies in human lactation: milk volumes in lactating women during the onset of lactation and full lactation. *American Journal of Clinical Nutrition, 48*(6), 1375-1386.

Newman, J., & Pitman, T. (2006). *The Ultimate Breastfeeding Book of Answers*. New York, New York: Three Rivers Press.

Nikodem, V. C., Danziger, D., Gebka, N., Gulmezoglu, A. M., & Hofmeyr, G. J. (1993). Do cabbage leaves prevent breast engorgement? A randomized, controlled study. *Birth, 20*(2), 61-64.

Noble, R., & Bovey, A. (1997). Therapeutic teat use for babies who breastfeed poorly. *Breastfeeding Review, 5*(2), 37-42.

Nommsen-Rivers, L. A., Heinig, M. J., Cohen, R. J., & Dewey, K. G. (2008). Newborn wet and soiled diaper counts and timing of onset of lactation as indicators of breastfeeding inadequacy. *Journal of Human Lactation, 24*(1), 27-33.

O'Callaghan, M. A. (1981). Atypical discharge from the breast during pregnancy and/or lactation. *Australian and New Zealand Journal of Obstetrics and Gynaecology, 21*(4), 214-216.

Ohene-Yeboah, M., & Amaning, E. (2008). Spectrum of complaints presented at a specialist breast clinic in kumasi, ghana. *Ghana Medical Journal, 42*(3), 110-113.

Olsen, C. G., & Gordon, R. E., Jr. (1990). Breast disorders in nursing mothers. *American Family Physician, 41*(5), 1509-1516.

Osterman, K. L., & Rahm, V. A. (2000). Lactation mastitis: bacterial cultivation of breast milk, symptoms, treatment, and outcome. *Journal of Human Lactation, 16*(4), 297-302.

Park, G. E., Hauch, M. A., Curlin, F., Datta, S., & Bader, A. M. (1996). The effects of varying volumes of crystalloid administration before cesarean delivery on maternal hemodynamics and colloid osmotic pressure. *Anesth Analg, 83*(2), 299-303.

Peters, F., Diemer, P., Mecks, O., & Behnken, L. L. (2003). Severity of mastalgia in relation to milk duct dilatation. *Obstetrics and Gynecology, 101*(1), 54-60.

Peterson, B. (2007). Incidence of MRSA in postpartum breast abscesses (abstract). *Breastfeeding Medicine, 2*(3), 190.

Pitanguy, I., Vaena, M., Radwanski, H. N., Nunes, D., & Vargas, A. F. (2007). Relative implant volume and sensibility alterations after breast augmentation. *Aesthetic Plastic Surgery, 31*(3), 238-243.

Powers, N. G. (1999). Slow weight gain and low milk supply in the breastfeeding dyad. *Clinics in Perinatology, 26*(2), 399-430.

Pringle, P. J., Stanhope, R., Hindmarsh, P., & Brook, C. G. (1988). Abnormal pubertal development in primary hypothyroidism. *Clinical Endocrinology, 28*(5), 479-486.

Ramsay, D. T., Kent, J. C., Hartmann, R. A., & Hartmann, P. E. (2005). Anatomy of the lactating human breast redefined with ultrasound imaging. *Journal of Anatomy, 206*(6), 525-534.

Ramsay, D. T., Kent, J. C., Owens, R. A., & Hartmann, P. E. (2004). Ultrasound imaging of milk ejection in the breast of lactating women. *Pediatrics, 113*(2), 361-367.

Rasmussen, L. B., Hansen, D. H., Kaestel, P., Michaelsen, K. F., Friis, H., & Larsen, T. (2008). Milk enzyme activities and subclinical mastitis among women in Guinea-Bissau. *Breastfeed Med, 3*(4), 215-219.

Riordan, J., & Hoover, K. (2010). Perinatal and intrapartum care. In J. Riordan & K. A. Wambach (Eds.), *Breastfeeding and Human Lactation* (4th ed., pp. 215-251). Boston, MA: Jones and Bartlett.

Riordan, J., & Wambach, K. A. (2010). Breast-related problems. In J. Riordan & K. A. Wambach (Eds.), *Breastfeeding and Human Lactation* (pp. 291-324). Boston MA: Jones and Bartlett.

Riordan, J. M., & Nichols, F. H. (1990). A descriptive study of lactation mastitis in long-term breastfeeding women. *Journal of Human Lactation, 6*(2), 53-58.

Roberts, K. L. (1995). A comparison of chilled cabbage leaves and chilled gelpaks in reducing breast engorgement. *Journal of Human Lactation, 11*(1), 17-20.

Roberts, K. L., Reiter, M., & Schuster, D. (1995). A comparison of chilled and room temperature cabbage leaves in treating breast engorgement. *Journal of Human Lactation, 11*(3), 191-194.

Roberts, K. L., Reiter, M., & Schuster, D. (1998). Effects of cabbage leaf extract on breast engorgement. *Journal of Human Lactation, 14*(3), 231-236.

Salgado, C. D., Farr, B. M., & Calfee, D. P. (2003). Community-acquired methicillin-resistant Staphylococcus aureus: a meta-analysis of prevalence and risk factors. *Clinical Infectious Diseases, 36*(2), 131-139.

Schlenz, I., Kuzbari, R., Gruber, H., & Holle, J. (2000). The sensitivity of the nipple-areola complex: an anatomic study. *Plastic and Reconstructive Surgery, 105*(3), 905-909.

Scott, J. A., Robertson, M., Fitzpatrick, J., Knight, C., & Mulholland, S. (2008). Occurrence of lactational mastitis and medical management: A prospective cohort study in Glasgow. *Int Breastfeed J, 3*, 21.

Semple, J. L., Lugowski, S. J., Baines, C. J., Smith, D. C., & McHugh, A. (1998). Breast milk contamination and silicone implants: preliminary results using silicon as a proxy measurement for silicone. *Plastic and Reconstructive Surgery, 102*(2), 528-533.

Sharma, Y., Bajpai, A., Mittal, S., Kabra, M., & Menon, P. S. (2006). Ovarian cysts in young girls with hypothyroidism: follow-up and effect of treatment. *Journal of Pediatric Endocrinology and Metabolism, 19*(7), 895-900.

Sickles, E. A., & Abele, J. S. (1981). Milk of calcium within tiny benign breast cysts. *Radiology, 141*(3), 655-658.

Snowden, H. M., Renfrew, M. J., & Woolridge, M. W. (2001). Treatments for breast engorgement during lactation. *Cochrane Database Syst Rev*(2), CD000046.

Souto, G. C., Giugliani, E. R., Giugliani, C., & Schneider, M. A. (2003). The impact of breast reduction surgery on breastfeeding performance. *Journal of Human Lactation, 19*(1), 43-49; quiz 66-49, 120.

Spear, S. (2006). *Surgeries of the Breast: Principles and Art*. Philadelphia, PA: Lippincott-Raven.

Stafford, I., Hernandez, J., Laibl, V., Sheffield, J., Roberts, S., & Wendel, G., Jr. (2008). Community-acquired methicillin-resistant Staphylococcus aureus among patients with puerperal mastitis requiring hospitalization. *Obstetrics and Gynecology, 112*(3), 533-537.

Strom, S. S., Baldwin, B. J., Sigurdson, A. J., & Schusterman, M. A. (1997). Cosmetic saline breast implants: a survey of satisfaction, breast-feeding experience, cancer screening, and health. *Plastic and Reconstructive Surgery, 100*(6), 1553-1557.

Stutte, P. C., Bowles, B. C., & Morman, G. Y. (1988). The effects of breast massage on volume and fat content of human milk. *Genesis, 10*, 22-25.

Teuber, S. S., & Gershwin, M. E. (1994). Autoantibodies and clinical rheumatic complaints in two children of women with silicone gel breast implants. *International Archives of Allergy and Immunology, 103*(1), 105-108.

Thomassen, P., Johansson, V. A., Wassberg, C., & Petrini, B. (1998). Breast-feeding, pain and infection. *Gynecol Obstet Invest, 46*(2), 73-74.

Thomsen, A. C., Espersen, T., & Maigaard, S. (1984). Course and treatment of milk stasis, noninfectious inflammation of the breast, and infectious mastitis in nursing women. *American Journal of Obstetrics and Gynecology, 149*(5), 492-495.

Thorley, V. (2005). Breast hypoplasia and breastfeeding: a case history. *Breastfeeding Review, 13*(2), 13-16.

Tokuda, Y., Kuriyama, K., Nakamoto, A., Choi, S., Yutani, K., Kunitomi, Y., et al. (2009). Evaluation of suspicious nipple discharge by magnetic resonance mammography based on breast imaging reporting and data system magnetic resonance imaging descriptors. *Journal of Computer Assisted Tomography, 33*(1), 58-62.

Trupiano, J. K., Sebek, B. A., Goldfarb, J., Levy, L. R., Hall, G. S., & Procop, G. W. (2001). Mastitis due to Mycobacterium abscessus after body piercing. *Clinical Infectious Diseases, 33*(1), 131-134.

Uematsu, T., Kasami, M., & Yuen, S. (2009). A cluster of microcalcifications: women with high risk for breast cancer versus other women. *Breast Cancer*.

Ulitzsch, D., Nyman, M. K., & Carlson, R. A. (2004). Breast abscess in lactating women: US-guided treatment. *Radiology, 232*(3), 904-909.

von Heimburg, D., Exner, K., Kruft, S., & Lemperle, G. (1996). The tuberous breast deformity: classification and treatment. *British Journal of Plastic Surgery, 49*(6), 339-345.

Walker, M. (2006). *Breastfeeding Management for the Clinician: Using the Evidence*. Boston, MA: Jones and Bartlett.

Wambach, K. A. (2003). Lactation mastitis: a descriptive study of the experience. *Journal of Human Lactation, 19*(1), 24-34.

West, D. (2001). *Defining Your Own Success: Breastfeeding after Breast Reduction Surgery*. Schaumburg, IL: La Leche League International.

West, D., & Hirsch, E. (2008). *Breastfeeding after Breast and Nipple Procedures*. Amarillo, TX: Hale Publishing.

West, D., & Marasco, L. (2009). *The Breastfeeding Mother's Guide to Making More Milk*. New York, NY: McGraw Hill.

WHO. (2000). *Mastitis: Causes and Management*. Retrieved. from.

Wilson-Clay, B. (2008). Case report of methicillin-resistant Staphylococcus aureus (MRSA) mastitis with abscess formation in a breastfeeding woman. *Journal of Human Lactation, 24*(3), 326-329.

Wilson-Clay, B., & Hoover, K. (2008). *The Breastfeeding Atlas* (4th ed.). Manchaca, TX: LactNews Press.

Wockel, A., Abou-Dakn, M., Beggel, A., & Arck, P. (2008). Inflammatory breast diseases during lactation: health effects on the newborn-a literature review. *Mediators of Inflammation, 2008*, 298760.

Wust, J., Rutsch, M., & Stocker, S. (1995). Streptococcus pneumoniae as an agent of mastitis. *European Journal of Clinical Microbiology and Infectious Diseases, 14*(2), 156-157.

Zocchi, M. L., & Zuliani, F. (2008). Bicompartmental breast lipostructuring. *Aesthetic Plastic Surgery, 32*(2), 313-328.

Health Issues—Mother

Chapter 19

BREASTFEEDING WITH HEALTH ISSUES

When a mother is ill, to help speed her recovery, those supporting her may look for ways to reduce her stress and workload. Sometimes others (including healthcare providers) assume that discontinuing breastfeeding will make an ill mother's life easier. Milk-making may seem like an unnecessary physical strain on her body, and it may seem to them that the time she spends breastfeeding is extra work, an inconvenience, or an interruption to her rest. However, the mother's feelings are more important. If she wants to continue breastfeeding, the following information may help her convey to those around her that breastfeeding can be good for her and for her recovery, as well as for her baby.

When a mother is ill, breastfeeding relieves stress; enhances her metabolism, immune system, and sleep; and provides a greater sense of control and normalcy.

Breastfeeding provides stress relief. Caring for a newborn can be intense and sometimes stressful (no matter how baby is fed). Research indicates, however, that not breastfeeding is more stressful for mothers than breastfeeding. The skin-to-skin contact and oxytocin release that occurs naturally during breastfeeding are no doubt factors, as Swedish research has found that higher oxytocin blood levels decrease blood pressure and levels of cortisol, a stress hormone (Jonas et al., 2008; Uvnas-Moberg, 1998) In one U.S. study of 24 women who both breastfed and bottle-fed, researchers assessed the study mothers' mood before and after breastfeeding and before and after bottle-feeding. Their findings indicated that the mothers were calmer after breastfeeding than after bottle-feeding. This study was significant because it eliminated one of the major problems in comparing breastfeeding and non-breastfeeding women: the often substantial differences between women who choose one feeding method over the other. Since the same mothers were studied after both breast and bottle, this potentially confounding factor was eliminated (Mezzacappa, Guethlein, & Katkin, 2002). The down-regulation of stress that breastfeeding provides is no doubt one reason research has linked longer breastfeeding duration to better cardiovascular outcomes in mothers later in life (Schwarz et al., 2009). For details, see the later section "Cardiac Issues/Hypertension."

Breastfeeding can enhance a mother's health when she is ill.

Breastfeeding enhances a mother's immune system and her mood. Another U.S. study of 181 mothers measured mothers' reactions to stress, including its effect on the immune system (measured by blood cytokine balance) and their mood (Groer & Davis, 2006). The researchers found that the immune systems of non-breastfeeding mothers were more depressed by life stressors, and these mothers developed more infections than the breastfeeding mothers. The non-breastfeeding mothers also had higher levels of anxiety and fatigue. Based on German research (Dimitrov, Lange, Fehm, & Born, 2004), Groer and Davis suggest that higher levels of blood prolactin stimulated by breastfeeding was related to more positive mood, greater immunity to infection, and decreased stress.

Breastfeeding mothers have greater metabolic efficiency. U.S. research has also found that a mother's body adapts to lactation by reducing the energy required to make milk, causing her metabolism to be more energy-efficient. During lactation, a mother's intestines enlarge and change to make digestion more efficient at absorbing nutrients (Hammond, 1997). After a meal, breastfeeding mothers were found to have greater metabolic efficiency than non-breastfeeding mothers (Illingworth, Jung, Howie, Leslie, & Isles, 1986). This greater metabolic efficiency has been found to continue long after breastfeeding ends and improve mothers' health outcomes later in life. A U.S. cross-sectional cohort analysis of 1,620 women found that duration of lactation was associated with a lower incidence later in life of the recently identified metabolic syndrome (Ram et al., 2008). For more details, see p. 761- "Type 2 (Non-Insulin Dependent) Diabetes Mellitus." One of these researchers wrote: "Lactation may prime the metabolic system by making it a more energy-efficient machine...." (Ram et al., 2008, p. 268).

Breastfeeding mothers sleep more and spend more time in deep sleep. Some think that if someone else feeds the baby at night the mother will get more sleep and sleep better, but in families with young babies, breastfeeding can help a mother get more sleep and improve the quality of her sleep. One U.S. study of 133 new mothers and fathers during the first 3 months postpartum found that mothers who exclusively breastfed averaged 40 to 45 minutes more sleep at night than those who breastfed and gave their babies formula (Doan, Gardiner, Gay, & Lee, 2007). Australian research found that breastfeeding mothers spent more time in deep sleep than non-breastfeeding mothers (Blyton, Sullivan, & Edwards, 2002). The exclusively breastfeeding mothers had "a marked alteration in their sleep architecture," giving them longer periods of slow-wave sleep (SWS), a type of deep sleep, than the formula-feeding mothers. For more details, see p. 86- "Sleep Patterns."

Breastfeeding can help give the mother a greater sense of normalcy and control. A very ill mother may be able to care for her baby at the breast, even when she can do little else for him. As one U.S. lactation consultant and author wrote:

> ...[E]vidence shows that the provision of breast milk provides a mechanism for the mother to regain an element of control over an overwhelming situation. Fear, grief, remorse, anger, and guilt can be refocused into activities that allow the mother to exercise her unique role in the intimate care of her [child] (Walker, 2006, p. 274).

If appropriate, discuss ways to make continued breastfeeding easier, such as bringing the young baby into bed while she recovers and breastfeeding while side-lying or semi-reclining, so she can rest. If she has an older, active baby, suggest closing her door and having toys available for him to play with while she rests. A toddler may be happy spending time with others, returning to mother every now and then to breastfeed and "touch base." For the mother with a disability or limitation, see that section (p. 773- "Basic Strategies for Mothers with Disabilities") for strategies for making breastfeeding easier and drawbacks to not breastfeeding.

In nearly all cases, continuing to breastfeed will be better for the baby.

Acute illness. Even before a mother exposed to an acute illness notices symptoms, she is already contagious. At this stage, one of her body's first responses is to make antibodies that pass into her milk specifically designed to protect her breastfeeding baby from her illness. By the time the mother starts to feel sick, her baby has already been exposed and is already receiving protection against her illness. When she keeps breastfeeding, she continues to protect her baby. Because of the antibodies he's receiving, if the breastfeeding baby does become ill, he almost always gets a milder case than he would have if he had weaned. In the case of a virus, most often immunity to that virus is transmitted through mother's milk. Exceptions include HIV and HTLV-1. For details, see the section later in this chapter.

Endocrine, metabolic, or autoimmune disorder. Some mothers worry that breastfeeding may transmit their chronic illness to their baby. If breastfeeding affects the baby's likelihood of having this disorder, usually the opposite is true. For example, when diabetic mothers exclusively breastfeed, their babies are less likely to develop diabetes than babies who are formula-fed (Sadauskaite-Kuehne, Ludvigsson, Padaiga, Jasinskiene, & Samuelsson, 2004). The same is true for rheumatoid arthritis, and many others. With a genetic disease, such as cystic fibrosis, if the baby has a genetic predisposition to this disorder, breastfeeding cannot prevent it, but it has been found to delay the onset of its symptoms (Colombo et al., 2007).

• •

Most medications and diagnostic tests are compatible with breastfeeding.

If a breastfeeding mother has concerns about whether she should take a medication prescribed for her health problem, check this drug in the most current edition of the book *Medications and Mothers' Milk* by Thomas W. Hale, RPh, PhD (Amarillo, TX: Hale Publishing). Another book often used to check a drug's compatibility with breastfeeding is *The Physician's Desk Reference* (*PDR*). However, the *PDR* is a compilation of package inserts from the drug manufacturers, whose main concern is avoiding lawsuits. In the *PDR,* weaning is recommended for many drugs research indicates are safe while breastfeeding. *Medications and Mothers' Milk,* on the other hand, provides information about the published research on each drug in breastfeeding mothers and assigns a "Lactation Risk Category" to simplify decisions:

- L1 (Safest) are drugs that have been taken by large numbers of breastfeeding mothers and controlled studies found no adverse effects in the baby, the possibility of risk is remote, or the drug is not orally bioavailable to the baby.
- L2 (Safer) are drugs for which studies exist in breastfeeding mothers without adverse effects on their baby and/or the risk during breastfeeding is remote.
- L3 (Moderately Safe) are new drugs with no research or existing drugs with no controlled studies in breastfeeding women, those with a possible risk of adverse effects in the baby, or controlled studies found minimal effects on the baby.
- L4 (Possibly Hazardous) are drugs for which evidence exists of risk to either the breastfeeding baby or the mother's milk production. If there are no alternative drugs available and the mother is seriously ill, the benefit may outweigh the risk.
- L5 (Contraindicated) are drugs that should not be taken while breastfeeding. Either studies have found a significant risk to the breastfeeding baby or the characteristics of the drug indicate the risks to the baby would outweigh the benefits to the mother.

For key points about breastfeeding and medications, see Table 19.1. The vast majority of medications and diagnostic tests are compatible with breastfeeding (AAP, 2001; Hale, 2010). This means that the health risks associated with feeding the baby infant formula are considered greater than the risks of continuing to breastfeed with a tiny amount of the drug (usually about 1%-2% of the maternal dose) in the mother's milk. However, because there are a few drugs that are not compatible with breastfeeding, the mother's medication should always be checked. Also, each drug needs to be evaluated by the families' healthcare providers in light of the mother's and baby's condition and health history. If an incompatible drug is recommended, there is often an alternative drug compatible with breastfeeding that can be substituted.

Table 19.1. Key Points about Breastfeeding and Medications

- Most drugs are safe in breastfeeding mothers. The hazards of using formula are well known and documented.
- Avoid using medications that are not necessary. Herbal drugs, high-dose vitamins, unusual supplements, etc. that are not necessary should be avoided.
- Medications used in the first 3 to 4 days are rarely of concern due to the limited volume of mother's milk the baby consumes.
- If the baby receives <10% of the mother's dose (Relative Infant Dose), the vast majority of medications are considered safe. For most drugs, the baby receives <1% of the mother's dose.
- Choose drugs for which there is published data, rather than new drugs, short-acting rather than long-acting drugs (short half-life), and drugs with high protein binding, low oral bioavailability, or high molecular weight.
- Be slightly more cautious with newborns and at-risk babies, such those ill or preterm. Be less concerned about older, heavier babies and those no longer exclusively breastfeeding.
- Recommend that mothers with symptoms of depression or other mental disorders seek treatment. Most of the medications used to treat them are safe.
- Temporary weaning may be required for hours or days for a few drugs and nearly all radioactive compounds. Follow published guidelines.

Adapted from (Hale, 2008). Used with permission.

• •

If the mother must wean temporarily or permanently due to illness or treatment, help her do so as gradually and comfortably as possible.

Continuing to breastfeed is nearly always the best option. But if the mother must wean her baby, either temporarily or permanently, discuss how to do this with the least amount of physical and emotional stress. Abrupt weaning during an illness can cause the mother intense discomfort from full breasts and put her at increased risk for mastitis. It can also upset the baby, making him difficult to console and increasing his odds of becoming ill.

If the weaning is temporary, discuss milk expression (see the chapter "Milk Expression and Storage"). Even if her milk cannot be fed to her baby, regular milk expression will prevent pain and mastitis and maintain her milk production until she is ready to breastfeed again. If weaning must be permanent, discuss her timing and help her wean as slowly and gradually as possible to make it easier for her and her baby. (For more details, see the chapter "Weaning from the Breast.")

BACTERIAL AND VIRAL ILLNESSES

When a breastfeeding mother is ill, first acknowledge her feelings and challenges, and then discuss her specific concerns.

A mother's illness can disrupt her whole household. In this situation, the mother must cope with her own health issues, along with any worries she has about the effect of her illness or treatment on her breastfeeding baby. If she has a serious illness, she may be afraid and grieving for her previous life. As identified by Dr. Elizabeth Kubler-Ross, stages of grief include denial, anger, bargaining, depression, and acceptance or resignation.

Whatever the mother's concerns and emotions, first acknowledge her feelings. Comments like "You're really having a difficult time" or "Don't worry about crying. You have so much to cope with" reassure her that she is being heard and that it is okay to express strong feelings. Feeling heard first may make it possible for her to better process information and make decisions. The following sections describe breastfeeding issues and specific illnesses.

Frequent hand-washing is important when mothers have a bacterial or viral illness.

When the mother is contagious, using good hygiene, such as frequent hand-washing, can reduce her baby's odds of catching her illness.

Most acute illnesses are transmitted through skin contact and nose or mouth secretions, not through breastfeeding. When a mother is ill, good personal hygiene, including regular hand-washing, can decrease the baby's chances of catching her illness. The mother can also try to avoid breathing on her baby by limiting face-to-face contact. In cases of a highly contagious or serious illness, wearing a face mask whenever holding the baby can help prevent transmission through breath or nose-and-mouth secretions.

Suggest any mother running a fever drink lots of fluids to stay well hydrated.

Fever can reduce the mother's body fluids, which increases her chances of becoming constipated and dehydrated. When she is feverish, encourage her to drink more fluids.

Common Illnesses

Cold, Virus, or Mild Infection

Interrupting breastfeeding during a cold, virus, or mild infection increases the baby's chance of getting sick.

See the previous sections. Before a mother notices symptoms of a cold, virus, or mild infection, she is already contagious. At this stage, her body begins producing antibodies, specifically designed to protect her breastfeeding baby, that pass into her milk. Continued breastfeeding helps protect the baby from catching the mother's illness or if he does catch it, the antibodies he receives usually makes his illness less severe.

Food Poisoning

Breastfeeding does not need to be interrupted when a mother has food poisoning.

Food poisoning is caused when the mother consumes a food or drink contaminated with specific bacteria or toxins. Bacteria that can cause food poisoning include botulism (*Clostridium botulinum*), listeriosis (*Listeria*), salmonella, *Shigella*, *E. coli*, and others.

Incubation period and symptoms. Incubation period varies by organism. Symptoms include vomiting, abdominal cramps, and diarrhea.

Food poisoning and the breastfeeding baby. Food poisoning should not affect the breastfeeding baby.

Food poisoning and the breastfeeding mother. Almost always, the mother will recover from food poisoning within a few days without further problems. If the mother has diarrhea and vomiting, suggest she drink enough liquids to avoid dehydration.

Treatments for food poisoning and breastfeeding. If a mother's food poisoning is so severe that she is prescribed antibiotics, its compatibility with breastfeeding should be checked (most antibiotics are compatible with breastfeeding). In severe cases, depending upon which bacteria are involved, precautions may be recommended to prevent airborne or skin-contact transmission between mother and baby, such as hand-washing and wearing a face mask while breastfeeding.

Seasonal Influenza (Flu)/H1N1

During influenza season, pregnant and breastfeeding mothers are encouraged to be vaccinated and follow recommended hygiene practices.

At this writing, the U.S. CDC recommends that pregnant women and anyone caring for a young infant be vaccinated for the flu (CDC, 2009a). To prevent its spread, recommended hygiene practices include frequent hand washing and covering mouth and nose when coughing or sneezing.

Mothers with seasonal influenza do not need to stop breastfeeding.

H1N1 flu and the breastfeeding mother and baby. At this writing, it is generally agreed that mothers who have been exposed to the seasonal flu, but do not have symptoms should continue breastfeeding, and when a baby becomes ill with the seasonal flu that he should continue breastfeeding (CDC, 2009a). There is controversy about recommendations for obviously ill breastfeeding mothers who have symptoms of the H1N1 virus but whose babies appear healthy. The baby cannot catch the flu from mother's milk, but some worry that if the mother breastfeeds, her baby will be exposed through touch and if the mother coughs or sneezes. Some U.S. public health groups have advised breastfeeding mothers with symptoms to keep their distance from their babies until they are no longer contagious and to arrange for their baby to be fed their expressed milk by someone else who is healthy (CDC, 2009a; CDC, 2009d). Because separation of mother and baby puts breastfeeding at risk, physicians Ruth Lawrence and John Bradley suggested as a compromise position in an American Academy of Pediatrics newsletter that mothers with flu symptoms continue breastfeeding while following these recommendations to minimize the chance their baby will catch the flu from them, especially after birth during their hospital stay (Lawrence & Bradley, 2009):

- Wash her hands well before touching her baby.
- Before breastfeeding, wash her breasts with mild soap and water, rinsing well.
- While holding or breastfeeding the baby, wear a surgical mask to protect the baby from contact with nasal secretions during coughing or sneezing.
- Use clean blankets or burp cloths at each feeding.
- Be sure everyone who touches the baby follows these precautions.

Treatments for the flu and breastfeeding. Lawrence and Bradley cited above also recommend that antiviral medications be chosen for breastfeeding mothers that are compatible with breastfeeding.

Bacterial Infections

Group B Streptococcus

One of the most common causes of newborn infection, *Group B Streptococcus,* is usually transmitted before or during birth and only rarely via mother's milk.

In the U.S., Group B Strep is a major cause of serious infections in mothers and newborns (AAP, 2009b). About 90% of newborn infection occurs within the first 6 days after birth, and the infected newborn is at risk of serious illness, such as pneumonia, meningitis, and blood-borne infection (sepsis). Mothers with Group B strep are at risk for blood-borne infection (bacteremia), endometritis, urinary tract infection, and mastitis.

Incubation period and symptoms. The incubation period for early-onset Group B strep after birth is fewer than 7 days (AAP, 2009b). As described above, Group B strep usually manifests as different illnesses and as infections throughout the body.

Prophylactic treatments for Group B strep. U.S. mothers are commonly tested for Group B strep during pregnancy, and if positive are treated with antibiotics. Many women who have not been tested but are considered at risk receive IV antibiotics for Group B strep during labor (Riordan, 2010). Some researchers have linked the use of prophylactic antibiotic treatment to the development of more virulent strains of Group B strep (Harris, Shelver, Bohnsack, & Rubens, 2003).

Group B strep and the breastfeeding baby. Although rare, it is possible for Group B strep to be transmitted to a very preterm or compromised baby through mother's milk (Dinger, Muller, Pargac, & Schwarze, 2002; Wang, Chen, Liu, & Wang, 2007). It is also possible for the Group B strep organism to be passed back and forth between mother and baby, unless both are treated effectively at the same time (Byrne, Miller, & Justus, 2006). If a mother's milk cultures positive for Group B strep and her baby is at risk, her milk may be heat-treated or discarded until the cultures are clear. Feeding babies formula in addition to mother's milk increases their risk of developing infections of all kinds (Ip, Chung, Raman, Trikalinos, & Lau, 2009). When the mother of a compromised baby in a hospital's special-care nursery develops mastitis or her baby becomes ill, culturing for Group B strep is recommended (Byrne et al., 2006; Riordan, 2010).

Treatments for Group B Strep and breastfeeding. The antibiotics used to treat Group B strep, such as penicillin, ampicillin, clindamycin, and erythromycin, are also used to treat babies and are considered compatible with breastfeeding (Hale, 2008).

Lyme Disease

No transmission of Lyme disease by breastfeeding has been reported, and antibiotic treatment is compatible with breastfeeding.

Lyme disease is caused by a type of spirochete bacterium (*Borrelia burgdorferi*) that lives in rodents and other small animals and is transmitted from animal to animal and to humans by tick bites. Most human cases occur in late spring and summer, when people spend more time outdoors.

Incubation period and symptoms. From the tick bites to the onset of symptoms is between 1 and 32 days, with an average of 11 days (AAP, 2009b). Symptoms usually start with a painless circular rash at the tick-bite site (usually appearing within 3 to 30 days after being bitten by an infected tick), which expands in size, reaching up to 12 inches (30 cm) in diameter. Symptoms may include fever, headache, chills, muscle and joint aches, and swollen lymph glands.

Lyme disease and the breastfeeding baby. Although the Lyme spirochete can be transmitted to an unborn baby in utero, there is no indication it can be transmitted by breastfeeding. According to the American Academy of Pediatrics Committee on Infectious Diseases: "No evidence exists that Lyme disease can be transmitted via human milk" (AAP, 2009b, p. 431). According to the U.S. Centers for Disease Control and Prevention, "There are no reports of Lyme disease transmission from breast milk" (CDC, 2007).

Treatments for Lyme disease and breastfeeding. Treatment of a breastfeeding mother with Lyme disease usually involves a several-week course of appropriate oral antibiotic, such as doxycycline, amoxicillin, and ceforoxime axetil, which are considered compatible with breastfeeding (Hale, 2008). Although most cases of Lyme disease treated early resolve completely, in some cases, symptoms like muscle and joint pain, sleep disturbance, and fatigue can continue long term.

Methicillin-Resistant Staphylococcus Aureus (MRSA)

When mother or baby is diagnosed with a methicillin-resistant *Staphylococcus aureas* (MRSA) infection, there is no benefit to separating them.

The *Staphylococcus aureus* bacterium (Staph aureus for short) is so common that during the 1950s by the 5th day after birth, 40% to 90% of newborns in hospital nurseries were colonized with it, not all of whom developed infections (Fairchild, Graber, Vogel, & Ingersoll, 1958). Over the years, with frequent use of antibiotics, virulent strains of methicillin-resistant Staph aureus (MRSA) have developed. "Methicillin-resistant" strains do not respond to the drugs typically used to treat Staph aureus infections. MRSA causes more severe illness and requires stronger antibiotics to eradicate. MRSA once existed only rarely in hospitals, but has become increasingly common—about 60% of Staph aureus infections in hospitals are now MRSA (AAP, 2009b)—and has also spread to some communities (Salgado, Farr, & Calfee, 2003; Stafford et al., 2008). Staph aureus infections are transmitted primarily by direct contact and can be harbored in the nose and throat.

Incubation period and symptoms. MRSA begins as a skin infection that may look like a spider bite, a boil, or an abscess. It is usually swollen, red, and painful and can progress to a fever, shortness of breath, a cough, and chills. The incubation period can be from 1 to 10 days, depending on its route of transmission.

MRSA and the breastfeeding baby. When a breastfeeding mother or baby contracts MRSA, some healthcare providers question whether it is risky to continue breastfeeding. However, *if a mother develops a MRSA infection, the baby has already been exposed to it before her symptoms become obvious, so there is no reason to stop breastfeeding unless the baby is ill or preterm.* If the baby's health is fragile, the mother's milk can be pasteurized before feeding (Gastelum, Dassey, Mascola, & Yasuda, 2005; Kim et al., 2007), or if that is not an option, her milk may need to be discarded until it is clear of infection, usually within 24 hours of starting treatment (Lawrence & Lawrence, 2005). Hand-washing and other routine hygiene practices are important to help stop the spread of infection. If a mother with MRSA has an open sore, precautions should be taken to prevent the baby from coming in contact with it.

Preventing MRSA in the baby after birth. A baby leaves the womb free from outside organisms, but is exposed to them in the birth canal. Japanese researchers suggest mother-baby skin-to-skin contact immediately after birth provides a defense against MRSA, colonizing newborns with their mother's normal flora, which decreases their susceptibility to MRSA colonization of their nose and throat that can lead to infection in the mother (Kitajima, 2003). To lower the risk of contracting MRSA in the hospital NICU, one Japanese report recommends, at the time of NICU admission, spreading mother's milk in and over the mouths of all extremely-low-birth-weight babies (Nakamura, 2001).

Treatment for MRSA and breastfeeding. The same antibiotics used to treat babies with MRSA are also used to treat mothers, making them compatible with breastfeeding (Hale, 2008).

Toxic Shock Syndrome

Breastfeeding can continue if the mother with toxic shock syndrome is well enough to do so.

Toxic shock syndrome occurs when a strain of staphyloccal or streptococcal bacteria release an enterotoxin (a protein-based toxin) into the bloodstream, infecting the body.

Incubation period and symptoms. When not associated with surgery, the incubation period for toxic shock syndrome is 1 to 10 days (AAP, 2009b). Symptoms include watery diarrhea, vomiting, muscle aches, and chills, fever of at least 102º F/38.9º C, and low blood pressure. About half of the cases occur in women using tampons during menstruation, but it can also occur after birth, after surgery, or in other circumstances (AAP, 2009b).

Toxic shock syndrome and the breastfeeding baby. Breastfeeding can continue. The enterotoxin associated with toxic shock syndrome was found in the milk of a U.S. mother who developed it after birth (Vergeront et al., 1982), but the toxin is inactivated by the acidic environment of a baby's stomach, so this presents no danger to the breastfeeding baby (Bergdoll, Crass, Reiser, Robbins, & Davis, 1981).

Toxic shock syndrome and the breastfeeding mother. If the mother is well enough, she can continue to breastfeed with careful attention to hand-washing and other standard precautions (Lawrence & Lawrence, 2005). If the mother becomes too ill to breastfeed, breastfeeding can be resumed later (Golden, 2003). During the most severe part of her illness, the mother may need help with breastfeeding or milk expression. If she stops breastfeeding during her illness, she can resume breastfeeding and increase her milk production when she's feeling better.

Treatments for toxic shock syndrome and breastfeeding. Most antibiotics used to treat toxic shock syndrome are considered compatible with breastfeeding (Hale, 2008; Lawrence & Lawrence, 2005).

Tuberculosis

When the mother with tuberculosis is well enough to hold her baby, she can breastfeed.

Tuberculosis is an infectious disease caused by the bacterium *Mycobacterium tuberculosis*, which is usually transmitted from person to person via droplets in the air from coughing. Tuberculosis bacteria usually attack the lungs, but can also spread to other parts of the body.

Incubation period and symptoms. The time from exposure to TB to a positive TB test is 2 to 10 weeks. Symptoms may not occur for 1 to 6 months and include weight loss, fever, cough, night sweats, and chills (AAP, 2009b).

Tuberculosis and the breastfeeding mother and baby. Mothers known to be contagious with active pulmonary tuberculosis are separated from their babies, no matter how they are fed, at least until they and their baby are started on drug therapy. Two U.S. physicians wrote:

> Initiation of prophylactic isoniazid [an antimicrobial drug] in the infant has been demonstrated to be effective in preventing TB infection and disease in the infant. Therefore, continued separation of the infant and mother is unnecessary once therapy in both mother and child has begun (Lawrence & Lawrence, 2005, p. 640).

This is common practice in many parts of the world.

If treatment of mother and baby after birth is delayed or healthcare providers recommend separation, suggest the mother establish her milk production using milk expression. (For details, see p. 466 in the chapter, "Milk Expression and Storage.") If a mother develops an active case of tuberculosis during pregnancy and receives appropriate drug therapy, she and her baby are unlikely to be separated after birth.

Treatments for tuberculosis and breastfeeding. Tubculosis requires long-term drug therapy. Anti-tubercular drugs—such as isoniazid, rifampin, and ethambutol—are considered compatible with breastfeeding (AAP, 2001; AAP, 2009b; Hale, 2008).

Viral Infections

Hepatitis A, B, C and Other Hepatic Diseases

Hepatitis A

When a mother contracts hepatitis A, her baby can be given its immune globulin and/or vaccine and breastfeeding can continue.

Hepatitis means "inflammation of the liver." Hepatitis A is liver inflammation caused by the hepatitis A virus (HAV), one of the three most common hepatitis viruses, which can be transmitted by contact with infected blood or feces. Hepatitis B and C (see next section) are chronic diseases, but hepatitis A is not. In most people, it resolves completely without long-term damage. A case of hepatitis A also confers life-long immunity to this illness.

Incubation period and symptoms. After exposure to hepatitis A, it may take 15 to 50 days for symptoms to develop (AAP, 2009b). During this illness, the liver becomes tender and swollen and bilirubin accumulates in the bloodstream, causing jaundice. Fever and nausea are also common symptoms.

Hepatitis A and the breastfeeding mother. If during the acute phase of hepatitis A a mother feels too ill to breastfeed, she can express her milk (which can be given to the baby) or rebuild her milk production after her symptoms subside. If she decides not to breastfeed, suggest, at a minimum, she express enough milk often enough to avoid uncomfortable breast fullness, as this could cause mastitis, complicating her health problems.

Hepatitis A and the breastfeeding baby. When the breastfeeding mother of a newborn contracts hepatitis A, the American Academy of Pediatrics Committee on Infectious Diseases recommends treating the baby with either the hepatitis A vaccine or immune globulin (AAP, 2009b) or both can be given (Lawrence &

Lawrence, 2005). Transmission of hepatitis A from mother to child is very rare, and there is no reason to stop breastfeeding.

Hepatitis A treatments and breastfeeding. Other than treatment of symptoms (such as fever-reducers or pain medication) Hepatitis A has no treatment.

Hepatitis B

Hepatitis B is the most common serious liver infection in the world and is caused by the hepatitis B virus (HBV).

If a mother has hepatitis B, her baby can be given its immune globulin and vaccine, and breastfeeding can continue.

Incubation period and symptoms. Acute symptoms usually appear between 45 and 160 days after exposure to hepatitis B (AAP, 2009b). Symptoms are similar to hepatitis A, but in about 5% to 10% of cases, hepatitis B becomes a chronic illness that may never completely resolve. It is spread whenever a body fluid (saliva, mucus, blood, etc.) containing the hepatitis B virus comes in contact with broken skin. It can also be transmitted from contaminated food and sexual contact. Some carriers of HBV do not become ill.

Hepatitis B at birth. When a mother giving birth has hepatitis B, the newborn may be exposed to it through contact with her body fluids during delivery. In this situation, the American Academy of Pediatrics Committee on Infectious Diseases recommended the baby of a hepatitis-B positive mother be given within 12 hours after birth both the first dose of the hepatitis-B vaccine and the hepatitis B immune globulin. There is no reason to delay breastfeeding after birth. The Committee wrote:

> Breastfeeding of the infant by an [hepatitis B-] positive mother poses no additional risk of acquisition of HBV infection by the infant with appropriate administration of hepatitis B vaccine and HBIG (AAP, 2009b, p. 354).

With treatments and/ or proper precautions, mothers with hepatitis can continue to breastfeed.

Hepatitis B and the breastfeeding mother and baby. If a breastfeeding mother contracts hepatitis B later, the same course of action is advised. Her baby (and other family members) should be vaccinated and breastfeeding should continue.

Treatment of hepatitis B and breastfeeding. Like hepatitis A, there are no treatments for hepatitis B, other than treating its symptoms.

Hepatitis C

The hepatitis C virus (HCV) causes this liver infection, which in many cases is chronic and incurable.

It is considered safe for mothers with hepatitis C, but without symptoms, to breastfeed. But breastfeeding with bleeding or cracked nipples is controversial.

Incubation period and symptoms. After transmission, the hepatitis C virus usually incubates for an average of 6 to 7 weeks before symptoms appear. It may start as a mild infection or there may be no symptoms at all. However, 75% to 85% of those who contract it develop chronic liver infections for which there is no cure and no treatment. Hepatitis C is transmitted through sexual contact and infected blood. It occurs most commonly in those who received blood transfusions or had an accidental needle stick in healthcare settings, babies infected during birth by infected mothers, and drug users who share needles (CDC, 2009c).

Hepatitis C and the breastfeeding mother and baby. The U.S. Centers for Disease Control and Prevention gave the following answer to the question "Is it safe for a mother infected with hepatitis C virus (HCV) to breastfeed her infant?"

> Yes. There is no documented evidence that breastfeeding spreads HCV. Therefore, having HCV-infection is not a contraindication to breastfeed. HCV is transmitted by infected blood, not by human breast milk. There are no current data to suggest that HCV is transmitted in human breast milk (CDC, 2009b, p. 1).

Hepatitis C and cracked and bleeding nipples. Because hepatitis C is transmitted via blood, controversy exists about whether an HCV-infected mother with cracked and bleeding nipples should stop breastfeeding until her nipples are healed. The American Academy of Pediatrics Committee on Infectious Diseases recommended temporarily interrupting breastfeeding until the mother's nipples are no longer bleeding (AAP, 2009a). However, at this writing, there are no documented cases of a baby contracting hepatitis C this way. The U.S. Centers for Disease Control and Prevention concluded:

> Data are insufficient to say yes or no. However, HCV is spread by infected blood. Therefore, if the HCV-positive mother's nipples and/or surrounding areola are cracked and bleeding, she should stop nursing temporarily. Instead, she should consider expressing and discarding her breast milk until her nipples are healed. Once her breasts are no longer cracked or bleeding, the HCV-positive mother may fully resume breastfeeding (CDC, 2009b).

According to Lawrence Gartner, MD, Professor Emeritus in Pediatrics at the University of Chicago (L. Gartner, personal communication, June 21, 2002):

> The issue of nipple bleeding as a risk for acquisition of hepatitis C is an entirely theoretical possibility for which there is no evidence that I have ever seen. There are now more than fifteen different studies comparing the incidence of hepatitis in infants who are either breastfed or formula-fed, and none have shown any difference. I must assume that some of these hepatitis C carrier mothers had bleeding nipples. Since human milk of some carrier mothers contains hepatitis C virus, the exposure should not be different whether the virus enters in a small amount of blood or a large volume of milk. The indirect evidence is that human milk protects the infant from becoming infected when ingesting the virus through its various protective agents, which either inactivate the virus or prevent its attachment to the intestinal mucosa. The fact is that there is no evidence that breastfeeding from a mother who is infected with hepatitis C increases the risk of the infant becoming infected.

Acute hepatitis C infection after birth and the breastfeeding mother. The rare exception is the mother who becomes infected with hepatitis C after birth and has acute symptoms while breastfeeding but before her levels of antibodies are high enough to provide protection for her baby. In this situation, suggest the mother talk to her healthcare provider about her options in light of her specific situation. One study done in Spain of 63 women and 73 babies found the rate of transmission of HCV and the level of the virus in the milk were higher (20% vs. 0% of the asymptomatic women) when the women had active HCV symptoms (Ruiz-Extremera et al., 2000). Another study of 65 HCV-infected mothers conducted in the United Arab Emirates found that when mothers were symptomatic, the level of virus in their milk increased along with the incidence of HCV transmission to their babies (Kumar & Shahul, 1998). If the symptomatic HCV-positive mother and her healthcare provider decide she should wean, offer to discuss milk expression with her to either maintain her milk production until her symptoms subside or decrease her milk production and wean comfortably (see the chapter "Milk Expression and Storage").

Treatments for hepatitis C and breastfeeding. At this writing, there are no treatments for hepatitis C.

Other Hepatic Diseases

Not much is known about other types of hepatitis and breastfeeding.

Hepatitis D virus causes a "double" infection only in those already infected with hepatitis B. Hepatitis E is transmitted primarily via contaminated food and water and has a high mortality rate when contracted during pregnancy (Lawrence & Lawrence, 2005). Hepatitis G is associated mainly with blood transfusions.

Breastfeeding and other types of hepatitis. Not much is known about the transmission of hepatitis D, E, or G through human milk. Because hepatitis D occurs only with hepatitis B infections, preventing hepatitis B by giving the baby hepatitis-B vaccine and immune globulin also provides protection from hepatitis D, making the risk from breastfeeding negligible (Lawrence & Lawrence, 2005). There is no evidence of transmission of hepatitis E or G through breastfeeding or mother's milk.

Herpes Viruses

Chickenpox

Breastfeeding can continue in the mother with chickenpox unless she becomes infected within days of giving birth.

Chickenpox is a common childhood illness that is highly contagious and caused by the same herpes varicella-zoster virus that causes shingles (see later section). Complications are rarely an issue if a baby catches it more than 10 days after birth, but it can be fatal in an unborn baby, a very preterm baby, and a newborn who contracted it in utero (congenital chickenpox). Its symptoms are usually more severe in adults than in children.

Incubation period and symptoms. Chickenpox is spread by contact with the lesions, or sores, or through inhaling droplets in the air from coughing or sneezing. The incubation period of chickenpox is from 10 to 21 days, and an infected person will be contagious for about 7 days, beginning about 2 days before the lesions appear. Chickenpox is no longer contagious when there are no new eruptions for 72 hours and all lesions are crusted.

Chickenpox and the pregnant or breastfeeding mother. If a pregnant woman is exposed to chickenpox and doesn't know if she had it as a child (which confers life-long immunity), a blood test can determine her immune status. When a breastfeeding mother who may not be immune to chickenpox is exposed to it, the American Academy of Pediatrics Committee on Infectious Diseases suggests contacting her healthcare provider about getting the varicella vaccine (AAP, 2009a).

In the rare case a mother becomes infected with chickenpox within a week of giving birth and her baby is not born with the disease, this situation is handled differently in different places. In the U.S., separation of mother and baby is recommended until the mother is no longer contagious, as this illness can be severe in the newborn (McCarter-Spaulding, 2001). In other parts of the world, however, mothers and babies are kept together. The position statement of the Australasian Society for Infectious Diseases recommended that when a mother develops chickenpox within the week before or after giving birth, her newborn receive an injection of the varicella zoster immune globulin (VZIG) and they be isolated together, away from other mothers and babies. According to this organization, "a mother with chickenpox or zoster does not need to be isolated from her own baby" (Heuchan & Isaacs, 2001, p. 290).

If the mother and her healthcare provider decide separation from the baby is the better course, offer to share milk-expression strategies with her so that she can establish her milk production. Any milk expressed can be fed to her baby. A varicella-zoster immune globulin (VZIG) injection can be given to the baby to help prevent transmission and lessen the severity of the infection. When the mother is no longer contagious, she and her baby can be reunited and begin breastfeeding.

If siblings at home are infected, the mother can keep them away from the baby to minimize the chances of transmission. If the mother has immunity to chickenpox, the baby received antibodies in utero, and the risk of the newborn catching chickenpox is greatly reduced.

Treatments for chickenpox and breastfeeding. Other than treating the mother's symptoms, no other treatments for chickenpox are available at this writing.

Cytomegalovirus (CMV)

Most mothers are CMV-positive, and breastfeeding provides immunity to full-term, healthy babies.

Cytomegalovirus (CMV) is the most widespread of the herpes viruses that infect humans. By 40 years of age, between 50% and 80% of U.S. adults are infected with CMV for life (CDC, 2006).

Incubation period and symptoms. The incubation period for person-to-person transmission of CMV is unknown (AAP, 2009b). Few who become infected experience symptoms, which may include fatigue, fever, and swollen lymph glands.

CMV and the full-term breastfeeding baby. In an infected mother, the CMV virus can be found in her urine, tears, saliva, and in her milk (Schleiss, 2006), and during pregnancy, the baby is exposed to both the virus and its antibodies in utero. In full-term healthy babies, mother's milk acts like a vaccine, with more than two-thirds of the full-term babies of CMV-positive mothers testing positive for it, despite having no symptoms (Dworsky, Yow, Stagno, Pass, & Alford, 1983).

CMV and the preterm or compromised baby. If at birth both mother and baby are CMV-negative or CMV-positive, there is no concern about the very preterm or immune-compromised baby breastfeeding or being fed his mother's expressed milk. But when a baby born at less than 1500 g (3 lbs. 5 oz.) is CMV-negative and his mother is CMV-positive, there is a small risk he could become seriously ill from exposure to the CMV virus in his mother's milk (Schanler, 2005). Being born CMV-negative means the baby did not receive antibodies to the virus in utero. An immature or compromised immune system makes a baby more vulnerable to infections of all kinds (Bryant, Morley, Garland, & Curtis, 2002). For more details and ways mother's milk can be treated to decrease the risk of CMV transmission in at-risk babies, see p. 356- "Cytomegalovirus (CMV) and Other Maternal Illnesses."

Treatments for CMV and breastfeeding. Other than the antiviral drugs or symptom treatments used in immune-compromised people, no treatments for CMV currently exist.

Herpes Simplex Viruses 1 & 2 (Cold Sores and Genital Herpes)

Breastfeeding should not be affected as long as the newborn does not come in contact with the mother's herpes sores.

Herpes simplex virus 1 (cold sores) and 2 (genital herpes) are two different herpes viruses spread by contact with the sores.

Incubation period and symptoms. When transmitted after the newborn period, the incubation period for herpes simplex viruses is between 2 days and 2 weeks (AAP, 2009b). Symptoms include small, painful, fluid-filled, red-rimmed blisters that dry after a few days and form a scab. Genital herpes sores can be spread by touching the sores and then touching the breast.

Herpes simplex 1 and 2 and the breastfeeding newborn. Herpes infection can be very dangerous (even fatal) to a newborn up to 3 weeks of age (Sullivan-Bolyai, Hull, Wilson, & Corey, 1983). If a pregnant woman or her partner has recurrent herpes, she should talk to a healthcare provider knowledgeable about herpes and breastfeeding to decide what precautions to take. If a sore on the nipple or breast is suspected of being herpes, a culture can be done and the results should be available within a few days.

If a mother is waiting for the results of her culture or herpes on the breast has been confirmed, she can continue to breastfeed if the sores can be covered so that the baby can't touch them. If the sores are on the nipple, areola, or anywhere else the baby might touch while breastfeeding, the mother should express milk from that breast until the sores heal, while continuing to breastfeed on the unaffected breast. If the mother's hand or breast-pump parts touch the sores while expressing milk, they may contaminate her milk with the virus, and the milk should be discarded. If the mother's hand (if hand-expressing) or breast-pump parts do not touch the sores, the baby may be fed the milk.

Herpes simplex 1 and 2 and the older breastfeeding baby. Although herpes simplex 1 and 2 can be dangerous to a baby within the first month of life, cases have been reported of older babies touching their mother's herpes sores while breastfeeding without developing complications. There is also a documented case of a breastfeeding 15-month-old with a cold sore in his mouth who passed herpes to his mother's breast (Sealander & Kerr, 1989). Although an older baby is not likely to develop life-threatening complications from herpes, suggest the mother take steps to avoid spreading it to her child, as the sores can be very painful for a week or more and may make eating and drinking difficult (Newman & Pitman, 2006, p. 215).

Treatments for herpes simplex 1 and 2 and breastfeeding. Antiviral drugs can be used to treat these herpes viruses (AAP, 2009b). The topical antiviral penicilovir has been found to be undetectable in the milk after application, making it "extremely unlikely that detectable amounts would transfer into human milk or be absorbable by an infant" (Hale, 2008, p. 747). Two oral antiviral drugs, acyclovir and famciclovir, are rated L2 (safer) in *Medications and Mothers' Milk*. Another commonly used antiviral, valacyclovir is rated L1 (safest).

Shingles

When a breastfeeding mother contracts shingles, the baby can be immunized.

The same virus responsible for chickenpox—varicella zoster—also causes shingles. It occurs most commonly in an adult who had a mild case of chickenpox as a child and didn't become completely immune to the virus, which lays dormant until it is reactivated later in life.

Incubation period and symptoms. Because shingles is caused by a virus that lived in the body after a previous chickenpox infection, it has no incubation period. Several days before the shingles rash erupts, the mother may notice burning pain and sensitive skin. The rash starts as small blisters on a red base that continue to form for 3 to 5 days. They often appear as a band- or belt-like pattern on an area of skin and can be very painful. The blisters will pop, ooze, crust over, and heal. The shingles episode may last 3 to 4 weeks from beginning to end.

Shingles and the breastfeeding baby. If a mother contracts shingles while she is breastfeeding, suggest she ask her healthcare provider about having her baby receive a varicella zoster immune globulin vaccination as soon as possible, as it is most effective when given soon after exposure (Isaacs, 2000).

Treatments for singles and breastfeeding. Antiviral drugs may be given (AAP, 2009b). See the section "Herpes Simplex 1 and 2" on p. 741- Herpes Simplex Viruses 1 & 2 (Cold Sores and Genital Herpes) for details on antiviral drugs and breastfeeding.

HIV

Breastfeeding recommendations for HIV-positive mothers vary by area.

A worldwide pandemic of human immunodeficiency virus (HIV) has caused the deaths of millions from Acquired Immune Deficiency Syndrome (AIDS), which destroys parts of the immune system, leaving those affected unable to fight off illness. HIV is transmitted by the exchange of body fluids from mother to child during pregnancy and birth, and from sexual contact, sharing needles, blood transfusions, and many believe through breastfeeding.

Transmission of HIV through breastfeeding. A 1992 U.K. research review estimated the rate of mother-to-child transmission of HIV after about 18 months of breastfeeding to be 14% (Dunn, Newell, Ades, & Peckham, 1992). Although effective strategies for reducing transmission rates to 1% have been developed (see later section), the drugs used as part of these strategies are not yet universally available. Mothers and children worldwide continue to die from this disease.

Breastfeeding recommendations for HIV-positive women in developed areas. Even with a small risk of transmission, this virus is potentially fatal, so the American Academy of Pediatrics recommends HIV-positive mothers in developed areas with good sanitation and low rates of infection refrain from breastfeeding and donating their milk (AAP, 2009a). See the later section on treating mother's milk as an alternative to infant formula.

Current guidelines state that mothers with HIV in developed countries should avoid breastfeeding.

Breastfeeding recommendations for HIV-positive women in developing areas. In areas where sanitation is poor and risk of infection is high, it is recommended that HIV-positive women breastfeed (AAP, 2009a; WHO, 2007). According to recent findings (Kuhn, Sinkala, Thea, Kankasa, & Aldrovandi, 2009), HIV transmission by breastfeeding can be dramatically reduced to about 1% with the following strategies:

1. **Breastfeed exclusively.** HIV-transmission rates are lower among exclusively breastfed babies and higher among babies "mixed fed," or receiving other liquids or solid foods (Becquet et al., 2008; Coutsoudis et al., 2001; Coutsoudis, Pillay, Spooner, Kuhn, & Coovadia, 1999; Iliff et al., 2005; Kuhn et al., 2007). From birth to 3 months of age, the

percentage of babies infected with HIV was about the same among those exclusively breastfed and exclusively formula-fed.

2. **Give triple antiretroviral drugs to the mother during pregnancy and breastfeeding and extended antiretroviral drugs to the baby during breastfeeding.** In some areas, these treatments are readily available, but unfortunately, not yet everywhere.

HIV+ mothers in developing countries should exclusively breastfeed.

Previous recommendations to reduce HIV transmission by breastfeeding included exclusive formula-feeding or weaning from the breast by 6 months. But research found that when HIV-infected mothers in developing areas chose not to breastfeed or weaned early, infant deaths increased six-fold in Uganda (Kagaayi et al., 2008) and doubled in Botswana (Thior et al., 2006). A Zambian study that followed babies of HIV-positive mothers from the age of 4 to 24 months (Kuhn, Aldrovandi et al., 2009) found:

> ...[T]he risk of uninfected child mortality to 24 months was increased about three-fold if women stopped breastfeeding early compared with breastfeeding for 18 months or longer....In other words, the benefit of HIV prevented was canceled out by the harm of uninfected child deaths caused by infectious diseases....
>
> ...['N]o benefit' does not mean the same thing as 'no harm.' A key point is that both of these examples are in the absence of effective antiretroviral regimens. When we provide antiretroviral drugs... postnatal transmission is substantially reduced. Viewed in this context, the elevations in uninfected child mortality caused by abstinence from breastfeeding or caused by early weaning are no longer justified by HIV prevention efforts. The numbers of HIV infections prevented are now considerably less than the numbers of replacement feeding-related deaths caused. When antiretroviral drugs are provided, what was previously 'no benefit' now becomes harm. This is not because the antiretroviral drugs are harmful, but because in the delicate risk-benefit balance, mortality caused by abstinence from breastfeeding or shortening the duration of breastfeeding is now greater than the amount of HIV prevented (Kuhn, Sinkala et al., 2009, p. 7).

These authors emphasized the importance to child survival that all information given to parents and health workers in these areas recommend continued breastfeeding.

In parts of the world where breastfeeding (but not necessarily exclusive breastfeeding) is the norm, promoting exclusive breastfeeding among HIV-positive mothers has been found to be more socially acceptable than promoting formula-feeding (Adejuyigbe, Orji, Onayade, Makinde, & Anyabolu, 2008; Hofmann, De Allegri, Sarker, Sanon, & Bohler, 2009). In these areas, addressing deep-rooted cultural beliefs underlying the customs of supplementing breastfeeding with other foods has been highlighted as an important component of breastfeeding promotion efforts (Fjeld et al., 2008). Breastfeeding peer counseling and the encouragement from the baby's father to breastfeed have been found to increase rates of exclusive breastfeeding (Matovu, Kirunda, Rugamba-Kabagambe, Tumwesigye, & Nuwaha, 2008; Nankunda, Tylleskar, Ndeezi, Semiyaga, & Tumwine, 2010). Lactation counseling is also recommended in these areas to help prevent some of the breastfeeding problems (such as mastitis and nipple trauma) that have been associated with higher rates of HIV transmission (Kuhn, Sinkala et al., 2009).

Treating mother's milk to kill the HIV virus. Alternatives to formula-feeding for HIV-positive mothers include the use of donor human milk and heat-treating their own expressed milk to kill the HIV virus (McDougal et al., 1985; Pennypacker, Perelson, Nys, Nelson, & Sessler, 1995). Heating expressed milk by using Holder pasteurization (heating milk to 73ºC for 30 minutes) is one option. Another option is flash-heating (also known as hot water baths), which involves placing a jar of expressed milk in a 450 mL container (a water jacket) in a pan of water over heat until the water boils, which was found to leave the milk's vitamin content mostly intact (Israel-Ballard et al., 2008). With some education, both of these methods were found acceptable among HIV-positive families in Zimbabwe (Israel-Ballard et al., 2006). Another way of treating mother's milk that does not involve heat is adding a colorless, tasteless, inexpensive microbicide (microbe-killing) substance, such as alkyl sulfates, to expressed milk (Hartmann, Berlin, & Howett, 2006).

Treatments for HIV and breastfeeding. The antiretroviral drugs given to breastfeeding mothers are considered compatible with breastfeeding (Hale, 2008). Many of these drugs (such as nevirapine and zidovudine) are also given to breastfeeding babies and children to prevent HIV infection.

HTLV-I

HTLV-I, rare in the U.S. and Europe, can be transmitted by long-term breastfeeding and may cause adult leukemia in a small percentage of those affected.

Discovered in 1980, human T-cell leukemia virus type I (HTLV-I) is spread through contact with body fluids from blood transfusions, through sexual contact, from mother to child during pregnancy and birth, and through breastfeeding. It is rare in the U.S. and Europe (CDC, 1987; Machuca et al., 2000), with most cases occurring in the Caribbean, Africa, South America, and southwestern Japan, where 10% of those older than 40 in one city are carriers of HTLV-I (Hino et al., 1997).

Incubation period and symptoms. Much later in life, 1% to 5% of those infected with HTLV-I develop adult T-cell leukemia and lymphoma, a very malignant, usually fatal disease (Tajima, 1988). Other possible illnesses associated with HTLV-I infection include infective dermatitis of children, swelling of the eye (uveitis), and infection of the spinal cord (Manns, Hisada, & La Grenade, 1999). When HTLV-I infection occurs during infancy, the 1% to 5% who eventually develop adult leukemia do not develop symptoms until adulthood.

HTLV-I and the breastfeeding baby. Lactoferrin in mother's milk appears to enhance transmission of this virus from mother to baby (Moriuchi & Moriuchi, 2006). In one Japanese study, about 30% of exclusively breastfed babies born to HTLV-I positive mothers became infected, as compared with 10% of the mixed-fed babies, and none of those exclusively formula-fed (Hino, 1989). Another Japanese study found 39% of the breastfed babies became infected as compared with none of the formula-fed babies (Tsuji et al., 1990).

Impact of breastfeeding duration on HTLV-I transmission. Breastfeeding duration makes a profound difference in infection rates. One Japanese study found that children breastfed for at least 12 months had the highest infection rate (16%), while only 4% of the formula-fed children became infected during their first year (Hino et al., 1997). Babies' breastfed for less than 6 months, however, were no more likely to develop HTLV-I infections than those that were formula-fed (Takezaki et al., 1997). As an explanation, Japanese researchers suggested the antibodies to HTLV-I in mother's milk may protect their babies from HTLV-I infection during the first 6 months.

Other Japanese retrospective and prospective studies of HTLV-I seropositive women found a significant difference between seroconversion rates of short-term (less than 7 months) and long-term (7 months or more) breastfed infants of 3.8% and 25%, respectively (Oki et al., 1992; Wiktor et al., 1993). Again, the short-term breastfeeding seroconversion rate was nearly equal to that of artificially fed infants. The overall prevalence of anti-HTLV-I antibodies among children breastfed more than 3 months was significantly higher (28%) than that of those breastfed for less than 3 months (5%) (Hirata et al., 1992). These studies found that over time 13% of formula-fed children born to carrier mothers became infected with HTLV-I.

Factors that increase risk of mother-baby transmission. Other factors that increase risk of transmission from mother to baby during breastfeeding are higher blood levels of the HTLV-I virus in the mother, older mother, and longer duration of breastfeeding (Hirata et al., 1992; Oki et al., 1992; Takahashi et al., 1991; Wiktor et al., 1993). Transmission was also more likely when infected cells appeared in the mother's blood and/or milk (Ichimaru, Ikeda, Kinoshita, Hino, & Tsuji, 1991). When no infected cells were found in the mother's blood or milk, no babies became infected.

In developing countries, it is safer for mothers with HTLV-1 infections to breastfeed.

Breastfeeding recommendations. Because this virus is relatively rare, most mothers are not routinely tested for HTLV-1. When a mother in a developed country is diagnosed with this infection, some recommend against breastfeeding (AAP, 2009a; Ichimaru et al., 1991). However, in areas where babies not breastfed are at greater risk of life-threatening infection and disease, breastfeeding is a better option for the HTLV-I positive mother. In some developing countries, even shortening breastfeeding duration to 6 months may be a greater health risk to the baby than acquiring HTLV-I (Nyambi et al., 1996). Because the risk of adult onset leukemia from HTLV-I infection is relatively small (1% to 5% of those infected), each carrier mother should discuss the risks with her baby's healthcare provider in light of their specific situation.

Milk treatment options to prevent HTLV-I transmission. If the HTLV-I positive mother wants to avoid any risk of transmission but wants her baby to receive her milk, studies have found that the HTLV-I virus is killed when mother's milk is frozen to -20 degrees C (-4° F) and thawed (Ando, Kakimoto et al., 1989; Ando, Saito et al., 1989). If an HTLV-I positive mother decides to exclusively express and treat her milk with this freeze-and-thaw method, offer to discuss milk-expression strategies to establish and maintain her milk production (see p. 466- "Establishing Full Milk Production After Birth").

Treatments for HTLV-1 and breastfeeding. At this writing, there are no treatments for this infection, other than treatments for symptoms.

Measles

Unless during birth the mother is contagious with measles, breastfeeding is not usually affected.

Like chickenpox, measles is usually less severe in children than in newborns and adults. When a baby contracts measles in utero, this can be fatal (congenital measles). If the baby becomes infected with measles after birth (symptoms will not appear until the baby is at least 14 days old), his illness is likely to be mild because the baby received antibodies from the mother (Lawrence & Lawrence, 2005).

Incubation period and symptoms. Measles are usually spread by contact with infectious droplets or in the air. In a person infected with measles, the incubation period before symptoms appear is usually 8 to 12 days (AAP, 2009b). During the first 3 to 4 days of this illness, there is no rash, and the symptoms are similar to a bad cold: fever, watery eyes, congestion, and cough. Typically, the rash appears on about the 4th day. Measles are no longer contagious when the rash and cold symptoms are gone, about 72 hours after the rash appeared. If the mother catches measles after the newborn period, the baby can be given the measles immune globulin. If separation of mother and baby is recommended, the baby can be fed the mother's expressed milk, which contains protective antibodies.

Exposure to measles during pregnancy. If a pregnant woman exposed to measles is unsure whether she had the vaccine or the illness (which gives her life-long immunity), her healthcare provider can order a blood test to determine her immune status. When she gives birth without symptoms, both she and her baby can be given the measles immune globulin.

Measles at birth in the breastfeeding mother. Because most women received the measles vaccine as a child, this is a rare situation. But if the mother gives birth with an acute case of the measles and the baby is born without the disease, the baby's healthcare provider may recommend separating mother and newborn until the mother is no longer contagious. About half of newborns in this situation will develop the disease despite the separation. If they are separated, offer to discuss with the mother milk-expression strategies to provide milk for her baby and to establish her milk production (see p. 466- "Establishing Full Milk Production after Birth"). The antibodies in the mother's milk will help prevent her baby from becoming ill or lessen the severity of her baby's illness. When the mother is no longer contagious, she can be reunited with her baby and they can begin breastfeeding. If siblings at home are infected and the mother is immune, the mother can keep them away from the baby to minimize the chances of transmission. If the mother has immunity to measles, the baby will receive antibodies in utero, and the risk of the newborn catching measles from his siblings is greatly reduced.

Measles treatments and breastfeeding. Other than treating the mother's symptoms, there are no treatments for measles.

Rubella or German Measles

Breastfeeding is not affected when a mother receives the rubella vaccine or if she has an active case of rubella.

Rubella is a mild infectious disease. The biggest risk of rubella is catching it during pregnancy (congenital rubella), when it can damage the unborn baby. At any other time, it is likely to be short-lived and without complications.

Incubation period and symptoms. Rubella is transmitted through contact with nose or mouth secretions, and the incubation period is 16 to 18 days. Symptoms include a generalized rash, swollen lymph glands, and a slight fever. Between one-quarter and half of its cases have no symptoms at all. The person with rubella (other than congenital rubella) is contagious for 2 to 7 days after the rash appears.

Rubella, the rubella vaccine, and the breastfeeding mother and baby. The breastfeeding baby of a mother with an active case of rubella has already been exposed to it before her symptoms appeared. Breastfeeding provides the baby with antibodies, so if he does become ill, he will likely have a milder case. If the mother previously had rubella or received the rubella vaccine, her milk may provide her baby a natural immunization to rubella (Hale, 2008; Losonsky, Fishaut, Strussenberg, & Ogra, 1982a; Losonsky, Fishaut, Strussenberg, & Ogra, 1982b). According to the American Academy of Pediatrics Committee on Infectious Diseases:

> ...[T]he presence of rubella virus in human milk has not been associated with significant disease in infants and transmission is more likely to occur via other routes. Women with rubella or women who have been immunized recently with live-attenuated rubella virus vaccine need not refrain from breastfeeding (AAP, 2009a, p. 122).

West Nile Virus

Mothers with the West Nile Virus can continue breastfeeding.

West Nile Virus, which can become a serious illness, is most often transmitted by mosquitoes, making it most common during summer and fall. But it can also be spread by blood transfusions, transplants, and from mother to child during pregnancy. It is not spread through touch or kissing.

Incubation period and symptoms. Its incubation period is usually 2 to 6 days, but may extend to 14 days. Symptoms of West Nile Virus include fever, headache, and neck stiffness. If severe, it can lead to disorientation, coma, tremors, vision loss, and paralysis.

West Nile Virus and the breastfeeding mother and baby. Although West Nile Virus has been found in the milk of infected mothers, none of their breastfed babies became ill (CDC, 2009e). In one U.S. case report, soon after birth a woman received a blood transfusion later found to contain the West Nile Virus. The mother developed symptoms of West Nile Virus when her baby was 11 days old and breastfed him for 6 more days. Testing revealed the mother's milk and the baby's blood were both positive for the West Nile Virus, but the baby stayed healthy and developed no symptoms. The CDC concluded: "these findings do not suggest a change in breastfeeding recommendations" (CDC, 2002, p. 878).

CANCER

A mother with cancer can continue to breastfeed through most diagnostic tests and surgeries. But some treatments require weaning.

Cancer occurs when cells in the body grow out of control. There are many kinds of cancer, but they all start with out-of-control growth of abnormal cells. Instead of eventually dying, like normal cells, cancer cells continue to grow and form new, abnormal cells. Cancer cells may invade other tissues, which normal cells cannot do. If found early and treated quickly, many types of cancer can be completely cured. As the cancerous cells spread from the original tumor through the body, the chances for a cure decrease.

Diagnostic tests, biopsy, surgery, and the breastfeeding mother. For details on diagnostic tests and breast biopsy in the breastfeeding mother, see p. 699- "Breast Lumps." Before having surgery, suggest the mother discuss with her surgeon that she is breastfeeding and ask if medications will be used that are most compatible with breastfeeding. For more details, see the later section "Surgery."

Radioactive tests and treatments and the breastfeeding mother. If the mother's healthcare provider recommends the use of radioactive materials to diagnose or treat her illness, which is common for thyroid cancer and other thyroid problems, suggest she ask what specific materials will be used. Some radioactive materials accumulate in mother's milk and temporary or permanent weaning may be necessary. After some tests or treatments, breastfeeding (or even holding the baby) may expose him to radioactivity. The specific substance, its form, and the dose will determine whether breastfeeding can continue. If weaning is necessary, it will also determine if the weaning must be permanent. If the weaning is temporary, this information will determine the length of time before the baby can resume breastfeeding. For example, when a radioactive iodine uptake test is performed, breastfeeding must be interrupted for a minimum of 12 to 24 hours. Of the various radioactive substances, technetium-99m pertechnetate has the shortest half-life (6.02 hours) and requires the shortest interruption of breastfeeding. For a listing of radioactive substances, their half-lives, and recommended length of weaning after use in diagnosis or treatment, see http://neonatal.ttuhsc.edu/lact/radioactive.pdf.

Mothers being treated with radioactive iodine ^{131}I cannot breastfeed.

Radioactive iodine ^{131}I and breastfeeding. Although some substances can be used for diagnostic tests without interrupting breastfeeding, when radioactive iodine ^{131}I is used for a thyroid scan or tumor imaging, a weaning of a minimum of several months is necessary due to potentially harmful effects on both mother and baby (Hale, 2008). Iodine radiation can directly affect baby's thyroid gland and increase his risk of thyroid cancer later in life. The mother needs to completely wean at least several weeks before the treatment because research indicates that about 40% of the radiation dose will be deposited in active breast tissue, putting the mother at higher risk for later breast cancer (Grunwald, Palmedo, & Biersack, 1995; Robinson et al., 1994). Weaning several weeks in advance gives her breast tissue time to involute, or revert back to its pre-pregnancy state, so it is no longer active during the treatment. After this treatment, it may be months before the radioactivity in the milk returns to safe levels.

Questions to ask. If the mother's healthcare provider recommends the use of radioactive materials and she does not want to wean, suggest she tell her healthcare provider her feelings and find out if there are any options that allow for continued breastfeeding. Suggest the mother find the answers to the following questions:

- Is the radioactive procedure for diagnosis or treatment?
- What will happen if the procedure is not done or it is postponed?
- Is there an alternative that would not involve weaning?
- If her baby is younger than 12 months, can the procedure be delayed until the mother can express enough milk for her baby during the temporary weaning?
- Was a radioactive material chosen that will clear the mother's milk in the shortest time possible? For example, a radioisotope in complexed form excretes less radioactivity into mother's milk than its uncomplexed form.
- Is there a local testing facility available to determine when the mother's milk is clear of radioactivity? With milk testing, some mothers resumed breastfeeding sooner than estimated (Saenz, 2000).

- Will the radioactive material be concentrated in one organ (i.e., the thyroid), and if so, will she need to keep her baby away from that part of her body for a while?

If the mother is not satisfied with her healthcare provider's answers, suggest she consider seeking a second opinion. See also the appendix, "Working with Healthcare Professionals."

Milk expression after radioactive procedures. If the mother decides to have the radioactive testing and wean temporarily, offer to discuss strategies for maintaining her milk production while she has to "pump and dump." Unlike medications, in most cases, milk expression will help the mother eliminate the radioactivity from her body more quickly (Rose, Prescott, & Herman, 1990).

Chemotherapy and breastfeeding. In most cases, if chemotherapy is needed to treat a mother's cancer, she will need to wean, as the drugs involved are not compatible with breastfeeding (Lawrence & Lawrence, 2005). For details about specific drugs and how long they remain in her system, see the book *Medications and Mother's Milk* (Hale, 2008).

Radiation therapy and breastfeeding. Like diagnostic x-rays, cancer radiation therapy does not make mother's milk radioactive, and breastfeeding can continue. During treatment for breast cancer, the unradiated breast will not be affected. The treated breast, however, is likely to undergo some changes. Radiation therapy of the breast damages a woman's breast tissue, which may affect breast development and lactation during treatment and with subsequent pregnancies (Neifert, 1992). One U.S. case report described the effects of breast radiation as "ductal shrinkage, condensation of cytoplasm in cells lining the ducts, atrophy of the lobules, and perilobar and periductal fibrosis" (David, 1985, p. 1425).

Mothers can continue breastfeeding during radiation therapy.

Mothers who breastfed after breast cancer radiation therapy. Most women found that radiation affected milk production in the affected breast. In one U.S. study of 21 women with previously irradiated breasts who later became pregnant and breastfed, all of the women had little or no breast tissue growth during pregnancy (Moran et al., 2005). After birth 56% lactated in the irradiated breast, although 80% reported their milk production was significantly less on that side. In another U.S. study of 13 pregnancies, in the 10 women who breastfed, the treated breast produced milk in four cases and produced no milk in six cases (Higgins & Haffty, 1994). Like the previous study, all reported little or no breast changes in the irradiated breast during pregnancy. In a third U.S. study, 18 of the 43 women (34%) reported some milk production from the irradiated breast and 13 (24.5%) breastfed, with five (9%) describing their treated breast as smaller (Tralins, 1995). Two-thirds of the nine women who commented on milk production in the treated breast described it as "less but adequate." One of these babies refused to breastfeed from the treated breast.

Because mothers can fully breastfeed twins, triplets, and quadruplets (Berlin, 2007), with frequent breastfeeding a mother with one breast treated with radiation therapy will probably produce enough milk to exclusively breastfeed. If not or if both breasts were treated, partial breastfeeding is an option.

Recommendations to wean. If weaning is suggested and there are no compelling medical reasons to do so, see the first section "Breastfeeding with Health Issues." If the mother does not want to stop breastfeeding or feels that weaning would not make her life easier, suggest she talk with her healthcare provider about her feelings.

Breastfeeding after breast cancer. The woman with a history of breast cancer who becomes pregnant may have many concerns and anxieties about breastfeeding. One Australian qualitative study of 13 women in this situation identified common issues (Connell, Patterson, & Newman, 2006). They worried that breastfeeding might cause their breast cancer to recur. They were concerned because the denser breast tissue that occurs during breastfeeding would make their mammograms more difficult to read (see p. 699- "Breast Lumps"). The researchers concluded that women in this situation would benefit from information and reassurance.

CARDIAC ISSUES/HYPERTENSION

Breastfeeding has a positive effect on cardiovascular health, and many treatments for cardiac problems and hypertension are compatible with breastfeeding.

Breastfeeding and cardiovascular health. If a breastfeeding mother is suffering from hypertension or cardiovascular problems, she may want to know that breastfeeding has been found to decrease both systolic and diastolic blood pressure (Jonas et al., 2008). Blood pressure was found to fall during breastfeeding. During the first 6 months postpartum, mothers' pre-feeding blood pressures were also lower than they were prepregnancy. A Korean cohort study examined the records of 177,749 women between 20-59 and found breastfeeding to be protective again hypertension among premenopausal women (Lee, Kim, Jee, & Yang, 2005).

Breastfeeding lowers women's lifetime of heart disease.

Breastfeeding appears to have a positive overall effect on cardiovascular health. One U.S. prospective cohort study found that women with a lifetime total of 2 or more years of breastfeeding had a 23% lower risk of coronary heart disease than women who had never breastfed. One U.S. retrospective study examined data from 139,681 postmenopausal mothers (Schwarz et al., 2009). After controlling for age, number of children, race, education, body mass index (BMI), and many other factors, women who breastfed for more than 12 months total were less likely than women who had never breastfed to have hypertension (39% vs. 42%), diabetes (4% vs. 5%), and cardiovascular disease (9% vs. 10%). Exploring this dynamic further, a U.S. cross-sectional analysis of 297 mothers found that those who had not breastfed were more likely to have vascular changes, such as calcifications in the aorta or heart, that are associated with an increased risk of cardiovascular disease (Schwarz et al., 2010).

Treatments for cardiac disease and hypertension in the breastfeeding mother. Diuretics are often used to treat hypertension by increasing the volume of urine and keeping fluid levels in the body down. High-dose diuretics can decrease milk production, but some low-dose diuretics are compatible with breastfeeding. Some beta-blockers and other drugs used for cardiovascular treatment are also considered compatible with breastfeeding (Hale, 2008; Lawrence & Lawrence, 2005).

DEPRESSION AND MENTAL HEALTH

Postpartum Depression and Psychosis

More than half of new mothers have occasional bouts of crying, irritability, and fatigue sometimes referred to as the "baby blues." Postpartum depression refers to more consistent and severe symptoms and is also relatively common, with some estimating the incidence within the first year of new motherhood to be 12% to 25% overall and 35% or more among high-risk mothers (CDC, 2008; Kendall-Tackett, 2010).

Depression puts breastfeeding mothers at risk of early weaning and their babies at risk of physical, emotional, and social issues.

Symptoms of postpartum depression include feelings of sadness, an absence of pleasure from activities once enjoyed (known as anhedonia), sleep problems unrelated to baby care, inability to focus, feelings of hopelessness, changes in appetite, anxiety, and greater anger or hostility, including thoughts of death. A mother with these symptoms may be difficult to listen to and conversations with her may feel draining because her sense of hopelessness may convince her that nothing can help her. Before considering treatment for depression, a mother should see her heathcare provider to rule out physical causes for her symptoms, such as thyroid problems and anemia. Symptoms considered *red flags that the mother needs immediate medical attention* include (Kendall-Tackett, 2009):

- Suicidal or bizarre statements: "My children would be better off without me" or "I'd like to give them away to strangers."
- Substance abuse
- Days without sleep
- Fast weight loss
- Lack of normal grooming
- Inability to get out of bed

See also the next point on postpartum psychosis.

Causes and risk factors for postpartum depression. Inflammation has recently been identified as the risk factor for depression that underlies all its other risk factors (Kendall-Tackett, 2007a). When the other risk factors are present—sleep disturbance, stress (a fussy baby, a household move away from family and friends), physical pain, psychological trauma, or a history of abuse or trauma (a traumatic birth)—these can cause the release of cells from the immune system (called "proinflammatory cytokines") that cause physical inflammation and depression. This can go both ways, with the mother who has inflammation from the other risk factors at increased risk for depression and the mother who is depressed releasing more of these inflammatory cells, causing more inflammation.

Nipple pain is one type of physical pain research has linked to depression. One Australian study that followed 65 breastfeeding mothers found 38% of the mothers with nipple pain rated as depressed compared to only 14% of those without pain (Amir, Dennerstein, Garland, Fisher, & Farish, 1997). When the mothers' nipple pain resolved, the percentage of depressed mothers in the two groups became comparable, so helping mothers increase breastfeeding comfort can resolve some cases of postpartum depression.

The value of a listening ear. A mother with postpartum depression may feel embarrassed, ashamed, or guilty and try to minimize her problem. This can make her feel even more isolated. She may imagine all other mothers as blissfully happy and in control of their lives and believe that she is the only one with negative feelings. Offer emotional support and praise for caring for her baby in spite of her feelings. Let her know that negative feelings are normal. Suggest she attend mother-support groups, so she can hear about other mothers' down moments. Let her know about some of the factors that can influence her feelings (unusual stress, a difficult birth, little support). Offer to brainstorm with her about how she can get more rest or the strategies (below) that can help alleviate depression. Encourage her to accept help and support from others.

Postpartum depression and breastfeeding. Breastfeeding lowers stress and increases sleep (see the first point in this chapter), which decreases a mother's risk of depression. When breastfeeding is going well, it can decrease inflammation and increase a mother's feelings of well-being. Overall, breastfeeding has been found to protect mothers' mental health. Although breastfeeding mothers have a lower risk of postpartum depression (Hatton et al., 2005; McCoy, Beal, Shipman, Payton, & Watson, 2006), breastfeeding is not a guarantee against depression. Research has also found that when a breastfeeding mother becomes depressed, she is at increased risk of breastfeeding less often and weaning earlier (Akman et al., 2008; Dennis & McQueen, 2009; Field, Hernandez-Reif, & Feijo, 2002).

Breastfeeding lowers women's risk of depression and protects women's mental health.

A depressed mother may describe breastfeeding in negative terms. One Finnish study found differences in mother-baby interactions during feedings when the mother was depressed (Tamminen & Salmelin, 1991). As compared with a group of breastfeeding mothers who were not depressed, the depressed mothers interpreted their baby's fussiness when hungry as a rejection of them or their milk rather than due to a physical cause. The depressed mothers also expressed less satisfaction in their interactions with their babies and appeared less sensitive to their babies' needs and cues (see below). A depressed mother may begin to believe that breastfeeding is the cause of her problems. If so, let her know that caring for a newborn can be stressful, and the challenges of a fussy baby, fatigue, and feeling overwhelmed are not confined to breastfeeding mothers.

Why treatment for postpartum depression is vital to mothers and babies. Depression negatively affects women's health, well being, and their relationships (Hammen & Brennan, 2002). But a mother's depression also affects her baby physically, emotionally, and socially, and can impair the way she interacts with her baby. Knowing this may motivate a mother to seek treatment sooner. But be careful how this information is shared with mothers. It is important never to imply that her depression has somehow "damaged" her baby, for mothers worry about this. Emphasize instead that when a mother seeks treatment it benefits both her and her baby.

When depressed, most mothers interact with their babies using one of two styles: avoidant or angry-intrusive (Kendall-Tackett, 2010). When avoidant, mothers ignore many of their baby's cues. This behavior is associated with high infant blood cortisol levels (a stress hormone) and abnormal EEG patterns (Field, 1995). If the mother's depression is chronic, these abnormal brain patterns may extend throughout infancy (Cicchetti & Toth, 1998), and their toddlers may experience developmental delays (Cornish et al., 2005). Depressed mothers who are angry-intrusive also ignore their babies' cues, but rather than being non-responsive, they take over the interactions. For example, if the baby looks or arches away because he doesn't like what his mother is doing, she may interpret this as a personal rejection and become hostile or abusive.

Long-term studies on children whose mothers were depressed when they were infants found that by school age they are less socially competent (Luoma et al., 2001), have lower IQs (Hay et al., 2001), and are at greater risk for depression (Murray, Woolgar, Cooper, & Hipwell, 2001). But one Dutch study found that if depressed mothers were breastfeeding, their babies were protected from the harmful effects of their depression (Jones, McFall, & Diego, 2004). To explain their findings, the authors noted that depressed, breastfeeding mothers did not disengage from their babies, but looked at, touched, and stroked their babies more often than mothers who were depressed but bottle-feeding. This type of interaction can be taught to mothers, but it's built into the breastfeeding relationship and is another good reason for depressed mothers to continue breastfeeding if possible.

Non-pharmacological treatments for postpartum depression. Many mothers are reluctant to seek treatment for depression due to fears that they might have to choose between treatment and breastfeeding (Kendall-Tackett, 2010). Fortunately, that's not the case. Most anti-depressant medications are compatible with breastfeeding (see next section). For mothers reluctant to use medications, there are many non-medication strategies that can effectively treat depression. The most important point to emphasize is that depression needs to be treated rather than ignored. Examples of non-pharmacologic treatments include:

There are a number of non-drug treatments for depression.

- **Long-chain omega-3 fatty acids.** These can be taken alone or with antidepressants. A review of the literature by a committee of the American Psychiatric Association found that DHA and EPA, which are anti-inflammatories, appears to have a protective effect on mood disorders (Freeman, Hibbeln, Wisner, Davis et al., 2006). DHA and EPA are considered safe during pregnancy and breastfeeding, even at high doses (Freeman, Hibbeln, Wisner, Brumbach et al., 2006). **Recommendation:** For the treatment of depression, take daily doses of 1000 mg of EPA and 200-400 mg of DHA (Kendall-Tackett, 2009). See www.USP.org for recommended brands.
- **Exercise** also lowers inflammation and improves mood in postpartum mothers (Heh, Huang, Ho, Fu, & Wang, 2008). U.S. research compared the effects of a placebo, exercise, and anti-depressant medication (sertraline) in 202 people with major depression (Blumenthal et al., 2007). Unlike the placebo, exercise (40 minutes three times per week) was found to be as effective at resolving depression as antidepressants. **Recommendation:** 20 to 30 minutes of exercise 2-3 times per week for moderate depression and 45 to 60 minutes of exercise 3-5 times per week for major depression (Kendall-Tackett, 2009).
- **Psychotherapy** has also been found to have an anti-inflammatory effect (Kendall-Tackett, 2010). Cognitive behavioral therapy (see www.nacbt.org) has been found to be as effective as medications in treating depression, with a lower incidence of relapse (Rupke, Blecke, & Renfrow, 2006). Interpersonal therapy (see www.interpersonalpsychotherapy.org) is another type of "talk therapy" found effective in both preventing and treating postpartum depression in high-risk groups (Weissman, 2007).

- **St. John's Wort.** The most widely used herbal antidepressant is St. John's wort (*Hypericum perforatum*), native to the U.K. and used for this purpose since the Middle Ages. Several studies have compared its effectiveness to the antidepressants imipramine (Philipp, Kohnen, & Hiller, 1999; Woelk, 2000), sertraline (HDTSG, 2002; van Gurp, Meterissian, Haiek, McCusker, & Bellavance, 2002), and paroxetine (Anghelescu, Kohnen, Szegedi, Klement, & Kieser, 2006; Szegedi, Kohnen, Dienel, & Kieser, 2005) and found St. John's wort as effective as prescribed antidepressants with fewer side effects. **Recommendation:** Take 300 mg of St. John's wort three times per day, standardized to 0.3% hypericin and/or 2% to 4% hyperforin (Kendall-Tackett, 2009).

Most antidepressants are compatible with breastfeeding.

Antidepressants and breastfeeding. Although most antidepressant medications are considered compatible with breastfeeding (see Table 19.2), one Canadian review article found that even after mothers were told this, they were still reluctant to take these medications due to concerns about addiction, side effects, possible harm to their breastfeeding baby, and the perceived stigma of taking antidepressants (Dennis & Chung-Lee, 2006). Suggest the mother discuss her concerns with her healthcare provider, as depending on her symptoms, her risk factors, and her preferences, prescribed medications may or may not be the best choice for her. When deciding what drug to use, several factors are important (Chaudron, 2007):

- Has the mother used an antidepressant before that worked well for her?
- Does she find particular side effects especially concerning?
- Is she taking any other medication that might interact with the drug?

If her healthcare provider recommends against breastfeeding, see Appendix C, "Working with Healthcare Professionals."

In early 2010, a U.S. study was published that found an association in first-time mothers between taking serotonin-disrupting drugs, such as Prozac (fluoxetine) and other selective serotonin reuptake inhibitors (SSRIs) listed in Table 19.2, and a delay in milk increase after birth (Marshall et al., 2010). However, only 8 of its 431 mothers took SSRIs during the study. Other studies have not found this association (Kendall-Tackett & Hale, 2009a).

Table 19.2. Antidepressants, Antipsychotics, and Their Lactation Risk Categories

Medication	Rated L2 (Safer, studies exist, risk to baby is remote)	Rated L3 (Moderately safe, no controlled studies, weigh risks/benefits)
SSRIs		
Sertraline (Zoloft)	X	
Paoxetine (Paxil)	X	
Escitalopram (Lexapro)	X	
Fluoxetine (Prozac)	X	
Citalopram (Celexa)	X	
Venlaxine (Efexor)		X
Older Antidepressants		
Buproprion (Wellbutrin)		X
Tricyclic Antidepressants		
Amitriptyline (Elavil)	X	
Imiprmine (Tofranil)	X	
Nortriptyline (Pamelor)	X	
Antipsychotics		
Risperidone		X
Clozapine		X
Olanzapine	X	

Adapted from (Kendall-Tackett, 2009) and (Hale, 2008).

Postpartum psychosis usually strikes during the first month after birth and is relatively rare, occurring in only 0.1% to 0.2% of mothers (Rapkin, Mikacich, Moatakef-Imani, & Rasgon, 2002). But when it occurs, the mother needs immediate help because both she and her baby are at risk of serious harm. A mother with postpartum psychosis may have a distorted perception of reality, hallucinations, delusions, and/or suicidal or homicidal thoughts. Immediate treatment is needed.

A mother with postpartum psychosis needs immediate medical attention.

Hospitalization. A mother with postpartum psychosis or a severe case of postpartum depression may require hospitalization. In England and some other countries, hospitals have mother-baby units where women can be treated, while caring for their babies (Nicholls & Cox, 1999). This allows a mother to get the help she needs without separation from her baby. Giving a hospitalized mother the option of keeping her baby with her can boost her often-fragile self-esteem, while recognizing her baby's need for her and her adequacy as a mother. It also allows breastfeeding to continue without interruption. Suggest the mother and her healthcare provider look into this possibility.

Medications. Many of the antipsychotic medications used to treat postpartum psychosis are considered compatible with breastfeeding (see Table 19.2).

If weaning is necessary. When a mother is unable to care for her baby or her medication is incompatible with breastfeeding, weaning carefully should be considered part of the mother's treatment. Physical, hormonal, and emotional changes take place during weaning that can affect the mother's mental and emotional state. Abrupt weaning increases a mother's risk for pain and mastitis, which increase inflammation. Weaning may also be experienced as an emotional loss, because for most women, breastfeeding is a way of giving and receiving love and comfort, as well as a way to feed their baby. Breastfeeding may be one of the few positive actions only the mother can do for her baby during a difficult time. Losing breastfeeding may leave her feeling useless and incompetent, interchangeable with any other caregiver. When weaning is necessary, offer to discuss ways to wean gradually. (See p. 186- "Gradual Weaning"). If the baby must stop breastfeeding abruptly, discuss milk-expression strategies that will allow her to reduce her milk production gradually and comfortably.

Past Sexual Abuse, Assault, or Childhood Trauma

A history of sexual trauma and other types of child abuse are common among new mothers and may or may not lead to breastfeeding difficulties.

About 25% of mothers have a history of sexual abuse or assault. It may have happened within their families, or they may have been assaulted by peers. In either case, it can affect their birth, breastfeeding, and early mothering experiences (Felitti et al., 1998; Kendall-Tackett, 2010). Childhood abuse is only rarely limited to one type. The more types of abuse and trauma children experience, the greater their long-term effects (Felitti, 2009; Felitti et al., 1998). In the Survey of Mothers' Sleep and Fatigue, which included 6410 new mothers worldwide, the following types of childhood abuse and trauma were reported (Kendall-Tackett & Hale, in press):

- 34% were hit or slapped hard enough to leave a mark
- 32% reported parental substance abuse
- 25% experienced sexual trauma as a child, teen, or adult
- 16% reported that their parent (usually their mother) had been hit, bitten, or kicked
- 13% were raped as a teen or adult

Sexual abuse and other types of adverse childhood experiences can influence a mother's breastfeeding experience.

Unfortunately, survivors of sexual abuse and assault have higher rates of other types of abuse or trauma, which can affect both their physical and mental health (Dong, Anda, Dube, Giles, & Felitti, 2003). For more on trauma and health, see www.UppityScienceChick.com.

Breastfeeding in mothers with a history of abuse. Although some assume that new mothers who are abuse survivors will not want to breastfeed, this is not the case. Two studies found that significantly more abuse survivors expressed the intention to breastfeed and actually initiated breastfeeding compared with their non-abused counterparts (Benedict, 1994; Prentice, Lu, Lange, & Halfon, 2002).

Some aspects of breastfeeding may be challenging for abuse and trauma survivors. For example, some find skin-to-skin contact too overwhelming to cope with. Some hate the visceral sensation of their babies' mouth on their breasts. Some have post-traumatic flashbacks during birth and breastfeeding. One of the most common challenges, however, is increased risk of depression (see previous section). But this may not affect their desire to breastfeed. After the fact, some of these mothers say they never learned to like breastfeeding, but they learned to tolerate it, which they considered an important goal. For others, breastfeeding was a positive and healing experience. There is a large range of possible reactions to breastfeeding these mothers may have.

When problems occur, be flexible about breastfeeding options. If a mother is having difficulties with breastfeeding related to her past experiences, talk with her about what might be triggering her negative reactions. If the mother is not sure, ask her to keep a diary for a few days. It may be possible to pinpoint the problem and modify what she's doing to increase her comfort with breastfeeding. (Can she reduce the amount of skin-to-skin contact? Is the problem only at night?). In some cases, the mother may find partial breastfeeding a workable solution. To avoid the intimate contact of breastfeeding, some mothers may feel the need to express their milk and bottle-feed it to their babies. Being flexible about options is important, keeping in mind that some breastfeeding is always better than none.

Encourage mothers with symptoms to seek treatment. There are a number of effective treatments for past trauma, most of which are compatible with breastfeeding, including (Kendall-Tackett, 2007b; Kendall-Tackett & Hale, 2009b):

Treatment for trauma symptoms and PTSD is usually compatible with breastfeeding.

- **Education and peer counseling.** This can help mothers understand their experiences and their reactions to trauma. Mothers learn how to avoid triggering reactions to the event, how to reduce their stress responses, and how to get ongoing support. By understanding that reactions after traumatic events are predictable, they are less likely to blame themselves and more likely to follow through on treatment.
- **Trauma-focused psychotherapy.** The following effective treatments for trauma symptoms are compatible with breastfeeding.
  - *Cognitive-behavioral therapy.* Its overall focus is to help identify faulty ways of thinking that increase the risk of depression and challenge those beliefs with more accurate interpretations. For trauma survivors, it targets distortions in their perceptions of threats and helps to desensitize them to reminders of the event.
  - *Eye movement desensitization and reprocessing (EMDR).* This highly effective therapy is approved for treating post-traumatic stress disorder by the American Psychiatric Association. The mother is asked to focus on the image, negative thought, and body sensations, while simultaneously moving her eyes back and forth, following the therapist's fingers. Sometimes sound or tactile stimulation is used instead. It allows mothers to think about their traumatic experiences without having to talk about them. For an international list of certified practitioners, see www.emdr.com or the EMDR International Association at www.emdria.com.
- **Medications.** Two U.S. articles reviewed the medications recommended for trauma symptoms, including some SSRIs, SNRIs, SARIs, and atypical antipsychotics, many of which (as described in the previous section) are compatible with breastfeeding (Alderman, McCarthy, & Marwood, 2009; Friedman, Davidson, & Stein, 2009).

ENDOCRINE, METABOLIC, AND AUTOIMMUNE DISORDERS

A mother with a chronic illness may be advised not to breastfeed to make her life easier.

A chronic illness or disorder may develop slowly over a long period of time, or it may be a condition the mother had at birth. Although many mothers with these disorders breastfeed—some at about the same rate as healthy mothers—keep in mind that the mother may be advised by healthcare providers or family not to breastfeed. Family or friends may tell her they want to help with the new baby to ease her fatigue or stress. This type of offer is usually made out of concern for the mother's well-being. But allowing others to take over her baby's care can undermine the mother's self-confidence and her relationship with her baby. For research on some of the many reasons breastfeeding may benefit the mother with a health issue, see the first point in this chapter.

Mothers with chronic illnesses often breastfeed at similar rates to healthy mothers.

Most of these mothers will have many of the same questions and concerns as healthy mothers. If the mother has questions about how her condition will affect breastfeeding, see the appropriate section. Keep in mind that most mothers are well-educated about their health issues, so if needed, feel free to ask her questions about her illness or limitations. For more details about a mother's illness, also check the informational websites available from the many national and international organizations that support those with chronic illnesses.

Cystic Fibrosis

Women with cystic fibrosis can breastfeed while carefully monitoring their diet and weight.

Cystic fibrosis is a genetic disease that causes the secretion of a thick, gluey mucus that clogs the bronchial tubes, interfering with breathing, and blocks digestive enzymes from leaving the pancreas, causing incomplete digestion. There are more than 1,000 mutations of the gene that causes cystic fibrosis, which means the mother may have a mild or severe form. Some cases of cystic fibrosis are so mild they can be detected only through laboratory tests, while some are serious enough to be life-threatening. Among pregnant mothers with cystic fibrosis, 25% deliver preterm (Gilljam et al., 2000).

Mothers with cystic fibrosis produce normal milk. According to several studies and case reports, mothers with cystic fibrosis with full milk production produce milk of normal composition and their babies grow normally (Kent & Farquharson, 1993; Michel & Mueller, 1994; Shiffman, Seale, Flux, Rennert, & Swender, 1989; Welch, Phelps, & Osher, 1981). An early case report found that one mother with cystic fibrosis produced milk with high sodium levels, but this mother was not breastfeeding and had expressed her milk only for research purposes (Alpert & Cormier, 1983). Milk sodium levels are usually elevated as milk production stops and the mother's breasts involute.

The mother's weight and nutrition. If a mother with cystic fibrosis has issues with incomplete digestion of food (called "pancreatic insufficiency" or "PI"), the nutrients in her food may not be well-absorbed and she may find it challenging to maintain a healthy weight. A mother like this is probably taking digestive enzymes to help break down her food more completely and may also be taking vitamin and mineral supplements. If so, this mother needs to carefully monitor her weight and nutritional needs while pregnant and breastfeeding (Edenborough et al., 2008). As long as she can maintain a healthy weight, breastfeeding can continue (Riordan, 2010).

Cystic fibrosis and the breastfeeding baby. As a genetic disease, a baby cannot "catch" cystic fibrosis by breastfeeding. In fact, babies born with cystic fibrosis who do not breastfeed have been found to have poorer health outcomes and earlier and more severe symptoms (Colombo et al., 2007; Parker, O'Sullivan, Shea, Regan, & Freedman, 2004). Also, mother's milk provides the baby with protection from the bacterial infections, such as *Staphylococcus aureus* and *Pseudomonas*, many mothers with cystic fibrosis regularly battle. For details about breastfeeding the baby with cystic fibrosis, see p. 301- "Cystic Fibrosis."

Treatments for cystic fibrosis and breastfeeding. Some mothers with cystic fibrosis decide not to breastfeed because they are concerned their medications may negatively affect their baby, but most drugs prescribed for these mothers are compatible with breastfeeding (Gilljam et al., 2000). One Italian case report documented a severe *Pseudomonas* lung infection in a breastfeeding mother with cystic fibrosis, which was treated with the IV antibiotic tobramycin (Festini et al., 2006). This medication was undetectable in her milk.

Diabetes Mellitus

Type-1 (Insulin-Dependent) Diabetes Mellitus

In the mother with Type-1 diabetes, milk increase after birth may be delayed a day or two, but formula-feeding is associated with more negative health outcomes.

Type-1 diabetes is also known as insulin-dependent diabetes mellitus (or IDDM). Only 5% to 10% of diabetics have this form of the disease. It occurs when the insulin-producing beta cells in the pancreas are destroyed, leaving the body unable to produce insulin, a hormone needed to convert sugar, starches, and other foods into fuel for the body. Without insulin, blood sugar can rise to dangerous levels and cause health complications. Mothers with Type-1 diabetes need to check their blood-sugar levels and receive daily insulin replacement therapy via injections or subcutaneous pump, so their blood sugar doesn't become dangerously high. Like other autoimmune disorders, Type-1 diabetes is thought to be caused by a combination of genetics and environmental triggers, such as viral infections (Tenconi et al., 2007), obesity (Viner, Hindmarsh, Taylor, & Cole, 2008), and early introduction of cereal or cow's milk (Skrodeniene et al., 2008).

Breastfeeding protects babies of diabetic mothers from developing diabetes.

Type-1 diabetes and the breastfeeding baby. Type-1 diabetes is not transmitted by breastfeeding. In fact, breastfeeding appears to be protective, reducing the baby's risk of developing Type-1 diabetes. Studies done worldwide have found longer duration of breastfeeding associated with lower incidence of Type-1 diabetes later in life (Holmberg, Wahlberg, Vaarala, & Ludvigsson, 2007; Karavanaki et al., 2008; Rosenbauer, Herzig, & Giani, 2008).

Type-1 diabetes and the early days after birth. Keeping the mother's blood sugar levels within a healthy range is vital to pregnancy outcomes and newborn health. When a mother has Type-1 diabetes, it increases her baby's risk of preterm birth, respiratory distress syndrome, heavier-than-average birthweight, exaggerated newborn jaundice, and low blood sugar (Cordero, Treuer, Landon, & Gabbe, 1998; Sirota, Ferrera, Lerer, & Dulitzky, 1992). One U.S. study found that 47% of these babies spent time after birth separated from their mothers in the special care nursery, which can delay and disrupt early breastfeeding. If possible, suggest the mother try to make arrangements before birth to minimize their separation and encourage early and frequent breastfeeding. (See p. 257- "Hypoglycemia" for details on its effects on a newborn's blood sugar.) One U.S. author suggested diabetic mothers plan to breastfeed within the first hour after birth and at least every hour for the first several hours until the baby's blood sugar stabilizes (Walker, 2006). After birth, diabetic mothers often experience major shifts in blood sugar levels, which also need to be closely monitored to help them quickly reestablish good control (Murtaugh, Ferris, Capacchione, & Reece, 1998).

Diabetes may delay lactogenesis-II.

Milk increase after birth can be delayed when early breastfeeding is postponed or limited, but Type-1 diabetes also has been found to delay milk increase after birth by a day or two (Hartmann & Cregan, 2001; Pang & Hartmann, 2007). If a mother has good blood-sugar control, she may be less likely to experience this delay (Neubauer et al., 1993). Because early exposure to cow's milk may be one of the environmental triggers of Type-1 diabetes (Perez-Bravo et al., 1996; Rosenbauer et al., 2008), if her milk production is delayed and her baby needs to be supplemented, she may want to avoid using cow's-milk-based infant formula. Alternatives include the mother's own colostrum expressed and stored during pregnancy (see p. 446- "Why Express Milk?"), donor human milk, or hypoallergenic infant formula (Greer, Sicherer, & Burks, 2008).

Breastfeeding increases insulin sensitivity, decreasing insulin needed. Breastfeeding has a healthy and long-term effect on a mother's insulin response (Diniz & Da Costa, 2004), increasing her insulin sensitivity (Butte, Hopkinson, Mehta, Moon, & Smith, 1999; McManus, Cunningham, Watson, Harker, & Finegood, 2001). Making milk "primes" a mother's metabolism, increasing its energy efficiency and reducing the amount of insulin needed by mothers with Type-1 diabetes by between 27% (Davies, Clark, Dalton, & Edwards, 1989) and 50% (Asselin & Lawrence, 1987; Riviello, Mello, & Jovanovic, 2009). So while she is exclusively breastfeeding, the mother should expect to need less insulin than she did before. Suggest the mother plan to have a snack each time she breastfeeds that includes protein and carbohydrates, as blood sugar often dips about an hour later (Walker, 2006). When the time comes for weaning, suggest it be done as gradually as possible to make maintaining blood-sugar control easier.

Long-term breastfeeding. When a mother's blood sugar is in good control, long-term milk production does not seem to be a problem. Similar rates of long-term breastfeeding were found in mothers with and without Type-1 diabetes in studies from Australia (Webster, Moore, & McMullan, 1995), the U.S. (Ferris et al., 1993), and Denmark (Stage, Norgard, Damm, & Mathiesen, 2006). However, since the mother with Type-1 diabetes is at greater risk of bacterial and fungal infections of all kinds, including mastitis and candida (thrush), suggest she learn how to prevent them, as well as recognize their signs and symptoms, so if needed, she can seek treatment immediately.

Treatments for Type-1 diabetes and breastfeeding. The insulin replacement needed daily by the mother with Type-1 diabetes does not affect her breastfeeding baby. Insulin molecules are too large to pass into her milk, but even if they did, they would be broken down in the baby's gut (Hale, 2008).

Type-2 (Non-Insulin Dependent) Diabetes Mellitus

Breastfeeding improves insulin sensitivity in the mother with Type-2 diabetes, which can reduce the severity of her illness.

Type-2 diabetes, also known as non-insulin dependent diabetes mellitus (NIDDM), accounts for about 90% of the diabetes cases. When a mother has Type-2 diabetes, either she does not produce enough insulin or her body's insulin receptors do not respond normally to it, known as insulin resistance. When sugar builds up in the blood instead being used as fuel by cells, this causes a variety of health complications that can affect the eyes, skin, feet, heart, and other systems. Type-2 diabetes is one part of the recently identified metabolic syndrome (which includes obesity, high cholesterol, and high blood pressure) that increases the risk of cardiovascular disease (Huang, 2009; Reaven, 2007).

Type-2 diabetes and the breastfeeding baby. Breastfed babies have a reduced risk of Type-2 diabetes and have lower blood sugar levels later in life, according to a U.K. review of 23 studies (Owen, Martin, Whincup, Smith, & Cook, 2006). However, like the babies of mothers with Type-1 diabetes, at birth these babies are at greater risk for hypoglycemia, or low blood sugar. Suggest the mother plan to breastfeed within the first hour and at least every hour thereafter until the baby's blood sugar is stable. One New Zealand study found that the main determinant of whether mothers with Type-2 diabetes were breastfeeding at hospital discharge was whether their baby's first feeding was at the breast or formula (Simmons, Conroy, & Thompson, 2005). Only 19% of those mothers whose babies received formula as their first feeding were breastfeeding at discharge compared with 78% whose first feeding was at the breast.

Type-2 diabetes and the breastfeeding mother. Lactation increases a woman's insulin sensitivity (Butte et al., 1999; McManus et al., 2001), which reduces the severity of Type-2 diabetes. One U.S. cohort study of 121,700 women found that longer duration of breastfeeding was associated with reduced incidence of Type-2 diabetes (Stuebe, Rich-Edwards, Willett, Manson, & Michels, 2005). For each additional year of breastfeeding, the study mothers had a decreased risk of contracting Type-2 diabetes over the next 15 years of 14% to 15%. Another U.K. review of 23 studies estimated that breastfeeding is associated with a 15% to 56% reduction in the risk for Type-2 diabetes (Owen et al., 2006). A U.S. cross-sectional cohort analysis of 1,620 women found that later in life duration of lactation was also associated with a lower prevalence of metabolic syndrome, of which Type-2 diabetes is a part (Ram et al., 2008). Breastfeeding was associated with better measures on all aspects of metabolic syndrome, including blood pressure, abdominal obesity, fasting glucose, cholesterol, and triglycerides. Not only does lactation increase a woman's insulin sensitivity while she is breastfeeding, it appears to positively program her metabolism for years afterwards. As one U.S. researcher wrote: "Lactation may prime the metabolic system by making it a more energy-efficient machine…." (Ram et al., 2008, p. 268).

Breastfeeding decreases insulin resistance.

Treatments for Type-2 diabetes and breastfeeding. During pregnancy, many mothers with Type-2 diabetes receive insulin to keep blood-sugar levels in the normal range. After birth, if needed, insulin may be continued (see the "Treatments" section in Type-1 diabetes) or hypoglycemic medications may be prescribed, along with diet and exercise. (Hale, 2008). A Canadian research review concluded that several hypoglycemic drugs commonly used to treat Type-2 diabetes, metformin (Glucophage), glyburide (Micronase), and glipizide (Melizide), were all compatible with breastfeeding (Feig, Briggs, & Koren, 2007).

Gestational Diabetes Mellitus

Mothers with gestational diabetes who do not breastfeed are twice as likely to develop other types of diabetes as those who breastfeed.

Gestational diabetes is a glucose intolerance that occurs in 4% of pregnancies. About 50% of the women who develop gestational diabetes will later develop one of the other types of diabetes (Hale & Berens, 2002).

Gestational diabetes and the breastfeeding mother. In these mothers, breastfeeding has been found to prevent or delay the development of other types of diabetes, no doubt due to increasing insulin sensitivity (see previous sections). One U.S. study of 809 women with gestational diabetes found that those doing any amount of breastfeeding between 4 and 12 weeks postpartum had significantly better glucose metabolism than those who were not breastfeeding (Kjos, Henry, Lee, Buchanan, & Mishell, 1993). The researchers found a "two-fold reduction in the development of diabetes mellitus in the lactating group compared to the nonlactating group…" (Kjos et al., 1993, p. 454).

Gestational diabetes and the breastfeeding baby. Like the babies of mothers with other types of diabetes, these babies are more likely to be admitted to the special-care nursery after birth (Cordero et al., 1998), so suggest the mother let her healthcare providers know that she will be breastfeeding and would like to minimize separation after birth. Suggest the mother plan to breastfeed within the first hour and at least every hour thereafter until the baby's blood sugar is stable.

Treatments for gestational diabetes and breastfeeding. See "Treatments" for the previously described types of diabetes for details on common diabetic treatments.

Galactosemia and PKU

Babies with galactosemia and PKU should not exclusively breastfeed, but mothers with these metabolic disorders can breastfeed their babies.

Individuals with galactosemia and phenylketonuria (PKU) are born unable to completely metabolize specific components of human milk. In the case of galactosemia, babies with this condition cannot metabolize galactose, a milk sugar, and its accumulation in their system causes severe health problems. With PKU, the essential amino acid phenylalanine is not well metabolized, also causing severe health issues unless diet is modified. As these babies grow, diet remains a life-long issue. For their entire lives, affected individuals must monitor their diets carefully to avoid dangerously high blood levels of these substances. In those with PKU, for example, too high levels of blood phenylalanine can lead to mental retardation. (See the sections on these metabolic disorders in the chapter "Health Issues—Baby" for details on how breastfeeding is affected in babies with these genetic disorders.)

When a girl with galactosemia or PKU reaches childbearing age, she can become pregnant and breastfeed. In pregnant mothers with PKU, careful dietary control of their blood levels of phenylalanine is critical, as too-high blood levels put them at greater risk of having a baby with birth defects similar to fetal alcohol syndrome (Matalon, Michals, & Gleason, 1986). During breastfeeding, the milk of these mothers is normal (Forbes, Barton, Nicholas, & Cook, 1988; Purnell, 2001). One U.S. case report documented identical twin mothers with PKU who breastfed their babies (Fox-Bacon, McCamman, Therou, Moore, & Kipp, 1997). After birth, the researchers found no association between the mothers' phenyalanine blood and milk levels. One Swedish mother with galactosemia breastfed two healthy babies, one for 8 months, with measures of her disorder staying within normal treatment levels (Ohlsson, Nasiell, & von Dobeln, 2007).

Gestational Ovarian Theca Lutein Cysts

After birth, mothers with gestational theca lutein cysts may have inhibited milk production, but most can eventually produce ample milk.

Gestational ovarian theca lutein cysts are benign cysts that develop on a woman's ovaries during pregnancy. They are more common among women who have undergone fertility treatments, but can also occur during a naturally-occurring pregnancy (Montz, Schlaerth, & Morrow, 1988). These cysts produce testosterone, sometimes at levels 10 to 150 times higher than normal. When testosterone levels are very high, body or facial hair may develop and the woman's voice may become deeper. If testosterone levels are elevated to more moderate levels, there may be no obvious symptoms, and a mother and her healthcare provider may be unaware she has this condition.

After birth, these cysts disappear without treatment, and within several weeks, a mother's testosterone levels return to normal. But during the first weeks after birth, her higher-than-normal testosterone levels may inhibit milk production. If a blood test reveals high testosterone levels (a "high normal" level is 67-70 ng/dL), an ultrasound can confirm the presence of the cysts. Some mothers with gestational ovarian theca lutein cysts have had blood testosterone levels as high as 711 ng/dL (Hoover, Barbalinardo, & Platia, 2002).

In one U.S. article, two mothers' experiences of breastfeeding with gestational ovarian theca lutein cysts were reported (Hoover et al., 2002). After birth, despite their lack of milk, both kept stimulating their breasts eight or more times per day either by breastfeeding (with an at-breast supplementer) or with a breast pump. When these mothers' testosterone blood level fell below 300 ng/dL, their milk finally "came in," one at 20 days postpartum and the other at 12 days postpartum. Another U.S. article reported two other mothers' experiences (Betzold, Hoover, & Snyder, 2004). With regular breast stimulation, these mothers achieved increased milk production, one at 10 days and the other at 31 days. One of these four mothers did not achieve full milk production, but the other three did.

Multiple Sclerosis

Exclusive breastfeeding appears to delay the postpartum recurrence of symptoms in a mother with multiple sclerosis.

Multiple sclerosis (or MS) is a chronic, often disabling disease that attacks the central nervous system. Symptoms may be mild, such as numbness in the limbs, or severe, such as paralysis or loss of vision. The development, severity, and symptoms of MS vary from person to person. Although the cause of MS is not yet known, it is thought by most to be a type of autoimmune disorder because the body's own defenses attack the fatty substance called myelin that surrounds and protects the nerves in the central nervous system. It may also damage the nerve fibers, which forms scar tissue (sclerosis) that gives the disease its name. When any part of the myelin sheath or nerve fiber is damaged or destroyed, nerve impulses traveling to and from the brain and spinal cord are distorted or interrupted, producing the variety of symptoms that can occur, such as numbness, fatigue, trouble walking, vision problems, pain, vertigo, and even paralysis.

In mild cases, the woman may completely recover after her symptoms have passed and have long periods of remission. In severe cases, her symptoms may become progressively worse and not subside, or she may have repeated relapses that leave her permanently and increasingly disabled.

Multiple sclerosis and the breastfeeding baby. Many mothers with chronic illnesses worry that breastfeeding will transmit their disease to their baby, but in this case, the opposite appears to be true. Multiple sclerosis cannot be transmitted by breastfeeding, and one Italian study found lower rates of multiple sclerosis among people breastfed for more than 6 months compared with those breastfed less than 6 months or never breastfed (Pisacane et al., 1994). The researchers suggested two possible reasons for this difference:

- Breastfeeding strengthens the immune system
- Possible differences in brain composition from differences in fatty acids in infant formula compared to human milk

Multiple sclerosis and the breastfeeding mother. During pregnancy, many women with multiple sclerosis enjoy a remission in their MS symptoms, especially during the third trimester (Vukusic & Confavreux, 2006). However, the first 3 months postpartum typically brings a significant increase in symptoms. Some of the early research from the U.S. and Ireland found no real difference in incidence of MS symptoms during the first months postpartum in breastfeeding and non-breastfeeding mothers (Confavreux, Hutchinson, Hours, Cortinovis-Tourniaire, & Moreau, 1998; Nelson, Franklin, & Jones, 1988). But these studies did not distinguish between exclusive and partial breastfeeding.

Breastfeeding may cause a remission of MS symptoms.

Studies that controlled for amount of breastfeeding found a significant difference. One U.S. study of 140 women with MS found that the lower the percentage of feedings at the breast, the more likely the mother was to suffer a relapse of MS symptoms (Gulick & Halper, 2002). A more recent U.S. prospective cohort study of 61 women (32 with MS) found a five-fold increase in relapse during the first year postpartum among mothers who breastfed partially or not at all compared with those who exclusively breastfed for the first 2 months (Langer-Gould et al., 2009). The researchers suggested one reason may have been the longer delay in the return of the mothers' menses in those exclusively breastfeeding. (For more details, see the chapter, "Sexuality, Fertility, and Contraception."). The difference in relapse rate was not related to the severity of illness, and the mothers' perception of their disease's severity was not related to their decision about breastfeeding.

Treatments for MS and breastfeeding. Most medications used as MS treatments are considered compatible with breastfeeding (Hale, 2008), such as interferon beta 1a (Avonex), rated L2 (safer) in *Medications and Mothers' Milk*, and interferon beta 1b (Betaseron), rated L3 (moderately safe). There are some exceptions, such as mixtoxantone (Novantrone), which is rated L5 (contraindicated). Those not familiar with the effect of breastfeeding in preventing postpartum relapse of MS symptoms may recommend mothers not breastfed in order to resume their medication more quickly after birth (Dwosh, Guimond, & Sadovnick, 2003). However, in most cases, mothers with MS can take their medications and breastfeed.

Polycystic Ovary Syndrome (PCOS)

Some women with PCOS produce overabundant milk, some have no milk production issues, and some have low milk production.

Polycystic ovary syndrome (PCOS) is not a disease but a syndrome (a constellation of symptoms) that is still poorly understood. It affects up to 15% of women and is one of the leading causes of infertility. Common symptoms of PCOS include:

- High levels of estrogen and androgens (testosterone and other male hormones), which can cause severe acne, skin discoloration, and excess hair growth
- High insulin levels, which contributes to the obesity that affects about

half of the women with PCOS

- Multiple ovarian cysts
- Menstrual abnormalities, which usually begin in adolescence and contribute to infertility

Many women with PCOS also develop Type-2 diabetes during their childbearing years. Insulin resistance (insulin receptors not responding normally to insulin in the body) appears to be a pivotal issue, as when insulin resistance is treated, it resolves many other PCOS symptoms (Glueck, Salehi, Aregawi, Sieve, & Wang, 2007).

PCOS and the breastfeeding mother. Because the hormonal disruptions in mothers with PCOS vary in type and degree, the effect of PCOS on breastfeeding is not consistent. Some women with PCOS produce overabundant milk, others have low milk production, and still others produce milk in the normal range. One Swedish radiological study that examined breast tissue in women with PCOS found that some had hypoplastic breasts, made mostly of fat with few milk-making glands (Balcar, Silinkova-Malkova, & Matys, 1972). A Brazilian study also found breast tissue abnormalities in women with PCOS (Fonseca, de Souza, Bagnoli, Celestino, & Salvatore, 1985). One U.S. article described the breastfeeding experiences of three women with PCOS, all of whom produced little milk despite expert help and the use of many usually effective strategies to increase milk production (Marasco, Marmet, & Shell, 2000). Insulin is known to affect breast growth and development during pregnancy and to play an important role in increasing milk production after birth (Czank, Henderson, Kent, Tat Lai, & Hartmann, 2007; Neville, McFadden, & Forsyth, 2002). When a mother's body does not respond normally to insulin, this has the potential to affect milk production.

The impact of PCOS on breastfeeding varies from woman to woman.

But not all women with PCOS have issues with breast function and milk production. A Norwegian study of 36 women with PCOS and 99 controls found that mothers with PCOS had a slightly reduced early breastfeeding rate, 75% vs. 89% among the control mothers, meaning three-quarters of the mothers with PCOS exclusively breastfed their babies (Vanky, Isaksen, Moen, & Carlsen, 2008). Another more recent Norwegian study found an association between the high androgen levels in many women with PCOS and reduced breastfeeding duration (Carlsen, Jacobsen, & Vanky, 2010). It is possible that higher levels of testosterone and other androgens during pregnancy may affect breast development. As with other breastfeeding red flags, when a mother has PCOS, this means she and her baby should be carefully monitored after birth without undermining her confidence in breastfeeding.

Treatments for PCOS and breastfeeding. A common treatment for PCOS, the hypoglycemic medication metformin, decreases the hormonal disruptions in some mothers, even those without insulin resistance (Baillargeon, Jakubowicz, Iuorno, Jakubowicz, & Nestler, 2004). This drug has helped some women overcome infertility, and during pregnancy, metformin has been found to reduce the incidence of miscarriages, gestational diabetes, hypertension, and preterm birth (Glueck, Wang, Goldenberg, & Sieve, 2004). Metformin is rated an L1 (safest) in *Medications and Mothers' Milk*, as several U.S. studies have found that little transfers into mother's milk (Hale, Kristensen, Hackett, Kohan, & Ilett, 2002), and when taken by mothers during pregnancy and breastfeeding, their babies grew normally and had no adverse effects (Glueck, Salehi, Sieve, & Wang, 2006). Some report that treatment with metformin through pregnancy and lactation has helped normalize milk production in some mothers with PCOS (Gabbay & Kelly, 2003). Doses start at about 500 mg per day and increase up to 1,000 to 2,500 mg per day (Glueck et al., 2006; West & Marasco, 2009).

Rheumatoid Arthritis and Systemic Lupus Erythematosus (Lupus)

Many breastfeeding mothers with rheumatoid arthritis and lupus have physical challenges and medication concerns.

Both rheumatoid arthritis and systemic lupus erythematosus (the most common type of lupus) are autoimmune disorders caused by the immune system attacking body tissues with unusual antibodies known as "autoantibodies." Autoimmune disorders are more common in women than men, with rheumatoid arthritis occurring in 2.5 women for every one man and lupus occurring in 10 women for every one man. These disorders often occur in periods of flares and remissions. During the flares, women may experience joint swelling, pain, fatigue, and fever. In women with lupus, neurological problems can occur and organ function may be affected. In severe cases, organ failure can occur.

Rheumatoid arthritis, lupus, and the breastfeeding baby. The baby cannot "catch" rheumatoid arthritis or lupus through breastfeeding. In fact, Swedish and U.S. research indicate that breastfed babies are less likely to contract these autoimmune disorders than babies not breastfed (Jacobsson, Jacobsson, Askling, & Knowler, 2003; Simard et al., 2008).

Rheumatoid arthritis, lupus, and the breastfeeding mother. Breastfeeding also appears to protect mothers from developing these autoimmune disorders, with longer-term breastfeeding providing greater protection than shorter-term breastfeeding (Costenbader, Feskanich, Stampfer, & Karlson, 2007; Karlson, Mandl, Hankinson, & Grodstein, 2004; Pikwer et al., 2009).

Mothers with RA or SLE may experience a relapse of their symptoms during breastfeeding.

Many mothers with rheumatoid arthritis experience a remission from their symptoms beginning in the second trimester of pregnancy and ending with their return about 3 to 4 months postpartum (Keeling & Oswald, 2009). When a chronic illness goes into remission during pregnancy and symptoms return during breastfeeding, the mother may think breastfeeding is the cause. If so, assure her that is not the case. In fact, for many mothers, the hormonal changes of breastfeeding actually help prolong their remission. After a long break from her symptoms, a mother may think they are worse than before. If so, gently explore with her the possibility that after a time of relief, she may have forgotten how severe her symptoms used to be. In mothers with lupus, symptoms during pregnancy are more unpredictable, and pregnancy may be a difficult time.

Physical challenges and breastfeeding. Many mothers with rheumatoid arthritis and lupus struggle with pain and fatigue. For practical strategies for making breastfeeding easier, see p. 773 for the later section "Basic Strategies for Mothers with Disabilities."

Treatments for rheumatoid arthritis and breastfeeding. Different types of medications are used in women with rheumatoid arthritis, many of which are compatible with breastfeeding, such as the non-steroidal anti-inflammatory drugs like ibruprofen (Advil) and aspirin. Acetaminophen (Tylenol) and meperidine are also considered compatible with breastfeeding and may sometimes be taken for pain. The disease-modifying antirheumatic drugs (DMARDs) include steroids, antimalarial medications, and others, many of which are compatible with breastfeeding. However, some cytotoxic drugs in this category, such as methotrexate, are questionable for breastfeeding mothers, because although only small amounts pass into the milk, they are believed to be retained in human tissues (Hale, 2008).

Treatments for lupus and breastfeeding. The medications used to treat lupus will depend on its severity and the organ involvement. Non-steroidal anti-inflammatories (mentioned above) may be used for inflammation and/or pain. The DMARDs mentioned may also be prescribed, many of which are compatible with breastfeeding (Hale, 2008).

Thyroid Disease

The physical changes that occur during pregnancy and lactation can affect thyroid function, which can affect a mother's health, mood, and milk production.

Located in the neck, the butterfly-shaped thyroid gland releases hormones (T_3 and T_4) that regulate much of the body's activities: metabolism, heat generation, brain and heart function, and more. When the thyroid gland becomes overactive (known as hyperthyroidism), it releases too much hormone. When it becomes underactive (known as hypothyroidism), it releases too little hormone. Both too much and too little thyroid hormone may affect the mother's mood and energy level, as well as her health and milk production. Encourage any mother with a history of thyroid problems to have her thyroid levels monitored every few weeks during pregnancy and after birth so that her medication can be adjusted as her hormonal levels change.

Postpartum Thyroiditis

Temporary changes in a mother's thyroid levels after birth are called postpartum thyroiditis.

In 7% to 11% of pregnancies, an autoimmune condition is triggered called postpartum thyroiditis, which can occur even in mothers without a history of thyroid problems (ATA, 2005; Shahbazian, Sarvghadi, & Azizi, 2001).

Symptoms and diagnosis of postpartum thyroiditis. This disorder usually starts with a period of overactive thyroid (thyrotoxicosis or hyperthyroidism), sometime between 1 and 4 months postpartum. Symptoms may include fast heartbeat, insomnia, anxiety, weight loss, and irritability. This overactive phase may last a few weeks to a few months, and then in some—but not all—mothers it is followed by a period of underactive thyroid (hypothyroidism), usually between 4 to 8 months postpartum. Symptoms in this phase may include weight gain, fatigue, dry skin, constipation, depression, and decrease in milk production. Postpartum thyroiditis may be diagnosed from its symptoms alone or blood tests may detect thyroid levels that are too high or too low. Depending on its severity, treatments described in the following two sections for hypo- and hyperthyroidism may be used to bring thyroid levels back into the normal range until the mother's thyroid function normalizes over time. In 80% of mothers with this condition, its symptoms resolve within 12 to 18 months after they began. If thyroid replacement therapy is used, it is tapered off gradually as the mother's thyroid begins functioning normally.

Postpartum hypothyroidism can cause symptoms similar to postpartum depression.

Postpartum thyroiditis may sometimes be mistaken for Graves' disease (for details, see later section "Hyperthyroidism"). According to two U.S. physicians, there are differences in these two conditions that distinguish them (Lawrence & Lawrence, 2005). For example, levels of thyroid stimulation immunoglobulins are high in those with Graves' disease and normal in those with postpartum thyroiditis. Symptoms are severe with Graves' disease and more modest with postpartum thyroiditis. The thyroid gland is usually more enlarged with Graves' disease, and those with Graves' disease have blood levels of thyroid hormone that are significantly high, as opposed to the more modestly elevated levels in those with postpartum thyroiditis.

Hypothyroidism

Treatments for underactive thyroid are compatible with breastfeeding and may boost milk production.

Causes of an underactive thryroid (hypothyroidism) include autoimmune disorders (such as Hashimoto's thyroiditis); medical treatments, such as surgery or radiation of the thyroid gland; medications; illness; and damage of the pituitary gland, the "master gland" that tells the thyroid how much hormone to release.

Symptoms and diagnosis of hypothyroidism. Less-than-normal levels of thyroid hormones cause symptoms that indicate the mother's body is slowing down. She may feel cold, a lack of energy, be forgetful, and depressed. Constipation and low milk production are other possible symptoms. Because the mother's symptoms may seem vague and start slowly, it is not unusual for hypothyroidism to be missed or misdiagnosed. This condition is usually diagnosed from a combination of symptoms, medical history, physical exam, and blood tests. If the mother's blood TSH (thyroid stimulating hormone) levels are high and her T_3 (triiodothyronine) and T_4 (thyrosine) levels are low, this indicates underactive thyroid. Two U.S. physicians specializing in breastfeeding medicine suggest that before any new mother is treated for depression, hypothyroidism first be ruled out (Lawrence & Lawrence, 2005). Taking St. John's wort (an herbal depression treatment) can mask hypothyroidism.

Treatments for hypothyroidism and breastfeeding. Hypothyroidism is usually treated with synthetic thyroid replacement hormones, such as levothyroxine (Synthroid), which bring the mother's levels up to normal by providing the hormones the mother should have produced naturally. In *Medications and Mothers' Milk,* this medication is rated an L1 (safest). Mothers with hypothyroidism often find that with this treatment they not only feel better, their milk production increases, sometimes dramatically.

Hyperthyroidism

Treatments for hyperthyroidism are compatible with breastfeeding unless radioactive iodine is used.

In more than 70% of people with overactive thyroid (hyperthyroidism), the cause is Graves' disease, an autoimmune disorder in which autoantibodies stimulate overproduction of the cells of the thyroid gland. It can also be caused by a nodes or lumps in the thyroid or a temporary condition called thyroiditis, which may be triggered by a virus.

Symptoms and diagnosis of hyperthyroidism. When a mother produces higher-than-normal thyroid levels, her symptoms indicate her body is running faster: racing heartbeat, anxiety, insomnia, irritability, more perspiration, and weight loss. Her eyes may bulge and her thyroid gland may swell into a visible lump (goiter) on her neck. Diagnosis is usually made first with a physical exam, which reveals a swollen thyroid gland, and confirmed by a blood test. When a mother's TSH (thyroid-stimulating hormone) levels are low and her T_3 and T_4 levels are high, this indicates an overactive thyroid.

Radioactive diagnostic tests and breastfeeding. Once hyperthyroidism has been confirmed, to determine its cause, the mother's healthcare provider may order a scan of the thyroid to see whether lumps are present. The radioactive iodine uptake test requires an interruption of breastfeeding until it clears the mother's system, usually at least 12 to 24 hours. If a radioactive scan is recommended, suggest the mother ask if technetium-99m pertechnetate can be used because it has the shortest half-life (6.02 hours), requiring the shortest interruption of breastfeeding (Hale, 2008). Hyperthyroidism can be a serious health problem that stresses a mother's heart, muscles, and nervous system, so if her condition is serious, quick treatment may be critical.

Hyperthyroidism medications and breastfeeding. Antithyroid medications, such as propylthioracil (PTU) and methimazole (Tapazole) and the beta-blocker propranolol (Inderal) are used to treat hyperthyroidism. All are considered compatible with breastfeeding (AAP, 2001; Azizi, 2006; Hale, 2008). In many cases of Graves' disease, medication alone for 12 to 18 months is enough to cause a remission of symptoms.

Radioactive iodine treatment, thyroid surgery, and breastfeeding. Unfortunately, the above medications are not always effective for all types of hyperthyroidism and in all women. Other treatment options include surgical removal of all or part of the thyroid gland, which is compatible with continued breastfeeding, or radioactive iodine treatment, which is not. For details on this last treatment option, see p. 748- "Cancer." Radioactive iodine is also used to treat thyroid cancer.

HEADACHES AND BREASTFEEDING

Rarely, headaches are associated with the hormonal changes of breastfeeding.

Some headaches, such as migraines, appear to be affected by a woman's hormonal fluctuations. For example, migraines tend to be less frequent during pregnancy and after menopause than during other times in a woman's life. In one Italian study of migraines during and after pregnancy, the researchers concluded that breastfeeding protected the mothers from migraine recurrence after birth (Sances et al., 2003). If a type of headache, such as a tension headache, is not affected by hormonal fluctuations, breastfeeding may have no effect (Marcus, Scharff, & Turk, 1999).

In rare cases, rather than preventing headaches, the hormonal changes of breastfeeding seem to trigger headaches. One U.S. article described four cases (out of a total of about 4500 lactation calls logged over a 6-year period) of mothers whose migraines became worse during breastfeeding. One breastfeeding mother got relief from her thrice-weekly migraines only when she weaned her 4-month-old twins (Wall, 1992). Another of these four mothers reported having migraines only during weaning, when her breasts became overly full. An Australian case report also described a mother whose headaches were related to feelings of breast fullness (Thorley, 1997a).

Australian author and lactation consultant Virginia Thorley wrote an overview of the cases described in the literature of mothers whose headaches appeared to be associated with breastfeeding (Thorley, 1997b). She noted two types of lactational headaches:

- One type occurred during the first milk ejection, such as the Swedish mother who developed a headache within 2 minutes of every breastfeeding session (Askmark & Lundberg, 1989).

- A second type occurred when mothers experienced full breasts, such as those described above.

HOSPITALIZATION AND SURGERY

Hospitalization

When discussing hospitalization, talk to the mother about her feelings, her situation and her breastfeeding goals.

A breastfeeding mother needing to be hospitalized may be as worried about her baby as she is about herself. Before discussing her options, first ask for some basic information.

- The reason for her hospitalization and/or surgery and how long she thinks she will be in the hospital
- The age of her breastfeeding child and any other children
- Her long- and short-term breastfeeding goals
- Plans for her breastfeeding child. Will he stay with her (with an adult helper)? If not, can he visit, and if so, for how much of the day? (Some hospitals will make exceptions to policies if asked.) Will he be cared for elsewhere?
- Available help from family and friends while in the hospital and after
- What her healthcare provider has said about breastfeeding
- Availability of lactation consultants and breast pumps at the hospital. If she needs help expressing her milk, is the nursing staff knowledgeable and willing?

With some planning and support, mothers can breastfeed or maintain their milk production while hospitalized.

To find out about the breastfeeding services and equipment available at the hospital, suggest the mother contact the lactation consultant or patient liaison. The mother—or her advocate—should explain to the hospital staff that breastfeeding or expressing her milk will help her avoid medical complications, such as mastitis. If the mother is told her child cannot stay with her, suggest she ask if arranging for a room in another area, such as the mother-baby unit, would make a difference. If the mother is discouraged from breastfeeding or expressing her milk due to health concerns, see the first point in this chapter for research on how breastfeeding can help a mother recover. If the mother's healthcare providers are concerned about her young baby being exposed to organisms in the hospital, explain that giving mother and baby a private room will decrease the risk and that whenever a mother is exposed to an organism, her body begins making antibodies that pass into her milk to protect her breastfeeding baby.

Her breastfeeding goals. If the mother's goal is to continue breastfeeding and she will be separated from her baby for all or part of her hospitalization, discuss milk-expression strategies for maintaining milk production (see p. 473- "Maintaining Full Milk Production"). If the mother wants to wean or wants to slow her milk production temporarily until she is feeling healthier, discuss how she can use milk expression to reduce milk production gradually and avoid painful breast fullness and mastitis (see p. 477- "Weaning from Exclusive Expression").

Suggest the mother ask for the names and spellings of all of her medications to check their compatibility with breastfeeding.

Suggest the mother make sure her healthcare providers know she's breastfeeding, so her medications' compatibility with breastfeeding can be evaluated. For the vast majority of drugs, the amount that passes into mother's milk is so small her child will not be affected. The older and heavier the child and the more other foods he eats, the less of a concern this is. If a drug is incompatible with breastfeeding, suggest she ask that alternatives be considered.

Suggest the book *Medications and Mothers' Milk* be used to determine her medications' compatibility with breastfeeding, as other resources, such as the *Physician's Desk Reference,* do not include the research and other specific information needed. If the mother is having difficulty discussing the situation with her healthcare providers, see Appendix C, "Working with Healthcare Professionals."

If the mother is concerned about her baby feeding well while they're separated or returning to breastfeeding later when they are reunited, discuss options and strategies.

The mother may be concerned about her exclusively breastfed baby accepting a bottle or other feeding method while they're apart. If so, for strategies see p. 586- "Introducing a Bottle." Also see the section "Alternative Feeding Methods" on p. 811 for the range of feeding options and their advantages and disadvantages.

If the mother is concerned her baby may refuse the breast when they are reunited, tell her most babies accept the breast after a separation, some willingly and others with coaxing. Tell her that even if her baby is reluctant to breastfeed at first, with patience and persistence, it is likely he can be persuaded to breastfeed again. For details on overcoming breast refusal, see p. 146- "Strategies to Achieve Settled Breastfeeding." Also reassure the mother that the loving care she gives her baby after they are reunited will allay any unhappiness he felt while she was in the hospital.

Surgery

Before surgery, suggest the mother ask what to expect afterwards, so she can make plans for breastfeeding.

After surgery, the mother's condition and level of pain will determine her ability and desire to breastfeed and care for her child. But if the mother can plan ahead, is motivated, and has help, it can be done. Suggest the mother ask her healthcare provider how she will feel after surgery. Depending on the procedure and the mother's condition, some mothers will be alert and in little pain, while others will be completely incapacitated and in need of intensive medical care. Knowing what to expect will help the mother decide how she wants to handle breastfeeding after her surgery. Some mothers may want to breastfeed as soon as possible, while others may want or need to wait several days. If there will be a wait, suggest the mother make arrangements to have a rental breast pump available, and if needed, help with expressing her milk.

In most cases after surgery, when the mother is alert and awake enough to hold her baby, it is safe for her to resume breastfeeding.

After surgery, according to the Academy for Breastfeeding Medicine's clinical protocol "Analgesia and Anesthesia for the Breastfeeding Mother":

> Mothers with normal term or older infants generally can resume breastfeeding as soon as they are awake, stable, and alert. Resumption of normal [alertness] is a hallmark that these medications have left the

> plasma compartment (and thus the milk compartment) and entered adipose and muscle tissue where they are slowly released. A single pumping and discarding of the mother's milk following surgery will significantly eliminate any drug retained in milk fat, although this is seldom necessary (Montgomery & Hale, 2006, p. 274).

An interruption of breastfeeding for 12 to 24 hours after surgery is recommended only for mothers whose babies are preterm or have apnea, low blood pressure, or weakness.

PHYSICAL IMPAIRMENT OR CHALLENGE

An illness or injury can make breastfeeding physically challenging for a mother, but bottle-feeding may be even more challenging.

A mother with a chronic illness or physical impairment may choose to breastfeed for the same reasons as other mothers. But there may be more. For many of these mothers, formula-feeding has even more significant drawbacks than those experienced by mothers without disabilities.

- Formula feeding requires buying and preparing bottles. Especially for the visually impaired mother, measuring and safely preparing bottles may be difficult.
- Statistically, babies who are not breastfed are sick more often, requiring more visits to the healthcare provider with ear infections, digestive issues, respiratory illnesses, and allergy. Mothers who do not breastfeed are also at greater risk of health problems later in life (Ip et al., 2009).
- Bottle-feeding requires an adult to be awake, alert, and upright for feedings, whereas the mother can breastfeed lying down and rest while her baby feeds.

Fatigue is a common symptom for many mothers with disabilities or chronic conditions.

Although many believe that breastfeeding "takes more energy" than bottle-feeding, research has found otherwise. For more details, see the first point in this chapter.

A physical limitation can be the result of an injury, an autoimmune disorder, or other chronic disease.

Physical limitations may occur after spinal cord injury, stroke, or the loss or absence of one or more limbs. Temporary or permanent loss of function, including swelling, weakness, numbness, and fatigue, can occur with autoimmune disorders, such as lupus, multiple sclerosis, myasthenia gravis (MG), and rheumatoid arthritis, as well as carpal tunnel syndrome.

A mother who lives with a physical limitation has probably learned how to set priorities, but offer to help her brainstorm.

One of the "blessings" described by some mothers with a chronic illness or physical disability is the necessity of carefully setting their priorities (for more insight, see the article "The Spoon Theory" at http://www.butyoudontlooksick.com/navigation/BYDLS-TheSpoonTheory.pdf). A mother in this situation has probably already found ways to simplify her routine and household tasks and adjusted her expectations of what really needs to be done to keep her household running. Even so, offer to brainstorm with her about ways other mothers have simplified their lives after the birth of a baby.

Especially during the early postpartum period, encourage her to accept offers of help from those supportive of breastfeeding. If family or friends are not available to help with housework and if finances allow, suggest she hire household help. What's most important in the early postpartum period is that her helpers focus on doing household chores, while the mother breastfeeds and establishes her relationship with her baby. Having others handle baby care simply postpones the mother acquiring the baby-care skills she'll need and distances her from her baby during this vulnerable time.

Basic Strategies for Mothers with Disabilities

Suggest the mother create a "breastfeeding nest" at home where everything is within easy reach and she can breastfeed comfortably.

No matter how a baby is fed and no matter how healthy or able the mother is, caring for a newborn can be challenging. To make breastfeeding easier for the mother with a physical limitation or impairment, it may help to designate an area of her home her "breastfeeding nest," where she can gather everything she needs during feedings. Items to have on hand include: water to drink, snacks, clean diapers, a container for used diapers, cleaning supplies for diaper changes, a safe area where she can lay her baby, her phone, a radio or television (with remote), and something to read. If she has other children, toys or other entertainment for them would also be a plus. Depending on the feeding positions she prefers, this area may include a comfortable chair, chaise lounge, or bed. Some mothers find it easiest to sit or lie on the floor, where dropping the baby is not a concern.

For some mothers, slings, pillows, and other tools may simplify baby care and breastfeeding.

Many mothers with physical limitations use "adaptive equipment," tools that allow them to more easily accomplish their goals. For a breastfeeding mother, this might include:

- A sling or baby carrier, so she can breastfeed without having to support the baby's weight with her arms
- Pillows or cushions for supporting the baby's weight in upright feeding positions
- A nursing bra with closures in front, rather than in back or velcro closures
- A bell to tie to the crawling baby's shoes to make his whereabouts known
- A prosthesis for missing arms and/or legs
- A stroller, where she can safely strap the baby while away from home

Suggest the mother who finds it difficult to support her baby's weight or who has chronic fatigue learn to breastfeed in the laid-back and side-lying breastfeeding positions described in Chapter 1. Some mothers have found it helpful to breastfeed their babies by leaning over an elevated surface (like a crib or the drawer of a tall dresser). This strategy would only work well if it was comfortable for the mother. If the mother is in a wheelchair, diaper/nappy changing areas and sleep surfaces need to be wheelchair accessible.

Use of a mirror for pumping in a mother with limited neck mobility. In one U.S. case report, a lactation consultant discovered that a mother who had limited neck movement from surgery as a child was unable to express milk using a rental breast pump because she could not see to center her nipple in the nipple tunnel (Drazin, 1995). The lactation consultant suggested using a mirror, which allowed the mother to see when her nipples were centered, and she was able to pump effectively.

Mothers with missing limbs have found creative ways to put their baby to breast.

A U.S. article described how a mother who was a triple amputee exclusively breastfed her baby, with her partner putting the baby to the breast (Dunne & Fuerst, 1995). When the baby's healthcare provider suggested switching to formula, the mother explained that bottle-feeding would be more difficult for her and involve her less in her baby's care.

An Australian article described the breastfeeding experience of a mother who was born without part of her lower left arm (Thomson, 1995). This mother breastfed two children, at first using a pillow to support her baby's weight, shaping her breast while leaning forward to put the breast in the baby's mouth. She later found another position that worked for her and her baby, with her baby straddling her thigh, while she leaned slightly forward.

Carpal Tunnel Syndrome

The breastfeeding mother with carpal tunnel syndrome may get relief from conservative treatments.

Carpal tunnel syndrome occurs when repetitive hand movements cause swelling in the tissues of the wrist, which compresses the nerves leading to the hand. Symptoms include hand numbness, tingling, and pain that can extend from the wrist to the shoulder.

When carpal tunnel syndrome develops during pregnancy, it usually resolves without treatment after birth, sometimes taking a month or two to resolve completely. A small number of women have developed carpal tunnel syndrome during the first month of breastfeeding, with symptoms that only completely resolved after weaning (Snell, Coysh, & Snell, 1980; Wand, 1989; Wand, 1990).

Carpal tunnel syndrome and the breastfeeding mother. If a breastfeeding mother finds it painful to support her breastfeeding baby's weight with her arms, suggest she breastfeed as much as possible on her side or using the laid-back breastfeeding positions described in Chapter 1. Suggest she use pillows or cushions as needed in upright breastfeeding positions or breastfeed her baby in a sling or baby carrier.

Treatments for carpal tunnel syndrome and breastfeeding. Most of the mothers who developed carpal tunnel syndrome while breastfeeding reported some relief from their symptoms by wearing a splint at night, keeping the hand elevated, and taking diuretic medications. Because these mothers had no symptoms later, continuing to breastfeed while using these conservative treatments is considered appropriate (Yagnik, 1987).

Epilepsy and Other Seizure Disorders

The breastfeeding mother with epilepsy can plan ahead to ensure her baby's safety in case of a seizure during feedings.

Epilepsy is a seizure disorder that affects about 1.1 million U.S. women of childbearing age, 20,000 of whom give birth each year (Pschirrer, 2004). Medication is usually so effective at preventing seizures that they are rare, but during pregnancy, many women experience more frequent seizures as their body changes and their usual dosage of medication becomes less effective (Yerby, Kaplan, & Tran, 2004).

Epilepsy and the breastfeeding baby. A baby cannot "catch" epilepsy by breastfeeding. In fact, one Canadian study that examined the records of all 124,207 children born between 1986 and 2000 in Nova Scotia found that not breastfeeding was associated with an increased incidence of epilepsy (Whitehead et al., 2006).

Epilepsy and the breastfeeding mother. To create a safe breastfeeding environment in case the mother has a seizure (which is important no matter how the baby is fed), suggest she choose a feeding area with padding to protect the baby, such as a bed or a chair with padded arms. If her chair doesn't have padded arms, she can fold two towels and wrap and secure them around the chair's arms. This creates a cushion for baby's head during a seizure. Padding and extra pillows may also help the mother avoid bruising. Other strategies include (Penovich, Eck, & Economou, 2004):

- In upright feeding positions, keep her feet elevated (i.e., use a footstool) so that if a seizure occurs the baby would roll back into her lap, not onto the floor.
- If she feeds her baby in bed, use guardrails and pillows for padding. A mattress or futon on the floor would be safer.
- Have a safe surface available on each level of her home, such as a pram, stroller, portable crib, or playyard, where the mother can lay the baby if she thinks she's about to have a seizure.
- Change the baby's diaper/nappy on the floor, or if using a changing table, strap the baby securely, and bathe the baby only when another adult is present.
- When babies and toddlers are crawling and walking, use gates at staircases and doorways to prevent accidents.
- When away from home, suggest the mother have a tag or sticker attached to her pram or stroller with information about her epilepsy, her baby's name, and contact information of a friend or relative to call who can care for the baby.

Treatments for epilepsy and breastfeeding. A major concern of many mothers is the compatibility of their medications with breastfeeding. However, the amount of the mother's medication the baby receives at the breast is much less than what he received while in utero. Although each mother and baby must be evaluated individually, "Most of these medications have been thoroughly studied and used in breastfeeding women for years…" (Hale & Berens, 2002, p. 254). Some anti-epileptic medications, such as phenobarbitol, have infrequently been associated with sedation in the newborn (Hale, 2008).

Spinal Cord Injury or Stroke

If a mother with a spinal cord injury has the use of her arms, breastfeeding is unlikely to be affected.

With a spinal cord injury, a mother's physical limitations will be determined by the location and extent of the spinal injury. In general, the lower a mother's spinal cord injury, the less her loss of function, and the higher and more complete the injury, the more function is lost (Cesario, 2002).

Lack of breast sensation. If a mother's spinal cord injury causes complete loss of breast sensation, milk ejection may be inhibited because the nerve pathways between breast and brain that trigger milk ejection are no longer functional (Craig, 1990; Walker, 2006). In this case, mental imagery can be used to help trigger milk ejection. One Canadian article described the experiences of three women with damaged nerve pathways between breast and brain. Because they were unable to feel the sensations of breastfeeding, they learned to trigger milk ejections with mental imagery while their babies were at the breast (Cowley, 2005). In some areas, nasal oxytocin spray is available from compounding pharmacies and can be used to help trigger milk ejection.

• •

A stroke can cause partial paralysis and affect the mother's vision and judgment.

The most common type of stroke associated with childbirth is caused by a clot that blocks blood flow to the brain (referred to as an "SSSVT" or superior sagittal sinus venous thrombus). When a mother giving birth suffers a stroke, breastfeeding is often sacrificed as the focus shifts to the mother's health and recovery (Flinn, 1995; Terhaar & Kaut, 1993). But a mother wanting to breastfeed in spite of a stroke deserves help. One U.S. article addressed some of the breastfeeding issues for these mothers (Halbert, 1998). The physical effects of the stroke will depend upon its severity and which side of the brain is affected. Suggestions for helping the breastfeeding mother include: letting the mother know when the baby needs to breastfeed, providing extra pillows for support, and if paralysis is involved, giving her help to hold her baby. One author suggests having the mother lie on her affected side so that she can use the unaffected arm and hand to help bring the baby to the breast (Walker, 2006). As with any disability, creativity and an open mind will be helpful in finding the strategies that work best.

Vision Impairment

Breastfeeding presents some challenges to vision-impaired mothers, but in general fewer than bottle-feeding.

In a mother with any type of sensory impairment, when one of her senses is unavailable, her other senses can be used to help her get closer to her baby. A sling or baby carrier can help the mother learn to read her baby's hunger cues through movements and changes in breathing. Keeping baby close also promotes strong attachment and responsive parenting.

The mother who is completely blind is likely to find breastfeeding easier to manage than formula-feeding, which involves (both at home and in unfamiliar places) measuring, preparing, pouring, and sterilizing.

To better help a vision-impaired mother, ask her about her vision limitations and how she accesses printed information. Some mothers have partial vision and can read large print materials or use magnifying lenses. Others use audio materials, Braille, or a computer screen reading program with a voice synthesizer (Good-Mojab, 1999). Braille materials and podcasts are available to vision-impaired mothers through La Leche League International (www.llli.org). When helping the mother put her baby to breast, remember that much printed material relies on photos and drawings to convey information, which the blind mother may not have been able to access. Use words and ask permission before touching her or her baby. For strategies for providing in-person breastfeeding help to vision-impaired mothers, see http://www.llli.org/llleaderweb/LV/LVJunJul99p51.html.

VACCINES

Nearly all vaccines given to the mother are compatible with breastfeeding.

According to the U.S. Centers for Disease Control and Prevention:

> Neither inactivated nor live vaccines administered to a lactating woman affect the safety of breastfeeding for women or their infants. Breastfeeding does not adversely affect immunization and is not a contraindication for any vaccine, with the exception of smallpox vaccine. Limited data indicate that breastfeeding can enhance the response to certain vaccine antigens (Kroger, Atkinson, Marcuse, & Pickering, 2006, p. 27).

See next point for more details.

Breastfeeding mothers can receive vaccinations.

Timing of the rubella vaccine. The rubella vaccine is not recommended for any woman who may become pregnant within the next 28 days, as the rubella virus is associated with birth defects when a mother contracts it during pregnancy (AAP, 2009b). In a mother without immunity to rubella (which can be measured with a blood test), often immunization after birth is recommended.

• •

When a breastfeeding mother is immunized, her baby also receives temporary protection from illness.

When a mother is exposed to an illness, as happens when she is immunized, her body produces antibodies to the illness that pass into her milk. Several studies have documented this effect in breastfeeding babies. In one U.S. study, mothers were immunized with a rotavirus vaccine during the first month postpartum, which provided the breastfeeding babies with passive protection from rotavirus diarrhea for their first 4 months (Pickering et al., 1995). A U.K. study found that vaccinating pregnant mothers against pneumoccoci (the leading cause of severe bacterial disease in children worldwide) resulted in passive immunization for their breastfed babies for up to 5 months (Shahid et al., 1995). These effects are temporary and do not take the place of immunizations for babies. (See p. 242-"Vaccines" for details on how breastfeeding enhances a baby's response to infant immunizations.)

• •

Breastfeeding is not affected when an Rh negative mother receives the Rh immune globulin (RhoGAM) after birth.

When an Rh-negative mother gives birth to an Rh-positive baby, an injection of Rh immune globulin (RhoGAM) is recommended to prevent complications in future pregnancies. Any Rh antibodies in the mother's milk are inactivated in the baby's stomach, so the mother should be encouraged to breastfeed, even when high doses are given (Lawrence & Lawrence, 2005).

REFERENCES

AAP. (2001). Transfer of drugs and other chemicals into human milk. *Pediatrics, 108*(3), 776-789.

AAP. (2009a). Recommendations for care of children in special circumstances. In L. K. Pickering, C. J. Baker, D. W. Kimberlin & S. S. Long (Eds.), *Red book: 2009 report of the Committee on Infectious Diseases* (Vol. 28th, pp. 105-201). Elk Grove Village, IL: American Academy of Pediatrics.

AAP. (2009b). Summaries of infectious diseases. In L. K. Pickering, C. J. Baker, D. W. Kimberlin & S. S. Long (Eds.), *Red book: 2009 report of the Committee on Infectious Diseases* (28th ed.). Elk Grove Village, IL: American Academy of Pediatrics.

Adejuyigbe, E., Orji, E., Onayade, A., Makinde, N., & Anyabolu, H. (2008). Infant feeding intentions and practices of HIV-positive mothers in southwestern Nigeria. *Journal of Human Lactation, 24*(3), 303-310.

Akman, I., Kuscu, M. K., Yurdakul, Z., Ozdemir, N., Solakoglu, M., Orhon, L., et al. (2008). Breastfeeding duration and postpartum psychological adjustment: role of maternal attachment styles. *Journal of Paediatrics and Child Health, 44*(6), 369-373.

Alderman, C. P., McCarthy, L. C., & Marwood, A. C. (2009). Pharmacotherapy for posttraumatic stress disorder. *Expert Review in Clinical Pharmacology, 2*, 77-86.

Alpert, S. E., & Cormier, A. D. (1983). Normal electrolyte and protein content in milk from mothers with cystic fibrosis: an explanation for the initial report of elevated milk sodium concentration. *Journal of Pediatrics, 102*(1), 77-80.

Amir, L. H., Dennerstein, L., Garland, S. M., Fisher, J., & Farish, S. J. (1997). Psychological aspects of nipple pain in lactating women. *Breastfeeding Review, 5*, 29-32.

Ando, Y., Kakimoto, K., Tanigawa, T., Furuki, K., Saito, K., Nakano, S., et al. (1989). Effect of freeze-thawing breast milk on vertical HTLV-I transmission from seropositive mothers to children. *Japanese Journal of Cancer Research, 80*(5), 405-407.

Ando, Y., Saito, K., Nakano, S., Kakimoto, K., Furuki, K., Tanigawa, T., et al. (1989). Bottle-feeding can prevent transmission of HTLV-I from mothers to their babies. *Journal of Infection, 19*(1), 25-29.

Anghelescu, I. G., Kohnen, R., Szegedi, A., Klement, S., & Kieser, M. (2006). Comparison of Hypericum extract WS 5570 and paroxetine in ongoing treatment after recovery from an episode of moderate to severe depression: results from a randomized multicenter study. *Pharmacopsychiatry, 39*(6), 213-219.

Askmark, H., & Lundberg, P. O. (1989). Lactation headache--a new form of headache? *Cephalalgia, 9*(2), 119-122.

Asselin, B. L., & Lawrence, R. A. (1987). Maternal disease as a consideration in lactation management. *Clinics in Perinatology, 14*(1), 71-87.

ATA. (2005). Postpartum Thyroiditis. Retrieved January 25, 2010, from http://www.thyroid.org/patients/brochures/Postpartum_Thyroiditis_brochure.pdf

Azizi, F. (2006). Treatment of post-partum thyrotoxicosis. *Journal of Endocrinological Investigation, 29*(3), 244-247.

Baillargeon, J. P., Jakubowicz, D. J., Iuorno, M. J., Jakubowicz, S., & Nestler, J. E. (2004). Effects of metformin and rosiglitazone, alone and in combination, in nonobese women with polycystic ovary syndrome and normal indices of insulin sensitivity. *Fertility and Sterility, 82*(4), 893-902.

Balcar, V., Silinkova-Malkova, E., & Matys, Z. (1972). Soft tissue radiography of the female breast and pelvic pneumoperitoneum in the Stein-Leventhal syndrome. *Acta Radiologica: Diagnosis, 12*(3), 353-362.

Becquet, R., Ekouevi, D. K., Menan, H., Amani-Bosse, C., Bequet, L., Viho, I., et al. (2008). Early mixed feeding and breastfeeding beyond 6 months increase the risk of postnatal HIV transmission: ANRS 1201/1202 Ditrame Plus, Abidjan, Cote d'Ivoire. *Preventive Medicine, 47*(1), 27-33.

Benedict, M. (1994). *Long-term effects of child sexual abuse on functioning in pregnancy and pregnancy outcome. Final report.* Washington, DC: National Center on Child Abuse and Neglect.

Bergdoll, M. S., Crass, B. A., Reiser, R. F., Robbins, R. N., & Davis, J. P. (1981). A new staphylococcal enterotoxin, enterotoxin F, associated with toxic-shock-syndrome Staphylococcus aureus isolates. *Lancet, 1*(8228), 1017-1021.

Berlin, C. M. (2007). "Exclusive" breastfeeding of quadruplets. *Breastfeeding Medicine, 2*(2), 125-126.

Betzold, C. M., Hoover, K. L., & Snyder, C. L. (2004). Delayed lactogenesis II: a comparison of four cases. *Journal of Midwifery & Women's Health, 49*(2), 132-137.

Blumenthal, J. A., Babyak, M. A., Doraiswamy, P. M., Watkins, L., Hoffman, B. M., Barbour, K. A., et al. (2007). Exercise and pharmacotherapy in the treatment of major depressive disorder. *Psychosomatic Medicine, 69*(7), 587-596.

Blyton, D. M., Sullivan, C. E., & Edwards, N. (2002). Lactation is associated with an increase in slow-wave sleep in women. *Journal of Sleep Research, 11*(4), 297-303.

Bryant, P., Morley, C., Garland, S., & Curtis, N. (2002). Cytomegalovirus transmission from breast milk in premature babies: does it matter? *Archives of Disease in Childhood. Fetal and Neonatal Edition, 87*(2), F75-77.

Butte, N. F., Hopkinson, J. M., Mehta, N., Moon, J. K., & Smith, E. O. (1999). Adjustments in energy expenditure and substrate utilization during late pregnancy and lactation. *American Journal of Clinical Nutrition, 69*(2), 299-307.

Byrne, P. A., Miller, C., & Justus, K. (2006). Neonatal group B streptococcal infection related to breast milk. *Breastfeeding Medicine, 1*(4), 263-270.

Carlsen, S. M., Jacobsen, G., & Vanky, E. (2010). Mid-pregnancy androgen levels are negatively associated with breastfeeding. *Acta Obstetricia et Gynecologica Scandinavica, 89*(1), 87-94.

CDC. (1987). Adult T-cell leukemia/lymphoma associated with human T-lymphotropic virus type I (HTLV-I) infection--North Carolina. *MMWR. Morbidity and Mortality Weekly Report, 36*(49), 804-806, 812.

CDC. (2002). Possible West Nile virus transmission to an infant through breast-feeding--Michigan, 2002. *MMWR. Morbidity and Mortality Weekly Report, 51*(39), 877-878.

CDC. (2006, February 9). About CMV. Retrieved January 10, 2010, from http://www.cdc.gov/cmv/facts.htm.

CDC (2007). Lyme disease transmission. *Journal.* Retrieved from http://www.cdc.gov/ncidod/dvbid/LYME/ld_transmission.htm.

CDC. (2008). Prevalence of self-reported postpartum depressive symptoms--17 states, 2004-2005. *MMWR Morbity and Mortality Weekly Report, 57*(14), 361-366.

CDC (2009a). 2009 H1N1 flu (Swine Flu) and feeding your baby: what parents should know, October 23, 2009. *Journal.* Retrieved from http://www.cdc.gov/h1n1flu/infantfeeding.htm?s_cid=h1n1Flu_outbreak_155.

CDC. (2009b, October 20, 2009). Hepatitis B and C infections. Retrieved January 14, 2010, from http://www.cdc.gov/breastfeeding/disease/hepatitis.htm.

CDC. (2009c, June 9, 2009). Hepatitis C FAQs for health professionals. Retrieved January 14, 2010, from http://www.cdc.gov/hepatitis/HCV/HCVfaq.htm.

CDC (2009d). Interim guidance: considerations regarding 2009 H1N1 Influenza in intrapartum and postpartum hospital settings, November 10, 2009. *Journal.* Retrieved from http://www.cdc.gov/h1n1flu/guidance/obstetric.htm.

CDC. (2009e, October 20, 2009). West Nile Virus. Retrieved January 14, 2010, from http://www.cdc.gov/breastfeeding/disease/west_nile_virus.htm.

Cesario, S. K. (2002). Spinal cord injuries. Nurses can help affected women & their families achieve pregnancy birth. *AWHONN Lifelines, 6*(3), 224-232.

Chaudron, L. H. (2007). Treating pregnant women with antidepressants: the gray zone. *J Womens Health (Larchmt), 16*(4), 551-553.

Cicchetti, D., & Toth, S. L. (1998). The development of depression in children and adolescents. *American Psychologist, 53*(2), 221-241.

Colombo, C., Costantini, D., Zazzeron, L., Faelli, N., Russo, M. C., Ghisleni, D., et al. (2007). Benefits of breastfeeding in cystic fibrosis: a single-centre follow-up survey. *Acta Paediatrica, 96*(8), 1228-1232.

Confavreux, C., Hutchinson, M., Hours, M. M., Cortinovis-Tourniaire, P., & Moreau, T. (1998). Rate of pregnancy-related relapse in multiple sclerosis. Pregnancy in Multiple Sclerosis Group. *New England Journal of Medicine, 339*(5), 285-291.

Connell, S., Patterson, C., & Newman, B. (2006). A qualitative analysis of reproductive issues raised by young Australian women with breast cancer. *Health Care for Women International, 27*(1), 94-110.

Cordero, L., Treuer, S. H., Landon, M. B., & Gabbe, S. G. (1998). Management of infants of diabetic mothers. *Archives of Pediatrics and Adolescent Medicine, 152*(3), 249-254.

Cornish, A. M., McMahon, C. A., Ungerer, J. A., Barnett, B., Kowalenko, N., & Tennant, C. (2005). Postnatal depression and infant cognitive and motor development in the seocnd postnatal year: the impact of depression chronicity and infant gender. *Infant Behavior and Development, 28*, 407-417.

Costenbader, K. H., Feskanich, D., Stampfer, M. J., & Karlson, E. W. (2007). Reproductive and menopausal factors and risk of systemic lupus erythematosus in women. *Arthritis and Rheumatism, 56*(4), 1251-1262.

Coutsoudis, A., Pillay, K., Kuhn, L., Spooner, E., Tsai, W. Y., & Coovadia, H. M. (2001). Method of feeding and transmission of HIV-1 from mothers to children by 15 months of age: prospective cohort study from Durban, South Africa. *AIDS, 15*(3), 379-387.

Coutsoudis, A., Pillay, K., Spooner, E., Kuhn, L., & Coovadia, H. M. (1999). Influence of infant-feeding patterns on early mother-to-child transmission of HIV-1 in Durban, South Africa: a prospective cohort study. South African Vitamin A Study Group. *Lancet, 354*(9177), 471-476.

Cowley, K. C. (2005). Psychogenic and pharmacologic induction of the let-down reflex can facilitate breastfeeding by tetraplegic women: a report of 3 cases. *Archives of Physical Medicine and Rehabilitation, 86*(6), 1261-1264.

Craig, D. I. (1990). The adaptation to pregnancy of spinal cord injured women. *Rehabilitation Nursing, 15*(1), 6-9.

Czank, C., Henderson, J. J., Kent, J. C., Tat Lai, C., & Hartmann, P. E. (2007). Hormonal control of the lactation cycle. In T. W. Hale & P. E. Hartmann (Eds.), *Hale & Hartmann's Textbook of Lactation* (pp. 89-111). Amarillo, TX: Hale Publishing.

David, F. C. (1985). Lactation following primary radiation therapy for carcinoma of the breast. *International Journal of Radiation Oncology, Biology, Physics, 11*(7), 1425.

Davies, H. A., Clark, J. D., Dalton, K. J., & Edwards, O. M. (1989). Insulin requirements of diabetic women who breast feed. *British Medical Journal, 298*(6684), 1357-1358.

Dennis, C. L., & Chung-Lee, L. (2006). Postpartum depression help-seeking barriers and maternal treatment preferences: a qualitative systematic review. *Birth, 33*(4), 323-331.

Dennis, C. L., & McQueen, K. (2009). The relationship between infant-feeding outcomes and postpartum depression: a qualitative systematic review. *Pediatrics, 123*(4), e736-751.

Dimitrov, S., Lange, T., Fehm, H. L., & Born, J. (2004). A regulatory role of prolactin, growth hormone, and corticosteroids for human T-cell production of cytokines. *Brain, Behavior, and Immunity, 18*(4), 368-374.

Dinger, J., Muller, D., Pargac, N., & Schwarze, R. (2002). Breast milk transmission of group B streptococcal infection. *Pediatric Infectious Disease Journal, 21*(6), 567-568.

Diniz, J. M., & Da Costa, T. H. (2004). Independent of body adiposity, breast-feeding has a protective effect on glucose metabolism in young adult women. *British Journal of Nutrition, 92*(6), 905-912.

Doan, T., Gardiner, A., Gay, C. L., & Lee, K. A. (2007). Breast-feeding increases sleep duration of new parents. *J Perinat Neonatal Nurs, 21*(3), 200-206.

Dong, M., Anda, R. F., Dube, S. R., Giles, W. H., & Felitti, V. J. (2003). The relationship of exposure to childhood sexual abuse to other forms of abuse, neglect, and household dysfunction during childhood. *Child Abuse and Neglect, 27*(6), 625-639.

Drazin, P. B. (1995). Use of a mirror to assist breast pumping. *Journal of Human Lactation, 11*(3), 219.

Dunn, D. T., Newell, M. L., Ades, A. E., & Peckham, C. S. (1992). Risk of human immunodeficiency virus type 1 transmission through breastfeeding. *Lancet, 340*(8819), 585-588.

Dunne, G., & Fuerst, K. (1995). Breastfeeding by a mother who is a triple amputee: a case report. *Journal of Human Lactation, 11*(3), 217-218.

Dworsky, M., Yow, M., Stagno, S., Pass, R. F., & Alford, C. (1983). Cytomegalovirus infection of breast milk and transmission in infancy. *Pediatrics, 72*(3), 295-299.

Dwosh, E., Guimond, C., & Sadovnick, A. D. (2003). Reproductive counselling for MS: a rationale. *International Multiple Sclerosis Journal, 10*(2), 52-59.

Edenborough, F. P., Borgo, G., Knoop, C., Lannefors, L., Mackenzie, W. E., Madge, S., et al. (2008). Guidelines for the management of pregnancy in women with cystic fibrosis. *Journal of Cystic Fibrosis, 7 Suppl 1*, S2-32.

Fairchild, J. P., Graber, C. D., Vogel, E. H., Jr., & Ingersoll, R. L. (1958). Flora of the umbilical stump; 2,479 cultures. *Journal of Pediatrics, 53*(5), 538-546.

Feig, D. S., Briggs, G. G., & Koren, G. (2007). Oral antidiabetic agents in pregnancy and lactation: a paradigm shift? *Annals of Pharmacotherapy, 41*(7), 1174-1180.

Felitti, V. J. (2009). Adverse childhood experiences and adult health. *Academic Pediatrics, 9*(3), 131-132.

Felitti, V. J., Anda, R. F., Nordenberg, D., Williamson, D. F., Spitz, A. M., Edwards, V., et al. (1998). Relationship of childhood abuse and household dysfunction to many of the leading causes of death in adults. The Adverse Childhood Experiences (ACE) Study. *American Journal of Preventive Medicine, 14*(4), 245-258.

Ferris, A. M., Neubauer, S. H., Bendel, R. B., Green, K. W., Ingardia, C. J., & Reece, E. A. (1993). Perinatal lactation protocol and outcome in mothers with and without insulin-dependent diabetes mellitus. *American Journal of Clinical Nutrition, 58*(1), 43-48.

Festini, F., Ciuti, R., Taccetti, G., Repetto, T., Campana, S., & De Martino, M. (2006). Breast-feeding in a woman with cystic fibrosis undergoing antibiotic intravenous treatment. *Journal of Maternal and Fetal Neonatal Medicine, 19*(6), 375-376.

Field, T. (1995). Infants of depressed mothers. *Infant Behavior and Development, 18*, 1-13.

Field, T., Hernandez-Reif, M., & Feijo, L. (2002). Breastfeeding in depressed mother-infant dyads. *Early Child Development and Care, 172*, 539-545.

Fjeld, E., Siziya, S., Katepa-Bwalya, M., Kankasa, C., Moland, K. M., & Tylleskar, T. (2008). 'No sister, the breast alone is not enough for my baby' a qualitative assessment of potentials and barriers in the promotion of exclusive breastfeeding in southern Zambia. *International Breastfeeding Journal, 3*, 26.

Flinn, N. (1995). A task-oriented approach to the treatment of a client with hemiplegia. *American Journal of Occupational Therapy, 49*(6), 560-569.

Fonseca, A. M., de Souza, A. Z., Bagnoli, V. R., Celestino, C. A., & Salvatore, C. A. (1985). Histologic and histometric aspects of the breast in polycystic ovary syndrome. *Archives of Gynecology, 237*, 380-381.

Forbes, G. B., Barton, L. D., Nicholas, D. L., & Cook, D. A. (1988). Composition of milk produced by a mother with galactosemia. *Journal of Pediatrics, 113*(1 Pt 1), 90-91.

Fox-Bacon, C., McCamman, S., Therou, L., Moore, W., & Kipp, D. E. (1997). Maternal PKU and breastfeeding: case report of identical twin mothers. *Clinical Pediatrics, 36*(9), 539-542.

Freeman, M. P., Hibbeln, J. R., Wisner, K. L., Brumbach, B. H., Watchman, M., & Gelenberg, A. J. (2006). Randomized dose-ranging pilot trial of omega-3 fatty acids for postpartum depression. *Acta Psychiatrica Scandinavica, 113*(1), 31-35.

Freeman, M. P., Hibbeln, J. R., Wisner, K. L., Davis, J. M., Mischoulon, D., Peet, M., et al. (2006). Omega-3 fatty acids: evidence basis for treatment and future research in psychiatry. *Journal of Clinical Psychiatry, 67*(12), 1954-1967.

Friedman, M. J., Davidson, J. R. T., & Stein, D. J. (2009). Psychopharmacotherapy for adults. In E. B. Foa, T. M. Keane, M. J. Friedman & J. A. Cohen (Eds.), *Practice guidelines from the International Society for Traumatic Stress Studies* (pp. 245-268). New York: Guilford.

Gabbay, M., & Kelly, H. (2003). Use of metformin to increase breast milk production in women with insulin resistance: case series. *ABM News and Views, 9*, 20.

Gastelum, D. T., Dassey, D., Mascola, L., & Yasuda, L. M. (2005). Transmission of community-associated methicillin-resistant Staphylococcus aureus from breast milk in the neonatal intensive care unit. *Pediatric Infectious Disease Journal, 24*(12), 1122-1124.

Gilljam, M., Antoniou, M., Shin, J., Dupuis, A., Corey, M., & Tullis, D. E. (2000). Pregnancy in cystic fibrosis. Fetal and maternal outcome. *Chest, 118*(1), 85-91.

Glueck, C. J., Salehi, M., Aregawi, D., Sieve, L., & Wang, P. (2007). Polycystic Ovary Syndrome: pathophysiology, endocrinopathy, treatment, and lactation. In T. W. Hale & P. E. Hartmann (Eds.), *Hale and Hartmann's Textbook of Lactation* (pp. 343-353). Amarillo, TX: Hale Publishing.

Glueck, C. J., Salehi, M., Sieve, L., & Wang, P. (2006). Growth, motor, and social development in breast- and formula-fed infants of metformin-treated women with polycystic ovary syndrome. *Journal of Pediatrics, 148*(5), 628-632.

Glueck, C. J., Wang, P., Goldenberg, N., & Sieve, L. (2004). Pregnancy loss, polycystic ovary syndrome, thrombophilia, hypofibrinolysis, enoxaparin, metformin. *Clinical and Applied Thrombosis/Hemostasis, 10*(4), 323-334.

Golden, S. (2003). Group A streptococcus and streptococcal toxic shock syndrome: a postpartum case report. *Journal of Midwifery & Women's Health, 48*(5), 357-359.

Good-Mojab, C. (1999). Helping the visually impaired or blind mother breastfeed. *Leaven, 35*(3), 51-56.

Greer, F. R., Sicherer, S. H., & Burks, A. W. (2008). Effects of early nutritional interventions on the development of atopic disease in infants and children: the role of maternal dietary restriction, breastfeeding, timing of introduction of complementary foods, and hydrolyzed formulas. *Pediatrics, 121*(1), 183-191.

Groer, M. W., & Davis, M. W. (2006). Cytokines, infections, stress, and dysphoric moods in breastfeeders and formula feeders. *Journal of Obstetric, Gynecologic, and Neonatal Nursing, 35*(5), 599-607.

Grunwald, F., Palmedo, H., & Biersack, H. J. (1995). Unilateral iodine-131 uptake in the lactating breast. *Journal of Nuclear Medicine, 36*(9), 1724-1725.

Gulick, E. E., & Halper, J. (2002). Influence of infant feeding method on postpartum relapse of mothers with MS. *International Journal of MS Care, 4*(4), 4-12.

Halbert, L. A. (1998). Breastfeeding in the woman with a compromised nervous system. *Journal of Human Lactation, 14*(4), 327-331.

Hale, T. (2008). *Medications and Mothers' Milk* (13 ed.). Amarillo, TX: Hale Publishing.

Hale, T. W., & Berens, P. (2002). *Clinical Therapy in Breastfeeding Patients* (2nd ed.). Amarillo, TX: Pharmasoft Publishing.

Hale, T. W., Kristensen, J. H., Hackett, L. P., Kohan, R., & Ilett, K. F. (2002). Transfer of metformin into human milk. *Diabetologia, 45*(11), 1509-1514.

Hammen, C., & Brennan, P. A. (2002). Interpersonal dysfunction in depressed women: impairments independent of depressive symptoms. *Journal of Affective Disorders, 72*(2), 145-156.

Hammond, K. A. (1997). Adaptation of the maternal intestine during lactation. *Journal of Mammary Gland Biology and Neoplasia, 2*(3), 243-252.

Harris, T. O., Shelver, D. W., Bohnsack, J. F., & Rubens, C. E. (2003). A novel streptococcal surface protease promotes virulence, resistance to opsonophagocytosis, and cleavage of human fibrinogen. *Journal of Clinical Investigation, 111*(1), 61-70.

Hartmann, P., & Cregan, M. (2001). Lactogenesis and the effects of insulin-dependent diabetes mellitus and prematurity. *Journal of Nutrition, 131*(11), 3016S-3020S.

Hartmann, S. U., Berlin, C. M., & Howett, M. K. (2006). Alternative modified infant-feeding practices to prevent postnatal transmission of human immunodeficiency virus type 1 through breast milk: past, present, and future. *Journal of Human Lactation, 22*(1), 75-88; quiz 89-93.

Hatton, D. C., Harrison-Hohner, J., Coste, S., Dorato, V., Curet, L. B., & McCarron, D. A. (2005). Symptoms of postpartum depression and breastfeeding. *Journal of Human Lactation, 21*(4), 444-449; quiz 450-444.

Hay, D. F., Pawlby, S., Sharp, D., Asten, P., Mills, A., & Kumar, R. (2001). Intellectual problems shown by 11-year-old children whose mothers had postnatal depression. *Journal of Child Psychology and Psychiatry and Allied Disciplines, 42*(7), 871-889.

HDTSG. (2002). Effect of Hypericum perforatum (St John's wort) in major depressive disorder: a randomized controlled trial. *Journal of the American Medical Association, 287*(14), 1807-1814.

Heh, S. S., Huang, L. H., Ho, S. M., Fu, Y. Y., & Wang, L. L. (2008). Effectiveness of an exercise support program in reducing the severity of postnatal depression in Taiwanese women. *Birth, 35*(1), 60-65.

Heuchan, A. M., & Isaacs, D. (2001). The management of varicella-zoster virus exposure and infection in pregnancy and the newborn period. Australasian Subgroup in Paediatric Infectious Diseases of the Australasian Society for Infectious Diseases. *Medical Journal of Australia, 174*(6), 288-292.

Higgins, S., & Haffty, B. G. (1994). Pregnancy and lactation after breast-conserving therapy for early stage breast cancer. *Cancer, 73*(8), 2175-2180.

Hino, S. (1989). Milk-borne transmission of HTLV-I as a major route in the endemic cycle. *Acta Paediatrica Japonica, 31*(4), 428-435.

Hino, S., Katamine, S., Miyata, H., Tsuji, Y., Yamabe, T., & Miyamoto, T. (1997). Primary prevention of HTLV-1 in Japan. *Leukemia, 11 Suppl 3*, 57-59.

Hirata, M., Hayashi, J., Noguchi, A., Nakashima, K., Kajiyama, W., Kashiwagi, S., et al. (1992). The effects of breastfeeding and presence of antibody to p40tax protein of human T cell lymphotropic virus type-I on mother to child transmission. *International Journal of Epidemiology, 21*(5), 989-994.

Hofmann, J., De Allegri, M., Sarker, M., Sanon, M., & Bohler, T. (2009). Breast milk as the "water that supports and preserves life"--socio-cultural constructions of breastfeeding and their implications for the prevention of mother to child transmission of HIV in sub-Saharan Africa. *Health Policy, 89*(3), 322-328.

Holmberg, H., Wahlberg, J., Vaarala, O., & Ludvigsson, J. (2007). Short duration of breast-feeding as a risk-factor for beta-cell autoantibodies in 5-year-old children from the general population. *British Journal of Nutrition, 97*(1), 111-116.

Hoover, K. L., Barbalinardo, L. H., & Platia, M. P. (2002). Delayed lactogenesis II secondary to gestational ovarian theca lutein cysts in two normal singleton pregnancies. *Journal of Human Lactation, 18*(3), 264-268.

Huang, P. L. (2009). A comprehensive definition for metabolic syndrome. *Disease Models and Mechanisms, 2*(5-6), 231-237.

Ichimaru, M., Ikeda, S., Kinoshita, K., Hino, S., & Tsuji, Y. (1991). Mother-to-child transmission of HTLV-1. *Cancer Detection and Prevention, 15*(3), 177-181.

Iliff, P. J., Piwoz, E. G., Tavengwa, N. V., Zunguza, C. D., Marinda, E. T., Nathoo, K. J., et al. (2005). Early exclusive breastfeeding reduces the risk of postnatal HIV-1 transmission and increases HIV-free survival. *AIDS, 19*(7), 699-708.

Illingworth, P. J., Jung, R. T., Howie, P. W., Leslie, P., & Isles, T. E. (1986). Diminution in energy expenditure during lactation. *British Medical Journal (Clinical Research Ed.), 292*(6518), 437-441.

Ip, S., Chung, M., Raman, G., Trikalinos, T. A., & Lau, J. (2009). A summary of the Agency for Healthcare Research and Quality's evidence report on breastfeeding in developed countries. *Breastfeeding Medicine, 4 Suppl 1*, S17-30.

Isaacs, D. (2000). Neonatal chickenpox. *Journal of Paediatrics and Child Health, 36*, 76-77.

Israel-Ballard, K. A., Abrams, B. F., Coutsoudis, A., Sibeko, L. N., Cheryk, L. A., & Chantry, C. J. (2008). Vitamin content of breast milk from HIV-1-infected mothers before and after flash-heat treatment. *Journal of Acquired Immune Deficiency Syndromes, 48*(4), 444-449.

Israel-Ballard, K. A., Maternowska, M. C., Abrams, B. F., Morrison, P., Chitibura, L., Chipato, T., et al. (2006). Acceptability of heat treating breast milk to prevent mother-to-child transmission of human immunodeficiency virus in Zimbabwe: a qualitative study. *Journal of Human Lactation, 22*(1), 48-60.

Jacobsson, L. T., Jacobsson, M. E., Askling, J., & Knowler, W. C. (2003). Perinatal characteristics and risk of rheumatoid arthritis. *British Medical Journal, 326*(7398), 1068-1069.

Jonas, W., Nissen, E., Ransjo-Arvidson, A. B., Wiklund, I., Henriksson, P., & Uvnas-Moberg, K. (2008). Short- and long-term decrease of blood pressure in women during breastfeeding. *Breastfeeding Medicine, 3*(2), 103-109.

Jones, N. A., McFall, B. A., & Diego, M. A. (2004). Patterns of brain electrical activity in infants of depressed mothers who breastfeed and bottle feed: the mediating role of infant temperament. *Biological Psychology, 67*(1-2), 103-124.

Kagaayi, J., Gray, R. H., Brahmbhatt, H., Kigozi, G., Nalugoda, F., Wabwire-Mangen, F., et al. (2008). Survival of infants born to HIV-positive mothers, by feeding modality, in Rakai, Uganda. *PLoS One, 3*(12), e3877.

Karavanaki, K., Tsoka, E., Karayianni, C., Petrou, V., Pippidou, E., Brisimitzi, M., et al. (2008). Prevalence of allergic symptoms among children with diabetes mellitus type 1 of different socioeconomic status. *Pediatric Diabetes, 9*(4 Pt 2), 407-416.

Karlson, E. W., Mandl, L. A., Hankinson, S. E., & Grodstein, F. (2004). Do breast-feeding and other reproductive factors influence future risk of rheumatoid arthritis? Results from the Nurses' Health Study. *Arthritis and Rheumatism, 50*(11), 3458-3467.

Keeling, S. O., & Oswald, A. E. (2009). Pregnancy and rheumatic disease: "by the book" or "by the doc". *Clinical Rheumatology, 28*(1), 1-9.

Kendall-Tackett, K. (2007a). A new paradigm for depression in new mothers: the central role of inflammation and how breastfeeding and anti-inflammatory treatments protect maternal mental health. *International Breastfeeding Journal, 2*, 6.

Kendall-Tackett, K. (2009). *Postpartum depression at a glance*. Amarillo, TX: Hale Publishing.

Kendall-Tackett, K. (2010). *Depression in new mothers: causes, consequences, and treatment alternatives* (2nd ed.). New York, NY: Routledge.

Kendall-Tackett, K., & Hale, T. (2009a). The use of antidepressants in pregnant and breastfeeding women: a review of recent studies. [online first pdf]. *Journal of Human Lactation*.

Kendall-Tackett, K. A. (2007b). Diagnosis and treatment of posttraumatic stress disorder (PTSD): compatibility of treatment choices with breastfeeding. *Medications & More, 23* ((October)), 1-3.

Kendall-Tackett, K. A., & Hale, T. W. (2009b). Medication use for trauma symptoms and ptsd in pregnant and breastfeeding women. *Trauma Psychology, 4*(2), 12-15.

Kent, N. E., & Farquharson, D. F. (1993). Cystic fibrosis in pregnancy. *Canadian Medical Association Journal, 149*(6), 809-813.

Kim, Y. H., Chang, S. S., Kim, Y. S., Kim, E. A., Yun, S. C., Kim, K. S., et al. (2007). Clinical outcomes in methicillin-resistant Staphylococcus aureus-colonized neonates in the neonatal intensive care unit. *Neonatology, 91*(4), 241-247.

Kitajima, H. (2003). Prevention of methicillin-resistant Staphylococcus aureus infections in neonates. *Pediatrics International, 45*(2), 238-245.

Kjos, S. L., Henry, O., Lee, R. M., Buchanan, T. A., & Mishell, D. R., Jr. (1993). The effect of lactation on glucose and lipid metabolism in women with recent gestational diabetes. *Obstetrics and Gynecology, 82*(3), 451-455.

Kroger, A. T., Atkinson, W. L., Marcuse, E. K., & Pickering, L. K. (2006). General recommendations on immunization: recommendations of the Advisory Committee on Immunization Practices (ACIP). *MMWR Recommendations and Reports, 55*(RR-15), 1-48.

Kuhn, L., Aldrovandi, G. M., Sinkala, M., Kankasa, C., Semrau, K., Kasonde, P., et al. (2009). Differential effects of early weaning for HIV-free survival of children born to HIV-infected mothers by severity of maternal disease. *PLoS One, 4*(6), e6059.

Kuhn, L., Sinkala, M., Kankasa, C., Semrau, K., Kasonde, P., Scott, N., et al. (2007). High uptake of exclusive breastfeeding and reduced early post-natal HIV transmission. *PLoS One, 2*(12), e1363.

Kuhn, L., Sinkala, M., Thea, D. M., Kankasa, C., & Aldrovandi, G. M. (2009). HIV prevention is not enough: child survival in the context of prevention of mother to child HIV transmission. *Journal of the International AIDS Society, 12*(1), 36.

Kumar, R. M., & Shahul, S. (1998). Role of breast-feeding in transmission of hepatitis C virus to infants of HCV-infected mothers. *Journal of Hepatology, 29*(2), 191-197.

Langer-Gould, A., Huang, S. M., Gupta, R., Leimpeter, A. D., Greenwood, E., Albers, K. B., et al. (2009). Exclusive breastfeeding and the risk of postpartum relapses in women with multiple sclerosis. *Archives of Neurology, 66*(8), 958-963.

Lawrence, R. A., & Bradley, J. S. (2009). Advice regarding breastfeeding for mothers with possible H1N1 infection. *AAP News*, aapnews.20091012-20091011.

Lawrence, R. A., & Lawrence, R. M. (2005). *Breastfeeding: A Guide for the Medical Profession* (6th ed.). Philadelphia, PA: Elsevier Mosby.

Lee, S. Y., Kim, M. T., Jee, S. H., & Yang, H. P. (2005). Does long-term lactation protect premenopausal women against hypertension risk? A Korean women's cohort study. *Preventive Medicine, 41*(2), 433-438.

Losonsky, G. A., Fishaut, J. M., Strussenberg, J., & Ogra, P. L. (1982a). Effect of immunization against rubella on lactation products. I. Development and characterization of specific immunologic reactivity in breast milk. *Journal of Infectious Diseases, 145*(5), 654-660.

Losonsky, G. A., Fishaut, J. M., Strussenberg, J., & Ogra, P. L. (1982b). Effect of immunization against rubella on lactation products. II. Maternal-neonatal interactions. *Journal of Infectious Diseases, 145*(5), 661-666.

Luoma, I., Tamminen, T., Kaukonen, P., Laippala, P., Puura, K., Salmelin, R., et al. (2001). Longitudinal study of maternal depressive symptoms and child well-being. *Journal of the American Academy of Child and Adolescent Psychiatry, 40*(12), 1367-1374.

Machuca, A., Tuset, C., Soriano, V., Caballero, E., Aguilera, A., & Ortiz de Lejarazu, R. (2000). Prevalence of HTLV infection in pregnant women in Spain. *Sexually Transmitted Infections, 76*(5), 366-370.

Manns, A., Hisada, M., & La Grenade, L. (1999). Human T-lymphotropic virus type I infection. *Lancet, 353*(9168), 1951-1958.

Marasco, L., Marmet, C., & Shell, E. (2000). Polycystic ovary syndrome: a connection to insufficient milk supply? *Journal of Human Lactation, 16*(2), 143-148.

Marcus, D. A., Scharff, L., & Turk, D. (1999). Longitudinal prospective study of headache during pregnancy and postpartum. *Headache, 39*(9), 625-632.

Marshall, A. M., Nommsen-Rivers, L. A., Hernandez, L. L., Dewey, K. G., Chantry, C. J., Gregerson, K. A., et al. (2010). Serotonin transport and metabolism in the mammary gland modulates secretory activation and involution. *Journal of Clinical Endocrinology and Metabolism, 95*(2), 837-846.

Matalon, R., Michals, K., & Gleason, L. (1986). Maternal PKU: strategies for dietary treatment and monitoring compliance. *Annals of the New York Academy of Sciences, 477*, 223-230.

Matovu, A., Kirunda, B., Rugamba-Kabagambe, G., Tumwesigye, N. M., & Nuwaha, F. (2008). Factors influencing adherence to exclusive breast feeding among HIV positive mothers in Kabarole district, Uganda. *East African Medical Journal, 85*(4), 162-170.

McCarter-Spaulding, D. E. (2001). Varicella infection in pregnancy. *Journal of Obstetric, Gynecologic and Neonatal Nursing, 30*(6), 667-673.

McCoy, S. J., Beal, J. M., Shipman, S. B., Payton, M. E., & Watson, G. H. (2006). Risk factors for postpartum depression: a retrospective investigation at 4-weeks postnatal and a review of the literature. *Journal of the American Osteopathic Association, 106*(4), 193-198.

McDougal, J. S., Martin, L. S., Cort, S. P., Mozen, M., Heldebrant, C. M., & Evatt, B. L. (1985). Thermal inactivation of the acquired immunodeficiency syndrome virus, human T lymphotropic virus-III/lymphadenopathy-associated virus, with special reference to antihemophilic factor. *Journal of Clinical Investigation, 76*(2), 875-877.

McManus, R. M., Cunningham, I., Watson, A., Harker, L., & Finegood, D. T. (2001). Beta-cell function and visceral fat in lactating women with a history of gestational diabetes. *Metabolism: Clinical and Experimental, 50*(6), 715-719.

Mezzacappa, E. S., Guethlein, W., & Katkin, E. S. (2002). Breast-feeding and maternal health in online mothers. *Annals of Behavioral Medicine, 24*(4), 299-309.

Michel, S. H., & Mueller, D. H. (1994). Impact of lactation on women with cystic fibrosis and their infants: a review of five cases. *Journal of the American Dietetic Association, 94*(2), 159-165.

Montgomery, A., & Hale, T. W. (2006). ABM clinical protocol #15: analgesia and anesthesia for the breastfeeding mother. *Breastfeeding Medicine, 1*(4), 271-277.

Montz, F. J., Schlaerth, J. B., & Morrow, C. P. (1988). The natural history of theca lutein cysts. *Obstetrics and Gynecology, 72*(2), 247-251.

Moran, M. S., Colasanto, J. M., Haffty, B. G., Wilson, L. D., Lund, M. W., & Higgins, S. A. (2005). Effects of breast-conserving therapy on lactation after pregnancy. *Cancer Journal, 11*(5), 399-403.

Moriuchi, M., & Moriuchi, H. (2006). Induction of lactoferrin gene expression in myeloid or mammary gland cells by human T-cell leukemia virus type 1 (HTLV-1) tax: implications for milk-borne transmission of HTLV-1. *Journal of Virology, 80*(14), 7118-7126.

Murray, L., Woolgar, M., Cooper, P., & Hipwell, A. (2001). Cognitive vulnerability to depression in 5-year-old children of depressed mothers. *Journal of Child Psychology and Psychiatry and Allied Disciplines, 42*(7), 891-899.

Murtaugh, M. A., Ferris, A. M., Capacchione, C. M., & Reece, E. A. (1998). Energy intake and glycemia in lactating women with type 1 diabetes. *Journal of the American Dietetic Association, 98*(6), 642-648.

Nakamura, T. (2001). Studies of colonization of MRSA and normal bacterial flora in the upper airway of extremely low birth weight infants. In *Annual Report: Risk Assessments and Preventive Measure for Nosocomial Infections Including MRSA One in Newborns and Infants* (pp. 27-30).

Nankunda, J., Tylleskar, T., Ndeezi, G., Semiyaga, N., & Tumwine, J. K. (2010). Establishing individual peer counselling for exclusive breastfeeding in Uganda: implications for scaling-up. *Maternal and Child Nutrition, 6*(1), 53-66.

Neifert, M. (1992). Breastfeeding after breast surgical procedure or breast cancer. *NAACOGS Clinical Issues in Perinatal and Womens Health Nursing, 3*(4), 673-682.

Nelson, L. M., Franklin, G. M., & Jones, M. C. (1988). Risk of multiple sclerosis exacerbation during pregnancy and breast-feeding. *Journal of the American Medical Association, 259*(23), 3441-3443.

Neubauer, S. H., Ferris, A. M., Chase, C. G., Fanelli, J., Thompson, C. A., Lammi-Keefe, C. J., et al. (1993). Delayed lactogenesis in women with insulin-dependent diabetes mellitus. *American Journal of Clinical Nutrition, 58*(1), 54-60.

Neville, M. C., McFadden, T. B., & Forsyth, I. (2002). Hormonal regulation of mammary differentiation and milk secretion. *Journal of Mammary Gland Biology and Neoplasia, 7*(1), 49-66.

Newman, J., & Pitman, T. (2006). *The Ultimate Breastfeeding Book of Answers*. New York, New York: Three Rivers Press.

Nicholls, K. R., & Cox, J. L. (1999). The provision of care for women with postnatal mental disorder in the United Kingdom: an overview. *Hong Kong Medical Journal, 5*(1), 43-47.

Nyambi, P. N., Ville, Y., Louwagie, J., Bedjabaga, I., Glowaczower, E., Peeters, M., et al. (1996). Mother-to-child transmission of human T-cell lymphotropic virus types I and II (HTLV-I/II) in Gabon: a prospective follow-up of 4 years. *Journal of Acquired Immune Deficiency Syndromes and Human Retrovirology, 12*(2), 187-192.

Ohlsson, A., Nasiell, J., & von Dobeln, U. (2007). Pregnancy and lactation in a woman with classical galactosaemia heterozygous for p.Q188R and p.R333W. *Journal of Inherited Metabolic Disease, 30*(1), 105.

Oki, T., Yoshinaga, M., Otsuka, H., Miyata, K., Sonoda, S., & Nagata, Y. (1992). A sero-epidemiological study on mother-to-child transmission of HTLV-I in southern Kyushu, Japan. *Asia-Oceania Journal of Obstetrics and Gynaecology, 18*(4), 371-377.

Owen, C. G., Martin, R. M., Whincup, P. H., Smith, G. D., & Cook, D. G. (2006). Does breastfeeding influence risk of type 2 diabetes in later life? A quantitative analysis of published evidence. *American Journal of Clinical Nutrition, 84*(5), 1043-1054.

Pang, W. W., & Hartmann, P. E. (2007). Initiation of human lactation: secretory differentiation and secretory activation. *Journal of Mammary Gland Biology and Neoplasia, 12*(4), 211-221.

Parker, E. M., O'Sullivan, B. P., Shea, J. C., Regan, M. M., & Freedman, S. D. (2004). Survey of breast-feeding practices and outcomes in the cystic fibrosis population. *Pediatric Pulmonology, 37*(4), 362-367.

Pennypacker, C., Perelson, A. S., Nys, N., Nelson, G., & Sessler, D. I. (1995). Localized or systemic in vivo heat inactivation of human immunodeficiency virus (HIV): a mathematical analysis. *Journal of Acquired Immune Deficiency Syndromes and Human Retrovirology, 8*(4), 321-329.

Penovich, P. E., Eck, K. E., & Economou, V. V. (2004). Recommendations for the care of women with epilepsy. *Cleveland Clinic Journal of Medicine, 71 Suppl 2*, S49-57.

Perez-Bravo, F., Carrasco, E., Gutierrez-Lopez, M. D., Martinez, M. T., Lopez, G., & de los Rios, M. G. (1996). Genetic predisposition and environmental factors leading to the development of insulin-dependent diabetes mellitus in Chilean children. *Journal of Molecular Medicine, 74*(2), 105-109.

Philipp, M., Kohnen, R., & Hiller, K. O. (1999). Hypericum extract versus imipramine or placebo in patients with moderate depression: randomised multicentre study of treatment for eight weeks. *British Medical Journal, 319*(7224), 1534-1538.

Pickering, L. K., Morrow, A. L., Herrera, I., O'Ryan, M., Estes, M. K., Guilliams, S. E., et al. (1995). Effect of maternal rotavirus immunization on milk and serum antibody titers. *Journal of Infectious Diseases, 172*(3), 723-728.

Pikwer, M., Bergstrom, U., Nilsson, J. A., Jacobsson, L., Berglund, G., & Turesson, C. (2009). Breast feeding, but not use of oral contraceptives, is associated with a reduced risk of rheumatoid arthritis. *Annals of the Rheumatic Diseases, 68*(4), 526-530.

Pisacane, A., Impagliazzo, N., Russo, M., Valiani, R., Mandarini, A., Florio, C., et al. (1994). Breast feeding and multiple sclerosis. *British Medical Journal, 308*(6941), 1411-1412.

Prentice, J. C., Lu, M. C., Lange, L., & Halfon, N. (2002). The association between reported childhood sexual abuse and breastfeeding initiation. *Journal of Human Lactation, 18*(3), 219-226.

Pschirrer, E. R. (2004). Seizure disorders in pregnancy. *Obstetrics and Gynecology Clinics of North America, 31*(2), 373-384, vii.

Purnell, H. (2001). Phenylketonuria and maternal phenylketonuria. *Breastfeeding Review, 9*(2), 19-21.

Ram, K. T., Bobby, P., Hailpern, S. M., Lo, J. C., Schocken, M., Skurnick, J., et al. (2008). Duration of lactation is associated with lower prevalence of the metabolic syndrome in midlife--SWAN, the study of women's health across the nation. *American Journal of Obstetrics and Gynecology, 198*(3), 268 e261-266.

Rapkin, A. J., Mikacich, J. A., Moatakef-Imani, B., & Rasgon, N. (2002). The clinical nature and formal diagnosis of premenstrual, postpartum, and perimenopausal affective disorders. *Curr Psychiatry Rep, 4*(6), 419-428.

Reaven, G. M. (2007). The individual components of the metabolic syndrome: is there a raison d'etre? *Journal of the American College of Nutrition, 26*(3), 191-195.

Riordan, J. (2010). Women's health and breastfeeding. In J. Riordan & K. Wambach (Eds.), *Breastfeeding and Human Lactation* (4th ed., pp. 519-549). Boston, MA: Jones and Bartlett.

Riviello, C., Mello, G., & Jovanovic, L. G. (2009). Breastfeeding and the basal insulin requirement in type 1 diabetic women. *Endocrine Practice, 15*(3), 187-193.

Robinson, P. S., Barker, P., Campbell, A., Henson, P., Surveyor, I., & Young, P. R. (1994). Iodine-131 in breast milk following therapy for thyroid carcinoma. *Journal of Nuclear Medicine, 35*(11), 1797-1801.

Rose, M. R., Prescott, M. C., & Herman, K. J. (1990). Excretion of iodine-123-hippuran, technetium-99m-red blood cells, and technetium-99m-macroaggregated albumin into breast milk. *Journal of Nuclear Medicine, 31*(6), 978-984.

Rosenbauer, J., Herzig, P., & Giani, G. (2008). Early infant feeding and risk of type 1 diabetes mellitus-a nationwide population-based case-control study in pre-school children. *Diabetes/Metabolism Research and Reviews, 24*(3), 211-222.

Ruiz-Extremera, A., Salmeron, J., Torres, C., De Rueda, P. M., Gimenez, F., Robles, C., et al. (2000). Follow-up of transmission of hepatitis C to babies of human immunodeficiency virus-negative women: the role of breast-feeding in transmission. *Pediatric Infectious Disease Journal, 19*(6), 511-516.

Rupke, S. J., Blecke, D., & Renfrow, M. (2006). Cognitive therapy for depression. *American Family Physician, 73*(1), 83-86.

Sadauskaite-Kuehne, V., Ludvigsson, J., Padaiga, Z., Jasinskiene, E., & Samuelsson, U. (2004). Longer breastfeeding is an independent protective factor against development of type 1 diabetes mellitus in childhood. *Diabetes/Metabolism Research and Reviews, 20*(2), 150-157.

Saenz, R. B. (2000). Iodine-131 elimination from breast milk: a case report. *Journal of Human Lactation, 16*(1), 44-46.

Salgado, C. D., Farr, B. M., & Calfee, D. P. (2003). Community-acquired methicillin-resistant Staphylococcus aureus: a meta-analysis of prevalence and risk factors. *Clinical Infectious Diseases, 36*(2), 131-139.

Sances, G., Granella, F., Nappi, R. E., Fignon, A., Ghiotto, N., Polatti, F., et al. (2003). Course of migraine during pregnancy and postpartum: a prospective study. *Cephalalgia, 23*(3), 197-205.

Schanler, R. J. (2005). CMV acquisition in premature infants fed human milk: reason to worry? *Journal of Perinatology, 25*(5), 297-298.

Schleiss, M. R. (2006). Acquisition of human cytomegalovirus infection in infants via breast milk: natural immunization or cause for concern? *Reviews in Medical Virology, 16*(2), 73-82.

Schwarz, E. B., McClure, C. K., Tepper, P. G., Thurston, R., Janssen, I., Matthews, K. A., et al. (2010). Lactation and maternal measures of subclinical cardiovascular disease. *Obstetrics and Gynecology, 115*(1), 41-48.

Schwarz, E. B., Ray, R. M., Stuebe, A. M., Allison, M. A., Ness, R. B., Freiberg, M. S., et al. (2009). Duration of lactation and risk factors for maternal cardiovascular disease. *Obstetrics and Gynecology, 113*(5), 974-982.

Sealander, J. Y., & Kerr, C. P. (1989). Herpes simplex of the nipple: infant-to-mother transmission. *American Family Physician, 39*(3), 111-113.

Shahbazian, H. B., Sarvghadi, F., & Azizi, F. (2001). Prevalence and characteristics of postpartum thyroid dysfunction in Tehran. *European Journal of Endocrinology / European Federation of Endocrine Societies, 145*(4), 397-401.

Shahid, N. S., Steinhoff, M. C., Hoque, S. S., Begum, T., Thompson, C., & Siber, G. R. (1995). Serum, breast milk, and infant antibody after maternal immunisation with pneumococcal vaccine. *Lancet, 346*(8985), 1252-1257.

Shiffman, M. L., Seale, T. W., Flux, M., Rennert, O. R., & Swender, P. T. (1989). Breast-milk composition in women with cystic fibrosis: report of two cases and a review of the literature. *American Journal of Clinical Nutrition, 49*(4), 612-617.

Simard, J. F., Karlson, E. W., Costenbader, K. H., Hernan, M. A., Stampfer, M. J., Liang, M. H., et al. (2008). Perinatal factors and adult-onset lupus. *Arthritis and Rheumatism, 59*(8), 1155-1161.

Simmons, D., Conroy, C., & Thompson, C. F. (2005). In-hospital breast feeding rates among women with gestational diabetes and pregestational Type 2 diabetes in South Auckland. *Diabetic Medicine, 22*(2), 177-181.

Sirota, L., Ferrera, M., Lerer, N., & Dulitzky, F. (1992). Beta glucuronidase and hyperbilirubinaemia in breast fed infants of diabetic mothers. *Archives of Disease in Childhood, 67*(1), 120-121.

Skrodeniene, E., Marciulionyte, D., Padaiga, Z., Jasinskiene, E., Sadauskaite-Kuehne, V., & Ludvigsson, J. (2008). Environmental risk factors in prediction of childhood prediabetes. *Medicina (Kaunas), 44*(1), 56-63.

Snell, N. J., Coysh, H. L., & Snell, B. J. (1980). Carpal tunnel syndrome presenting in the puerperium. *Practitioner, 224*(1340), 191-193.

Stafford, I., Hernandez, J., Laibl, V., Sheffield, J., Roberts, S., & Wendel, G., Jr. (2008). Community-acquired methicillin-resistant Staphylococcus aureus among patients with puerperal mastitis requiring hospitalization. *Obstetrics and Gynecology, 112*(3), 533-537.

Stage, E., Norgard, H., Damm, P., & Mathiesen, E. (2006). Long-term breast-feeding in women with type 1 diabetes. *Diabetes Care, 29*(4), 771-774.

Stuebe, A. M., Rich-Edwards, J. W., Willett, W. C., Manson, J. E., & Michels, K. B. (2005). Duration of lactation and incidence of type 2 diabetes. *Journal of the American Medical Association, 294*(20), 2601-2610.

Sullivan-Bolyai, J,Z., Fife, K.H., Jacobs, R.F., Miller, Z., & Corey L. (1983). Disseminated neonatal herpes simplex virus type 1 from a maternal breast lesion. *Pediatrics,* 71:455-57.

Sullivan-Bolyai, J., Hull, H. F., Wilson, C., & Corey, L. (1983). Neonatal herpes simplex virus infection in King County, Washington, increasing incidence and epidemiologic correlates. *Journal of the American Medical Association, 250*(22), 3059-3062. Szegedi, A., Kohnen, R., Dienel, A., & Kieser, M. (2005). Acute treatment of moderate to severe depression with hypericum extract WS 5570 (St John's wort): randomised controlled double blind non-inferiority trial versus paroxetine. *British Medical Journal, 330*(7490), 503.

Tajima, K. (1988). Malignant lymphomas in Japan: epidemiological analysis of adult T-cell leukemia/lymphoma (ATL). *Cancer and Metastasis Reviews, 7*(3), 223-241.

Takahashi, K., Takezaki, T., Oki, T., Kawakami, K., Yashiki, S., Fujiyoshi, T., et al. (1991). Inhibitory effect of maternal antibody on mother-to-child transmission of human T-lymphotropic virus type I. The Mother-to-Child Transmission Study Group. *International Journal of Cancer, 49*(5), 673-677.

Takezaki, T., Tajima, K., Ito, M., Ito, S., Kinoshita, K., Tachibana, K., et al. (1997). Short-term breast-feeding may reduce the risk of vertical transmission of HTLV-I. The Tsushima ATL Study Group. *Leukemia, 11 Suppl 3*, 60-62.

Tamminen, T. M., & Salmelin, R. K. (1991). Psychosomatic interaction between mother and infant during breast feeding. *Psychotherapy and Psychosomatics, 56*(1-2), 78-84.

Tenconi, M. T., Devoti, G., Comelli, M., Pinon, M., Capocchiano, A., Calcaterra, V., et al. (2007). Major childhood infectious diseases and other determinants associated with type 1 diabetes: a case-control study. *Acta Diabetologica, 44*(1), 14-19.

Terhaar, M. F., & Kaut, K. (1993). Perinatal superior sagittal sinus venous thrombosis. *Journal of Perinatal and Neonatal Nursing, 7*(1), 35-48.

Thior, I., Lockman, S., Smeaton, L. M., Shapiro, R. L., Wester, C., Heymann, S. J., et al. (2006). Breastfeeding plus infant zidovudine prophylaxis for 6 months vs formula feeding plus infant zidovudine for 1 month to reduce mother-to-child HIV transmission in Botswana: a randomized trial: the Mashi Study. *Journal of the American Medical Association, 296*(7), 794-805.

Thomson, V. M. (1995). Breastfeeding and mothering one-handed. *Journal of Human Lactation, 11*(3), 211-215.

Thorley, V. (1997a). Lactational headache: a lactation consultant's diary. *Journal of Human Lactation, 13*(1), 51-53.

Thorley, V. (1997b). Lactational headaches. *Breastfeeding Review, 5*(1), 23-25.

Tralins, A. H. (1995). Lactation after conservative breast surgery combined with radiation therapy. *American Journal of Clinical Oncology, 18*(1), 40-43.

Tsuji, Y., Doi, H., Yamabe, T., Ishimaru, T., Miyamoto, T., & Hino, S. (1990). Prevention of mother-to-child transmission of human T-lymphotropic virus type-I. *Pediatrics, 86*(1), 11-17.

Uvnas-Moberg, K. (1998). Antistress Pattern Induced by Oxytocin. *News in Physiological Sciences, 13*, 22-25.

van Gurp, G., Meterissian, G. B., Haiek, L. N., McCusker, J., & Bellavance, F. (2002). St John's wort or sertraline? Randomized controlled trial in primary care. *Canadian Family Physician, 48*, 905-912.

Vanky, E., Isaksen, H., Moen, M. H., & Carlsen, S. M. (2008). Breastfeeding in polycystic ovary syndrome. *Acta Obstetricia et Gynecologica Scandinavica, 87*(5), 531-535.

Vergeront, J. M., Evenson, M. L., Crass, B. A., Davis, J. P., Bergdoll, M. S., Wand, P. J., et al. (1982). Recovery of staphylococcal enterotoxin F from the breast milk of a woman with toxic-shock syndrome. *Journal of Infectious Diseases, 146*(4), 456-459.

Viner, R. M., Hindmarsh, P. C., Taylor, B., & Cole, T. J. (2008). Childhood body mass index (BMI), breastfeeding and risk of Type 1 diabetes: findings from a longitudinal national birth cohort. *Diabetic Medicine, 25*(9), 1056-1061.

Vukusic, S., & Confavreux, C. (2006). Pregnancy and multiple sclerosis: the children of PRIMS. *Clinical Neurology and Neurosurgery, 108*(3), 266-270.

Walker, M. (2006). *Breastfeeding Management for the Clinician: Using the Evidence*. Boston, MA: Jones and Bartlett.

Wall, V. R. (1992). Breastfeeding and migraine headaches. *Journal of Human Lactation, 8*(4), 209-212.

Wand, J. S. (1989). The natural history of carpal tunnel syndrome in lactation. *Journal of the Royal Society of Medicine, 82*(6), 349-350.

Wand, J. S. (1990). Carpal tunnel syndrome in pregnancy and lactation. *Journal of Hand Surgery. British Volume, 15*(1), 93-95.

Wang, L. Y., Chen, C. T., Liu, W. H., & Wang, Y. H. (2007). Recurrent neonatal group B streptococcal disease associated with infected breast milk. *Clinical Pediatrics, 46*(6), 547-549.

Webster, J., Moore, K., & McMullan, A. (1995). Breastfeeding outcomes for women with insulin dependent diabetes. *Journal of Human Lactation, 11*(3), 195-200.

Weissman, M. M. (2007). Recent non-medication trials of interpersonal psychotherapy for depression. *International Journal of Neuropsychopharmacology, 10*(1), 117-122.

Welch, M. J., Phelps, D. L., & Osher, A. B. (1981). Breast-feeding by a mother with cystic fibrosis. *Pediatrics, 67*(5), 664-666.

West, D., & Marasco, L. (2009). *The Breastfeeding Mother's Guide to Making More Milk*. New York, NY: McGraw Hill.

Whitehead, E., Dodds, L., Joseph, K. S., Gordon, K. E., Wood, E., Allen, A. C., et al. (2006). Relation of pregnancy and neonatal factors to subsequent development of childhood epilepsy: a population-based cohort study. *Pediatrics, 117*(4), 1298-1306.

WHO. (2007). *Guidance on Global Scale-Up of the Prevention of Mother-to-Child Transmission of HIV*. Geneva, Switzerland: World Health Organization.

Wiktor, S. Z., Pate, E. J., Murphy, E. L., Palker, T. J., Champegnie, E., Ramlal, A., et al. (1993). Mother-to-child transmission of human T-cell lymphotropic virus type I (HTLV-I) in Jamaica: association with antibodies to envelope glycoprotein (gp46) epitopes. *Journal of Acquired Immune Deficiency Syndromes, 6*(10), 1162-1167.

Woelk, H. (2000). Comparison of St John's wort and imipramine for treating depression: randomised controlled trial. *British Medical Journal, 321*(7260), 536-539.

Yagnik, P. M. (1987). Carpal tunnel syndrome in nursing mothers. *Southern Medical Journal, 80*(11), 1468.

Yerby, M. S., Kaplan, P., & Tran, T. (2004). Risks and management of pregnancy in women with epilepsy. *Cleveland Clinic Journal of Medicine, 71 Suppl 2*, S25-37.

Techniques

Appendix A

REVERSE PRESSURE SOFTENING

Developed by U.S. lactation consultant and nurse Jean Cotterman, Reverse Pressure Softening (or RPS for short) can be used any time a mother's areola is so firm that breastfeeding or milk expression is challenging (Cotterman, 2004). This technique is used most often in the early days after birth when a mother's breasts are swollen from excess IV fluids received during labor or when she is engorged (see p. 677- "Engorgement"). But RPS can also be used any time a mother's breasts feel very full or to trigger milk ejection before milk expression.

Reverse Pressure Softening can be used to ease engorgement and help the baby achieve deep breastfeeding.

Reverse Pressure Softening applies gentle pressure to the mother's areola to soften it by moving the swelling (edema) farther back into the breast. With the areola soft and the swelling out of the way, the baby can take the breast deeper and the mother has easier access to her milk during milk expression.

NOTE: The one-page handout on p. 796 was written by Jean Cotterman for those helping breastfeeding mothers.

The two-sided handout on pages 797-798 was written for mothers.

Both of the handouts can be photocopied freely and distributed without further permission needed as long as the request at the end of the handout is honored.

Reverse Pressure Softening

-developed by K. Jean Cotterman RNC-E, IBCLC (mellomom@gmail.com)

Try this if pain, swelling, or fullness creates problems during the early weeks of learning to breastfeed.

The key is making the areola very soft right around the base of the nipple for better latching.

- A softer areola protects the nipple deep in baby's mouth, helping his tongue remove milk better.
- Mothers say curved fingers work best (Fig. A.1 or A.2).
- Press inward toward the chest wall and count slowly to 50.
- Pressure should be steady and firm, and gentle enough to avoid pain.
- If mom wishes, someone else may help, using thumbs (Fig. A.3).
- (For long fingernails, try another way shown below.)
- If breasts are quite large or very swollen, count very slowly, with mom lying down on her back. This delays return of swelling to the areola, giving more time to latch.
- Soften the areola right before each feeding (or pumping) till swelling goes away. For some mothers, this takes 2-4 days.
- Make any pumping sessions short, with pauses to re-soften the areola if needed.
- Use medium or low vacuum, to reduce the return of swelling into the areola.

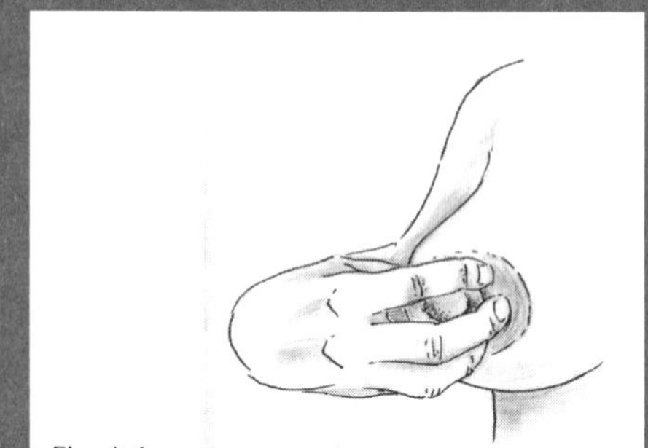

Fig. A.1

One handed "flower hold": Fingernails short, Fingertips curved, placed where baby's tongue will go.

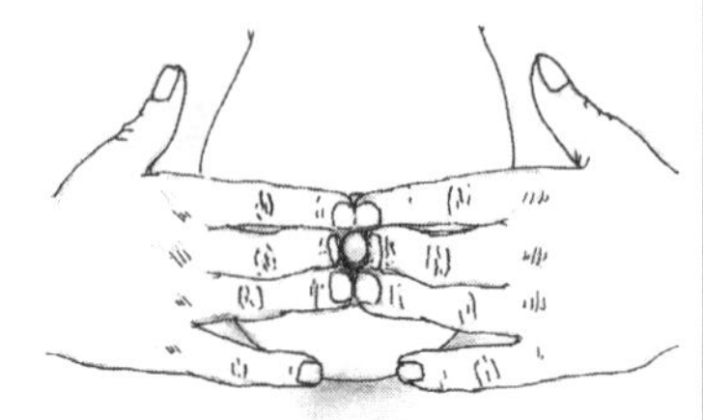

Fig. A.2

Two handed, one-step method: Fingernails short, Fingertips curved, each one touching the side of the nipple.

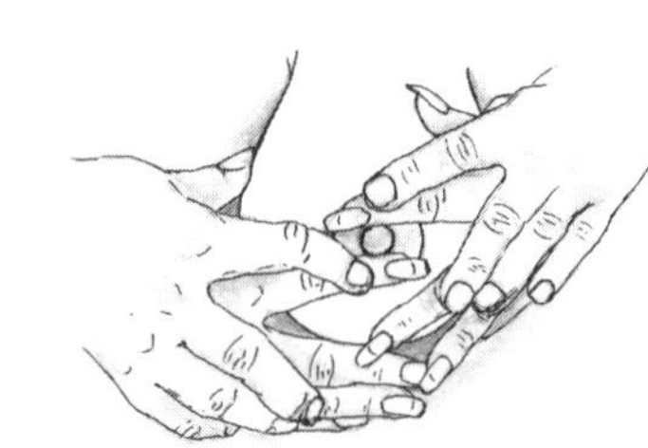

Fig. A.3

You may ask someone to help press by placing fingers or thumbs on top of yours.

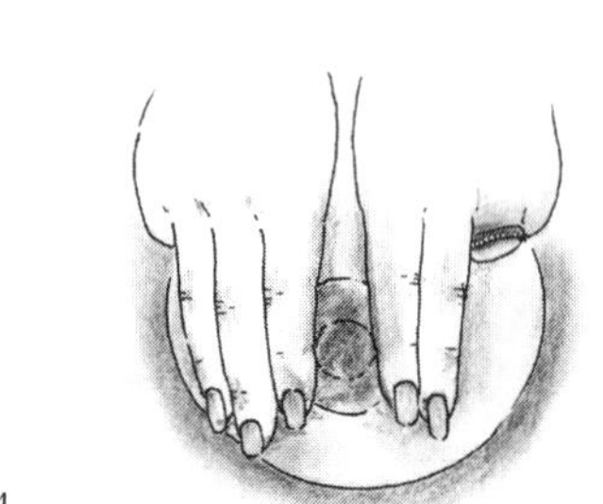

Fig. A.4

Two step method, two hands: using 2 or 3 straight fingers each side, first knuckles touching nipple. Move ¼ turn, repeat above & below nipple.

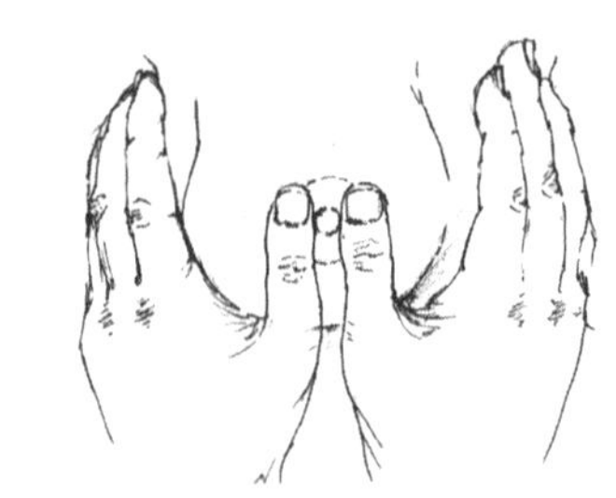

Fig. A.5

Two step method, two hands: using straight thumbs, base of thumbnail at side of nipple. Move ¼ turn, repeat, thumbs above & below nipple.

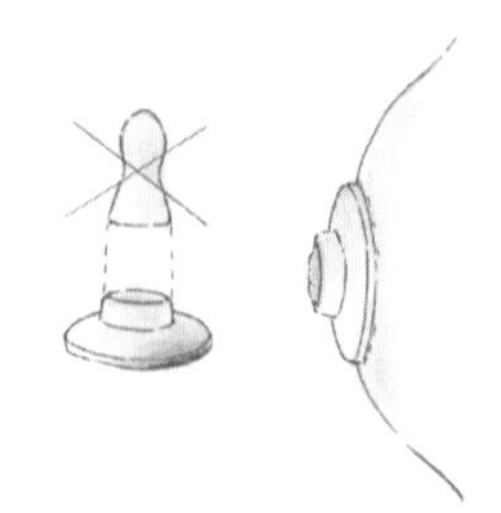

Fig. A.6

Soft ring method: Cut off bottom half of an artificial nipple to place on areola to press with fingers.

Reverse Pressure Softening

K. Jean Cotterman RNC, IBCLC, (mellomom@juno.com)

What is it?

REVERSE PRESSURE SOFTENING is a new way to soften the **circle around your nipple (the a-re-o-la)** to make latching and getting your milk out easy while your baby and you are learning. **LATCHING SHOULDN'T BE PAINFUL.** If your **areola** is soft enough to **change shape** while feeding, it helps your baby **gently extend your nipple deep inside his mouth,** so his tongue and jaws can press on milk ducts under the **areola**.

(**These motions differ from those which artificial nipples force a baby to use.**)

This new method is **NOT THE SAME** as removing milk with your fingers. **DON'T EXPECT MILK TO COME FROM YOUR NIPPLE** while you soften your **areola** this way. (But it's OK if some milk does come out.)

When is it helpful?

Try **REVERSE PRESSURE SOFTENING** in the early days after birth if you begin to notice firmness of the **areola**, latch pain or breast fullness. (This full feeling is **only partly due to milk.** Delayed or skipped feedings may also cause **the tissue around your milk ducts** to hold extra fluid much like a sponge does**. This fluid never goes to your baby.**) **Intravenous (IV) fluids**, or drugs such as **pitocin** may cause even more retained tissue fluid, which often takes **7-14 days** to go away**. Avoid long pumping sessions and high vacuum settings on breast pumps to prevent extra swelling of the areola itself.**

Feel your **areola and the tissue deeper inside it**. Is it soft and easy to squeeze, like **your earlobe or your lip?** Or does it feel **FIRMER and harder to compress, like your chin?** If so, it's time to try **REVERSE PRESSURE SOFTENING** just before each time you offer your baby your breast. (Some mothers soften their **areola** before feeding, for a week or longer, till swelling goes down, baby can be heard swallowing milk regularly, and latching is always painfree without softening first.)

Why does it work?

REVERSE PRESSURE SOFTENING briefly moves some swelling **backward and upward into your breast** to soften your **areola** so it can change shape and extend your nipple. It sends a **special signal to the back of your breasts to start moving milk forward (let-down reflex)** where your baby's tongue can reach it. It also makes it easy to remove milk with your fingertips or with **SHORT PERIODS OF SLOW GENTLE PUMPING,** combined with gentle forward massage of the upper breast, if you need to remove milk for your baby.

Where should I press?

It is most important to soften the **areola** in the whole **1-inch area all around where it joins your nipple.** Soften even more of the **areola** if you wish. You may also want to soften a place where your baby's chin will be able to move easily against the breast. **REVERSE PRESSURE SOFTENING** should cause **NO DISCOMFORT.**

(OVER)

How do I do REVERSE PRESSURE SOFTENING?

K. Jean Cotterman RNC, IBCLC (mellomom@juno.com)
Illustrations by Kyle Cotterman, Dayton, Ohio

- You (or your helper, from in front, or behind you) choose one of the patterns pictured.
- Place the fingers/thumbs on the circle **touching the nipple.**
- (If swelling is very firm, lie down on your back, and/or ask someone to help by pressing his or her fingers on top of your fingers.)
- Push **gently but firmly** straight inward toward your ribs.
- Hold the pressure **steady** for a period of **1 to 3 full minutes.**
- Relax, breathe easy, sing a lullaby, listen to a favorite song or have someone else watch a clock or set a timer. To see your **areola** better, try using a hand mirror.
- It's OK to repeat the inward pressure again as often as you need. Deep "dimples" may form, lasting long enough for easy latching. Keep testing how soft your **areola** feels.
- You may also press with a soft ring made by cutting off half of an artificial nipple.
- Offer your baby your breast promptly while the circle is soft.

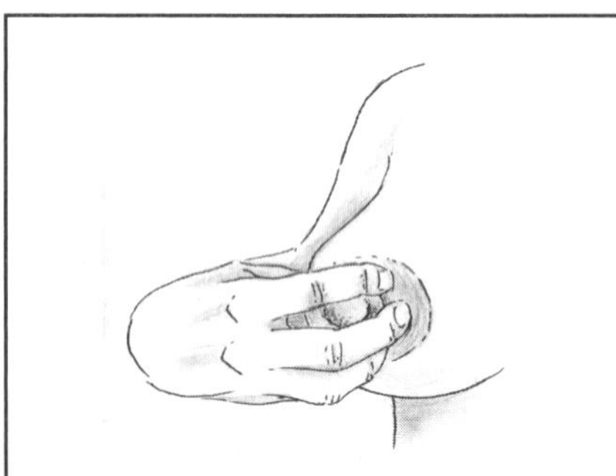

One handed "flower hold": Fingernails short, Fingertips curved, placed where baby's tongue will go

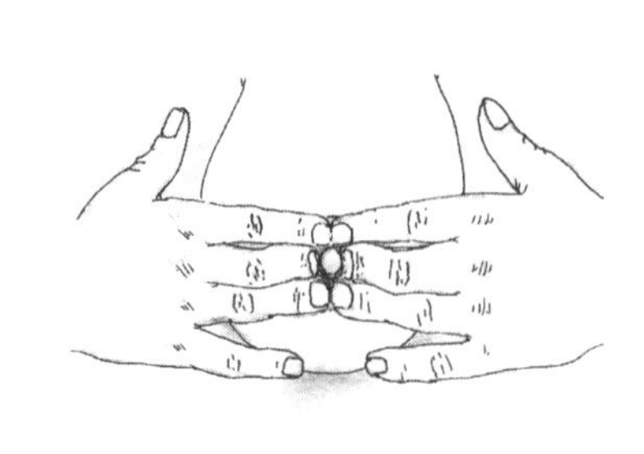

Two handed, one-step method: Fingernails short, Fingertips curved, each one touching the side of the nipple

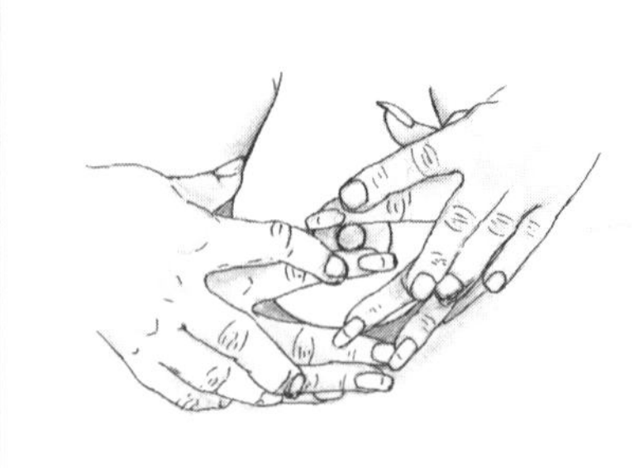

You may ask someone to help press by placing fingers or thumbs on top of yours

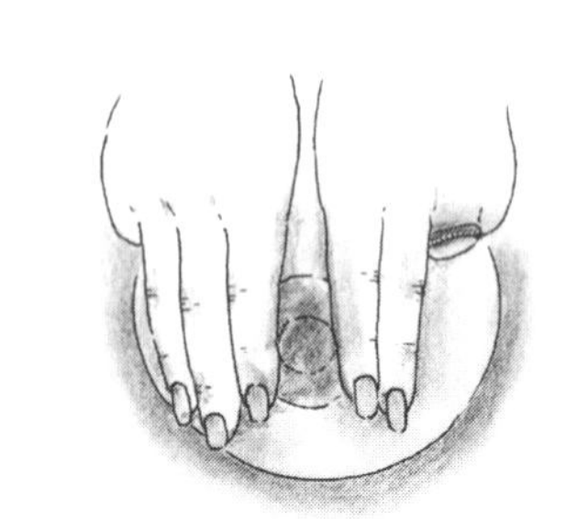

Two step method, two hands: using 2 or 3 straight fingers each side, first knuckles touching nipple. Move ¼ turn, repeat above & below nipple

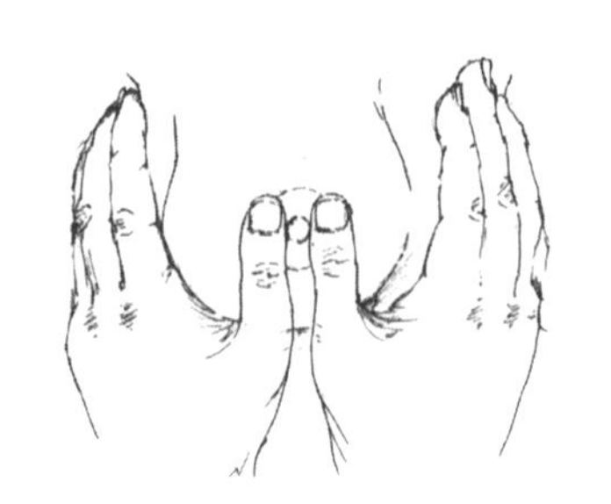

Two step method, two hands: using straight thumbs, base of thumbnail at side of nipple. Move ¼ turn, repeat, thumbs above & below nipple

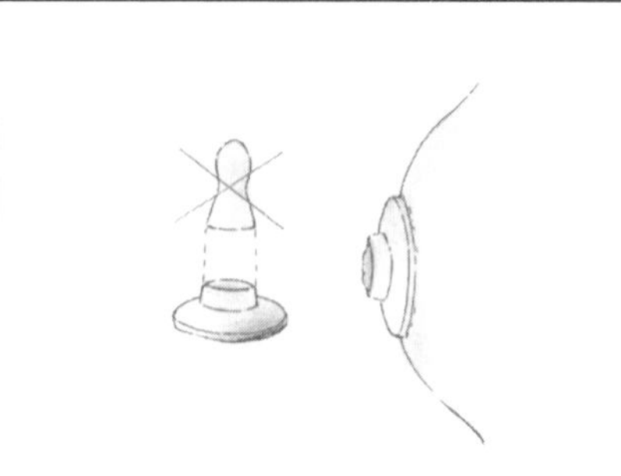

Soft ring method: Cut off bottom half of an artificial nipple to place on areola to press with fingers

ASYMMETRICAL LATCH

When a baby is breastfeeding deeply and well, on average, the mother's nipple extends to within 5 mm of where the baby's hard and soft palates meet (Jacobs, Dickinson, Hart, Doherty, & Faulkner, 2007). Some call this area in the back of the baby's mouth the "comfort zone," because in most cases, when the nipple reaches this area, breastfeeding is comfortable and effective (Mohrbacher & Kendall-Tackett, 2010).

The "asymmetrical latch" is one strategy used to achieve deep breastfeeding, but it is only used and makes sense in parts of the world where the "centered" or "bull's-eye" latch was once taught, such as the U.S. and Canada. In Australia and the U.K., for example, asymmetrical latch (or attachment) is assumed, because mothers and breastfeeding supporters never taught mothers to center their nipple in the baby's mouth.

The "working jaw." During an "asymmetrical latch," the baby takes the breast "off-center," with his lower jaw taking more breast than his upper jaw (Figure A.7). This allows the nipple to extend deeper into the baby's mouth, which makes breastfeeding more comfortable and effective. One Japanese study found that shallow breastfeeding drained the breast unevenly, with some lobes left fuller, while others were well-drained. Deep breastfeeding, on the other hand, drained the breast evenly (Mizuno et al., 2008).

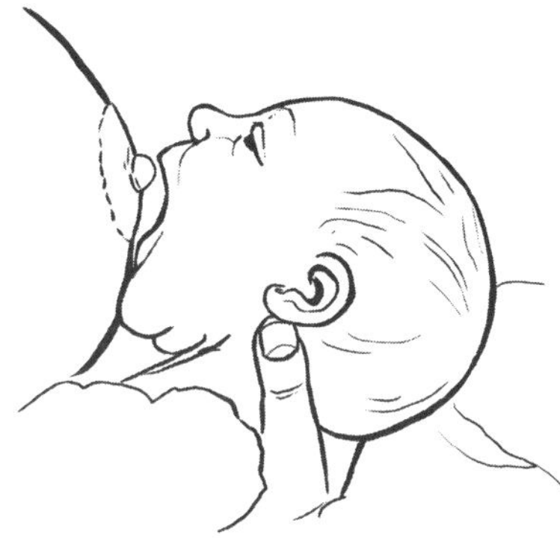

Figure A.7. Baby's lower jaw lands on the breast off-center for an asymmetrical latch.

©2010 Anna Mohrbacher, used with permission.

To understand this better, notice how only the lower jaw moves during talking or eating. The same is true during breastfeeding, which is why some refer to the lower jaw as the "working jaw" (Wiessinger, 1998). The lower jaw does all the work of feeding, while the upper jaw simply keeps the breast in place. The further away from the nipple the lower jaw lands when baby takes the breast, the further back in his mouth the nipple can extend.

The lower jaw does all the work during feeding.

As described in Chapter 1, the breastfeeding positions a mother uses can make achieving deep breastfeeding easier or more difficult, especially during the early weeks. When a mother leans back in semi-reclined positions with the baby tummy down on her body, gravity naturally keeps baby's head, chin, and torso in constant contact with hers (Figure A.8). This mother-baby body contact is the trigger for baby's inborn feeding behaviors, including rooting, opening wide, and taking the breast. In these laid-back positions, when the baby opens wide and takes the breast, gravity pulls the baby's head down to help him get further onto the breast, making it easier for the nipple to extend into the comfort zone.

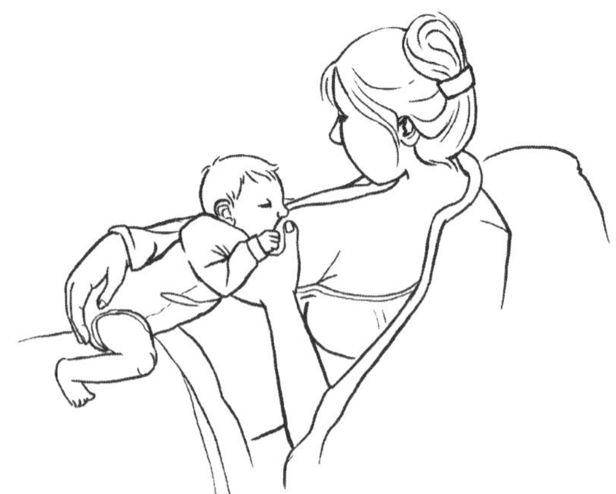

Figure A.8. Laid-back breastfeeding (semi-reclined).

©2010 Anna Mohrbacher, used with permission.

The laid-back breastfeeding position can help the baby acheive deeper breastfeeding.

In a semi-reclined breastfeeding position, the baby is completely supported tummy down on his mother's body, so he can take an active role in going to the breast and adjust his body position until he's in a good relationship to the nipple (Colson, Meek, & Hawdon, 2008). In an upright feeding position, gravity pulls the baby's body away from the breast, so the mother needs to provide much more help. Taking the breast in an upright position can be trickier, especially during the early weeks. The mother needs to support the baby's body, either with her arms or with pillows. She needs to make sure his body is in good alignment with the breast (see below). She needs to keep his body pressed against hers to trigger his inborn feeding behaviors, so he opens wide. And as he opens wide and takes the breast, she needs to provide a gentle push at just the right moment to help him further onto the breast so that her nipple reaches the comfort zone.

To achieve deep breastfeeding in an upright position, suggest the mother:

1. Start by aligning the baby's body with the breast so that the baby is "nose to nipple" (Figure A.9), supporting the baby's shoulders and neck, so his head can tilt back slightly (the "instinctive feeding position").
2. Make sure the baby's chin, torso, hips, legs, and feet are pulled in close with the baby's whole body touching the mother (no gaps between them).
3. Wait until the stimulation of the baby's chin and torso against the breast triggers a wide open mouth (Figure A.10).
4. As the baby moves toward the breast, apply gentle pressure on the baby's back and shoulders (avoid pushing on baby's head) to help him get onto the breast deeply, so the nipple extends back to the comfort zone (Figure A.11).

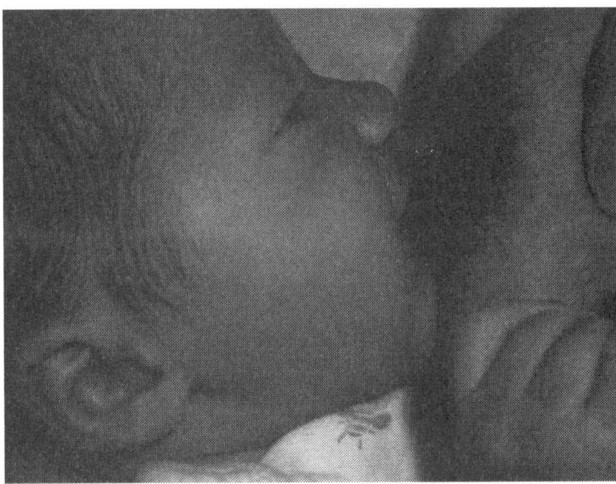

Figure A.9. Nose to nipple.

©Catherine Watson Genna, BS, IBCLC, used with permission

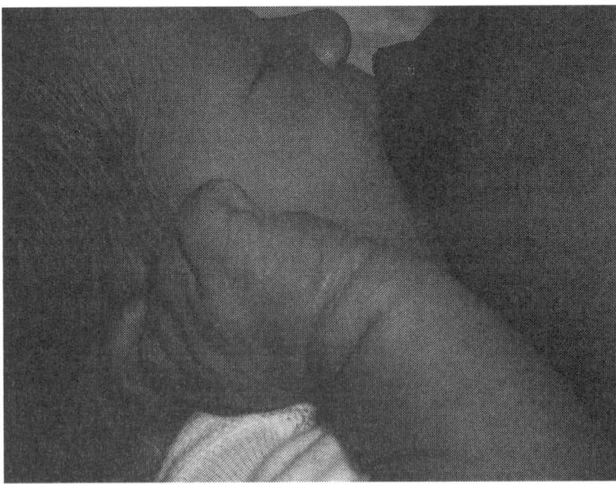

Figure A.10. Baby's lower jaw lands on the breast off-center, well away from the nipple.

©Catherine Watson Genna, BS, IBCLC, used with permission

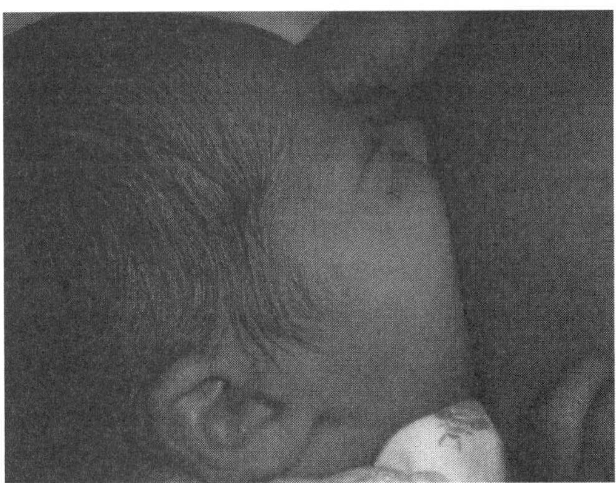

Figure A.11. Baby takes a big mouthful of breast.

©Catherine Watson Genna, BS, IBCLC, used with permission

Approaching the breast "nose to nipple" allows the baby to take enough of the areola below the nipple (3 to 4 cm) into his mouth so that the nipple can extend back into the comfort zone (Glover & Wiessinger, 2008). If the baby takes the breast with his lower jaw at nipple level, shallow breastfeeding is more likely, because at that angle, the nipple can't stretch back far enough. The baby who approaches the breast with his head tilted forward instead of slightly back is at the same disadvantage, because this angle tilts his lower jaw away from the breast.

BREAST SHAPING

Breast shaping can also help the baby take the breast more deeply.

When a baby has trouble taking the breast deeply, breast-shaping techniques can sometimes make it easier for him to get a bigger mouthful of breast so the nipple can extend into the comfort zone (see previous section). Breast sandwich and nipple tilting are two breast-shaping techniques that can help some mothers and babies.

Breast Sandwich

Using this technique, the mother shapes her breast by gently squeezing the tissue near the areola (fingers on one side of the breast and thumb on the other) to narrow the shape of the breast and make it easier for the baby's lower jaw to land further back (Wilson-Clay & Hoover, 2008). This technique can be especially helpful for the mother with firm breast tissue, either naturally occurring or from engorgement or breast swelling from excess IV fluids during labor. It can also be helpful during the newborn period for any mother and baby having breastfeeding difficulties.

For the breast sandwich technique to help, the oval of the compressed breast must match the oval of the baby's mouth—wider at the corners and narrower between upper and lower lips. If the directions of these two ovals do not match, breast shaping can make breastfeeding more difficult rather than easier.

There are a couple of ways to explain where to gently squeeze the breast that may make this concept easier for mothers to grasp. Suggest the mother:

- Imagine how she takes a bite out of a sandwich. First she lines it up horizontally with her mouth, so its narrowest part runs parallel to her lips to make it easier to take a big bite (Wiessinger, 1998). Think about how much harder it would be to take a bite if the mother rotated the sandwich 90º and it was perpendicular to her mouth. The same is true with the breast.
- Think of either her thumb or fingers (whichever is closest to where her baby's upper lip will land) as a "mustache" for her baby. In other words, for the breast and mouth ovals to align in the same direction, her thumb and fingers should run parallel to the baby's lips (Figure A.12).

When forming a "breast sandwich," it's also important for the mother to keep her fingers far enough back on the breast, so they don't get in baby's way as he latches on.

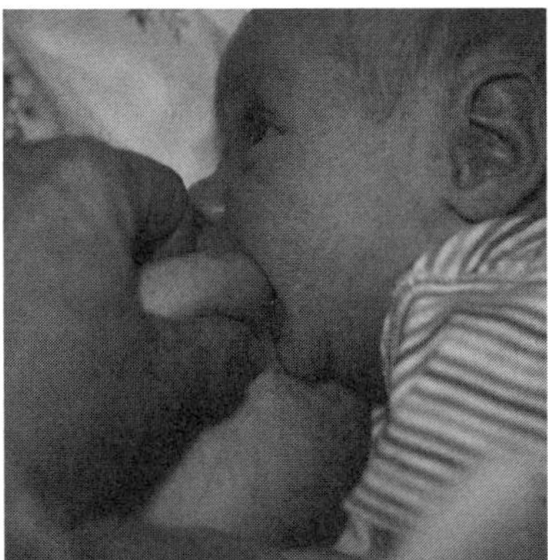

Figure A.12. Breast sandwich can help baby's lower jaw take more breast.

©Wilson-Clay and Hoover, The Breastfeeding Atlas, 4th ed. 2008

Nipple Tilting

"Nipple tilting" (sometimes called "The Flipple") is a breast-shaping strategy developed by Rebecca Glover, an Australian midwife and lactation consultant, which can sometimes make it easier for the baby's lower "working" jaw to land further back on the breast for deeper breastfeeding (Glover & Wiessinger, 2008). To use this technique:

- With the baby's body pulled in close to the mother and his chin touching the breast, the mother presses on her breast just above the nipple with a thumb or finger running parallel to the baby's upper lip, pointing the nipple up and away from the baby (Figure A.13).
- The touch of the breast on her baby's chin triggers a wide-open mouth (gape).
- The mother then presses this thumb or finger into the breast to help roll the underside of the breast into baby's wide-open mouth.
- As the breast enters the baby's mouth, she can use this finger to gently push the nipple inside the baby's upper gum before removing her finger.

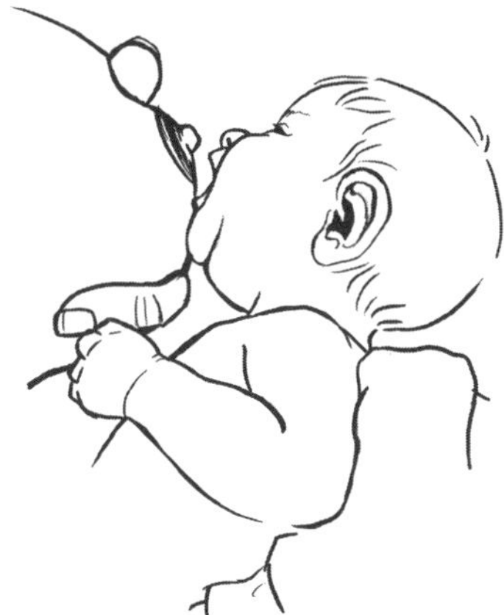

Figure A.13. Nipple tilting

©2010 Anna Mohrbacher, used with permission

BREAST COMPRESSION

Breast compression and alternate breast massage are simple techniques a mother can use to help keep her breastfeeding baby actively suckling longer to increase milk intake, which also increases her milk's fat content (Stutte, 1988). This can be useful for the healthy baby who is gaining weight slowly, the newborn with hypoglycemia or exaggerated jaundice, and the baby with cardiac problems or any other health or neurological problems that compromise baby's weight gain or growth. It can also be helpful for the mother trying to increase her milk production.

Breast compression can keep a baby active at the breast and is useful for babies who are gaining weight slowly.

This technique was popularized by Canadian pediatrician Jack Newman (Newman & Pitman, 2006, pp. 72-73). Here's how he described the technique (used with permission):

1. The mother needs to know when the baby is getting milk (open mouth wide—pause—close mouth type of sucking.
2. When the baby is drinking milk actively, the mother does not need to use any breast compression.
3. Once the baby is sucking, but no longer drinking, just nibbling, the mother should start with the breast compression.
4. The baby should be sucking, but not actually drinking (open mouth wide—pause—close type of sucking). As the baby sucks, the mother, who is holding her breast with one hand, the thumb on one side and her other fingers on the other side of the breast, with a good amount of breast in her hand, should just bring her thumb and fingers together, compressing the breast. This should be done firmly, but not so hard that it hurts.
5. The baby may start to drink again (open mouth wide—pause—close mouth type of sucking). If so, the mother should keep up the pressure until the baby is back to nibbling. Once the baby is nibbling only, the mother should release the pressure on the breast so her hand does not get tired, and allow milk to start flowing again.
6. When the mother releases the pressure, a young baby, say under 2 or 3 weeks of age, will stop sucking. He will restart sucking when he tastes milk again. An older baby may continue to suck. If the baby drinks, fine. If he sucks but does not drink, the mother should restart the compression.
7. If the compression has no effect at a particular moment, this does not mean the mother must immediately switch sides. Sometimes compression will work, other times not. But as the baby has nursed longer and longer, it will work less and less, as the flow of milk slows. This means not that the breast is "empty," but that the baby is getting less and less. Babies respond to flow of milk.
8. If the compression is no longer having an effect and the baby is getting sleepy, or starting to fuss because flow is slow, the mother should take the baby off the breast and offer the other side. She should then repeat the process.

9. The mother should experiment....The mother should do whatever works best for them. As long as it does not hurt the mother to compress the breast, and the baby gets milk, the technique is working.

DANCER HAND POSITION

The Dancer Hand Position was named after U.S. midwife Sarah DANner and physician Edward CERutti (Danner & Cerutti, 1984). It provides jaw support and reduces the space inside baby's mouth during breastfeeding, which increases the vacuum a special-needs baby can generate. Enough (but not too much) vacuum is vital to milk transfer during breastfeeding (Geddes, Kent, Mitoulas, & Hartmann, 2008). The Dancer Hand Position may help the preterm baby, the baby with a cleft palate, or the baby with high or low tone who (Marmet & Shell, 2008):

The Dancer Hand Position can help special needs babies feed at the breast by increasing the vaccuum they can generate.

- Has trouble maintaining an air seal on the breast
- Suckles weakly (may have unusually wide jaw movements)
- Has difficulty staying on the breast

To use the Dancer Hand Position, suggest the mother (Figure A.14):

1. Support her breast with her hand, thumb on one side, and four fingers on the other.
2. Slide this hand forward, supporting the breast with her palm and her middle, ring, and little fingers. Her index finger and thumb should now be free in front of her nipple.
3. Bend her index finger slightly as the baby takes the breast, so her finger gently presses the baby's cheek on one side, while the thumb presses the other cheek. The baby's chin rests on the bottom of the "U."
4. Maintain this hand position during breastfeeding, using this position with the other hand when the baby changes breasts.

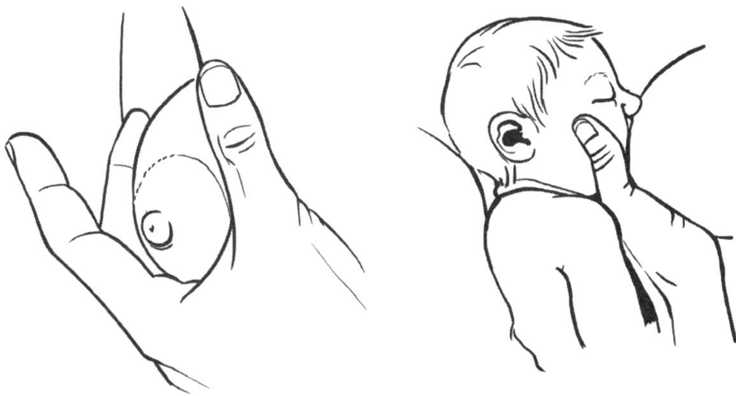

Figure A.14. Dancer Hand Position

©2010 Anna Mohrbacher, used with permission

TONGUE EXERCISES

When a baby has difficulty breastfeeding due to high or low muscle tone (or due to sensory processing or neurological impairment), mouth and tongue exercises may help. But to be effective, they should be tailored to the baby's specific issues. Some babies having breastfeeding problems become more organized when oral exercises are used and some become less organized. There is a wide range of possible tongue and mouth exercises, but choosing an oral exercise should be done by someone familiar with the underlying cause of the baby's problem and the techniques that best address it (Genna, Fram, & Sandora, 2008). Unless the person providing skilled breastfeeding help is trained in oral-motor evaluation and therapy, she/he should consider referring the mother and baby to someone with this training, especially if the baby has difficulty feeding at both breast and bottle. The following websites list local people trained in oral-motor evaluation and therapy. Because many in these fields were trained using bottle-feeding norms, ask if they are familiar with the breastfeeding baby.

Tongue exercises can help babies with high or low muscle tone effectively feed at the breast.

- www.asha.org – The U.S. website of the American Speech and Hearing Association, where parents can find a U.S. speech pathologist trained in assessing and treating feeding problems.
- www.ndta – The U.S. website of the Neuro-Developmental Treatment Association, where parents can find a therapist who uses a neuro-developmental (whole child) approach.

Mouth and tongue exercises should always be enjoyable for everyone. The baby should be actively involved, and because his mouth is a private space, the baby should be the one to decide if others can enter it and for how long (Genna et al., 2008). It is important to model sensitivity to the baby's responses. To avoid overstimulation, in some cases, these exercises may be best timed before the baby shows feeding cues or when switching breasts.

Walking Back on the Tongue

- Wash hands well with soap and water. Trim the fingernail of the index finger to be used.
- Touch baby's cheek lightly with the index finger and move it against the baby's skin to his lips, brushing his lips several times to trigger an open mouth.
- When he opens, massage the outside of his gums with the index finger, starting at the middle of the upper or low gum and moving toward either side.
- As he opens wide, use the fingertip to press down firmly near the tip of the baby's tongue and count slowly to three before releasing the pressure, keeping the finger in the baby's mouth.
- Move this finger a little farther back on his tongue, pressing again to a count of three.
- Move farther back on the baby's tongue once or twice more.

- Avoid making the baby gag. If he gags, avoid going that far back on the tongue the next time.
- If the baby enjoys this exercise, repeat it three or four times. If not, stop.

Pushing the Tongue Down and Out

- Wash and rinse hands well and trim the index finger to be used.
- Insert an index finger, pad side up, gently into the baby's mouth, pressing gently on his tongue.
- Leave the finger in that position for about 30 seconds while the baby sucks on it.
- Turn the finger over, so it is pad side down on the baby's tongue, and push down gently, while gradually pulling the finger out of his mouth.
- Repeat several times, then put baby to the breast.

REFERENCES

Colson, S. D., Meek, J. H., & Hawdon, J. M. (2008). Optimal positions for the release of primitive neonatal reflexes stimulating breastfeeding. *Early Human Development, 84*(7), 441-449.

Cotterman, K. J. (2004). Reverse pressure softening: a simple tool to prepare areola for easier latching during engorgement. *Journal of Human Lactation, 20*(2), 227-237.

Danner, S., & Cerutti, E. (1984). *Nursing your neurologically impaired baby.* . Rochester, NY: Childbirth Graphics.

Geddes, D. T., Kent, J. C., Mitoulas, L. R., & Hartmann, P. E. (2008). Tongue movement and intra-oral vacuum in breastfeeding infants. *Early Human Development, 84*(7), 471-477.

Genna, C. W., Fram, J. L., & Sandora, L. (2008). Neurological issues and breastfeeding. In C. W. Genna (Ed.), *Supporting sucking skills in breastfeeding infants* (pp. 253-303). Boston, MA: Jones and Bartlett.

Glover, R., & Wiessinger, D. (2008). The infant-mother breastfeeding conversation: Helping when they lose the thread. In C. W. Genna (Ed.), *Supporting sucking skills in breastfeeding infants* (pp. 97-129). Boston, MA: Jones and Bartlett.

Jacobs, L. A., Dickinson, J. E., Hart, P. D., Doherty, D. A., & Faulkner, S. J. (2007). Normal nipple position in term infants measured on breastfeeding ultrasound. *Journal of Human Lactatation, 23*(1), 52-59.

Marmet, C., & Shell, E. (2008). Therapeutic positioning for Breastfeeding. In C. W. Genna (Ed.), *Supporting sucking skills in breastfeeding infants* (pp. 305-325). Boston, MA: Jones and Bartlett.

Mizuno, K., Nishida, Y., Mizuno, N., Taki, M., Murase, M., & Itabashi, K. (2008). The important role of deep attachment in the uniform drainage of breast milk from mammary lobe. *Acta Paediatrica, 97*(9), 1200-1204.

Mohrbacher, N., & Kendall-Tackett, K. (2010). *Breastfeeding made simple: seven natural laws for nursing mothers, 2nd edition*. Oakland, CA: New Harbinger Publications.

Newman, J., & Pitman, T. (2006). *The ultimate breastfeeding book of answers*. New York, New York: Three Rivers Press.

Stutte, P. (1988). the effects of breast massage on volume and fat content of human milk. *Genesis, 10*(2), 22-25.

Wiessinger, D. (1998). A breastfeeding teaching tool using a sandwich analogy for latch-on. *Journal of Human Lactation, 14*(1), 51-56.

Wilson-Clay, B., & Hoover, K. (2008). *The breastfeeding atlas* (4th ed.). Manchaca, TX: LactNews Press.

Tools and Products

Appendix B

ALTERNATIVE FEEDING METHODS

Indications for Use

An alternative to the breast is needed when the mother and baby are separated at feeding times or the baby can't breastfeed effectively or at all.

Choosing a Method

The mother and her partner should be the final decision-makers on feeding method, ideally after reviewing each method's pros and cons, which are listed in Table B.1. According to U.S. lactation consultants Barbara Wilson-Clay and Kay Hoover, any feeding method should have the following characteristics (Wilson-Clay & Hoover, 2008):

- It cannot harm the baby.
- It is a good match for the baby's size and condition.
- It is accessible and affordable.
- It is easy to use and clean.
- It is suitable for the length of time needed.
- It promotes the transition to breastfeeding.

The mother and her partner should be the final decision-makers on feeding method.

In addition, it is important that the mother and others feeding the baby are comfortable with the feeding method. All of the methods described require instruction and practice, including feeding bottles. But most can be mastered quickly and get easier over time with practice.

Comparative Research

Much of the research comparing feeding methods was focused on preterm babies. Some may not apply to full-term healthy babies.

NG Tube Versus Feeding Bottles

In many hospitals, small preterm babies receive their first oral feedings by tube. One type of tube-feeding is done by nasogastric tube, NG tube for short. Using this method, the milk flows through a thin tube inserted through the baby's nose directly into his stomach. An advantage of supplementing a baby this way is there is no exposure to artificial nipples/teats. Some babies transition from NG-tube feedings directly to the breast without the use of feeding bottles. One U.S. randomized controlled trial found that preterm babies supplemented only by NG tube were 4.5 times more likely to be breastfeeding at hospital discharge and more than 9.0 times more likely to be exclusively breastfed than the babies who had been supplemented by bottle (Kliethermes, Cross, Lanese, Johnson, & Simon, 1999). At 3 months, the babies supplemented by NG tube were 3.0 times more likely to be breastfeeding and 3.0 times more likely to be fully breastfeeding than the preemies who were supplemented by bottle.

Cups Versus Feeding Bottles

Research done internationally has compared breastfeeding outcomes and babies' stability when supplemented by cup and bottle. Several studies found supplementing preterm babies by cup rather than by bottle led to higher breastfeeding rates at hospital discharge (Abouelfettoh, Dowling, Dabash, Elguindy, & Seoud, 2008; Collins et al., 2004; Lang, Lawrence, & Orme, 1994). One study that followed preemies long term found that after 6 weeks, those fed by cup had "significantly more mature breastfeeding behaviors" when compared with those fed by bottle (Abouelfettoh et al., 2008). An early U.K. study comparing 85 preterm babies found that they could feed successfully by cup as young as 30 weeks gestation, earlier than they could bottle-feed (Lang et al., 1994). More of the babies fed by cup were fully breastfeeding at hospital discharge than those fed by bottle (81% vs. 63%). During cup-feedings, the preemies maintained satisfactory heart rate, breathing, and oxygen levels, whereas during bottle-feeding, they were compromised (Blaymore Bier et al., 1997). Not all studies comparing cup and bottle found this, but study parameters varied. In one Australian study of 319 preemies, 56% of those in its cup-feeding group were also bottle-fed, leading to an underestimation of the effect of cup-feeding on breastfeeding outcomes (Collins et al., 2004).

One possible reason cup-feeding might ease the transition to breastfeeding among preemies is the differences in the oral muscles used. A Brazilian study found that babies use the same mouth and facial muscles during cup-feeding and breastfeeding, whereas different facial muscles were used during bottle-feeding (Gomes, Thomson, & Cardoso, 2009; Gomes, Trezza, Murade, & Padovani, 2006).

Two Cochrane reviews concluded there was no benefit to choosing cup over bottle, in part because no long-term differences in breastfeeding outcomes were found (Collins, Makrides, Gillis, & McPhee, 2008; Flint, New, & Davies, 2007). But a later U.K. review of the literature noted that staff training in cup-feeding technique and mothers' acceptance of the cup as a feeding method appeared to be key to research results (Renfrew et al., 2009). This article concluded that cup feeding may increase breastfeeding rates at discharge and reduce frequency of oxygen desaturation in preterm babies. Several studies found that among preterm babies, feeding bottles produced up to a ten-fold greater frequency of oxygen desaturation (Marinelli, Burke, & Dodd, 2001; Rocha, Martinez, & Jorge, 2002).

Two reviews concluded there was no advantage to choosing cup over bottles for feeding preterm infants.

Drawbacks to cup feeding in one study included a 10-day delay in hospital discharge compared to bottle-fed preemies (Collins et al., 2004); however, no difference in hospital length of stay was found in other studies. One U.S. study found that nearly 40% of the milk taken from the cup was recovered on the baby's bib (Dowling, Meier, DiFiore, Blatz, & Martin, 2002). In some studies, preemies fed by cup took longer to feed than preemies fed by bottle, while other studies found no difference (Marinelli et al., 2001; Rocha et al., 2002). Some studies found preterm babies fed by cup took less milk at each feeding than those fed by bottle (Dowling et al., 2002; Malhotra, Vishwambaran, Sundaram, & Narayanan, 1999; Marinelli et al., 2001). However, feeding time and amount of milk taken can also vary by gestational age. Some studies included babies as young as 30 weeks, while others included only older preemies.

Full-term babies may react differently than preterm babies to cup- and bottle-feeding. A Taiwanese study of 138 full-term babies found that although breastfeeding outcomes were virtually the same between the groups supplemented by cup and bottle, those supplemented by bottle were more fretful at the breast in the early days than those supplemented by cup (Huang, Gau, Huang, & Lee, 2009). The researchers also noted that the mothers who supplemented by bottle were more likely to believe they had insufficient milk compared with mothers who supplemented by cup. A U.S. study found no difference in milk intake and feeding time among full-term babies supplemented by cup or bottle or later breastfeeding rates (Howard et al., 1999). Another U.S. study found that cup-feeding improved breastfeeding outcomes only among mothers who gave birth by cesarean section and babies who received more than two supplemental feedings in the hospital (Howard et al., 2003).

Paladai Versus Cup Versus Feeding Bottle

One type of feeding cup used traditionally in India is the "paladai," which is a low bowl with a small spout that is shaped like "Aladdin's lamp." During feedings, the milk is poured from its spout into the baby's mouth. In a study done in India of 100 babies (which included full-term, growth retarded, and preterm babies), those fed by paladai had the greatest milk intake in the shortest time and were quiet longer after feedings than babies fed by cup or bottle (Malhotra et al., 1999). This study found higher rates of milk spillage with a cup compared to a paladai or a bottle. Technique is obviously important when feeding with a paladai. A study of preterm babies in the U.K.—where the paladai is not traditionally used—found longer feeding times, more milk spillage, and more stress cues among the babies fed by a paladai (Aloysius & Hickson, 2007).

Finger Feeding Versus Feeding Bottles

Not much research has been done on finger feeding. One Australian study examined the effect of feeding method on the transition to breastfeeding among preterm babies in its special-care nursery (Oddy & Glenn, 2003). This study hospital charted breastfeeding rates at discharge among preterm babies before and after it became Baby Friendly, which involved other changes in practice. Before becoming Baby Friendly, preterm babies were supplemented by bottle. After becoming Baby Friendly, finger feeding was substituted using the Lactation Aid developed by Canadian pediatrician Jack Newman (Newman & Pitman, 2006). Breastfeeding rates at discharge among preterm babies were 44% during the time babies were supplemented by bottles and 71% after supplements were given exclusively by finger feeding.

Table B.1. Advantages and Disadvantages of Alternative Feeding Methods

Feeding Method	Advantages	Disadvantages
At-Breast Supplementer	Reinforces breastfeeding Reduces or eliminates the need to feed baby again after breastfeeding Can improve suckling skills in some babies If breastfeeding deeply, stimulates milk production	Mothers may find it stressful and time-consuming Babies may suck on tubing like a straw If latching with tubing in place, may add stress to taking the breast If tape is used often, can cause skin damage Some are expensive
Feeding Bottles	Culturally acceptable and readily available in the West Familiar to parents Some babies took more milk in a shorter time Relatively inexpensive	Can replace breastfeeding Fast flow causes more oxygen desaturation in preemies May complicate transition to breast if used for >2 feedings or after a c-sec Uses different mouth muscles; long-term regular use increases risk of oral malformations Fast flow may cause overfeeding; long-term, regular use increases risk of obesity
Finger-Feeding	May make transition to the breast easier Can be used to improve suckling in some babies Viewed as temporary	Unfamiliar to many parents Finger-feeding equipment may not be easily available to parents
Sipping/lapping Methods (cup, bowl, spoon, paladai, eyedropper, and syringe)	Easy to clean Readily available Inexpensive In preemies, less oxygen desaturation and more breastfeeding at discharge May make transition to the breast easier Oral-muscle activity more like breastfeeding Viewed as temporary	When milk is poured during cup-feeding, some may be lost from spillage If hospital staff or parents are not well trained, can lead to feeding problems Feedings may take longer In one study (but not others) led to 10-day longer hospital stays

For research citations, see earlier and later sections.

At-Breast Supplementers

Sometimes called "feeding-tube devices," "tube-feeding devices," or "nursing supplementers," an at-breast supplementer delivers extra milk to the baby during breastfeeding through a thin tube. The baby's natural response to a swallow is to suckle. Some babies learn to suckle more effectively when the steady milk flow from the tube stimulates more active and consistent suckling and swallowing. When a baby takes the breast deeply and suckles longer or more vigorously, he also takes more milk directly from the breast and stimulates the mother's milk production. An at-breast supplementer can allow a mother with low milk production to feed her baby exclusively at the breast, eliminating the need to feed him again afterwards. Unlike other feeding methods, supplementing a baby at the breast provides positive reinforcement for breastfeeding.

There are commercially manufactured versions of at-breast supplementers, and there are makeshift versions. One easy-to-make "lactation aid" functions as a siphon and consists of a bottle with a hole cut in the nipple to insert one end of a feeding tube into the milk and the other end into the breastfeeding baby's mouth (Newman & Pitman, 2006). These devices can be used alone or with a nipple shield. One U.S. lactation consultant suggests that if used with a nipple shield to choose a device with softer tubing, so positioning the tubing inside the shield is less likely to disrupt the shield from the breast (Genna, 2009).

An at-breast supplementer can allow a mother with low milk production to feed her baby exclusively at the breast.

Indications for Use

At-breast supplementers may be a good choice if the mother's milk production is low or baby is gaining weight slowly. It can provide a faster, more consistent milk flow during relactation or induced lactation. This immediate milk flow may help some babies transition to the breast from other feeding methods. It can provide extra milk for babies with special needs, such as those with cardiac issues, neurological impairment, cleft palate, Down syndrome, and prematurity, which—depending on the issue—can sometimes help a baby with challenges learn to breastfeed more effectively.

The Two Types of At-Breast Supplementers

At-breast supplementers fall into two general categories:

- **Suction required.** These devices can be makeshift or manufactured. They include a container to hold the supplement, which hangs around the mother's neck, clips to her clothing, or is set on or hung from a nearby surface. When the baby takes the breast, he also takes its thin tubing, and as he suckles, milk flows through the tubing. When used effectively, the breastfeeding baby receives both the supplement through the tubing and milk directly from the mother's breast.
- **Suction not required.** These makeshift devices (at this writing, no manufactured versions are commercially available) consist of either a periodontal syringe or a syringe with needle removed attached by port to a thin feeding tube. With these supplementers, the feeder controls milk flow, and the baby does not need to generate suction.

The "suction-required" at-breast supplementers are only a useful tool if the baby can generate enough suction to pull the supplement through the tubing.

The "suction-not-required" supplementers can be used with babies who can't generate suction, such as those with a cleft palate or who are weakened from underfeeding. The "suction-not-required" devices should be used with caution with babies who have cardiac defects and respiratory problems. These babies must breathe more times per minute to maintain adequate oxygen levels. If a faster milk flow generated by the feeder forces them to swallow more often, this can compromise their oxygen levels (Genna, Fram, & Sandora, 2008).

What Research Says About At-Breast Supplementers

Some mothers find at-breast supplementers difficult and cumbersome.

Little research is available on these devices. One U.S. survey of 22 mothers who used a suction-required at-breast supplementer reported very mixed feelings about their experiences (Borucki, 2005). Some mothers considered it a "necessary evil" that allowed them to maintain the breastfeeding relationship. Some described it as "cumbersome, timing-consuming, compromising, artificial, complicated, and messy" (Borucki, 2005, p. 435). One mother used the device twice for a short-term issue; another mother used it continuously for 13 months. Five of the 22 mothers stopped breastfeeding within a week due to struggles with the device. Sixteen of the mothers breastfed longer than 6 months and one breastfed for 4.5 years. Mother-related reasons for using this device included insufficient milk production, delay in milk increase after birth, nipple pain and trauma, history of breast-reduction surgery, and adoption. Baby-related reasons included shallow latch, weak suck, slow weight gain, and prematurity-related feeding problems.

Milk in the Container

If the mother is using infant formula as a supplement, suggest she use either the concentrate or ready-to-feed form, as powdered formula can clump and clog the thin tubing. To make sure a compromised baby gets the milk he needs, suggest the mother add enough milk to the container so that about a half-ounce (15 mL) is left after every feeding. If all is taken, add more at that feeding and start the next feeding with 1 ounce (30 mL) more. If more than a half-ounce (15 mL) is left consistently, decrease the amount of milk in the supplementer at the next feeding. If the baby is not compromised, see Table B.2 for milk-volume suggestions. Unless the mother is using disposable tubing, suggest she either wash the tubing immediately after the feeding or immerse it in a container of water, so the milk doesn't dry. Tubing with dried milk inside would need to be replaced.

Latching to Breast and Tubing

One of the challenges mothers report when using an at-breast supplementer is achieving a deep latch with the tubing in place. Another common problem is that babies sometimes learn to take the breast shallowly and suck the tubing like a straw without stimulating the breast. If this happens, the mother will not see wide jaw movements during breastfeeding. If taking the breast deeper doesn't correct this, this device will not be helpful.

To make it easier to get a deep latch with both breast and tubing, some suggest latching first, and then pushing the firmer tubing included with some models into the corner of the baby's mouth until milk starts to flow (Newman & Pitman,

2006). Some devices include surgical tape to keep the tubing in place while baby latches. Usually the tubing is taped just behind the areola to keep it out of baby's way, with the tape running lengthwise on the tubing and the tubing tip extending about a quarter-inch (6 mm) past the nipple. Finding a good spot to tape the tubing so it doesn't get in the baby's way can be a challenge.

There are several ways milk flow can be adjusted using an at-breast supplementer.

An alternative to tape is for the mother to place a self-adhesive bandage on the appropriate place on her breast after bathing and leave it there until she bathes again. At each feeding, the bandage can be pinched to allow the tubing to extend through it. Although some devices recommend positioning the tubing on top of the breast when baby latches on, some suggest instead positioning it on the underside of the breast so that it rests against baby's tongue during feedings (Figure B.1). Some babies find it irritating when the tubing rubs against their palate during breastfeeding (Genna, 2009).

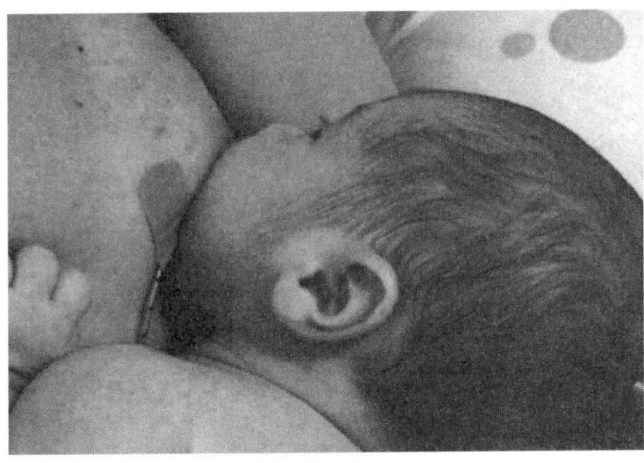

Figure B.1. Note the bandage holding the supplementer tubing under the breast.

©2010 Catherine Watson Genna, BS, IBCLC, used with permission.

Adjusting the Milk Flow of an At-Breast Supplementer

To provide good breast stimulation with this feeding method, the goal is for feedings to last 20 to 40 minutes. To achieve this, suggest the mother adjust the device's milk flow so that at each breastfeeding, the baby suckles actively for about 10 to 15 minutes per breast, switching breasts about halfway through. If the milk flow is too fast, the baby may finish before 20 minutes. If the milk flow is too slow, feedings may take more than 45 minutes, which can be difficult for the mother or the baby may lose interest quickly. There are several ways milk flow can be adjusted in suction-required at-breast supplementers so it can be tailored to baby's needs:

- **Raise or lower the container.** These devices work as a siphon, with a higher container providing faster flow and a lower container providing slower flow.
- **Increase or decrease tubing diameter.** Some at-breast supplementers include different size tubing (small, medium, large). Larger diameter tubing provides faster flow; smaller diameter tubing provides slower flow.

- **Open or close one tube.** At-breast supplementers with a closed container and two tubes can be set up with either both tubes open or one or both closed. Both tubes open provides faster milk flow; one tube closed provides slower milk flow.

If the baby begins to breastfeed more effectively and/or the mother's milk production increases, adjustments can be made to the supplementer to maintain feeding times.

Determining Amount of Supplement Needed

The baby who is compromised by low milk intake needs to be encouraged to take as much milk as possible to increase his energy for more effective breastfeeding. But when a baby's weight gain is just a little slow, a balance needs to be found between providing him with the milk he needs to gain normally and not giving him so much supplement that he takes less from the breast. For the baby younger than 4 months, U.S. lactation consultant Catherine Watson Genna developed Table B.2 to describe the amount of supplement needed to increase a baby's weight gain to reach the average weight gain of 7 ounces (198 g.) per week (WHO, 2006).

Table B.2. Amount of Supplement Needed to Increase Weight Gain

Weekly Weight Gain	6 oz. (170 g)	5 oz. (142 g)	4 oz. (113 g)	3 oz. (85 g)	2 oz. (57 g)	1 oz. (28 g)	0 oz. (0 g)
Weekly Weight Deficit	1 oz. (28 g)	2 oz. (57 g)	3 oz. (85 g)	4 oz. (113 g)	5 oz. (142 g)	6 oz. (170 g)	7 oz. (198 g)
Daily Supplement Needed	2 oz. (60 mL)	4 oz. (120 mL)	6 oz. (180 mL)	8 oz. (240 mL)	10 oz. (300 mL)	12 oz. (360 mL)	14 oz. (420 mL)

Adapted from (Genna, 2009)

Weaning from an At-Breast Supplementer

If during her baby's first 6 months a mother's milk production cannot be increased enough to fully meet her baby's needs, such as the mother with inadequate glandular tissue or the mother with a history of breast-reduction surgery, the supplementer may be needed until solid foods eventually reduce baby's need for milk to match the mother's production. In most cases, though, this device will be needed short-term until the baby's breastfeeding effectiveness improves and/or the mother's milk production increases.

If the baby begins feeding more effectively, he may start to take all of the supplement in a shorter time. If the baby finishes feeding in less than 20 minutes and the at-breast supplementer has multiple tubing sizes, suggest the mother switch to a smaller size tubing to slow the flow and increase feeding time for better breast stimulation.

If the mother wants to know how much milk the baby is taking directly from the breast, she can do a test-weigh (see last section) and subtract the amount the baby took from the supplementer from his total milk intake at the feeding. As the baby takes more milk from the breast, the following strategies can be used to gradually wean from the device:

- Lower the height of the container to slow milk flow.
- Clamp the tubing shut before baby takes the breast and wait to unclamp it until the sound of baby's swallowing stops.
- Try breastfeeding without the supplementer at the first morning feeding, which is usually when the most milk is available in the breast.
- Use the supplementer at gradually fewer feedings each day.

As the mother weans the baby from the supplement, she should expect the baby will want to breastfeed more often. Some mothers use their baby's behavior as a guide. As one U.S. mother said, "When I really felt like he didn't have a good feeding, and he really seemed like he was hungry, I would put it on" (Borucki, 2005, p. 433). Suggest the mother have her baby weighed regularly as she weans from the supplementer to ensure he gets enough milk.

Some mothers have a difficult time emotionally weaning from the supplementer, considering it a kind of "security blanket." As one U.S. mother said:

> I think that, towards the end, I might have tried to do plain breastfeeding without the system, but he never wanted to do that. I wasn't too supportive of that anyway, because I had lost confidence in my ability to do it on my own (Borucki, 2005, pp. 433-434).

Support, encouragement, and the use of test-weighing to provide objective reassurance of baby's milk intake may be helpful in convincing mothers the at-breast supplementer is no longer needed.

Feeding Bottles

What Research Says About Feeding Bottles

Bottle-feeding may cause problems for preterm and full-term infants.

Most likely due, at least in part, to their fast flow, research has found preterm babies have more frequent oxygen desaturation and more breathing and heart irregularities during bottle-feeding than breastfeeding (Blaymore Bier et al., 1997; Chen, Wang, Chang, & Chi, 2000; Meier & Anderson, 1987; Poets, Langner, & Bohnhorst, 1997). For more details, see p. 358- "Feeding Methods." Supplementation of preterm babies with bottles has also been associated with lower breastfeeding rates at hospital discharge (see previous section "Comparative Research").

In full-term babies, two Swedish studies found an association between early use of feeding bottles and pacifiers/dummies and the development of "superficial nipple sucking," which may lead to nipple pain (Righard, 1998; Righard & Alade, 1997). One Italian study of 219 mothers found the use of a pacifier or feeding bottles in the hospital was associated with nipple pain at discharge (Centuori et al., 1999). Another Swedish study found that when mothers of full-term babies supplemented their babies by bottle after birth, the reason for the supplementation affected breastfeeding outcomes (Ekstrom, Widstrom, & Nissen, 2003). When the supplements were given for medical reasons, breastfeeding outcomes were not affected. But when there were no medical reasons, it was associated with a shorter duration of breastfeeding. Researchers suggested that mothers' lack of self-confidence about breastfeeding may have a greater effect than bottle-feeding on breastfeeding duration. Some more recent research found no difference in breastfeeding outcomes among full-term babies supplemented by bottle or cup after birth. Others found a difference only among babies who received more than two bottles in the hospital and among mothers who gave birth by cesarean. For more details, see the previous section "Comparative Research." Regular, long-term bottle-feeding has been associated with oral malformations, such as crossbite and maxillary atresia (Carrascoza, Possobon Rde, Tomita, & Moraes, 2006; Kobayashi, Scavone, Ferreira, & Garib, 2010).

In *The Breastfeeding Atlas,* U.S. authors Barbara Wilson-Clay and Kay Hoover suggest the mother's anatomy may also play a role in a baby's response to a bottle teat. They wrote: "If women have erectile nipples with good elasticity, their babies may not be vulnerable...." (Wilson-Clay & Hoover, 2008, p. 41). In other words, bottles may pose a greater risk of feeding problems in babies whose mothers have flat or inverted nipples. They suggest the fast flow of the bottle and the firm teat provide a "supernormal stimulus" in the baby's mouth, which may lead to feeding problems for mothers with non-protruding nipples.

When considering the bottle as a long-term feeding option, research has found a risk of overfeeding. Because milk flows more consistently from the bottle than the breast (which has a natural ebb and flow of milk due to milk ejections), on average, babies consume more milk from the bottle at a feeding (Li, Fein, & Grummer-Strawn, 2008; Taveras et al., 2006). When used regularly and long-term, babies fed by bottle are at greater risk of overweight and obesity. One large, prospective, randomized, controlled trial (16,755 babies in Belarus) compared volume of milk per feeding in formula-fed and breastfed babies (Kramer et al., 2004). At each feeding, the bottle-fed babies took 49% more milk at 1 month, 57% more at 3 months, and 71% more at 5 months as compared with the breastfeeding babies.

Feeding-Bottle Options

There are many aspects of bottle-feeding that can affect a baby's response and potentially make the transition to the breast easier. If the mother plans to use a feeding bottle, suggest she consider teat flow rate, shape, and feeding techniques. For a detailed description of teat-flow, teat shape, and feeding techniques, see the book, *Balancing Breast & Bottle Reaching Your Breastfeeding Goals* by Amy Peterson and Mindy Harmer (2010). In general, by choosing the options that are more like breastfeeding, the mother may reduce the risk her baby will grow to prefer the bottle. However, not all babies are the same and she should use her baby's response as her guide.

Teat Flow Rate

Suggest that mothers choose a bottle nipple/teat with a slow flow.

In general, suggest the mother choose a bottle nipple/teat that flows as slowly as possible. The slow flow will help minimize overfeeding, leaving the baby feeling full with less milk. This can be especially helpful for the mother away from her baby regularly at feeding times because it reduces the amount of expressed milk needed. A slower flow also makes it easier for a compromised baby to coordinate sucking, swallowing, and breathing. At this writing in the U.S., there is no standardized system for rating teat flow, and flow rates vary greatly by brand. Some teats labeled slow flow may actually flow faster than others not labeled slow flow. Suggest the mother buy several brands of slow-flow teats. To determine which has the slowest flow, fill the bottle with water and turn them upside down over a drain. If a bottle-feeding takes less than about 20 minutes, suggest the mother try to find a slower-flow teat. The mother will know the flow is too slow for her baby if he seems frustrated, disinterested, or feedings take longer than 20 minutes, and she will know that it is too fast if he gasps, coughs, and cries (Peterson & Harmer, 2010).

Teat Shape

When a baby takes a wide-based nipple into his mouth by opening wide and closing his lips on its wide base rather than the nipple shaft, this mimics the wider gape of a baby at the breast. However, one size does not fit all. Australian authors and clinicians Robyn Noble and Anne Bovey describe their positive experiences when using a long, narrow-based teat with babies with breastfeeding problems (Noble & Bovey, 1997). Because babies are different, U.S. lactation consultants Barbara Wilson-Clay and Kay Hoover recommend experimenting with teat shape:

Teat length and shape should be based on the baby's response as the internal contours of babies' mouths vary.

> Some infants require a narrow based teat owing to poor lip tone and inability to seal to a wider base. Some infants will gag if the teat is too long. Other infants seem not to respond if the teat is too short.... (Wilson-Clay & Hoover, 2008, p. 114).

Teat length and shape should be based on the baby's response, as the internal contours of babies' mouths vary. To understand the differences in babies mouths, Wilson-Clay took measurements of the mouths of 98 babies from 35-week-old preemies to 3-month-old full-term babies (Wilson-Clay & Hoover, 2008). She offered each baby her gloved finger, pad side up, and allowed them to draw in her finger to the depth that triggered sucking. She then marked with a pen on her glove the spot where the babies' lips closed and considered the measurement from the tip of her finger to the pen mark as each baby's "oral reach," that baby's ideal teat length. In these 98 babies, the range was 1.9 cm to 3.1 cm.

According to U.S. clinicians Amy Peterson and Mindy Harmer (2010), a bottle teat is too short if the baby's lips touch the bottle collar that keeps the teat in place, and it is too long if the baby gags or he can only feed comfortably when his lips close on the narrow "length" of teat, rather than on its wider base. The nipple shape may not be a good fit for a baby if he retracts or humps his tongue while bottle-feeding. Regular tongue retraction during bottle-feeding can make it more difficult to transition back to the breast because using this movement during breastfeeding will push the breast out of baby's mouth.

Feeding Techniques

If a mother supplements her baby by bottle, encourage her to use techniques that reinforce breastfeeding. U.S. lactation consultant Dee Kassing described how the mother can use bottle-feeding techniques that mimic breastfeeding to make the transition from bottle to breast easier. For example, rather than inserting the bottle nipple into the baby's mouth, hold the baby on the feeder's lap in a semi-upright position with the bottle held horizontally and brush the bottle nipple lightly against the baby's lips, waiting for a wide gape before allowing the baby to draw it in (Kassing, 2002).

Paced Bottle-Feeding

Paced bottle feeding can make bottle feeding less stressful for babies.

For preterm or compromised babies who struggle at feedings and find the flow of the bottle overwhelming, paced bottle-feeding can make feedings more manageable. To gauge whether this might be helpful, count how many times a baby sucks and swallows before taking a breath. If he still hasn't taken a breath within three to five sucks, the feeder stops the milk flow (Law-Morstatt, Judd, Snyder, Baier, & Dhanireddy, 2003). Some other signs of respiratory problems during bottle-feeding include flaring nostrils, milk dribbling from the corners of baby's mouth, wide eyes, and/or blue around the lips. The purpose of paced bottle-feeding is for the feeder to give the baby as much control as possible over the feeding (Wilson-Clay, 2005). This can be done in two ways. To provide a pause, the feeder can remove the bottle teat from the baby's mouth, resting it lightly on the baby's upper lip, and wait for signs he wants to continue feeding. If the baby resists the withdrawal of the teat, the feeder can instead lower the level of the bottle so that milk leaves the teat. When the baby starts to suck again, the feeder can raise the bottle so milk flows back into the teat (Wilson-Clay & Hoover, 2008).

Specialty Feeding Bottles

Most feeding bottles flow freely. Another way to give a compromised baby more control over milk flow during feedings is to use a specialty feeding bottle, such as the Haberman Feeder, which doesn't rely on suction and only flows when the baby compresses the teat. Babies who might benefit from these devices include those with special needs. The baby with a cleft palate, for example, can easily become overwhelmed when milk flows through the opening in their palate into their nasal cavity and ear tubes.

Finger Feeding

Finger feeding involves feeding milk to a baby while he's sucking on an adult's finger.

Indications for Use

It can be used with any baby to provide extra milk and can be used therapeutically to teach more normal sucking to babies with poor oral-motor skills by rewarding them with milk when they make correct feeding movements (Genna, 2009).

What Research Says About Finger-Feeding

See the previous section "Comparative Research" for a description of a study of preterm babies that compared finger feeding to bottle-feeding.

Tools and Strategies for Finger-Feeding

Whichever of the following tools is used to finger feed, tell the feeder the first step is to wash her hands well and to be sure the finger used to feed the baby has a closely-trimmed nail:

- Any at-breast supplementer can be used to finger feed by placing its tubing along an adult's finger, pad side up, and extending it about a quarter-inch (6 mm) past the fingertip. If desired, the tubing can be taped to the finger, ideally lengthwise, so the baby can't suck the tape into his mouth. Tap baby's lips and wait until he opens. Allow baby to draw the finger into his mouth to the area where active sucking is triggered.
- Periodontal syringes, which typically hold 10 to 20 mL of milk each, can be used by pulling back on the plunger to draw milk into the syringe and resting the curved tip against the feeder's finger and just inside the corner of the baby's mouth (about 1/16th of an inch or 2 mm). The plunger should be depressed slowly only while the baby sucks. When the baby pauses, the feeder pauses to avoid overwhelming the baby.
- Commercial finger-feeding devices are also available.

Sipping and Lapping Methods

Feeding methods that require the baby to sip or lap the milk (as opposed to sucking) include cup, bowl, spoon, eyedropper, and syringe.

What Research Says About Sipping/Lapping Methods

As one Swedish researcher wrote, "Cup feeding has been used for feeding infants and young children as far back in history as we have any insight" (Nyqvist & Ewald, 2006, p. 85). In many parts of the developing world, cups and spoons are considered the only safe alternatives to breastfeeding, because clean water for washing feeding utensils is not always available and dangerous bacteria can grow in the cracks and crevices of feeding bottles, spreading illness (Bergman & Jurisoo, 1994). In the 1980s, journal articles described cup-feeding of low birthweight babies in Kenya (Armstrong, 1987) and a UNICEF video was widely distributed, increasing interest in cup feeding in the U.K. and spurring research. Research in both India and the U.K. found that very preterm babies as young as 30 weeks gestation could effectively cup-feed even before they could bottle-feed (Gupta, Khanna, & Chattree, 1999; Lang et al., 1994; Malhotra et al., 1999). In some developed countries, cups are recommended over bottles for hospitalized babies (Cloherty, Alexander, Holloway, Galvin, & Inch, 2005; Nyqvist & Ewald, 2006). Brazilian research has found that unlike bottle-feeding, the feeding behaviors babies use while cup-feeding are similar to breastfeeding (Gomes et al., 2009; Gomes et al., 2006). See the earlier section "Comparative Research" (p. 811) for the effects of cup-feeding on infant stability and breastfeeding outcomes compared with other feeding methods.

In the developing world, cup and spoon feeding are considered the only safe alternatives.

Feeding with a Cup, Bowl, Spoon, Eyedropper, or Syringe

Technique is key when feeding a baby with a sipping or lapping method. If cup-feeding, any small cup can be used, such as a shot glass or the plastic cup included with children's liquid medicines. Commercial baby feeding cups are also available, some with snap-on lids and some with valves that regulate the baby's access to milk. If a bowl is used for feeding, a small, flexible bowl may be easier to manage than a rigid one. But any clean cup, glass, or bowl can be used, even those that are adult-sized. Spoon-feeding can also be used when supplements are needed after birth. In some hospitals, breastfeeding specialists help mothers express colostrum into a plastic spoon (like those available in the hospital cafeteria) and feed it to their non-breastfeeding baby. Any spoon can be used. Other sipping/lapping tools include an eyedropper or a syringe (with needle removed) for dripping milk into baby's mouth.

While the baby and the feeder are learning this feeding method, it is best to go slowly. As both have more practice, feedings are often quick. No matter what container is used, when starting out:

- Make sure baby is awake and alert before feeding.
- Wrap the baby's hands securely to prevent them from bumping the feeding container, and use a bib or cloth to protect baby's clothes from spills.
- Hold the baby in a sitting position (Figure B.2).

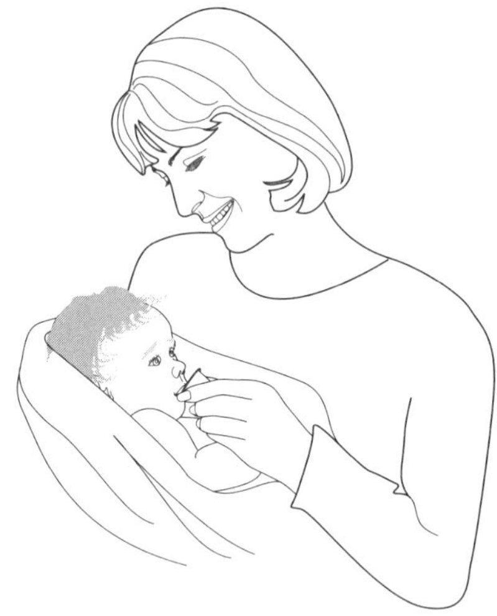

Figure B.2. Sit a baby upright when using a sipping/lapping feeding method

©2010 Ameda Breastfeeding Products, used with permission.

When cup-feeding:

- Raise the cup and rest its rim lightly on baby's lower lip.
- Tip the cup so the milk just touches his lips and he can sip or lap it in, but not so much that it pours into his mouth.
- Let the baby set his own sipping or lapping rhythm, pausing when needed, until he finishes. Some babies prefer the cup be tilted away between swallows, others prefer to feed continuously. Some use their tongue to lap the milk, others sip it in.

A variation of the cup is a feeding device used traditionally in India, called the paladai, which is shaped like "Aladdin's lamp." When feeding with the paladai, milk is poured from its small spout into the baby's mouth. See the earlier section "Comparative Research" for studies comparing the paladai with cup and feeding bottle.

When spoon-feeding:

- Fill the spoon with a mouthful of milk.
- Rest the spoon lightly on baby's lower lip and tilt it so the milk touches his lips.
- Either pour the milk into baby's mouth or allow him to sip or lap it, whichever he prefers.
- Give the baby time to swallow, refill the spoon, and repeat until baby is done.

When feeding with an eyedropper or syringe:

- Fill the eyedropper or syringe with a mouthful of milk.
- Raise it and drip the milk into baby's mouth at a slow enough pace so that he can swallow it before more is given.

BREAST PUMPS

Indications for Use

See p. 445- "Why Express Milk?" for the many reasons mothers give for expressing milk. Although hand expression is an option for most mothers and is used exclusively for milk expression in some parts of the world, there are some situations, such as establishing milk production after birth when baby is not yet breastfeeding, in which a breast pump may be a better choice. Research conducted in Nigeria and Kenya found breast pumps were more effective at stimulating more milk production sooner than hand expression (Slusher et al., 2007). Work settings in which a mother has very limited milk expression time may be another situation in which a breast pump might be a better choice, as double-pumping can cut milk expression time in half. In some cultures, mothers prefer to use breast pumps over hand expression (Binns, Win, Zhao, & Scott, 2006; Labiner-Wolfe, Fein, Shealy, & Wang, 2008).

A breast pump may be a better choice than hand expression when mothers need to establish a milk supply.

What Research Says About Breast Pumps

One of the first breast pump studies was done by Swedish civil engineer Einar Egnell and published in 1956 in the journal of the Swedish medical association (Egnell, 1956). In the early 1940s, Egnell spent three years developing a better breast pump because the U.S. Abt pumps available at the time caused skin rupture in one-third of the mothers who used them. In his landmark article, Egnell described the science behind the suction and cycling parameters he developed, which are still used today to gauge breast-pump safety and efficacy. By decreasing pump vacuum and increasing the number of suction-and-release cycles per minute, Egnell created a breast pump that was both comfortable and effective. Since then, many breast pump studies have been published. Although significant improvements have been made in pump fit and portability, as yet no one has improved upon Egnell's basic pump design.

That said, however, mothers vary in their response to pump stimulation, and subtle differences between brands and models may produce different results. For this reason, those who work with breastfeeding mothers should be familiar with locally available equipment and their differences. Be aware that some pumps start at lower vacuum levels, which may make them a better choice for mothers who are engorged or in pain. It is also important to be aware of available "fit" options (see next section) when a pump's nipple tunnel is too large or too small for a mother. As U.S. lactation consultant Catherine Watson Genna wrote:

> The take-home message here is that mothers differ…and so far no one pump has been developed that works optimally for absolutely all mothers (Genna, 2009, p. 124).

Pump Fit

Pumping should feel comfortable.

This is based on how well the mother's nipple fits into the pump's nipple tunnel, the opening the breast is drawn into during pumping. Pump companies call this pump piece the "flange" or "breastshield." Mothers sometime refer to it as the "horn" or "funnel." A good pump fit is key to the mother's comfort and milk flow, and her fit can change over time. For mothers pumping often, a less-than-optimal fit can lead to pain, trauma, and reduced milk flow, putting milk production at risk.

Nipple tunnel diameter varies slightly by brand, with 24 or 25 mm the standard size of most brands. The best way to gauge pump fit is to watch a mother pump or to have her compare what she sees during pumping to the images below. When a mother has a good fit (Figure B.3), space should be visible around her nipple as she pumps. Pumping should feel comfortable, and if she has ample milk production, she should see good milk flow.

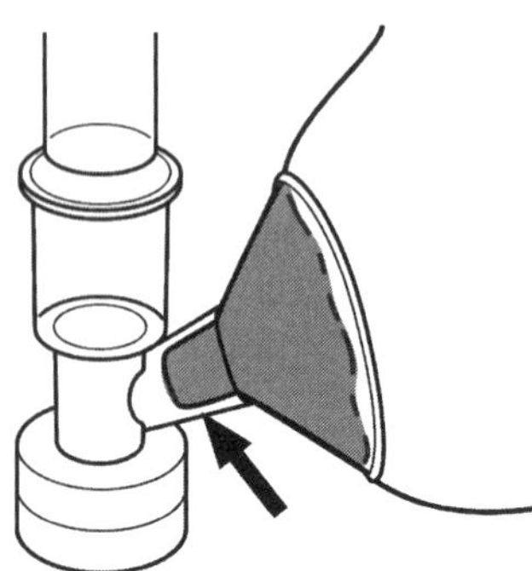

Figure B.3. With a good pump fit, a mother sees space around her nipple.
©2010 Ameda, used with permission.

When a breast pump is too tight, the mother's nipple is squeezed by the nipple tunnel, which compresses her milk ducts, preventing milk from flowing freely (Figure B.4).

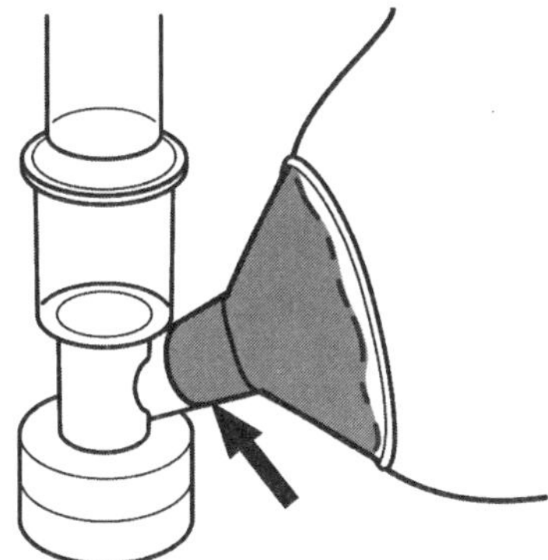

Figure B.4. With a tight fit, her nipple rubs along the tunnel.
©2010 Ameda, used with permission.

In some cases, part of her nipple may also blanch, or turn white. Friction from rubbing can cause pain and skin trauma, which may appear as a crack at the base of the nipple or a ring around the nipple after pumping. Mothers can see online photos illustrating a good fit and a tight fit at http://www.ameda.com/breastpumping/most/fit.aspx.

Larger nipple tunnels have become available in recent years from the pump manufacturers Ameda and Medela, and a significant percentage of mothers pump more comfortably and effectively with them. In one U.K. study, 36 mothers with babies in the NICU pumped with a standard 25 mm nipple-tunnel opening to establish milk production, and the researchers noted that the opening was too small for 28%:

> If the [opening] is too small, pressure is highest on the nipple tissue, which can cause sore nipples and ineffective drainage (Jones, Dimmock, & Spencer, 2001, p. F94).

In a U.S. NICU study, a different brand of pump with a 24 mm standard opening was used. When both milk flow and comfort were assessed, a much greater percentage of mothers had better results with a larger nipple tunnel:

> [W]e found that 51.4%--or about half—of the 35 mothers who served as subjects in the research initially required either the 27 or 30 mm shield in order to achieve optimal, pain-free nipple and areolar movement during milk expression. As lactation progressed, 77.1%--or slightly over three quarters—of the mothers eventually found they needed these larger shields (Meier, Motykowski, & Zuleger, 2004, p. 8).

Pumping causes mother's nipple to expand, influencing pump fit.

This study was the first to note that pump fit can change over time. U.S. lactation consultants Barbara Wilson-Clay and Kay Hoover used an engineer's template to measure mothers' nipples before and after pumping and found that pumping causes nipples to increase in size. They wrote: "Pre- and post-pumping measurements taken with a circle template reveal that nipple size can increase 3 to 4 millimeters" (Wilson-Clay & Hoover, 2008, p. 75). With regular pumping, this expansion of nipple size may continue. For this reason, encourage mothers to recheck their pump fit from time to time.

As an easy gauge of which mothers have an obvious need for larger nipple-tunnel openings, some U.S. public health departments suggested mothers compare their nipple with the width of a U.S. nickel (22 mm). Due to nipple swelling during pumping, if a mother's nipples at rest are wider than a U.S. nickel, this agency recommends starting with a larger-than-standard nipple tunnel.

But the breast is dynamic and changes during pumping, so if a mother's nipples are smaller than a nickel, this does not completely rule out the need for a larger opening. Some women have wide underlying tissue in their breasts that is drawn out during pumping, causing rubbing along the nipple tunnel, and these mothers also benefit from larger nipple tunnels. The most reliable way to help a mother gauge pump fit is to observe a pumping or to ask her to compare what she sees with the "Good Fit/Tight Fit" photos.

Not all mothers need to go larger for a better pump fit. Mothers who need smaller openings are in the minority, but a good fit is just as vital to them, as rubbing too much of the areola can also cause discomfort. See Table B.3 for signs that pump fit may need adjusting.

Table B.3. Signs a Mother Needs a Larger or Smaller Nipple Tunnel

Suggest a larger nipple-tunnel opening if a mother reports:
• Nipple rubs along the tunnel, despite efforts to center it. • Nipple blanches, or turns white. • Nipple does not move freely in the nipple tunnel. • Discomfort, even on low suction settings. • Slow milk flow or less milk expressed than expected.
Suggest a smaller nipple-tunnel opening if a mother reports:
• More than about 1/8 inch (25 mm) of the areola is pulled into the nipple tunnel. • Nipple bounces in and out of the tunnel. • Difficulty maintaining an air seal.

Breast Pump Vacuum (Suction)

Many mothers assume that "more is better" when it comes to pump vacuum. But expressing milk with a pump is not like sucking a drink through a straw. For a pump to be effective, milk ejections (ideally more than one) need to occur. When vacuum levels become high enough to be uncomfortable, this may actually inhibit milk ejection, resulting in less milk expressed. Suggest the mother set her pump at the highest vacuum that is truly comfortable for her, and this setting will vary by mother.

Vaccuum levels that are too high may inhibit milk ejection.

Australian breast pump research found that when mothers set their breast pump vacuum at their highest comfortable setting, during the first milk ejection, on average, a little less than half of their available milk was expressed (Kent et al., 2008). As the volume of milk in the breast decreases, milk flow slows, and less milk is expressed with each subsequent milk ejection. In one study of 21 breastfeeding mothers using a hospital-grade double electric breast pump, the mothers expressed from both breasts after two milk ejections, on average, about 76% of their available milk, or an average milk volume of about 90 mL (about 3 ounces). This was 10% more than the 67% a baby takes, on average, during a breastfeeding (Kent et al., 2006). With four milk ejections, on average, mothers expressed about 99% of the available milk. After four milk ejections, the amount of milk expressed continues to decrease. The fifth and sixth milk ejections yielded only 7 mL, or about one-quarter ounce each. (See p. 452 for a table illustrating this.)

Breast Pump Cycles

Pump "cycles per minute" (cpm) is the unit used to describe this pump feature, which refers to the number of times every minute the pump vacuum builds, peaks, and releases. This variable distinguishes, in part, more effective from less effective breast pumps. Most mothers using their pump daily to replace missed feedings will get better milk yields with an automatic pump that generates at least 40 to 60 cpm (Alekseev, Omel'ianuk, & Talalaeva, 2000). A pump that can cycle in this range is generally considered most effective at establishing and maintaining milk production. Breast pumps that generate fewer than 40 cpm usually cost less and are considered appropriate for "occasional use" (replacing a feeding less often than once per day).

Breast pumps with 40 to 60 cpm lead to better milk yield.

Some costlier breast pumps (marketed as"2-phase" pumps) cycle in their first phase at 120 cpm, but Australian research found that 86% of mothers express no milk at all during this very fast first phase (Ramsay et al., 2006). If the mother is using one of these "2-phase" pumps, suggest she minimize any time spent at that cycle setting. Before milk ejection at 120 cpm, mothers average only 1 to 2.7 mL of milk (Kent et al., 2008) compared with 10 mL (about 1/3 oz.) at 60 cpm (Ramsay, Mitoulas, Kent, Larsson, & Hartmann, 2005).

Research comparing time to milk ejection has been mixed. One small Australian study of 28 mothers found that mothers experienced milk ejection about 30 seconds faster with a "2-phase" pump, but expressed slightly less milk overall than a pump cycling at a set 50 cpm (Kent, Ramsay, Doherty, Larsson, & Hartmann, 2003). However, one larger U.S. study of 100 mothers of preterm babies who initiated lactation after birth with a breast pump providing a set 50 cpm cycle speed reported that when the mothers were switched to a "2-phase" pump, their milk ejection was delayed by an average of nearly a minute compared with the slower "single-phase" pump (Meier et al., 2008). The researchers suggested this was because milk ejection is a conditioned response, and these mothers had become conditioned to the feel of the "single-phase" pump. In this study, the mothers using the "single-phase" pump (with a set 50 cpm) also expressed more milk overall, but the difference was not statistically significant. In other words, since a mother's milk ejection will respond faster to any type of pump she becomes conditioned to, there is no advantage to the "2-phase" pump in terms of speed to milk ejection or overall amount of milk expressed.

Interestingly, the mothers in this study rated the programmable pump set to mimic the 50 cpm of the older model as "more comfortable" than the older model pump, even though they functioned identically. The researchers suggested other factors, such as the difference in the pumps' sound quality, may have influenced the mothers' perception of comfort.

Doubt has been raised on the effectiveness of "2-phase" pumps in establishing milk production in the early days after birth. A U.S. study described online but not yet published at this writing indicates that a "2-phase" pump may be much less effective at establishing milk production than other types of hospital-grade pumps during the first 14 days after birth (http://www.medelabreastfeedingus.com/preemie-plus-researchstudy). Mothers using the "2-phase" pump did not exceed the "borderline" amount of milk produced by Day 14, expressing, on average, less than 500 mL of milk per day. Pumps that cycle in the 40 to 60 cpm range, on the other hand, have been found to yield, on average, more than 700 mL per day by Day 14 (Rosen, Shuster, & Barber, 2001). A Japanese study compared the volume of colostrum expressed by hand (by a midwife) during the first 48 hours after birth with milk yield from a "2-phase" hospital-grade pump (Ohyama, 2007). Hand-expression yielded more than 3 times more colostrum (2 mL vs. 0.6 mL) at each session.

Choosing a Breast Pump

For the mother pumping daily for missed feedings, choosing the right type of pump can affect her ability to meet her breastfeeding goals. If a mother asks which pump is best for her, the answer will depend on her situation and her means. Suggest the mother consider her choice carefully if a breast pump plays a major role in maintaining milk production. This would include a mother whose baby is not breastfeeding at all and the mother away from her baby and missing feedings 30 hours or more per week. For more details on choosing a pump by type, see p. 458.

The following characteristics distinguish pumps designed for regular use from those more appropriate for occasional use:

- **Vacuum and cycle options**. Those designed for regular use generate automatically at least 40-60 cpm per minute and provide vacuum in the range considered safe and effective: about 50 to 250 millimeters of mercury (mmHg).
- **Comfort.** To maintain milk production with frequent use, a pump must be comfortable. Several factors affect comfort: 1) availability of different size nipple tunnels (see previous "Fit" section), 2) vacuum adjustability (more possible vacuum settings within the right range permit mothers to fine-tune vacuum levels for greater comfort and effectiveness), and 3) waveform shape (the waveform is a visual representation of how pump suction builds, peaks, and releases), with a smooth waveform being more effective and comfortable than a sharp one (Mitoulas, Lai, Gurrin, Larsson, & Hartmann, 2002).
- **Reliability.** Pumps designed for regular use are built to withstand at least three to four pumpings per day (i.e., mothers employed full-time) and have at least a 1-year warranty on their motor.

Recommend a pump designed for regular use for the mother who is exclusively pumping or employed full-time, as her pump substitutes for her baby for many of his daily feedings.

BREAST SHELLS AND NIPPLE EVERTERS

Breast Shells

These hard-plastic cups are worn in the mother's bra during pregnancy or between breastfeedings to either protect painful nipples from pressure and clothing friction or draw out flat or inverted nipples. Most versions include a dome (usually with holes for air circulation) and a backing (either hard plastic or silicone). In some versions only one type of backing (one size opening) is included. In other versions, two different backings are included that can both be snapped onto the dome. The backing with the smaller opening is designed to apply pressure to the areola and draw out non-protruding nipples. The backing with the larger opening is designed to protect painful nipples from pressure and clothing friction.

Indications for Use

When used to draw out flat or inverted nipples, breast shells may be worn during the last trimester of pregnancy for increasing amounts of time each day or in the early postpartum period for about 30 minutes before feedings. If they are used after the mother's milk has increased, be sure the mother's bra cups are large enough to accommodate them without putting too much pressure on the breast. If her bra cup is too small, consistent pressure on the breast increases her risk of mastitis.

What Research Says About Breast Shells

Breast shells may cause more breastfeeding problems than they solve.

Although breast shells have been recommended for decades to draw out flat or inverted nipples, research has found they may cause more breastfeeding problems than they solve. Two U.K. studies found that identifying flat or inverted nipples during pregnancy and "treating" them with either breast shells or the Hoffman technique (using the fingers to pull back on the areolae to draw out the nipples) resulted in fewer women breastfeeding (Alexander, Grant, & Campbell, 1992; MAIN, 1994). The first of these two studies, which followed 96 first-time mothers with flat or inverted nipples, found that more of those in the treatment group either decided not to breastfeed or stopped breastfeeding earlier than those whose nipples were not treated. The researchers expressed concern that telling a pregnant woman her nipples could be problematic may act as a disincentive to successful breastfeeding because it calls into question her ability to breastfeed. They concluded that during pregnancy recommending breast shells may reduce the chances of successful breastfeeding (Alexander et al., 1992). The second study, which followed 463 mothers with flat or inverted nipples, found that babies whose mothers did *not* receive treatment during pregnancy had fewer problems taking the breast than babies whose mothers received treatment. They therefore recommended that healthcare professionals stop screening mothers during pregnancy for flat or inverted nipples. Due to these research findings, the U.K. Royal College of Midwives warned against focusing on "inadequate nipples," encouraging a focus instead on making sure the baby takes the breast deeply after birth.

Nipple Everters

The purpose of these devices is to physically pull out a mother's flat or inverted nipples to make them easier for the baby to grasp for breastfeeding.

Indications for Use

This device may be helpful for the mother with flat or inverted nipples that are not caused by shortened milk ducts (tethered) and whose baby is having difficulty taking the breast (Genna, 2009).

What Research Says about Nipple Everters

Nipple everters can help mothers with flat or inverted nipples breastfeed.

In the one published study in which a makeshift version of this device was used, mothers gently pulled on its piston for about 30 to 60 seconds a couple of times each day and right before putting baby to breast (Kesaree, Banapurmath, Banapurmath, & Shamanur, 1993). This small study followed eight mothers from India who had inverted nipples and whose babies were unable to take the breast. When the study started, they had been bottle-feeding for 28 to 103 days. To create this device, the researchers transformed a 10 or 20 mL syringe (depending on nipple size) into a small suction device. After receiving positioning help and using the modified syringe before feedings, seven of eight babies took the breast. Within 4 to 6 weeks of breastfeeding often, six of the eight women were exclusively breastfeeding.

To transform a 10 or 20 mL syringe into a nipple suction device:

1. Remove the piston from the syringe and cut off the nozzle with a sharp blade.
2. Reinsert the piston through the cut end of the syringe so that the piston is pulled away from the smooth end of the syringe.
3. Put the smooth end of the syringe over the nipple and onto the areola.
4. Gently pull the piston to maintain steady but gentle pressure for 30 to 60 seconds, adjusting the pressure to comfort.

Commercial Nipple Everters

Along with the makeshift device described above, there are also available in some areas manufactured products specifically designed to perform this function. Examples of these types of products include Evert-It™, Niplette™, Supple Cups™ (can be used for tethered or untethered inverted nipples), and LatchAssist™. For a complete description of each with advantages and disadvantages, see the book *Selecting and Using Breastfeeding Tools* by U.S. lactation consultant Catherine Watson Genna.

NIPPLE CREAMS, OINTMENTS, AND PADS

Indications for Use

Nipple creams, ointments, and hydrogel pads may be used to speed the healing of traumatized nipples and reduce nipple pain. Canadian research found topical ointments ineffective treatments for bacterial infections of the nipple (Livingstone & Stringer, 1999; Livingstone, Willis, & Berkowitz, 1996). If a mother's nipples show signs of infection, such as visible pus, see p. 651- "Bacterial Infections."

What Research Says About Moist Wound Healing

Researchers in the wound-care field found nearly 50 years ago that wounds heal 50% faster when the internal moisture of the skin is maintained and scabbing and crusting are avoided (Hinman & Maibach, 1963). To maintain internal moisture, a moisture barrier must cover the broken skin to prevent evaporation, drying, and scab formation. Scabbing slows healing because it reduces the flow of nutrients to the wound and acts as a barrier to new cells, which must burrow under the scab. One drawback of scabbing unique to the breastfeeding mother is that nipple scabs pull off when baby breastfeeds, requiring the healing process to begin all over again.

Wounds heal faster when internal moisture is maintained.

Maintaining a normal moisture balance has also been found to decrease pain because it keeps the nerve endings in a more normal environment and protected from outside stimuli (Mann Mertz, 1990). To maintain a moisture barrier, the mother can use a product such as USP-modified anhydrous lanolin or hydrogel pads. If the moisture barrier is not used continuously other than when she's breastfeeding and the skin dries, healing will slow. See p. 646- "Treatments by Stages of Trauma" for treatments to consider for different stages of nipple trauma. Expressed milk, warm compresses, and tea bags have been recommended for nipple trauma in the past, but these treatments do not provide a moisture barrier, and studies have not found them to be effective at speeding healing (Akkuzu & Taskin, 2000; Lavergne, 1997; Melli et al., 2007).

USP-Modified Anhydrous Lanolin

What makes this type of lanolin different from the lanolins used in the past is that impurities that caused the skin reactions previously thought to be due to "wool allergy" (such as free alcohols, detergents, and pesticides) have been removed. Different brands of this type of lanolin contain different levels of these impurities. The lower the levels of these impurities, the less likely the product will cause a skin reaction (Clark, Blondeel, Cronin, Oleffe, & Wilkinson, 1981). USP-modified anhydrous lanolin is considered safe for the baby to ingest, so it does not have to be washed off before breastfeeding.

When using this type of lanolin, suggest the mother take care not use too much or too little. To provide a moist-wound-healing environment, enough lanolin must be applied after every breastfeeding to keep the broken skin moist. Several studies have found that when this lanolin is not applied after every breastfeeding, it does not speed healing (Mohammadzadeh, Farhat, & Esmaeily, 2005; Pugh et al., 1996). On the other hand, applying too much lanolin can make it more difficult for babies to take the breast (Dodd & Chalmers, 2003).

Other Over-the-Counter Nipple Topicals

Other nipple creams and ointments have possible drawbacks. Some need to be washed off before feedings. Some have tastes babies dislike. Some have ingredients like petroleum jelly that can clog skin pores. Some contain alcohol, which is drying. Some contain numbing ingredients that can delay the mother's milk ejection. Those containing vitamin E can cause elevated blood levels in the baby and trigger allergic reactions. Olive oil has anti-inflammatory properties, but does not provide a moist-wound-healing environment, and allergic reactions in mother or baby are possible.

All-Purpose Nipple Ointment (APNO)

Developed by Canadian pediatrician Jack Newman (see p. 649), this ointment requires a prescription and is created by a pharmacist by mixing antibiotic, anti-fungal, and anti-inflammatory medications to form a topical that is applied after every feeding to the affected nipple (Newman & Pitman, 2006). Once the pain is gone, the mother weans from it gradually over the course of a week. Because the ingredients are absorbed into the mother's skin, the mother does not need to remove it before the next breastfeeding. Although this nipple topical has been widely used in many countries, there is no published research on its use.

Glycerin-Based Hydrogel Pads

Hydrogel pads can decrease pain in mothers with nipple trauma.

Hydrogel pads, which are worn in the bra like a breast pad between feedings, have been used for decades to speed healing of all types of wounds, but they were not recommended for breastfeeding mothers until the late 1990s (Cable, Stewart, & Davis, 1997). Shortly after, a U.S. study found an association between the use of hydrogel pads in breastfeeding mothers with nipple trauma and an increased incidence of infection (Brent, Rudy, Redd, Rudy, & Roth, 1998). This study of 42 women was stopped early because the mothers using the glycerin-based pads developed significantly more infections than women in the group using USP-modified lanolin and breast shells. This was unexpected because the wound-healing literature indicated that hydrogel pads decrease the rate of infection. In another study of 94 breastfeeding mothers in Latvia, no infections developed, but the mothers in the glycerin-pad group healed no faster and had no less pain than the mothers using USP-modified lanolin or no products at all (Cadwell, Turner-Maffei, Blair, Brimdyr, & Maja McInerney, 2004).

Water-Based Hydrogel Pads

In a U.S. multi-centered, prospective, randomized controlled clinical trial with 106 breastfeeding mothers, researchers found that water-based hydrogel pads provided more pain relief and were used for a shorter time as compared with

USP-modified anhydrous lanolin (Dodd & Chalmers, 2003). None of the mothers in the hydrogel group developed infections.

Choosing a Product

If a mother wants to buy a USP-modified lanolin, suggest she choose a product with the lowest level of impurities, as it will be less likely to cause skin reactions. When choosing a hydrogel pad, suggest she choose one without adhesive on the pad (which can cause skin damage when removed for breastfeeding) and with the longest wear time, as this will be more cost-effective and indicates a greater product integrity. Cloth backing on a hydrogel pad indicates lower product integrity and shorter wear time.

NIPPLE SHIELDS

Unlike breast shells, nipple shields are worn over the nipple during breastfeeding, with the baby taking milk through the holes in the tip. Most are made of silicone and consist of a thin "brim" that covers all or part of the mother's areola and a firmer, protruding "tip" that fits over her nipple and has several holes through which milk flows. During the last few decades, the pendulum has swung to both extremes regarding nipple shield use. After a time of being used often in hospitals during the early postpartum period, their use was strongly discouraged (Mohrbacher & Stock, 1996; Newman & Pitman, 2006). However, the research and case reports cited in the following sections indicate that in the right situations, nipple shields can be a useful tool to support breastfeeding.

Nipple shields can be a useful tool to support breastfeeding.

Indications for Use

Nipples shields can be used as a tool to help preserve breastfeeding in some situations. In one U.S. retrospective telephone survey of 202 breastfeeding mothers who used nipple shields, the mothers used them for the following reasons (Powers & Tapia, 2004):

- Flat or inverted nipples (62%)
- Disorganized infant suck (43%)
- Sore nipples (23%)
- Engorgement (15%)
- Prematurity (12%)
- Tongue tie (1%)

In a mother with flat or inverted nipples, the tip of the nipple shield can provide the firm feeling deep in his mouth a baby is looking for, especially when bottles and/or pacifiers have altered his expectations (Wilson-Clay & Hoover, 2008). For this same reason, a shield may help a newborn take an engorged breast or transition a reluctant bottle-feeding baby to the breast (Wilson-Clay, 1996). For mothers with traumatized nipples, temporary use of a nipple shield may provide just enough pain relief to avoid interrupting breastfeeding. For the baby with high muscle tone or tongue tie, the firm shield can help push the breast past a retracted or humped tongue to trigger active suckling (Genna et al., 2008). For some preterm babies, use of a nipple shield may improve milk intake at the breast and avoid the need for supplementation (Clum & Primomo, 1996; Meier et al., 2000). For a mother with a breastfeeding problem, using a nipple shield can allow her baby to feed directly from the breast, simplifying her life by minimizing the need to express her milk and feed it to her baby another way.

That said, whenever possible, it is always better to solve a breastfeeding problem by improving feeding dynamics than by using a nipple shield. Like any tool, nipple shields can be used appropriately or misused. Examples of misuse of a nipple shield include offering it to a mother as the first solution to a breastfeeding problem or giving it to her as an alternative to spending time improving breastfeeding dynamics.

What Research Says About Nipple Shields

The literature features many case reports in which nipple shields have helped to preserve breastfeeding (Bodley & Powers, 1996; Brigham, 1996; Clum & Primomo, 1996; Elliott, 1996; Sealy, 1996; Wilson-Clay, 1996; Woodworth & Frank, 1996).

Some preterm babies have benefited from using a nipple shield. In one U.S. study, nipple shields were used with 34 preemies who were slipping off the nipple during pauses or falling asleep early in feedings (Meier et al., 2000). Milk transfer was greater for all 34 babies, with a mean increase of 14.4 mL or about a half-ounce. With the shield at the breast, the babies suckled for longer bursts and stayed awake at the breast longer. These preterm babies used the shield for a mean of 32.5 days (with a range of 2 to 171 days) out of a mean breastfeeding duration of 169 days (with a range of 14 to 365 days), so overall the mothers used the shield for about 24% of their time breastfeeding. The babies who were previously unable to transfer milk without the shield used it longer than the babies who took some milk from the bare breast. There was no association between the length of time the shield was used and duration of breastfeeding. The reason the shield helps some preemies is not yet fully understood, but some think its firmer tip may push deeper into baby's mouth triggering more active suckling (Hurst & Meier, 2010).

For a mother whose baby is not taking the breast well, using a nipple shield may make breastfeeding less stressful. It can also eliminate the need to supplement and shorten the time to exclusive breastfeeding. If a nipple shield helps increase milk intake at the breast, encourage the mother to use it for as long as needed. The preterm babies who benefit from using a nipple shield have been found to take more milk on average until they reach their full-term corrected age of about 40 weeks (Meier et al., 2000).

Choosing a Nipple Shield Style

There are two general nipple shield styles. Both are made of ultra-thin silicone and have a firm, protruding tip surrounded by a soft brim that lays flat on the mother's areola. One, referred to as a "regular" nipple shield, has a completely circular brim and is preferred by some mothers and their helpers because on some mothers it stays on the breast better during feedings. One U.S. lactation

A nipple shield will only be effective if it is a good fit for mother and baby.

consultant suggested that the more spherical the mother's breast, the better the regular style seems to fit (Genna, 2009). The other style, referred to as a "contact" nipple shield, has a cutout area on its brim that can be positioned for skin-to-skin contact with the baby's nose or chin. Some prefer this second style because of this increased skin-to-skin contact and because aligning the cutout with the baby's nose prevents the shield brim from bending back into the baby's face during breastfeeding. Because the anatomies and preferences of mothers and helpers vary, it may be wise to suggest a mother start with one of each style and see which works better for her.

Fitting a Nipple Shield

A nipple shield will only be an effective tool if is a good fit for both mother and baby. If the shield is too large for the baby, it can cause gagging (which can lead to feeding aversion), and if his jaws close on its tip rather than its soft brim, it can prevent effective milk transfer. A too-small shield may fail to stimulate active suckling because it doesn't extend deep enough into the baby's mouth. At one time, nipple shield length varied from between 1.9 and 6.4 cm (Drazin, 1998). After measuring 98 babies, one U.S. lactation consultant found the length of a young baby's "oral reach" (from mouth closure to the area in his mouth that triggers suckling) varied from 1.9 to 3.1 cm (Wilson-Clay & Hoover, 2008).

Most of the major brands of nipple shields have tips very close to the same length. The measurement that varies most, which is sometimes listed on the package, is the diameter of the tip opening. To fit the mother, the tip opening must be wide enough to comfortably accommodate her nipple. At this writing, the nipple shield sizes with narrower tip openings (16 mm and 20 mm) are most often chosen for preterm babies and newborns. Those with wider tip openings (24 mm) are most often chosen for older or larger babies. But the size of the baby is unrelated to the width of his mother's nipple, which means the nipple shield that is a good fit for a baby may not be a good fit for the mother, and vice versa. The mother's nipples may not fit comfortably in the shield (which can slow milk flow like a too-small pump opening) and the shield that fits the mother may not fit comfortably in the baby's mouth. In this case, a nipple shield would not be a helpful tool.

Applying a Nipple Shield

There are several different strategies for applying a nipple shield to the breast. Some simply place the shield over the mother's breast with the mother's nipple centered inside the tip. To keep it in place, the mother can place her thumb on one side of the brim's border and her fingers on the other side. Figures B.5, B.6, and B.7 illustrate one way to apply the shield that pulls the nipple farther in to the tip, reducing the work of the baby and helping it stay on the breast more easily:

1. Turn most of the shield tip inside out (Figure B.5).
2. Place the shield over the mother's nipple (Firgure B.6).
3. When the shield is slowly turned right side out and smoothed into place, the nipple is drawn into the tip (Figure B.7).

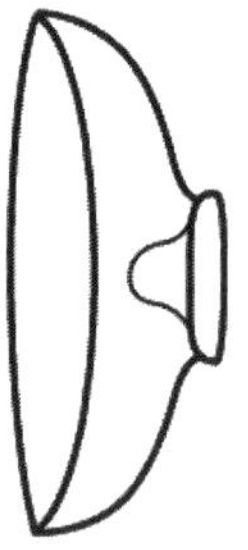

Figure B.5. To apply nipple shield, first turn tip partly inside out.
©2010 Ameda, used with permission.

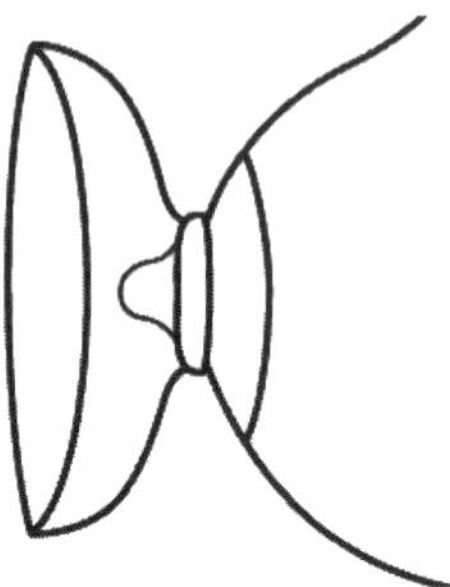

Figure B.6. Place shield over nipple.
©2010 Ameda, used with permission.

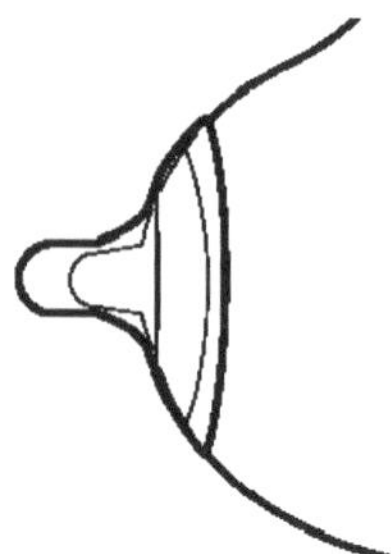

Figure B.7. As shield is smoothed onto breast, nipple is drawn into tip.
©2010 Ameda, used with permission.

Other ways to help keep the shield in place during breastfeeding include running hot or warm water over it before applying it or applying a small amount of USP-modified lanolin to the inside borders of the brim to help it stick to the skin.

Taking the Breast with the Nipple Shield

In addition to a well-fitting shield and good application to the breast, the mother needs to be sure the baby latches on deeply to the shield for effective breastfeeding (see Figure B.8). If the baby's jaws close on the shield's tip instead of its brim (see Figure B.9), it is less likely to trigger active suckling. As with any breastfeeding baby, the baby needs to open wide and take the breast deeply. If the mother can see any part of the firmer tip of the shield while the baby breastfeeds, suggest she take the baby off the breast and try again, making sure his mouth is open very wide as he takes the breast. U.S. lactation consultant Catherine Watson Genna wrote:

> Infants who are repeatedly allowed to slide down the teat with pursed lips are being set up for failure once the shield is removed. Sliding pursed lips along the soft human nipple pushes it out of the mouth. LCs always want to consider that any movement provides for future normal function of the infant and promote as close to normal as the infant can perform (Genna, 2009, p. 55).

Genna suggests starting baby in a "nose-to-nipple" position with both lips on the underside of the shield to help mimic what he will do later at the bare breast.

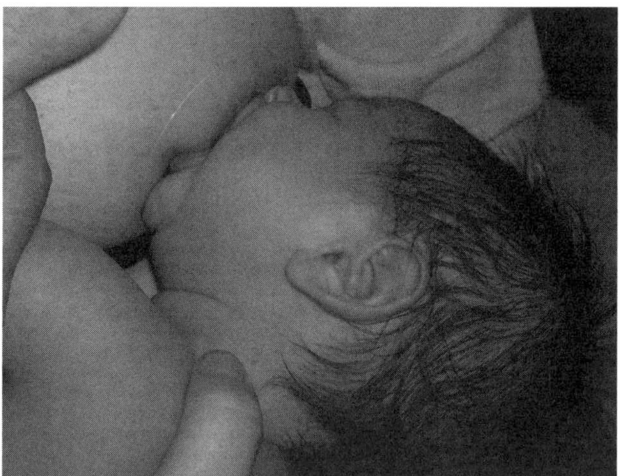

Figure B.8. Baby latched deeply with a nipple shield (wide gape, no tip showing)
©Catherine Watson Genna, used with permission

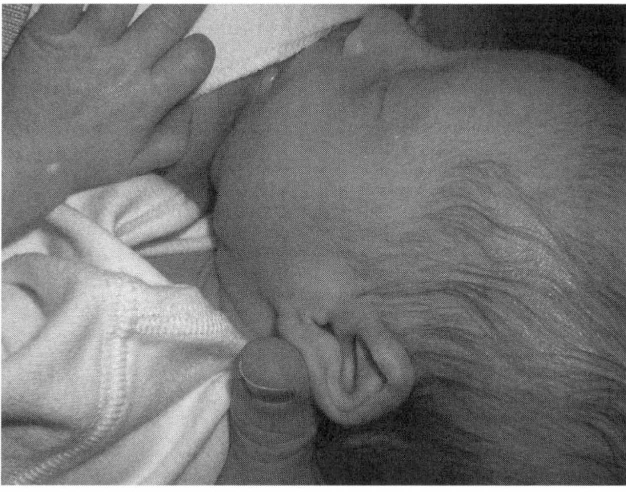

Figure B.9. Baby latched shallowly with a nipple shield (narrower gape, tip showing)
©Catherine Watson Genna, used with permission

Assessing Feeding Effectiveness with the Nipple Shield

After each feeding, suggest the mother look for signs of effective breastfeeding, such as milk in the tip of the shield and a decrease in breast fullness. The baby's behavior can also provide clues. A satisfied baby will release the breast when he's full. He may rest his head on the breast or be quietly alert, hands will be relaxed, and he will not begin to fuss right away if the mother lays him down. As a precaution, it is wise to have the baby's weight checked after a day or two on the shield, and weekly after that, to be sure he is getting enough milk and stimulating the mother's milk production.

Should the Mother Express Milk When Using a Nipple Shield?

Mothers do not need to express milk while using a nipple shield.

The original recommendation to express milk when using a nipple shield was made after research found reduced milk transfer with a nipple shield. One early U.K. study found that thick nipple shields altered babies' suckling patterns and the babies took less milk from the breast (Woolridge, Baum, & Drewett, 1980). The babies using the thick rubber "Mexican Hat" nipple shields took 58% less milk, and those using the thinner latex nipple shields took 22% less milk. However, the babies in the study had been breastfeeding well without the shield, and the change in suckling may have been simply because the shield was a new experience. The same dynamic may also have been at work in a Swedish study that found no difference in mothers' blood prolactin and cortisol levels when breastfeeding with or without a thin latex nipple shield, but also found a 42% decrease in milk transfer during breastfeeding (Amatayakul et al., 1987). A U.S. study used a breast pump with a nipple shield and also found reduced milk transfer, but pumping with the shield is not comparable to breastfeeding (Auerbach, 1990).

More recent U.S. research looked at weight gain in 54 breastfeeding babies using a nipple shield whose mothers were not expressing milk after feedings and found no statistically significant difference in weight gain at 2 weeks, 1 month, and 2 months between babies using a nipple shield at the breast and babies who were not (Chertok, 2009). U.S. lactation consultant Catherine Watson Genna wrote:

> Many LCs encourage mothers using a nipple shield to pump. I originally followed the 'party line' and encouraged mothers to express milk while using a nipple shield, but soon found that some mothers were developing uncomfortable hyperlactation and recurrent plugged ducts. Now instructions are individualized. If the infant feeds efficiently and effectively with the nipple shield, the mother is encouraged to watch the baby for normal energy, copious stools, and sated behaviors. If the infant is sleepier than usual, has fewer than four or five stools per day in the early weeks, or is unsettled, she is encouraged to express and feed sufficient milk to the infant to resolve these concerns (Genna, 2009, p. 57).

In some situations, expressing after feeding makes sense, such as when a mother's milk production is low or if she is unsure whether her baby is draining her breasts effectively with the shield. Regular weight checks are recommended until it is clear milk expression is not needed. Other signs a mother can use between weight checks include looking for milk in the tip of the shield after feedings and a decrease in breast fullness after feedings.

Weaning from the Nipple Shield

The right time to wean from the shield will depend in large part on the reason it was used. For example, if it is used to help a baby who has been bottle-feeding recognize the breast as a source of milk, it may only be useful at one feeding. But if mother and baby have been struggling with breastfeeding for some time and the baby considers the breast a source of frustration, a longer time of easier breastfeeding to build positive associations may be better. The preterm baby using the nipple shield to improve breastfeeding effectiveness may need to grow and mature for several weeks before he can feed well without the shield (Meier et al., 2000).

In one U.S. retrospective telephone survey of 202 mothers who used a nipple shield, 67% eventually weaned from the shield and breastfed without it, with the length of shield use ranging from 1 day to 5 months and the median duration 2 weeks (Powers & Tapia, 2004). Of the 33% who used the shield for the duration of breastfeeding, 11% said the baby would have breastfed without it at any time, but they continued using it because breastfeeding was more comfortable with it. One mother used the nipple shield for the entire 15 months she and her baby breastfed.

When a mother uses the shield because her baby has had trouble taking the breast, suggest she start breastfeeding with the shield, and after she has a milk ejection and hears her baby swallowing, try removing the shield quickly and putting baby back to breast. If the baby takes the breast, she can use this strategy whenever needed to move from shield to bare breast. Usually, as the baby becomes more coordinated and more practiced, the shield will be needed at fewer and fewer feedings.

If this strategy doesn't work, suggest the mother continue using the shield throughout the feedings and try again a few days later when she and the baby are feeling relaxed, perhaps at a time when the baby is not too hungry. Suggest the mother always strive to keep the breast a pleasant place for her baby and avoid the stress of trying to breastfeed without the shield at every feeding.

The mother should be encouraged to use the shield as long as it helps the baby breastfeed more effectively. In general, as the baby matures, his coordination increases, and as he develops more practice and positive associations at the breast, the easier it will be to wean him off the shield. A baby may need the shield for one feeding, a few feedings, a few days, a few weeks, or very rarely, a few months. If the baby is unable or unwilling to breastfeed without the shield, chances are the problem that caused the baby to need the nipple shield is not yet completely resolved. Encourage the mother to follow her baby's cues, but keep trying to offer the breast without the shield every few days.

The mother should be encouraged to use the shield as long as it helps the baby breastfeed effectively.

Although it was once recommended to wean a baby from a nipple shield by gradually cutting off more of the tip of the shield until it is gone, this strategy is not recommended for the ultra-thin silicone shields used today. When cut, silicone has sharp edges that can hurt the baby.

SCALES FOR TEST-WEIGHING

Indications for Use with Preterm Babies

Test-weighing allows mothers to monitor their babies' intake.

Test-weighing can be a helpful tool to determine milk intake when a preterm baby begins breastfeeding. This can also prevent delays in initiating breastfeeding, as some healthcare providers are reluctant to allow early breastfeeding when a preterm baby's milk intake cannot be accurately measured. Knowing how much milk a preterm baby takes at the breast can prevent oversupplementation, which can delay the transition to full breastfeeding (Hurst, Meier, Engstrom, & Myatt, 2004). Knowing how effectively a preterm baby breastfeeds can also affect discharge plans, as feeding competence is usually one of the determining criteria (McCain, Gartside, Greenberg, & Lott, 2001; Nye, 2008).

Indications for Use with Any Baby

Test-weighing can allow a mother to monitor milk intake while her baby transitions from other feeding methods to exclusive breastfeeding, which can prevent oversupplementation. It can also be useful to know a baby's milk intake at the breast while determining the cause of a breastfeeding problem. When a mother is very anxious about her baby's milk intake, test-weighing can provide reassurance that her baby is getting what he needs from the breast. It can also reveal when a baby is breastfeeding ineffectively so that supplements can be started before the baby becomes unduly stressed.

What Research Says About Scales for Test-Weighing

Research has found that the baby scales typically found in healthcare offices are not accurate enough to assess milk intake at the breast (Savenije & Brand, 2006). Only scales accurate to at least 2 g (0.1 ounce) are precise enough for this purpose. Most research on test-weighing relates to its use with preterm babies. U.S. research had found that neither mothers nor lactation consultants could accurately estimate preterm babies' milk intake at the breast by observing behaviors used to gauge milk intake in full-term healthy babies, such as audible swallowing and wide jaw movements (Meier, Engstrom, Fleming, Streeter, & Lawrence, 1996). But doing pre- and post-feed weights with a scale accurate to 2 g was found to be a reliable way to measure milk intake at the breast (Meier et al., 1994). Even when babies have leads attached to them to connect them to medical equipment, test-weighing has been found to be reliable in measuring milk intake during breastfeeding (Haase, Barreira, Murphy, Mueller, & Rhodes, 2009).

Mothers' Reactions to Test-Weighing

Some assume that test-weighing will increase mothers' anxiety. While that may be true of a small percentage of mothers, one U.S. study examined mothers' reactions to either using or not using a scale as they transitioned their preterm baby to breastfeeding (Hurst et al., 2004). All the mothers who used the scale found it either very or extremely helpful, and 75% of the mothers who didn't use the scale reported it would have been somewhat to extremely helpful to them to know exactly how much milk their baby was taking at the breast. Another U.S. study found that there was no significant difference in confidence among mothers who transitioned to the breast using a scale for test-weighs and those who didn't (Hall, Shearer, Mogan, & Berkowitz, 2002). If a mother finds test-weighing stressful or low milk intake leaves her feeling discouraged, as an alternative, she can reduce her baby's supplement gradually, while carefully monitoring his weight and growth at regular check-ups (Flacking, Nyqvist, Ewald, & Wallin, 2003).

Avoiding Weight Errors

Although the scales suitable for test-weighing are accurate to 2 g, common mistakes sometimes affect results. For example, to get an accurate estimate of milk intake, the baby must be dressed identically during the before and after weights. If a sock falls off or the baby's diaper is changed, the weight will not be accurate. Milk dripped onto the baby's clothes either from dribbling during feeding or milk leaked onto the baby from the other breast will also throw off the weight. The extension of a blanket or baby's arm or leg over the side of the scale basket is another variable that can affect the weight.

Weigh Small Babies Tummy Down

Newborns feel very insecure on their backs and may find being weighed in that position upsetting. Most small babies find being weighed much less stressful if they are placed on the scale basket tummy down.

Newborns should be weighed while prone.

Where to Find Scales for Test-Weighing

These scales are available in many hospitals, clinics, and lactation consultant offices. In some areas, they can be rented for home use, usually from medical supply companies or breast pump rental businesses. The scales commonly used featuring buttons that allow the difference between the before and after weights to be automatically calculated are made by the Japanese company Tanita. These scales are also available through other companies that rebrand them and sell them at a higher price, but they are available more economically from the manufacturer.

RESOURCES FOR PARENTS

Books

Genna, C.W. (2009). *Selecting and using breastfeeding tools: Improving care and outcomes.* Amarillo, TX: Hale Publishing.

Peterson, A. & Harmer, M. *Balancing breast & bottle: Reaching your breastfeeding goals.* Amarillo, TX: Hale Publishing, 2010.

REFERENCES

Abouelfettoh, A. M., Dowling, D. A., Dabash, S. A., Elguindy, S. R., & Seoud, I. A. (2008). Cup versus bottle feeding for hospitalized late preterm infants in Egypt: a quasi-experimental study. *International Breastfeeding Journal, 3*, 27.

Akkuzu, G., & Taskin, L. (2000). Impacts of breast-care techniques on prevention of possible postpartum nipple problems. *Professional Care of Mother and Child, 10*(2), 38-41.

Alekseev, N. P., Omel'ianuk, E. V., & Talalaeva, N. E. (2000). [Dynamics of milk ejection reflex during continuous rhythmic stimulation of areola-nipple complex of the mammary gland]. *Rossiiskii Fiziologicheskii Zhurnal Imeni I. M. Sechenova, 86*(6), 711-719.

Alexander, J. M., Grant, A. M., & Campbell, M. J. (1992). Randomised controlled trial of breast shells and Hoffman's exercises for inverted and non-protractile nipples. *British Medical Journal, 304*(6833), 1030-1032.

Aloysius, A., & Hickson, M. (2007). Evaluation of paladai cup feeding in breast-fed preterm infants compared with bottle feeding. *Early Human Development, 83*(9), 619-621.

Amatayakul, K., Vutyavanich, T., Tanthayaphinant, O., Tovanabutra, S., Yutabootr, Y., & Drewett, R. F. (1987). Serum prolactin and cortisol levels after suckling for varying periods of time and the effect of a nipple shield. *Acta Obstetricia et Gynecologica Scandinavica, 66*(1), 47-51.

Armstrong, H. C. (1987). Breastfeeding low birthweight babies: advances in Kenya. *Journal of Human Lactation, 3*(2), 34-37.

Auerbach, K. G. (1990). The effect of nipple shields on maternal milk volume. *Journal of Obstetric, Gynecologic, and Neonatal Nursing, 19*(5), 419-427.

Bergman, N. J., & Jurisoo, L. A. (1994). The 'kangaroo-method' for treating low birth weight babies in a developing country. *Tropical Doctor, 24*(2), 57-60.

Binns, C. W., Win, N. N., Zhao, Y., & Scott, J. A. (2006). Trends in the expression of breastmilk 1993-2003. *Breastfeeding Review, 14*(3), 5-9.

Blaymore Bier, J. A., Ferguson, A. E., Morales, Y., Liebling, J. A., Oh, W., & Vohr, B. R. (1997). Breastfeeding infants who were extremely low birth weight. *Pediatrics, 100*(6), E3.

Bodley, V., & Powers, D. (1996). Long-term nipple shield use--a positive perspective. *Journal of Human Lactation, 12*(4), 301-304.

Borucki, L. C. (2005). Breastfeeding mothers' experiences using a supplemental feeding tube device: finding an alternative. *Journal of Human Lactation, 21*(4), 429-438.

Brent, N., Rudy, S. J., Redd, B., Rudy, T. E., & Roth, L. A. (1998). Sore nipples in breast-feeding women: a clinical trial of wound dressings vs conventional care. *Archives of Pediatrics and Adolescent Medicine, 152*(11), 1077-1082.

Brigham, M. (1996). Mothers' reports of the outcome of nipple shield use. *Journal of Human Lactation, 12*(4), 291-297.

Cable, B., Stewart, M., & Davis, J. (1997). Nipple wound care: a new approach to an old problem. *Journal of Human Lactation, 13*(4), 313-318.

Cadwell, K., Turner-Maffei, C., Blair, A., Brimdyr, K., & Maja McInerney, Z. (2004). Pain reduction and treatment of sore nipples in nursing mothers. *Journal of Perinatal Education, 13*(1), 29-35.

Carrascoza, K. C., Possobon Rde, F., Tomita, L. M., & Moraes, A. B. (2006). Consequences of bottle-feeding to the oral facial development of initially breastfed children. *Jornal de Pediatria, 82*(5), 395-397.

Centuori, S., Burmaz, T., Ronfani, L., Fragiacomo, M., Quintero, S., Pavan, C., et al. (1999). Nipple care, sore nipples, and breastfeeding: a randomized trial. *Journal of Human Lactation, 15*(2), 125-130.

Chen, C. H., Wang, T. M., Chang, H. M., & Chi, C. S. (2000). The effect of breast- and bottle-feeding on oxygen saturation and body temperature in preterm infants. *Journal of Human Lactation, 16*(1), 21-27.

Chertok, I. R. (2009). Reexamination of ultra-thin nipple shield use, infant growth and maternal satisfaction. *Journal of Clinical Nursing, 18*(21), 2949-2955.

Clark, E. W., Blondeel, A., Cronin, E., Oleffe, J. A., & Wilkinson, D. S. (1981). Lanolin of reduced sensitizing potential. *Contact Dermatitis, 7*(2), 80-83.

Cloherty, M., Alexander, J., Holloway, I., Galvin, K., & Inch, S. (2005). The cup-versus-bottle debate: a theme from an ethnographic study of the supplementation of breastfed infants in hospital in the United Kingdom. *Journal of Human Lactation, 21*(2), 151-162; quiz 163-156.

Clum, D., & Primomo, J. (1996). Use of a silicone nipple shield with premature infants. *Journal of Human Lactation, 12*(4), 287-290.

Collins, C. T., Makrides, M., Gillis, J., & McPhee, A. J. (2008). Avoidance of bottles during the establishment of breast feeds in preterm infants. *Cochrane Database of Systematic Reviews*(4), CD005252.

Collins, C. T., Ryan, P., Crowther, C. A., McPhee, A. J., Paterson, S., & Hiller, J. E. (2004). Effect of bottles, cups, and dummies on breast feeding in preterm infants: a randomised controlled trial. *British Medical Journal, 329*(7459), 193-198.

Dodd, V., & Chalmers, C. (2003). Comparing the use of hydrogel dressings to lanolin ointment with lactating mothers. *Journal of Obstetric, Gynecologic, and Neonatal Nursing, 32*(4), 486-494.

Dowling, D. A., Meier, P. P., DiFiore, J. M., Blatz, M., & Martin, R. J. (2002). Cup-feeding for preterm infants: mechanics and safety. *Journal of Human Lactation, 18*(1), 13-20; quiz 46-19, 72.

Drazin, P. (1998). Taking nipple shields out of the closet. *Birth Issues, 7*(2), 41-47.

Egnell, E. (1956). The mechanics of different methods of emptying the female breast. *Svenska Lakartidningen*(40), 1-7.

Ekstrom, A., Widstrom, A. M., & Nissen, E. (2003). Duration of breastfeeding in Swedish primiparous and multiparous women. *Journal of Human Lactation, 19*(2), 172-178.

Elliott, C. (1996). Using a silicone nipple shield to assist a baby unable to latch. *Journal of Human Lactation, 12*(4), 309-313.

Flacking, R., Nyqvist, K. H., Ewald, U., & Wallin, L. (2003). Long-term duration of breastfeeding in Swedish low birth weight infants. *Journal of Human Lactation, 19*(2), 157-165.

Flint, A., New, K., & Davies, M. W. (2007). Cup feeding versus other forms of supplemental enteral feeding for newborn infants unable to fully breastfeed. *Cochrane Database of Systematic Reviews*(2), CD005092.

Genna, C. W. (2009). *Selecting and using breastfeeding tools: improving care and outcomes*. Amarillo, TX: Hale Publishing.

Genna, C. W., Fram, J. L., & Sandora, L. (2008). Neurological issues and breastfeeding. In C. W. Genna (Ed.), *Supporting sucking skills in breastfeeding infants* (pp. 253-303). Boston, MA: Jones and Bartlett.

Gomes, C. F., Thomson, Z., & Cardoso, J. R. (2009). Utilization of surface electromyography during the feeding of term and preterm infants: a literature review. *Developmental Medicine and Child Neurology, 51*(12), 936-942.

Gomes, C. F., Trezza, E. M., Murade, E. C., & Padovani, C. R. (2006). Surface electromyography of facial muscles during natural and artificial feeding of infants. *Jornal de Pediatria, 82*(2), 103-109.

Gupta, A., Khanna, K., & Chattree, S. (1999). Cup feeding: an alternative to bottle feeding in a neonatal intensive care unit. *Journal of Tropical Pediatrics, 45*(2), 108-110.

Haase, B., Barreira, J., Murphy, P. K., Mueller, M., & Rhodes, J. (2009). The Development of an Accurate Test Weighing Technique for Preterm and High-Risk Hospitalized Infants. *Breastfeed Med.*

Hall, W. A., Shearer, K., Mogan, J., & Berkowitz, J. (2002). Weighing preterm infants before & after breastfeeding: does it increase maternal confidence and competence? *MCN; American Journal of Maternal Child Nursing, 27*(6), 318-326; quiz 327.

Hinman, C. D., & Maibach, H. (1963). Effect of Air Exposure and Occlusion on Experimental Human Skin Wounds. *Nature, 200*, 377-378.

Howard, C. R., de Blieck, E. A., ten Hoopen, C. B., Howard, F. M., Lanphear, B. P., & Lawrence, R. A. (1999). Physiologic stability of newborns during cup- and bottle-feeding. *Pediatrics, 104*(5 Pt 2), 1204-1207.

Howard, C. R., Howard, F. M., Lanphear, B., Eberly, S., deBlieck, E. A., Oakes, D., et al. (2003). Randomized clinical trial of pacifier use and bottle-feeding or cupfeeding and their effect on breastfeeding. *Pediatrics, 111*(3), 511-518.

Huang, Y. Y., Gau, M. L., Huang, C. M., & Lee, J. T. (2009). Supplementation with cup-feeding as a substitute for bottle-feeding to promote breastfeeding. *Chang Gung Medical Journal, 32*(4), 423-431.

Hurst, N. M., & Meier, P. P. (2010). Breastfeeding the preterm infant. In J. Riordan (Ed.), *Breastfeeding and human lactation* (4th ed., pp. 425-470). Boston, MA: Jones and Bartlett.

Hurst, N. M., Meier, P. P., Engstrom, J. L., & Myatt, A. (2004). Mothers performing in-home measurement of milk intake during breastfeeding of their preterm infants: maternal reactions and feeding outcomes. *J Hum Lact, 20*(2), 178-187.

Jones, E., Dimmock, P. W., & Spencer, S. A. (2001). A randomised controlled trial to compare methods of milk expression after preterm delivery. *Archives of Disease in Childhood. Fetal and Neonatal Edition, 85*(2), F91-95.

Kassing, D. (2002). Bottle-feeding as a tool to reinforce breastfeeding. *Journal of Human Lactation, 18*(1), 56-60.

Kent, J. C., Mitoulas, L. R., Cregan, M. D., Geddes, D. T., Larsson, M., Doherty, D. A., et al. (2008). Importance of vacuum for breastmilk expression. *Breastfeeding Medicine, 3*(1), 11-19.

Kent, J. C., Mitoulas, L. R., Cregan, M. D., Ramsay, D. T., Doherty, D. A., & Hartmann, P. E. (2006). Volume and frequency of breastfeedings and fat content of breast milk throughout the day. *Pediatrics, 117*(3), e387-395.

Kent, J. C., Ramsay, D. T., Doherty, D., Larsson, M., & Hartmann, P. E. (2003). Response of breasts to different stimulation patterns of an electric breast pump. *Journal of Human Lactation, 19*(2), 179-186; quiz 187-178, 218.

Kesaree, N., Banapurmath, C. R., Banapurmath, S., & Shamanur, K. (1993). Treatment of inverted nipples using a disposable syringe. *Journal of Human Lactation, 9*(1), 27-29.

Kliethermes, P. A., Cross, M. L., Lanese, M. G., Johnson, K. M., & Simon, S. D. (1999). Transitioning preterm infants with nasogastric tube supplementation: increased likelihood of breastfeeding. *Journal of Obstetric, Gynecologic, and Neonatal Nursing, 28*(3), 264-273.

Kobayashi, H. M., Scavone, H., Jr., Ferreira, R. I., & Garib, D. G. (2010). Relationship between breastfeeding duration and prevalence of posterior crossbite in the deciduous dentition. *American Journal of Orthodontics and Dentofacial Orthopedics, 137*(1), 54-58.

Kramer, M. S., Guo, T., Platt, R. W., Vanilovich, I., Sevkovskaya, Z., Dzikovich, I., et al. (2004). Feeding effects on growth during infancy. *Journal of Pediatrics, 145*(5), 600-605.

Labiner-Wolfe, J., Fein, S. B., Shealy, K. R., & Wang, C. (2008). Prevalence of breast milk expression and associated factors. *Pediatrics, 122 Suppl 2*, S63-68.

Lang, S., Lawrence, C. J., & Orme, R. L. (1994). Cup feeding: an alternative method of infant feeding. *Archives of Disease in Childhood, 71*(4), 365-369.

Lavergne, N. A. (1997). Does application of tea bags to sore nipples while breastfeeding provide effective relief? *Journal of Obstetric, Gynecologic, and Neonatal Nursing, 26*(1), 53-58.

Law-Morstatt, L., Judd, D. M., Snyder, P., Baier, R. J., & Dhanireddy, R. (2003). Pacing as a treatment technique for transitional sucking patterns. *Journal of Perinatology, 23*(6), 483-488.

Li, R., Fein, S. B., & Grummer-Strawn, L. M. (2008). Association of breastfeeding intensity and bottle-emptying behaviors at early infancy with infants' risk for excess weight at late infancy. *Pediatrics, 122 Suppl 2*, S77-84.

Livingstone, V., & Stringer, L. J. (1999). The treatment of Staphyloccocus aureus infected sore nipples: a randomized comparative study. *Journal of Human Lactation, 15*(3), 241-246.

Livingstone, V. H., Willis, C. E., & Berkowitz, J. (1996). Staphylococcus aureus and sore nipples. *Canadian Family Physician, 42*, 654-659.

MAIN. (1994). Preparing for breast feeding: treatment of inverted and non-protractile nipples in pregnancy. The MAIN Trial Collaborative Group. *Midwifery, 10*(4), 200-214.

Malhotra, N., Vishwambaran, L., Sundaram, K. R., & Narayanan, I. (1999). A controlled trial of alternative methods of oral feeding in neonates. *Early Human Development, 54*(1), 29-38.

Mann Mertz, P. (1990). Intervention: Dressing effects on wound healing. In W. H. Eaglstein (Ed.), Wound care manual: New directions in wound healing (pp. 83-96). Princeton, NJ: ConvaTec.

Marinelli, K. A., Burke, G. S., & Dodd, V. L. (2001). A comparison of the safety of cupfeedings and bottlefeedings in premature infants whose mothers intend to breastfeed. *Journal of Perinatology, 21*(6), 350-355.

McCain, G. C., Gartside, P. S., Greenberg, J. M., & Lott, J. W. (2001). A feeding protocol for healthy preterm infants that shortens time to oral feeding. *Journal of Pediatrics, 139*(3), 374-379.

Meier, P., & Anderson, G. C. (1987). Responses of small preterm infants to bottle- and breast-feeding. *MCN; American Journal of Maternal Child Nursing, 12*(2), 97-105.

Meier, P., Motykowski, J. E., & Zuleger, J. L. (2004). Choosing a correctly-fitted breastshield for milk expression. *Medela Messenger, 21,* 8-9.

Meier, P. P., Brown, L. P., Hurst, N. M., Spatz, D. L., Engstrom, J. L., Borucki, L. C., et al. (2000). Nipple shields for preterm infants: effect on milk transfer and duration of breastfeeding. *Journal of Human Lactation, 16*(2), 106-114; quiz 129-131.

Meier, P. P., Engstrom, J. L., Crichton, C. L., Clark, D. R., Williams, M. M., & Mangurten, H. H. (1994). A new scale for in-home test-weighing for mothers of preterm and high risk infants. *Journal of Human Lactation, 10*(3), 163-168.

Meier, P. P., Engstrom, J. L., Fleming, B. A., Streeter, P. L., & Lawrence, P. B. (1996). Estimating milk intake of hospitalized preterm infants who breastfeed. *Journal of Human Lactation, 12*(1), 21-26.

Meier, P. P., Engstrom, J. L., Hurst, N. M., Ackerman, B., Allen, M., Motykowski, J. E., et al. (2008). A comparison of the efficiency, efficacy, comfort, and convenience of two hospital-grade electric breast pumps for mothers of very low birthweight infants. *Breastfeeding Medicine, 3*(3), 141-150.

Melli, M. S., Rashidi, M. R., Nokhoodchi, A., Tagavi, S., Farzadi, L., Sadaghat, K., et al. (2007). A randomized trial of peppermint gel, lanolin ointment, and placebo gel to prevent nipple crack in primiparous breastfeeding women. *Medical Science Monitor, 13*(9), CR406-411.

Mitoulas, L. R., Lai, C. T., Gurrin, L. C., Larsson, M., & Hartmann, P. E. (2002). Effect of vacuum profile on breast milk expression using an electric breast pump. *Journal of Human Lactation, 18*(4), 353-360.

Mohammadzadeh, A., Farhat, A., & Esmaeily, H. (2005). The effect of breast milk and lanolin on sore nipples. *Saudi Med J, 26*(8), 1231-1234.

Mohrbacher, N., & Stock, J. (1996). *The Breastfeeding answer book* (2nd ed.). Schaumburg, IL: La Leche League International.

Newman, J., & Pitman, T. (2006). *The ultimate breastfeeding book of answers*. New York, New York: Three Rivers Press.

Noble, R., & Bovey, A. (1997). Therapeutic teat use for babies who breastfeed poorly. *Breastfeeding Review, 5*(2), 37-42.

Nye, C. (2008). Transitioning premature infants from gavage to breast. *Neonatal Network, 27*(1), 7-13.

Nyqvist, K. H., & Ewald, U. (2006). Surface electromyography of facial muscles during natural and artificial feeding of infants: identification of differences between breast-, cup- and bottle-feeding. *Jornal de Pediatria, 82*(2), 85-86.

Oddy, W. H., & Glenn, K. (2003). Implementing the Baby Friendly Hospital Initiative: the role of finger feeding. *Breastfeeding Review, 11*(1), 5-10.

Ohyama, M. (2007). Which is more effective, manual- or electric-expression in the first 48 hours after delivery in a setting of mother-infant separation? Preliminary report. [abstract]. *Breastfeeding Medicine, 2*(3), 179.

Peterson, A., & Harmer, M. (2010). *Balancing breast & bottle: reaching your breasrtfeeding goals*. Amarillo, TX: Hale Publishing.

Poets, C. F., Langner, M. U., & Bohnhorst, B. (1997). Effects of bottle feeding and two different methods of gavage feeding on oxygenation and breathing patterns in preterm infants. *Acta Paediatrica, 86*(4), 419-423.

Powers, D., & Tapia, V. B. (2004). Women's experiences using a nipple shield. *Journal of Human Lactation, 20*(3), 327-334.

Pugh, L. C., Buchko, B. L., Bishop, B. A., Cochran, J. F., Smith, L. R., & Lerew, D. J. (1996). A comparison of topical agents to relieve nipple pain and enhance breastfeeding. *Birth, 23*(2), 88-93.

Ramsay, D. T., Mitoulas, L. R., Kent, J. C., Cregan, M. D., Doherty, D. A., Larsson, M., et al. (2006). Milk flow rates can be used to identify and investigate milk ejection in women expressing breast milk using an electric breast pump. *Breastfeeding Medicine, 1*(1), 14-23.

Ramsay, D. T., Mitoulas, L. R., Kent, J. C., Larsson, M., & Hartmann, P. E. (2005). The use of ultrasound to characterize milk ejection in women using an electric breast pump. *Journal of Human Lactation, 21*(4), 421-428.

Renfrew, M. J., Craig, D., Dyson, L., McCormick, F., Rice, S., King, S. E., et al. (2009). Breastfeeding promotion for infants in neonatal units: a systematic review and economic analysis. *Health Technology Assessment, 13*(40), 1-146, iii-iv.

Righard, L. (1998). Are breastfeeding problems related to incorrect breastfeeding technique and the use of pacifiers and bottles? *Birth, 25*(1), 40-44.

Righard, L., & Alade, M. O. (1997). Breastfeeding and the use of pacifiers. *Birth, 24*(2), 116-120.

Rocha, N. M., Martinez, F. E., & Jorge, S. M. (2002). Cup or bottle for preterm infants: effects on oxygen saturation, weight gain, and breastfeeding. *Journal of Human Lactation, 18*(2), 132-138.

Rosen, L., Shuster, K., & Barber, C. C. (2001). Does the Ameda Elite breast pump have the ability to bring in and maintain the milk supply of mothers whose babies are in the Neonatal Intensive Care (NICU)? Poster session ILCA 2001, Acapulco, Mexico: Stormont -Vail HealthCare.

Savenije, O. E., & Brand, P. L. (2006). Accuracy and precision of test weighing to assess milk intake in newborn infants. *Archives of Disease in Childhood. Fetal and Neonatal Edition, 91*(5), F330-332.

Sealy, C. N. (1996). Rethinking the use of nipple shields. *Journal of Human Lactation, 12*(4), 299-300.

Slusher, T., Slusher, I. L., Biomdo, M., Bode-Thomas, F., Curtis, B. A., & Meier, P. (2007). Electric breast pump use increases maternal milk volume in African nurseries. *Journal of Tropical Pediatrics, 53*(2), 125-130.

Taveras, E. M., Rifas-Shiman, S. L., Scanlon, K. S., Grummer-Strawn, L. M., Sherry, B., & Gillman, M. W. (2006). To what extent is the protective effect of breastfeeding on future overweight explained by decreased maternal feeding restriction? *Pediatrics, 118*(6), 2341-2348.

WHO. (2006). Breastfeeding in the WHO Multicentre Growth Reference Study. *Acta Paediatrica. Supplement, 450*, 16-26.

Wilson-Clay, B. (1996). Clinical use of silicone nipple shields. *Journal of Human Lactation, 12*(4), 279-285.

Wilson-Clay, B. (2005). External pacing techniques: protecting respiratory stability during feeding. In *Independent Study Module*. Amarillo, TX: Hale Publishing.

Wilson-Clay, B., & Hoover, K. (2008). *The Breastfeeding Atlas* (4th ed.). Manchaca, TX: LactNews Press.

Woodworth, M., & Frank, E. (1996). Transitioning to the breast at six weeks: use of a nipple shield. *Journal of Human Lactation, 12*(4), 305-307.

Woolridge, M. W., Baum, J. D., & Drewett, R. F. (1980). Effect of a traditional and of a new nipple shield on sucking patterns and milk flow. *Early Human Development, 4*(4), 357-364.

Working with Health Professionals

Appendix

C

IN A HOSPITAL SETTING

Ask if a lactation consultant or other breastfeeding specialist is available to help. Most hospitals have someone on staff dedicated to helping breastfeeding mothers and babies. Whether mother and her baby are on the mother-baby unit or not, suggest she ask to see the breastfeeding specialist. In some hospitals, lactation professionals can only be seen when specifically requested.

When the mother has questions or concerns, suggest she seek out the hospital personnel who are most supportive of her and of breastfeeding. Most mothers find there are one or two people at the hospital who are especially good at listening and explaining the sometimes intimidating terminology and high-tech equipment.

IN ALL SETTINGS

Suggest the mother be clear about her breastfeeding goals from the start. This can help avoid conflict later. Knowing the importance of breastfeeding to a mother may motivate the healthcare providers working with that family to be more willing to try different approaches. She might say, for example, "Let's discuss treatments (strategies, approaches) that will be most supportive of breastfeeding."

Mothers who are concerned about advice they've received from healthcare providers may want you to offer them research citations.

If actions are suggested that could negatively affect breastfeeding or are counter to the research, offer citations to share. When discussing options with the mother, keep in mind she may not have understood everything about the situation and there may be more going on than she describes. Also, it is important for the mother to come to an agreement with her healthcare provider. Openly disagreeing with the healthcare provider's advice may make their situation more difficult and may confuse the mother.

One way to phrase this to a mother is: "Some medical professionals do use that approach, but research has found…" and then ask the mother if she would like some references she can pass along. For the appropriate citations, see the chapter that covers their situation. Medical articles should be easy for health professionals to access either online or through their medical library.

Example: The neonatologist tells the mother he does not want her to breastfeed her preterm baby because he will not know how much milk the baby takes at the breast. Possible response: "I appreciate your concern for my baby. I understand, though, that my baby's milk intake at the breast can be measured using an electronic scale accurate to 2 g. Research has found that by weighing my baby on this scale before and after breastfeeding, we can chart the amount of milk he took at the breast, even when he is wearing his leads." Share with the mother the following citations:

Meier, P. P., Engstrom, J. L., Crichton, C. L., Clark, D. R., Williams, M. M., & Mangurten, H. H. (1994). A new scale for in-home test-weighing for mothers of preterm and high risk infants. *Journal of Human Lactation, 10*(3), 163-168.

Haase, B., Barreira, J., Murphy, P. K., Mueller, M., & Rhodes, J. (2009). The development of an accurate test weighing technique for preterm and high-risk hospitalized infants. *Breastfeeding Medicine, 4*(3): 151-156.

Example: A full-term, healthy newborn has a blood bilirubin level of 14 mg/dL on Day 4. The baby's pediatrician recommends the mother stop breastfeeding and feed formula for the next 48 hours. One possible response: "I'd like to look over with you the American Academy of Pediatrics' recommendations for newborns with jaundice so that you can explain why you want to make my baby's case an exception to continuing to breastfeed." Share with the mother the following citation:

AAP. (2004). Management of hyperbilirubinemia in the newborn infant 35 or more weeks of gestation. *Pediatrics, 114*(1), 297-316.

If a mother is uncomfortable with recommendations from healthcare professionals, offer to discuss other tactful ways to raise her concerns with them. Most people find it stressful to be in conflict, but this can be even more difficult for an emotional new mother when she or her baby has health problems. When the breastfeeding baby is hospitalized, some mothers hesitate to question or disagree for fear they will alienate their baby's healthcare providers and his care will suffer (Weimers, Svensson, Dumas, Naver, & Wahlberg, 2006). Offer to practice these basic approaches with her:

- **Practice** what she wants to say before talking to the healthcare professionals.
- **Ask for more information** about the treatment/strategy and the reasons for it. If the mother is unsure about the reasons, suggest she ask the healthcare professional to take the time needed to give her a fuller explanation. One question she might consider asking is: "Is this your usual recommendation or is this specific to me (or my baby)?"

Provide mothers with strategies about how to talk with their healthcare providers.

- **Repeat her goals**. By repeating her position calmly to each response, this may help to reinforce her message. For a slow-gaining baby: "I appreciate your concern, but I'd like to first try improving our breastfeeding dynamics and check his weight in a few more days before giving supplements." For a jaundiced newborn: "I understand your concern about my newborn's bilirubin level, but I can feel that my milk has increased and I'd like to try breastfeeding more often for another day before giving supplements."
- **Paraphrase what she is told to clarify her understanding.**
- **Describe her goals and the reasons for them.** Parents' preferences vary, and her baby's healthcare provider needs to know hers. For example, she might say, "My family has a history of allergies so I feel strongly about my baby receiving only my milk. Are there ways to make this possible?" Or for a preterm baby, "I know my baby is still small, but I'd like to give him more practice at the breast so that he can learn to breastfeed more effectively."
- **Be friendly and project confidence** while being willing to consider alternatives.
- **Word statements positively**. "I'd like to try breastfeeding my baby more often to lower his bilirubin levels (raise his blood sugar/increase his weight gain/etc.)," rather than "I don't want my baby to have formula."

- **Acknowledge everyone's good intentions**. "Thank you for your concern about my baby's health. I understand, though, that breastfeeding does not usually need to be interrupted during jaundice treatment (when baby is gaining slowly, when a baby has low blood sugar, when a breastfeeding mother has x-rays or a scan using radiocontrast agents, etc.)."
- **Be tactful and respectful and expect this in return.** If a healthcare professional recommends a treatment that runs counter to the mother's goals, ask for the research that supports this and be willing to listen. "I understand that my hyperthyroidism needs to be treated. Would it be possible to consider treating it with medication rather than starting with radioactive iodine, which requires that I wean my baby?"
- **Be honest with all healthcare providers.** The health of mother and baby hinges on an honest working relationship between parents and healthcare providers. If the mother and her healthcare providers disagree, encourage her to continue to discuss the issues and try to separate fact from feelings.
- **Be aware that the parents have the ultimate responsibility** for the baby's health and will live with the consequences of any decisions. To emphasize this, the mother might say, "You'd like my permission to..." or "You recommend...."
- **If the mother is not satisfied, encourage her to ask for a second opinion**, which is common practice and is her right. If she is unsure who to approach for a second opinion, suggest she ask the hospital breastfeeding specialist for the name of a healthcare provider who is supportive of breastfeeding.

REFERENCES

Weimers, L., Svensson, K., Dumas, L., Naver, L., & Wahlberg, V. (2006). Hands-on approach during breastfeeding support in a neonatal intensive care unit: a qualitative study of Swedish mothers' experiences. *International Breastfeeding Journal, 1*, 20.

World Health Organization Growth Charts

Appendix D

INTRODUCTION

In 2006, the World Health Organization (WHO) released growth charts that accurately reflected the normal growth of the breastfed baby, based on data from its Multicentre Growth Reference Study. (For details, see p. 208 "Growth Charts.") This study's goal was to define optimal growth in six culturally and ethnically diverse countries (Brazil, Ghana, India, Norway, Oman, and the U.S.) over a 6-year period. About 8,500 children—including about 300 newborns—participated in the study. The mothers of these babies followed healthy practices by breastfeeding exclusively, not smoking, and adding appropriate solid foods to their babies' diet at the recommended age.

Researchers found that no matter where these mothers and children lived, and no matter what their ethnic background, average growth was nearly identical in all six countries. The charts developed from this research for children aged 0-60 months are free and downloadable online at: http://www.who.int/childgrowth/standards/en/ and include weight for age, weight for length, weight for height, length/height for age, body mass index, and motor development milestones. Some of these charts are included in this appendix.

These WHO growth charts reflect breastfeeding norms and differ from the earlier growth charts, which were a reflection of how mostly formula-fed children grew in a particular time and place. In contrast, the data used to create these WHO growth charts were compiled internationally among families using optimal feeding practices, making them a benchmark of how all children *should* grow. They are a standard that can be used to judge childhood growth anywhere in the world.

Table D.1.

1-month weight increments (g) BOYS
Birth to 12 months (percentiles)

World Health Organization

Interval	1st	3rd	5th	15th	25th	50th	75th	85th	95th	97th	99th
0 - 4 wks	182	369	460	681	805	1023	1229	1336	1509	1575	1697
4 wks - 2 mo	528	648	713	886	992	1196	1408	1524	1724	1803	1955
2 - 3 mo	307	397	446	577	658	815	980	1071	1228	1290	1410
3 - 4 mo	160	241	285	403	476	617	764	845	985	1041	1147
4 - 5 mo	70	150	194	311	383	522	666	746	883	937	1041
5 - 6 mo	-17	61	103	217	287	422	563	640	773	826	927
6 - 7 mo	-76	0	42	154	223	357	496	573	706	758	859
7 - 8 mo	-118	-43	-1	111	181	316	457	535	671	724	827
8 - 9 mo	-153	-77	-36	77	148	285	429	508	646	701	806
9 - 10 mo	-183	-108	-66	48	120	259	405	486	627	683	790
10 - 11 mo	-209	-132	-89	27	100	243	394	478	623	680	791
11 - 12 mo	-229	-150	-106	15	91	239	397	484	635	695	811

WHO Growth Velocity Standards

28.35 grams (g) = 1 ounce (oz) To convert g to oz. divide g by 28.35.

Table D.2.

1-month weight increments (g) GIRLS
Birth to 12 months (percentiles)

World Health Organization

Interval	1st	3rd	5th	15th	25th	50th	75th	85th	95th	97th	99th
0 - 4 wks	280	388	446	602	697	879	1068	1171	1348	1418	1551
4 wks - 2 mo	410	519	578	734	829	1011	1198	1301	1476	1545	1677
2 - 3 mo	233	321	369	494	571	718	869	952	1094	1150	1256
3 - 4 mo	133	214	259	376	448	585	726	804	937	990	1090
4 - 5 mo	51	130	172	286	355	489	627	703	833	885	983
5 - 6 mo	-24	52	93	203	271	401	537	611	739	790	886
6 - 7 mo	-79	-4	37	146	214	344	480	555	684	734	832
7 - 8 mo	-119	-44	-2	109	178	311	450	526	659	711	811
8 - 9 mo	-155	-81	-40	70	139	273	412	489	623	675	776
9 - 10 mo	-184	-110	-70	41	110	245	385	464	598	652	754
10 - 11 mo	-206	-131	-89	24	95	233	378	459	598	653	759
11 - 12 mo	-222	-145	-102	15	88	232	383	467	612	670	781

WHO Growth Velocity Standards

28.35 grams (g) = 1 ounce (oz) To convert g to oz. divide g by 28.35.

Table D.3.

Weight-for-age BOYS

Birth to 2 years (percentiles)

World Health Organization

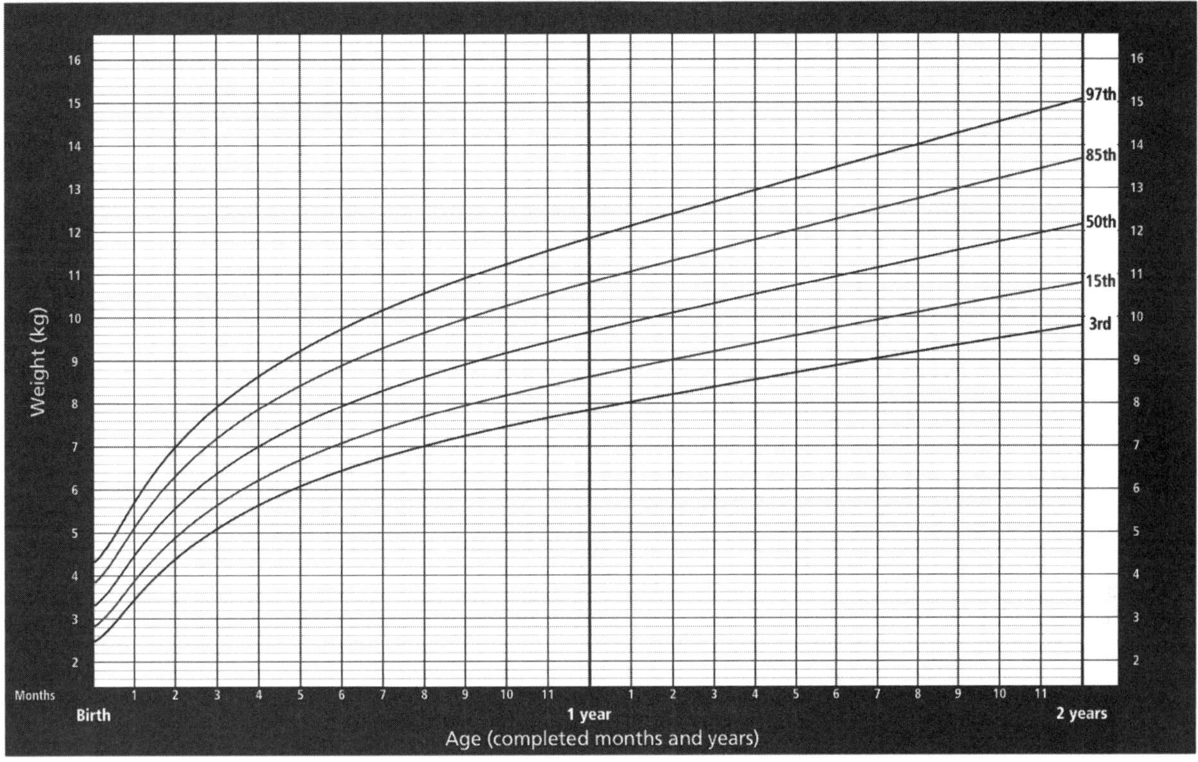

0.035274 kilograms (kg) = 1 ounce (oz) To convert kg to oz., multiply kg by 35.274

WHO Child Growth Standards

Table D.4.

Weight-for-age GIRLS

Birth to 2 years (percentiles)

World Health Organization

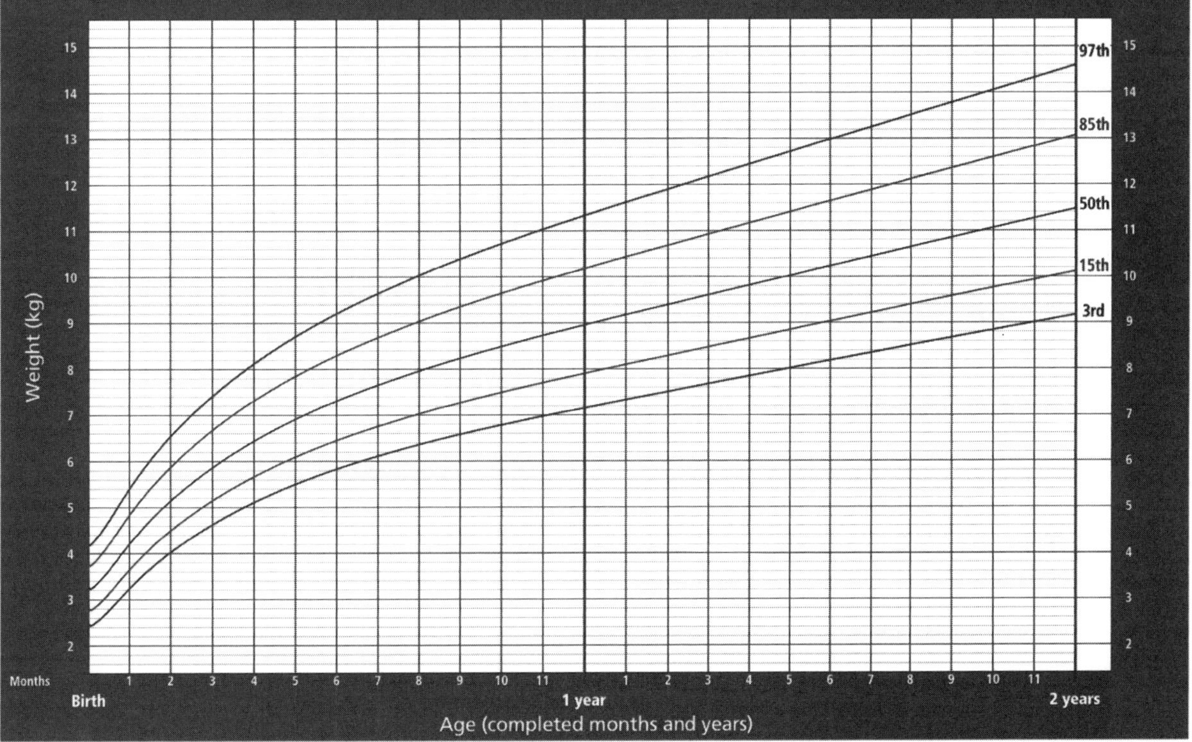

0.035274 kilograms (kg) = 1 ounce (oz) To convert kg to oz., multiply kg by 35.274

WHO Child Growth Standards

Table D.5.

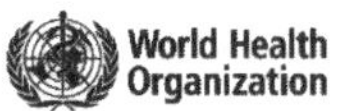

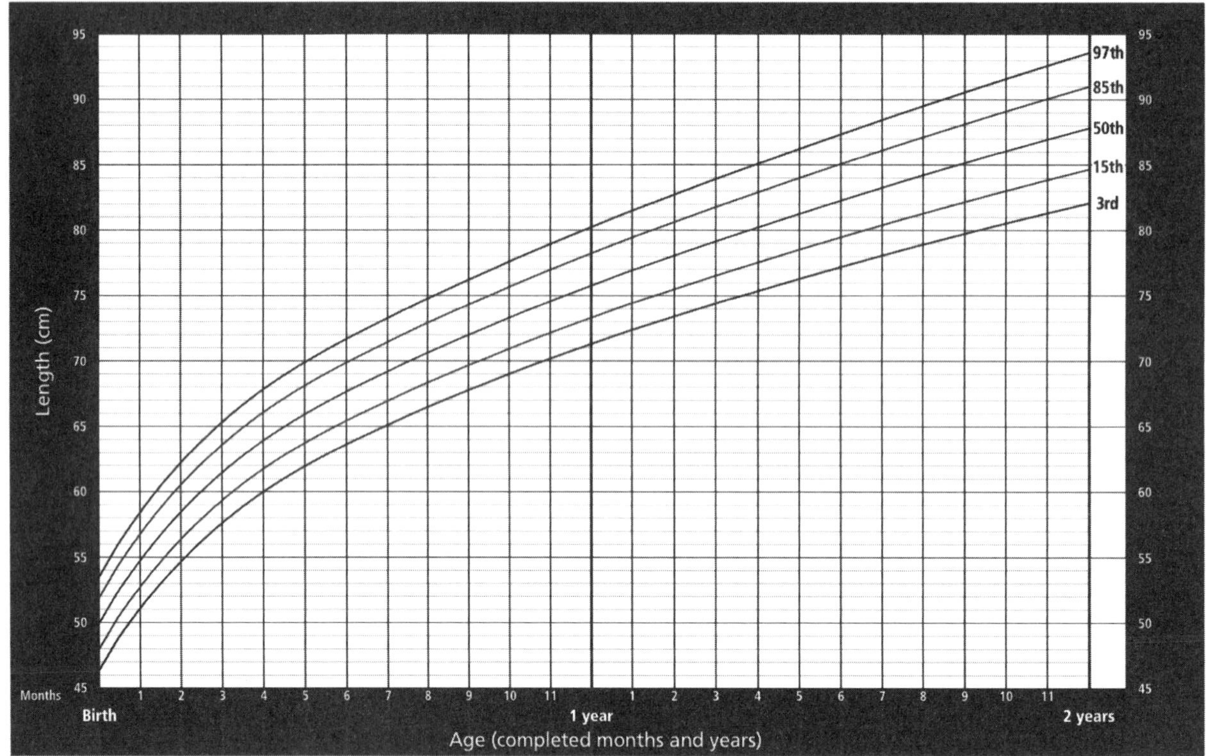

0.3937 centimeters (cm) = 1 inch To convert cm to inches, multiply cm by 0.3937

WHO Child Growth Standards

Table D.6.

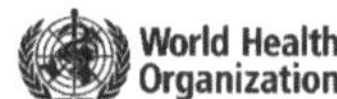

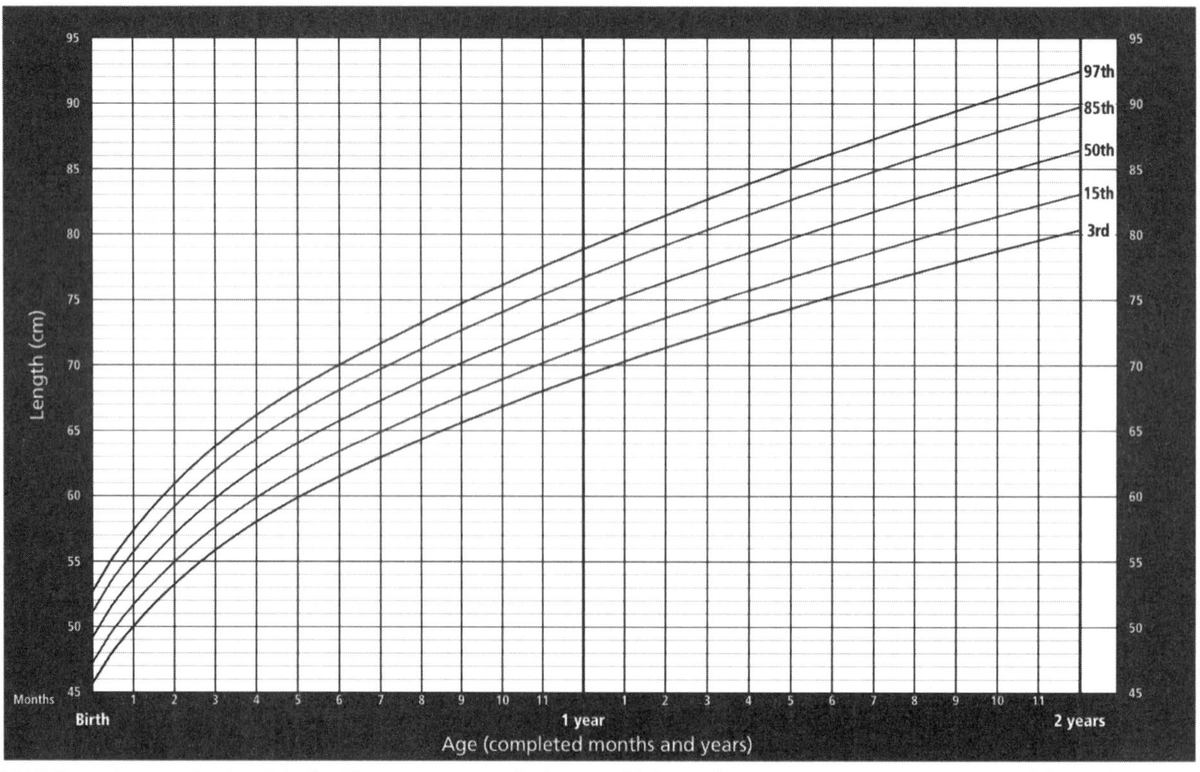

0.3937 centimeters (cm) = 1 inch To convert cm to inches, multiply cm by 0.3937

WHO Child Growth Standards

Table D.7.

Weight-for-length BOYS

Birth to 2 years (percentiles)

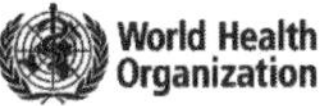

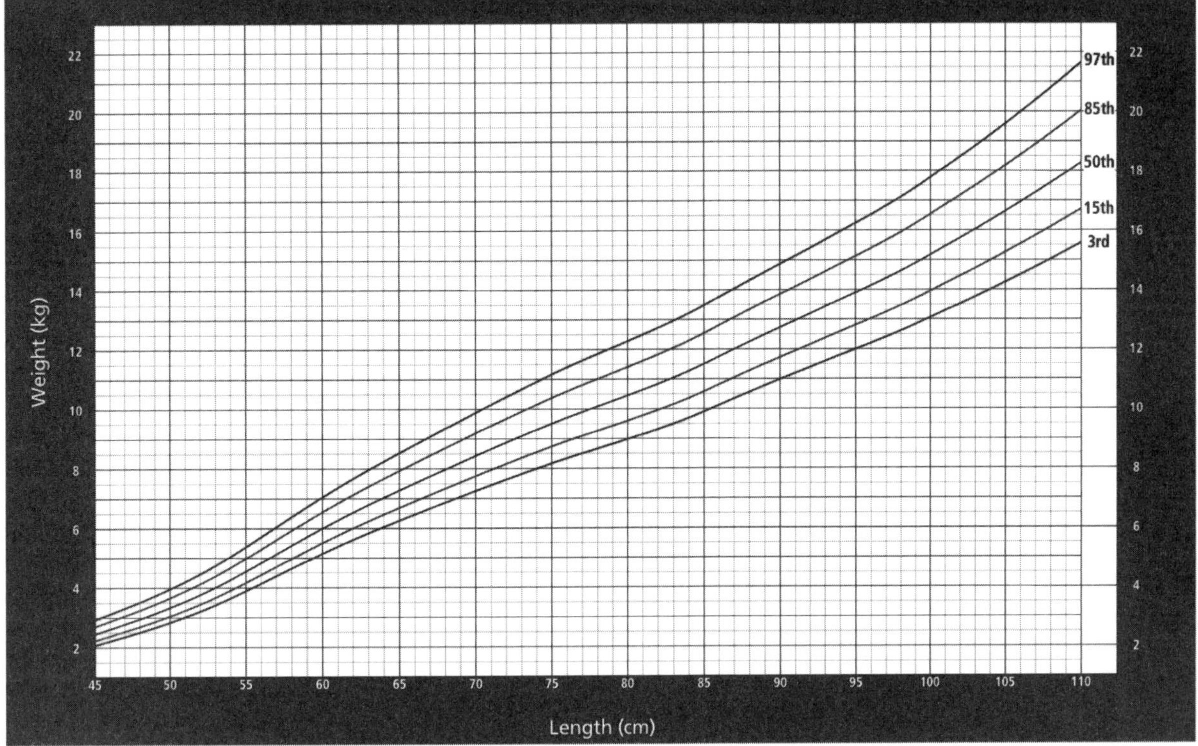

0.3937 centimeters (cm) = 1 inch To convert cm to inches, multiply cm by 0.3937
0.035274 kilograms (kg). = 1 ounce (oz.) To convert kg to oz., multiply kg by 35.274

WHO Child Growth Standards

Table D.8.

Weight-for-length GIRLS

Birth to 2 years (percentiles)

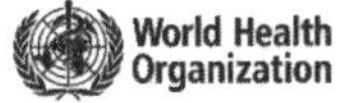

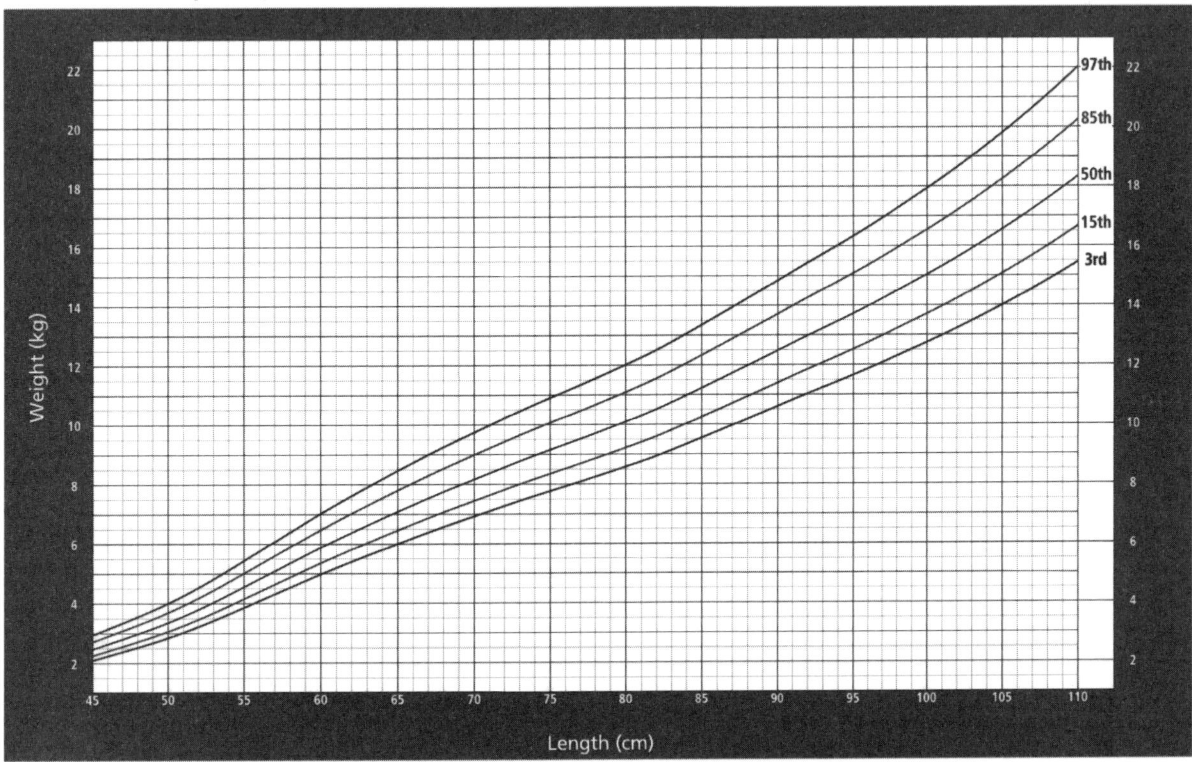

0.3937 centimeters (cm) = 1 inch To convert cm to inches, multiply cm by 0.3937
0.035274 kilograms (kg). = 1 ounce (oz.) To convert kg to oz., multiply kg by 35.274

WHO Child Growth Standards

Table D.9.

Windows of Achievement

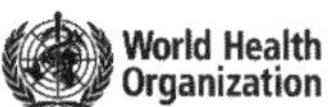

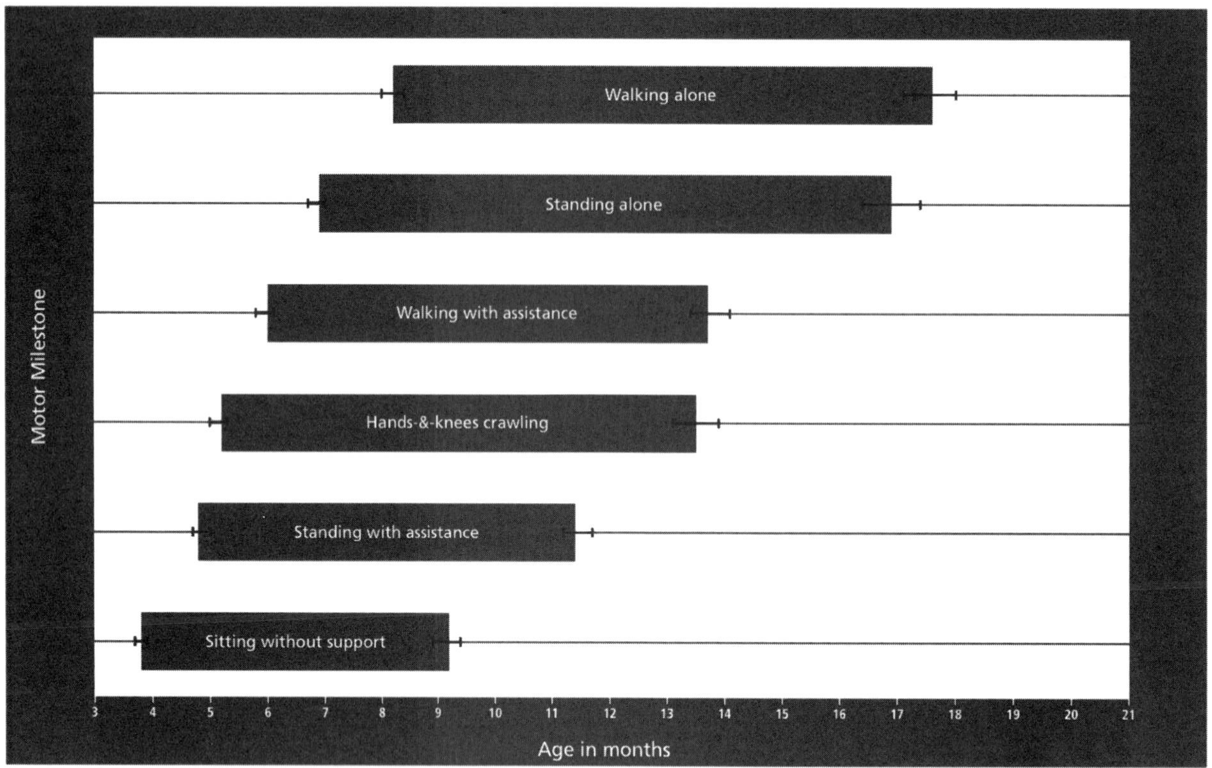

WHO Child Growth Standards

INDEX

A

B

E

G

H

I

J

N

O

P

Q

R

T

U

V

W

Y

Z

About the Author

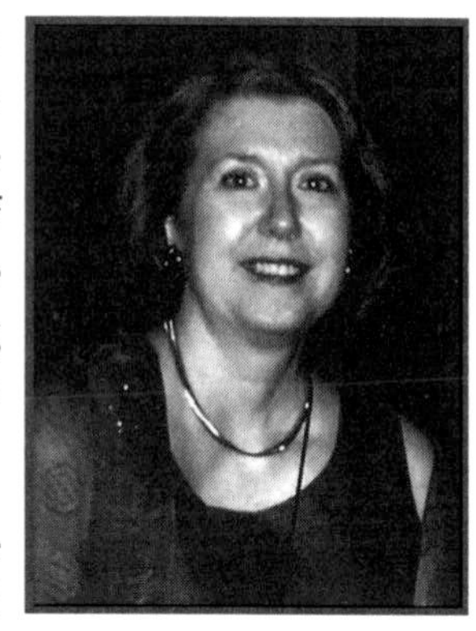

Nancy Mohrbacher, IBCLC, FILCA, is best known as coauthor of *The Breastfeeding Answer Book*, a research-based counseling guide that has sold more than 130,000 copies worldwide, and co-author of the best-selling guide for parents, *Breastfeeding Made Simple*. She has been working with breastfeeding mothers since 1982 and currently works as a Lactation Consultant for Ameda Breastfeeding Products.

For 10 years, Nancy founded and maintained a large private practice in the Chicago area, where she worked one-on-one with thousands of breastfeeding families. She has written for many publications and spoken at breastfeeding conferences around the world.

In 2008 the International Lactation Consultant Association (ILCA) officially recognized Nancy's contributions to the field by awarding her the designation FILCA, which stands for Fellow of the International Lactation Consultant Association. Nancy was one of the first group of 16 to be recognized for their lifetime achievements in breastfeeding.

Ordering Information

Hale Publishing, L.P.
1712 N. Forest Street
Amarillo, Texas, USA 79106

8:00 am to 5:00 pm CST

Call » 806.376.9900
Sales » 800.378.1317
Fax » 806.376.9901

Online Web Orders
www.ibreastfeeding.com